RED BOOK®
Atlas of Pediatric Infectious Diseases

5th Edition

Editor
Tina Q. Tan, MD, FAAP

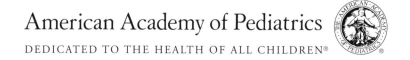

American Academy of Pediatrics
DEDICATED TO THE HEALTH OF ALL CHILDREN®

American Academy of Pediatrics Publishing Staff

Mary Lou White, *Chief Product and Services Officer/SVP, Membership, Marketing, and Publishing*
Mark Grimes, *Vice President, Publishing*
Heather Babiar, MS, *Senior Editor, Professional/Clinical Publishing*
Theresa Wiener, *Production Manager, Clinical and Professional Publications*
Amanda Helmholz, *Medical Copy Editor*
Peg Mulcahy, *Manager, Art Direction and Production*
Mary Louise Carr, MBA, *Marketing Manager, Clinical Publications*

Published by the American Academy of Pediatrics
345 Park Blvd
Itasca, IL 60143
Telephone: 630/626-6000
Facsimile: 847/434-8000
www.aap.org

The American Academy of Pediatrics is an organization of 67,000 primary care pediatricians, pediatric medical subspecialists, and pediatric surgical specialists dedicated to the health, safety, and well-being of all infants, children, adolescents, and young adults.

While every effort has been made to ensure the accuracy of this publication, the American Academy of Pediatrics does not guarantee that it is accurate, complete, or without error.

The recommendations in this publication do not indicate an exclusive course of treatment or serve as a standard of medical care. Variations, taking into account individual circumstances, may be appropriate.

Statements and opinions expressed are those of the authors and not necessarily those of the American Academy of Pediatrics.

Any websites, brand names, products, or manufacturers are mentioned for informational and identification purposes only and do not imply an endorsement by the American Academy of Pediatrics (AAP). The AAP is not responsible for the content of external resources. Information was current at the time of publication.

The publishers have made every effort to trace the copyright holders for borrowed materials. If they have inadvertently overlooked any, they will be pleased to make the necessary arrangements at the first opportunity.

This publication has been developed by the American Academy of Pediatrics. The contributors are expert authorities in the field of pediatrics. No commercial involvement of any kind has been solicited or accepted in the development of the content of this publication. Dr Tan disclosed financial relationships with Merck and Sanofi Pasteur advisory boards, a principal investigator research relationship and an advisory board relationship with GSK, and an advisory board relationship with Pfizer.

Every effort has been made to ensure that the drug selection and dosages set forth in this publication are in accordance with the current recommendations and practice at the time of publication. It is the responsibility of the health care professional to check the package insert of each drug for any change in indications or dosage and for added warnings and precautions.

Every effort is made to keep *Red Book Atlas of Pediatric Infectious Diseases* consistent with the most recent advice and information available from the American Academy of Pediatrics.

Please visit www.aap.org/errata for an up-to-date list of any applicable errata for this publication.

Special discounts are available for bulk purchases of this publication. Email Special Sales at nationalaccounts@aap.org for more information.

© 2023 American Academy of Pediatrics

All rights reserved. No part of this publication may be reproduced, stored in a retrieval system, or transmitted in any form or by any means—electronic, mechanical, photocopying, recording, or otherwise—without prior permission from the publisher (locate title at https://publications.aap.org/aapbooks and click on © Get Permissions; you may also fax the permissions editor at 847/434-8780 or email permissions@aap.org). First edition published 2010; second, 2013; third, 2017; fourth, 2020; fifth, 2023.

Printed in the United States of America

9-481/1022   1 2 3 4 5 6 7 8 9 10
MA1066
ISBN: 978-1-61002-630-7
eBook: 978-1-61002-631-4

Library of Congress Control Number: 2022900419

Equity, Diversity, and Inclusion Statement

The American Academy of Pediatrics is committed to principles of equity, diversity, and inclusion in its publishing program. Editorial boards, author selections, and author transitions (publication succession plans) are designed to include diverse voices that reflect society as a whole. Editor and author teams are encouraged to actively seek out diverse authors and reviewers at all stages of the editorial process. Publishing staff are committed to promoting equity, diversity, and inclusion in all aspects of publication writing, review, and production.

Contents

Preface xi

1. Actinomycosis 1
2. Adenovirus Infections 4
3. Amebiasis 7
4. Amebic Meningoencephalitis and Keratitis (*Naegleria fowleri*, *Acanthamoeba* species, and *Balamuthia mandrillaris*) 14
5. Anthrax 18
6. Arboviruses (Including Colorado tick fever, Eastern equine encephalitis, Heartland, Jamestown Canyon, Japanese encephalitis, La Crosse, Powassan, St Louis encephalitis, tickborne encephalitis, and yellow fever viruses) 26
7. *Arcanobacterium haemolyticum* Infections 35
8. *Ascaris lumbricoides* Infections 37
9. Aspergillosis 41
10. Astrovirus Infections 47
11. Babesiosis 49
12. *Bacillus cereus* Infections and Intoxications 54
13. Bacterial Vaginosis 56
14. *Bacteroides*, *Prevotella*, and Other Anaerobic Gram-Negative Bacilli Infections 59
15. *Balantidium coli* Infections (Balantidiasis) 61
16. *Bartonella henselae* (Cat-Scratch Disease) 63
17. *Baylisascaris* Infections 68
18. Infections With *Blastocystis* Species 72
19. Blastomycosis 75
20. Bocavirus 78
21. *Borrelia* Infections Other Than Lyme Disease (Relapsing Fever) 79
22. Brucellosis 82
23. *Burkholderia* Infections 85
24. *Campylobacter* Infections 88
25. Candidiasis 91
26. Chancroid and Cutaneous Ulcers 100

27	Chikungunya	103
28	Chlamydial Infections (*Chlamydia pneumoniae*)	105
29	*Chlamydia psittaci* (Psittacosis, Ornithosis, Parrot Fever)	107
30	*Chlamydia trachomatis*	110
31	Botulism and Infant Botulism (*Clostridium botulinum*)	115
32	Clostridial Myonecrosis (Gas Gangrene)	120
33	*Clostridioides difficile* (formerly *Clostridium difficile*)	122
34	*Clostridium perfringens* Foodborne Illness	127
35	Coccidioidomycosis	129
36	Coronaviruses, Including SARS-CoV-2 and MERS-CoV	137
37	*Cryptococcus neoformans* and *Cryptococcus gattii* Infections (Cryptococcosis)	143
38	Cryptosporidiosis	146
39	Cutaneous Larva Migrans	151
40	Cyclosporiasis	153
41	Cystoisosporiasis (formerly Isosporiasis)	155
42	Cytomegalovirus Infection	158
43	Dengue	166
44	Diphtheria	171
45	*Ehrlichia, Anaplasma,* and Related Infections (Human Ehrlichiosis, Anaplasmosis, and Related Infections Attributable to Bacteria in the Family *Anaplasmataceae*)	177
46	Serious Neonatal Bacterial Infections Caused by *Enterobacteriaceae* (Including Septicemia and Meningitis)	185
47	Enterovirus (Nonpoliovirus) (Group A and B Coxsackieviruses, Echoviruses, Numbered Enteroviruses)	192
48	Epstein-Barr Virus Infections (Infectious Mononucleosis)	197
49	*Escherichia coli* Diarrhea (Including Hemolytic-Uremic Syndrome)	202
50	Other Fungal Diseases	208
51	*Fusobacterium* Infections (Including Lemierre Syndrome)	216
52	*Giardia duodenalis* (formerly *Giardia lamblia* and *Giardia intestinalis*) Infections (Giardiasis)	219
53	Gonococcal Infections	224

54	Granuloma Inguinale (Donovanosis)	232
55	*Haemophilus influenzae* Infections	234
56	Hantavirus Pulmonary Syndrome	245
57	*Helicobacter pylori* Infections	249
58	Hemorrhagic Fevers Caused by Arenaviruses	253
59	Hemorrhagic Fevers Caused by Bunyaviruses	255
60	Hemorrhagic Fevers Caused by Filoviruses: Ebola and Marburg	259
61	Hepatitis A	265
62	Hepatitis B	269
63	Hepatitis C	277
64	Hepatitis D	281
65	Hepatitis E	283
66	Herpes Simplex	285
67	Histoplasmosis	296
68	Hookworm Infections (*Ancylostoma duodenale* and *Necator americanus*)	301
69	Human Herpesviruses 6 (Including Roseola) and 7	306
70	Human Herpesvirus 8	311
71	Human Immunodeficiency Virus Infection	313
72	Human Papillomaviruses	331
73	Influenza	335
74	Kawasaki Disease	345
75	*Kingella kingae* Infections	353
76	*Legionella pneumophila* Infections	355
77	Leishmaniasis	360
78	Leprosy	367
79	Leptospirosis	372
80	*Listeria monocytogenes* Infections (Listeriosis)	377
81	Lyme Disease (Lyme Borreliosis, *Borrelia burgdorferi* sensu lato Infection)	381
82	Lymphatic Filariasis (Bancroftian, Malayan, and Timorian)	393
83	Lymphocytic Choriomeningitis Virus	398
84	Malaria	400

85	Measles	411
86	Meningococcal Infections	419
87	Human Metapneumovirus	428
88	Microsporidia Infections (Microsporidiosis)	430
89	Molluscum Contagiosum	434
90	*Moraxella catarrhalis* Infections	437
91	Mumps	439
92	*Mycoplasma pneumoniae* and Other *Mycoplasma* Species Infections	444
93	Nocardiosis	449
94	Norovirus and Sapovirus Infections	453
95	Onchocerciasis (River Blindness, Filariasis)	456
96	Paracoccidioidomycosis (Formerly Known as South American Blastomycosis)	460
97	Paragonimiasis	463
98	Parainfluenza Viral Infections	467
99	Parasitic Diseases	470
100	Parechovirus Infections	480
101	Parvovirus B19 (Erythema Infectiosum, Fifth Disease)	483
102	*Pasteurella* Infections	488
103	Pediculosis Capitis (Head Lice)	490
104	Pediculosis Corporis (Body Lice)	495
105	Pediculosis Pubis (Pubic Lice, Crab Lice)	497
106	Pelvic Inflammatory Disease	499
107	Pertussis (Whooping Cough)	503
108	Pinworm Infection (*Enterobius vermicularis*)	510
109	Pityriasis Versicolor (Formerly Tinea Versicolor)	513
110	Plague	516
111	*Pneumocystis jirovecii* Infections	522
112	Poliovirus Infections	528
113	Polyomaviruses (BK, JC, and Other Polyomaviruses)	533
114	Prion Diseases: Transmissible Spongiform Encephalopathies	536
115	*Pseudomonas aeruginosa* Infections	540

116	Q Fever (*Coxiella burnetii* Infection)	543
117	Rabies	546
118	Rat-Bite Fever	552
119	Respiratory Syncytial Virus	555
120	Rhinovirus Infections	559
121	Rickettsial Diseases	561
122	Rickettsialpox	563
123	Rocky Mountain Spotted Fever	565
124	Rotavirus Infections	571
125	Rubella	573
126	*Salmonella* Infections	579
127	Scabies	588
128	Schistosomiasis	593
129	*Shigella* Infections	599
130	Smallpox (Variola)	603
131	Sporotrichosis	610
132	Staphylococcal Food Poisoning	614
133	*Staphylococcus aureus*	616
134	Coagulase-Negative Staphylococcal Infections	631
135	Group A Streptococcal Infections	633
136	Group B Streptococcal Infections	647
137	Non–group A or B Streptococcal and Enterococcal Infections	652
138	*Streptococcus pneumoniae* (Pneumococcal) Infections	657
139	Strongyloidiasis (*Strongyloides stercoralis*)	667
140	Syphilis	670
141	Tapeworm Diseases (Taeniasis and Cysticercosis)	689
142	Other Tapeworm Infections (Including Hydatid Disease)	695
143	Tetanus (Lockjaw)	700
144	Tinea Capitis (Ringworm of the Scalp)	704
145	Tinea Corporis (Ringworm of the Body)	708
146	Tinea Cruris (Jock Itch)	712

147	Tinea Pedis and Tinea Unguium (Onychomycosis) (Athlete's Foot, Ringworm of the Feet)	714
148	Toxocariasis	717
149	*Toxoplasma gondii* Infections (Toxoplasmosis)	720
150	Trichinellosis (*Trichinella spiralis* and Other Species)	730
151	*Trichomonas vaginalis* Infections (Trichomoniasis)	734
152	Trichuriasis (Whipworm Infection)	739
153	African Trypanosomiasis (African Sleeping Sickness)	742
154	American Trypanosomiasis (Chagas Disease)	745
155	Tuberculosis	750
156	Nontuberculous Mycobacteria (Environmental *Mycobacteria*, *Mycobacteria* other than *Mycobacterium tuberculosis*)	777
157	Tularemia	786
158	Louseborne Typhus (Epidemic or Sylvatic Typhus)	793
159	Murine Typhus (Endemic or Fleaborne Typhus)	796
160	*Ureaplasma urealyticum* and *Ureaplasma parvum* Infections	798
161	Varicella-Zoster Virus Infections	801
162	Cholera (*Vibrio cholerae*)	812
163	Other *Vibrio* Infections	816
164	West Nile Virus	818
165	*Yersinia enterocolitica* and *Yersinia pseudotuberculosis* Infections (Enteritis and Other Illnesses)	824
166	Zika	828
Index		835

Preface

The American Academy of Pediatrics (AAP) *Red Book Atlas of Pediatric Infectious Diseases*, 5th Edition, summarizes key disease information from the AAP *Red Book: 2021–2024 Report of the Committee on Infectious Diseases*. It is intended to be a study guide and visual resource for students, residents, practicing physicians, and other health care professionals who care for infants and children.

The compilation of images of common and unusual features of infants and children with a broad range of infectious diseases can provide diagnostic clues that are not found in the print version of the *Red Book*. It is my hope that the juxtaposition of these images against text summarizing the clinical manifestations, epidemiological factors, diagnostic methods, and treatment information will be effective as a teaching tool and a quick reference. The *Red Book Atlas* is not meant to detail information on treatment and management of a disease but instead provide a big-picture approach that can be refined, as desired, by reference to authoritative textbooks, original articles, or infectious diseases specialists. Complete disease and treatment information from the AAP can be found in the electronic version of the *Red Book* at https://publications.aap.org/redbook.

The *Red Book Atlas* would not exist without the incredible support and assistance provided by Heather Babiar, Amanda Helmholz, and Theresa Wiener at the AAP and the generosity of the physicians who photographed disease manifestations in their patients and shared these with the AAP. Some diseases have disappeared in the world (ie, smallpox), and others are rare in the United States (eg, diphtheria, tetanus, congenital rubella syndrome) because of effective prevention strategies, especially immunization. Although photographs cannot replace hands-on familiarity, they are very helpful in considering the likelihood of alternative diagnoses, and I hope that this will be so for the reader. I also want to thank the many individuals at the Centers for Disease Control and Prevention who generously provided many images of etiologic agents, vectors, and life cycles of parasites and protozoa relevant to some of these infections.

The study and practice of pediatric infectious diseases, through the dynamic nature of the specialty and the challenges that this brings, has brought me incredible fulfilment and joy. Simply put, it is one of the "best jobs in the world." To be able to interact with patients and their families; gather physical examination, laboratory, and radiographic data; and put the pieces together to assign a diagnosis and develop a treatment plan leading to the complete recovery of the patient is one of the most exciting and gratifying parts of the job. Solving the medical puzzle peaks your curiosity and provides you with exposure to many diverse resources, intellectual stimulation, and immense satisfaction when you are able to help a patient and their family as they are dealing with the illness. It is my hope that readers will experience a bit of the enthusiasm that I have for infectious diseases after reading the fifth edition of the *Red Book Atlas*.

Tina Q. Tan, MD, FAAP
Editor

CHAPTER 1
Actinomycosis

CLINICAL MANIFESTATIONS

Actinomycosis results from pathogen introduction following a breakdown in mucocutaneous protective barriers. Spread within the host are, by direct invasion of adjacent tissues, typically forming sinus tracts that cross tissue planes. The most common species causing human disease is *Actinomyces israelii*.

There are 3 common anatomical sites of infection. **Cervicofacial** is most common, often occurring after tooth extraction, oral surgery, or other oral/facial trauma or even from carious teeth. Localized pain and induration may progress to cervical abscess and "woody hard" nodular lesions ("lumpy jaw"), which can develop draining sinus tracts, usually at the angle of the jaw or in the submandibular region. Infection may contribute to recurrent or persistent tonsillitis. **Thoracic** disease is most commonly secondary to aspiration of oropharyngeal secretions but may be an extension of cervicofacial infection. It occurs rarely after esophageal disruption secondary to surgery or nonpenetrating trauma. Thoracic manifestation includes pneumonia, which can be complicated by abscesses, empyema, and, rarely, pleurodermal sinuses. Focal or multifocal mediastinal and pulmonary masses may be mistaken for tumors. **Abdominal** actinomycosis is usually attributable to penetrating trauma or intestinal perforation. The appendix and cecum are the most common sites; symptoms are like those of appendicitis. Slowly developing masses may simulate abdominal or retroperitoneal neoplasms. Intra-abdominal abscesses and peritoneal-dermal draining sinuses occur eventually. Chronic localized disease often forms draining sinus tracts with purulent discharge. **Other sites** of infection include the liver, pelvis (which, in some cases, has been linked to use of intrauterine devices), heart, testicles, and brain (which is usually associated with a primary pulmonary focus). Noninvasive primary cutaneous actinomycosis has occurred.

ETIOLOGY

A israelii and at least 5 other *Actinomyces* species cause human disease. All are slow-growing, microaerophilic or facultative anaerobic, gram-positive, filamentous branching bacilli. They can be part of normal oral, gastrointestinal tract, or vaginal flora. *Actinomyces* species are frequently copathogens in tissues harboring multiple other anaerobic and/or aerobic species. Isolation of *Aggregatibacter* (*Actinobacillus*) *actinomycetemcomitans*, frequently detected with *Actinomyces* species, may predict the presence of actinomycosis.

EPIDEMIOLOGY

Actinomyces species occur worldwide. *Actinomyces* species are opportunistic pathogens in the setting of disrupted mucosal barriers. Infection is uncommon in infants and children, with 80% of cases occurring in adults. The male-to-female ratio in children is 1.5:1. Although microbiologically confirmed infections caused by *Actinomyces* species are now less common, there are reports from patients who have undergone a transplant or are receiving biologics.

The **incubation period** varies from several days to several years.

DIAGNOSTIC TESTS

Microscopic demonstration of beaded, branched, gram-positive bacilli in purulent material or tissue specimens suggests the diagnosis. Only specimens from normally sterile sites should be submitted for culture. Specimens must be obtained, transported, and cultured anaerobically on semiselective (kanamycin-vancomycin) media such as the modified Thayer-Martin agar or buffered charcoal–yeast extract agar. Acid-fast testing can distinguish *Actinomyces* species, which are acid-fast negative, from *Nocardia* species, which are variably acid-fast positive staining. Yellow sulfur granules visualized microscopically or macroscopically in drainage or loculations of purulent material suggest the diagnosis. A Gram stain of sulfur granules discloses a dense aggregate of bacterial filaments mixed with inflammatory debris. *A israelii* forms spiderlike microcolonies on culture medium after 48 hours. *Actinomyces* species can be identified in tissue specimens by using polymerase chain reaction assay and sequencing of the 16S ribosomal RNA.

TREATMENT

Initial therapy should include intravenous penicillin G or ampicillin for 4 to 6 weeks followed by high doses of oral penicillin (up to 2 g/day for adults), usually for a total of 6 to 12 months depending on the extent of disease and success of surgical management (when indicated). Treatment of mild disease can be initiated with oral therapy. Amoxicillin and doxycycline are alternative antimicrobial choices. Amoxicillin-clavulanate, piperacillin-tazobactam, ceftriaxone, clarithromycin, linezolid, and imipenem-meropenem also show high activity in vitro, but the latter antimicrobials have extended spectrums, which may not always be required. All *Actinomyces* species appear to be resistant to ciprofloxacin and metronidazole. Doxycycline is not typically recommended for children younger than 8 years when therapy will continue beyond 21 days.

Surgical drainage is often a necessary adjunct to medical management and may shorten, but does not obviate, antimicrobial therapy.

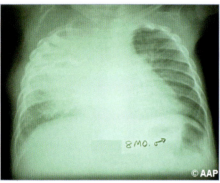

Image 1.1
An 8-month-old boy with pulmonary actinomycosis, an uncommon infection in infancy that may follow aspiration. As in this infant, most cases of actinomycosis are caused by *Actinomyces israelii*.

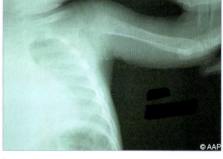

Image 1.2
Periosteal reaction along the left humeral shaft (diaphysis) in the 8-month-old boy in Image 1.1, with pulmonary actinomycosis. The presence of clubbing with this chronic suppurative pulmonary infection and the absence of heart disease suggest that pulmonary fibrosis contributed to this infant's pulmonary hypertrophic osteoarthropathy. Courtesy of Edgar O. Ledbetter, MD, FAAP.

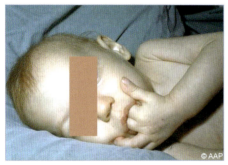

Image 1.3
Clubbing of the thumb and fingers of the 8-month-old boy in images 1.1 and 1.2, with chronic pulmonary actinomycosis. Results from blood cultures were repeatedly negative without clinical signs of endocarditis. Courtesy of Edgar O. Ledbetter, MD, FAAP.

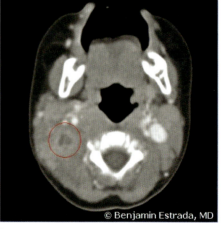

Image 1.4
Actinomyces cervical abscess (circled) in a 6-month-old girl. Courtesy of Benjamin Estrada, MD.

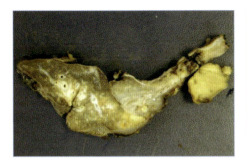

Image 1.5
The resected right lower lobe, diaphragm, and portion of the liver in a 3-year-old previously healthy girl with an unknown source for her pulmonary actinomycosis. Courtesy of Carol J. Baker, MD, FAAP.

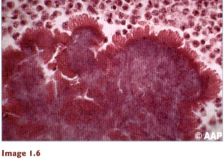

Image 1.6
A sulfur granule from an actinomycotic abscess (hematoxylin-eosin stain). While pathognomonic of actinomycosis, granules are not always present. A Gram stain of sulfur granules shows a dense reticulum of filaments.

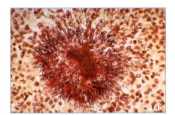

Image 1.7
Tissue showing filamentous branching rods of *Actinomyces israelii* (Brown-Brenn tissue Gram stain). *Actinomyces* species have fastidious growth requirements. Staining of a crushed sulfur granule reveals branching bacilli.

CHAPTER 2

Adenovirus Infections

CLINICAL MANIFESTATIONS

Adenovirus infections of the upper respiratory tract are common and often subclinical; when symptomatic, adenoviruses may cause common cold symptoms, pharyngitis, tonsillitis, otitis media, and pharyngoconjunctival fever. Adenoviruses occasionally cause a pertussis-like syndrome, croup, bronchiolitis, influenzalike illness, exudative tonsillitis, and hemorrhagic cystitis. Ocular adenovirus infections may manifest as follicular conjunctivitis or as epidemic keratoconjunctivitis. Enteric adenoviruses are an important cause of childhood gastroenteritis. Life-threatening disseminated infection, lower respiratory tract infection (eg, severe pneumonia, bronchiolitis obliterans), hepatitis, meningitis, and encephalitis occur occasionally, especially in young infants and immunocompromised people.

ETIOLOGY

Adenoviruses are double-stranded, nonenveloped DNA viruses of the *Adenoviridae* family and *Mastadenovirus* genus, with more than 80 recognized types and multiple genetic variants divided into 7 species (A–G) that infect humans. Some adenovirus types are associated primarily with respiratory tract disease (types 1–5, 7, 14, and 21), epidemic keratoconjunctivitis (types 8, 19, and 37), or gastroenteritis (types 40 and 41).

EPIDEMIOLOGY

Infection in children can occur at any age. Adenoviruses causing respiratory tract infections are usually transmitted by respiratory tract secretions through person-to-person contact, airborne droplets, and fomites. Adenoviruses are hardy viruses, can survive on environmental surfaces for long periods, and are not easily inactivated by many disinfectants. Outbreaks of febrile respiratory tract illness attributable to adenoviruses can be a significant problem in military trainees, college students, and residents of long-term care facilities. Community outbreaks of adenovirus-associated pharyngoconjunctival fever have been attributed to water exposure from contaminated swimming pools and fomites, such as shared towels. Health care–associated transmission of adenovirus infections can occur in hospitals, residential institutions, and nursing homes from exposures to infected health care personnel, patients, or contaminated equipment. Adenovirus infections in solid organ transplant recipients can occur from donor tissues. Epidemic keratoconjunctivitis commonly occurs by direct contact and has been associated with equipment used during eye examinations. Enteric strains of adenoviruses are transmitted by the fecal-oral route. Adenoviruses do not demonstrate the marked seasonality of other respiratory tract viruses and instead circulate throughout the year. Enteric disease occurs year round and primarily affects children younger than 4 years. Adenovirus infections are most communicable during the first few days of an acute illness, but persistent and intermittent shedding for longer periods, even months, can occur, especially in people with weakened immune systems. In healthy people, infection with one adenovirus type should confer type-specific immunity or at least lessen symptoms associated with reinfection, which forms the basis of adenovirus vaccines used in new recruits in the military.

The **incubation period** for respiratory tract infection varies from 2 to 14 days; for gastroenteritis, the **incubation period** is 3 to 10 days.

DIAGNOSTIC TESTS

Methods for diagnosis of adenovirus infection include molecular detection, isolation in cell culture, and antigen detection. Molecular assays (eg, polymerase chain reaction) are the preferred diagnostic method for detection of adenoviruses, and these assays are widely available commercially. However, the persistent and intermittent shedding that commonly follows an acute adenovirus infection can complicate the clinical interpretation of a positive molecular test result. Quantitative adenovirus assays can be useful for management of immunocompromised patients, such as hematopoietic stem cell and solid organ transplant recipients. Adenoviruses associated with respiratory tract and ocular disease can be isolated by culture from respiratory specimens (eg, nasopharyngeal swab, oropharyngeal swab, nasal wash, sputum) and eye secretions in standard susceptible cell lines. Enteric adenoviruses types 40 and 41 usually require specialized cell lines for successful isolation. Rapid antigen-detection techniques, including immunofluorescence and enzyme immunoassay, have been used to detect virus in respiratory tract secretions, conjunctival swabs, and stool, but these methods lack sensitivity. Adenovirus typing by molecular methods is available from some reference laboratories. Although its clinical utility is limited, typing can help establish an etiologic association with disease and help investigate clusters of adenovirus-associated illness. Serodiagnosis is used primarily for epidemiological studies and has no clinical utility.

TREATMENT

Treatment of adenovirus infection is primarily supportive. In immunocompromised patients, immunosuppressive therapy should be reduced whenever possible. There are no antivirals approved by the US Food and Drug Administration for the treatment of adenovirus infections. Reports on the successful use of cidofovir and ribavirin in immunocompromised patients with severe adenoviral disease have been published.

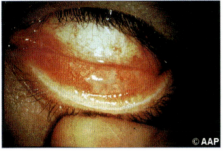

Image 2.1
Acute follicular adenovirus conjunctivitis. Adenoviruses are resistant to alcohol, detergents, and chlorhexidine and may contaminate ophthalmologic solutions and equipment. Instruments can be disinfected by steam autoclaving or immersion in 1% sodium hypochlorite for 10 minutes.

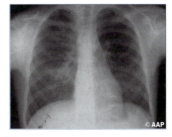

Image 2.2
Adenoviral pneumonia in an 8-year-old girl with diffuse pulmonary infiltrate occurring bilaterally. Most adenoviral infections in the normal host are self-limited and require no specific treatment. Lobar consolidation is unusual.

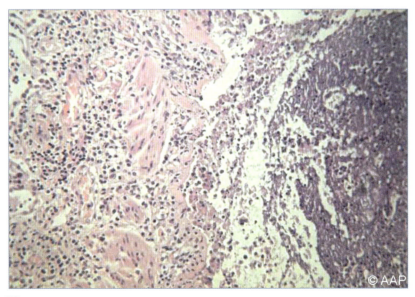

Image 2.3
Histopathologic features of the lung with bronchiolar occlusion in an immunocompromised child who died with adenoviral pneumonia. Note interstitial mononuclear cell infiltration and hyaline membranes. Adenoviruses types 3 and 7 can cause necrotizing bronchitis and bronchiolitis. Courtesy of Edgar O. Ledbetter, MD, FAAP.

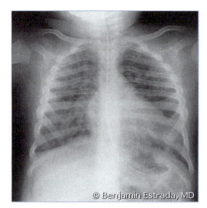

Image 2.4
Adenovirus pneumonia in a 4-year-old boy. Courtesy of Benjamin Estrada, MD.

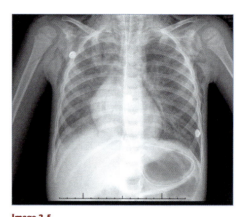

Image 2.5
This previously healthy 3-year-old boy presented with respiratory failure requiring intensive care for adenovirus type 7 pneumonia. He eventually recovered with some mild impairment noted in pulmonary function studies. Note the pneumomediastinum. Courtesy of Carol J. Baker, MD, FAAP.

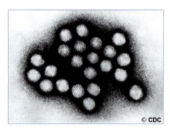

Image 2.6
Transmission electron micrograph of adenovirus. Adenoviruses have a characteristic icosahedral structure. Courtesy of Centers for Disease Control and Prevention.

CHAPTER 3

Amebiasis

CLINICAL MANIFESTATIONS

Most individuals with *Entamoeba histolytica* have asymptomatic noninvasive intestinal tract infection. When present, symptoms associated with *E histolytica* infection generally include cramps, watery or bloody diarrhea, and weight loss. Occasionally, the parasite may spread to other organs, most commonly the liver (liver abscess), and cause fever and right upper quadrant pain. Disease is more severe in very young children, elderly people, malnourished people, pregnant women, and people who receive corticosteroids. People with symptomatic intestinal amebiasis generally have gradual onset of symptoms over 1 to 3 weeks. The mildest form of intestinal tract disease is nondysenteric colitis. Amebic dysentery is the most common clinical manifestation of amebiasis and generally includes diarrhea with either gross or microscopic blood or mucus in the stool, lower abdominal pain, and tenesmus. Weight loss is common because of the gradual onset, but fever occurs in a minority of patients (8%–38%). Symptoms may be chronic, with periods of diarrhea and intestinal spasms alternating with periods of constipation. The manifestation may mimic that of inflammatory bowel disease. Progressive involvement of the colon may produce toxic megacolon, fulminant colitis, ulceration of the colon and perianal area, and, rarely, perforation. Colonic progression may occur at multiple sites and has a high fatality rate. Progression may occur in patients inappropriately treated with corticosteroids or antimotility drugs. An amebic granuloma (ameboma) may form as an annular lesion of the colon and may manifest as a palpable mass on physical examination. Amebomas can occur in any area of the colon but are most common in the cecum and may be mistaken for colonic carcinoma. Amebomas usually resolve with antiamebic therapy and do not require surgery.

Extraintestinal disease occurs in a small proportion of patients. The liver is the most common extraintestinal site, and infection may spread from there to the pleural space, lungs, and pericardium. Liver abscess may be acute, with fever, abdominal pain, tachypnea, liver tenderness, and hepatomegaly, or may be chronic, with weight loss and vague abdominal symptoms. Liver abscess can also be asymptomatic and discovered only on abdominal imaging that is performed for other reasons. Rupture of abscesses into the abdomen or chest may lead to death. Evidence of recent or concurrent intestinal tract infection is usually absent in extraintestinal disease. Infection may spread from the colon to the genitourinary tract and the skin. The organism may spread hematogenously to the brain and other areas of the body.

ETIOLOGY

The genus *Entamoeba* includes 6 species that live in the human intestine. Four of these species are identical morphologically: *E histolytica, Entamoeba dispar, Entamoeba moshkouskii,* and *Entamoeba bangladeshi. Dientamoeba fragilis* can also lead to asymptomatic infection and intraluminal intestinal disease. Not all *Entamoeba* species are virulent. *E dispar* and *Entamoeba coli* are generally recognized as commensals, and although *E moshkouskii* was generally believed to be nonpathogenic, it may be associated with diarrhea in infants. The pathogenic potential of *E bangladeshi* is unclear. *Entamoeba* and *Dientamoeba* organisms are excreted as cysts or trophozoites in stool of infected people.

EPIDEMIOLOGY

E histolytica can be found worldwide but is more prevalent among people with lower income who live in resource-limited countries, where prevalence of amebic infection may be as high as 50% in some communities. Groups with risk factors for infection in industrialized countries include immigrants from or long-term visitors to areas with endemic infection, people in institutions, and men who have sex with men. Intestinal and asymptomatic infections are distributed equally across the sexes, but incidence of invasive disease, especially liver abscess, is significantly higher among men.

E histolytica is transmitted via ingestion of infective amebic cysts, through fecally contaminated food or water, or oral-anal sexual practices. Transmission can also occur via direct rectal inoculation through colonic irrigation devices. Ingested cysts, which are unaffected by gastric acid, undergo excystation in the alkaline small intestine and produce trophozoites that can cause invasive disease in the colon. Cysts that develop subsequently are the source of transmission, especially from asymptomatic cyst excreters. Infected patients excrete cysts intermittently, sometimes for years if untreated. Cysts can remain viable in the environment for weeks to months, are relatively resistant to chlorine, and, by ingestion of a single cyst, are sufficient to cause disease.

The **incubation period** is variable, ranging from a few days to months or years, but is commonly 2 to 4 weeks.

DIAGNOSTIC TESTS

Intestinal amebiasis can be diagnosed by molecular tests, direct microscopy, and antigen detection tests. Stool polymerase chain reaction (PCR) tests have the highest sensitivity and specificity, are available in US Food and Drug Administration (FDA)–approved multiplex assays, and can differentiate *E histolytica* from other *Entamoeba* species. Traditionally, diagnosis of intestinal tract infection was made by identifying trophozoites or cysts in stool specimens, either on wet mount or after fixing and staining. This technique is still used in some laboratories but is labor intensive and has a sensitivity lower than for PCR testing and the requirement to review multiple stool specimens. Microscopy also does not differentiate between *E histolytica* and less pathogenic species, although trophozoites containing ingested red blood cells are more likely to be *E histolytica*. Antigen test kits are available in some clinical laboratories for testing of *E histolytica* directly from stool specimens. Examination of biopsy specimens, endoscopy scrapings (not swabs), and abscess aspirates by using microscopy or antigen detection is not typically fruitful; PCR assay is preferred, when available, but is FDA approved only for stool specimens. Some monoclonal antibody-based antigen detection assays can also differentiate *E histolytica* from other *Entamoeba* species. *D fragilis* is diagnosed by microscopy.

The indirect hemagglutination test has been replaced by commercially available enzyme immunoassay (EIA) kits for routine serodiagnosis of amebiasis, especially in countries without endemic disease. The EIA detects antibodies specific for *E histolytica* in about 95% or more of patients with extraintestinal amebiasis, 70% of patients with active intestinal tract infection, and 10% of asymptomatic people who are passing cysts of *E histolytica*. Patients may continue to have positive serological test results even after adequate therapy. Diagnosis of an *E histolytica* liver abscess and other extraintestinal infections is aided by serological testing, because stool tests and abscess aspirations are frequently nondiagnostic.

Ultrasonography, computed tomography, and magnetic resonance imaging can be used to presumptively identify liver abscesses presumptively; those caused by *E histolytica* are typically solitary and smooth walled. Imaging can also be used to identify other extraintestinal sites of infection.

TREATMENT

Treatment should be prioritized for all patients with *E histolytica*, including those who are asymptomatic, given the propensity of this organism to spread among family members and other contacts and to cause invasive infection. When tests to distinguish species are unavailable, treatment should be administered to symptomatic people on the basis of positive results of microscopic examination. A treatment plan should include directed therapy to eliminate invading trophozoites as well as organisms carried in the intestinal lumen, including cysts. Corticosteroids and antimotility drugs should not be used because they can worsen symptoms and aggravate the disease process. The following treatment regimens and follow-up are recommended:

- **Asymptomatic cyst excreters (intraluminal infections):** Treat with an intraluminal amebicide alone (paromomycin, diiodohydroxyquinoline-iodoquinol, or diloxanide furoate [diloxanide furoate is not currently available in the United States]). Metronidazole and tinidazole are ineffective against cysts.

- **Patients with invasive colitis manifesting as mild, moderate, or severe intestinal tract symptoms or extraintestinal disease (including liver abscess):** Treat with metronidazole or tinidazole, followed by an intraluminal amebicide: diiodohydroxyquinoline-iodoquinol, diloxanide furoate, or, in absence of intestinal obstruction, paromomycin. Nitazoxanide may be effective for mild to moderate intestinal amebiasis, although it is not approved by the FDA for this indication.

- **Additional considerations for patients with hepatic abscess, pleural or pericardial abscess, or other severe complications:** Percutaneous or surgical aspiration of large liver abscesses may occasionally be required when response of the abscess to medical therapy is unsatisfactory or there is risk of rupture. In most cases of liver abscess, however, drainage is not required and does not speed recovery. Although patients typically improve symptomatically within days, it may take months for a liver abscess to resolve on ultrasonography. Rupture into the peritoneal or pleural space usually requires drainage. For patients who have peritonitis attributable to intestinal perforation, broad-spectrum antibacterial therapy should be used in addition to an amebicide. In cases with toxic megacolon, colectomy may be necessary.

Follow-up stool examination is recommended after completion of therapy for intestinal disease, because no pharmacological regimen is completely effective in eradicating intestinal tract infection. Household members and other suspected contacts should undergo adequate stool examinations and should be treated if results are positive for *E histolytica*.

E dispar and *E coli* are generally considered nonpathogenic and do not necessarily require treatment. The pathogenic significance of finding *E moshkovskii* and *E bangladeshi* is unclear; treatment of symptomatic infection is reasonable. *D fragilis* is treated with iodoquinol, paromomycin, or metronidazole.

ISOLATION OF THE HOSPITALIZED PATIENT

Standard precautions are considered adequate for hospitalized patients; nosocomial transmission is rare.

CONTROL MEASURES

Careful hand hygiene after defecation, sanitary disposal of fecal material, and treatment of drinking water will control spread of infection. Sexual transmission may be controlled by use of condoms and avoidance of sexual activity with those who have diarrhea or who recently recovered from diarrhea. Because of the risk of shedding infectious cysts, people diagnosed with amebiasis should refrain from using recreational water venues (eg, swimming pools, water parks) until their course of luminal chemotherapy is completed and diarrhea has resolved. Some states prohibit return to work or school for food handlers or children until symptoms have resolved.

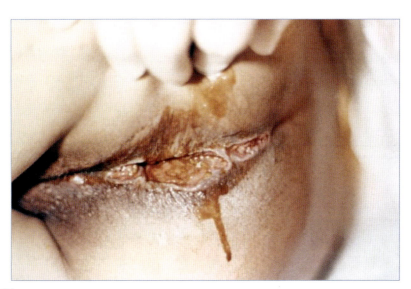

Image 3.1
This patient with amebiasis presented with tissue destruction and granulation of the anoperineal region caused by an *Entamoeba histolytica* infection. Courtesy of Centers for Disease Control and Prevention.

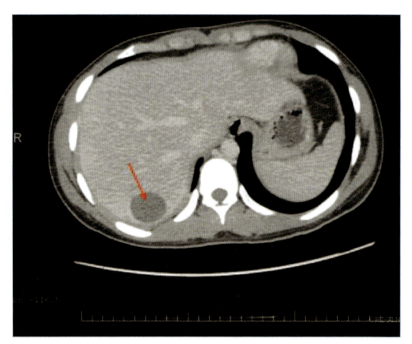

Image 3.2
Computed tomographic scan of the abdomen showing a peripherally enhancing low-density lesion in the posterior aspect of the right hepatic lobe. Amebic liver abscess amebiasis, caused by the intestinal protozoal parasite *Entamoeba histolytica*, remains a global health problem, infecting about 50 million people and resulting in 40,000–100,000 deaths per year. Prevalence may be as high as 50% in tropical and subtropical countries where overcrowding and poor sanitation are common. In the United States, *E histolytica* infection is found most commonly in immigrants from developing countries, long-term travelers to endemic areas (most frequently, Mexico or Southeast Asia), individuals in institutions, and men who have sex with men. In 1993, the previously known species *E histolytica* was reclassified into 2 genetically and biochemically distinct but morphologically identical species: the pathogenic *E histolytica* and the nonpathogenic commensal *Entamoeba dispar*. Courtesy of *Pediatrics in Review*.

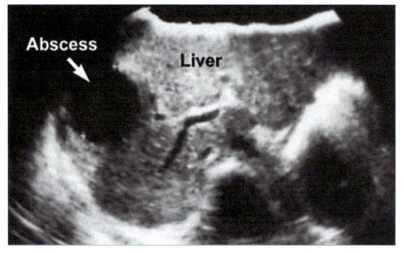

Image 3.3
Abdominal ultrasound showing a liver abscess caused by *Entamoeba histolytica*.

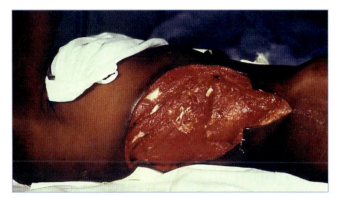

Image 3.4
This patient presented with invasive extraintestinal amebiasis affecting the cutaneous region of the right flank. Courtesy of Centers for Disease Control and Prevention.

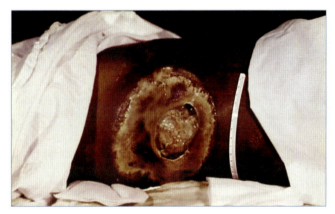

Image 3.5
This patient, also shown in Image 3.4, presented with invasive extraintestinal amebiasis affecting the cutaneous region of the right flank and causing severe tissue necrosis. Photographed is the site of tissue destruction, pre-debridement. Courtesy of Centers for Disease Control and Prevention/Kerrison Juniper, MD, and George Healy, PhD, DPDx.

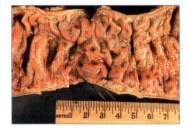

Image 3.6
Gross pathological features of intestinal ulcers caused by amebiasis. Courtesy of Centers for Disease Control and Prevention.

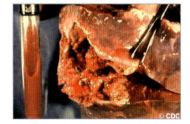

Image 3.7
Gross pathological features of amebic (*Entamoeba histolytica*) abscess of liver; tube of chocolate-like pus from abscess. Amebic liver abscesses are usually singular and large and in the right lobe of the liver. Bacterial hepatic abscesses are more likely to be multiple. Courtesy of Centers for Disease Control and Prevention.

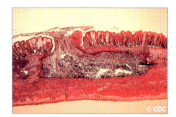

Image 3.8
Histopathologic features of a typical flask-shaped ulcer of intestinal amebiasis in a kitten. Courtesy of Centers for Disease Control and Prevention.

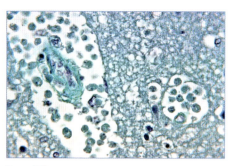

Image 3.9
This micrograph of a brain tissue specimen reveals the presence of *Entamoeba histolytica* amoebae (magnification ×500). In more serious cases of amebiasis, amoebae can cause an infection of tissue outside the intestinal tract. Courtesy of Centers for Disease Control and Prevention.

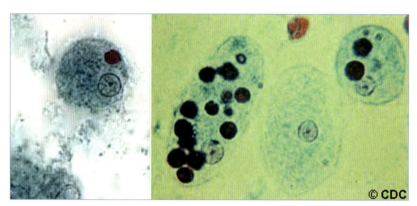

Image 3.10
Trophozoites of *Entamoeba histolytica* with ingested erythrocytes (trichrome stain). The ingested erythrocytes appear as dark inclusions. Erythrophagocytosis is the only characteristic that can be used to morphologically differentiate *E histolytica* from the nonpathogenic *Entamoeba dispar*. In these specimens, the parasite nuclei have the typical small, centrally located karyosome and thin, uniform peripheral chromatin. Courtesy of Centers for Disease Control and Prevention.

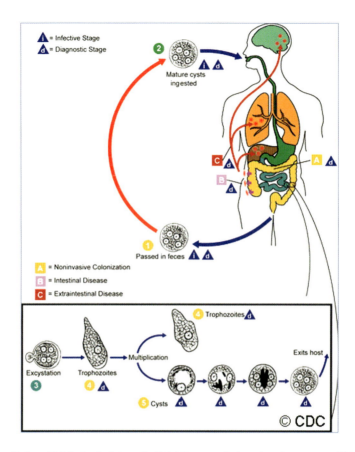

Image 3.11
Cysts are passed in feces (1). Infection by *Entamoeba histolytica* occurs by ingestion of mature cysts (2) in fecally contaminated food, water, or hands. Excystation (3) occurs in the small intestine and trophozoites (4) are released, which migrate to the large intestine. The trophozoites multiply by binary fission and produce cysts (5), which are passed in feces (1). Because of the protection conferred by their walls, the cysts can survive days to weeks in the external environment and are responsible for transmission. (Trophozoites can also be passed in diarrheal stools but are rapidly destroyed once outside the body and, if ingested, would not survive exposure to the gastric environment.) In many cases, trophozoites remain confined to the intestinal lumen (A, noninvasive colonization) of individuals who are asymptomatic carriers, passing cysts in their stool. In some patients, trophozoites invade the intestinal mucosa (B, intestinal disease) or, through the bloodstream, extraintestinal sites, such as the liver, brain, and lungs (C, extraintestinal disease), with resultant pathological manifestations. It has been established that invasive and noninvasive forms represent 2 separate species, *E histolytica* and *Entamoeba dispar*, respectively; however, not all people infected with *E histolytica* have invasive disease. These 2 species are morphologically indistinguishable. Transmission can also occur through fecal exposure during sexual contact (from which not only cysts but also trophozoites could prove infective). Courtesy of Centers for Disease Control and Prevention.

CHAPTER 4

Amebic Meningoencephalitis and Keratitis

(*Naegleria fowleri*, *Acanthamoeba* species, and *Balamuthia mandrillaris*)

CLINICAL MANIFESTATIONS

Naegleria fowleri can cause a rapidly progressive, almost always fatal, primary amebic meningoencephalitis (PAM). Early symptoms include fever, headache, vomiting, and, sometimes, disturbances of smell and taste. The illness progresses rapidly to signs of meningoencephalitis, including nuchal rigidity, lethargy, confusion, personality changes, and altered level of consciousness. Seizures are common, and death generally occurs within a week of onset of symptoms. No distinct clinical features differentiate this disease from fulminant bacterial meningitis.

Granulomatous amebic encephalitis (GAE) caused by *Acanthamoeba* species and *Balamuthia mandrillaris* has a more insidious onset than PAM and develops as a subacute or chronic disease. In general, patients with GAE die several weeks to months after onset of symptoms. Signs and symptoms may include altered mental status, personality changes, seizures, headaches, ataxia, cranial nerve palsies, hemiparesis, and other focal neurological deficits. Fever is often low-grade and intermittent. The course may resemble that of a bacterial brain abscess or a brain tumor. Chronic granulomatous skin lesions (pustules, nodules, and ulcers) may be present without central nervous system (CNS) involvement, particularly in patients with AIDS, and lesions may be present for months before brain involvement in immunocompetent hosts.

The most common symptoms of amebic keratitis, a vision-threatening infection usually caused by *Acanthamoeba* species, are pain (often out of proportion to clinical signs), photophobia, tearing, and foreign body sensation. Characteristic clinical findings include radial keratoneuritis and stromal ring infiltrate. *Acanthamoeba* keratitis generally follows an indolent course and may initially resemble herpes simplex or bacterial keratitis; delay in diagnosis is associated with worse outcomes.

ETIOLOGY

N fowleri, *Acanthamoeba* species, and *B mandrillaris* are free-living amebae that exist as motile, infectious trophozoites and environmentally hardy cysts.

EPIDEMIOLOGY

N fowleri is found in warm fresh water and moist soil. Most infections with *N fowleri* have been associated with swimming in natural bodies of warm fresh water, such as ponds, lakes, and hot springs, but other sources have included tap water from household plumbing systems and geothermal sources as well as poorly chlorinated swimming pools and municipal water. Disease has been reported worldwide but is uncommon. In the United States, infection occurs primarily in the summer and usually affects children and young adults. The recent northward extension of reported cases may be the result of climatic changes. Disease has followed use of tap water for sinus rinses or exposures related to recreational activities (eg, tap water used for a backyard waterslide). Trophozoites of the amebae invade the brain directly from the nose along the olfactory nerves via the cribriform plate. *Acanthamoeba* species are distributed worldwide and are found in soil; dust; cooling towers of electric and nuclear power plants; heating, ventilating, and air conditioning units; fresh and brackish water; whirlpool baths; and physiotherapy pools. The environmental niche of *B mandrillaris* is not delineated clearly, although it has been isolated from soil. CNS infection attributable to *Acanthamoeba* occurs primarily in debilitated and immunocompromised people. Some patients, and all reported children infected with *B mandrillaris*, have had no demonstrable underlying disease or defect. CNS infection by both amebae probably occurs most commonly by inhalation or direct contact with contaminated soil or water. The primary foci of these infections are most likely respiratory tract or skin, followed by hematogenous spread to the brain. Fatal encephalitis caused by *Balamuthia* species transmitted by the donated organ has been reported in recipients of organ transplants. *Acanthamoeba* keratitis occurs primarily in people who wear contact lenses, although it has also been associated with corneal trauma. Poor contact lens hygiene and/or disinfection practices as well as swimming with contact lenses are risk factors.

The **incubation period** for *N fowleri* infection is typically 3 to 7 days.

The **incubation periods** for *Acanthamoeba* and *Balamuthia* GAE are unknown. It is believed to take several weeks or months to develop the first symptoms of CNS disease following exposure to the amebae. Chronic progression (1–2 years) to CNS symptoms has been reported in children. Patients exposed to *Balamuthia* through a solid organ transplant can develop symptoms of *Balamuthia* GAE more quickly, within a few weeks.

The **incubation period** for *Acanthamoeba* keratitis is unknown but believed to range from several days to several weeks.

DIAGNOSTIC TESTS

In *N fowleri* infection, computed tomographic scans of the head without contrast are unremarkable or show only cerebral edema, but with contrast, they might show meningeal enhancement of the basilar cisterns and sulci. These changes, however, are nonspecific for amebic infection. Cerebrospinal fluid (CSF) pressure is usually elevated (300 to >600 mm water), and CSF indices may show a polymorphonuclear pleocytosis, an increased protein concentration, and a normal to very low glucose concentration. Motile trophozoites may be visualized by microscopic examination of CSF on a wet mount. If structures resembling trophozoites are visualized but no motility is observed, smears of CSF should be stained with Giemsa, trichrome, or Wright stain to verify the trophozoites. Gram stain is negative in *N fowleri* CNS infection. Trophozoites, but not cysts, can be visualized in sections of brain during autopsy. Microscopic images containing suspicious amebic structures can be evaluated by the morphology experts at the Centers for Disease Control and Prevention (CDC) DPDx (Laboratory Identification of Parasites of Public Health Concern; **www.cdc.gov/dpdx/index.html**). Polymerase chain reaction (PCR) and immunofluorescence assays performed on CSF and biopsy material to identify the organism are available through the CDC, as are consultation services for diagnosis and management (telephone: 770/488-7100).

In infection with *Acanthamoeba* species and *B mandrillaris*, trophozoites and cysts can be visualized in sections of brain, lungs, and skin; in *Acanthamoeba* keratitis, they can also be visualized in corneal scrapings and by confocal microscopy in vivo in the cornea on examination by an expert ophthalmologist. In GAE infections, CSF indices typically reveal a lymphocytic pleocytosis and an increased protein concentration, with normal or low glucose concentration but no organisms. Computed tomography and magnetic resonance imaging of the head may show single or multiple space-occupying, ring-enhancing lesions that can mimic brain abscesses, neurocysticercosis, tumors, cerebrovascular accidents, or other diseases. As on *N fowleri*, PCR and immunofluorescence assays can be performed on clinical specimens to identify *Acanthamoeba* species and *Balamuthia* species; these tests are available through the CDC.

TREATMENT

The most current guidance for treatment of PAM can be found by visiting the CDC website (**www.cdc.gov/parasites/naegleria/treatment-hcp.html**) or by contacting the CDC (telephone: 770/488-7100). Early diagnosis and institution of combination high-dose drug therapy is believed to be important for optimizing outcome. If meningoencephalitis possibly caused by *N fowleri* is suspected, treatment should not be withheld pending confirmation. Presence of amebic organisms in CSF is valuable for probable diagnosis, but confirmatory diagnostic tests should still be performed. Although an effective treatment regimen for PAM has not been identified, amphotericin B is the drug of choice in combination with other agents. In vitro testing indicates that *N fowleri* is highly susceptible to amphotericin B. Miltefosine, which is approved for treatment of leishmaniasis, has been used successfully to treat PAM caused by *N fowleri*. The CDC no longer provides miltefosine for treatment of free-living ameba infections; miltefosine is available commercially in the United States (**www.impavido.com**). There have been 4 US survivors of PAM, and on the basis of most recent cases, treatment with the combination of amphotericin B, azithromycin, fluconazole, miltefosine, and rifampin is recommended. These patients also received dexamethasone to control cerebral edema.

Effective treatment of infections caused by *Acanthamoeba* species and *B mandrillaris* has not been established. Several patients with *Acanthamoeba* GAE and *Acanthamoeba* cutaneous infections without CNS involvement have been treated successfully with a multidrug regimen consisting of various combinations of pentamidine, sulfadiazine, flucytosine, either fluconazole or itraconazole (voriconazole is not active against *Balamuthia* species), trimethoprim-sulfamethoxazole, and topical application of chlorhexidine gluconate and ketoconazole for skin lesions. Voriconazole, miltefosine, and azithromycin might also be of some value in treating *Acanthamoeba* infections. For patients with *B mandrillaris* infection, combination therapy, such as with pentamidine, sulfadiazine, fluconazole, either azithromycin or clarithromycin, and flucytosine, in addition to surgical resection of the CNS lesions, has been reported to be successful. Miltefosine has amebicidal activity against *B mandrillaris* in vitro.

Patients with *Acanthamoeba* keratitis should be evaluated by an ophthalmologist. Early diagnosis and therapy are important for a good outcome.

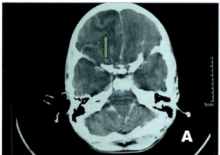

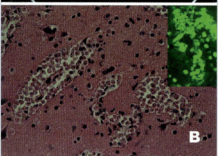

Image 4.1
A, Computed tomographic scan; note the right frontobasal collection (arrow) with a midline shift from right to left. B, Brain histological features; 3 large clusters of amebic vegetative forms can be observed (hematoxylin-eosin stain, magnification ×250). Inset: positive indirect immunofluorescent analysis on tissue section with anti–*Naegleria fowleri* serum. Courtesy of *Emerging Infectious Diseases*.

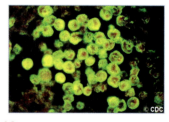

Image 4.2
This photomicrograph of brain tissue reveals free-living amoebas. Courtesy of Centers for Disease Control and Prevention.

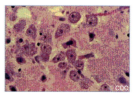

Image 4.3
Histopathologic features of amebic meningoencephalitis caused by *Naegleria fowleri* (direct fluorescent antibody stain). Courtesy of Centers for Disease Control and Prevention.

Image 4.4
Balamuthia mandrillaris trophozoites in brain tissue. Courtesy of Centers for Disease Control and Prevention.

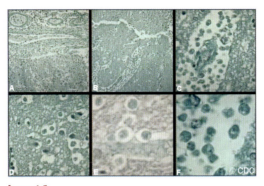

Image 4.5
A–F, *Naegleria fowleri* in brain tissue (trichrome stain). Courtesy of Centers for Disease Control and Prevention.

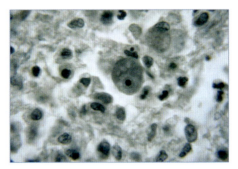

Image 4.6
This photomicrograph of a brain tissue specimen depicts the cytoarchitectural changes associated with a free-living amebic infection, which may have been caused by either *Naegleria fowleri* or *Acanthamoeba* species. Courtesy of Centers for Disease Control and Prevention.

CHAPTER 5
Anthrax

CLINICAL MANIFESTATIONS

Anthrax resulting from natural infection or secondary to a bioterror event can occur in multiple forms, depending on the route of infection: cutaneous, inhalation, ingestion, or injection. Manifestations of anthrax are mainly from the 2 primary toxins, lethal toxin and edema toxin. **Cutaneous** anthrax accounts for 95% of all human infections and begins as a pruritic papule or vesicle that progresses over 2 to 6 days to an ulcerated lesion with subsequent formation of a central black eschar. The lesion is characteristically painless and has surrounding edema and hyperemia. Patients may have associated fever.

Inhalation anthrax is a frequently lethal form of the disease and is a medical emergency. The initial manifestation is nonspecific and usually includes fever, malaise, and nonproductive cough. Many patients also report chest pain, headache, nausea, vomiting, and abdominal pain; sweating may be profuse. Illness usually progresses to the fulminant phase within 2 to 5 days. Illness has been noted to sometimes be biphasic, with a period of improvement between prodromal symptoms and overwhelming illness. Significant vital sign abnormalities are often present early, and fulminant manifestations include hypotension, dyspnea, hypoxia, cyanosis, and shock. Most patients with inhalation anthrax fulfill sepsis criteria, and up to half develop meningitis. Imaging abnormalities noted at presentation include pleural effusions in most, widened mediastinum in up to half, and infiltrates in many.

Ingestion anthrax can manifest as either of 2 distinct clinical syndromes—gastrointestinal or oropharyngeal. Patients with the gastrointestinal form often have nausea, anorexia, vomiting, and fever that progress to severe abdominal pain, often accompanied by marked ascites. Vomiting and diarrhea, which are not always present, may be bloody. Although gastrointestinal tract involvement at multiple sites may occur following hematogenous spread, the cecum and terminal ileum are often involved when the disease is primary. Patients with oropharyngeal anthrax may have dysphagia accompanied by posterior oropharyngeal necrotic ulcers. There may be marked, often unilateral neck swelling, regional lymphadenopathy, fever, and sepsis. Evidence of coagulopathy is common.

Injection anthrax occurs primarily in adults injecting drugs, associated with anthrax-contaminated heroin, and has not been reported in children. Smoking and snorting contaminated heroin have also been identified as exposure routes.

Any route of infection can lead to bacteremia and sepsis. Patients with inhalation, ingestion, or injection anthrax should be considered to have systemic illness. So should patients with cutaneous anthrax if they have tachycardia, tachypnea, hypotension, hyperthermia, hypothermia, or leukocytosis or have lesions that involve the head, neck, or upper torso or that are large, bullous, multiple, or surrounded by edema. Anthrax meningitis or hemorrhagic meningoencephalitis can occur in any patient with systemic illness and in patients without other apparent routes of infection. Therefore, lumbar puncture should be performed to rule out central nervous system (CNS) infection whenever clinically indicated. With appropriate treatment and supportive care, case-fatality rates range from less than 2% for cutaneous anthrax to 45% for inhalation anthrax and 92% for anthrax meningitis.

ETIOLOGY

Bacillus anthracis is an aerobic, gram-positive, encapsulated, spore-forming, nonhemolytic, nonmotile rod. *B anthracis* has 3 major virulence factors: an antiphagocytic capsule and 2 exotoxins, called *lethal toxin* and *edema toxin*. The toxins are responsible for most of the morbidity associated with anthrax and clinical manifestations of hemorrhage, edema, and necrosis.

EPIDEMIOLOGY

Anthrax is a zoonotic disease that most commonly affects domestic and wild herbivores and occurs in many rural regions of the world. *B anthracis* spores can remain viable in the soil for decades, representing a potential source of infection for livestock or wildlife through ingestion of spore-contaminated vegetation or water. In susceptible hosts, spores germinate to become viable bacteria. Natural infection of humans occurs through contact with infected animals or contaminated animal products, including carcasses, hides, hair, wool, meat, and bonemeal. Outbreaks of ingestion anthrax have occurred after consumption of meat from infected animals. Historically, more than 95% of anthrax cases in the United States were cutaneous infections in animal handlers or mill workers. The incidence of naturally occurring human anthrax decreased in the United States from an estimated 130 cases annually in the early 1900s to 0 to 2 cases per year from 1979 through 2011. Only one anthrax case (cutaneous) was confirmed in the United States from 2012–2018. Inhalation, cutaneous, and ingestion (gastrointestinal) anthrax have occurred in drum makers working with animal hides contaminated with B anthracis spores and in people participating in events where spore-contaminated drums were played. Severe soft tissue infections in adults injecting heroin, including disseminated systemic infection, have been reported in Europe.

B anthracis is one of the agents most likely to be used as a biological weapon, because (1) its spores are highly stable; (2) spores can infect via the respiratory route; and (3) the resulting inhalation anthrax has a high mortality rate. In 1979, an unintentional release of B anthracis spores from a military microbiology facility in the former Soviet Union resulted in at least 68 deaths. In 2001, 22 cases of anthrax (11 inhalation, 11 cutaneous) were identified in the United States after intentional contamination of the mail; 5 (45%) of the inhalation anthrax cases were fatal. In addition to aerosolization, B anthracis spores introduced into food products or water supplies could theoretically pose a risk to the public's health. Use of B anthracis in a biological attack would require immediate response and mobilization of public health resources (**www.cdc.gov/anthrax/ bioterrorism/index.html**).

Although the **incubation periods** for both cutaneous and ingestion anthrax are typically less than 1 week, rare cases for both have been reported more than 2 weeks after exposure. Because of spore dormancy (persistence of viable spores that have not yet germinated) and slow clearance of spores from the lungs, the **incubation period** for inhalation anthrax may be prolonged and has been reported to range from 2 days to 6 weeks in humans and up to 2 months in experimental nonhuman primates. Discharge from cutaneous lesions is potentially infectious, but person-to-person transmission has only rarely been reported, and other forms of anthrax are not associated with person-to person transmission. Both inhalation and cutaneous anthrax have occurred in laboratory workers.

DIAGNOSTIC TESTS

Depending on the clinical manifestation, Gram stain, culture, and polymerase chain reaction (PCR) testing for B anthracis should be performed with the assistance of state or local health departments on specimens of blood, pleural fluid, cerebrospinal fluid, and tissue biopsy specimens and on swabs of vesicular fluid or eschar material from cutaneous or oropharyngeal lesions, rectal swabs, or stool (**www.cdc.gov/anthrax/lab-testing/ index.html**). Acute sera may be tested for lethal factor (either of the 2 exotoxins of anthrax). Whenever possible, specimens for these tests should be obtained before initiating antimicrobial therapy because previous treatment with antimicrobial agents makes isolation by culture unlikely and decreases the sensitivity of PCR testing on both blood and tissue samples. Traditional microbiological methods can be used to presumptively identify B anthracis isolated readily on routine agar media (blood and chocolate) used in clinical laboratories. Definitive identification of suspected B anthracis isolates can be performed via the Laboratory Response Network in each state, accessed through state and local health departments. Additional diagnostic tests for anthrax are available through state health departments and the Centers for Disease Control and Prevention (CDC), including bacterial DNA detection in specimens by PCR assay, tissue immunohistochemistry, an enzyme immunoassay that measures immunoglobulin G antibodies against B anthracis protective antigen in paired sera, and a MALDI-TOF (matrix-assisted laser desorption/ionization–time-of-flight) mass spectrometry assay measuring lethal factor activity in sera. A commercially available enzyme-linked immunosorbent assay (QuickELISA Anthrax-PA kit) can be used for screening but not for definitive diagnosis. This assay detects antibodies to protective antigen protein of B anthracis in human serum from individuals with clinical history or symptoms consistent with anthrax. Clinical evaluation of patients with suspected inhalation anthrax should include a chest radiograph and/or computed tomographic scan to evaluate for widened mediastinum, pleural effusion, and/or pulmonary infiltrates. Lumbar punctures should be performed whenever feasible on systemically ill patients with any type of anthrax to rule out meningitis and to guide therapy.

TREATMENT

A high index of suspicion and rapid administration of appropriate antimicrobial therapy to people suspected of being infected, along with access to critical care support, are essential for effective treatment of anthrax. No controlled trials in humans have been performed to validate current treatment recommendations for anthrax, and there is limited clinical experience. Case reports suggest that naturally occurring localized or uncomplicated cutaneous disease can be treated effectively with 7 to 10 days of a single oral antimicrobial agent. First-line agents include a fluoroquinolone or doxycycline. Clindamycin is an alternative, as are penicillins, if the isolate is known to be penicillin susceptible, which is likely to occur with environmental isolates. For bioterrorism-associated cutaneous disease in adults or children lacking signs and symptoms of systemic illness (ie, localized cutaneous disease), oral ciprofloxacin or oral doxycycline is recommended for initial treatment until antimicrobial susceptibility data are available. Doxycycline can be used regardless of patient age. Because of the risk of concomitant inhalational exposure and subsequent spore dormancy in the lungs, the antimicrobial regimen for patients with bioterrorism-associated cutaneous anthrax or with exposure to other sources of aerosolized spores should be continued for a total of 60 days to provide postexposure prophylaxis (PEP), in conjunction with administration of vaccine if available (see Control Measures).

On the basis of in vitro data and animal studies, parenteral ciprofloxacin is recommended as the primary antimicrobial component of an initial multidrug regimen for treatment of all forms of systemic anthrax until results of antimicrobial susceptibility testing are known. Levofloxacin and moxifloxacin are considered equivalent alternatives to ciprofloxacin. CNS involvement should be suspected in all cases of inhalation anthrax and other systemic anthrax; thus, until this has been ruled out, treatment of systemic anthrax should include at least 2 other agents with known CNS penetration, in conjunction with ciprofloxacin. There appears to be a benefit to the use of a second bactericidal agent and a theoretical benefit to the use of a protein synthesis-inhibiting agent as the additional drugs in this combination. Meropenem is recommended as the second bactericidal antimicrobial, and if meropenem is unavailable, imipenem-cilastatin and meropenem-vaborbactam are considered alternatives; if the strain is known to be susceptible, penicillin G and ampicillin are equivalent alternatives. Linezolid is recommended as the preferred protein synthesis inhibitor if CNS involvement is suspected. Clindamycin and rifampin are alternatives.

If CNS penetration is less important because meningitis has been ruled out, treatment may consist of 2 antimicrobial agents, including a bactericidal and a protein synthesis-inhibiting agent. Ciprofloxacin is the preferred bactericidal agent, with meropenem, levofloxacin, imipenem-cilastatin, and vancomycin being alternatives; if the strain is known to be susceptible, penicillin G and ampicillin are equivalent alternatives. In this instance, clindamycin is the preferred protein synthesis inhibitor, and linezolid, doxycycline, and rifampin are acceptable alternatives. Because of intrinsic resistance, cephalosporins and trimethoprim-sulfamethoxazole should not be used.

For patients with systemic disease, treatment should continue for at least 14 days or longer, depending on patient condition. Intravenous therapy can be changed to oral therapy when progression of symptoms ceases and clinical symptoms are improving. There is risk of spore dormancy in the lungs in people with bioterrorism-associated cutaneous or systemic anthrax or people with exposure to other sources of aerosolized spores. In these cases, one of the PEP antimicrobials mentioned later in this chapter should be continued for a total of 60 days, in conjunction with administration of vaccine (see Control Measures).

For patients with anthrax and evidence of systemic illness, such as fever, tachypnea, tachycardia, or shock, polyclonal anthrax immune globulin intravenous or either of the monoclonal *B anthracis* antitoxins, obiltoxaximab or raxibacumab, should be considered in consultation with the CDC. Supportive symptomatic (intensive care) treatment is important. Aggressive pleural fluid or ascites drainage is critical if effusions exist, because drainage appears to be associated with improved survival. Obstructive airway disease resulting from associated edema may complicate cutaneous anthrax of the face or neck and can require aggressive monitoring for airway compromise.

ISOLATION OF THE HOSPITALIZED PATIENT

Standard precautions are recommended. In addition, contact precautions should be implemented when draining cutaneous lesions are present. Cutaneous lesions become sterile within 24 hours of starting appropriate antimicrobial therapy. Patients with cutaneous illness pose minimal risk for transmission if the wound is kept covered during the first day of antimicrobial therapy. Contaminated dressings and bedclothes should be incinerated or steam sterilized (121 °C [250 °F] for 30 minutes) to destroy spores. Terminal cleaning of the patient's room can be accomplished with an Environmental Protection Agency–registered hospital-grade disinfectant and should follow standard facility practices typically used for all patients. Autopsies performed on patients with systemic anthrax require special precautions.

CONTROL MEASURES

BioThrax (anthrax vaccine adsorbed [AVA]), the only anthrax vaccine currently licensed in the United States for use in humans, is prepared from a cell-free culture filtrate. The vaccine's efficacy for prevention of anthrax is based on animal studies, a single placebo-controlled human trial of the alum-precipitated precursor of the current AVA, observational data from humans, and immunogenicity data from humans and other mammals. In a human trial in adult mill workers, the alum-precipitated precursor to AVA demonstrated 93% efficacy for preventing cutaneous and inhalation anthrax. Multiple reviews and publications evaluating AVA safety have shown that adverse events are usually local injection site reactions, with rare systemic symptoms, including fever, chills, muscle aches, and hypersensitivity.

Recommendations for the response to possible exposure to anthrax through bioterrorism are available on the CDC website (**www.cdc.gov/anthrax/bioterrorism/index.html**). In the event of a bioterrorism event, information for health care professionals and the public relevant to that exposure will be posted on the CDC anthrax website (**www.cdc.gov/anthrax/index.html**). Within 48 hours of exposure to *B anthracis* spores, public health authorities plan to provide a 10-day course of antimicrobial prophylaxis to the local population, including children likely to have been exposed to spores. Within 10 days of exposure, public health authorities plan to further define those who have had a clear and significant exposure and will require additional antimicrobial PEP and a 3-dose anthrax vaccine (AVA) series.

PEP is recommended only for select groups of workers at continued risk of infection.

PEP for previously unvaccinated people older than 18 years who have been exposed to aerosolized *B anthracis* spores consists of up to 60 days of appropriate antimicrobial prophylaxis combined with 3 subcutaneous doses of AVA (administered at 0, 2, and 4 weeks postexposure). AVA is not licensed for use in pregnant women; however, in a postevent setting that poses a high risk of exposure to aerosolized *B anthracis* spores, pregnancy is neither a precaution nor a contraindication to its use in PEP. Similarly, AVA is not licensed for use in pediatric populations and has not been studied in children. Until there are sufficient data to support US Food and Drug Administration (FDA) approval, AVA is likely to be made available for children at the time of an event as an investigational vaccine under an appropriate regulatory mechanism that will require institutional review board approval, including the use of appropriate informed consent documents. Information on the process required for use of AVA in children will be available on the CDC website at the time of an event (**www.cdc.gov/anthrax/index.html**), as well as through the American Academy of Pediatrics (AAP) and the FDA. All exposed children 6 weeks and older should receive 3 doses of AVA at 0, 2, and 4 weeks in addition to 60 days of antimicrobial chemoprophylaxis. The recommended route of vaccine administration in children is subcutaneous. Children younger than 6 weeks should immediately begin antimicrobial prophylaxis, but initiation of the vaccine series should be delayed until they reach 6 weeks of age.

When no information is available about antimicrobial susceptibility of the implicated strain of *B anthracis*, ciprofloxacin and doxycycline are equivalent first-line antimicrobial agents for initial PEP for adults or children. Levofloxacin and clindamycin are second-line antimicrobial agents for PEP. Safety data on extended use of levofloxacin in any population for longer than 28 days are limited; however, the benefits of using levofloxacin as PEP for anthrax likely outweigh the risk. When the antimicrobial susceptibility profile demonstrates appropriate sensitivity to amoxicillin (minimum inhibitory concentration, ≤0.125 µg/mL), public health authorities may recommend changing PEP antimicrobial therapy for children to oral amoxicillin. Because of the lack of data on amoxicillin dosages for treating anthrax (and the associated high mortality rate), the AAP recommends a higher-than-usual dosage of oral amoxicillin, 75 mg/kg per day, divided into 3 daily doses administered every 8 hours (each dose not to exceed 1 g). Because of intrinsic resistance, cephalosporins and trimethoprim-sulfamethoxazole should not be used for prophylaxis.

Case Reporting

Anthrax meets the definition of a nationally and immediately notifiable condition, as specified by the US Council of State and Territorial Epidemiologists; therefore, every suspected case should be reported **immediately** to the state or local health department.

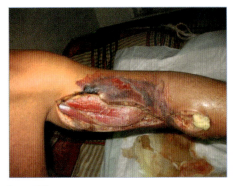

Image 5.2
Generalized cutaneous anthrax infection acquired from an ill cow. The infection began as a papule and was thought to be a simple furuncle. Following an attempt at drainage, the infection aggressively spread. Antibiotic therapy was started, and the patient survived. Courtesy of Mariam Svanidze, MD.

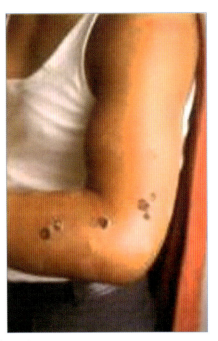

Image 5.1
Cutaneous anthrax. Notice edema and typical lesions. Courtesy of Centers for Disease Control and Prevention.

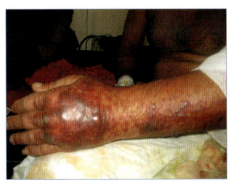

Image 5.3
Generalized cutaneous anthrax infection acquired from an ill cow. The infection began as a papule and was thought to be a simple furuncle. Following an attempt at drainage, the infection aggressively spread. Antibiotic therapy was started, and the patient survived. Courtesy of Mariam Svanidze, MD.

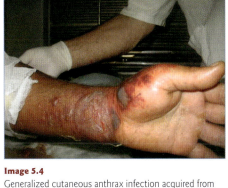

Image 5.4
Generalized cutaneous anthrax infection acquired from an ill cow. The infection began as a papule and was thought to be a simple furuncle. Following an attempt at drainage, the infection aggressively spread. Antibiotic therapy was started, and the patient survived. Courtesy of Mariam Svanidze, MD.

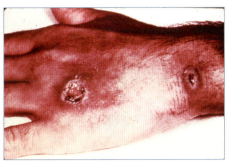

Image 5.5
Anthrax ulcers on the hand and wrist of an adult. The cutaneous eschar of anthrax had been misdiagnosed as a brown recluse spider bite. Edema is common and suppuration is absent.

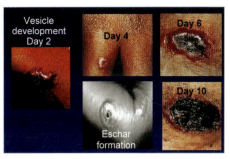

Image 5.6
Cutaneous anthrax. Vesicle development occurs from day 2–day 10 of progression. Courtesy of Centers for Disease Control and Prevention.

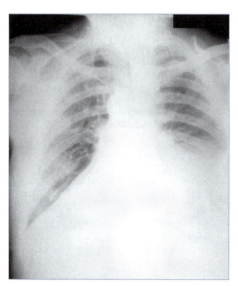

Image 5.7
Posteroanterior chest radiograph taken on the fourth day of illness, which shows a large pleural effusion and marked widening of the mediastinal shadow. Courtesy of Centers for Disease Control and Prevention.

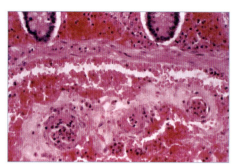

Image 5.8
This micrograph reveals submucosal hemorrhage in the small intestine in a case of fatal human anthrax (hematoxylin-eosin stain, magnification ×240). The first symptoms of gastrointestinal tract anthrax are nausea, loss of appetite, bloody diarrhea, and fever, followed by severe stomach pain. One-fourth to more than half of gastrointestinal anthrax cases lead to death. Note the associated arteriolar degeneration. Courtesy of Centers for Disease Control and Prevention.

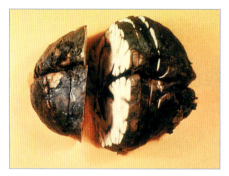

Image 5.9
Gross pathological features of fixed, cut brain showing hemorrhagic meningitis secondary to inhalational anthrax. Courtesy of Centers for Disease Control and Prevention.

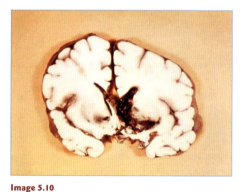

Image 5.10
This is a brain section through the ventricles revealing an interventricular hemorrhage. The 3 virulence factors of *Bacillus anthracis* are edema toxin, lethal toxin, and an antiphagocytic capsular antigen. The toxins are responsible for the primary clinical manifestations of hemorrhage, edema, and necrosis. Courtesy of Centers for Disease Control and Prevention.

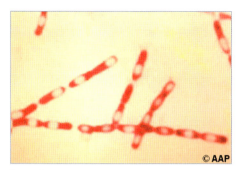

Image 5.11
Sporulation of *Bacillus anthracis*, a gram-positive, nonmotile, encapsulated bacillus.

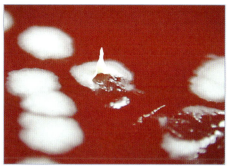

Image 5.12
Bacillus anthracis tenacity positively reacting on sheep blood agar. *B anthracis* colony characteristics: consistency, sticky (tenacious). When teased with loop, colony stands up like a beaten egg white. Courtesy of Centers for Disease Control and Prevention.

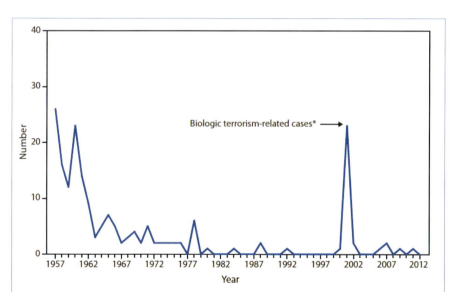

*Twenty-two bioterrorism-associated cases were reported from Connecticut, Florida, Maryland, New Jersey, Pennsylvania, and Virginia in 2001, and one naturally occurring epizootic-associated case was reported from Texas.

Naturally occurring anthrax epizootics occur annually among U.S. wildlife and livestock populations. In 2012, these were reported in states that routinely experience such outbreaks including Texas, North Dakota, and Nevada; however, livestock outbreaks additionally occurred in 2012 in Mississippi, Oregon, and Colorado, where anthrax outbreaks were not reported in livestock for ≥2 decades. These outbreaks were associated with exposures in persons handling and disposing of affected livestock and collecting diagnostic specimens. Although no human infections resulted, these exposures reflect the importance of timely recognition of anthrax in susceptible animals and the use of appropriate protective measures to prevent human exposures.

Image 5.13
Anthrax. Number of naturally occurring and biological terrorism–related cases reported, by year—United States, 1957–2012. There have been ≤2 cases of naturally occurring anthrax per year in the United States over the past 30 years. Courtesy of *Morbidity and Mortality Weekly Report*.

CHAPTER 6

Arboviruses

(Including Colorado tick fever, eastern equine encephalitis, Heartland, Jamestown Canyon, Japanese encephalitis, La Crosse, Powassan, St Louis encephalitis, tickborne encephalitis, and yellow fever viruses)

CLINICAL MANIFESTATIONS

Most infections with arthropodborne viruses (arboviruses) are subclinical. Symptomatic illness usually manifests as 1 of 3 primary clinical syndromes: generalized febrile illness, neuroinvasive disease, or hemorrhagic fever (Table 6.1).

- **Generalized febrile illness.** Most arboviruses are capable of causing a nonspecific febrile illness that often includes headache, arthralgia, myalgia, and rash. Some arboviruses can cause more characteristic clinical manifestations, such as neuroinvasive disease (see Chapter 164, West Nile Virus), severe polyarthralgia (see Chapter 27, Chikungunya), thrombocytopenia and leukopenia (eg, Heartland virus), or jaundice (eg, yellow fever virus). With some arboviruses, fatigue, malaise, and weakness can linger for weeks following the initial infection.

- **Neuroinvasive disease.** Many arboviruses cause neuroinvasive disease, including aseptic meningitis, encephalitis, or myelitis. Less common neurological manifestations (eg, Guillain-Barré syndrome) can also occur. Illness often manifests with a prodrome like that of the systemic febrile illness followed by neurological symptoms, although in some cases, neurological findings may be the initial indication of infection. Specific symptoms vary by virus but can include vomiting, stiff neck, mental status changes, seizures, or focal neurological deficits. Some viruses (eg, West Nile and Japanese encephalitis viruses) can cause a syndrome of acute flaccid paralysis, either in conjunction with meningoencephalitis or as an isolated finding. Severity and long-term outcome of the

Table 6.1
Clinical Manifestations for Selected Domestic and International Arboviral Diseases

Virus	Generalized Febrile Illness	Neuroinvasive Disease[a]	Hemorrhagic Fever
Domestic			
Colorado tick fever	Yes	Rare	No
Eastern equine encephalitis	Yes	Yes	No
Heartland[b]	Yes	No	No
Jamestown Canyon	Yes	Yes	No
La Crosse	Yes	Yes	No
Powassan	Yes	Yes	No
St Louis encephalitis	Yes	Yes	No
West Nile	Yes	Yes	No
International			
Chikungunya[c]	Yes	Rare	No
Dengue[c]	Yes	Rare	Yes
Japanese encephalitis	Yes	Yes	No
Tickborne encephalitis	Yes	Yes	No
Yellow fever	Yes	No	Yes
Zika[c]	Yes	Yes	No

[a] Meningitis, encephalitis, or myelitis.
[b] As of 2019, no pediatric infections documented; however, testing of children has been limited.
[c] Endemic with periodic outbreaks in US territories (Puerto Rico, US Virgin Islands, and American Samoa); local mosquitoborne transmission of chikungunya, dengue, and Zika viruses previously identified in Florida and Texas; local transmission of dengue virus also previously identified in Hawaii.

illness vary by etiologic agent and the underlying characteristics of the host, such as age, immune status, and preexisting medical conditions.

- **Hemorrhagic fever.** Hemorrhagic fever can be caused by some arboviruses, such as dengue (see Chapter 43, Dengue) and yellow fever viruses. After several days of nonspecific febrile illness, the patient may develop overt signs of hemorrhage (eg, petechiae, ecchymoses, bleeding from the nose and gums, hematemesis, melena) and shock (eg, decreased peripheral circulation, azotemia, tachycardia, hypotension). Hemorrhagic fever and shock caused by yellow fever virus have a high mortality rate and may be confused with other viral hemorrhagic fevers that can occur in the same geographic areas (eg, Argentine hemorrhagic fever, Bolivian hemorrhagic fever, Ebola, Lassa fever, or Marburg). Although dengue may be associated with severe hemorrhage, the shock is attributable primarily to a capillary leak syndrome, which, if properly treated with fluids, has a good prognosis. For information on other potential infections causing hemorrhagic manifestations, see Chapter 43, Dengue; Chapter 58, Hemorrhagic Fevers Caused by Arenaviruses; Chapter 59, Hemorrhagic Fevers Caused by Bunyaviruses; and Chapter 60, Hemorrhagic Fevers Caused by Filoviruses: Ebola and Marburg.

ETIOLOGY

Arboviruses are RNA viruses that are transmitted to humans primarily through bites of infected arthropods (mosquitoes, ticks, sand flies, and biting midges). More than 100 arboviruses are known to cause human disease. The viral families responsible for most arboviral infections in humans are *Flaviviridae* (genus *Flavivirus*), *Togaviridae* (genus *Alphavirus*), *Peribunyaviridae* (genus *Orthobunyavirus*), and *Phenuiviridae* (genus *Phlebovirus*). *Reoviridae* (genus *Coltivirus*) are also responsible but for fewer human arboviral infections (eg, Colorado tick fever) (Table 6.2).

EPIDEMIOLOGY

Most arboviruses maintain enzootic cycles of transmission between birds or small mammals and arthropod vectors. Humans and domestic animals are usually infected incidentally as dead-end hosts (Table 6.2). Important exceptions are chikungunya, dengue, yellow fever, and Zika viruses, which can be spread from person to arthropod to person (anthroponotic transmission). For other arboviruses, humans do not usually develop a sustained or high enough level of viremia to infect biting arthropod vectors. Direct person-to-person spread of some arboviruses has been documented to occur through blood transfusion, organ transplant, sexual transmission, intrauterine transmission, perinatal transmission, and human milk. Transmission through percutaneous, mucosal, or aerosol exposure to some arboviruses has occurred rarely in laboratory and occupational settings.

Arboviral infections occur in the United States primarily from late spring through early fall, when mosquitoes and ticks are most active. The number of domestic or imported arboviral disease cases reported in the United States varies greatly by specific etiology and year. Underdiagnosis of milder disease makes an accurate determination of the number of cases difficult.

In general, the risk of developing severe clinical disease for most arboviral infections in the United States is higher among adults than among children. One notable exception is La Crosse virus infection, for which children are at highest risk of severe neurological disease and possible long-term sequelae. Eastern equine encephalitis virus causes a low incidence of disease but a high case-fatality rate (40%) across all age-groups.

The **incubation periods** for arboviral diseases typically range between 2 and 15 days. Longer incubation periods can occur in immunocompromised people and with tickborne viruses, such as Colorado tick fever, Powassan, and tickborne encephalitis viruses.

DIAGNOSTIC TESTS

Arboviral infections are confirmed most frequently by detection of virus-specific antibody in serum or cerebrospinal fluid (CSF). Acute-phase serum specimens should be tested for virus-specific immunoglobulin M (IgM) antibody. With clinical and epidemiological correlation, a positive IgM test result has good diagnostic predictive value, but cross-reaction between related arboviruses from the same viral family can occur (eg, West Nile and St Louis encephalitis viruses, both of which are flaviviruses). For most arboviral infections, IgM is detectable within a week after onset of illness and persists for 30 to 90 days, but longer persistence has been documented, especially with West Nile and Zika viruses. Therefore, a positive serum IgM test result may occasionally reflect a prior infection. Serum collected within 10 days of illness onset may not have detectable IgM, and the test should be repeated on a convalescent-phase serum sample. Immunoglobulin G antibody is generally detectable in serum shortly after IgM and persists for years. A plaque-reduction neutralization test can be performed to measure virus-specific neutralizing antibodies and to discriminate between cross-reacting antibodies in primary arboviral infections. Either seroconversion or a 4-fold or greater increase in virus-specific neutralizing antibodies between acute- and convalescent-phase serum specimens collected 2 to 3 weeks apart is diagnostic of recent infection. In patients who have been immunized against or infected with another arbovirus from the same virus family in the past (ie, secondary infection), cross-reactive antibodies in both the IgM and neutralizing antibody assays might make it difficult to identify which arbovirus is causing the patient's current illness. For some arboviral infections (eg, Colorado tick fever or Heartland virus disease), the immune response may be delayed, with IgM antibodies not appearing until 2 to 3 weeks after onset of illness and neutralizing antibodies taking up to a month to develop. Patients with significant immunosuppression (eg, patients who have received a solid organ transplant or recent chemotherapy) may have a delayed or blunted serological response,

and nucleic acid amplification tests (NAATs) may be indicated in these cases. Immunization and travel history, date of symptom onset, and information regarding other arboviruses known to circulate in the geographic area that may cross-react in serological assays should be considered when interpreting results.

Viral culture and NAATs for RNA detection can be performed on acute-phase serum, CSF, or tissue specimens. Arboviruses that are more likely to be detected by using culture or NAATs early in the illness include Colorado tick fever, dengue, Heartland, yellow fever, and Zika viruses. For other arboviruses, results of these tests are often negative, even early in the clinical course, because of the relatively short duration of viremia. Immunohistochemical (IHC) staining can detect specific viral antigen in fixed tissue.

Antibody testing for common domestic arboviral diseases is performed in most state public health laboratories and many commercial laboratories. Confirmatory plaque-reduction neutralization tests, viral culture, NAATs, IHC staining, and testing for less common domestic and international arboviruses are performed at the Centers for Disease Control and Prevention (telephone: 970/221-6400) and selected other reference laboratories. Confirmatory testing is typically arranged through local and state health departments.

TREATMENT

The primary treatment of all arboviral disease is supportive care. Although various antiviral and immunologic therapies have been evaluated for several arboviral diseases, none have shown clear benefit.

Table 6.2
Genus, Geographic Location, and Vectors for Selected Domestic and International Arboviral Diseases

Virus	Genus	Predominant Geographic Locations United States	Predominant Geographic Locations Non–United States	Vector
Domestic				
Colorado tick fever	Coltivirus	Rocky Mountain and western states	Western Canada	Ticks
Eastern equine encephalitis	Alphavirus	Eastern and Gulf coast states	Americas	Mosquitoes
Heartland	Phlebovirus	Central and Southeast	None	Ticks
Jamestown Canyon	Orthobunyavirus	Widespread	Canada	Mosquitoes
La Crosse	Orthobunyavirus	Midwest and Appalachia	Canada	Mosquitoes
Powassan	Flavivirus	Northeast and Midwest	Canada, Russia	Ticks
St Louis encephalitis	Flavivirus	Widespread	Americas	Mosquitoes
West Nile	Flavivirus	Widespread	Americas, Europe, Africa, Asia	Mosquitoes
International				
Chikungunya	Alphavirus	Imported and periodic local transmission[a]	Worldwide in tropical and subtropical areas	Mosquitoes
Dengue	Flavivirus	Imported and periodic local transmission[a]	Worldwide in tropical and subtropical areas	Mosquitoes
Japanese encephalitis	Flavivirus	Imported only	Asia	Mosquitoes
Tickborne encephalitis	Flavivirus	Imported only	Europe, northern Asia	Ticks
Yellow fever	Flavivirus	Imported only	South America, Africa	Mosquitoes
Zika	Flavivirus	Imported and periodic local transmission[a]	Worldwide in tropical and subtropical areas	Mosquitoes

[a] Endemic with periodic outbreaks in US territories (Puerto Rico, US Virgin Islands, and American Samoa); local mosquitoborne transmission of chikungunya, dengue, and Zika viruses previously identified in Florida and Texas; local transmission of dengue virus also previously identified in Hawaii.

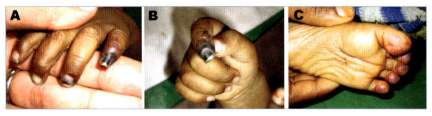

Image 6.1
Digital gangrene in an 8-month-old girl during week 3 of hospitalization. She was admitted to the hospital with fever, multiple seizures, and a widespread rash; chikungunya virus was detected in her plasma. A, Little finger of the left hand; B, index finger of the right hand; C, 4 toes on the right foot. Courtesy of Centers for Disease Control and Prevention/*Emerging Infectious Diseases*.

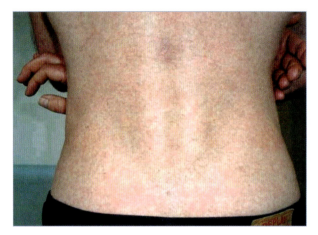

Image 6.2
Cutaneous eruption of chikungunya virus infection, a generalized exanthema comprising noncoalescent lesions, occurs during the first week of the disease, as found in this patient with erythematous maculopapular lesions with islands of normal skin. Courtesy of Centers for Disease Control and Prevention/*Emerging Infectious Diseases* and Patrick Hochedez.

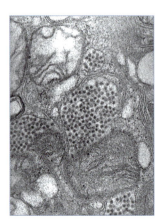

Image 6.3
An electron micrograph of eastern equine encephalomyelitis virus in a mosquito salivary gland; *Alphavirus*, eastern equine encephalomyelitis. Courtesy of Centers for Disease Control and Prevention.

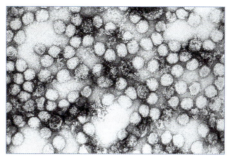

Image 6.4
An electron micrograph of yellow fever virus virions. Virions are spheroidal, uniform in shape, and 40–60 nm in diameter. The name *yellow fever* comes from the ensuing jaundice that affects some patients. The vector is the *Aedes aegypti* or *Haemagogus* species mosquito. Courtesy of Centers for Disease Control and Prevention.

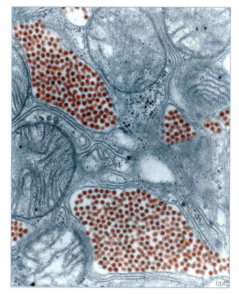

Image 6.5
This colorized transmission electron micrograph depicts a salivary gland that had been extracted from a mosquito, which was infected by the eastern equine encephalitis virus, which has been colorized red (magnification ×83,900). Courtesy of Centers for Disease Control and Prevention/Fred Murphy, MD, and Sylvia Whitfield.

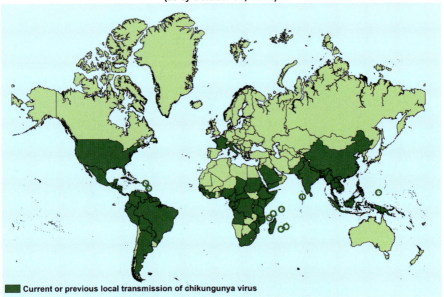

Countries and territories where chikungunya cases have been reported* (*as of October 30, 2020*)

■ Current or previous local transmission of chikungunya virus

*Does not include countries or territories where only imported cases have been documented.

Data table: Countries and territories where chikungunya cases have been reported

AFRICA	ASIA	AMERICAS	
Angola	Bangladesh	Anguilla	Panama
Benin	Bhutan	Antigua and Barbuda	Paraguay
Burundi	Cambodia	Argentina	Peru
Cameroon	China	Aruba	Puerto Rico
Central African Republic	India	Bahamas	Saint Barthelemy
Chad	Indonesia	Barbados	Saint Kitts and Nevis
Cote d'Ivoire	Laos	Belize	Saint Lucia
Dem. Republic of the	Malaysia	Bolivia	Saint Martin
Djibouti	Maldives	Brazil	Saint Vincent & the
Equatorial Guinea	Myanmar (Burma)	British Virgin Islands	Sint Maarten
Eritrea	Nepal	Cayman Islands	Suriname
Ethiopia	Pakistan	Colombia	Trinidad and Tobago
Gabon	Philippines	Costa Rica	Turks and Caicos Islands
Guinea	Saudi Arabia	Cuba	United States
Kenya	Singapore	Curacao	US Virgin Islands
Madagascar	Sri Lanka	Dominica	Venezuela
Malawi	Taiwan	Dominican Republic	
Mauritius	Thailand	Ecuador	
Mayotte	Timor-Leste	El Salvador	**OCEANIA/PACIFIC ISLANDS**
Mozambique	Vietnam	French Guiana	American Samoa
Nigeria	Yemen	Grenada	Cook Islands
Republic of the Congo		Guadeloupe	Federal States of Micronesia
Reunion		Guatemala	Fiji
Senegal	**EUROPE**	Guyana	French Polynesia
Seychelles	France	Haiti	Kiribati
Sierra Leone	Italy	Honduras	Marshall Islands
Somalia		Jamaica	New Caledonia
South Africa		Martinique	Papua New Guinea
Sudan		Mexico	Samoa
Tanzania		Montserrat	Tokelau
Uganda		Nicaragua	Tonga
Zimbabwe			

Image 6.6
Countries and territories where chikungunya has been reported (as of October 30, 2020).

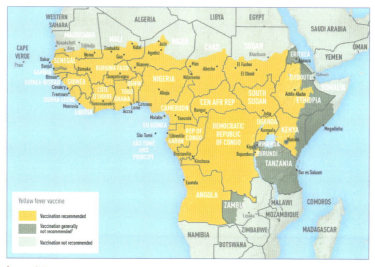

Image 6.7
Yellow fever vaccine recommendations in Africa. Courtesy of Centers for Disease Control and Prevention.

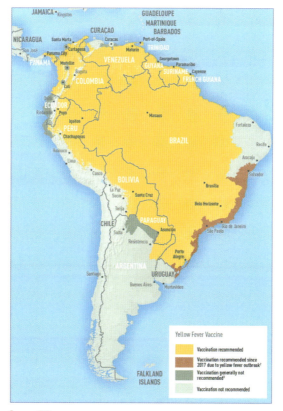

Image 6.8
Yellow fever vaccine recommendations in the Americas. Courtesy of Centers for Disease Control and Prevention.

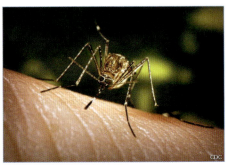

Image 6.10
A close-up anterior view of a *Culex tarsalis* mosquito as it was about to begin feeding. The epidemiological importance of *C tarsalis* lies in its ability to spread western equine encephalomyelitis, St Louis encephalitis, and California encephalitis, and *C tarsalis* is currently the main vector of West Nile virus in the western United States. Courtesy of Centers for Disease Control and Prevention/James Gathany.

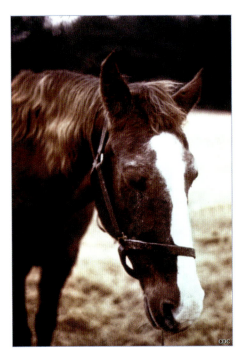

Image 6.9
This horse was displaying symptoms of the arboviral disease Venezuelan equine encephalomyelitis. Etiologic pathogens responsible for equine encephalitic diseases are transmitted to horses by mosquitoes, with reservoirs being various bird species. Courtesy of Centers for Disease Control and Prevention.

CHAPTER 7
Arcanobacterium haemolyticum Infections

CLINICAL MANIFESTATIONS

Acute pharyngitis attributable to *Arcanobacterium haemolyticum* is often indistinguishable from group A streptococcal pharyngitis. *A haemolyticum* has been associated with fever, pharyngeal erythema and exudates, cervical lymphadenopathy, and rash but not with palatal petechiae and strawberry tongue. A morbilliform or scarlatiniform exanthem is present in half of cases, beginning on extensor surfaces of the distal extremities; spreading to the torso, back, and neck; and sparing the face, palms, and soles. Rash typically develops 1 to 4 days after onset of sore throat, although rash preceding pharyngitis can occur; desquamation can occur. Respiratory tract infections that mimic diphtheria include membranous pharyngitis and peritonsillar and pharyngeal abscesses. Skin and soft tissue infections, including chronic ulcers, cellulitis, paronychia, and wound infection, have been attributed to *A haemolyticum*. Rarely, invasive infections have been reported, including Lemierre syndrome, bacteremia, sepsis, endocarditis, brain abscess, orbital cellulitis, and pyogenic arthritis. Nonsuppurative sequelae have not been reported.

ETIOLOGY

A haemolyticum is a catalase-negative, weakly acid-fast, facultatively anaerobic, hemolytic, gram-positive to gram-variable, slender, sometimes club-shaped bacillus.

EPIDEMIOLOGY

Humans are the primary reservoir of *A haemolyticum*, and spread is person to person, presumably via droplet respiratory secretions. Severe disease occurs almost exclusively in immunocompromised people. *Arcanobacterium* pharyngitis occurs primarily in adolescents and young adults and only rarely in young children. *A haemolyticum* accounts for approximately 0.5% of pharyngeal infections overall and up to 2.5% of pharyngeal infections in 15- to 25-year-olds. Isolation of the bacterium from the nasopharynx of asymptomatic people is rare. Person-to-person spread is inferred from family studies.

The **incubation period** is unknown.

DIAGNOSTIC TESTS

A haemolyticum grows on blood-enriched agar, but colonies are small, have narrow bands of beta hemolysis, and may not be visible for 48 to 72 hours. The organism is not detected by rapid antigen tests for group A streptococci. Detection is enhanced by culture on rabbit or human blood agar rather than on sheep blood agar, which yields larger colony size and wider zones of hemolysis. Presence of 5% carbon dioxide enhances growth. *A haemolyticum* may be missed in routine throat cultures on sheep blood agar if laboratory personnel are not specifically trained to identify the organism. Pits characteristically form under colonies on blood agar plates. Two biotypes of *A haemolyticum* have been identified: a rough colonial biotype predominates in respiratory tract infections; a smooth biotype typically predominates in skin and soft tissue infections.

TREATMENT

Optimal treatment of patients with *A haemolyticum* pharyngitis has not been determined, and symptoms can resolve without antibiotic treatment. Erythromycin and azithromycin are drugs of choice for *A haemolyticum* tonsillopharyngitis, but no controlled trials have been performed. *A haemolyticum* is generally susceptible in vitro to macrolides, clindamycin, cephalosporins, ciprofloxacin, vancomycin, and gentamicin. Treatment failures with penicillin despite predicted susceptibility from in vitro testing occur and may be attributable to tolerance. Resistance to trimethoprim-sulfamethoxazole is common. In rare cases of invasive infection, susceptibility tests should be performed and treatment should be individualized. While awaiting results, initial empirical combination therapy can be initiated by using a parenteral β-lactam agent, with or without gentamicin or a macrolide and with consideration of metronidazole if *Fusobacterium* infection is suspected.

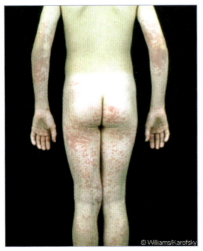

Image 7.1
Arcanobacterium haemolyticum was isolated on pharyngeal culture from this 12-year-old boy with an erythematous rash that was followed by mild desquamation. Copyright Williams/Karofsky.

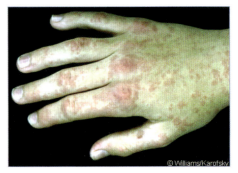

Image 7.2
Arcanobacterium haemolyticum–associated rash on dorsal surface of the hand in the 12-year-old boy in images 7.1, 7.3, and 7.4. Copyright Williams/Karofsky.

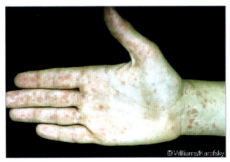

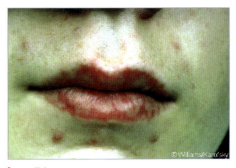

Image 7.3
Note that the palms are affected in this patient, although they are often spared. Copyright Williams/Karofsky.

Image 7.4
Although not present in this patient with facial skin lesions associated with Arcanobacterium haemolyticum pharyngitis, a pharyngeal membrane similar to that of diphtheria may occur with A haemolyticum pharyngeal infection. Copyright Williams/Karofsky.

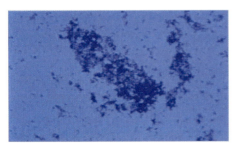

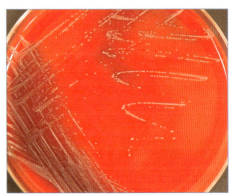

Image 7.5
Arcanobacterium haemolyticum (Gram stain). A haemolyticum appears strongly gram positive in young cultures but becomes more gram variable after 24 hours of incubation. Copyright Noni MacDonald, MD, FAAP.

Image 7.6
Arcanobacterium haemolyticum on blood agar. Colonies are small and produce beta hemolysis on blood agar. Courtesy of Julia Rosebush, DO; Robert Jerris, PhD; and Theresa Stanley, M(ASCP).

CHAPTER 8

Ascaris lumbricoides Infections

CLINICAL MANIFESTATIONS

Most infections with *Ascaris lumbricoides* are asymptomatic, although moderate to heavy infections may lead to nonspecific gastrointestinal tract symptoms, malnutrition, and growth delay. During the larval migratory phase, an acute transient pneumonitis (Löffler syndrome) associated with cough, substernal discomfort, shortness of breath, fever, and marked eosinophilia may occur. Acute intestinal obstruction has been associated with heavy infections. Children are prone to this complication because of the small diameter of the intestinal lumen and their propensity to acquire large worm burdens. Heavy worm burdens can also affect nutritional status, intellectual development, cognitive performance, and growth. Worm migration can cause peritonitis secondary to intestinal wall perforation as well as appendicitis or common bile duct obstruction resulting in biliary colic, cholangitis, or pancreatitis. Adult worms can be stimulated to migrate by stressful conditions (eg, fever, illness, anesthesia) and by some anthelmintic drugs.

ETIOLOGY

Following ingestion of embryonated eggs, usually from contaminated soil, larvae hatch in the small intestine, penetrate the mucosa, and are transported passively by portal blood to the liver and lungs. After migrating from alveolar capillaries into the small airways, larvae ascend through the tracheobronchial tree to the pharynx, are swallowed, and mature into adults in the small intestine. Female worms produce approximately 200,000 eggs per day, which are excreted in stool and must incubate in soil to become infectious. Adult worms can live in the lumen of the small intestine for up to 18 months. Female worms are longer than male worms and can measure 40 cm (>15 inches) in length and 6 mm in diameter.

EPIDEMIOLOGY

A lumbricoides is the most prevalent of all human intestinal nematodes (roundworms), with approximately 800 million people infected worldwide. Infection with *A lumbricoides* is most common in resource-limited countries, including rural and urban communities characterized by poor sanitation. Direct person-to-person transmission does not occur. *Ascaris suum*, a pig roundworm like *A lumbricoides*, also causes human disease and is associated with raising pigs and using their stool for fertilizer.

The **incubation period** (interval between ingestion of eggs and development of egg-laying adults) is approximately 9 to 11 weeks.

DIAGNOSTIC TESTS

Ascariasis is diagnosed by examining a fresh or preserved stool specimen for eggs via light microscopy. Adult worms may also be passed from the rectum, through the nares, or from the mouth, usually in vomitus. Imaging of the gastrointestinal tract or biliary tree by using computed tomography or ultrasonography may detect adult *Ascaris* worms, which can cause filling defects following administration of oral contrast.

TREATMENT

Albendazole (taken with food in a single dose), mebendazole (taken in a single dose or taken twice daily for 3 days), and pyrantel pamoate are first-line agents for treatment of ascariasis. Ivermectin (taken on an empty stomach in a single dose) and nitazoxanide are alternative therapies. Cure rates range from 90% with pyrantel pamoate to 100% with albendazole. Albendazole, pyrantel pamoate, ivermectin, and nitazoxanide are not approved by the US Food and Drug Administration for treatment of ascariasis, although albendazole has become the drug of choice for most soil-transmitted nematode infections, including ascariasis. Studies in children as young as 1 year of age suggest that albendazole can be administered safely to this population. The safety of ivermectin in children weighing less than 15 kg and in pregnant women has not been established. Reexamination of stool specimens may be performed at approximately 2 weeks after deworming to document cure and again at 2 to 3 months to account for migrating larvae from new infections (which are resistant to anthelmintics) at the time of treatment. Patients who remain infected should be re-treated, preferably with albendazole or the multidose regimen of mebendazole, and the reasons for the repeated infections should be explored and addressed.

Conservative management of small-bowel obstruction, including nasogastric suction, intravenous fluids, and repletion of electrolytes, may alleviate symptoms before administration of anthelmintic therapy. Use of mineral oil or diatrizoate meglumine and diatrizoate sodium solution, either orally or by nasogastric tube, may also cause relaxation of a bolus of worms. Endoscopic retrograde cholangiopancreatography has been used successfully for extraction of worms from the biliary tree. Surgical intervention (eg, laparotomy) is indicated for intestinal or biliary tract obstruction that does not resolve with conservative therapy or for volvulus or peritonitis secondary to perforation.

ISOLATION OF THE HOSPITALIZED PATIENT

Standard precautions are recommended.

CONTROL MEASURES

Sanitary disposal of human feces prevents transmission. Vegetables cultivated in areas where human feces are used as fertilizer must be washed thoroughly and cooked before eating.

Preventive chemotherapy (deworming) administered once or twice annually with albendazole or single-dose mebendazole and targeting high-risk groups, most notably preschool and school-aged children and pregnant women (after the first trimester), is recommended by the World Health Organization for control of *A lumbricoides* and other soil-transmitted nematodes in communities with 20% or more baseline prevalence of infection. Reinfection is common in high-prevalence areas, and additional public health measures, including improved sanitation, safe drinking water, and health education, will likely be required to eliminate these infections.

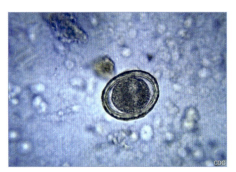

Image 8.1
This micrograph reveals a fertilized egg of the roundworm *Ascaris lumbricoides* (magnification ×400). Fertilized eggs are round with a thick shell, whereas unfertilized eggs are elongate with a larger, thinner shell, and covered by a more visible mammillated layer, which is sometimes covered by protuberances. Courtesy of Centers for Disease Control and Prevention/Mae Melvin, MD.

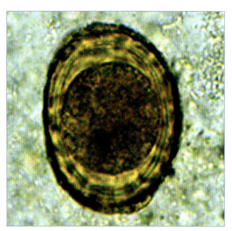

Image 8.2
A fertilized ascaris egg, still at the unicellular stage, which is the usual stage when the eggs are passed in the stool (complete development of the larva requires 18 days under favorable conditions). Courtesy of Centers for Disease Control and Prevention.

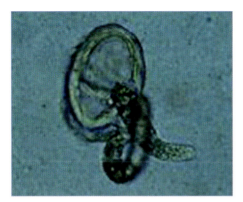

Image 8.3
Larva hatching from an ascaris egg. Hatching occurs in the small intestine. Courtesy of Centers for Disease Control and Prevention.

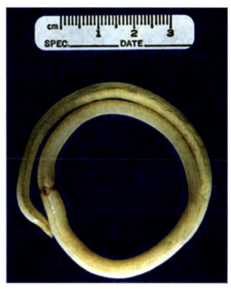

Image 8.4
An adult ascaris. Diagnostic characteristics: tapered ends; length, 15–35 cm (females tend to be larger). This worm is a female, as evidenced by the size and genital girdle (the dark circular groove at the left side of the image). Courtesy of Centers for Disease Control and Prevention.

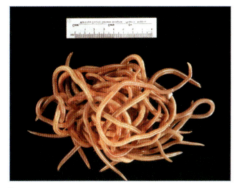

Image 8.5
A mass of large roundworms (*Ascaris lumbricoides*) from infestation in a human.

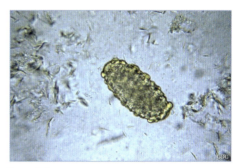

Image 8.6
This micrograph reveals an unfertilized egg of the roundworm *Ascaris lumbricoides* (magnification ×400). Fertilized eggs are round with a thick shell, whereas unfertilized eggs are elongate with a larger, thinner shell, and covered by a more visible mammillated layer, which is sometimes covered by protuberances, as in this case. Courtesy of Centers for Disease Control and Prevention/ Mae Melvin, MD.

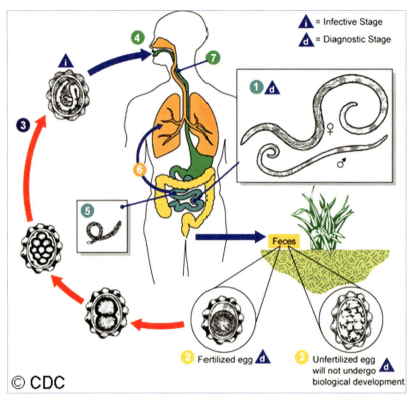

Image 8.7
Adult worms (1) live in the lumen of the small intestine. A female may produce approximately 200,000 eggs per day, which are passed with the feces (2). Unfertilized eggs may be ingested but are noninfective. Fertile eggs embryonate and become infective after 18 days to several weeks (3), depending on the environmental conditions (optimum: moist, warm, shaded soil). After infective eggs are swallowed (4), the larvae hatch (5), invade the intestinal mucosa, and are carried via the portal and then via systemic circulation to the lungs (6). The larvae mature further in the lungs (10–14 days), penetrate the alveolar walls, ascend the bronchial tree to the throat, and are swallowed (7). On reaching the small intestine, they develop into adult worms (8). Between 2 and 3 months is required from ingestion of the infective eggs to oviposition by the adult female. Adult worms can live 1–2 years. Courtesy of Centers for Disease Control and Prevention.

CHAPTER 9
Aspergillosis

CLINICAL MANIFESTATIONS

Aspergillosis manifests as 5 principal clinical entities: invasive aspergillosis, aspergilloma, allergic bronchopulmonary aspergillosis, allergic sinusitis, and chronic pulmonary aspergillosis. Colonization of the respiratory tract is common. The clinical manifestations and severity depend on host immune status (either immunocompromised or atopic).

- Invasive aspergillosis occurs mostly in immunocompromised patients with prolonged neutropenia, graft-versus-host disease, or impaired phagocyte function (eg, chronic granulomatous disease) or those who have received T-lymphocyte immunosuppressive therapy (eg, corticosteroids, calcineurin inhibitors, tumor necrosis factor–α inhibitors). Children with highest risk include those with new-onset acute myelogenous leukemia, relapse of hematologic malignancy, aplastic anemia, chronic granulomatous disease, and allogeneic hematopoietic stem cell and certain types (eg, heart, lung) of solid organ transplants. Invasive infection usually involves pulmonary, sinus, cerebral, or cutaneous sites. Rarely, endocarditis, osteomyelitis, meningitis, peritonitis, infection of the eye or orbit, and esophagitis occur. The hallmark of invasive aspergillosis is angioinvasion with resulting thrombosis, dissemination to other organs, and, occasionally, erosion of the blood vessel wall with catastrophic hemorrhage. Invasive aspergillosis in patients with chronic granulomatous disease is unique in that it is more indolent and displays a general lack of angioinvasion. Invasive aspergillosis has also been described in intensive care patients with severe influenza, with and without underlying immunocompromise.

- Aspergillomas and otomycosis are 2 syndromes of nonallergic colonization by *Aspergillus* species in immunocompetent children. Aspergillomas ("fungal balls") grow in preexisting pulmonary cavities or bronchogenic cysts without invading pulmonary tissue; almost all patients have underlying lung disease, such as cystic fibrosis or tuberculosis. Patients with otomycosis have chronic otitis media with colonization of the external auditory canal by a fungal mat that produces a dark discharge.

- Allergic bronchopulmonary aspergillosis is a hypersensitivity lung disease that manifests as episodic wheezing, expectoration of brown mucus plugs, low-grade fever, eosinophilia, and transient pulmonary infiltrates. This form of aspergillosis occurs most commonly in immunocompetent children with asthma or cystic fibrosis and can be a trigger for asthmatic flares.

- Allergic sinusitis is a far less common allergic response to colonization by *Aspergillus* species than is allergic bronchopulmonary aspergillosis. Allergic sinusitis occurs in children with nasal polyps or previous episodes of sinusitis or in children who have undergone sinus surgery. Allergic sinusitis is characterized by symptoms of chronic sinusitis with dark plugs of nasal discharge and is different from invasive *Aspergillus* sinusitis.

- Chronic aspergillosis typically affects patients who are not immunocompromised or are less immunocompromised, although exposure to corticosteroids is common, and patients often have underlying pulmonary conditions. Diagnosis of chronic aspergillosis requires at least 3 months of chronic pulmonary symptoms or chronic illness or progressive radiological abnormalities, along with an elevated *Aspergillus* immunoglobulin G concentration or other microbiological evidence. Because of the ubiquitous nature of *Aspergillus* species, a positive sputum culture alone is not diagnostic.

ETIOLOGY

Aspergillus species are molds that grow on decaying vegetation and in soil and are very common in the environment. *Aspergillus fumigatus* is the most common (>75%) cause of invasive aspergillosis, with *Aspergillus flavus* being the next most common. Several other major species, including *Aspergillus terreus*, *Aspergillus nidulans*, and *Aspergillus niger*, also cause invasive human infections. *A nidulans* is the second most encountered mold in patients with chronic granulomatous disease, causing an almost exclusively invasive infection in this specific host characterized by its aggressive behavior including lung infection that invades the chest wall with contiguous osteomyelitis and chest wall abscesses. Of increasing concern are emerging *Aspergillus* species that are resistant to antifungals, such as *A fumigatus,* which harbors environmentally acquired resistance mutations to azole antifungals; *A terreus,* which is intrinsically resistant to amphotericin B; and *Aspergillus calidoustus,* which is often resistant to most antifungals.

EPIDEMIOLOGY

The principal route of transmission is inhalation of conidia (spores) originating from multiple environmental sources (eg, plants, vegetables, dust from construction or demolition), soil, and water supplies (eg, showerheads). Incidence of disease in hematopoietic stem cell transplant recipients is highest during periods of neutropenia or during treatment of graft-versus-host disease. In solid organ transplant recipients, the risk is highest approximately 6 months after transplant or during periods of increased immunosuppression. Disease has followed use of contaminated marijuana in the immunocompromised host. Health care–associated outbreaks of invasive pulmonary aspergillosis in susceptible hosts have occurred in which the probable source of the fungus was a nearby construction site or faulty ventilation system, but the source of health care–associated aspergillosis is frequently unknown. Cutaneous aspergillosis occurs less frequently and usually involves sites of skin injury, such as sites of an intravenous catheter (including in neonates), sites of traumatic inoculation, and sites associated with occlusive dressings, burns, or surgery. Transmission by direct inoculation of skin abrasions or wounds is less likely. Person-to-person spread does not occur.

The **incubation period** is unknown and may be variable.

DIAGNOSTIC TESTS

Dichotomously branched and septate hyphae, identified by microscopic examination of 10% potassium hydroxide wet preparations or of Grocott-Gomori methenamine–silver nitrate stain of tissue or bronchoalveolar lavage (BAL) specimens, are suggestive of the diagnosis. Isolation of *Aspergillus* species or molecular testing with specific reagents is required for definitive diagnosis. The organism is usually not recoverable from blood (except in catheter-related infections) but is isolated readily from lung, sinus, and skin biopsy specimens when cultured on Sabouraud dextrose agar or brain-heart infusion media (without cycloheximide). *Aspergillus* species can be associated with colonization or may be a laboratory contaminant, but when results from immunocompromised patients are evaluated, recovery of this organism frequently indicates infection. Biopsy can be used to establish the diagnosis, but *Aspergillus* hyphae are like other hyaline molds (eg, *Fusarium*). Care should be taken to distinguish aspergillosis from mucormycosis, which can appear similar by diagnostic imaging studies but is pauci-septate (few septa) and requires a different treatment regimen.

An enzyme immunosorbent assay for detection of galactomannan, a molecule found in the cell wall of *Aspergillus* species, from serum or BAL fluid is available commercially and may be useful in children and adults with hematologic malignancies or hematopoietic stem cell transplants. A test result of 0.5 or greater from the serum or 1.0 or greater from BAL fluid supports a diagnosis of invasive aspergillosis, and monitoring of serum antigen concentrations twice weekly in periods of highest risk (eg, neutropenia and active graft-versus-host disease) if the patient is not receiving mold-active antifungal prophylaxis may be useful for early detection of invasive aspergillosis in these patients. False-positive test results have been reported and can be related to consumption of food products containing galactomannan (eg, rice and pasta), other invasive fungal infections (eg, *Fusarium, Histoplasma capsulatum*), and colonization of the gut of neonates with *Bifidobacterium* species. Previous cross-reactivity with antimicrobial agents derived from fungi, especially piperacillin-tazobactam, no longer occurs because of manufacturing changes.

A negative galactomannan test result does not exclude diagnosis of invasive aspergillosis, and its greatest utility may be in monitoring response to disease rather than in being used as a diagnostic marker. False-negative galactomannan test results consistently occur in patients with chronic granulomatous disease, so the test should not be used in these patients. Galactomannan is not recommended for routine screening in patients receiving mold-active antifungal therapy or prophylaxis.

Galactomannan is not recommended for screening in solid organ transplant recipients because of very poor sensitivity.

Limited data suggest that testing for other non-specific fungal biomarkers, such as 1,3-β-D-glucan, may be useful in the diagnosis of aspergillosis. This test is nonspecific for aspergillosis, and specificity may be reduced in a variety of clinical settings, including exposure to certain antibiotics, hemodialysis, and coinfection with certain bacteria. *Aspergillus* polymerase chain reaction testing is promising, but its clinical utility remains controversial. Unlike adults, children do not frequently manifest cavitation or the air crescent or halo signs on chest radiography, and lack of these characteristic signs does not exclude the diagnosis of invasive aspergillosis.

In allergic aspergillosis, diagnosis is suggested by a typical clinical syndrome with elevated total concentrations of immunoglobulin E (IgE; ≥1,000 ng/mL) and *Aspergillus*-specific serum IgE, eosinophilia, and a positive result from a skin test for *Aspergillus* antigens. In people with cystic fibrosis, the diagnosis is more difficult because wheezing, eosinophilia, and a positive skin test result not associated with allergic bronchopulmonary aspergillosis are often present.

TREATMENT

Voriconazole is the drug of choice for all clinical forms of invasive aspergillosis, except in neonates, for whom amphotericin B deoxycholate in high doses is recommended because of voriconazole's potential visual adverse effects, and perhaps for chronic granulomatous disease, in which posaconazole appears to be superior to voriconazole. Voriconazole has been shown to be superior to amphotericin B in a large, randomized trial in adults. Immune reconstitution is paramount; decreasing immunosuppression, if possible (specifically, corticosteroid dose), is critical to disease control. The diagnostic workup needs to be aggressive to confirm disease, but it should never delay antifungal therapy in the setting of true concern for invasive aspergillosis. Therapy is continued for a minimum of 6 to 12 weeks, but treatment duration should be individualized on the basis of degree and duration of immunosuppression. Monitoring of serum galactomannan concentrations in those with significant elevation at onset may be useful to assess response to therapy concomitant with clinical and radiological evaluation.

Close monitoring of voriconazole serum trough concentrations is critical for both efficacy and safety, and most experts agree that for children, voriconazole trough concentrations should be between 2 μg/mL and 6 μg/mL. It is important to individualize dosing in patients following initiation of voriconazole therapy, because there is high interpatient variability in metabolism. Certain *Aspergillus* species (*A calidoustus*) are inherently resistant to azoles, and isolation of azole-resistant *A fumigatus* is increasing and may be related to environmental acquisition through use of agricultural fungicides in previously azole-naïve patients. Resistance can also develop in patients receiving long-term azole therapy.

Alternative therapies include liposomal amphotericin B, isavuconazole, posaconazole, or other lipid formulations of amphotericin B. Primary therapy with an echinocandin alone (ie, caspofungin, micafungin) is not recommended, but an echinocandin can be used when an azole or amphotericin B is contraindicated. The pharmacokinetics and safety of posaconazole have not been evaluated fully in younger children. Posaconazole absorption is improved significantly with use of the extended-release tablet rather than the oral suspension. Isavuconazole is an alternative therapy in adults but has not been studied in children. Combination antifungal therapy with voriconazole and an echinocandin may be considered in select patients with documented invasive aspergillosis. In areas with high azole resistance, empirical therapy until antifungal susceptibilities are obtained should include voriconazole plus an echinocandin, or liposomal amphotericin B monotherapy.

If primary antifungal therapy fails, general strategies for salvage therapy include (a) changing the class of antifungal, (b) tapering or reversal of underlying immunosuppression when feasible, (c) susceptibility testing of any *Aspergillus* isolates recovered, and (d) surgical resection of necrotic lesions in selected cases. In pulmonary disease, surgery is indicated only when a mass is impinging on a great vessel.

Allergic bronchopulmonary aspergillosis is treated with antifungal therapy, usually with itraconazole or another mold-active azole; in addition, corticosteroids are a cornerstone of therapy for exacerbations. Itraconazole has a demonstrable corticosteroid-sparing effect. Allergic sinus aspergillosis is also treated with corticosteroids, and surgery has been reported to be beneficial in many cases. Antifungal therapy has not been found to be useful but could be considered for refractory infection and/or relapsing disease. There may be an emerging role for immunotherapy. Guidelines specific to treatment of allergic bronchopulmonary aspergillosis in patients with cystic fibrosis are available (**www.cff.org/Care/Clinical-Care-Guidelines/Infection-Prevention-and-Control-Clinical-Care-Guidelines/Allergic-Bronchopulmonary-Aspergillosis-Clinical-Care-Guidelines**).

ISOLATION OF THE HOSPITALIZED PATIENT

Standard precautions are recommended.

CONTROL MEASURES

Outbreaks of invasive aspergillosis and *Aspergillus* colonization have occurred among hospitalized patients during construction in hospitals and at nearby sites. Environmental measures reported to be effective include erecting of suitable barriers between patient care areas and construction sites, routine cleaning of air-handling systems, repair of faulty airflow, and replacement of contaminated air filters. High-efficiency particulate air filters and laminar flow rooms markedly decrease the risk of exposure to conidia in patient care areas. Plants and flowers may be reservoirs for *Aspergillus* and should be avoided in intensive care units and immunocompromised patient care settings. Use of high-efficiency respirators during transport away from protective environment rooms has been associated with reduced incidence of invasive pulmonary aspergillosis during hospital construction.

Posaconazole has been shown to be effective in 2 randomized controlled trials as prophylaxis against invasive aspergillosis for patients 13 years and older who have undergone hematopoietic stem cell transplant and have graft-versus-host disease as well as in patients with hematologic malignancies with prolonged neutropenia, although breakthrough disease has been reported in those with gastrointestinal tract issues (eg, graft-versus-host disease) affecting drug bioavailability. Low-dose amphotericin B, itraconazole, voriconazole, or posaconazole prophylaxis has been reported for other patients with high risk, but controlled trials have not been completed in pediatric patients.

Patients with risk for invasive infection should avoid high environmental exposure (eg, gardening) following discharge from the hospital. People with allergic aspergillosis should take measures to reduce exposure to *Aspergillus* species in the home.

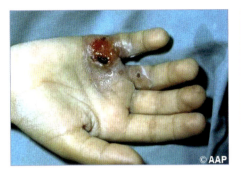

Image 9.1
Aspergilloma of the hand in a 7-year-old boy with chronic granulomatous disease.

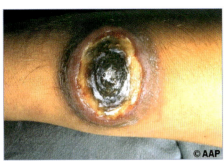

Image 9.2
Aspergilloma at intravenous catheter site in a 9-year-old boy with acute lymphoblastic leukemia.

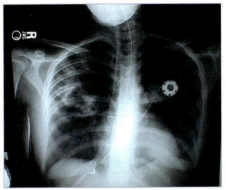

Image 9.3
Aspergillus pneumonia, bilateral, in a 16-year-old boy with acute myelogenous leukemia. Note pulmonary cavitation in the right lung field and perihilar and retrocardiac densities in the left lung field. Copyright Michael Rajnik, MD, FAAP.

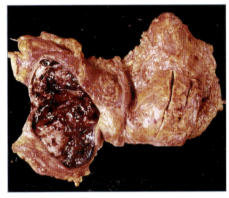

Image 9.4
Pulmonary aspergillosis in a patient with acute lymphatic leukemia. Courtesy of Dimitris P. Agamanolis, MD.

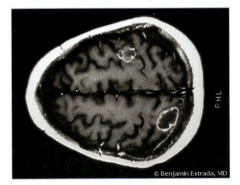

Image 9.5
Aspergillomas in a 10-year-old with Hodgkin-type lymphoma. Courtesy of Benjamin Estrada, MD.

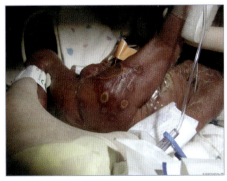

Image 9.6
Cutaneous aspergillosis in a 23-weeks' gestation preterm neonate. Courtesy of David Kaufman, MD.

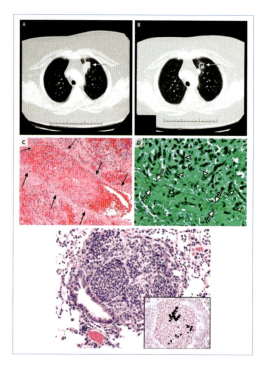

Image 9.7
A, Computed tomographic scan of the chest of a patient with neutropenia who has invasive aspergillosis (arrow). A positive result from a serum galactomannan test established the diagnosis of probable invasive aspergillosis, which averted the need for an invasive diagnostic procedure. B, Cavitation of the lesion after a successful response to therapy and neutrophil recovery (arrow). C, Vascular invasive aspergillosis can occur in patients with other conditions, such as in this case of fatal aspergillosis in a recipient of an allogeneic hematopoietic stem cell transplant with severe graft-versus-host disease. A low-power micrograph shows vascular thrombosis (with an arterial vessel outlined by arrows) (hematoxylin-eosin stain). D, A high-power micrograph shows hyphae (arrowheads) transverse to the blood vessel wall (outlined by arrows) and intravascular invasion (Grocott-Gomori methenamine–silver nitrate stain, with hyphal walls staining dark). The septate hyphae are morphologically consistent with *Aspergillus* species. E, Experimental aspergillosis in a knockout mouse model of chronic granulomatous disease, an inherited disorder of NADPH oxidase. Densely inflammatory pyogranulomatous pneumonia without vascular invasion or tissue infarction is visible (hematoxylin-eosin stain), with invasive hyphae in the lung as observed with silver staining (inset). Copyright *New England Journal of Medicine*.

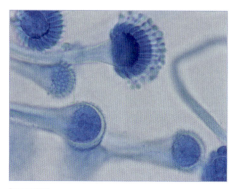

Image 9.8
Aspergillus fumigatus. Courtesy of H. Cody Meissner, MD, FAAP.

CHAPTER 10
Astrovirus Infections

CLINICAL MANIFESTATIONS

Astrovirus illness is most commonly manifested as 2 to 5 days of acute watery diarrhea accompanied by low-grade fever, malaise, and nausea; less commonly, by vomiting and mild dehydration. Illness in an immunocompetent host is self-limited, lasting a median of 5 to 6 days. Asymptomatic infections are common. Astrovirus infections have also been associated with encephalitis and meningitis, particularly in immunocompromised individuals.

ETIOLOGY

Members of the family *Astroviridae*, astroviruses are nonenveloped, single-stranded RNA viruses with a subset of particles (10%) having a characteristic starlike appearance when visualized by electron microscopy. Astroviruses are classified into 2 genera: *Mamastrovirus* (MAstV), which infects mammals, and *Avastrovirus*, which infects birds. Four MAstV species have been identified in humans: MAstV 1, MAstV 6, MAstV 8, and MAstV 9. MAstV 1 includes the 8 antigenic types of classic human astroviruses (HAstV types 1–8), whereas MAstV 6, MAstV 8, and MAstV 9 are novel astroviruses that have been identified in recent years and include Melbourne and Virginia/human-mink-ovine–like strains.

EPIDEMIOLOGY

HAstVs have a worldwide distribution. Multiple antigenic types co-circulate in the same geographic region. HAstVs have been detected in as many as 5% to 17% of sporadic cases of nonbacterial gastroenteritis in young children in the community but appear to cause a lower proportion of cases of more severe childhood gastroenteritis requiring hospitalization (2.5%–9%). HAstV infections occur predominantly in children younger than 4 years and have a seasonal peak during the late winter and spring in the United States. Transmission is via the fecal-oral route through contaminated food or water, person-to-person contact, or contaminated surfaces. Outbreaks tend to occur among closed populations of young children and elderly people, particularly among children in hospitals (health care–associated infections) and children in child care centers. In general, virus is shed 1 to 2 days before illness and lasts a median of 5 days after onset of symptoms, but asymptomatic excretion after illness can last for several weeks in healthy children. Persistent excretion may occur in immunocompromised hosts. MAstV 6, MAstV 8, and MAstV 9 have been detected sporadically in stool samples, blood, respiratory samples, cerebrospinal fluid, and brain tissue of immunocompromised patients with acute encephalitis.

The **incubation period** is 3 to 4 days.

DIAGNOSTIC TESTS

Commercial tests for diagnosis have not been available in the United States until recently, although enzyme immunoassays are available in many other countries. There are several US Food and Drug Administration approved multiplex nucleic acid–based assays for the detection of gastrointestinal tract pathogens, at least 2 of which include astrovirus (MAstV 1). These multiplex tests are more sensitive and are replacing traditional tests to detect fecal viral pathogens. Interpretation of assay results may be complicated by the frequent detection of viruses in fecal samples from asymptomatic children and the detection of multiple viruses in a single sample. A few research and reference laboratories test stool samples by enzyme immunoassay for detection of viral antigen and/or real-time reverse transcriptase–quantitative polymerase chain reaction assay for detection of viral RNA in stool.

TREATMENT

No specific antiviral therapy is available. Oral or parenteral fluids and electrolytes are given to prevent and correct dehydration.

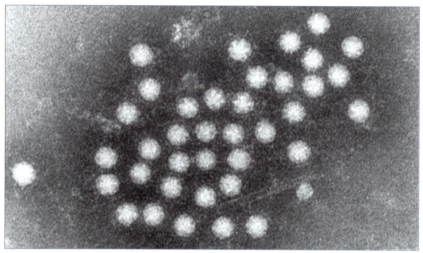

Image 10.1
Electron micrograph of astrovirus obtained from stool of a child with gastroenteritis. Note the characteristic starlike appearance. Courtesy of Centers for Disease Control and Prevention.

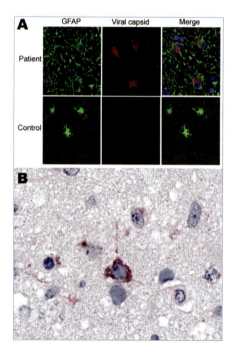

Image 10.2
Astrovirus encephalitis in a boy with X-linked agammaglobulinemia. Encephalitis is a major cause of death worldwide. Although >100 pathogens have been identified as causative agents, the pathogen is not determined for up to 75% of cases. This diagnostic failure impedes effective treatment and underscores the need for better tools and new approaches for detecting novel pathogens or determining new manifestations of known pathogens. Although astroviruses are commonly associated with gastroenteritis, they have not been associated with central nervous system disease. With unbiased pyrosequencing, astrovirus was determined to be the causative agent for encephalitis in a 15-year-old boy with agammaglobulinemia. Courtesy of *Emerging Infectious Diseases*.

CHAPTER 11
Babesiosis

CLINICAL MANIFESTATIONS

Babesia infection is often asymptomatic or associated with mild, nonspecific symptoms. The infection can also be severe and life threatening, particularly in people who are asplenic, immunocompromised, or elderly. When symptomatic, babesiosis, like malaria, is characterized by fever and hemolytic anemia. Clinical manifestations of babesiosis include malaise, anorexia, and fatigue, followed by fever, chills, sweats, myalgia, arthralgia, headache, and nausea. Severe babesiosis may require hospitalization for management of marked anemia, adult respiratory distress syndrome, disseminated intravascular coagulation, renal impairment, shock, or splenic rupture. Congenital infection with nonspecific manifestations suggestive of sepsis has been reported.

Babesiosis should be considered in a patient who resides in or traveled to an endemic area and develops compatible symptoms and characteristic laboratory abnormalities, including anemia, thrombocytopenia, and evidence of intravascular hemolysis (abnormal aspartate aminotransferase, alanine aminotransferase, alkaline phosphatase, lactate dehydrogenase, and total and direct bilirubin concentrations, and reduced haptoglobin). Thrombocytopenia is common; disseminated intravascular coagulation can be a complication of severe babesiosis. If untreated, the infection can last for several weeks or months.

ETIOLOGY

Babesia species are intraerythrocytic protozoa that are transmitted mostly by the bite of a hard-bodied tick. The etiologic agents of human babesiosis in the United States include *Babesia microti*, which causes most reported cases, and, less commonly, *Babesia duncani* and *Babesia divergens*.

EPIDEMIOLOGY

Babesiosis is predominantly a tickborne zoonosis. *Babesia* parasites can also be transmitted via blood transfusion, via organ transplant, and perinatally. The primary reservoir host for *B microti* in the United States is the white-footed mouse (*Peromyscus leucopus*), and the tick vector is *Ixodes scapularis*, which can transmit other pathogens, such as *Borrelia burgdorferi*, the causative agent of Lyme disease, and *Anaplasma phagocytophilum*, the causative agent of human granulocytic anaplasmosis. The tick bite is often not noticed, in part because at the nymphal stage, the tick is about the size of a poppy seed. White-tailed deer (*Odocoileus virginianus*) serve as hosts for blood meals by the tick but are not reservoir hosts of *B microti*. An increase in the deer population in some geographic regions, including some suburban areas, during the past few decades is thought to be a major factor in the spread of *I scapularis*. The reported vectorborne cases of *B microti* infection have been acquired in the Northeast (in parts of Connecticut, Massachusetts, New Jersey, New York, and Rhode Island, as well as other states, including Maine and New Hampshire) and in the upper Midwest (Wisconsin and Minnesota). Most cases are in the New England and Mid-Atlantic regions (**www.cdc.gov/parasites/babesiosis/data-statistics/maps/maps.html**). Most US vectorborne cases of babesiosis occur during late spring, summer, or fall; transfusion-associated cases can occur year round. More than 2,000 cases of babesiosis are reported annually to the Centers for Disease Control and Prevention (CDC), but the number of cases is likely to be higher.

The **incubation period** typically ranges from approximately 1 week to 5 weeks following a tick bite. A study of transfusion-associated cases showed a median incubation period following a contaminated blood transfusion of 37 days (range, 11–176 days), but it may be longer (eg, latent infection might become symptomatic after splenectomy).

DIAGNOSTIC TESTS

Acute, symptomatic cases of babesiosis are typically diagnosed by microscopic identification of *Babesia* parasites on Giemsa- or Wright-stained blood smears. If the diagnosis of babesiosis is being considered, manual (nonautomated) review of blood smears for parasites should be requested explicitly. If found, the tetrad (Maltese-cross) form is pathognomonic. *B microti* and other *Babesia* species can be difficult to distinguish from the *Plasmodium falciparum* trophozoite; examination of blood smears by a reference laboratory should be considered for confirmation of the diagnosis.

When blood smear examination is negative but index of suspicion for babesiosis remains high, molecular testing by polymerase chain reaction (PCR) offers increased sensitivity in settings of low-level B microti parasitemia; PCR results may remain positive for several months after successful treatment. PCR testing is now available at some clinical and public health laboratories as well as at the CDC.

Serological tests for Babesia antibody detection on a single serum specimen should not be used to diagnose acute disease because of difficulty distinguishing acute disease from previous infection. Real-time PCR assays are typically species specific, but most laboratories offer only B microti PCR (**www.cdc.gov/dpdx/babesiosis/index.html**). In geographic areas where both B microti and B burgdorferi are endemic, approximately one-tenth of patients with early Lyme disease experience concurrent babesiosis coinfection and approximately half of patients with babesiosis are coinfected with B burgdorferi. When coinfection is documented, patients should receive therapies appropriate for each infection.

TREATMENT

Atovaquone (administered orally) plus azithromycin (administered orally in ambulatory patients with mild to moderate disease and intravenously in hospitalized patients with severe disease) for 7 to 10 days is the regimen of choice. Oral or intravenous clindamycin plus oral quinine may be used for patients who do not respond to atovaquone and azithromycin, although quinine commonly causes severe adverse effects. Severe babesiosis can be life threatening despite antimicrobial therapy. Limited data suggest that exchange transfusion has potential benefits that may outweigh potential adverse effects, particularly in patients with high levels of parasitemia. In severely immunocompromised patients, treatment for at least 6 weeks or longer, with negative blood smears for 2 weeks or longer before discontinuing therapy, is recommended. Limited data are available for treatment of infection caused by B duncani or B divergens, but most reported patients have been treated with intravenous clindamycin plus oral quinine.

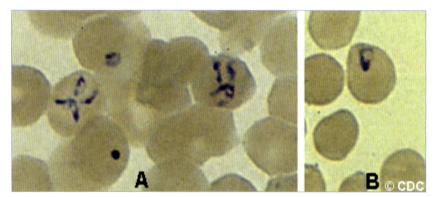

Image 11.1
Infection with Babesia in a 6-year-old girl after a splenectomy was performed because of hereditary spherocytosis (Giemsa-stained thin smears). A, The tetrad (left side of the image), a dividing form, is pathognomonic for Babesia. Note also the variation in size and shape of the ring stage parasites (compare A and B) and the absence of pigment. Courtesy of Centers for Disease Control and Prevention.

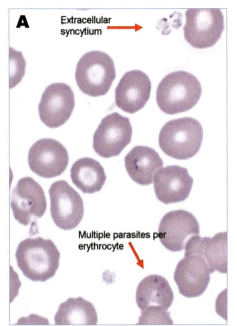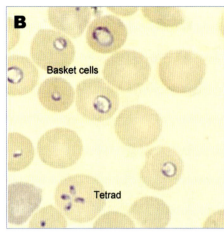

Image 11.2
Giemsa-stained (A) and Wright-stained (B) peripheral blood smear from a newborn with probable *Babesia microti* infection. Parasitemia was estimated in this newborn at approximately 15% on the basis of the number of parasites per 200 leukocytes counted. The smear demonstrated thrombocytopenia and parasites of variable size and morphological appearance and an absence of pigment (magnification ×1,000). Courtesy of Centers for Disease Control and Prevention/*Emerging Infectious Diseases*.

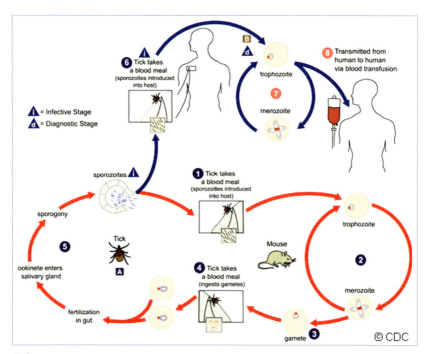

Image 11.3
The *Babesia microti* life cycle involves 2 hosts, including a rodent, primarily the white-footed mouse (*Peromyscus leucopus*). During a blood meal, a *Babesia*-infected tick introduces sporozoites into the mouse host (1). Sporozoites enter erythrocytes and undergo asexual reproduction (budding) (2). In the blood, some parasites differentiate into male and female gametes, although these cannot be distinguished at the light microscope level (3). The definitive host is a tick, in this case the deer tick (*Ixodes scapularis*). Once ingested by an appropriate tick (4), gametes unite and undergo a sporogonic cycle, resulting in sporozoites (5). Transovarial transmission (also known as vertical, or hereditary, transmission) has been documented for "large" *Babesia* species but not for the "small" *Babesia* species, such as *B microti* (A). Humans enter the cycle when bitten by infected ticks. During a blood meal, a *Babesia*-infected tick introduces sporozoites into the human host (6). Sporozoites enter erythrocytes (B) and undergo asexual replication (budding) (7). Multiplication of the blood stage parasites is responsible for clinical manifestations of the disease. Humans are, for all practical purposes, dead-end hosts, and there is probably little, if any, subsequent transmission that occurs from ticks feeding on infected persons. However, human-to-human transmission is well recognized to occur through blood transfusions (8). Note: Deer are the hosts on which the adult ticks feed and are indirectly part of the *Babesia* cycle, because they influence the tick population. When deer populations increase, tick population also increases, thus heightening the potential for transmission. Courtesy of Centers for Disease Control and Prevention.

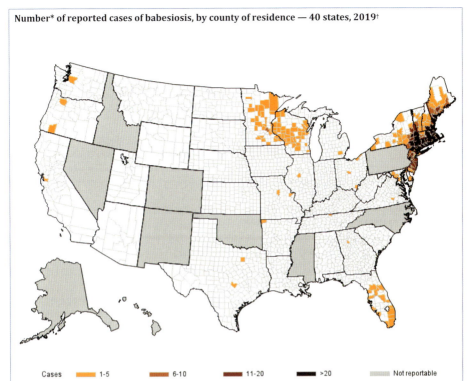

Image 11.4
Number of reported cases of babesiosis, by patient's county of residence—40 states, 2019. Courtesy of Centers for Disease Control and Prevention.

CHAPTER 12

Bacillus cereus Infections and Intoxications

CLINICAL MANIFESTATIONS

Bacillus cereus is associated primarily with 2 toxin-mediated foodborne illnesses, emetic and diarrheal, but it can also cause invasive extraintestinal infection. The **emetic syndrome** develops after a short incubation period, as staphylococcal foodborne illness does. It is characterized by nausea, vomiting, and abdominal cramps, and diarrhea may follow in up to one-third of patients. The **diarrheal syndrome** has a longer incubation period, is more severe, and resembles Clostridium perfringens foodborne illness. It is characterized by moderate to severe abdominal cramps and watery diarrhea, vomiting in approximately 25% of patients, and, occasionally, low-grade fever. Both illnesses are usually short-lived, about 24 hours, but the emetic toxin is occasionally associated with fulminant liver failure.

Invasive extraintestinal infection can be severe and includes wound and soft tissue infections; sepsis and bacteremia, including central catheter–associated bloodstream infection; endocarditis; osteomyelitis; purulent meningitis and ventricular shunt infection; pneumonia; and ocular infections (endophthalmitis and keratitis). Infection can be acquired through use of contaminated blood products, especially platelets. B cereus is a leading cause of bacterial endophthalmitis following penetrating ocular trauma. Endogenous endophthalmitis can result from bacteremic seeding. Other ocular manifestations include an indolent keratitis related to corneal abrasions.

ETIOLOGY

B cereus is an aerobic and facultative anaerobic, spore-forming, gram-positive or gram-variable bacillus.

EPIDEMIOLOGY

B cereus is ubiquitous in the environment because of the high resistance of its endospores to extreme conditions, including heat, cold, desiccation, salinity, and radiation, and is commonly present in small numbers in raw, dried, and processed foods and in the feces of healthy people. The organism is a common cause of foodborne illness in the United States but may be underrecognized, because few people seek care for mild illness and physicians and clinical laboratories do not routinely test for B cereus. Several confirmed outbreaks were reported to the Centers for Disease Control and Prevention in recent years. A wide variety of food vehicles have been implicated.

Spores of B cereus are heat resistant and can survive pasteurization, brief cooking, boiling, and high saline concentrations. Spores germinate to vegetative forms that produce enterotoxins over a wide range of temperatures, in foods and in the gastrointestinal tract. The diarrheal syndrome is caused by several distinct toxins that are ingested before formation or are produced after spores germinate in the gastrointestinal tract. The diarrheal toxins are heat labile and can be destroyed by heating. The emetic syndrome occurs after eating contaminated food containing a preformed toxin called cereulide. The best known association of the emetic syndrome is with ingestion of fried rice made from boiled rice stored at room temperature overnight, because B cereus can be present in uncooked rice. However, a wide variety of foods, especially starchy foods (including cereals), cheese products, meats, and vegetables, have been implicated. Foodborne illness caused by B cereus is not transmissible from person to person.

Risk factors for invasive disease attributable to B cereus include history of injection drug use, presence of indwelling intravascular catheters or implanted devices, neutropenia or immunosuppression, and preterm birth. B cereus endophthalmitis has occurred after penetrating ocular trauma and injection drug use. Hospital outbreaks have been associated with contaminated medical equipment.

The **incubation period** for foodborne illness is 0.5 to 6 hours for the emetic syndrome and 6 to 15 hours for the diarrheal syndrome.

DIAGNOSTIC TESTS

Diagnostic testing is not recommended for sporadic cases. For foodborne outbreaks, isolation of B cereus from the stool or vomitus of 2 or more ill people and not from control patients, or isolation of 10^5 colony-forming units/g or greater from epidemiologically implicated food, suggests that B cereus causes the outbreak. Because the organism can be recovered from stool specimens from some well people, the presence of B cereus in feces or vomitus of ill people is not definitive evidence of infection. Food samples must be tested for both types of diarrheal enterotoxins, because either alone can cause illness. B cereus colonies isolated from food or specimens of ill individuals may be tested by polymerase chain reaction assay for the emetic toxin gene in diagnostic laboratories.

In patients with risk factors for invasive disease (eg, preterm infants, people with immunosuppressing conditions), isolation of B cereus from wounds or from blood or other sterile body fluids is significant. The common perception of Bacillus species as "contaminants" may delay recognition and treatment of serious B cereus infections.

TREATMENT

B cereus foodborne illness usually requires only supportive treatment, including rehydration. Antimicrobial therapy is indicated for patients with invasive disease. Prompt removal of any potentially infected foreign bodies, such as central catheters or implants, is essential. For intraocular infections, an ophthalmologist should be consulted regarding surgical management and use of intravitreal antimicrobial therapy in addition to systemic therapy. B cereus is usually resistant to β-lactam antibiotics and often to clindamycin but is susceptible to vancomycin, which is the drug of choice. Alternative drugs, including linezolid, clindamycin, aminoglycosides, erythromycin, tetracyclines, and fluoroquinolones, may be considered depending on susceptibility results.

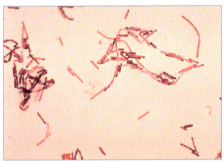

Image 12.1
Bacillus cereus subspecies mycoides (Gram stain). B cereus is a known cause of toxin-induced food poisoning. These organisms may appear gram variable, as shown here. Courtesy of Centers for Disease Control and Prevention.

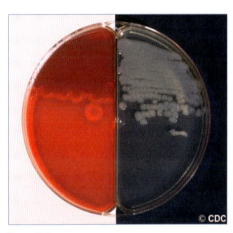

Image 12.2
Blood agar and bicarbonate agar plate cultures of Bacillus cereus (negative result from encapsulation test). Rough colonies of B cereus on blood and bicarbonate agars. Courtesy of Centers for Disease Control and Prevention.

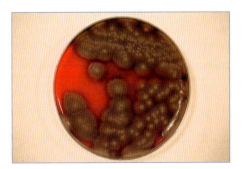

Image 12.3
Bacillus cereus on sheep blood agar. Large, circular β-hemolytic colonies are noted. The greenish color and ground-glass appearance are typical characteristics of this organism on culture media. Courtesy of Julia Rosebush, DO; Robert Jerris, PhD; and Theresa Stanley, M(ASCP).

CHAPTER 13

Bacterial Vaginosis

CLINICAL MANIFESTATIONS

Bacterial vaginosis (BV) is a polymicrobial clinical syndrome characterized by changes in vaginal flora, with a reduction in normally abundant *Lactobacillus* species and acquisition of a diverse community of anaerobic and facultative bacteria. Vaginal lactobacilli act as an important host-defense mechanism by secreting substances that inhibit the growth of microbial pathogens and indigenous anaerobes. BV is diagnosed primarily in sexually active postpubertal females. Symptoms may include vaginal irritation, vaginal discharge, and/or vaginal odor. However, studies have shown that up to 50% of females who meet microbiological criteria for a diagnosis of BV are asymptomatic. Classic signs, when present, include a thin white or grey, homogenous, adherent vaginal discharge with a fishy odor. Symptoms of pruritus, dysuria, or abdominal pain are not typically associated with BV but can be suggestive of mixed vaginitis. In pregnant females, BV has been associated with adverse outcomes, including chorioamnionitis, premature rupture of membranes, preterm delivery, and postpartum endometritis.

Vaginitis and vulvitis in prepubertal girls rarely, if ever, are manifestations of BV. Vaginitis in prepubertal girls is frequently nonspecific. Possible causes of vaginitis in this population include foreign bodies and infections attributable to group A streptococci, *Escherichia coli*, herpes simplex virus, *Neisseria gonorrhoeae*, *Chlamydia trachomatis*, *Trichomonas vaginalis*, or enteric bacteria, including *Shigella* species. In any prepubertal girl who has symptoms of BV, a full history and workup should be considered to rule out sexual abuse and/or a sexually transmitted infection (STI). If sexual abuse is suspected, those who are mandated to report need to follow their state regulations for immediate reporting.

ETIOLOGY

The microbiological cause of BV has not been delineated fully. Hydrogen peroxide and lactic acid–producing *Lactobacillus* species, particularly *Lactobacillus crispatus*, predominate among vaginal flora and play a protective role by maintaining a low vaginal pH level. In females with BV, these species are largely replaced by commensal facultative and strict anaerobes including *Gardnerella vaginalis*, *Prevotella bivia*, *Atopobium vaginae*, *Mycoplasma hominis*, *Megasphaera* types, and *Mobiluncus* species.

G vaginalis, present in 95% to 100% of BV cases, was originally believed to be the primary BV pathogen. However, *G vaginalis* is also found in sexually active women with normal vaginal flora, and colonization with *G vaginalis* does not always lead to BV. Thus, microbiological identification of *G vaginalis* is not, by itself, sufficient for the diagnosis of BV, even in a symptomatic individual.

EPIDEMIOLOGY

BV is the most common cause of vaginal discharge in sexually active adolescents and women. BV occurs more frequently in females with a new sexual partner or a higher number of sexual partners and is also associated with douching and not using condoms. BV may be the sole cause of the symptoms, or it may accompany other conditions associated with vaginal discharge, such as trichomoniasis or cervicitis secondary to other STIs. BV can increase the risk of acquisition of other STIs, including HIV, herpes simplex virus, *Mycoplasma genitalium*, *N gonorrhoeae*, *C trachomatis*, and *T vaginalis*, and increase the risk of infectious complications following gynecologic surgeries. It can also increase the risk of HIV transmission to male partners.

Although the exact etiology of BV remains unknown, an **incubation period** of around 4 days (as with other bacterial STIs such as *N gonorrhoeae*) has been suggested in recent studies. Recurrence is common, with more than 50% of women experiencing BV within 12 months after treatment.

DIAGNOSTIC TESTS

BV is most commonly diagnosed clinically by using the Amsel criteria, requiring that 3 or more of the following symptoms or signs are present:

- Homogenous, thin grey or white vaginal discharge that smoothly coats the vaginal walls

- Vaginal fluid pH greater than 4.5

- A fishy (amine) odor of vaginal discharge before or after addition of 10% potassium hydroxide (ie, the "whiff test")

- Clue cells (squamous vaginal epithelial cells covered with bacteria, which cause a stippled or granular appearance and ragged "moth-eaten" borders) representing at least 20% of the total vaginal epithelial cells visualized on microscopic evaluation of vaginal fluid

An alternative method for diagnosing BV is the Nugent score, which is used widely as the gold standard for making the diagnosis in the research setting. A Gram stain of the vaginal fluid is evaluated, and a numerical score is generated on the basis of the apparent quantity of lactobacilli relative to BV-associated bacteria (*G vaginalis* and *Mobiluncus* species). The score is interpreted as normal (0–3), intermediate (4–6), or BV (7–10). Douching, recent intercourse, menstruation, and coexisting infection can alter findings on Gram stain.

Over-the-counter vaginal pH test kits have been marketed as home screening or testing options for BV. Despite diagnostic claims for such basic pH test kits, formal clinical evaluation and targeted laboratory-based diagnostic testing are warranted for patients reporting a positive home test result before any therapeutic interventions are instituted.

There are a wide variety of diagnostic laboratory assays available to diagnose BV, ranging from point-of-care tests that typically identify a single agent, commonly *G vaginalis*, to multiplex molecular assays in which diagnosis is based on algorithms of relative quantifications of both favorable and detrimental vaginal organisms. Clinicians need to consider costs, result turnaround time, and accuracy in their decision to select a particular assay to test for BV in symptomatic females. No recommendations exist to screen asymptomatic females for BV. Culture for *G vaginalis* is not recommended as a diagnostic tool, because it is not specific, and Papanicolaou testing is not recommended because of its extremely low sensitivity. Although the microscopy-based wet mount is advantageous for its low cost and immediate results, the multiplex polymerase chain reaction assays might be more useful, particularly in the diagnostic workup of symptomatic females with recurrent or refractory vaginitis.

Sexually active females with BV should be evaluated for coinfection with other STIs, including syphilis, gonorrhea, chlamydia, trichomoniasis, and HIV infection. If the hepatitis B and human papillomavirus vaccine series have not been completed, these immunizations should be offered.

TREATMENT

Symptomatic patients with BV should be treated. The goals of treatment are to relieve the symptoms and signs of infection and to potentially decrease the risk of acquiring other STIs. Treatment considerations should include patient preference for oral versus intravaginal treatment, possible adverse effects, and the presence of coinfections.

Nonpregnant females may be treated orally with metronidazole or topically with metronidazole gel, 0.75%, or clindamycin cream, 2%. Alternative regimens include oral tinidazole, oral clindamycin, oral secnidazole, or clindamycin intravaginal ovules. Patients should refrain from sexual intercourse or use condoms appropriately during treatment, keeping in mind that clindamycin cream is oil based and can weaken latex condoms and diaphragms for up to 5 days after completion of therapy. There is no evidence that treatment of sexual partners affects treatment response or risk of recurrence. Follow-up is unnecessary if symptoms resolve.

Pregnant females with symptoms of BV should be treated because they have high risk for having preterm or low birth weight infants, premature rupture of membranes, intra-amniotic infections, and postpartum endometriosis. Symptomatic pregnant females can be treated with either oral or vaginal metronidazole or clindamycin regimens recommended for nonpregnant females. Tinidazole should be avoided during pregnancy, because animal studies have shown teratogenic effects.

Breastfeeding mothers with symptoms of BV should be treated. Topical metronidazole is preferred for treating breastfeeding mothers.

Approximately 30% of appropriately treated females have a recurrence within 3 months. Re-treatment with the same regimen or an alternative regimen is a reasonable option for treating persistent or recurrent BV after the first occurrence. For females with multiple recurrences (>3 in the previous 12 months), either metronidazole gel, 0.75%, or metronidazole vaginal suppository at 750 mg twice weekly for at least 3 months has been shown to reduce recurrences, although this benefit does not persist when suppressive therapy is discontinued.

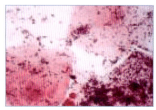

Image 13.1
Mobiluncus species (Gram stain), an anaerobe commonly found in bacterial vaginosis along with other anaerobes, especially *Prevotella* species. Copyright Yamajiku.co.jp.

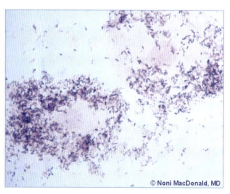

Image 13.2
Clue cells are squamous epithelial cells covered with bacteria found in bacterial vaginosis. Copyright Noni MacDonald, MD.

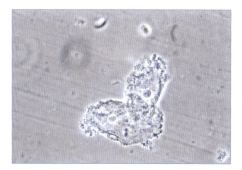

Image 13.3
This photomicrograph reveals bacteria adhering to vaginal epithelial cells known as clue cells. Clue cells are epithelial cells that have had bacteria adhere to their surface, obscuring their borders and imparting a stippled appearance. The presence of such clue cells is a sign that the patient has bacterial vaginosis. Courtesy of Centers for Disease Control and Prevention.

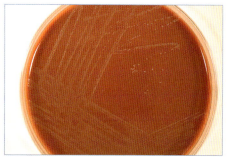

Image 13.4
Gardnerella vaginalis on chocolate agar. Colonies are small, circular, gray, and convex. Courtesy of Julia Rosebush, DO; Robert Jerris, PhD; and Theresa Stanley, M(ASCP).

CHAPTER 14

Bacteroides, Prevotella, and Other Anaerobic Gram-Negative Bacilli Infections

CLINICAL MANIFESTATIONS

Bacteroides, Prevotella, and other anaerobic gram-negative bacilli (AGNB) organisms from the oral cavity can cause chronic sinusitis, chronic otitis media, parotitis, dental infection, peritonsillar abscess, cervical adenitis, retropharyngeal space infection, aspiration pneumonia, lung abscess, pleural empyema, or necrotizing pneumonia. Species from the gastrointestinal tract are recovered in patients with peritonitis, intra-abdominal abscess, pelvic inflammatory disease, Bartholin cyst abscess, tubo-ovarian abscess, endometritis, acute and chronic prostatitis, prostatic and scrotal abscesses, scrotal gangrene, postoperative wound infection, and vulvovaginal and perianal infections. Invasion of the bloodstream from the oral cavity or intestinal tract can lead to brain abscess, meningitis, endocarditis, arthritis, or osteomyelitis. Skin and soft tissue infections include bacterial gangrene and necrotizing fasciitis; omphalitis in newborns; cellulitis at the site of fetal monitors, human bite wounds, or burns; infections adjacent to the mouth or rectum; and infected decubitus ulcers. Neonatal infections, including conjunctivitis, pneumonia, bacteremia, or meningitis, rarely occur. In most cases in which *Bacteroides*, *Prevotella*, and other AGNB are implicated, the infections are polymicrobial, with between 5 and 10 different organisms present.

ETIOLOGY

Most *Bacteroides*, *Prevotella*, *Porphyromonas*, and *Fusobacterium* organisms associated with human disease are pleomorphic, non–spore-forming, facultatively AGNB.

EPIDEMIOLOGY

Bacteroides, *Prevotella*, and other AGNB are part of the normal flora of the mouth, gastrointestinal tract, and female and male genital tracts. Members of the *Bacteroides fragilis* group predominate in the gastrointestinal tract flora; enterotoxigenic *B fragilis* may be a cause of diarrhea. Members of the *Prevotella melaninogenica* (formerly *Bacteroides melaninogenicus*) and *Prevotella oralis* (formerly *Bacteroides oralis*) groups are more common in the oral cavity. These species cause infection as opportunists, usually after an alteration in skin or mucosal membranes in conjunction with other endogenous species, and are often associated with chronic injury. Rates of upper respiratory tract, head, and neck infections associated with AGNB are higher among children. Endogenous infection results from aspiration, bowel perforation, or damage to mucosal surfaces from trauma, surgery, or chemotherapy. Mucosal injury or granulocytopenia predisposes to infection. Except in infections resulting from human bites, no evidence of person-to-person transmission exists.

The **incubation period** is variable and depends on the inoculum and the site of involvement but is usually 1 to 5 days.

DIAGNOSTIC TESTS

Anaerobic culture media are necessary for recovery of *Bacteroides*, *Prevotella*, and other AGNB species. Because infections are usually polymicrobial, aerobic and anaerobic cultures should be obtained. A putrid odor, with or without gas in the infected site, suggests anaerobic infection. Use of an anaerobic transport tube or a sealed syringe is recommended for collection of clinical specimens.

TREATMENT

Abscesses should be drained when feasible; abscesses involving the brain, liver, and lungs may resolve with effective antimicrobial therapy alone. Necrotizing soft tissue lesions should be debrided surgically.

The choice of antimicrobial agent(s) is based on anticipated or known in vitro susceptibility testing and local antimicrobial resistance patterns. *Bacteroides* infections of the mouth and respiratory tract are generally susceptible to penicillin G, ampicillin, and clindamycin. However, some species of *Bacteroides* and almost 50% of *Prevotella* species produce β-lactamase, and penicillin treatment failure has emerged as a consequence, so penicillin is not recommended for empirical coverage or for treatment of severe oropharyngeal or pleuropulmonary infections or of any abdominopelvic infections. A β-lactam penicillin active against *Bacteroides* species combined with a β-lactamase inhibitor (ampicillin-sulbactam, amoxicillin-clavulanate, or piperacillin-tazobactam) can be used to treat these infections. *Bacteroides* species of the gastrointestinal tract are often resistant to penicillin G but are typically susceptible to metronidazole, β-lactam plus β-lactamase inhibitors, carbapenems, and chloramphenicol, but resistance is emerging to clindamycin. More than 80% of isolates are susceptible to cefoxitin and linezolid. Tigecycline has demonstrated in vitro activity against *Prevotella* and *Bacteroides* species but has limited pediatric dosing and safety data available, particularly for children younger than 8 years. Moxifloxacin may be an alternative for anaerobic infections in children with severe β-lactam allergies, although emerging resistance to *Bacteroides* species is a concern. Cefuroxime, cefotaxime, and ceftriaxone are not reliably effective.

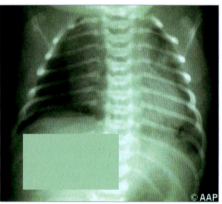

Image 14.1
Bacteroides fragilis pneumonia in a newborn (*B fragilis* isolated from the placenta and blood culture from the newborn). Anaerobic cultures were obtained because of a fecal odor in the amniotic fluid.

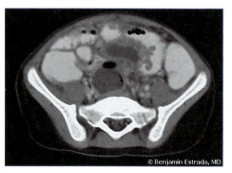

Image 14.2
Bacteroides fragilis abdominal abscess in a 9-year-old boy. Courtesy of Benjamin Estrada, MD.

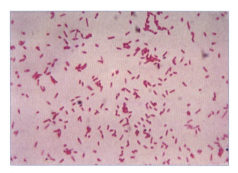

Image 14.3
This photomicrograph shows *Bacteroides fragilis* after being cultured in a thioglycolate medium for 48 hours. *B fragilis* is a gram-negative rod that constitutes 1%–2% of the normal colonic bacterial microflora in humans. It is associated with extraintestinal infections such as abscesses and soft tissue infections, as well as diarrheal diseases. Courtesy of Centers for Disease Control and Prevention.

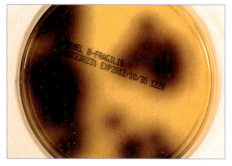

Image 14.4
Bacteroides fragilis on bacteroid bile-esculin agar. This organism not only grows in 20% bile but also hydrolyzes esculin, causing the browning of the agar. Courtesy of Julia Rosebush, DO; Robert Jerris, PhD; and Theresa Stanley, M(ASCP).

CHAPTER 15
Balantidium coli Infections
(Balantidiasis)

CLINICAL MANIFESTATIONS

Most human infections are asymptomatic. Symptomatic infection is characterized by acute onset of bloody or watery mucoid diarrhea with abdominal pain or by chronic or intermittent episodes of diarrhea, anorexia, and weight loss. Inflammation of the gastrointestinal tract and local lymphatic vessels can result in bowel dilation, ulceration, perforation, and extraintestinal spread or secondary bacterial invasion. Colitis produced by *Balantidium coli* can mimic that of *Entamoeba histolytica* or noninfectious causes. Fulminant disease can occur in malnourished or otherwise debilitated or immunocompromised patients.

ETIOLOGY

B coli, a ciliated protozoan, is the largest pathogenic protozoan known to infect humans.

EPIDEMIOLOGY

Pigs are the primary host reservoir of *B coli*, but the parasite has also been found in other primates and domestic animals. Infections have been reported in most areas of the world but are more common in tropical and subtropical areas or areas with poor sanitation systems. Cysts excreted in feces can be transmitted directly from hand to mouth or indirectly through fecally contaminated water or food. Excysted trophozoites infect the colon. A person is infectious as long as cysts are excreted in stool. Cysts may remain viable in the environment for months.

The **incubation period** is not established but may be several days.

DIAGNOSTIC TESTS

Diagnosis is usually made by demonstrating trophozoites (or, less frequently, cysts) in stool or tissue by scraping lesions via sigmoidoscopy or colonoscopy, histological examination of intestinal biopsy specimens, or ova and parasite examination of stool. Stool examination is less sensitive; repeated examination may be necessary, because shedding of organisms can be intermittent. Because trophozoites degenerate rapidly, fresh diarrheal stools require either prompt microscopic examination or placement into stool fixation medium.

TREATMENT

The drug of choice is tetracycline. Alternative drugs are metronidazole (or tinidazole), iodoquinol, and nitazoxanide.

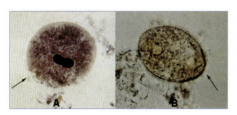

Image 15.1
Balantidium coli trophozoites are characterized by their large size (40 to >70 μm); on the cell surface, the presence of cilia, which are particularly visible (B); a cytostome (arrows); a bean-shaped macronucleus that is often visible (A); and a smaller, less conspicuous micronucleus. Courtesy of Centers for Disease Control and Prevention.

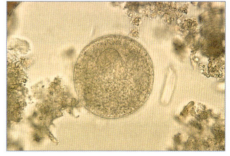

Image 15.2
Balantidium coli cyst in stool preparation. Courtesy of Centers for Disease Control and Prevention.

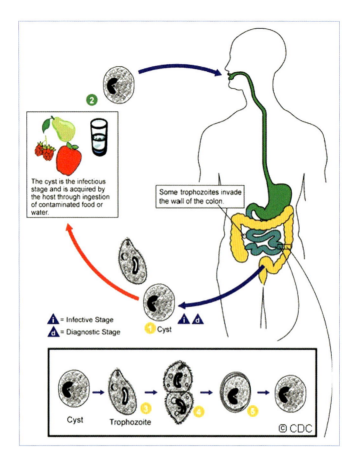

Image 15.3
Cysts are the parasite stage responsible for transmission of balantidiasis (1). The host most often acquires the cyst through ingestion of contaminated food or water (2). Following ingestion, excystation occurs in the small intestine, and the trophozoites colonize the large intestine (3). The trophozoites reside in the lumen of the large intestine of humans and animals, where they replicate by binary fission, during which conjugation may occur (4). Trophozoites undergo encystation to produce infective cysts (5). Some trophozoites invade the wall of the colon and multiply. Some return to the lumen and disintegrate. Mature cysts are passed with feces (1). Courtesy of Centers for Disease Control and Prevention.

CHAPTER 16

Bartonella henselae (Cat-Scratch Disease)

CLINICAL MANIFESTATIONS

Cat-scratch disease (CSD), the predominant clinical manifestation of *Bartonella henselae* infection, manifests in 85% to 90% of children as a localized cutaneous and regional lymphadenopathy disorder. A skin papule or pustule develops within 12 days at the presumed site of inoculation in approximately two-thirds of cases and usually precedes development of lymphadenopathy by 1 to 2 weeks (range, 7–60 days). Lymphadenopathy occurs in nodes that drain the site of inoculation, typically axillary, but cervical, submandibular, submental, epitrochlear, or inguinal nodes can be involved. Low-grade fever lasting several days develops in 30% of patients. The skin overlying affected lymph nodes can be normal or tender, warm, erythematous, and indurated, and approximately 10% to 20% of affected nodes suppurate. Typically, lymphadenopathy resolves spontaneously in 2 to 4 months.

Less common manifestations of *B henselae* infection likely reflect bloodborne disseminated disease and include culture-negative endocarditis, encephalopathy, osteolytic lesions, glomerulonephritis, pneumonia, thrombocytopenic purpura, erythema nodosum, and prolonged fever with granulomata in the liver and spleen.

Ocular manifestations occur in 5% to 10% of patients. The most classic and frequent manifestation of ocular *B henselae* infection is Parinaud oculoglandular syndrome, which consists of follicular conjunctivitis and ipsilateral preauricular lymphadenopathy. Another occasional ocular manifestation is neuroretinitis, which is characterized by abrupt unilateral (and, rarely, bilateral) painless vision impairment, granulomatous optic disc swelling, and macular edema, with lipid exudates (macular star). Rare manifestations include retinochoroiditis, anterior uveitis, vitritis, pars planitis, retinal vasculitis, retinitis, branch retinal arteriolar or venular occlusions, macular hole, or retinal detachments (extraordinarily rare).

ETIOLOGY

B henselae not only is a fastidious, slow-growing, gram-negative bacillus but also is the causative agent of bacillary angiomatosis (vascular proliferative lesions of skin and subcutaneous tissue) and bacillary peliosis (reticuloendothelial lesions in visceral organs, primarily the liver). The last 2 manifestations of infection are reported in immunocompromised patients, primarily those with HIV infection. Additional species, such as *Bartonella clarridgeiae*, have also been found to cause CSD. *B henselae* is related closely to *Bartonella quintana*, the agent of human body louseborne trench fever that caused significant disease in troops during World War I and now affects homeless people lacking adequate sanitation and hygiene. *B quintana* can also cause bacillary angiomatosis and endocarditis.

EPIDEMIOLOGY

B henselae commonly causes regional lymphadenopathy in children. The highest incidence (9 per 100,000 population) is found in children 5 to 9 years of age; infections occur more often during the fall and winter. Cats are the natural reservoir for *B henselae*, with a seroprevalence of 30% to 40% in domestic and adopted shelter cats in the United States. Other animals, including dogs, can be infected and are rarely associated with human illness. Cat-to-cat transmission occurs via the cat flea (*Ctenocephalides felis*), with feline infection resulting in bacteremia that is usually asymptomatic and lasts weeks to months. Fleas acquire the organism when feeding on a bacteremic cat and then shed infectious organisms in their feces. The bacteria are transmitted to humans by inoculation through a scratch, lick, or bite from a bacteremic cat. Most patients with CSD have a history of recent contact with apparently healthy cats, especially kittens. Kittens are nearly 5 times as likely to be bacteremic with *B henselae* as older cats. Cats obtained from shelters or adopted as strays also have high rates of bacteremia. There is no convincing evidence that ticks are a competent vector for transmission of *Bartonella* organisms to humans. No evidence of person-to-person transmission exists.

The **incubation period** from the time of the scratch to the appearance of the primary cutaneous lesion is 3 to 12 days; the median period from the appearance of the primary lesion to the appearance of lymphadenopathy is 12 days (range, 7–60 days).

DIAGNOSTIC TESTS

Both enzyme immunoassay (EIA) and indirect immunofluorescent antibody (IFA) platforms for detection of immunoglobulin M (IgM) and immunoglobulin G (IgG) serum antibodies to antigens of *Bartonella* species are available for diagnosis of CSD. Both formats have limitations in sensitivity and specificity. With both types of tests, cross-reactivity with other infectious agents (such as *Chlamydia pneumoniae, Coxiella burnetii,* and especially other *Bartonella* species) is common. Elevated IgM titers may suggest recent infection, but both false-positive and false-negative IgM test results occur. In adults, there is a high rate of anti–*B henselae* IgG seroprevalence in the general population attributable to prior exposure. Generally, if an IFA or EIA IgG titer is less than 1:64, the patient does not have acute infection. Titers between 1:64 and 1:256 may represent past or acute infection, and follow-up titers in 2 to 4 weeks should be considered. An IgG titer of 1:256 or greater or a 4-fold increase in IgG titer is consistent with acute infection.

Polymerase chain reaction (PCR) assays are available in some commercial and research laboratories for testing of tissue or body fluids. *Bartonella* PCR assay is highly specific and fairly sensitive for use on tissue, although some assays do not distinguish between the various *Bartonella* species. *Bartonella* PCR assay is very insensitive for testing blood, however, and it is not generally recommended for this specimen.

B henselae is a fastidious organism; recovery by routine culture requires prolonged incubation (>10 days) and rarely succeeds.

If tissue (eg, lymph node) specimens are available, bacilli may occasionally be visualized by using a silver stain (eg, Warthin-Starry or Steiner stain); however, these stains are nonspecific for *B henselae*. Early histological changes in lymph node specimens consist of lymphocytic infiltration with epithelioid granuloma formation. Later changes consist of polymorphonuclear leukocyte infiltration with granulomas that become necrotic and resemble granulomas from patients with tularemia, brucellosis, or mycobacterial infections.

TREATMENT

Management of localized uncomplicated CSD is primarily aimed at relief of symptoms, because the disease is self-limited, resolving spontaneously in 2 to 4 months. No antibiotic regimen has been shown to improve the clinical cure rate, and in most cases, antibiotic therapy is not indicated. Painful suppurative nodes can be treated with needle aspiration for relief of symptoms. Incision and drainage should be avoided, because this may facilitate fistula formation; surgical excision is generally unnecessary.

Some experts recommend antimicrobial therapy in acutely or severely ill immunocompetent patients with systemic symptoms, particularly people with retinitis, hepatic or splenic involvement, osteomyelitis, or painful adenitis. Several antimicrobial agents (azithromycin, clarithromycin, ciprofloxacin, doxycycline, trimethoprim-sulfamethoxazole, ceftriaxone, gentamicin, and rifampin) have in vitro activity against *B henselae*. However, outcomes for most forms of CSD are generally excellent with or without therapy.

Doxycycline plus rifampin is often used for patients with neuroretinitis. Doxycycline may be used regardless of patient age. Reports in the literature note that a large majority of such patients experience significant visual recovery to 20/40 or better. Corticosteroids should be considered in conjunction with ophthalmology consultation.

Antimicrobial therapy is recommended for all immunocompromised people, because treatment of bacillary angiomatosis and bacillary peliosis has been shown to be beneficial. Azithromycin or doxycycline is effective for treatment of these conditions; therapy should be administered for 3 months for bacillary angiomatosis and for 4 months for bacillary peliosis to prevent relapse. In these patients, doxycycline can be used for short durations (ie, ≤21 days) without regard to patient age; for the longer treatment durations required for *Bartonella* infection in immunocompromised people, for whom the alternative treatment of azithromycin exists, doxycycline is not recommended in children younger than 8 years.

For patients with unusual manifestations of *Bartonella* infection (eg, culture-negative endocarditis, neuroretinitis, disease in immunocompromised patients), consultation with a pediatric infectious diseases expert is recommended.

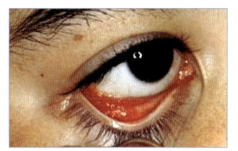

Image 16.1
Clinical manifestations of cat-scratch disease include Parinaud oculoglandular syndrome, which results when inoculation of the eye conjunctiva causes conjunctivitis.

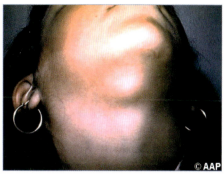

Image 16.2
Submental lymphadenitis caused by cat-scratch disease.

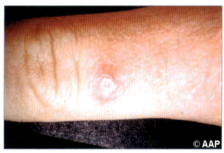

Image 16.3
Cat-scratch granuloma of the finger of a 6-year-old boy. This is a typical inoculation site lesion, which was noted about 10 days before the development of regional lymphadenopathy.

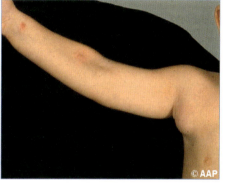

Image 16.4
Cat-scratch granuloma of the wrist with anterior axillary lymphadenitis in a 4-year-old boy. Cat-scratch disease is a common cause of prolonged lymphadenopathy in children.

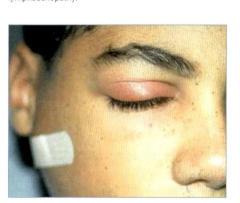

Image 16.5
Parinaud oculoglandular syndrome (inoculation of the conjunctivae with ipsilateral preauricular adenopathy) in a 6-year-old boy.

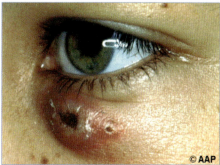

Image 16.6
Papules at inoculation sites on the face of a patient with cat-scratch disease.

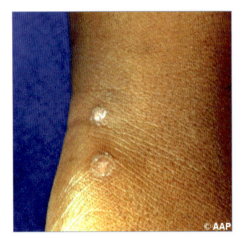

Image 16.7
A papule at each of 2 inoculation sites on the arm of a patient with cat-scratch disease.

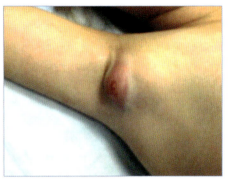

Image 16.8
A 2-year-old with suppurative right axillary lymphadenopathy secondary to cat-scratch disease. Copyright Michael Rajnik, MD, FAAP.

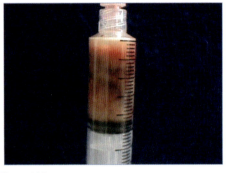

Image 16.9
Sanguinopurulent exudate aspirated from the axillary node of the patient in Image 16.8 with cat-scratch disease. Copyright Michael Rajnik, MD, FAAP.

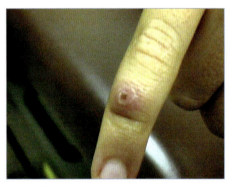

Image 16.10
Cat-scratch disease granuloma of the finger in a 12-year-old boy with epitrochlear node involvement (see Image 16.11). Copyright Michael Rajnik, MD, FAAP.

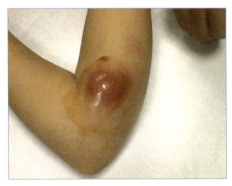

Image 16.11
Epitrochlear suppurative adenitis of cat-scratch disease in the boy in Image 16.10, with a cat-scratch granuloma of the finger. Copyright Michael Rajnik, MD, FAAP.

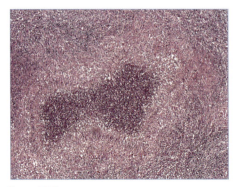

Image 16.12
Stellate microabscess and silver-stained coccobacillary forms of *Bartonella henselae* within the inflammatory infiltrate of the involved lymph node (hematoxylin-eosin stain; original magnification ×12.5). Courtesy of Christopher Paddock, MD.

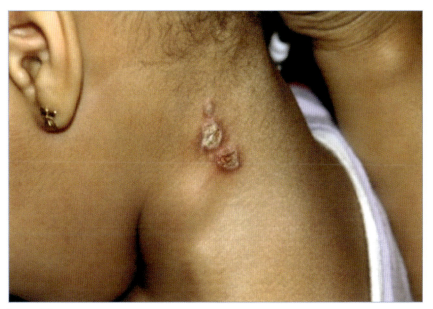

Image 16.13
This 3-year-old was previously scratched on the left side of her neck by a kitten. She developed raised red bumps around the scratch on day 5. This area ulcerated slightly and was slow to heal. No fever was noted, although she was less active for the next several days and shared that her arms and legs were sore. She developed swollen posterior cervical lymph nodes about 1 week later. Physical examination indicated two 8-mm ulcerations with raised borders and a papule near an enlarged minimally tender posterior cervical node. Result from the serological test was positive for *Bartonella henselae*. She improved with time following a course of azithromycin. Courtesy of Will Sorey, MD.

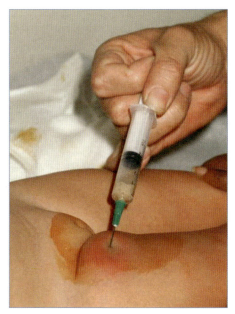

Image 16.14
Needle aspiration of purulent material caused by cat-scratch disease. Courtesy of Ed Fajardo, MD.

CHAPTER 17
Baylisascaris Infections

CLINICAL MANIFESTATIONS

Infection with *Baylisascaris procyonis*, a raccoon roundworm, can manifest with nonspecific signs such as nausea, fever, and fatigue. Other clinical manifestations include neural larval migrans, ocular larval migrans, and visceral larval migrans. Acute central nervous system (CNS) disease (eg, altered mental status and seizures) accompanied by peripheral and/or cerebrospinal fluid (CSF) eosinophilia are manifestations of neural larval migrans (eosinophilic meningoencephalitis) and can occur 2 to 4 weeks after infection. Severe neurological sequelae or death is the usual outcome. Ocular larval migrans can result in diffuse unilateral subacute neuroretinitis; direct visualization of larvae in the retina is sometimes possible. Visceral larval migrans can manifest with nonspecific signs such as macular rash, pneumonitis, and hepatomegaly. Like visceral larval migrans caused by *Toxocara* species, subclinical or asymptomatic infection is thought to be the most common outcome of infection.

ETIOLOGY

B procyonis is a 10- to 25-cm long roundworm (nematode) with a direct life cycle usually limited to its definitive host, the raccoon. Domestic dogs and some less commonly owned pets, such as kinkajous and ringtails, can serve as definitive hosts and are potential sources of human disease.

EPIDEMIOLOGY

B procyonis is distributed focally throughout the United States; in areas where disease is endemic, 22% to 80% of raccoons can harbor the parasite in their intestines. Reports of infections in dogs raise concern that infected dogs may be able to spread the disease. Embryonated eggs containing infective larvae are ingested from the soil by raccoons, rodents, and birds. When infective eggs or an infected host is eaten by a raccoon, the larvae grow to maturity in the small intestine, where adult female worms shed millions of eggs per day. Eggs become infective after 2 to 4 weeks in the environment and may persist over the long term in the soil. Cases of raccoon infection have been reported in many parts of the United States. Risk of human infection is greatest in areas where significant raccoon populations live in peridomestic settings. Fewer than 30 cases of *Baylisascaris* CNS disease have been documented in the United States, although cases may be undiagnosed or underreported.

Risk factors for *Baylisascaris* infection include contact with raccoon latrines (communal defecation sites often found at or on the base of trees; raised flat surfaces such as tree stumps, logs, rocks, decks, and rooftops; or unsealed attics or garages), geophagia/pica, age younger than 4 years, and, in older children, developmental delay. Most reported cases of CNS disease have been in males.

The **incubation period** is usually 1 to 4 weeks.

DIAGNOSTIC TESTS

Baylisascaris infection is confirmed by identification of larvae in biopsy specimens. A presumptive diagnosis of CNS disease can be made on the basis of clinical (meningoencephalitis, diffuse unilateral subacute neuroretinitis, or pseudotumor), epidemiological (raccoon exposure), and laboratory (blood and CSF eosinophilia) findings. Serological testing (ie, serum, CSF) for patients with clinical symptoms is available at the Centers for Disease Control and Prevention. Neuroimaging results can be normal initially, but as larvae grow and migrate through CNS tissue, focal abnormalities are found in periventricular white matter and elsewhere. In ocular disease, ophthalmologic examination can reveal chorioretinal lesions or, rarely, larvae. Stool examination is not helpful because eggs are not shed in human feces. The disease is not transmitted from person to person.

TREATMENT

Albendazole, in conjunction with high-dose corticosteroids, has been advocated most widely on the basis of CNS and CSF penetration and in vitro activity. Treatment with anthelmintic agents and corticosteroids may not affect clinical outcome once severe CNS disease manifestations are evident. Treatment should be initiated while the diagnostic evaluation is being completed if infection is suspected. Preventive therapy with albendazole should be considered for children with a history of ingestion of soil potentially contaminated with raccoon feces but no definitive preventive dosing regimen established. Studies in children as young as 1 year of age suggest that albendazole can be administered safely to this population. Larvae

localized to the retina may be killed by direct photocoagulation.

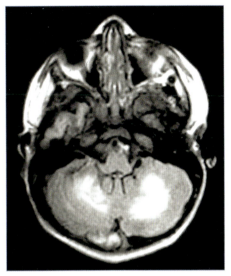

Image 17.1
Neuroimaging of human *Baylisascaris procyonis* neural larval migrans. In acute neural larval migrans, axial flair magnetic resonance image (at the level of the posterior fossa) demonstrates abnormal hyperintense signal of cerebellar white matter.

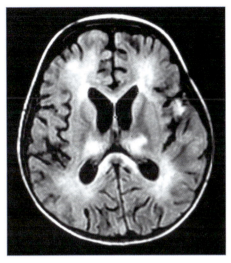

Image 17.2
Neuroimaging of human *Baylisascaris procyonis* neural larval migrans. Axial T2-weighted magnetic resonance image (at the level of the lateral ventricles) demonstrates abnormal patchy hyperintense signal of periventricular white matter and basal ganglia.

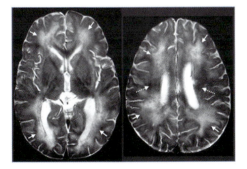

Image 17.3
Biopsy-proven *Baylisascaris procyonis* encephalitis in a 13-month-old boy. Axial T2-weighted magnetic resonance images obtained 12 days after symptom onset show an abnormally high signal throughout most of the central white matter (arrows) compared with the dark signal expected at this age (broken arrows). Courtesy of *Emerging Infectious Diseases*.

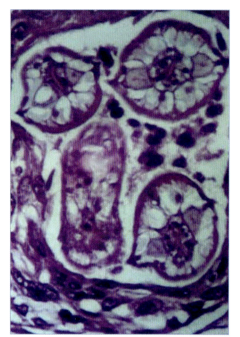

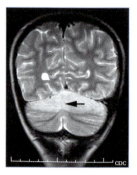

Image 17.5
Coronal T2-weighted magnetic resonance image of the brain in a 4-year-old with *Baylisascaris procyonis* eosinophilic meningitis. Arrow shows diffuse edema of the superior cerebellar hemispheres (scale bar increments in centimeters). Courtesy of Centers for Disease Control and Prevention/*Emerging Infectious Diseases* and Poulomi J. Pai.

Image 17.4
Cross section of *Baylisascaris procyonis* larva in tissue section of brain, demonstrating characteristic diagnostic features including prominent lateral alae and excretory columns. Courtesy of *Emerging Infectious Diseases*.

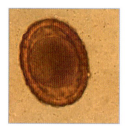

Image 17.6
Unembryonated egg of *Baylisascaris procyonis*. *B procyonis* eggs are 80–85 μm × 65–70 μm, thick shelled, and usually slightly oval. They are similar morphologically to fertile eggs of *Ascaris lumbricoides*, although eggs of *A lumbricoides* are smaller (55–75 μm × 35–50 μm). The definitive host for *B procyonis* is the raccoon, although dogs may also serve as definitive hosts. Because humans do not serve as definitive hosts for *B procyonis*, eggs are not considered a diagnostic finding and are not excreted in human feces. Courtesy of Cheryl Davis, MD, Western Kentucky University.

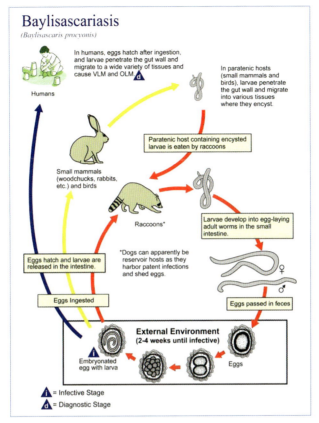

Image 17.7
This illustration depicts the life cycle of *Baylisascaris procyonis*, the causal agent of *Baylisascaris* disease. OLM indicates ocular larval migrans; VLM, visceral larva migrans. Courtesy of Centers for Disease Control and Prevention.

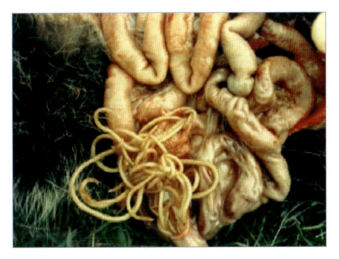

Image 17.8
Baylisascaris is raccoon roundworm that may cause ocular and neural larval migrans and encephalitis in humans. Photo used with permission of Michigan Department of Natural Resources.

CHAPTER 18
Infections With *Blastocystis* Species

CLINICAL MANIFESTATIONS

The importance of *Blastocystis* species as a cause of gastrointestinal tract disease is controversial. The asymptomatic carrier state is well-documented. Clinical symptoms reported include bloating, flatulence, acute or chronic watery diarrhea without fecal leukocytes or blood, constipation, abdominal pain, nausea, anorexia, weight loss, and poor growth; fever is generally absent. Some case series and reports have noted an association between infection with *Blastocystis* and chronic urticaria and irritable bowel syndrome. When *Blastocystis* organisms are identified in stool from symptomatic patients, other causes of this symptom complex, particularly *Giardia duodenalis* and *Cryptosporidium parvum*, should be investigated before assuming that blastocystosis causes the signs and symptoms. Polymerase chain reaction fingerprinting suggests that some *Blastocystis* subtypes are disease associated and others are not.

ETIOLOGY

Blastocystis species (previously referred to as *Blastocystis hominis*) consists of several species that reside in the gastrointestinal tracts of humans as well as other mammals, reptiles, amphibians, and fish. Some *Blastocystis* species believed to be specific to other animals are now recognized as being transmissible to humans. Previously classified as a protozoan, the organism is now characterized as a stramenopile (a eukaryote) because of more recent molecular studies. Multiple forms have been described: vacuolar, which is observed most commonly in clinical specimens; granular, which is found rarely in fresh stools; amoeboid; and cystic.

EPIDEMIOLOGY

Blastocystis infection is observed commonly throughout the world, although prevalence among countries and communities varies. In the United States, Europe, and Japan, *Blastocystis* species are recovered from 1% to 20% of stool specimens examined for ova and parasites, whereas prevalence of 100% has been observed among school-aged children in countries without modern sanitation. Because transmission is believed to occur via the fecal-oral route, presence of the organism may be a marker for presence of other pathogens spread by fecal contamination. *Blastocystis* infection is more common in people who have pets or live near farm animals; however, exposure is insufficient for infection because pathogenicity appears related to subtype, host immunocompetence, and other factors. Organisms may remain in the gastrointestinal tract for years.

The **incubation period** has not been established.

DIAGNOSTIC TESTS

Stool specimens should be preserved in polyvinyl alcohol and stained with trichrome or iron-hematoxylin before microscopic examination. Small round cysts, the most common form, vary markedly in size, from 6 to 40 μm, and are characterized by a large central body (like a large vacuole) surrounded by multiple nuclei. The parasite may be present in varying numbers, and infections may be reported as light to heavy. The presence of 5 or more organisms per high-power (×400 magnification) field can indicate heavy infection, which to some experts suggests causation when other enteropathogens are absent. Other experts consider the presence of 10 or more organisms per 10 oil immersion fields (×1,000 magnification) to represent heavy infection.

TREATMENT

Indications for treatment are not established. Some experts recommend that treatment be reserved for patients who have persistent symptoms and in whom no other pathogen or process is found to explain the gastrointestinal tract symptoms. Randomized controlled treatment trials with both metronidazole and nitazoxanide have demonstrated benefit in symptomatic patients, although microbiological resolution does not always occur. Tinidazole is an alternative that may be tolerated better than metronidazole.

INFECTIONS WITH *BLASTOCYSTIS* SPECIES

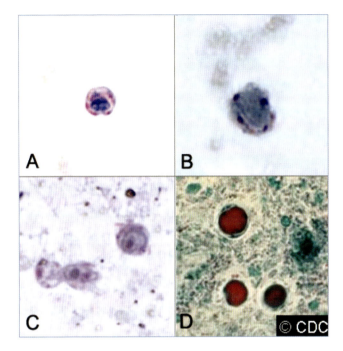

Image 18.1
A–D, *Blastocystis hominis* cystlike forms (trichrome stain). The sizes vary from 4–10 µm. The vacuoles stain variably from red to blue. The nuclei in the peripheral cytoplasmic rim are clearly visible, staining purple (B) (4 nuclei). Specimens in A–C contributed by Ray Kaplan, MD, SmithKline Beecham Diagnostic Laboratories, Atlanta, GA. D, Courtesy of Centers for Disease Control and Prevention.

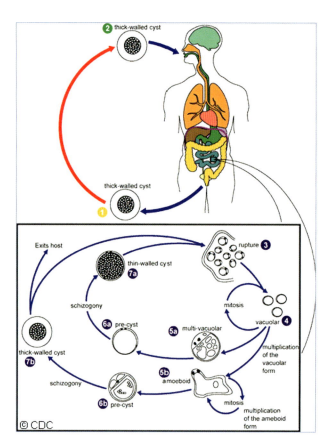

Image 18.2
Knowledge of the life cycle and transmission are still under investigation; therefore, this is a proposed life cycle for *Blastocystis hominis*. The classic form found in human stools is the cyst, which varies tremendously in size from 6 to 40 μm (1). The thick-walled cyst present in the stools (1) is believed to be responsible for external transmission, possibly by the fecal-oral route through ingestion of contaminated water or food (2). The cysts infect epithelial cells of the digestive tract and multiply asexually (3, 4). Vacuolar forms of the parasite give origin to multivacuolar (5a) and ameboid (5b) forms. The multivacuolar form develops into a precyst (6a) that gives origin to a thin-walled cyst (7a) thought to be responsible for autoinfection. The ameboid form gives origin to a precyst (6b), which develops into thick-walled cyst by schizogony (7b). *B hominis* stages were reproduced from Singh M, Suresh K, Ho LC, Ng GC, Yap EH. Elucidation of the life cycle of the intestinal protozoan *Blastocystis hominis*. *Parasitol Res.* 1995;81(5):449. Permission granted by M Singh and Springer-Verlag.

CHAPTER 19
Blastomycosis

CLINICAL MANIFESTATIONS

Infections can be acute, chronic, or fulminant but are asymptomatic in up to 50% of infected people. The most common clinical manifestation of blastomycosis in children is cough (often productive) accompanying pulmonary disease, with fever, chest pain, and nonspecific symptoms such as fatigue and myalgia. Rarely, patients may develop acute respiratory distress syndrome. Typical radiographic patterns include consolidation, patchy pneumonitis, a mass-like infiltrate, or nodules. Blastomycosis can be misdiagnosed as bacterial pneumonia, tuberculosis, sarcoidosis, or malignant neoplasm. Disseminated blastomycosis, which can occur in up to 25% of symptomatic cases, most commonly involves the skin and osteoarticular structures. Cutaneous manifestations can be verrucous, nodular, ulcerative, or pustular. Abscesses are usually subcutaneous but can involve any organ. Erythema nodosum, which is common in patients with histoplasmosis and coccidioidomycosis, is rare in blastomycosis. Central nervous system (CNS) infection is less common, and intrauterine or congenital infection is rare.

ETIOLOGY

Blastomycosis is caused by *Blastomyces* species (*Blastomyces dermatitidis, Blastomyces gilchristii,* and *Blastomyces helicus*), which are thermally dimorphic fungi existing in the yeast form at 37 °C (98 °F) in infected tissues and in a mycelial form at room temperature and in soil. Conidia, produced from hyphae of the mycelial form, are infectious.

EPIDEMIOLOGY

Infection is acquired through inhalation of conidia from the environment. Increased mortality rates for patients with pulmonary blastomycosis have been associated with advanced age, chronic obstructive pulmonary disease, cancer, and Black race. Person-to-person transmission does not occur. In the United States, blastomycosis is endemic in the central states, with most cases occurring in the Ohio and Mississippi river valleys, the southeastern states, and states that border the Great Lakes; however, sporadic cases have occurred outside these areas. Like *Histoplasma capsulatum*, *Blastomyces* species can grow in bird and animal excreta. Occupational and recreational activities associated with infection often involve environmental disruption such as construction of homes or roads, boating and canoeing, tubing on a river, fishing, exploration of beaver dams and underground forts, and a community compost pile.

The **incubation period** ranges from approximately 2 weeks to 3 months.

DIAGNOSTIC TESTS

Definitive diagnosis of blastomycosis is based on microscopic identification of characteristic thick-walled, broad-based, single budding yeast cells either by culture at 37 °C (98 °F) or in histopathologic specimens. The organism may be seen in sputum, tracheal aspirates, cerebrospinal fluid (CSF), urine, or histopathologic specimens from lesions processed with 10% potassium hydroxide or a silver stain. Children with pneumonia who are unable to produce sputum may require bronchoalveolar lavage or open biopsy to establish the diagnosis. Bronchoalveolar lavage is high yield, even in patients with bone or skin manifestations. Organisms can be cultured on brain-heart infusion media and Sabouraud dextrose agar at 25 to 30 °C (77–86 °F) as a mold; identification can be confirmed by conversion to yeast phase at 37 °C (98 °F). Chemiluminescent DNA probes are available for identification of *B dermatitidis*. Polymerase chain reaction assay can be used directly on certain clinical specimens but is not widely performed.

Because serological tests (immunodiffusion and complement fixation) lack adequate sensitivity, they are generally not useful for diagnosis. An enzyme immunoassay that detects *Blastomyces* antigen in urine has replaced classic serological studies and performs well for the diagnosis of disseminated and pulmonary disease as well as for the monitoring of response to antifungal therapy. Antigen testing of urine performs better than antigen testing of serum, and antigen testing of bronchoalveolar lavage fluid or CSF is also available. Significant cross-reactivity occurs in patients with other endemic mycoses (specifically, *H capsulatum, Paracoccidioides brasiliensis,* and *Talaromyces marneffei*); clinical and epidemiological considerations often aid with interpretation.

TREATMENT

Because of the high risk of dissemination, some experts recommend that all cases of blastomycosis in children be treated. Amphotericin B deoxycholate or an amphotericin B lipid formulation is recommended for initial therapy for severe pulmonary disease for 1 to 2 weeks or until improvement, followed by 6 to 12 months of itraconazole therapy. Oral itraconazole is recommended for 6 to 12 months for mild to moderate infection. Some experts suggest 12 months of therapy for patients with osteoarticular disease. For CNS infection, a lipid formulation of amphotericin B is recommended for 4 to 6 weeks, followed by an azole for at least 12 months and until resolution of all CSF abnormalities. The preferred azole for prolonged CNS infection treatment is voriconazole, given the limited CNS penetration of itraconazole. Itraconazole is indicated for treatment of non–life-threatening infection outside the CNS in adults and is recommended in children. Serum trough concentrations of itraconazole should be 1 to 2 μg/mL. Concentrations should be checked after several days of therapy to ensure adequate drug exposure. When measured by high-pressure liquid chromatography, both itraconazole and its bioactive hydroxyitraconazole metabolite are reported, the sum of which should be considered in assessing drug concentrations. The itraconazole oral solution formulation is preferred because of improved absorption and should be taken on an empty stomach.

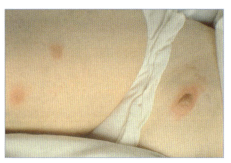

Image 19.1
Nodular skin lesions of blastomycosis, one of which is a bullous lesion on top of a nodule. Aspiration of the bulla revealed yeast forms of *Blastomyces dermatitidis*. Courtesy of Centers for Disease Control and Prevention.

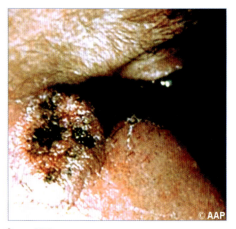

Image 19.2
Cutaneous blastomycosis (face). Cutaneous lesions are nodular, verrucous, or ulcerative, as in this man. Most cutaneous lesions are caused by hematogenous spread from a pulmonary infection. Courtesy of Edgar O. Ledbetter, MD, FAAP.

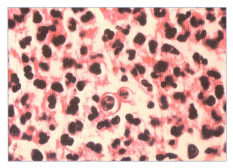

Image 19.3
Histopathologic features of blastomycosis of skin. Budding cell of *Blastomyces dermatitidis* surrounded by neutrophils. Multiple nuclei are visible. Courtesy of Centers for Disease Control and Prevention.

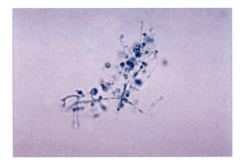

Image 19.4
Photomicrograph of *Blastomyces dermatitidis* by use of a cotton blue–staining technique. Blastomycosis caused by *B dermatitidis* can be asymptomatic or associated with acute, chronic, or fulminant disease. Courtesy of Centers for Disease Control and Prevention.

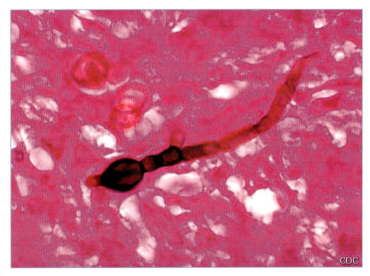

Image 19.5
This micrograph shows histopathologic changes that reveal the presence of the fungal agent *Blastomyces dermatitidis*. Courtesy of Centers for Disease Control and Prevention/Libero Ajello, MD.

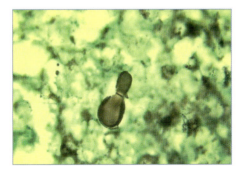

Image 19.6
Histopathologic features of blastomycosis. Yeast cell of *Blastomyces dermatitidis* undergoing broad-base budding (methenamine silver stain). Courtesy of Centers for Disease Control and Prevention.

CHAPTER 20
Bocavirus

CLINICAL MANIFESTATIONS

Human bocavirus (HBoV) was first identified in 2005 from a cohort of children with acute respiratory tract symptoms. Pneumonia, bronchiolitis, exacerbations of asthma, the common cold, and acute otitis media have been attributed to HBoV. Symptoms may include cough, rhinorrhea, wheezing, and fever. HBoV has been identified in 5% to 33% of all children with acute respiratory tract infections in various settings (eg, inpatient facilities, outpatient facilities, child care centers). High rates of HBoV subclinical infections have been documented, complicating etiologic association with disease. The role of HBoV as a pathogen in human infection is further confounded by simultaneous detection of other viral pathogens in patients in whom HBoV is identified, with coinfection rates ranging from 20% to as high as 80%. However, a number of lines of evidence support the role of HBoV as a pathogen, at least during primary infection. These include longitudinal cohort studies showing an association of primary infection with symptomatic illness and case-control studies showing associations of illness with monoinfection, high viral load, and detection of HBoV messenger RNA (mRNA).

Infection with HBoV appears to be ubiquitous, because nearly all children develop serological evidence of previous HBoV infection by 5 years of age.

ETIOLOGY

HBoV is a nonenveloped, single-stranded DNA virus classified in the family *Parvoviridae*, subfamily *Parvovirinae*, genus *Bocaparvovirus*, on the basis of its genetic similarity to the closely related **bo**vine parvovirus 1 and **ca**nine minute virus, from which the name "**boca**virus" was derived. Four distinct genotypes have been described (HBoV types 1–4), although there are no data regarding antigenic variation or distinct serotypes. HBoV 1 replicates primarily in the respiratory tract and has been associated with upper and lower respiratory tract illness. HBoV 2, HBoV 3, and HBoV 4 have been found predominantly in stool, without clear association with any clinical illness.

EPIDEMIOLOGY

Detection of HBoV has been described only in humans. Transmission is presumed to be from respiratory tract secretions, although fecal-oral transmission may be possible because of finding of HBoV in stool specimens from children, including symptomatic children with diarrhea.

The frequent codetection of other viral pathogens of the respiratory tract in association with HBoV has led to speculation about the pathological role played by HBoV; it may be a true pathogen or copathogen, and emerging evidence seems to support both roles. Codetection of HBoV with other respiratory viruses is more common when HBoV is present at lower viral loads ($\leq 10^4$ copies/mL). Extended and intermittent shedding of HBoV has been reported for up to a year after initial detection, with median shedding duration of approximately 2 months. Because HBoV may be shed for long periods after primary infection and because of the possibility of reactivation during subsequent viral infections and the high rate of detection in healthy people, clinical interpretation of HBoV detection is difficult.

HBoV circulates worldwide and year round. In temperate climates, seasonal clustering in the spring associated with increased transmission of other respiratory tract viruses has been reported.

DIAGNOSTIC TESTS

Commercial molecular diagnostic assays for HBoV are available. HBoV quantitative polymerase chain reaction (respiratory and serum specimens), detection of HBoV mRNA in the respiratory tract, and detection of HBoV-specific immunoglobulin M and immunoglobulin G antibody are also used by research laboratories to detect virus and infection. A positive laboratory test does not necessarily imply etiology, in part because of prolonged shedding and codetection of other respiratory pathogens.

TREATMENT

No specific therapy is available.

CHAPTER 21
Borrelia Infections Other Than Lyme Disease
(Relapsing Fever)

CLINICAL MANIFESTATIONS

Two types of relapsing fever occur in humans: tickborne and louseborne. Both are characterized by sudden onset of high fever, shaking chills, sweats, headache, muscle and joint pain, altered sensorium, and nausea. A fleeting macular rash of the trunk and petechiae of the skin and mucous membranes sometimes occur but are uncommon. Findings and complications can differ between types of relapsing fever and include hepatosplenomegaly, jaundice, thrombocytopenia, iridocyclitis, cough with pleuritic pain, pneumonitis, Bell palsy, meningitis, and myocarditis. Mortality rates are 10% to 70% in untreated louseborne relapsing fever (possibly related to comorbidities in refugee-type settings, where this disease is typically found) and 4% to 10% in untreated tickborne relapsing fever. Death occurs predominantly in infants, older adults, and people with underlying illnesses. Early treatment reduces mortality to less than 5%. Untreated, an initial febrile period of 2 to 6 days terminates spontaneously and is followed by an afebrile period of several days to weeks, then by 1 relapse or more (0–13 for tickborne, 1–5 for louseborne). Relapses typically become shorter and progressively milder as afebrile periods lengthen. Relapse is associated with expression of new borrelial antigens, and resolution of symptoms is associated with production of antibody specific to those new antigenic determinants. Infection during pregnancy is often severe and can result in spontaneous abortion, preterm birth, stillbirth, or neonatal infection.

ETIOLOGY

Relapsing fever is caused by certain spirochetes of the genus *Borrelia*. Worldwide, at least 14 *Borrelia* species cause tickborne (endemic) relapsing fever, including *Borrelia hermsii, Borrelia turicatae,* and *Borrelia parkeri* in North America. *Borrelia miyamotoi* is associated with a similar but distinct tickborne acute febrile illness in the United States. Louseborne (epidemic) relapsing fever is cause by *Borrelia recurrentis*.

EPIDEMIOLOGY

Endemic tickborne relapsing fever is distributed widely throughout the world. Most species, including *B hermsii, B turicatae,* and *B parkeri,* are transmitted through the bite of soft-bodied ticks (*Ornithodoros* species). *B miyamotoi*, which only recently has been recognized as a cause of human illness, is transmitted through the bite of hard-bodied ticks (*Ixodes* species). Vector ticks become infected by feeding on rodents or other small mammals and transmit infection via their saliva during subsequent blood meals. Ticks may serve as reservoirs of infection through transovarial and trans-stadial transmission. Because of differences in the distribution, life cycle, and feeding habits of soft- and hard-bodied ticks, the epidemiology differs somewhat for infections transmitted by these 2 classes of ticks.

Soft-bodied ticks typically live within rodent nests. They inflict painless bites and feed briefly (seconds to 30 minutes), usually at night, so people are often unaware of having been bitten. In the United States, vector soft-bodied ticks are found most often in mountainous areas of the West. Human infection typically follows sleeping in rustic, rodent-infested cabins, although cases have been associated with primary residences and luxurious rental properties. Cases occur sporadically or in small clusters in families or cohabiting groups. *B hermsii* is the most common cause of these infections. *B turicatae* infections occur less frequently; most cases have been reported from Texas and are associated with tick exposures in rodent-infested caves. Clinically apparent human infections with *B parkeri* in the United States are rare; the tick infected with this *Borrelia* species is associated with arid areas or grasslands in the western United States.

The hard-bodied ticks *Ixodes scapularis* and *Ixodes pacificus* transmit *B miyamotoi* in North America. These ticks are better known as vectors of Lyme disease, anaplasmosis, and babesiosis; coinfections have been reported. It is likely that risk factors described for Lyme disease are similar for *B miyamotoi*. Unlike Lyme disease, *B miyamotoi* can be transmitted within the first 24 hours of tick attachment, and probability of transmission increases with prolonged attachment. Most known cases of *B miyamotoi* infection have occurred in July or August, later than most Lyme disease cases. This suggests that *B miyamotoi* transmission more often occurs through the bite of larval, rather than nymphal, *Ixodes* ticks.

Louseborne epidemic relapsing fever had previously been widespread but is now mainly restricted to Ethiopia, Eritrea, Somalia, and Sudan, especially in refugee and displaced populations. Epidemic transmission occurs when body lice (*Pediculus humanus*) become infected by feeding on humans with spirochetemia; infection is transmitted when infected lice are crushed and their body fluids contaminate a bite wound or skin abraded by scratching.

Infected body lice and ticks may remain alive and infectious for several years to decades without feeding. Relapsing fever is not transmitted between individual humans, but perinatal transmission from an infected mother to her infant occurs and can result in preterm birth, stillbirth, and neonatal death.

The **incubation period** is 2 to 18 days, with a mean of 7 days.

DIAGNOSTIC TESTS

Spirochetes can be observed by dark-field microscopy and in Wright-, Giemsa-, or acridine orange–stained preparations of thin or dehemoglobinized thick smears of peripheral blood or in stained buffy-coat preparations. Organisms can often be visualized in blood obtained while the person is febrile, particularly during initial febrile episodes; organisms are less likely to be recovered from subsequent relapses. Direct detection by polymerase chain reaction is available at some commercial and reference laboratories. Spirochetes can be cultured in specialized media from blood obtained before treatment. Serum antibodies to *Borrelia* species can be detected by enzyme immunoassay and Western immunoblot analysis at some reference and commercial specialty laboratories. Serum tested early in infection may be negative, so it is important to also obtain a serum sample for serological testing during the convalescent period (at least 21 days after symptom onset); development of an immunoglobulin G response in the convalescent sample supports a tickborne relapsing fever diagnosis. Early antibiotic treatment may limit the antibody response. Antibody tests are not standardized and are affected by antigenic variations among and within *Borrelia* species and strains. Serological cross-reactions can occur with other spirochetes, including *Borrelia burgdorferi*, *Treponema pallidum*, and *Leptospira* species.

TREATMENT

Treatment of tickborne relapsing fever with a 5- to 10-day course of doxycycline produces prompt clearance of spirochetes and remission of symptoms; doxycycline can be used regardless of patient age. For pregnant women, penicillin and erythromycin are the preferred drugs. Penicillin G procaine or intravenous penicillin G is recommended as initial therapy for people who cannot tolerate oral therapy, although low-dose penicillin G has been associated with a higher frequency of relapse. A Jarisch-Herxheimer reaction (an acute febrile reaction accompanied by headache, myalgia, respiratory distress in some cases, and an aggravated clinical picture lasting <24 hours) is commonly observed during the first few hours after initiating antimicrobial therapy. Because this reaction is sometimes associated with transient hypotension attributable to decreased effective circulating blood volume (especially in louseborne relapsing fever), patients should be hospitalized and monitored closely, particularly during the first 4 hours of treatment. The Jarisch-Herxheimer reaction in children may be milder and can typically be managed with antipyretic agents alone.

Physicians have treated patients infected with *B miyamotoi* successfully with a 2- to 4-week course of doxycycline. Amoxicillin and ceftriaxone have also been used.

For louseborne relapsing fever, single-dose treatment by using doxycycline, penicillin, or erythromycin is effective.

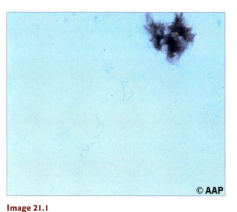

Image 21.1
Borrelia in peripheral blood smear. The spirochetes can be observed with darkfield microscopy and in Wright-, Giemsa-, or acridine orange–stained smears.

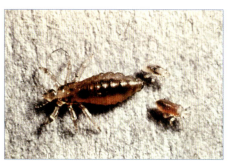

Image 21.2
This image depicts an adult female body louse, *Pediculus humanus*, and 2 larval young. *P humanus* has been shown to serve as a vector for diseases such as typhus, caused by *Rickettsia prowazekii*; trench fever, caused by *Bartonella* (formerly *Rochalimaea*) *quintana*; and relapsing fever, caused by *Borrelia recurrentis*. Courtesy of Centers for Disease Control and Prevention.

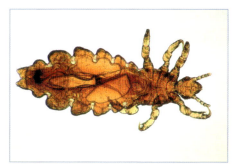

Image 21.3
Dorsal view of a female head louse, *Pediculus humanus capitis*. The body louse, *Pediculus humanus* subspecies *humanus*, is the vector of 3 human pathogens: *Rickettsia prowazekii*, the agent of epidemic typhus; *Borrelia recurrentis*, the agent of relapsing fever; and *Bartonella quintana*, the agent of trench fever, bacillary angiomatosis, endocarditis, chronic bacteremia, and chronic lymphadenopathy. Courtesy of Centers for Disease Control and Prevention.

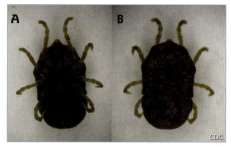

Image 21.4
Ventral (A) and dorsal (B) views of *Ornithodoros tholozani*. Tickborne relapsing fever is transmitted to humans by the *Ornithodoros* species soft ticks and is distributed widely throughout the world. This tick is prevalent in central Asia and the Middle East. Courtesy of Centers for Disease Control and Prevention/*Emerging Infectious Diseases* and Marc Victor Assous.

CHAPTER 22
Brucellosis

CLINICAL MANIFESTATIONS

Onset of brucellosis in children can be acute or insidious. Manifestations are nonspecific and include fever, night sweats, weakness, malaise, anorexia, weight loss, arthralgia, myalgia, back pain, abdominal pain, and headache. Physical findings may include lymphadenopathy, hepatosplenomegaly, and arthritis. Abdominal pain and peripheral arthritis are reported more frequently in children than in adults. Neurological deficits, ocular involvement, epididymo-orchitis, and liver or spleen abscesses are reported. Anemia, leukopenia, thrombocytopenia, or, less frequently, pancytopenia and hemophagocytosis are hematologic findings that might suggest the diagnosis. Serious complications include meningitis, endocarditis, spondylitis, osteomyelitis, and, less frequently, pneumonitis and aortic involvement. A detailed history including travel; exposure to animals; food habits, including ingestion of unpasteurized milk or cheese; and occupation should be obtained if brucellosis is considered. Chronic disease is less common in children than in adults, although the rate of relapse has been found to be similar. Brucellosis in pregnancy is associated with risk of spontaneous abortion, preterm delivery, miscarriage, and intrauterine infection with fetal death.

ETIOLOGY

Brucella bacteria are small, nonmotile, gram-negative coccobacilli. The species that are commonly known to infect humans are *Brucella abortus, Brucella melitensis, Brucella suis,* and, rarely, *Brucella canis.* However, human infections with *Brucella ceti, Brucella pinnipedialis, Brucella inopinata,* and *Brucella neotomae* have also been identified. *B abortus* strain RB51 is a live attenuated cattle vaccine strain that can be shed in milk and can cause infections in humans.

EPIDEMIOLOGY

Brucellosis is a zoonotic disease of wild and domestic animals. It is transmissible to humans by direct or indirect exposure to aborted fetuses or to tissues or fluids of infected animals. Transmission occurs by inoculation through mucous membranes or cuts and abrasions in the skin, inhalation of contaminated aerosols, or ingestion of unpasteurized dairy products. People in occupations such as farming, ranching, and veterinary medicine, as well as abattoir workers, meat inspectors, and laboratory personnel, have increased risk. Clinicians should alert the laboratory if they anticipate that *Brucella* organisms might grow from microbiological specimens, so appropriate laboratory precautions can be taken. In the United States, approximately 100 to 120 cases of brucellosis are reported annually, and 3% to 10% of cases occur in people younger than 19 years. Most pediatric cases reported in the United States result from ingestion of unpasteurized dairy products, commonly acquired from outside the United States. Human-to-human transmission is rare. Mother-to-child transmission is possible by transplacental transmission or via human milk. Other less common modes of transmission include blood transfusion, hematopoietic stem cell transplant, and sexual transmission.

The **incubation period** varies from 5 days to 6 months, but most people become ill within 2 to 4 weeks of exposure.

DIAGNOSTIC TESTS

A definitive diagnosis is established by recovery of *Brucella* species from blood, bone marrow, or other tissue specimens. A variety of media will support growth of *Brucella* species, but the physician should contact laboratory personnel and ask that cultures be incubated for a minimum of 14 days. Newer BACTEC systems have greater reliability and can detect *Brucella* species within 7 days with no need to prolong incubation.

In patients with a clinically compatible illness, serological testing by using the serum agglutination test can confirm the diagnosis with a 4-fold or greater increase in antibody titers between acute and convalescent phase serum specimens collected at least 2 weeks apart. The serum agglutination test, the gold standard test for serological diagnosis, will detect antibodies against *B abortus, B suis,* and *B melitensis* but not *B canis* or *B abortus* strain RB51. Although a single titer is nondiagnostic, most patients with active infection in an area where brucellosis is not endemic will have a titer of 1:160 or greater within 2 to 4 weeks of clinical disease onset. Lower titers may be found early in the course of infection. Enzyme immunoassay (EIA) is a sensitive method for determining total or specific immunoglobulin G (IgG), immunoglobulin A, and immunoglobulin M (IgM) anti–*Brucella* antibody titers. Until better standardization is established, EIA should be used only for evaluation of patients with suspected cases with negative serum agglutination test results or for evaluation of patients with suspected chronic brucellosis, reinfection, or complicated cases.

When interpreting serological results, it is important to take into consideration exposure history, because a serological response for *B canis* and *B abortus* strain RB51 will not be detected by commercially available tests. *Brucella* antibodies also cross-react with antibodies against other gram-negative bacteria, such as *Yersinia enterocolitica* serotype 09, *Francisella tularensis*, *Escherichia coli* O116 and O157, *Salmonella urbana*, *Vibrio cholerae*, *Xanthomonas maltophilia*, and *Afipia clevelandensis*. The timing of exposure and symptom development will assist in determining the classes of antibodies expected. IgM antibodies are produced within the first week, followed by a gradual increase in IgG synthesis. Low IgM titers may persist for months or years after initial infection. Increased concentrations of IgG agglutinins are found in acute infection, chronic infection, and relapse.

If a laboratory is unavailable to perform diagnostic testing for *Brucella* species, the physician should contact the local or state health department for assistance.

TREATMENT

Prolonged antimicrobial therapy is imperative for achieving a cure. Relapses are generally not associated with development of *Brucella* resistance but rather with premature discontinuation of therapy, localized infection, or monotherapy. Because monotherapy is associated with a high rate of relapse, combination therapy is recommended as standard treatment. Most combination regimens include oral doxycycline or trimethoprim-sulfamethoxazole plus rifampin.

Oral doxycycline is the drug of choice and should be administered for a minimum of 6 weeks. Because of this prolonged duration of therapy, doxycycline is not recommended for children younger than 8 years; these children (<8 years) should receive oral trimethoprim-sulfamethoxazole for at least 6 weeks. Rifampin should be added to doxycycline or trimethoprim-sulfamethoxazole. Failure to complete the full 6-week course of therapy may result in relapse.

For treatment of serious infections or complications, including endocarditis, meningitis, spondylitis, and osteomyelitis, a 3-drug regimen should be used, with gentamicin included for the first 7 to 14 days of therapy, in addition to doxycycline (or trimethoprim-sulfamethoxazole, if doxycycline is not used) and rifampin for a minimum of 6 weeks. For life-threatening complications of brucellosis, such as meningitis or endocarditis, the duration of therapy is often extended for 4 to 6 months. Surgical intervention should be considered in patients with complications, such as deep tissue abscesses, endocarditis, mycotic aneurysm, and foreign body infections.

Because of antibiotic resistance with *B abortus* strain RB51, rifampin and penicillin should not be used for treatment of infection caused by this cattle vaccine strain.

The benefit of corticosteroids for people with neurobrucellosis is unproven.

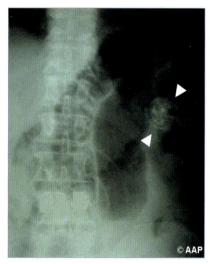

Image 22.1
A calcified *Brucella* granuloma in the spleen of a man with fever of several years' duration. *Brucella* organisms that survive the action of polymorphonuclear leukocytes are ingested by macrophages and become localized in the organs of the reticuloendothelial system.

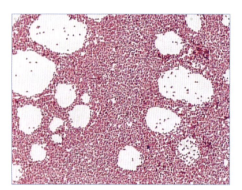

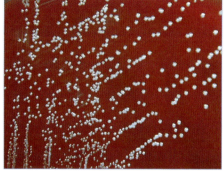

Image 22.2
Brucella species (Gram stain). Typical gram-negative coccobacilli. Courtesy of Robert Jerris, PhD.

Image 22.3
Brucella melitensis colonies. *Brucella* species colony characteristics: fastidious organism and colonies not usually visible at 24 hours. *Brucella* grows slowly on most standard laboratory media (eg, sheep blood, chocolate, and trypticase soy agars). Pinpoint, smooth, translucent, nonhemolytic colonies are shown at 48 hours of incubation. Courtesy of Centers for Disease Control and Prevention.

CHAPTER 23
Burkholderia Infections

CLINICAL MANIFESTATIONS

Species within the *Burkholderia cepacia* complex have been primarily associated with infections in individuals with cystic fibrosis (CF) or chronic granulomatous disease (CGD). Infections have also been reported in people with hemoglobinopathies and malignant neoplasms and in preterm infants. Airway infections of *B cepacia* in people with CF usually occur later in the course of disease, after respiratory epithelial damage and bronchiectasis have occurred. Patients with CF can become chronically infected with little change in the rate of pulmonary decompensation, or they can experience an accelerated decline in pulmonary function or an unexpectedly rapid deterioration in clinical status that results in death. In patients with CGD, pneumonia is the most common manifestation of *B cepacia* complex infection; lymphadenitis also occurs. Disease onset is insidious, with low-grade fever occurring early in the course and systemic effects occurring 3 to 4 weeks later. Pleural effusions are common, and lung abscesses can occur. Health care–associated infections including wound and urinary tract infections and pneumonia have been reported, and clusters of disease have been associated with contaminated pharmaceutical products, including nasal sprays, mouthwash, sublingual probes, prefilled saline flush syringes, and oral docusate sodium.

Burkholderia pseudomallei causes melioidosis. Its geographic range is expanding, and disease is now known to be endemic in Southeast Asia, northern Australia, areas of the Indian Subcontinent, southern China, Hong Kong, Taiwan, several Pacific and Indian Ocean Islands, and some areas of South and Central America. Melioidosis can occur in patients in the United States, usually in travelers returning from areas with endemic disease. Melioidosis can be asymptomatic or can manifest as a localized infection or as fulminant septicemia with or without pneumonia. Approximately 50% of adults with melioidosis are bacteremic on admission to hospital; bacteremia is less common in children. Pneumonia is the most commonly reported clinical manifestation of melioidosis in adults. Localized cutaneous disease is the most common manifestation in immunocompetent children. Genitourinary infections, including prostatic abscesses; septic arthritis and osteomyelitis; and central nervous system involvement, including brain abscesses, also occur. Acute suppurative parotitis is a manifestation that occurs frequently in children in Thailand and Cambodia but is less common in other areas with endemic infection. In severe cutaneous infection, necrotizing fasciitis has been reported. In disseminated infection, hepatic and splenic abscesses can occur, as can disseminated cutaneous abscesses, and relapses are common without prolonged therapy.

ETIOLOGY

The *Burkholderia* genus comprises more than 115 diverse species that are oxidase- and catalase-producing, non–lactose-fermenting, gram-negative bacilli. *B cepacia* complex comprises at least 22 species. Additional members of the complex continue to be identified but are rare human pathogens. Other clinically important species of *Burkholderia* include *B pseudomallei*, *Burkholderia mallei* (the agent responsible for glanders), *Burkholderia gladioli*, *Burkholderia thailandensis*, and *Burkholderia oklahomensis*.

EPIDEMIOLOGY

Burkholderia species are environmentally derived waterborne and soilborne organisms that can survive for prolonged periods in a moist environment. Depending on the species, transmission may occur from other people (person to person), from contact with contaminated fomites, and from exposure to environmental sources. Epidemiological studies of recreational camps and social events attended by people with CF from different geographic areas have documented person-to-person spread of *B cepacia* complex. The source of acquisition of *B cepacia* complex by patients with CGD has not been clearly identified, although environmental sources seem likely. *B cepacia* complex can persist in the environment and spread through lapses in infection control, including indirect contact via environmental surfaces. Health care–associated spread of *B cepacia* complex has been associated with contamination of disinfectant solutions used to clean reusable patient equipment, such as bronchoscopes and pressure transducers, or to disinfect skin. Its intrinsic resistance to preservatives enables it to contaminate many types of aqueous medical and personal care products, leading to large outbreaks. Contaminated mouthwash, liquid docusate sodium, and inhaled medications have been identified as causes of multistate outbreaks of colonization and infection. *B gladioli* is also isolated from sputum of people with CF and may be mistaken for *B cepacia*. *B gladioli* may be associated with transient or more prolonged chronic infection in patients with CF; poor outcomes have been noted in lung transplant recipients who have *B gladioli* infection.

In areas of high endemicity, children may be exposed to *B pseudomallei* early in life, with the highest seroconversion rates occurring between 6 months and 4 years of age. Melioidosis is seasonal in countries with endemic infection, with more than 75% of cases occurring during the rainy season. Disease can be acquired by direct inhalation of aerosolized organisms or dust particles containing organisms, by percutaneous or wound inoculation with contaminated soil or water, or by ingestion of contaminated soil, water, or food. People can also become infected from laboratory exposures when proper techniques and/or proper personal protective equipment guidelines are not followed. Symptomatic infection can occur in children 1 year or younger, with pneumonia and parotitis reported in infants as young as 8 months; in addition, 2 cases of human milk transmission from mothers with mastitis have been reported. Risk factors for melioidosis include frequent contact with soil and water as well as underlying chronic disease, such as diabetes mellitus, renal insufficiency, chronic pulmonary disease, thalassemia, and immunosuppression not related to HIV infection. *B pseudomallei* has also been reported to cause pulmonary infection in people with CF and septicemia in children with CGD.

The **incubation period** for melioidosis is 1 to 21 days, with a median of 9 days, but can be prolonged (years).

DIAGNOSTIC TESTS

Culture is the appropriate method to diagnose *B cepacia* complex infection. In CF airway infection, culture of sputum on selective agar is recommended to decrease the potential for overgrowth by mucoid *Pseudomonas aeruginosa*. Confirmation of identification of *B cepacia* complex species by mass spectrometry or by polymerase chain reaction assay is recommended.

Definitive diagnosis of melioidosis is made by isolation of *B pseudomallei* from blood or other specimens. The likelihood of successfully isolating the organism is increased by culture of sputum, throat, rectum, and ulcer or skin lesion specimens, in addition to blood. Serological testing is inadequate for diagnosis in areas with endemic infection because of high background seropositivity. However, a positive result by the indirect hemagglutination assay for a traveler who has returned from an area with endemic infection may support the diagnosis of melioidosis; definitive diagnosis still requires isolation of *B pseudomallei* from blood or other specimens.

Suspected isolates of *B mallei* and *B pseudomallei* should be referred to local or state public health Laboratory Response Network laboratories. If laboratory personnel are suspected to have been exposed to these pathogens while conducting initial diagnostic testing, occupational exposure in the original clinical laboratory should be reviewed and evaluated.

TREATMENT

Drugs that may have activity against *B cepacia* complex include trimethoprim-sulfamethoxazole, ceftazidime, minocycline, fluoroquinolones, carbapenems, and newer β-lactam/β-lactamase inhibitor combinations. Some experts recommend combinations of antimicrobial agents that provide synergistic activity against *B cepacia* complex in vitro. Most *B cepacia* complex isolates are intrinsically resistant to aminoglycosides and polymyxins and are resistant to many β-lactam agents such as penicillin, ampicillin, carboxypenicillins, and first- and second-generation cephalosporins.

The drugs of choice for initial treatment of melioidosis depend on the type of clinical infection, susceptibility testing, and presence of comorbidities in the patient (eg, diabetes mellitus, liver or renal disease, cancer, hemoglobinopathies, CF). Treatment of severe invasive infection should include meropenem or ceftazidime (rare resistance) for a minimum of 10 to 14 days, with prolonged therapy (>4 weeks) for deep-seated and complicated infections. After acute therapy is completed, oral eradication therapy with trimethoprim-sulfamethoxazole for 3 to 6 months is recommended to reduce recurrence. Amoxicillin-clavulanate is considered a second-line oral agent and may be associated with a higher rate of relapse.

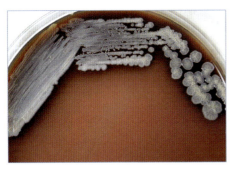

Image 23.1
This photograph depicts the colonial morphological features displayed by gram-negative *Burkholderia pseudomallei* bacteria, which was grown on a medium of chocolate agar, for a 72-hour period, at a temperature of 37 °C (98.6 °F). Courtesy of Centers for Disease Control and Prevention.

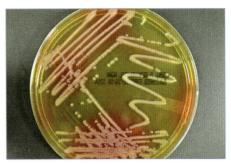

Image 23.2
Burkholderia cepacia on *Burkholderia* selective agar. With vancomycin, gentamicin, and polymyxin B, this agar is used for the isolation of *B cepacia* complex from respiratory secretions of patients with cystic fibrosis. Growth of the organism turns the medium from orange to yellow, and colonies are surrounded by a pink-yellow zone in the medium. Growth may require up to 72 hours of incubation. Courtesy of Julia Rosebush, DO; Robert Jerris, PhD; and Theresa Stanley, M(ASCP).

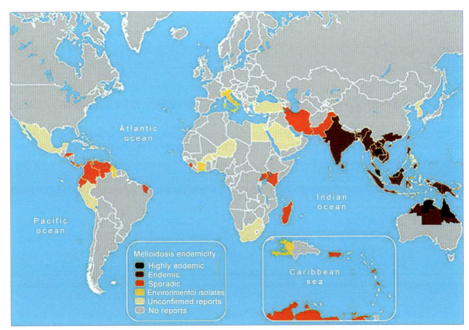

Image 23.3
Endemicity of melioidosis infection. Courtesy of Centers for Disease Control and Prevention.

CHAPTER 24

Campylobacter Infections

CLINICAL MANIFESTATIONS

Predominant symptoms of *Campylobacter* infection include diarrhea, abdominal pain, malaise, and fever. Stools can contain visible or occult blood. In neonates and young infants, bloody diarrhea without fever can be the only manifestation of infection. Pronounced fevers in children can result in febrile seizures that occur before gastrointestinal tract symptoms. Abdominal pain can mimic appendicitis or intussusception. Mild infection lasts 1 or 2 days and resembles viral gastroenteritis. Most patients recover in less than 1 week, but 10% to 20% have a relapse or a prolonged or severe illness. Severe or persistent infection can mimic acute inflammatory bowel disease. Bacteremia is uncommon but can occur in elderly patients and in patients with underlying conditions. Immunocompromised hosts can have prolonged, relapsing, or extraintestinal infections, especially with *Campylobacter fetus* and other *Campylobacter* species. Immunoreactive complications, such as Guillain-Barré syndrome (occurring in 1:1,000), Miller Fisher variant of Guillain-Barré syndrome (ie, ophthalmoplegia, areflexia, ataxia), reactive arthritis (with the classic triad, formerly known as Reiter syndrome, consisting of arthritis, urethritis, and bilateral conjunctivitis), myocarditis, pericarditis, and erythema nodosum, can occur during convalescence.

ETIOLOGY

Campylobacter species are motile, comma-shaped, gram-negative bacilli that cause gastroenteritis. There are 25 species within the genus *Campylobacter*, but *Campylobacter jejuni* and *Campylobacter coli* are the species isolated most commonly from patients with diarrhea. *C fetus* predominantly causes systemic illness in neonates and debilitated hosts. Other *Campylobacter* species, including *Campylobacter upsaliensis*, *Campylobacter lari*, and *Campylobacter hyointestinalis*, can cause similar diarrheal or systemic illnesses in children.

EPIDEMIOLOGY

Campylobacter is associated with an estimated 1.3 million illnesses each year in the United States. Although incidence decreased in the early 2000s, data from the Foodborne Diseases Active Surveillance Network indicate that in recent years, the incidence has increased, and the 2018 incidence of infections with *Campylobacter* was 19.6 infections per 100,000 population. This increased incidence likely resulted from the increased use and sensitivity of culture-independent diagnostic tests (CIDTs). The highest rates of infection occur among children younger than 5 years. Most cases of *Campylobacter* infection are acquired domestically, but it is also a very common cause of laboratory-confirmed diarrhea in returning international travelers. In susceptible people, as few as 500 *Campylobacter* organisms can cause infection.

The gastrointestinal tracts of domestic and wild birds and animals are reservoirs of the bacteria. *C jejuni* and *C coli* have been isolated from feces of 30% to 100% of healthy chickens, turkeys, and waterfowl. Poultry carcasses are commonly contaminated. Many farm animals, pets, and meat sources can harbor the organism and are potential sources of infection. Transmission of *C jejuni* and *C coli* occurs by ingestion of contaminated food or water or by direct contact with fecal material from infected animals or people. Improperly cooked poultry, untreated or contaminated water, and unpasteurized milk have been the main vehicles of transmission. *Campylobacter* infections are usually sporadic; outbreaks are rare but have occurred among school children participants in field trips to dairy farms where they consumed unpasteurized milk and among people who had contact with pet store puppies (**www.cdc.gov/campylobacter/outbreaks/outbreaks.html**). Person-to-person spread occurs occasionally, particularly among very young children, and risk is greatest during the acute phase of illness. Person-to-person transmission has occurred in neonates of infected mothers and has resulted in health care–associated outbreaks in nurseries. In perinatal infection, *C jejuni* and *C coli* usually cause neonatal gastroenteritis, whereas *C fetus* often causes neonatal septicemia or meningitis. Enteritis occurs in people of all ages. Excretion of *Campylobacter* organisms typically lasts 2 to 3 weeks without antimicrobial treatment but can be as long as 7 weeks.

The **incubation period** is usually 2 to 5 days but can be longer.

DIAGNOSTIC TESTS

C jejuni and *C coli* can be recovered from feces, and *Campylobacter* species, including *C fetus*, can be recovered from blood. Isolation of *C jejuni* and *C coli* from stool specimens requires selective media, microaerobic conditions, and an incubation temperature of 42 °C (108 °F). Molecular and antigen CIDTs can provide rapid diagnostic testing; however, these tests will not provide antibiotic susceptibilities. It should be noted that false-positive results from antigen-based tests have been reported, and molecular tests detect bacterial DNA, which may not reflect viable organism; therefore, clinical correlation is advised. Additionally, some of these tests may not distinguish between *C jejuni* and *C coli* and may not detect other *Campylobacter* species. Referral of isolates and CIDT positive specimens to state public health laboratories is based on state regulations. Molecular analysis of isolates is important for national *Campylobacter* surveillance and outbreak monitoring.

TREATMENT

Rehydration is the mainstay of treatment for all children with diarrhea. Most patients do not require antimicrobial therapy. Azithromycin and erythromycin shorten the duration of illness and excretion of susceptible organisms (2% of *C jejuni* isolates are resistant to erythromycin and azithromycin, and 17% of *C coli* are resistant to erythromycin; 18%, to azithromycin) and may prevent relapse when administered early in gastrointestinal tract infection. Treatment with azithromycin (10 mg/kg/day, for 3 days) or erythromycin (40 mg/kg/day, in 4 divided doses, for 5 days) usually eradicates the organism from stool within 2 or 3 days. A fluoroquinolone, such as ciprofloxacin, may be effective, but resistance to ciprofloxacin is common (found in 28% of isolates in 2017 [**www.cdc.gov/DrugResistance/Biggest-Threats.html**]; see also **www.cdc.gov/NARMS**). Resistance to fluoroquinolones is more common in low- to middle-income countries. Antimicrobial susceptibility testing of the isolate or epidemiological data from the location of acquisition can help guide appropriate therapy. If antimicrobial therapy is administered for treatment of gastroenteritis, the recommended duration is 3 to 5 days. *C fetus* is generally susceptible to aminoglycosides, extended-spectrum cephalosporins, meropenem, imipenem, ampicillin, and erythromycin. Antimotility agents are generally not recommended in children because of their limited benefit and reports of adverse outcomes in those who received these agents as monotherapy.

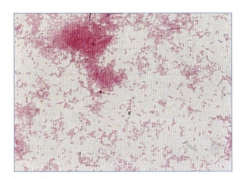

Image 24.1
Campylobacter jejuni (Gram stain) faintly staining short, curved, or spiral-shaped gram-negative rods from a culture of the organism. Courtesy of Robert Jerris, PhD.

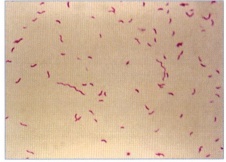

Image 24.2
This image of a Gram-stained specimen shows the spiral rods of *Campylobacter fetus* subspecies *fetus* taken from an 18-hour brain-heart infusion with a 7% addition of rabbit blood agar plate culture. Courtesy of Centers for Disease Control and Prevention.

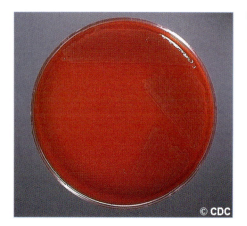

Image 24.3
Blood agar plate culture of *Campylobacter fetus* subspecies *intestinalis*. *C fetus* causes prolonged, relapsing, or extraintestinal illness in hosts with immunocompromise. During convalescence, *C fetus* infections have been associated with immunoreactive complications such as Guillain-Barré syndrome, reactive arthritis, and erythema nodosum. Courtesy of Centers for Disease Control and Prevention.

CHAPTER 25
Candidiasis

CLINICAL MANIFESTATIONS

Mucocutaneous infection results in oropharyngeal (thrush) or vaginal or cervical candidiasis; intertriginous lesions of the gluteal folds, buttocks, neck, groin, and axilla; paronychia; and onychia. Dysfunction of T lymphocytes, other immunologic disorders, and endocrinologic diseases are associated with chronic mucocutaneous candidiasis. Chronic or recurrent oral candidiasis can be the manifesting sign of HIV infection or primary immunodeficiency. Esophageal and laryngeal candidiasis can occur in immunocompromised patients. Disseminated candidiasis has a predilection for extremely preterm neonates and immunocompromised or debilitated hosts, can involve virtually any organ or anatomical site, and can be rapidly fatal. Candidemia can occur with or without associated end-organ disease in patients with indwelling central vascular catheters, especially in patients receiving prolonged intravenous infusions with parenteral alimentation or lipids. Peritonitis can occur in patients undergoing peritoneal dialysis, especially in patients receiving prolonged broad-spectrum antimicrobial therapy. Candiduria can occur in patients with indwelling urinary catheters, focal renal infection, or disseminated disease.

ETIOLOGY

Candida species are yeasts that reproduce by budding. *Candida albicans* and several other species form long chains of elongated yeast forms called *pseudohyphae*. *C albicans* causes most infections, but in some regions and patient populations, non-*albicans Candida* species now account for more than half of invasive infections. Other species, including *Candida tropicalis, Candida parapsilosis, Candida glabrata, Candida krusei, Candida guilliermondii, Candida lusitaniae*, and *Candida dubliniensis*, can cause serious infections, especially in immunocompromised and debilitated hosts. *C parapsilosis* is second only to *C albicans* as a cause of systemic candidiasis in pediatric and neonatal populations. *Candida auris*, a *Candida* species that is often multidrug resistant, is virtually always found in immunocompromised hosts or those requiring high-acuity care. It is generally acquired in health care settings, especially high-acuity postacute care settings such as long-term acute care hospitals and skilled nursing facilities that provide care for patients on ventilators.

EPIDEMIOLOGY

Like other *Candida* species, *C albicans* is present on skin and in the mouth, intestinal tract, and vagina of immunocompetent people. Vulvovaginal candidiasis is associated with pregnancy, and newborns can acquire the organism in utero, during passage through the vagina, or postnatally. Mild mucocutaneous infection is common in healthy infants. Person-to-person transmission occurs rarely for most *Candida* species but is common for *C auris*. Invasive disease typically occurs in those with impaired immunity, with infection usually arising endogenously from colonized sites. Factors such as extreme prematurity, neutropenia, or treatment with corticosteroids or cytotoxic chemotherapy increase the risk of invasive infection. People with diabetes mellitus generally have localized mucocutaneous lesions. People with neutrophil defects, such as chronic granulomatous disease or myeloperoxidase deficiency, have increased risk. People undergoing intravenous alimentation or receiving broad-spectrum antimicrobial agents, especially extended-spectrum cephalosporins, carbapenems, and vancomycin, or requiring long-term indwelling central venous or peritoneal dialysis catheters, have increased susceptibility to infection. Postsurgical patients can have risk, particularly after cardiothoracic or abdominal procedures.

The **incubation period** is unknown.

DIAGNOSTIC TESTS

Presumptive diagnosis of mucocutaneous candidiasis or thrush can usually be made clinically, but other organisms or trauma can cause clinically similar lesions. Yeast cells and pseudohyphae can be found in *C albicans*–infected tissue and are identifiable by microscopic examination of scrapings prepared with Gram, calcofluor white, or fluorescent antibody stains or in a potassium hydroxide suspension, 10% to 20%. Endoscopy is useful for diagnosis of esophagitis. Although ophthalmologic examination can reveal typical retinal lesions attributable to hematogenous dissemination, the yield of routine ophthalmologic evaluation in affected patients is low. Lesions in the brain, kidney, liver, heart, or spleen can be detected by ultrasonography, computed tomography (CT), or magnetic resonance imaging, but these lesions are typically not detected by imaging until late in the course of disease or after neutropenia has resolved.

A definitive diagnosis of invasive candidiasis requires isolation of the organism from a normally sterile body site (eg, blood, cerebrospinal fluid [CSF], bone marrow) or demonstration of organisms in a tissue biopsy specimen. Negative results of culture for *Candida* species do not exclude invasive infection in immunocompromised hosts; in some settings, blood culture is less than 50% sensitive. Special fungal culture media are not needed to grow *Candida* species. A presumptive species identification of *C albicans* can be made by demonstrating germ tube formation, and molecular fluorescence in situ hybridization testing can rapidly distinguish *C albicans* from non-*albicans Candida* species. *C auris* may be misidentified as another *Candida* species. Recovery of the organism is expedited by using automated blood culture systems or a lysis-centrifugation method. Peptide nucleic acid fluorescent in situ hybridization probes cleared by the US Food and Drug Administration and multiplex polymerase chain reaction assays have been developed for rapid detection of *Candida* species directly from positive blood culture bottles.

Patient serum can be tested by using the assay for 1,3-β-D-glucan from fungal cell walls, which does not distinguish *Candida* species from other fungi. Data on use of this assay for children are more limited than for adults, and there are a significant number of false-positive results. The diagnostic cut point for this assay is not well established in children.

Testing for azole susceptibility is recommended for all bloodstream and other clinically relevant *Candida* isolates. Testing for echinocandin susceptibility should be considered in patients who have had prior treatment with an echinocandin and in those who have infection with *C glabrata*, *C parapsilosis*, or *C auris* (confirmed or suspected).

TREATMENT

Mucous Membrane and Skin Infections

Oral candidiasis in immunocompetent hosts is treated with oral nystatin suspension, clotrimazole troches applied to lesions, or miconazole mucoadhesive buccal tablets. Troches should not be used in infants. Fluconazole may be more effective than oral nystatin or clotrimazole troches and may be considered if other treatments fail. Fluconazole can benefit immunocompromised patients with oropharyngeal candidiasis. For fluconazole-refractory disease, itraconazole, voriconazole, posaconazole, amphotericin B deoxycholate oral suspension, or intravenous echinocandins (ie, caspofungin, micafungin) is an alternative.

Esophagitis caused by *Candida* species is generally treated with oral fluconazole. Intravenous fluconazole, an echinocandin, or amphotericin B should be used for patients who cannot tolerate oral therapy. For disease refractory to fluconazole, itraconazole solution, voriconazole, posaconazole, or an echinocandin is recommended. The recommended duration of therapy is 14 to 21 days but depends on severity of illness and patient factors, such as age and degree of immunocompromise. Changing from intravenous to oral therapy with fluconazole is recommended when the patient is able to tolerate oral intake. Suppressive therapy with fluconazole (3 times weekly) is recommended for recurrent infections.

Skin infections are treated with topical nystatin, miconazole, clotrimazole, naftifine, ketoconazole, econazole, or ciclopirox. Nystatin is usually effective and is the least expensive of these drugs.

Vulvovaginal candidiasis is treated effectively with many topical formulations, including clotrimazole or miconazole (available over the counter). Such topically applied azole drugs are more effective than nystatin. Oral azole agents are also effective and should be considered for recurrent or refractory cases. Azole treatment of *C glabrata* vulvovaginal candidiasis is ineffective; nystatin intravaginal suppositories have been effective.

Nipple and ductal breast infections with candidiasis have been described in breastfeeding mothers. Topical treatment as for vulvovaginal candidiasis may be adequate for nipple infection, but systemic treatment with fluconazole is often used in breast infections, with continuation of breastfeeding.

For chronic mucocutaneous candidiasis, fluconazole, itraconazole, and voriconazole are effective drugs. Low-dose amphotericin B administered intravenously is effective in severe cases. Relapses are common with any of these agents once therapy is terminated, and treatment should be viewed as a lifelong process that generally requires intermittent pulses of antifungal agents. Invasive infections in patients with this condition are rare.

For management of asymptomatic candiduria, elimination of predisposing factors, such as indwelling bladder catheters, is strongly recommended. Antifungal treatment is not recommended unless patients have high risk for candidemia, such as neutropenic patients and preterm infants. If candiduria occurs in a preterm infant, evaluation should be performed (blood cultures, CSF evaluation, ophthalmologic examination, brain imaging, and abdominal ultrasonography) and treatment should be initiated. For patients with symptomatic *Candida* cystitis, elimination of predisposing factors, such as indwelling bladder catheters, is strongly recommended, in addition to use of fluconazole for 2 weeks. Repeated bladder irrigations with amphotericin B (50 μg/mL of sterile water) have been used to treat patients with candidal cystitis, but this procedure does not treat disease beyond the bladder and is not recommended routinely. Urinary catheters, if unable to be removed, should be replaced promptly in patients with candidiasis. Echinocandins have poor urinary concentration.

Keratomycosis is treated with corneal baths of voriconazole, 1%, and always in conjunction with systemic therapy. Vision-threatening infections (near the macula or into the vitreous) require intravitreal injection of antifungal agents, usually amphotericin B or voriconazole, with or without vitrectomy, in addition to systemic antifungal agents.

Invasive Disease

General Recommendations

Most *Candida* species are susceptible to amphotericin B, although *C lusitaniae, C auris*, and some strains of *C glabrata* and *C krusei* exhibit decreased susceptibility or resistance. *C auris* is often drug resistant, and echinocandins should be used as initial therapy because most *C auris* strains have been susceptible to echinocandins; susceptibility testing should be performed and patients should be monitored carefully for treatment effectiveness. Investigation for a deep focus of infection should be conducted for all patients with candidemia, regardless of species, when candidemia persists despite appropriate therapy.

C krusei is resistant to fluconazole, and more than 50% of *C glabrata* and approximately 90% of *C auris* isolates can be resistant. Although voriconazole is effective against *C krusei*, it is often ineffective against *C glabrata* and *C auris*. All the echinocandins (caspofungin, micafungin, and anidulafungin) are active in vitro against most *Candida* species and are recommended first-line drugs for *Candida* infections in severely ill or neutropenic patients. Echinocandin resistance is extremely rare in *C parapsilosis*. Removal of infected devices (eg, ventriculostomy drains, shunts, nerve stimulators, prosthetic reconstructive devices) is absolutely necessary in addition to antifungal treatment. Breastfeeding may continue during maternal treatment of candidiasis.

Neonatal Candidiasis

Infants are more likely than older children and adults to have meningitis as a manifestation of candidiasis. Although meningitis can occur in association with candidemia, approximately half of infants with *Candida* meningitis do not have a positive blood culture. Central nervous system (CNS) disease in the infant typically manifests as meningoencephalitis and should be assumed to be present in the infant with candidemia and signs and symptoms of meningoencephalitis, because of the high incidence of this complication. Lumbar puncture, brain imaging, and dilated retinal examination are recommended for all infants with cultures positive for *Candida* in the blood and/or urine. CT or ultrasonography of the genitourinary tract, liver, and spleen should also be performed.

Amphotericin B deoxycholate (first choice for infants), fluconazole (for infants who have not been receiving fluconazole prophylaxis), or an echinocandin (generally reserved for salvage therapy) can be used in infants with systemic candidiasis. Amphotericin B deoxycholate, 1 mg/kg, intravenously, daily, is recommended for initial treatment. Fluconazole, 25 mg/kg loading dose followed by 12 mg/kg daily, may be used for isolates susceptible to fluconazole. Therapy for candidemia without metastatic disease should continue for 2 weeks after documented clearance of *Candida* species from the bloodstream and resolution of signs attributable to candidemia. Therapy for CNS infection is at least 3 weeks and should be continued until all signs, symptoms, and CSF and radiological abnormalities, if present, have resolved. CT or ultrasonography of the genitourinary tract, liver, heart, and spleen should be performed or repeated if blood cultures are persistently positive for *Candida* species.

Lipid formulations of amphotericin B should be used with caution in infants, particularly in infants with urinary tract involvement. Retrospective evidence suggests that treatment of infants with lipid formulations of amphotericin may be associated with worse outcomes than that with amphotericin B deoxycholate or fluconazole. Published reports indicate that lipid-associated amphotericin B preparations have failed to eradicate renal candidiasis, because these large-molecule drugs may not penetrate well into the renal parenchyma. It is unclear whether this is the reason for the inferior outcomes reported with the lipid formulations. Flucytosine is not recommended routinely for infants because of concerns regarding toxicity.

Older Children and Adolescents

In neutropenic or nonneutropenic children and adults, an echinocandin (caspofungin, micafungin, or anidulafungin) is preferred according to guidelines, but fluconazole may be considered in those who not only are considered clinically stable but also are unlikely to have a fluconazole-resistant isolate. Transition from an echinocandin to fluconazole (usually in 5–7 days) is indicated in patients who are clinically stable, have isolates that are susceptible to fluconazole, and have negative blood cultures since initiation of antifungal therapy. Amphotericin B deoxycholate or lipid formulations are alternative therapies. In nonneutropenic patients with candidemia and no metastatic complications, treatment should continue for 2 weeks after documented clearance of *Candida* organisms from the bloodstream and resolution of clinical manifestations associated with candidemia.

In neutropenic patients who are not critically ill, fluconazole is the alternative treatment for patients who have not had recent azole exposure, but voriconazole can be considered when additional mold coverage is desired. Duration of treatment of candidemia without metastatic complications is 2 weeks after documented clearance of *Candida* organisms from the bloodstream and resolution of symptoms attributable to candidemia. Avoidance or reduction of systemic immunosuppression is advised when feasible.

For chronic disseminated candidiasis (hepatosplenic infection), initial therapy with lipid formulation amphotericin B or an echinocandin for several weeks is recommended, followed by oral fluconazole. Discontinuation of therapy is recommended once lesions have resolved on repeated imaging.

Management of Indwelling Catheters

Prompt removal of any infected vascular or peritoneal catheters is strongly recommended, although this recommendation is weaker for neutropenic children, because the source of candidemia in these patients is more likely to be gastrointestinal and it is difficult to determine the relative contribution of the catheter. Immediate replacement of a catheter over a wire in the same catheter site is not recommended.

Additional Assessments

Nonneutropenic patients with candidemia should have a dilated ophthalmologic examination within the first week after diagnosis. In neutropenic patients, dilated fundoscopic examinations should be performed within the first week after counts have recovered, because ophthalmologic findings of choroidal and vitreal infection are minimal until recovery from neutropenia is achieved.

Chemoprophylaxis

Invasive candidiasis in infants is associated with prolonged hospitalization and neurodevelopmental impairment or death in almost 75% of affected infants with extremely low birth weight ($<$1,000 g). The poor outcomes, despite prompt diagnosis and therapy, make prevention of invasive candidiasis in this population desirable. Adherence to optimal infection control practices, including "bundles" for intravascular catheter insertion and maintenance and antimicrobial stewardship, can diminish infection rates and should be optimized before implementation of chemoprophylaxis as standard practice in a neonatal intensive care unit. Fluconazole is the preferred agent for prophylaxis and is recommended for extremely low birth weight infants (<1,000 g) cared for in neonatal intensive care units with high (≥10%) rates of invasive candidiasis. The recommended regimen for extremely low birth weight infants is to initiate fluconazole treatment intravenously during the first 48 to 72 hours after birth at a dose of 6 mg/kg and then to administer it twice a week for 6 weeks. Once infants tolerate enteral feedings, fluconazole oral absorption is good, even in preterm infants. This chemoprophylaxis regimen has not been associated with emergence of fluconazole-resistant *Candida* species in randomized trials.

Fluconazole prophylaxis can decrease the risk of mucosal (eg, oropharyngeal and esophageal) candidiasis in patients with advanced HIV disease. Adults undergoing allogeneic hematopoietic stem cell transplant have significantly fewer *Candida* infections when receiving fluconazole, but limited data are available for children. Micafungin has been used for prophylaxis. Among patients without HIV infection receiving prophylaxis with fluconazole, an increased incidence of infections attributable to *C krusei* (which is intrinsically resistant to fluconazole) has been reported. Prophylaxis should be considered for children undergoing allogenic hematopoietic stem cell transplant and other highly myelosuppressive chemotherapy during the period of neutropenia. Prophylaxis is not recommended routinely for other immunocompromised children, including children with HIV infection.

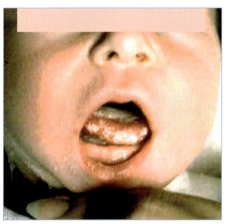

Image 25.1
Candida albicans infection (thrush) in a 1-week-old. Copyright James Brien, DO.

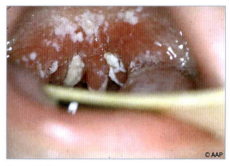

Image 25.2
Candida albicans infection (thrush) of the tonsils and uvula of an otherwise healthy 6-month-old. The white exudate may resemble curds of milk. Courtesy of Edgar O. Ledbetter, MD, FAAP.

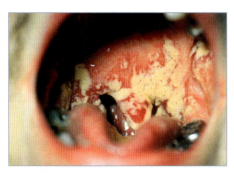

Image 25.3
Oral thrush covering the soft palate and uvula. Courtesy of Centers for Disease Control and Prevention.

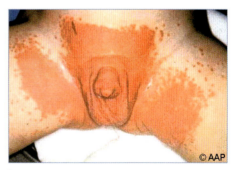

Image 25.4
Candida rash with typical satellite lesions in an infant boy.

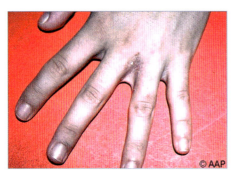

Image 25.5
Intertriginous lesions caused by *Candida albicans*.
Courtesy of James Brien, DO.

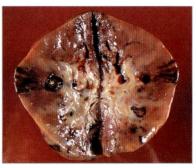

Image 25.6
Disseminated *Candida* infection in a patient with acute lymphocytic leukemia. Hemorrhagic necrotic lesions of the kidney are shown. Courtesy of Dimitris P. Agamanolis, MD.

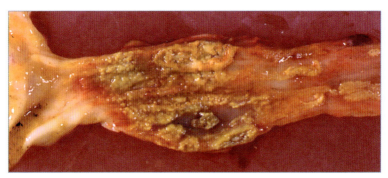

Image 25.7
Candida esophagitis with abscesses and ulceration of the mucosa. Courtesy of Dimitris P. Agamanolis, MD.

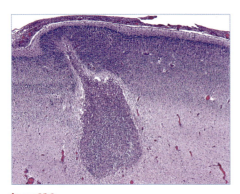

Image 25.8
Disseminated neonatal candidiasis. *Candida* microabscess in the brain. Courtesy of Dimitris P. Agamanolis, MD.

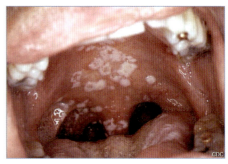

Image 25.9
This patient with HIV/AIDS presented with secondary oral pseudomembranous candidiasis. Courtesy of Centers for Disease Control and Prevention/Sol Silverman Jr, DDS.

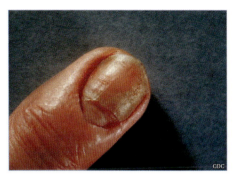

Image 25.10
Candidiasis of the fingernail bed. Courtesy of Centers for Disease Control and Prevention/Sherry Brinkman.

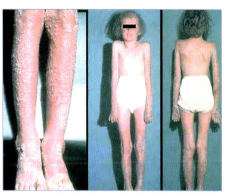

Image 25.11
Chronic mucocutaneous candidiasis in a preadolescent girl with immunodeficiency.

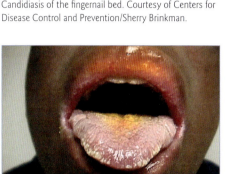

Image 25.12
Candida albicans in a 9-year-old boy with chronic mucocutaneous candidiasis. Courtesy of Benjamin Estrada, MD.

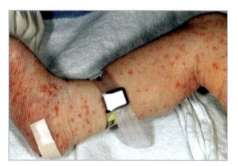

Image 25.13
Congenital candidiasis is characterized by widespread erythematous papules or pustules. Courtesy of Anthony J. Mancini, MD, FAAP.

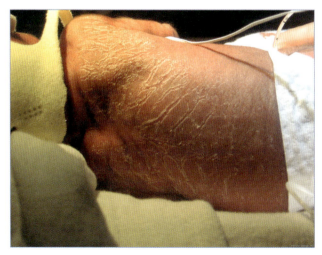

Image 25.14
Neonate with extremely low birth weight (<1,000 g) and congenital cutaneous candidiasis of varying manifestations (results from all skin cultures positive for *Candida albicans*). Courtesy of David Kaufman, MD.

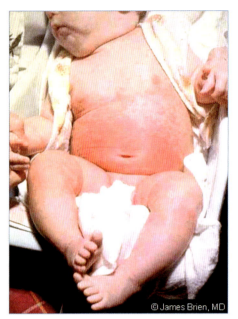

Image 25.15
Cutaneous candidiasis in a 5-week-old. Courtesy of James Brien.

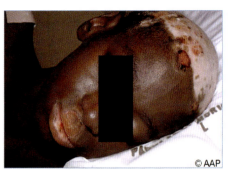

Image 25.16
Chronic mucocutaneous candidiasis in a 15-year-old boy with immunodeficiency. Impaired T-cell function predisposes patients to this infection. Courtesy of David Clark.

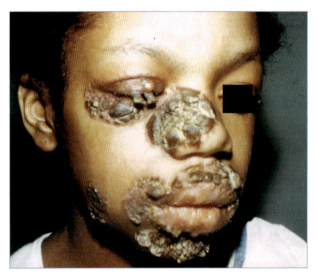

Image 25.17
A 5-year-old boy with immunocompromise and multiple *Candida* granulomatous lesions, a rare response to an invasive cutaneous infection. These crusted, verrucous plaques and hornlike projections require systemic candicidal agents for eradication or palliation. Courtesy of George Nankervis, MD.

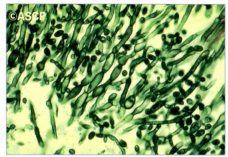

Image 25.18
Histopathologic features of *Candida albicans* infection. Pseudohyphae and true hyphae (methenamine silver stain) found in a tissue biopsy. Copyright American Society for Clinical Pathology.

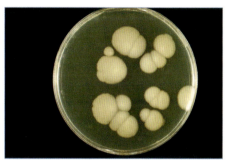

Image 25.19
Sabhi agar plate culture of the fungus *Candida albicans* grown at 20 °C (68 °F). Courtesy of Centers for Disease Control and Prevention.

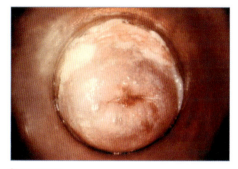

Image 25.20
This girl presented with *Candida* infection of the cervix. *Candida albicans* lives in or on numerous parts of the body as normal flora. However, when an imbalance occurs, such as when antibiotics are administered, *C albicans* can multiply, resulting in a mucosal or skin infection. Courtesy of Centers for Disease Control and Prevention.

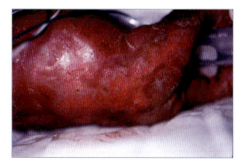

Image 25.21
Photograph of a neonate who has very low birth weight and developed invasive fungal dermatitis of the back caused by *Candida albicans*. This is an uncommon manifestation that is often accompanied by disseminated infection. The diagnosis is established by skin biopsy that reveals invasion of the yeast into the dermis and culture that grows the yeast on routine culture media within 2–4 days. Courtesy of Carol J. Baker, MD, FAAP.

CHAPTER 26
Chancroid and Cutaneous Ulcers

CLINICAL MANIFESTATIONS

Chancroid is an acute ulcerative disease of the genitalia that occurs primarily in sexually active adolescents and adults. A painful genital ulcer and tender suppurative inguinal lymphadenopathy should raise suspicion for chancroid. An ulcer begins as an erythematous papule that becomes pustular and erodes over several days, forming a sharply demarcated, somewhat superficial lesion with a serpiginous border. The base of the ulcer is friable and can be covered with a gray or yellow purulent exudate. Single or multiple ulcers can be present. Unlike a syphilitic chancre, which is painless and indurated, the chancroidal ulcer is often painful and nonindurated and can be associated with painful, inguinal suppurative adenitis (bubo) ipsilateral to the lesion. Without treatment, ulcer(s) can spontaneously resolve, cause extensive erosion of the genitalia, or lead to scarring and, in men, phimosis, a painful inability to retract the foreskin.

In most males, chancroid manifests as a genital ulcer with or without inguinal tenderness; edema of the prepuce is common. In females, most lesions are at the vaginal introitus, and symptoms include dysuria, dyspareunia, and vaginal discharge. Both men and women with anal infection may have pain on defecation or anal bleeding. Constitutional symptoms are unusual.

ETIOLOGY

Chancroid and cutaneous ulcers are caused by *Haemophilus ducreyi*, a gram-negative coccobacillus.

EPIDEMIOLOGY

Chancroid is a sexually transmitted infection (STI). Chancroid is endemic in some parts of Africa and the tropics but is uncommon in the United States, and when it does occur, it is usually imported from areas with endemic infection. Coinfection with syphilis or herpes simplex virus (HSV) occurs in as many as 17% of patients. Chancroid is a well-established cofactor for acquisition and transmission of HIV.

Because sexual contact is the major primary route of transmission in the United States, the diagnosis of chancroid ulcers in infants and young adults, especially in the genital or perineal region, is highly suggestive of sexual abuse. However, *H ducreyi* is recognized as a major cause of non–sexually transmitted cutaneous ulcers in children in tropical regions and, specifically, countries with endemic yaws. The acquisition of a lower extremity ulcer attributable to *H ducreyi* in a child or young adult without genital ulcers and reported travel to a region with endemic yaws should not be considered evidence of sexual abuse.

For both chancroid and cutaneous ulcers, the **incubation period** is 1 to 10 days.

DIAGNOSTIC TESTS

Chancroid is usually diagnosed on the basis of clinical findings (≥1 painful genital ulcers with tender suppurative inguinal adenopathy) and by excluding other genital ulcerative diseases, such as syphilis, HSV infection, or lymphogranuloma venereum. Cutaneous ulcers can be diagnosed on the basis of clinical findings described, but clinical findings overlap, and mixed infections with *H ducreyi* and *Treponema pallidum* subspecies (subsp) *pertenue* are common. Confirmation is made by isolation of *H ducreyi* from an ulcer or lymph node aspirate, although culture sensitivity is less than 80%. Because special culture media and conditions are required for isolation, laboratory personnel should be informed of the suspicion of *H ducreyi*. Approximately 30% to 40% of lymph node aspirates are culture positive. Polymerase chain reaction assays can provide a specific diagnosis but are not widely available.

TREATMENT

Genital strains of *H ducreyi* have been uniformly susceptible only to third-generation cephalosporins, macrolides, and quinolones. Recommended regimens include azithromycin orally in a single dose, ceftriaxone intramuscularly in a single dose, erythromycin orally for 7 days, or ciprofloxacin orally for 3 days. Patients with HIV infection and men who are uncircumcised do not respond as well to treatment and may need repeated or longer courses of therapy. Syndromic management of genital ulcer disease usually includes treatment of syphilis.

Clinical improvement occurs 3 to 7 days after initiation of therapy, and healing is complete in approximately 2 weeks. Adenitis is often slow to resolve and can require needle aspiration or surgical incision. Patients should be reexamined 3 to 7 days after initiating therapy to verify healing. If healing has not begun, the diagnosis may be incorrect or the patient may have an additional STI, both of which necessitate further testing. Slow clinical improvement and relapses can occur after therapy, especially in HIV-infected people. Close clinical follow-up is recommended; re-treatment with the original regimen is usually effective in patients who experience a relapse.

Patients with chancroid should be evaluated for other STIs, including syphilis, HSV infection, chlamydia, gonorrhea, and HIV infection, at the time of diagnosis. All people who had sexual contact with patients with chancroid within 10 days before onset of the patient's symptoms need to be examined and treated, even if they are asymptomatic.

Cutaneous ulcers are treated with single-dose azithromycin (30 mg/kg, maximum 2 g) to cover both *T pallidum* subsp *pertenue* and *H ducreyi*. Cutaneous ulcers attributable to *H ducreyi* respond to single-dose azithromycin within 14 days.

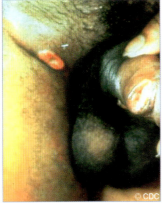

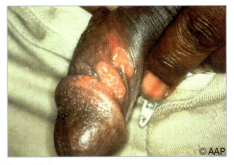

Image 26.2
Haemophilus ducreyi. Chancroid ulcerations of the penis in the same patient as in Image 26.1. Courtesy of Centers for Disease Control and Prevention.

Image 26.1
Penile and inguinal chancroid caused by *Haemophilus ducreyi*, a gram-negative coccobacillus. This sexually transmitted infection is endemic in some areas of the United States and also occurs in discrete outbreaks. Courtesy of Centers for Disease Control and Prevention.

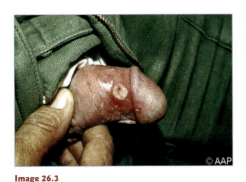

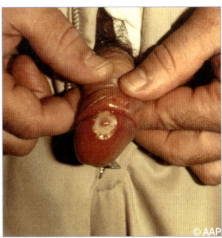

Image 26.3
Ulcerative chancroid lesions with inflammation of the shaft and glans penis caused by *Haemophilus ducreyi*. Chancroid lesions are irregular in shape, painful, and soft (nonindurated) to touch. Courtesy of Hugh Moffet, MD.

Image 26.4
Chancroid ulcer on the glans penis. Coinfection with syphilis or human herpesvirus occurs in as many as 10% of patients. Courtesy of Hugh Moffet, MD.

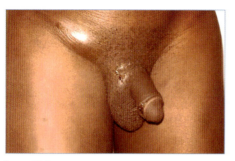

Image 26.5
This adolescent boy presented with a chancroid lesion of the groin and penis affecting the ipsilateral inguinal lymph nodes. First signs of infection typically appear 3–5 days after exposure, although symptoms can take up to 2 weeks to appear. Courtesy of Centers for Disease Control and Prevention.

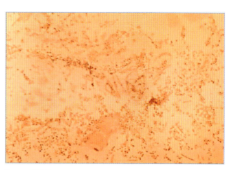

Image 26.6
Haemophilus ducreyi is a gram-negative coccobacillus, as shown in this preparation. Courtesy of Centers for Disease Control and Prevention.

CHAPTER 27

Chikungunya

CLINICAL MANIFESTATIONS

Most people infected with chikungunya virus become symptomatic. The disease is most often characterized by acute onset of high fever (typically >39 °C [102 °F]) and polyarthralgia. Other symptoms may include headache, myalgia, arthritis, conjunctivitis, nausea, vomiting, or maculopapular rash. Fever typically lasts for several days to a week and can be biphasic. Rash usually occurs after onset of fever, can be pruritic, and typically involves the trunk and extremities, but the palms, soles, and face may be affected. Joint symptoms are often severe and debilitating, are usually bilateral and symmetrical, and occur most commonly in the hands and feet but can affect more proximal joints. Clinical laboratory findings can include lymphopenia, thrombocytopenia, elevated creatinine level, and elevated hepatic aminotransferase levels. Acute symptoms typically resolve within 7 to 10 days. Rare complications include meningoencephalitis, myelitis, Guillain-Barré syndrome, cranial nerve palsies, uveitis, retinitis, myocarditis, hepatitis, nephritis, bullous skin lesions, and hemorrhage. In infants, acrocyanosis without hemodynamic instability, symmetrical vesiculobullous lesions, and edema of the lower extremities may occur. People with risk for severe disease include neonates exposed perinatally, older adults (eg, >65 years), and people with underlying medical conditions (eg, hypertension, diabetes, cardiovascular disease, and kidney disease). Some patients might have relapse of rheumatologic symptoms (polyarthralgia, polyarthritis, and tenosynovitis) in the months following acute illness. Studies report variable proportions of patients with persistent joint pains for months to years. Risk factors for chronic arthralgia are age older than 50 years, arthritis during the acute phase, and severe or prolonged initial infection. Mortality is rare.

ETIOLOGY

Chikungunya virus is a single-stranded RNA virus in the *Alphavirus* genus of the *Togaviridae* family.

EPIDEMIOLOGY

Chikungunya virus is primarily transmitted to humans through the bites of infected mosquitoes, predominantly *Aedes aegypti* and *Aedes albopictus*. Humans are the primary host of chikungunya virus during epidemic periods. Once a person has been infected, they are likely to be protected from future infections. Bloodborne transmission is possible; cases have been documented among laboratory personnel handling infected blood and a health care worker drawing blood from an infected patient. Rare in utero transmission has been documented, mostly during the second trimester. Intrapartum transmission has also been documented when the mother was viremic around the time of delivery.

Before 2013, outbreaks of chikungunya infection were reported from countries in Africa, Asia, Europe, and the Indian and Pacific oceans. In 2013, chikungunya virus was found for the first time in the Americas on islands in the Caribbean. The virus then spread rapidly throughout the Americas, with local transmission reported from 44 countries and territories, and more than 1 million suspected cases reported by the end of 2014. Chikungunya virus disease cases were reported in US travelers returning from affected areas in the Americas beginning in 2014, and local transmission was identified in Florida, Puerto Rico, Texas, and the US Virgin Islands. Updated reports of cases in the United States can be found at **www.cdc.gov/chikungunya/geo/index.html**.

The **incubation period** is typically between 3 and 7 days (range, 1–12 days).

DIAGNOSTIC TESTS

Preliminary diagnosis is based on the patient's clinical features, places and dates of travel, and activities. Laboratory diagnosis is generally accomplished by testing serum to detect virus, viral nucleic acid, or virus-specific immunoglobulin M (IgM) and neutralizing antibodies. During the first week after onset of symptoms, chikungunya virus infection can often be diagnosed by performing reverse transcriptase–polymerase chain reaction on serum. Chikungunya virus–specific IgM and neutralizing antibodies normally develop toward the end of the first week of illness. A plaque-reduction neutralization test can be performed to quantitate virus-specific neutralizing antibodies and to discriminate between cross-reacting antibodies (eg, Mayaro and o'nyong nyong viruses). IgM antibodies usually persist for 30 to 90 days, but longer persistence has been documented. Therefore, a positive IgM test result on serum may occasionally reflect a past infection. Immunohistochemical staining can detect specific viral antigen in fixed tissue.

Routine molecular and serological testing for chikungunya virus is performed at commercial laboratories, several state health department laboratories, and Centers for Disease Control and Prevention (CDC) laboratories. Plaque-reduction neutralization tests and immunohistochemical staining are performed at CDC and selected other reference laboratories.

TREATMENT

There is no antiviral treatment available for chikungunya. The primary treatment is supportive care and includes rest, fluids, analgesics, and antipyretics. In areas where dengue is endemic, acetaminophen is the preferred treatment of fever and joint pain until a dengue diagnosis is excluded to reduce the risk of hemorrhagic complications. Patients with persistent joint pain may benefit from the use of nonsteroidal anti-inflammatory drugs, corticosteroids, and physiotherapy.

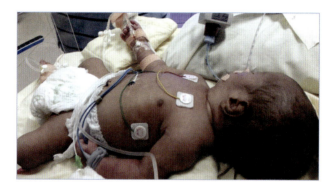

Image 27.1
A newborn with chikungunya. Appearance on day 3 of admission shows hyperpigmentation of the skin. Reprinted with permission from Reddy VS, Jinka DR. A case of neonatal thrombocytopenia and seizures: diagnostic value of hyperpigmentation. *NeoReviews*. 2018;19(8):e502–e506.

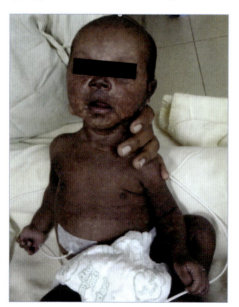

Image 27.2
Generalized hyperpigmentation of chikungunya is shown, with a distinctly prominent pigmentation of the patient's nose. Reprinted with permission from Reddy VS, Jinka DR. A case of neonatal thrombocytopenia and seizures: diagnostic value of hyperpigmentation. *NeoReviews*. 2018;19(8):e502–e506.

CHAPTER 28

Chlamydial Infections
(*Chlamydia pneumoniae*)

CLINICAL MANIFESTATIONS

Patients may be asymptomatic or mildly to moderately ill with a variety of respiratory tract diseases caused by *Chlamydia pneumoniae*, including pneumonia, acute bronchitis, prolonged cough, and, less commonly, pharyngitis, laryngitis, otitis media, and sinusitis. In some patients, a sore throat precedes the onset of cough by a week or more. The clinical course can be biphasic, culminating in atypical pneumonia. *C pneumoniae* can manifest as severe community-acquired pneumonia in immunocompromised hosts and has been associated with onset or acute exacerbation of respiratory symptoms in patients with asthma, cystic fibrosis, and acute chest syndrome in children with sickle cell disease. Rare cases of meningoencephalitis and myocarditis have been attributed to *C pneumoniae*.

Physical examination may reveal nonexudative pharyngitis, pulmonary rales, and bronchospasm. Chest radiography may reveal findings ranging from pleural effusion and bilateral infiltrates to a single patchy subsegmental infiltrate. Illness can be prolonged and cough can persist for 2 to 6 weeks or longer.

ETIOLOGY

C pneumoniae is an obligate intracellular bacterium for which entry into mucosal epithelial cells is necessary for intracellular survival and growth. It exists in both an infectious nonreplicating extracellular form called an *elementary body* and a replicating intracellular form called a *reticulate body*. Reticulate bodies replicate within a protective intracellular membrane-bound vesicle called an *inclusion*.

EPIDEMIOLOGY

C pneumoniae infection is presumed to be transmitted from person to person via infected respiratory tract secretions. It is unknown whether there is an animal reservoir. The disease occurs worldwide but occurs earlier in life in tropical and less developed areas than in industrialized countries in temperate climates. The timing of initial infection peaks between 5 and 15 years of age; however, studies have shown that the prevalence rate of infection among children beyond early infancy is like that among adults. In the United States, approximately 50% of adults have *C pneumoniae*–specific serum antibody by 20 years of age, indicating previous infection by the organism. Recurrent infection is common, especially in adults. Clusters of infection have been reported in groups of children and adults. There is no evidence of seasonality.

The mean **incubation period** is 21 days.

DIAGNOSTIC TESTS

Nucleic acid amplification tests, such as real-time polymerase chain reaction (PCR) assays, are the preferred method for the diagnosis of an acute *C pneumoniae* infection because of their utility for rapid and accurate detection. Multiplex PCR assays have been cleared by the US Food and Drug Administration for the diagnosis of *C pneumoniae* by using nasopharyngeal swab specimens. The tests appear to have high sensitivity and specificity. However, nasopharyngeal shedding can occur for months after acute disease, even with treatment.

Serological testing for *C pneumoniae* is problematic. The microimmunofluorescent antibody test is the most sensitive and specific serological test for acute infection, but it is technically complex and interpretation is subjective. A 4-fold increase in immunoglobulin G (IgG) titer between acute and convalescent sera provides evidence of acute infection. Use of a single IgG titer in diagnosis of acute infection is not recommended, because IgG antibody may not appear until 6 to 8 weeks after onset of illness during primary infection and increases within 1 to 2 weeks with reinfection. In primary infection, IgM antibody appears approximately 2 to 3 weeks after onset of illness, and an IgM titer of 1:16 or greater supports an acute infection. However, caution is advised when interpreting a single IgM antibody titer for diagnosis, because a single result can be either falsely positive because of cross-reactivity with other *Chlamydia* species or falsely negative in reinfection. Early antimicrobial therapy may suppress antibody response. Past exposure is indicated by a stable IgG titer of 1:16 or greater.

C pneumoniae is difficult to culture but can be isolated from swab specimens obtained from the nasopharynx or oropharynx or from sputum, bronchoalveolar lavage, or tissue biopsy specimens. Specimens should be placed into appropriate transport media and stored at 4 °C (39 °F) until inoculation into cell culture; specimens that cannot be processed within 24 hours should be frozen and stored at –70 °C (–94 °F).

TREATMENT

Most respiratory tract infections believed to be caused by *C pneumoniae* are treated empirically. For suspected *C pneumoniae* infections, treatment with macrolides (eg, azithromycin, erythromycin, or clarithromycin) is recommended. Doxycycline can be used for short durations (ie, ≤21 days) without regard to patient age. Tetracycline may be used but should not be administered routinely to children younger than 8 years. Fluoroquinolones (levofloxacin and moxifloxacin) are alternative drugs for patients who are unable to tolerate macrolide antibiotic agents, but these drugs should not be used as first-line treatment. In vitro data suggest that *C pneumoniae* is nonsusceptible to sulfonamides.

Duration of therapy is typically 10 to 14 days for erythromycin, clarithromycin, tetracycline, or doxycycline. With azithromycin, the treatment duration is typically 5 days. Duration of therapy for levofloxacin is 7 to 14 days; for moxifloxacin, 10 days.

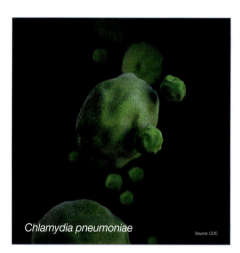

Image 28.1
Three-dimensional computer-generated image of a group of gram-negative *Chlamydia pneumoniae* bacteria. The artistic re-creation was based on scanning electron microscopic imagery. Courtesy of Centers for Disease Control and Prevention.

CHAPTER 29
Chlamydia psittaci
(Psittacosis, Ornithosis, Parrot Fever)

CLINICAL MANIFESTATIONS

Psittacosis (ornithosis) is an acute respiratory tract infection with systemic symptoms and signs that often include fever, nonproductive cough, dyspnea, headache, myalgia, chills, and malaise. Less common symptoms include pharyngitis, diarrhea, constipation, nausea and vomiting, abdominal pain, arthralgia, rash, and altered mental status. Extensive interstitial pneumonia can occur, with radiographic changes characteristically more severe than would be expected from physical examination findings. Rarely, infection with *Chlamydia psittaci* has been reported to affect organ systems other than the respiratory tract, resulting in arthritis, endocarditis, myocarditis, pericarditis, dilated cardiomyopathy, thrombophlebitis, nephritis, hepatitis, cranial nerve palsy (including sensorineural hearing loss), transverse myelitis, meningitis, and encephalitis. Infection in pregnancy may be life threatening to the mother and cause fetal loss.

ETIOLOGY

C psittaci is a gram-negative, obligate intracellular bacterial pathogen that exists in 2 forms. The extracellular form is called an *elementary body* and is infectious. The elementary body enters the epithelial host cell through receptor-mediated endocytosis, then differentiates into a replicating reticulate body within a membrane-bound vesicle called an *inclusion*. Reticulate bodies require host cell nutrients to multiply and later differentiate to produce new elementary bodies that are released from the host cell to infect neighboring cells.

EPIDEMIOLOGY

Birds are the major reservoir of *C psittaci*. The term **psittacosis** is commonly used, although the term **ornithosis** more accurately describes the potential for nearly all domestic and wild birds to spread this infection, not just psittacine birds (eg, parakeets, parrots, macaws, cockatoos). In the United States, a variety of birds including psittacine birds, poultry birds (eg, chickens, ducks, turkeys, pheasants), and pigeons have been reported as sources of human disease. Infected birds, whether they appear healthy or ill, may transmit the organism. Infection is usually acquired by direct contact or inhalation of aerosolized excrement or respiratory secretions from the eyes or beaks of infected birds. Once dry, the organism remains viable for months, particularly at room temperature. Importation and illegal trafficking of exotic birds may be associated with disease in humans, because shipping, crowding, and other stress factors may increase shedding of the organism in birds with latent infection. Handling of plumage and mouth-to-beak contact are the modes of exposure described most frequently, although transmission has been reported through exposure to aviaries, poultry slaughter plants, bird exhibits, and lawn mowing. Excretion of *C psittaci* from birds may be intermittent or continuous for weeks or months. Pet bird owners and breeders, veterinarians, and workers at poultry slaughter plants, poultry farms, and pet shops may have increased risk for infection. Laboratory personnel working with *C psittaci* also have risk. Psittacosis is worldwide in distribution and tends to occur sporadically in any season.

The **incubation period** is usually 5 to 14 days but may be longer.

DIAGNOSTIC TESTS

The diagnosis of *C psittaci* disease has historically been based on clinical manifestation and a positive serological test result from microimmunofluorescence (MIF) with paired sera. Although the MIF test is generally more sensitive and specific than complement fixation tests, MIF still displays cross-reactivity with other *Chlamydia* species in some instances. Because of this, a titer less than 1:128 should be interpreted with caution. Paired acute- and convalescent-phase serum specimens should be obtained at least 2 to 4 weeks apart and sent to the same laboratory to ensure consistency in sample analysis. Treatment with antimicrobial agents may suppress the antibody response, and in such cases, a third serum sample obtained 4 to 6 weeks after the acute-phase sample may be useful in confirming the diagnosis. Although serological testing is more commonly used and available than molecular testing, serological test results can often be ambiguous, subjective in their interpretation, and misleading because of the inherent limitations of this approach.

Nucleic acid amplification tests have been developed that can distinguish *C psittaci* from other chlamydial species. Real-time polymerase chain reaction assays are now available within specialized laboratories (**www.cdc.gov/laboratory/specimen-submission/detail.html?CDCTestCode=CDC-10153**). Because the organism is difficult to recover in culture and because laboratory-acquired cases have been reported, culture is not generally recommended and should be attempted only by experienced personnel in laboratories in which strict containment measures to prevent spread of the organism are used.

TREATMENT

Doxycycline is the drug of choice and can be used for short durations (ie, ≤21 days) without regard to patient age. Erythromycin and azithromycin are alternative agents and are recommended for pregnant women. Therapy should continue for 10 to 14 days after fever abates. Most *C psittaci* infections are responsive to antimicrobial agents within 1 to 2 days. In patients with severe infection, intravenous doxycycline may be considered.

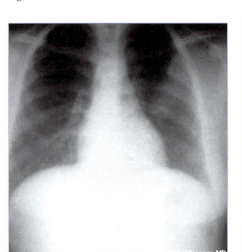

Image 29.1
Chlamydophila psittaci pneumonia in a 16-year-old girl with a cough of 3 weeks' duration. The family had several parrots in the home that were purchased from a roadside stand near the Texas-Mexico border. Interstitial pneumonia, most prominent in the lower lobe of the left lung, is shown. Complement fixation titer for *C psittaci* is 1:128. Copyright David Waagner, MD.

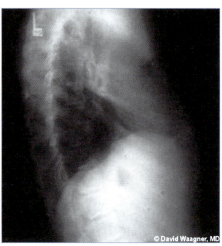

Image 29.2
Lateral chest radiograph of the patient in Image 29.1. Copyright David Waagner, MD.

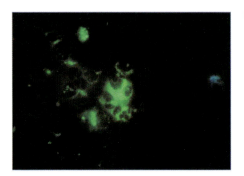

Image 29.3
This mouse-brain impression smear stained with direct fluorescent antibody reveals the presence of the bacterium *Chlamydophila psittaci*. Psittacosis is acquired by inhaling dried secretions from birds infected with *C psittaci*. Although all birds are susceptible, pet birds and poultry are most frequently involved in transmission to humans. Courtesy of Centers for Disease Control and Prevention/Vester Lewis, MD.

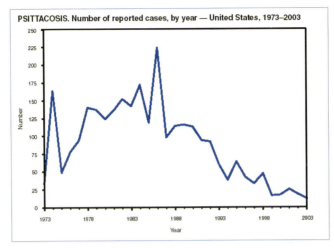

Image 29.4
Number of US cases of psittacosis reported per year, 1973–2003. Courtesy of *Morbidity and Mortality Weekly Report*.

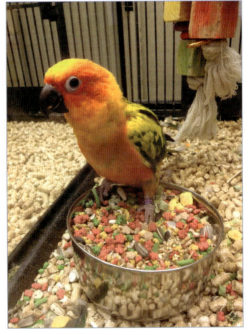

Image 29.5
Chlamydia psittaci is a type of bacteria that often infects birds. These bacteria can infect people and cause psittacosis. Psittacosis can cause mild illness or pneumonia. To help prevent this illness, precautions should be taken when handling and cleaning birds and cages. Courtesy of Centers for Disease Control and Prevention.

CHAPTER 30
Chlamydia trachomatis

CLINICAL MANIFESTATIONS

Chlamydia trachomatis is associated with a range of clinical manifestations, including neonatal conjunctivitis, nasopharyngitis, and pneumonia in young infants as well as genital tract infection, lymphogranuloma venereum (LGV), and trachoma in children, adolescents, and adults.

- **Neonatal chlamydial conjunctivitis** is characterized by ocular congestion, edema, and discharge developing a few days to several weeks after birth and lasting for 1 to 2 weeks and sometimes longer. In contrast to trachoma, scars and pannus formation (vascularization of the normally avascular cornea) are rare.

- **Pneumonia** in young infants is usually an afebrile illness of insidious onset occurring between 2 and 19 weeks after birth. A repetitive staccato cough, tachypnea, and rales in an afebrile 1-month-old infant are characteristic but not always present. Wheezing is uncommon. Hyperinflation usually accompanies infiltrates visualized on chest radiographs. Nasal stuffiness and otitis media may occur. Untreated disease can linger or recur. Severe chlamydial pneumonia has occurred in infants and some immunocompromised adults.

- **Genitourinary tract** manifestations can occur, such as vaginitis in prepubertal females; urethritis, cervicitis, endometritis, salpingitis, and pelvic inflammatory disease, with or without perihepatitis (Fitz-Hugh–Curtis syndrome) in postpubertal females; urethritis and epididymitis in males; and reactive arthritis (with the classic triad, formerly known as Reiter syndrome, consisting of arthritis, urethritis, and bilateral conjunctivitis). Infection can persist for months to years. Reinfection is common.

- **Proctocolitis** may occur in women or men who engage in receptive anal intercourse. Symptoms can resemble those of inflammatory bowel disease, including mucoid or hemorrhagic rectal discharge, constipation, tenesmus, and/or anorectal pain. Stricture or fistula formation can follow severe or inadequately treated infection. Infection is often asymptomatic in females.

- **LGV** is classically an invasive lymphatic infection with an initial ulcerative lesion on the genitalia accompanied by tender, suppurative inguinal and/or femoral lymphadenopathy that is typically unilateral. The ulcerative lesion often resolves by the time the patient seeks care for the adenopathy.

- **Trachoma** is a chronic follicular keratoconjunctivitis with pannus formation that results from repeated and chronic infection. Blindness secondary to extensive local scarring and inflammation occurs in 1% to 15% of people with trachoma.

ETIOLOGY

C trachomatis is an obligate intracellular bacterial agent with at least 15 serological variants (serovars) divided between the following biological variants (biovars): oculogenital (serovars A–K) and LGV (serovars L1–L3). Trachoma is usually caused by serovars A through C, and genital and perinatal infections are caused by serovars B and D through K.

EPIDEMIOLOGY

C trachomatis is the most commonly reported notifiable condition in the United States, with highest rates among sexually active adolescents and young adult women (aged 15–24 years). A significant proportion of female patients are asymptomatic, providing an ongoing reservoir for infection. Among sexually active 14- to 24-year-old females participating in the 2013–2016 cycles of the National Health and Nutrition Examination Survey, the estimated prevalence was 4.3% (5.5% among 14- to 19-year-olds and 3.6% among 20- to 24-year-olds). Among men, infection rates are highest for those 20 to 24 years of age. Among men who have sex with men (MSM) tested for chlamydial infection through the STD Surveillance Network of the Centers for Disease Control and Prevention, 27.8% of those 19 years and younger and 26.1% of 20- to 24-year-olds tested positive for *C trachomatis*. Racial disparities are significant, with higher rates among Black, American Indian/Alaska Native, Native Hawaiian/Other Pacific Islander, and Hispanic populations than among white people.

Oculogenital serovars of *C trachomatis* can be transmitted from the genital tract of infected mothers to their infants during birth. Acquisition occurs in approximately 50% of infants born vaginally to infected mothers and in some infants born by cesarean delivery with membranes intact. For infants who contract *C trachomatis*, the risk of conjunctivitis is 25% to 50% and the risk of pneumonia is 5% to 30%. The nasopharynx is the anatomical site most commonly infected. Asymptomatic infection of the nasopharynx, conjunctivae, vagina, and rectum can be acquired at birth, and cultures from these sites of perinatal infection may remain positive for 2 to 3 years. Infection is not known to be communicable among infants and children. The degree of contagiousness of pulmonary disease is unknown but seems low.

Genital tract infection in adolescents and adults is sexually transmitted. The possibility of sexual abuse should always be considered in prepubertal children beyond infancy who have vaginal, urethral, or rectal chlamydial infection.

LGV biovars are worldwide in distribution but are particularly prevalent in tropical and subtropical areas. Although disease occurs rarely in the United States, reports of outbreaks of LGV proctocolitis have been increasing among MSM. Perinatal transmission is rare. LGV is infectious during active disease. Little is known about the prevalence or duration of asymptomatic carriage.

Although rarely observed in the United States since the 1950s, trachoma is the leading infectious cause of blindness worldwide, causing up to 3% of the world's blindness. Trachoma is transmitted by transfer of ocular discharge and is generally confined to poor populations in resource-limited nations in Africa, the Middle East, Asia, and Latin America; the Pacific Islands; and remote aboriginal communities in Australia.

The **incubation period** of chlamydial illness is variable, depending on the type of infection, but is usually at least 1 week.

DIAGNOSTIC TESTS

Among **postpubertal individuals,** *C trachomatis* nucleic acid amplification tests (NAATs) are the most sensitive tests and are recommended for laboratory diagnosis. NAATs have been cleared for testing vaginal (provider or patient collected), endocervical, male intraurethral, throat, and rectal swabs; male and female first-catch urine specimens placed into appropriate transport devices; and liquid cytology specimens. *C trachomatis* urogenital infections are diagnosed in women by vaginal or cervical swabs or first-catch urine. Patient-collected vaginal swabs are equivalent in sensitivity and specificity to those collected by a clinician by using NAATs. Diagnosis of *C trachomatis* urethral infection in men is made by testing first-catch urine or a urethral swab. Patient collection of a meatal swab for *C trachomatis* testing may be a reasonable approach for men who are either unable to provide urine or prefer to collect their own meatal swab over providing urine. NAATs have been demonstrated to have improved sensitivity and specificity when compared with culture for the detection of *C trachomatis* at rectal and oropharyngeal sites. Data indicate that performance of NAATs on self-collected rectal swabs is comparable to that with clinician-collected rectal swabs. The clinical significance of oropharyngeal *C trachomatis* infection is unclear, and testing in asymptomatic individuals is not recommended.

Specimen collection for diagnosis of **neonatal chlamydial ophthalmia** must contain conjunctival cells, not eye discharge alone. Sensitive and specific methods used for diagnosis include both cell culture and nonculture tests (eg, direct fluorescent antibody [DFA] and NAAT). DFA is the only culture-independent method that is US Food and Drug Administration (FDA) approved for the detection of chlamydia from conjunctival swabs; NAATs are not FDA cleared for the detection of chlamydia from conjunctival swabs.

For diagnosing **infant pneumonia** caused by *C trachomatis,* specimens for chlamydial testing should be collected from the posterior nasopharynx. Isolation of the organism in cell culture is the definitive standard diagnostic test for chlamydial pneumonia. Culture-independent tests (eg, DFA and NAAT) can be used. DFA is the only culture-independent FDA-approved test for the detection of *C trachomatis* from nasopharyngeal specimens. DFA testing of nasopharyngeal specimens has a lower sensitivity and specificity than culture. Tracheal aspirates and lung biopsy specimens, if collected, should be tested for *C trachomatis* by cell culture.

Diagnosis of genitourinary tract chlamydial disease in a child should prompt examination for **other sexually transmitted infections,** including syphilis, gonorrhea, trichomoniasis, HIV infection, hepatitis B virus infection, and hepatitis C virus infection, and investigation of sexual abuse.

Serological testing has little, if any, value in diagnosing uncomplicated genital *C trachomatis* infection. In **children with pneumonia,** an acute microimmunofluorescent serum titer of *C trachomatis*–specific immunoglobulin M of 1:32 or greater is diagnostic.

A definitive **diagnosis of LGV** can be made only with LGV-specific molecular testing. (eg, polymerase chain reaction–based genotyping). Genital or oral lesions, rectal swab, and lymph node specimens (lesion swab or bubo aspirate) can be tested for *C trachomatis* by NAAT or culture. NAAT is the preferred approach to testing because these tests can detect both LGV strains and non-LGV *C trachomatis* strains. Chlamydia serology (complement fixation or microimmunofluorescence) should not be routinely used to diagnose LGV because the diagnostic utility of these serological methods has not been established and interpretation has not been standardized.

Diagnosis of **ocular trachoma** is usually made clinically in countries with endemic infection.

TREATMENT

- **Infants with chlamydial conjunctivitis or pneumonia** are treated with oral erythromycin base or ethylsuccinate (50 mg/kg/day in 4 divided doses daily) for 14 days or with azithromycin (20 mg/kg as a single daily dose) for 3 days. Because the efficacy of erythromycin treatment of either disease is approximately 80%, a second course of therapy might be required. Clinical follow-up of infants treated with either drug is recommended to determine whether initial treatment was effective. A diagnosis of *C trachomatis* infection in an infant should prompt treatment of the mother and her sexual partner(s). Neonates with documented chlamydial infection should be evaluated for possible gonococcal infection. An association between orally administered erythromycin and azithromycin and infantile hypertrophic pyloric stenosis (IHPS) has been reported in infants younger than 6 weeks. Infants treated with either of these antimicrobial agents should be followed up for signs and symptoms of IHPS.

- Infants born to mothers known to have untreated chlamydial infection have high risk for infection; however, prophylactic antimicrobial treatment is not indicated.

- For treatment of **chlamydial infections in infants and children: For children who weigh less than 45 kg,** the recommended regimen is oral erythromycin base or ethylsuccinate, 50 mg/kg/day, divided into 4 doses daily for 14 days. Data are limited on the effectiveness and optimal dose of azithromycin for treatment of chlamydial infections in infants and children who weigh less than 45 kg. **For children who weigh 45 kg or greater but who are younger than 8 years,** the recommended regimen is azithromycin, 1 g, orally, in a single dose. **For children 8 years and older,** the recommended regimen is azithromycin, 1 g, orally, in a single dose, or doxycycline, 100 mg, orally, twice a day for 7 days.

- For uncomplicated ***C trachomatis* anogenital tract infection in adolescents or adults,** oral doxycycline (100 mg, twice daily) for 7 days is recommended. Alternatives include oral azithromycin in a single 1-g dose, or levofloxacin (500 mg orally, once daily) for 7 days. **For pregnant females,** the recommended treatment is azithromycin (1 g, orally, as a single dose), with amoxicillin (500 mg, orally, 3 times/day for 7 days) as an alternative regimen.

Follow-up Testing

Test of cure immediately following treatment is not recommended for **nonpregnant adult or adolescent** patients treated for uncomplicated chlamydial infection unless adherence is in question, symptoms persist, or reinfection is suspected. Reinfection is common after initial infection and treatment, and all infected adolescents and adults should be retested for *C trachomatis* approximately 3 months following initial treatment, regardless of whether patients believe their sexual partners were treated. If retesting at 3 months is not possible, patients should be retested when they next present for health care in the 12 months after initial treatment. Test of cure (preferably by NAAT) is recommended approximately 4 weeks after treatment of **pregnant females.** In addition, all pregnant females who have diagnosed chlamydia should be retested 3 months after treatment.

- For **LGV,** doxycycline (100 mg, orally, twice daily for 21 days) is the preferred treatment. Azithromycin (1 g, once weekly for 3 weeks) and erythromycin (500 mg, orally, 4 times daily for 21 days) are alternative regimens. Because azithromycin has not been rigorously validated, a test of cure with *C trachomatis* NAAT 4 weeks after completion of treatment can be considered.

- Treatment of **trachoma** is azithromycin, orally, as a single dose of 20 mg/kg (maximum dose of 1 g), as recommended by the World Health Organization for all people diagnosed with trachoma as well as for all their household contacts.

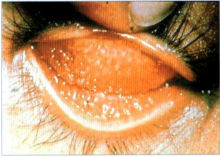

Image 30.1
Conjunctivitis in an infant caused by *Chlamydia trachomatis*. The risk of neonatal conjunctivitis is 25% to 50% for infants of mothers who are infected and untreated. Copyright James Brien, DO.

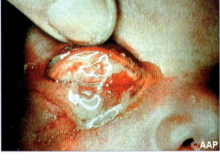

Image 30.2
Conjunctivitis caused by *Chlamydia trachomatis*, the most common cause of ophthalmia neonatorum. This is the same infant as in Image 30.1.

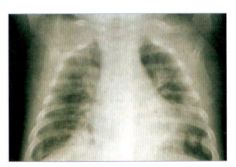

Image 30.3
Chlamydia trachomatis pneumonia, severe and bilateral, in a 5-week-old. Courtesy of Edgar O. Ledbetter, MD, FAAP.

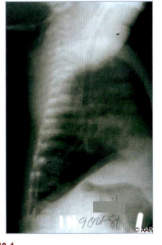

Image 30.4
Left lateral radiograph of the infant in Image 30.3, with *Chlamydia trachomatis* pneumonia. Note the characteristic hyperinflation. Courtesy of Edgar O. Ledbetter, MD, FAAP.

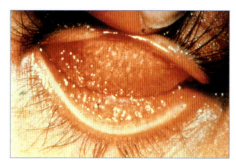

Image 30.5
Chlamydia trachomatis. Copyright James Brien, DO.

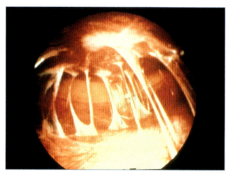

Image 30.6
Chlamydia trachomatis. Copyright James Brien, DO.

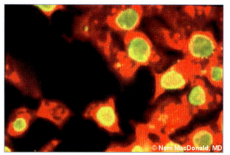

Image 30.7
Infected HeLa cells (fluorescent antibody stain). *Chlamydia trachomatis* is the most common reportable sexually transmitted infection in the United States, with high rates of infection among sexually active adolescents and young adults. Copyright Noni MacDonald, MD.

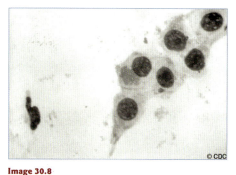

Image 30.8
Photomicrograph of *Chlamydia trachomatis* taken from a urethral scrape (iodine-stained inclusions in McCoy cell line, magnification ×200). Untreated, chlamydia can cause severe, costly reproductive and other health problems, including short- and long-term consequences (eg, pelvic inflammatory disease, infertility, potentially fatal tubal pregnancy). Courtesy of Centers for Disease Control and Prevention.

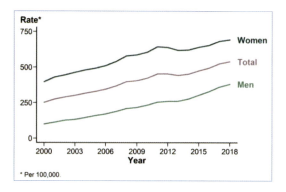

Image 30.9
Rates of reported cases of chlamydia in the United States by sex from 2000–2018. In 2018, a total of 1,758,668 chlamydial infections were reported to the Centers for Disease Control and Prevention in 50 states and the District of Columbia. This case count corresponds to a rate of 539.9 cases per 100,000 population. In 2018, 1,145,063 cases of chlamydia were reported among females for a rate of 692.7 cases per 100,000 females. Among males, 610,447 cases of chlamydia were reported for a rate of 380.6 cases per 100,000 males. Courtesy of Centers for Disease Control and Prevention.

CHAPTER 31
Botulism and Infant Botulism
(*Clostridium botulinum*)

CLINICAL MANIFESTATIONS

Botulism is a neuroparalytic disorder characterized by an acute, afebrile, symmetrical, descending, flaccid paralysis that can progress to respiratory distress or failure. Paralysis is caused by blockade of neurotransmitter release at the voluntary motor and autonomic neuromuscular junctions. Four naturally occurring forms of human botulism exist: infant, foodborne, wound, and adult intestinal colonization. Cases of iatrogenic botulism, which result from injection of excess therapeutic or cosmetic botulinum toxin, have been reported, and botulinum neurotoxins are considered a potential agent of bioterrorism. Symptoms of botulism can occur abruptly, within hours of exposure, or evolve gradually over several days and may include diplopia, dysphagia, dysphonia, and dysarthria. Cranial nerve palsies are followed by symmetrical, descending, flaccid paralysis of somatic musculature in patients who remain fully alert. Infant botulism, which occurs predominantly in infants younger than 6 months (range, 1 day–12 months), is preceded by or begins with constipation and manifests as decreased movement, loss of facial expression, poor feeding, weak cry, diminished gag reflex, ocular palsies, loss of head control, and progressive descending generalized weakness and hypotonia. Some reports suggest that sudden infant death could result from rapidly progressing infant botulism.

ETIOLOGY

Botulism occurs after absorption of botulinum toxin into the circulation from a mucosal or wound surface. At least 7 antigenic toxin types (A–G) of *Clostridium botulinum* are known. An eighth toxin type (H) has been reported, but its identity as a distinct serotype remains controversial. Non-*botulinum* species of *Clostridium* may rarely produce these neurotoxins and cause disease. The most common botulinum toxin serotypes associated with naturally occurring illness are types A, B, E, and, rarely, F. Most cases of infant botulism result from toxin types A and B, but a few cases of types E and F have been caused by *Clostridium butyricum* (type E), *C botulinum* (type E), and *Clostridium baratii* (type F). *C botulinum* spores are ubiquitous in soils and dust worldwide and have been isolated from the home environment and vacuum cleaner dust of infant botulism cases.

EPIDEMIOLOGY

Infant botulism results after ingested spores of *C botulinum* or related neurotoxigenic clostridial species germinate, multiply, and produce botulinum toxin in the large intestine through transient colonization of the intestinal microflora. Cases may occur in breastfed infants before or after the first introduction of nonhuman milk substances; the source of spores is not usually identified. Honey has been identified as an avoidable source of spores. No case of infant botulism has been proven to be from consumption of corn syrup. Rarely, intestinal botulism can occur in older children and adults, usually after intestinal surgery and exposure to antimicrobial agents.

Foodborne botulism results when food that carries spores of *C botulinum* is preserved or stored improperly under anaerobic conditions that permit germination, multiplication, and toxin production. Illness follows ingestion of the food containing preformed botulinum toxin. Home processing of foods is the most common cause of foodborne botulism in the United States, followed by rare outbreaks associated with commercially processed foods, restaurant-associated foods, and wine produced in prisons ("pruno" and "hooch").

Wound botulism results when *C botulinum* contaminates traumatized tissue, germinates, multiplies, and produces toxin. Gross trauma or crush injury can be a predisposing event. In recent years, skin-popping and self-injection of contaminated black tar heroin have been associated with most cases.

Immunity to botulinum toxin does not develop in botulism. Botulism is not transmitted from person to person. The usual **incubation period** for foodborne botulism is 12 to 48 hours (range, 6 hours–10 days). In infant botulism, the **incubation period** is estimated at 3 to 30 days from the time of ingestion of spores. For wound botulism, the **incubation period** is 4 to 14 days from the time of injury until onset of symptoms.

DIAGNOSTIC TESTS

A toxin neutralization bioassay in mice and an in vitro mass spectrometry assay can be used to detect botulinum toxin in serum, stool, enema fluid, gastric aspirate, or suspect foods. Enriched selective media are required to isolate *C botulinum* from stool and foods. The diagnosis of infant botulism is made by demonstrating botulinum toxin in serum or feces or botulinum toxin–producing organisms in feces or enema fluid. Wound botulism is confirmed by demonstrating botulinum toxin–producing organisms in the wound or tissue or toxin in the serum. Foodborne botulism is confirmed by demonstrating botulinum toxin in food, serum, or stool or botulinum toxin–producing organism in stool. To increase the likelihood of diagnosis in foodborne botulism, all suspect foods should be collected, and serum and stool or enema specimens should be obtained from all people with suspected illness. In foodborne cases, the length of time that serum specimens may be positive for toxin varies and, in some cases, can be longer than 10 days after illness onset. Although toxin can be demonstrated in serum in some infants with botulism (13% in one large study), stool is the best specimen for diagnosis; enema effluent can also be useful. Because results of laboratory testing may require several days, treatment with antitoxin should be initiated urgently for all forms of botulism on the basis of clinical suspicion. The most prominent electromyographic finding is an incremental increase of evoked muscle potentials at high-frequency nerve stimulation (20–50 Hz). In addition, a characteristic pattern of brief, small-amplitude, overly abundant motor action potentials may be visible after stimulation of muscle, but its absence does not exclude the diagnosis.

TREATMENT

Meticulous Supportive Care

Meticulous supportive care, in particular respiratory and nutritional support, constitutes a fundamental aspect of therapy in all forms of botulism. Recovery from botulism may take weeks to months.

Antitoxin for Infant Botulism

Human-derived antitoxin should be administered immediately. Human botulism immune globulin for intravenous use (which goes by the brand name BabyBIG) is licensed by the US Food and Drug Administration for treatment of infant botulism caused by *C botulinum* type A or type B. BabyBIG is produced and distributed by the California Department of Public Health (24-hour telephone number: 510/231-7600; **www.infantbotulism.org**). BabyBIG significantly decreases days of mechanical ventilation, days of intensive care unit stay, and total length of hospital stay by almost 1 month and is cost saving. BabyBIG is first-line therapy for naturally occurring infant botulism. Equine-derived heptavalent botulinum antitoxin (BAT; see the next section in this chapter) is available through the Centers for Disease Control and Prevention (CDC). BAT has been used to treat type F infant botulism patients, where the antitoxin is not contained in BabyBIG.

As with other immune globulin intravenous preparations, routine live-virus vaccines should be delayed for 6 months after receipt of BabyBIG because of potential interference with immune responses.

Antitoxin for Noninfant Forms of Botulism

Immediate administration of antitoxin is the key to successful therapy, because antitoxin treatment ends the toxemia and stops further uptake of toxin. However, because botulinum neurotoxin becomes internalized in the nerve ending, administration of antitoxin does not reverse paralysis. If foodborne or other botulism is suspected, the state health department should be contacted immediately to discuss and report the case. BAT is the only botulinum antitoxin released in the United States for treatment of noninfant botulism. BAT contains antitoxins against botulinum toxin types A through G and is provided by the CDC.

Antimicrobial Agents

Antimicrobial therapy is not prescribed in infant botulism unless clearly indicated for a concurrent infection. Aminoglycoside agents can potentiate the paralytic effects of the toxin and should be avoided. Given theoretical concerns of toxin release from antibiotic-induced bacterial cell death, providers should consider delaying the use of antibiotics in wound botulism until after antitoxin is administered, depending on the clinical situation. The role for antimicrobial therapy in the adult intestinal colonization form of botulism, if any, has not been established.

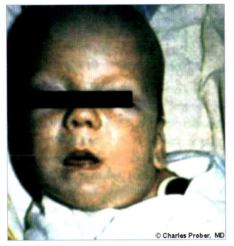

Image 31.1
An infant with mild botulism causing the loss of facial expression. This infant also had a weak cry, poor feeding, diminished gag reflex, and hypotonia. Infant botulism occurs most often in infants <6 months of age. Copyright Charles Prober, MD.

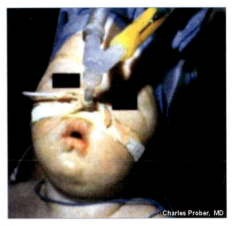

Image 31.2
An infant with severe botulism. This infant required ventilatory support for survival. The source of the toxin producing clostridia was not determined. Copyright Charles Prober, MD.

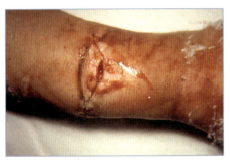

Image 31.3
Wound botulism in the compound fracture of the right arm of a 14-year-old boy. The patient fractured his right ulna and radius and subsequently developed wound botulism. Courtesy of Centers for Disease Control and Prevention.

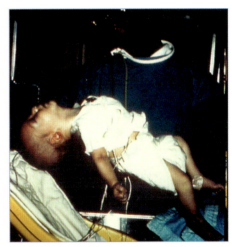

Image 31.4
A 6-week-old with botulism, which is evident as marked loss of muscle tone, especially in the region of the head and neck. Courtesy of Centers for Disease Control and Prevention.

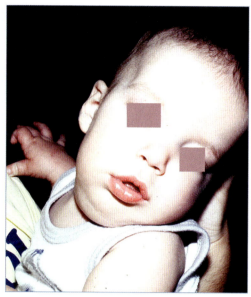

Image 31.5
Infant botulism in a 4-month-old boy with a 6-day history of progressive weakness, constipation, decreased appetite, and weight loss. The infant had been afebrile, was breastfed, and had not received honey. He was intubated within 24 hours of admission and remained ventilated for 26 days. Stool specimens were positive for *Clostridium botulinum* type A. Copyright Larry I. Corman.

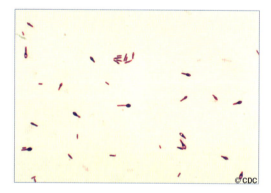

Image 31.6
A photomicrograph of spore forms of *Clostridium botulinum* type A (Gram stain). These *C botulinum* bacteria were cultured in thioglycolate broth for 48 hours at 35 °C (95 °F). The bacterium *C botulinum* produces a nerve toxin that causes the rare but serious paralytic illness botulism. Courtesy of Centers for Disease Control and Prevention.

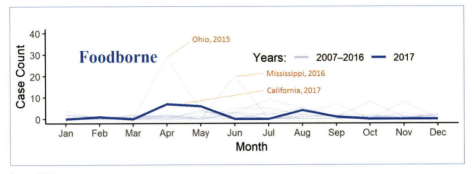

Image 31.7
Confirmed foodborne botulism cases by month of onset—United States, 2007–2017. Courtesy of Centers for Disease Control and Prevention.

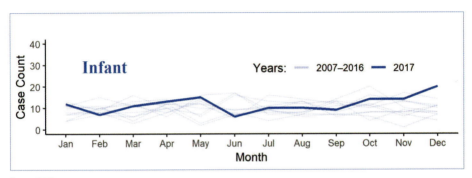

Image 31.8
Confirmed infant botulism cases by month of onset—United States, 2007–2017. Courtesy of Centers for Disease Control and Prevention.

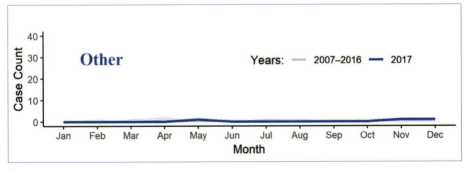

Image 31.9
Confirmed other botulism cases by month of onset—United States, 2007–2017. Courtesy of Centers for Disease Control and Prevention.

CHAPTER 32

Clostridial Myonecrosis
(Gas Gangrene)

CLINICAL MANIFESTATIONS

Disease onset is heralded by acute and progressive pain at the site of the wound, followed by edema, increasing exquisite tenderness, and exudate. Systemic findings initially include tachycardia disproportionate to the degree of fever, pallor, and diaphoresis. Crepitus is suggestive but not pathognomonic of *Clostridium* infection and is not always present. Tense bullae containing thin, serosanguineous or dark fluid develop in the overlying skin, and areas of green-black cutaneous necrosis appear. Fluid in the bullae has a foul odor. Disease can progress rapidly with development of hypotension, renal failure, and alterations in mental status. Diagnosis is based on clinical manifestations, including the characteristic appearance of necrotic muscle at surgery. Untreated clostridial myonecrosis, also known as gas gangrene, can lead to disseminated myonecrosis, suppurative visceral infection, septicemia, and death within hours.

Nontraumatic gas gangrene is usually caused by *Clostridium septicum* and is a complication of bacteremia, which results from an occult gastrointestinal mucosal lesion (most commonly colon cancer) or a complication of neutropenic colitis, leukemia, or diabetes mellitus.

ETIOLOGY

Clostridial myonecrosis is caused by *Clostridium* species, most often *Clostridium perfringens*. Other *Clostridium* species (eg, *Clostridium sordellii, C septicum, Clostridium novyi*) have also been associated with myonecrosis. These organisms are large, gram-positive, spore-forming, anaerobic bacilli with blunt ends. Disease manifestations are caused by potent clostridial exotoxins. Mixed infection with other gram-positive and gram-negative bacteria is common.

EPIDEMIOLOGY

Clostridial myonecrosis usually results from contamination of deep open wounds. The sources of *Clostridium* species are soil, contaminated foreign bodies, and human and animal feces. Dirty surgical or traumatic wounds, particularly those with retained foreign bodies or significant amounts of devitalized tissue, predispose to disease. Cases have occurred in people who inject drugs, in association with contaminated black tar heroin. Rarely, nontraumatic gas gangrene occurs in immunocompromised people, most frequently in those with underlying malignancy, neutrophil dysfunction, or diseases associated with bowel ischemia.

The **incubation period** from the time of injury is 6 hours to 4 days.

DIAGNOSTIC TESTS

Anaerobic cultures of wound exudate, involved soft tissue and muscle, and blood should be performed. MALDI-TOF (matrix-assisted laser desorption/ionization–time-of-flight) devices have an approved indication from the US Food and Drug Administration to identify *C perfringens*. Because *Clostridium* species are ubiquitous, their recovery from a wound is nondiagnostic unless typical clinical manifestations are present. A Gram-stained smear of wound discharge demonstrating characteristic gram-positive bacilli and few, if any, polymorphonuclear leukocytes suggests clostridial infection. Tissue specimens (not swab specimens) for anaerobic culture must be obtained to confirm the diagnosis. Because some pathogenic *Clostridium* species are exquisitely sensitive to oxygen, care should be taken during the collection and processing of a sample to optimize anaerobic growth conditions. A radiograph of the affected site might demonstrate gas in the tissue, but this is a nonspecific finding that is not always present. Occasionally, blood cultures are positive and are considered diagnostic.

TREATMENT

- Prompt and complete surgical excision of necrotic tissue and removal of foreign material are essential. Repeated surgical debridement may be required to ensure complete removal of all infected tissue. Vacuum-assisted wound closure can be used following multiple debridements.

- Management of shock, fluid and electrolyte imbalance, hemolytic anemia, and other complications is crucial.

- High-dose penicillin G should be administered intravenously. Clindamycin, metronidazole, meropenem, ertapenem, and chloramphenicol can be considered as alternative drugs for patients with a serious penicillin allergy or for treatment of polymicrobial infections. The combination of penicillin G and clindamycin may be superior to penicillin alone because of the theoretical benefit of clindamycin inhibiting toxin synthesis.

- Hyperbaric oxygen may be beneficial, but efficacy data from adequately controlled clinical studies are unavailable.

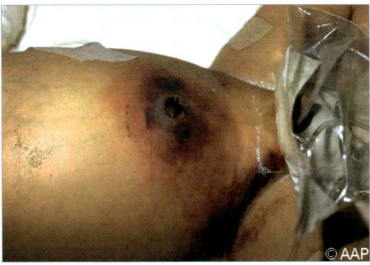

Image 32.1
Clostridial omphalitis in an infant with myonecrosis of the abdominal wall (periumbilical). Early and complete surgical excision of necrotic tissue and careful management of shock, fluid balance, and other complications are crucial for survival.

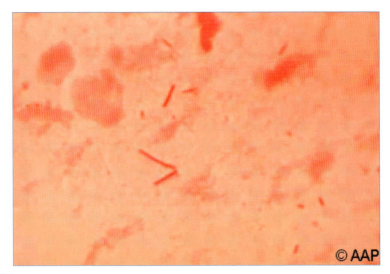

Image 32.2
Gram stain of a tissue aspirate from a patient with clostridial omphalitis showing the characteristic morphological features of *Clostridia* bacilli, erroneously stained gram negative, and sparse polymorphonuclear leukocytes.

CHAPTER 33
Clostridioides difficile (formerly Clostridium difficile)

CLINICAL MANIFESTATIONS

Clostridioides difficile (formerly Clostridium difficile) is associated with a spectrum of gastrointestinal illness as well as with asymptomatic colonization that is common, especially in young infants. Mild to moderate illness is characterized by watery diarrhea, low-grade fever, and abdominal pain. Symptoms may occur in hospitalized and nonhospitalized children. Pseudomembranous colitis is characterized by diarrhea with mucus in feces, abdominal cramps and pain, fever, and systemic toxicity. Toxic megacolon (acute dilatation of the colon) should be considered in children who develop marked abdominal tenderness and distension with minimal diarrhea and may be associated with hemodynamic instability. Other complications of C difficile disease include intestinal perforation, hypotension, shock, and death. Complicated infections are less common in children than adults. Severe or fatal disease is more likely to occur in neutropenic children with leukemia, infants with Hirschsprung disease, and patients with inflammatory bowel disease. Extraintestinal manifestations of C difficile infection are uncommon but can include bacteremia, wound infections, and reactive arthritis. Clinical illness attributable to C difficile is considered very rare in children younger than 12 months. In infants, C difficile should not be considered until other infectious and noninfectious causes of diarrhea have been excluded.

ETIOLOGY

C difficile is a spore-forming, obligate anaerobic, gram-positive bacillus. Some strains produce exotoxins (toxins A and B), which are responsible for the clinical manifestations of disease when there is overgrowth of C difficile in the intestine.

EPIDEMIOLOGY

C difficile is shed in feces. People can acquire infection from the stool of other colonized or infected people through the fecal-oral route. Any surface (including hands), device, or material that has become contaminated with feces may also transmit C difficile spores. Hospitals, nursing homes, and child care facilities are major reservoirs for C difficile. Risk factors for acquisition of the bacterium include prolonged hospitalization and exposure to an infected person in the hospital or in the community. Risk factors for C difficile disease include antimicrobial therapy, repeated enemas, proton pump inhibitor therapy, prolonged nasogastric tube placement, gastrostomy and jejunostomy tube placement, underlying bowel disease, gastrointestinal tract surgery, renal insufficiency, and immunocompromised state. C difficile colitis has been associated with exposure to almost every antimicrobial agent; cephalosporins and fluoroquinolones are considered the highest-risk antibiotic agents, particularly for recurrent C difficile disease and infections with epidemic strains. The ribotype 027 (formerly known as NAP-1) strain is a virulent strain of C difficile because of increased toxin production and is associated with an increased risk of severe disease. Ribotype 027 strains of C difficile have emerged as a cause of outbreaks among adults and are reported sporadically in children.

Recent data suggest that the incidence of pediatric community-associated C difficile disease may be twice as frequent as that of health care–associated disease.

Asymptomatic intestinal colonization with C difficile (including toxin-producing strains) is common in children younger than 2 years and is most common in infants younger than 1 year (up to 50%). The rate of asymptomatic colonization with C difficile in hospitalized adults is upward of 26%.

The **incubation period** is unknown; colitis usually develops 5 to 10 days after initiation of antimicrobial therapy but can occur on the first day of treatment and up to 10 weeks after therapy cessation.

DIAGNOSTIC TESTS

Endoscopic findings of pseudomembranes (2- to 5-mm yellowish raised plaques) and hyperemic, friable rectal mucosa suggesting pseudomembranous colitis are highly correlated with C difficile disease. More commonly, the diagnosis of C difficile disease is based on laboratory methods including the detection of C difficile toxin(s) or toxin gene(s) in a diarrheal stool specimen. In general, laboratory tests for *C difficile* should not be ordered for a patient who is passing formed stools unless ileus or toxic megacolon is suspected. There is presently no generally agreed on gold standard laboratory test method for the diagnosis of *C difficile* disease.

Molecular assays via nucleic acid amplification tests (NAATs) are commonly used for toxigenic strains of *C difficile*. NAATs detect genes responsible for the production of toxins A and B, rather than free toxins A and B in the stool, which are detected by enzyme immunoassay (EIA). EIAs are rapid, performed easily, and highly specific for diagnosis of *C difficile* disease, but their sensitivity is relatively low. The cell culture cytotoxicity assay, which also tests for toxin in stool, is more sensitive than the EIA but is labor intensive and has a long turnaround time, limiting its usefulness in the clinical setting.

NAATs combine excellent sensitivity and analytic specificity and provide results to clinicians in times comparable to those of EIAs. However, detecting toxin gene(s) in patients who are colonized only with *C difficile* is common and likely contributes to misdiagnosis of *C difficile* disease in children with other causes of diarrhea. Several steps can be taken to reduce the likelihood of misdiagnosis of *C difficile* disease related to use of highly sensitive NAATs. Age should be considered, because colonization with *C difficile* in infants is common and symptomatic infection in this age-group is not believed to occur; therefore, *C difficile* diagnostic testing on samples from children younger than 12 months is discouraged. Likewise, testing should not be performed routinely in toddlers with diarrhea who are 1 to 2 years of age unless other infectious or noninfectious causes have been excluded. For children older than 2 years, testing is recommended if there is new onset of prolonged and worsening diarrhea and risk factors (eg, inflammatory bowel disease, immunocompromising condition) or recent course of antibiotics or health care exposures. Because shedding of *C difficile* in the stool can persist for several months after treatment and symptom resolution and because sensitivity of NAAT testing is nearly 100%, tests of cure are discouraged.

A 2- or 3-stage approach increases the positive predictive value versus 1-stage testing. Multistep algorithms have been suggested by the Infectious Diseases Society of America guidelines that incorporate testing for stool toxin (EIA); testing for glutamate dehydrogenase (GDH), an enzyme expressed by both toxigenic and nontoxigenic strains of *C difficile;* and NAAT depending on whether the laboratory has a policy with screening symptoms incorporated. For such a policy, the testing could include NAAT alone or EIA as part of a multistep algorithm (GDH plus EIA, GDH plus EIA arbitrated by NAAT, or NAAT plus toxin). If a screening policy is not incorporated, the testing would include EIA as part of a multistep algorithm as outlined above (and not NAAT alone).

TREATMENT

A central tenet to control *C difficile* disease is the discontinuation of precipitating antimicrobial therapy. Stopping these agents will allow competing gut flora to reemerge and, thus, crowd out *C difficile* within the intestine. A variety of therapies are available; use of a particular treatment modality is dependent on severity of illness, the number of recurrences of infection, tolerability of adverse effects, and cost. Recommended therapies for first occurrence, first recurrence, and second recurrence are provided in Table 33.1. Drugs that decrease intestinal motility should not be administered. Asymptomatic patients should not be treated.

To reduce costs, some experts recommend oral administration of the intravenous formulation of vancomycin. Intravenously administered vancomycin is ineffective for *C difficile* disease.

Fidaxomicin is approved for treatment of *C difficile*–associated diarrhea in adults and children 6 months and older. Studies have demonstrated equivalent efficacy to oral vancomycin, although participants with life-threatening and fulminant infection, hypotension, septic shock, peritoneal signs, significant dehydration, or toxic megacolon were excluded. No comparative data of fidaxomicin to metronidazole are available.

Up to 20% of patients experience a recurrence after discontinuing therapy, but infection usually responds to a second course of the same

Table 33.1
Treatments for *Clostridioides difficile* Disease

Severity	Recommendation
First Occurrence	
Mild-moderate	Metronidazole, 30 mg/kg/day, orally, every 6 h (preferred), or IV, every 6 h for 10 days (maximum 500 mg/dose)
	If failure to respond in 5–7 days: Consider switch to vancomycin, 40 mg/kg/day, orally, every 6 h for 10 days (maximum 125 mg/dose).
	For pregnant/breastfeeding or metronidazole-intolerant patients: Vancomycin, 40 mg/kg/day, orally, every 6 h for 10 days (maximum 125 mg/dose)
	In patients whose oral therapy cannot reach the colon: To above regimen, **ADD** vancomycin, 500 mg/100 mL normal saline enema, as needed every 8 h until improvement.
Severe[a]	Vancomycin, 40 mg/kg/day, orally, every 6 h for 10 days (maximum 125 mg/dose)
Severe and complicated[b]	If no abdominal distension (use both for 10 days): Vancomycin, 40 mg/kg/day, orally, every 6 h (maximum 125 mg/dose) **PLUS** metronidazole, 30 mg/kg/day, IV, every 6 h (maximum 500 mg/dose)
	If complicated with ileus or toxic colitis and/or significant abdominal distension (use all for 10 days): Vancomycin, 40 mg/kg/day, orally, every 6 h (maximum 500 mg/dose) **PLUS** metronidazole, 30 mg/kg/day, IV, every 6 h (maximum 500 mg/dose) **PLUS** vancomycin, 500 mg/100 mL normal saline enema, as needed every 8 h until improvement
First Recurrence	
Mild-moderate	Same regimen as for first occurrence (See above.)
Severe	Vancomycin, 40 mg/kg/day, orally, every 6 h (maximum 125 mg/dose)
Second Recurrence	
All	DO NOT USE METRONIDAZOLE.
	Vancomycin, orally, as pulsed or prolonged tapered dose (See text for options.)

IV indicates intravenously.
[a] Severe: not well-defined in children but should be considered in the presence of leukocytosis, leukopenia, or worsening renal function.
[b] Severe and complicated: intensive care unit admission, hypotension or shock, pseudomembranous colitis by endoscopy, ileus, toxic megacolon.

treatment. Metronidazole should not be used for treatment of a second recurrence or for prolonged therapy, because neurotoxicity is possible. A variety of tapered or pulsed regimens of vancomycin have been used to treat recurrent disease, including the following regimens:

- Vancomycin, orally, 10 mg/kg/dose (maximum 125 mg/dose), 4 times a day for 7 days, then 3 times a day for 7 days, then twice a day for 7 days, then once daily for 7 days, then once every other day for 7 days, then every 72 hours for 7 days

- Vancomycin, orally, 10 mg/kg/dose (maximum 125 mg/dose), 4 times a day for 14 days, then twice a day for 7 to 14 days, then once daily for 7 to 14 days, then every 2 to 3 days for 2 to 8 weeks

- Vancomycin, orally, 10 mg/kg/dose (maximum 125 mg/dose), 4 times a day for 14 days, then either

  ○ Rifaximin, orally, 400 mg, 3 times a day for 14 days (Note that rifaximin dosing in pediatric patients is not well described; it is poorly water soluble and minimally absorbed and should be avoided if the patient has recently received rifaximin for C difficile disease or another indication.)

OR

- Nitazoxanide, orally, 100 mg, twice a day (1–3 years of age), 200 mg, twice a day (4–11 years of age), or 500 mg, twice a day (≥12 years of age) for 10 days

Fecal transplant (intestinal microbiota transplant) appears to be effective in adults, but there are limited data in pediatrics. No pediatric data are available evaluating use of human monoclonal antibodies (against toxins A and B). Cholestyramine is not recommended. Other potential adjunctive therapies of unclear efficacy include immune globulin therapy and probiotics (particularly *Saccharomyces boulardii* and kefir).

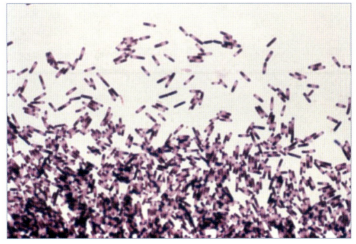

Image 33.1
Clostridioides difficile (formerly *Clostridium difficile*) is a gram-positive, spore-forming bacteria that can be part of the normal intestinal flora in as many as 50% of children <2 years of age. It is a cause of pseudomembranous enterocolitis and antibiotic-associated diarrhea in older children and adults. Courtesy of *AAP News*.

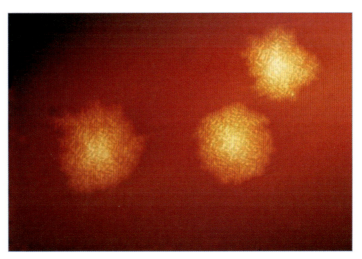

Image 33.2
This photograph depicts *Clostridioides difficile* (formerly *Clostridium difficile*) colonies after 48 hours' growth on a blood agar plate (magnification ×4.8). Courtesy of Centers for Disease Control and Prevention.

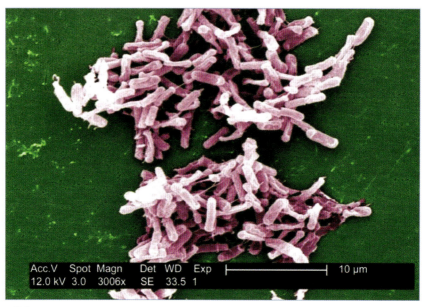

Image 33.3
This micrograph depicts gram-positive *Clostridioides difficile* (formerly *Clostridium difficile*) from a stool sample culture obtained with a 0.1-µm filter. People can become infected if they touch items or surfaces that are contaminated with *C difficile* spores and then touch their mouths or mucous membranes. Health care workers can spread the bacteria to other patients or contaminate surfaces through hand contact. Courtesy of Centers for Disease Control and Prevention/Lois S. Wiggs.

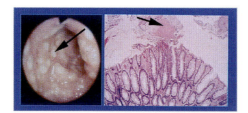

Image 33.4
The right-hand panel shows the typical pseudomembranes of *Clostridioides difficile* (formerly *Clostridium difficile*) colitis; the left-hand panel shows the histological features, with the pseudomembrane structure at the top middle (arrows). Courtesy of Carol J. Baker, MD, FAAP.

CHAPTER 34
Clostridium perfringens Foodborne Illness

CLINICAL MANIFESTATIONS

Clostridium perfringens foodborne illness is characterized by a sudden onset of watery diarrhea and moderate to severe crampy, midepigastric pain. Symptoms usually resolve within 24 hours. The shorter incubation period, shorter duration of illness, and absence of fever in most patients differentiates C perfringens foodborne disease from shigellosis and salmonellosis. C perfringens foodborne illness is infrequently associated with vomiting. Diarrheal illness caused by Bacillus cereus diarrheal enterotoxins can be indistinguishable from that caused by C perfringens. Necrotizing colitis and death have been described in patients with disease attributable to type A C perfringens who received antidiarrheal medications resulting in constipation. Enteritis necroticans (also known as pigbel) results from hemorrhagic necrosis of the midgut and causes severe illness and death attributable to C perfringens infection caused by contamination with Clostridium strains carrying a beta toxin. Rare cases have been reported in the highlands of Papua New Guinea and in Thailand; protein malnutrition is an important risk factor. Additionally, enteritis necroticans has been reported in a child with poorly controlled diabetes in the United States who consumed chitterlings (pig intestine).

ETIOLOGY

Typical infection is caused by a heat-labile C perfringens enterotoxin, produced during sporulation in the small intestine. C perfringens type F (formerly cpe-positive type A), which produces alpha toxin and enterotoxin, commonly causes foodborne illness. Enteritis necroticans is caused by C perfringens type C, which produces a beta toxin that causes necrotizing small-bowel inflammation.

EPIDEMIOLOGY

C perfringens is a gram-positive, spore-forming bacillus that is ubiquitous in the environment and the intestinal tracts of humans and animals and is commonly present in raw meat and poultry. Spores of C perfringens that survive cooking can germinate and multiply rapidly during slow cooling, in storage at temperatures from 20 to 60 °C (68–140 °F), and during inadequate reheating. At an optimum temperature, C perfringens has one of the fastest rates of growth of any bacterium. Illness results from consumption of food containing high numbers of vegetative organisms ($>10^5$ colony-forming units [CFUs]/g) that produce enterotoxin in the intestine of the consumer.

Ingestion of the organism is most commonly associated with foods prepared by restaurants or caterers or in institutional settings (eg, schools and camps) where food is prepared in large quantities, cooled slowly, and stored inappropriately for prolonged periods. Beef, poultry, gravies, and dried or precooked foods are the most commonly implicated sources. Illness is not transmissible from person to person.

The **incubation period** is 6 to 24 hours, usually 8 to 12 hours.

DIAGNOSTIC TESTS

Because the fecal flora of healthy people commonly includes C perfringens, counts of C perfringens of 10^6 CFUs/g of feces or greater obtained within 48 hours of onset of illness support the diagnosis in ill people. The diagnosis can also be supported by detection of enterotoxin in stool. C perfringens can be confirmed as the cause of an outbreak if 10^6 CFUs/g are isolated from stool, enterotoxin is demonstrated in the stool of 2 or more ill people, or the concentration of organisms is at least 10^5 CFUs/g in the implicated food. Although C perfringens is an anaerobe, special transport conditions are unnecessary. Whole stool, rather than rectal swab specimens, should be obtained, transported in ice packs, and tested within 24 hours. For enumeration and enterotoxin testing, obtaining stool specimens in bulk without added transport media is required.

TREATMENT

C perfringens foodborne illness is typically self-limited. Oral rehydration or, occasionally, intravenous fluid and electrolyte replacement may be indicated to prevent or treat dehydration. Antimicrobial agents are not indicated.

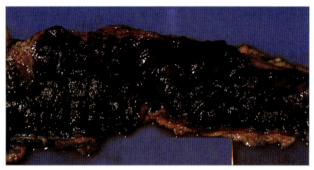

Image 34.1
This slide shows hemorrhagic necrosis of the intestine in a patient with *Clostridium perfringens* sepsis. Courtesy of Dimitris P. Agamanolis, MD.

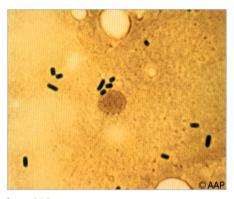

Image 34.2
Clostridium perfringens, an anaerobic, gram-positive, spore-forming bacillus, causes a broad spectrum of pathological effects, including food poisoning. In Papua New Guinea, *C perfringens* is a cause of severe illness and death called *necrotizing enteritis necroticans* (locally known as pigbel). Courtesy of Hugh Moffet, MD.

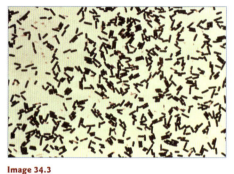

Image 34.3
This photomicrograph reveals numbers of *Clostridium perfringens* bacteria grown in Schaedler broth and subsequently stained with Gram stain (magnification ×1,000). *C perfringens* is a spore-forming, heat-resistant bacterium that can cause foodborne disease. The spores persist in the environment and often contaminate raw food materials. These bacteria are found in mammalian feces and soil. Courtesy of Centers for Disease Control and Prevention/Don Stalons.

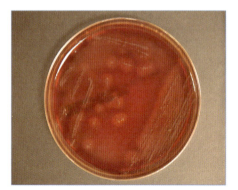

Image 34.4
Clostridium perfringens on phenylethyl alcohol–blood agar. A double zone of hemolysis is often observed as surrounding individual colonies. Courtesy of Julia Rosebush, DO; Robert Jerris, PhD; and Theresa Stanley, M(ASCP).

CHAPTER 35

Coccidioidomycosis

CLINICAL MANIFESTATIONS

Coccidioidomycosis, also called *valley fever*, is an infection caused by the fungus *Coccidioides*. Primary pulmonary infection is acquired by inhaling fungal conidia and is asymptomatic or self-limited in 60% to 65% of infected children and adults. Constitutional symptoms, including extreme fatigue and weight loss, are common and can persist for weeks or months. Symptomatic disease can resemble influenza or community-acquired pneumonia, with malaise, fever, cough, myalgia, arthralgia, headache, and chest pain. Pleural effusion, empyema, and mediastinal involvement are more common in children.

Acute infection may be associated only with cutaneous abnormalities, such as erythema multiforme, an erythematous maculopapular rash, or erythema nodosum manifesting as bilateral symmetrical violaceous nodules usually overlying the shins. Chronic pulmonary lesions are rare, but approximately 5% of infected people develop asymptomatic pulmonary radiographic residua (eg, cysts, nodules, cavitary lesions, coin lesions).

Nonpulmonary primary infection is rare and usually follows trauma associated with contamination of wounds by arthroconidia. Cutaneous lesions and soft tissue infections are often accompanied by regional lymphadenitis.

Disseminated (extrapulmonary) infection occurs in less than 0.5% of infected people; common sites of dissemination include skin, bones, joints, and the central nervous system (CNS). Meningitis is invariably fatal if untreated. Congenital infection is rare.

ETIOLOGY

Coccidioides species are dimorphic fungi. In soil, *Coccidioides* organisms exist in the mycelial phase as mold that grows as branching, septate hyphae. Infectious arthroconidia (ie, spores) produced from hyphae become airborne, infecting the host after inhalation or, rarely, inoculation. In tissues, arthroconidia enlarge to form spherules; mature spherules release hundreds to thousands of endospores that develop into new spherules and continue the tissue cycle. Molecular studies have divided the genus *Coccidioides* into 2 species: *Coccidioides immitis*, confined mainly to California, and *Coccidioides posadasii*, encompassing the remaining areas of distribution of the fungus within certain deserts of the southwestern United States, northern Mexico, and areas of Central and South America.

EPIDEMIOLOGY

Coccidioides species are found mostly in soil in areas of the southwestern United States with endemic infection, including California, Arizona, New Mexico, West and South Texas, southern Nevada, and Utah; in northern Mexico; and throughout certain parts of Central and South America.

In areas with endemic coccidioidomycosis, clusters of cases can follow dust-generating events, such as storms, seismic events, archaeological digging, and recreational and construction activities, including building of solar farms. Most cases occur without a known preceding event.

Infection is believed to provide lifelong immunity. Person-to-person transmission of coccidioidomycosis does not occur except in rare instances of cutaneous infection with actively draining lesions, donor-derived transmission via an infected organ, or congenital infection following in utero exposure. People with impairment of T-lymphocyte–mediated immunity caused by a congenital immune defect or HIV infection or those receiving immune-modulating medications (eg, tumor necrosis factor–α antagonists) have major risk for severe primary coccidioidomycosis, disseminated disease, or relapse of past infection. Other people with elevated risk for severe or disseminated disease include people of African or Filipino ancestry, women in the third trimester of pregnancy and those postpartum, and children younger than 1 year.

The **incubation period** is typically 1 to 3 weeks in primary infection. Disseminated infection may develop years after primary infection.

DIAGNOSTIC TESTS

Diagnosis of coccidioidomycosis is best established by using serological, histopathologic, and culture methods. Nucleic acid amplification tests have been developed but are not widely available.

Serological tests are useful in the diagnosis and management of infection. One approach is to test first with enzyme immunoassay (EIA), then perform immunodiffusion testing if the EIA result is positive. The former is more sensitive; the latter, more specific. The immunoglobulin M (IgM) response can be detected by EIA or immunodiffusion methods. In approximately 50% of primary infections, IgM is detected in the first week; approximately 90%, the third week. Immunoglobulin G response can be detected by immunodiffusion, EIA, or complement fixation (CF) tests. Immunodiffusion is considered more specific, whereas CF is more sensitive. Serum antibodies detected by CF are usually of low titer and are transient if the disease is asymptomatic or mild; persistent high titers ($\geq$1:16) occur with severe disease and are almost always measured in disseminated infection. Cerebrospinal fluid (CSF) antibodies are also detectable by immunodiffusion or CF testing. Increasing serum and CSF titers indicate progressive disease, and decreasing titers usually suggest improvement. Antibody titers detected by CF may not be reliable in immunocompromised patients; low or nondetectable titers in immunocompromised patients should be interpreted with caution.

Spherules are as large as 80 μm in diameter and can be visualized with 100× to 400× magnification in infected body fluid specimens (eg, pleural fluid, bronchoalveolar lavage) and biopsy specimens of skin lesions or organs. Use of silver or period acid–Schiff staining is helpful for biopsy specimens. The presence of a mature spherule with endospores is pathognomonic of infection. Isolation of *Coccidioides* species in culture establishes the diagnosis, even in patients with mild symptoms. Culture of organisms is possible on a variety of artificial media but is hazardous to laboratory personnel, because spherules can convert to arthroconidia-bearing mycelia on culture plates. A DNA probe can identify *Coccidioides* species in cultures.

At least one commercial laboratory offers an EIA test for urine, serum, plasma, CSF, or bronchoalveolar lavage fluid for detection of *Coccidioides* antigen. Antigen may be positive in patients with more severe forms of disease (sensitivity, 71%). Cross-reactions occur in patients with histoplasmosis, blastomycosis, or paracoccidioidomycosis.

TREATMENT

Antifungal therapy is not recommended routinely for uncomplicated asymptomatic primary infection in people without risk factors for severe disease. Although most mild cases resolve without therapy, some experts believe that treatment may reduce illness duration or risk of severe complications. Most experts recommend treatment of coccidioidomycosis with fluconazole for 3 to 6 months for people with risk for severe disease or people with severe primary infection. During pregnancy, amphotericin B (including lipid formulations) is the treatment of choice over fluconazole and other azole antifungals, because fluconazole has been demonstrated to be a teratogen in early pregnancy. Follow-up every 1 to 3 months for up to 2 years, to document radiographic resolution or to identify residual abnormalities or pulmonary or extrapulmonary complications, is recommended. For diffuse pneumonia, defined as bilateral reticulonodular or miliary infiltrates, amphotericin B or high-dose fluconazole is recommended. Amphotericin B is used more frequently in the presence of severe hypoxemia or rapid clinical deterioration. The total length of therapy for diffuse pneumonia is 1 year.

Oral fluconazole or itraconazole is the recommended initial therapy for disseminated infection not involving the CNS. Amphotericin B is recommended as alternative therapy if lesions are progressing or are in critical locations, such as the vertebral column, or in fulminant infections because it is believed to result in more rapid improvement.

Consultation with a specialist for treatment of patients with CNS disease caused by *Coccidioides* species is recommended. High-dose oral fluconazole (adult dose: 400–1,200 mg/day) is recommended for treatment of patients with CNS infection. Patients who respond to azole therapy should continue this treatment indefinitely (for the remainder of life). For CNS infections that are unresponsive to oral azoles or are associated with severe basilar inflammation, intrathecal amphotericin B deoxycholate therapy can be used to augment the azole therapy. A subcutaneous reservoir can facilitate administration into the cisternal space or lateral ventricle. Hydrocephalus is a common complication of coccidioidal meningitis and nearly always requires a shunt for decompression.

There are reports of success with voriconazole, posaconazole, and isavuconazole in treatment of coccidioidomycosis, but this has not been established in children.

The duration of antifungal therapy is variable and depends on the site(s) of involvement, clinical response, and mycological and immunologic test results. In general, therapy is continued until clinical and laboratory evidence indicates that active infection has resolved. Treatment of disseminated coccidioidomycosis is at least 6 months but for some patients may be extended to 1 year or longer. The role of subsequent suppressive azole therapy is uncertain, except for patients with CNS infection, osteomyelitis, or underlying HIV infection or for solid organ transplant recipients. Coccidioidal meningitis requires lifelong therapy. The duration of suppressive therapy may also be lifelong for other groups with high risk. Women should be advised to avoid pregnancy while receiving fluconazole, which is known to be teratogenic.

Surgical debridement or excision of lesions in bone, pericardium, and lung has been advocated for localized, symptomatic, persistent, resistant, or progressive lesions. In some localized infections with sinuses, fistulae, or abscesses, amphotericin B has been instilled locally or used for irrigation of wounds. Antifungal prophylaxis for solid organ transplant recipients may be considered if they reside in areas with endemicity and have prior serological evidence or a history of coccidioidomycosis.

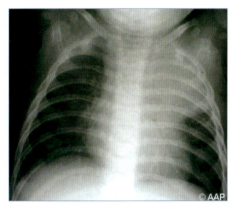

Image 35.1
Pneumonia caused by *Coccidioides immitis* in the upper lobe of the left lung of a 5½-month-old. The organism was isolated from gastric aspirate, and the result from the complement fixation test was elevated.

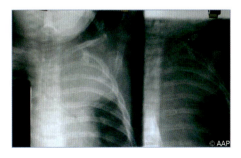

Image 35.2
Coccidioidomycosis of the upper lobe of the left lung of a 1-year-old boy, proven by gastric aspirate culture that tested positive for *Coccidioides immitis*. Courtesy of Edgar O. Ledbetter, MD, FAAP.

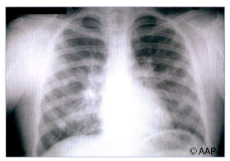

Image 35.3
Primary pulmonary coccidioidomycosis in an 11-year-old boy who recovered spontaneously. The acute disease is usually self-limited in otherwise healthy children. The patient also had erythema nodosum lesions over the tibial area.

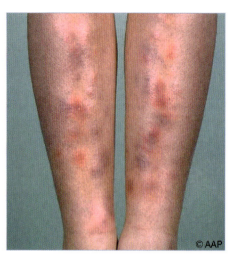

Image 35.4
Erythema nodosum in a preadolescent girl with primary pulmonary coccidioidomycosis.

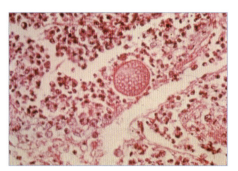

Image 35.5
Histopathologic features of coccidioidomycosis of lung. Mature spherule with endospores of *Coccidioides immitis* and intense infiltrate of neutrophils (hematoxylin-eosin stain). Courtesy of Centers for Disease Control and Prevention.

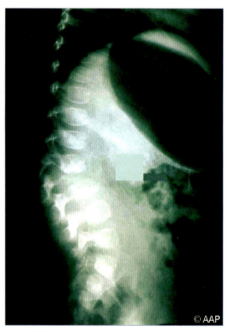

Image 35.6
Spondylitis caused by *Coccidioides immitis* in a 2-year-old boy with disseminated disease.

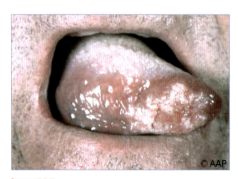

Image 35.7
Coccidioidomycosis of the tongue in a male adult. Courtesy of Edgar O. Ledbetter, MD, FAAP.

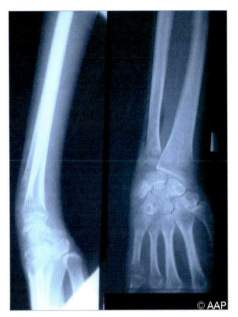

Image 35.8
Disseminated coccidioidomycosis with osteomyelitis of the distal radius and ulna in a preadolescent boy.

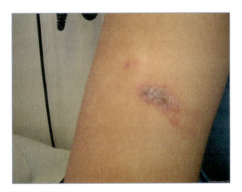

Image 35.10
A 15-year-old girl who originally presented with forehead lesions without other symptoms. At the third visit, she had disseminated coccidioidomycosis disease and had developed extensive cutaneous lesions all over her body with severe nasal involvement. Courtesy of Sabiha Hussain, MD.

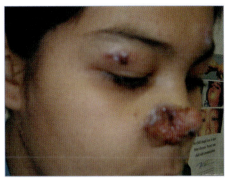

Image 35.9
A 15-year-old girl who originally presented with forehead lesions without other symptoms. At the third visit, she had disseminated coccidioidomycosis disease and had developed extensive cutaneous lesions all over her body with severe nasal involvement. Courtesy of Sabiha Hussain, MD.

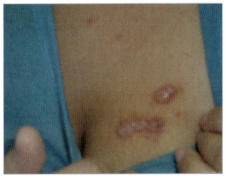

Image 35.11
A 15-year-old girl who originally presented with forehead lesions without other symptoms. At the third visit, she had disseminated coccidioidomycosis disease and had developed extensive cutaneous lesions all over her body with severe nasal involvement. Courtesy of Sabiha Hussain, MD.

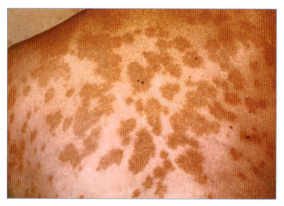

Image 35.12
Erythema nodosum lesions on skin of the back caused by hypersensitivity to antigens of *Coccidioides immitis*.
Courtesy of Centers for Disease Control and Prevention/Lucille K. Georg, MD.

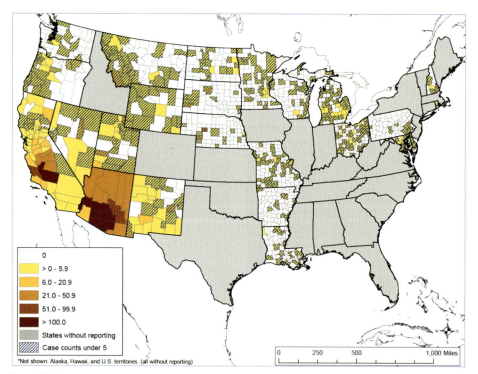

Image 35.13
This map shows the average incidence of reported Valley fever per 100,000 people, by county, during 2011–2017.
Courtesy of Centers for Disease Control and Prevention.

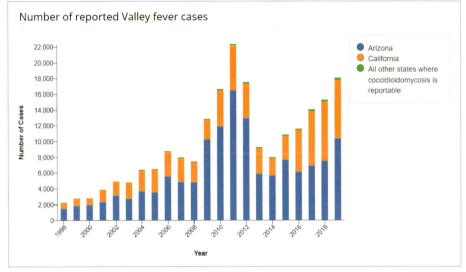

Image 35.14
Number of reported Valley fever cases from 1998–2019. Courtesy of Centers for Disease Control and Prevention.

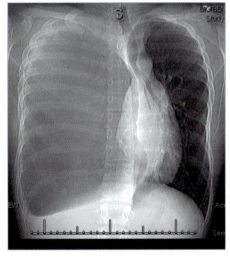

Image 35.15
Chest radiograph of a previously healthy 14-year-old boy who had a several months' history of intermittent fever, weight loss, and chest pain and recent onset of exercise intolerance. His pyopneumothorax was caused by *Coccidioides immitis*. He lived in West Texas near the Mexican border. Courtesy of Jeffrey R. Starke, MD.

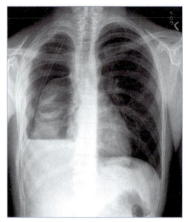

Image 35.16
A chest tube was inserted emergently in the patient in Image 35.15, and his right lung was expanded. Courtesy of Jeffrey R. Starke, MD.

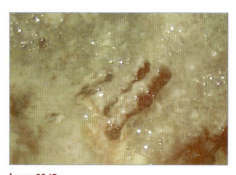

Image 35.17
After 7 days of hospitalization, the patient in images 35.15 and 35.16 underwent a video-assisted thoracostomy followed by an open thoracotomy for decortication procedure. This photograph demonstrates the copious fluid and thick fibrinous exudate of a chronic empyema found at surgery. Courtesy of Jeffrey R. Starke, MD.

CHAPTER 36

Coronaviruses, Including SARS-CoV-2 and MERS-CoV

CLINICAL MANIFESTATIONS

Novel COVID-19, caused by SARS-CoV-2, emerged in China in late 2019. The most common manifesting symptoms of COVID-19 in children are fever and cough; other symptoms can include shortness of breath, sore throat, headache, myalgia, fatigue, and, less frequently, rhinorrhea. Gastrointestinal symptoms such as nausea, vomiting, diarrhea, and poor appetite may occur, with or without respiratory symptoms. Less frequently, infected people can experience anosmia (loss of smell) or ageusia (loss of taste); these occur more commonly in adolescents than in younger children. Conjunctivitis and rashes have also been reported. Children generally have mild disease or may be asymptomatic, although severe and even fatal cases have occurred. Children with obesity or medical comorbidities have risk for more severe disease. Children from racial or ethnic minority groups may have higher risk for severe illness. Complications include respiratory failure, acute cardiac injury, acute kidney injury, shock, coagulopathy, and multiorgan failure. Diabetic ketoacidosis and intussusception have also been reported. Laboratory findings may be normal or may include lymphopenia, leukopenia, elevated C-reactive protein or procalcitonin level, and elevated alanine aminotransferase and aspartate aminotransferase levels. Chest imaging may be normal or there may be unilateral or bilateral lung involvement with multiple areas of consolidation and ground-glass opacities.

Multisystem inflammatory syndrome in children (MIS-C) may manifest during or weeks following SARS-CoV-2 infection. Children present with fever, severe disease of 2 or more organ systems (cardiac, gastrointestinal tract, skin, kidney, neurological, hematologic, or respiratory tract), and laboratory evidence of inflammation. The case definition from the Centers for Disease Control and Prevention (CDC; www.cdc.gov/mis-c/hcp) includes no alternative diagnosis in addition to evidence of recent or concurrent SARS-CoV-2 infection or exposure to someone with known or suspected COVID-19 within the past 4 weeks. Children with MIS-C often present with severe abdominal pain, and many have features that can be like those of Kawasaki disease. Children with MIS-C may have echocardiographic abnormalities, including myocarditis and coronary artery abnormalities.

Human coronaviruses (HCoVs) 229E, OC43, NL63, and HKU1 are associated most frequently with an upper respiratory tract infection characterized by rhinorrhea, nasal congestion, sore throat, sneezing, and cough that may be associated with mild fever. Symptoms are self-limited and typically peak on day 3 or 4 of illness. These HCoV infections may also be associated with acute otitis media or asthma exacerbations. Less frequently, they are associated with lower respiratory tract infections, including bronchiolitis, croup, and pneumonia, primarily in infants and children and adults who are immunocompromised.

MERS-CoV, the virus associated with the Middle East respiratory syndrome (MERS), can cause severe disease, but asymptomatic infections and mild disease may occur. Most cases have been identified in men with comorbidities. Infections in children are uncommon and are typically milder. Patients initially present with fever, myalgia, and chills followed by a nonproductive cough and dyspnea a few days later. Approximately 25% of patients may experience vomiting, diarrhea, or abdominal pain. Rapid deterioration of oxygenation with progressive unilateral or bilateral airspace infiltrates on chest imaging may follow, requiring mechanical ventilation and often associated with acute renal failure. The case-fatality rate is high, estimated at 36%, but may partially reflect surveillance bias for more severe disease. Laboratory abnormalities may include thrombocytopenia, lymphopenia, and increased lactate dehydrogenase concentration, particularly in severely infected individuals.

SARS-CoV-1 was responsible for the 2002–2003 global outbreak of severe acute respiratory syndrome (SARS), which was associated with severe symptoms, although a spectrum of disease including asymptomatic infections and mild disease occurred. Infections in children were less severe than in adults and typically manifested with fever, cough, and rhinorrhea. Adolescents with SARS had clinical courses more closely resembling those of adult disease, manifesting with fever, myalgia, headache, and chills. No deaths in children or adolescents from SARS-CoV-1 infection were documented.

ETIOLOGY

Coronaviruses are enveloped, nonsegmented, single-stranded, positive-sense RNA viruses named after their crown- or Latin *corona*-like surface projections observed on electron microscopy that correspond to large surface spike proteins. Coronaviruses are classified in the *Nidovirales* order. Coronaviruses are host specific and can infect humans as well as a variety of different animals, causing diverse clinical syndromes. Four distinct genera have been described: *Alphacoronavirus, Betacoronavirus, Gammacoronavirus,* and *Deltacoronavirus.* HCoVs 229E and NL63 belong to the genus *Alphacoronavirus.* HCoVs OC43 and HKU1 belong to lineage A, SARS-CoV-1 and SARS-CoV-2 belong to lineage B, and MERS-CoV belongs to lineage C of the genus *Betacoronavirus.*

EPIDEMIOLOGY

SARS-CoV-2 emerged in Wuhan, China, near the end of 2019. Infection rapidly spread throughout Hubei province and across China. In January 2020, cases were detected outside of China (the first US case was reported on January 21, 2020). The World Health Organization (WHO) declared SARS-CoV-2 a "public health emergency of international concern" on January 30, 2020, and the United States declared a "public health emergency" the following day. A global pandemic was declared by the WHO on March 11, 2020. By March 2021, more than 112 million cases and 2.5 million deaths were reported globally, with approximately 28 million cases and 500,000 deaths in the United States. Children constitute approximately 10% of US cases. MIS-C is a rare diagnosis, with just over 2,000 cases and approximately 30 deaths in the United States by early February 2021; most cases occurred in children and teens aged 1 to 14 years, with an average age of 8 years. Additional information on COVID-19 and the fast-moving pandemic can be found at **www.cdc.gov/coronavirus/2019-ncov/index.html.**

SARS-CoV-2 is transmitted efficiently between people, including from presymptomatic, symptomatic, and asymptomatic people. Infection is believed to be primarily through transmission of large and small respiratory droplets and particles among people in close proximity (generally within 2 m [6 feet]), although transmission can occur at larger distances. Aerosol transmission, which is essentially spread from very small droplets that can remain suspended in the air for longer periods, can also occur. Crowded, enclosed, and poorly ventilated spaces are particularly concerning environments for the transmission of SARS-CoV-2. Infected people are believed to be infectious 2 days before symptom onset through 10 days after symptom onset, with viral loads being higher earlier in the course of infection and with decreasing infectivity as time progresses. Patients with severe disease or severe immunocompromise may shed viable virus for longer than 10 days. Health care–associated transmission occurs with SARS-CoV-2, and strict adherence to infection prevention guidance is necessary. Outbreaks of SARS-CoV-2 infection occur readily in congregate settings (eg, long-term care facilities, group homes, prisons, shelters, congregate workplaces, dormitories) and households.

HCoVs 229E, OC43, NL63, and HKU1 can be found worldwide. They cause most disease in the winter and spring months in temperate climates. Seroprevalence data for these HCoVs suggest that exposure is common in early childhood, with approximately 90% of adults being seropositive for HCoVs 229E, OC43, and NL63 and 60% being seropositive for HCoV HKU1. The modes of transmission for HCoVs 229E, OC43, NL63, and HKU1 have not been well studied. However, on the basis of studies of other respiratory tract viruses, it is likely that transmission occurs primarily via a combination of droplet and direct and indirect contact spread.

MERS-CoV likely evolved from bat coronaviruses and infected dromedary camels, which now demonstrate seroprevalence and infection with MERS-CoV in parts of the Middle East and Africa. MERS-CoV cases continue mostly in the Middle East, primarily linked to close contact with camels or an infected person. Human-to-human transmission occurs generally in health care settings and less frequently in household settings and is believed to occur most commonly through droplet and contact spread, although airborne spread may occur. Updated figures on global cases can be found on the WHO website (**www.who.int/emergencies/mers-cov/en**).

SARS-CoV-1 likely evolved from a natural reservoir of SARS-CoV–like viruses in horseshoe bats through civet cats or intermediate animal hosts in wet markets of China. Public health interventions ultimately aborted the epidemic. SARS-CoV-1 was last reported with human disease in 2004 from laboratory-acquired infections.

The **incubation period** for SARS-CoV-2 is 2 to 14 days (median, 5 days). The **incubation period** for HCoV 229E is 2 to 5 days (median, 3 days). The **incubation period** for MERS-CoV is estimated to be 2 to 14 days (median, 5 days).

DIAGNOSTIC TESTS

Acute SARS-CoV-2 infection can be diagnosed by detection of viral RNA from a respiratory source from the upper or lower airway (eg, nasopharynx, oropharynx, nose, saliva, trachea) through reverse transcriptase–polymerase chain reaction (RT-PCR) assay (some may be multiplex assays) or through direct antigen testing for SARS-CoV-2 from a nasopharyngeal or nasal specimen. Serological testing is not helpful for the diagnosis of acute SARS-CoV-2 infection but can be used in the diagnosis of MIS-C.

Multiplex assays for respiratory pathogens are commercially available that include HCoVs 229E, OC43, NL63, and HKU1 as targets. State public health departments should be contacted for evaluation of suspected cases of MERS-CoV with RT-PCR assay.

TREATMENT

Treatment of COVID-19 is evolving rapidly. The National Institutes of Health (**www.covid19treatmentguidelines.nih.gov**) and the Infectious Diseases Society of America (**www.idsociety.org/practice-guideline/covid-19-guideline-treatment-and-management**) have updated information on treatment of COVID-19 on their websites. As of the end of February 2021, remdesivir has received US Food and Drug Administration approval for use in children 12 years and older (≥40 kg) and adults hospitalized with COVID-19, in whom the medication shortens hospitalization, and has received emergency use authorization (EUA) for use in younger children. In adults, use of dexamethasone in COVID-19 hospitalized patients requiring oxygen or invasive mechanical ventilation has improved survival. Use of convalescent plasma in children with COVID-19 is under investigation. A number of monoclonal antibody therapies are under investigation, with at least 3 (bamlanivimab, as monotherapy or in combination with etesevimab, and the combination of casirivimab and imdevimab) receiving EUA for use in infected non-hospitalized children 12 years and older (≥40 kg) and adults with high risk for severe COVID-19.

For the treatment of MIS-C, the American Academy of Pediatrics (**https://services.aap.org/en/pages/2019-novel-coronavirus-covid-19-infections/clinical-guidance/multisystem-inflammatory-syndrome-in-children-mis-c-interim-guidance**), CDC (**www.cdc.gov/mis-c/hcp**), and American College of Rheumatology have developed interim guidance. As of March 2021, there are no trials evaluating efficacy of treatment options. A multidisciplinary approach, with the involvement of pediatric specialists in cardiology, rheumatology, infectious disease, hematology, immunology, and critical care, is recommended to guide individual management. In addition to supportive care, therapies have included immune globulin intravenous (1–2 g/kg), steroids, biologics (anakinra), and prophylaxis or treatment of thromboses.

Infections attributable to HCoVs HKU1, OC43, 229E, and NL63 are treated with supportive care. No controlled trials have been conducted for treatment of MERS-CoV.

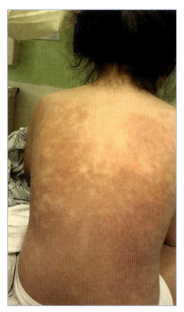

Image 36.1
Rash on the back of a 7-year-old girl who tested positive for severe acute respiratory syndrome coronavirus 2 (SARS-CoV-2) with reverse transcription polymerase chain reaction (RT-PCR) testing. From Spencer R, Closson, RC, Gorelik M, et al. COVID-19 inflammatory syndrome with clinical features resembling Kawasaki disease. *Pediatrics.* 2020;146(3):e20201845.

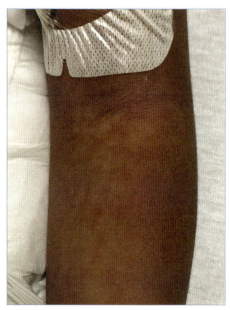

Image 36.2
Rash on the arm of an 11-year-old boy in whom novel coronavirus disease 2019 (COVID-19) was diagnosed on the basis of RT-PCR testing for SARS-CoV-2. From Spencer R, Closson, RC, Gorelik M, et al. COVID-19 inflammatory syndrome with clinical features resembling Kawasaki disease. *Pediatrics.* 2020;146(3):e20201845.

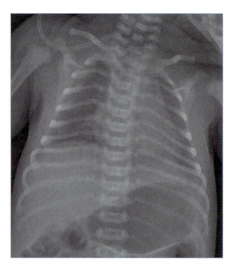

Image 36.3
Chest radiograph of a newborn with SARS-CoV-2 infection, obtained on day 3 after birth. The image shows mild bilateral ground-glass opacities, which caused silent hypoxemia and necessitated respiratory support. From Sinelli M, Paterlini G, Citterio M, et al. Early neonatal SARS-CoV-2 infection manifesting with hypoxemia requiring respiratory support. *Pediatrics.* 2020;146(1):e20201121.

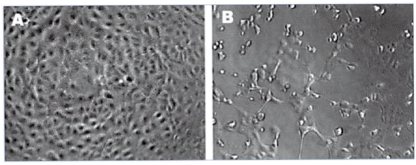

Image 36.4
Microscopic appearance of control (A) and infected (B) Vero E6 cells, demonstrating cytopathic effects. The cytopathic effect of severe acute respiratory syndrome coronavirus on Vero E6 cells was evident within 24 hours after infection. Courtesy of Centers for Disease Control and Prevention.

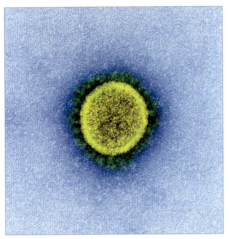

Image 36.5
Electron micrograph of a coronavirus. Pleomorphic virions average 100 nm in diameter and are covered with club-shaped knobs. Courtesy of NIAID.

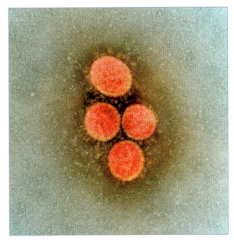

Image 36.6
Coronaviruses are a group of viruses that have a halo or crownlike (corona) appearance when viewed in an electron microscope. SARS-CoV-2, pictured, is the coronavirus that is the etiologic agent of the COVID-19 pandemic. Additional specimens are being tested to learn more about this coronavirus. Courtesy of NIAID.

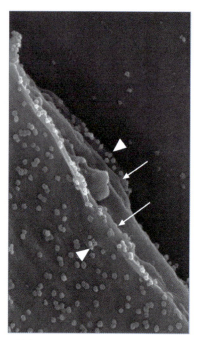

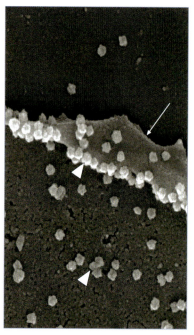

Image 36.7
This scanning electron micrograph (SEM) revealed the thickened, layered edge of severe acute respiratory syndrome–infected Vero E6 culture cells. The thickened edges of the infected cells were ruffled and appeared to comprise layers of folded plasma membranes. Note the layered cell edge (arrows) on SEM. Virus particles (arrowheads) are extruded from the layered surfaces. Courtesy of Centers for Disease Control and Prevention.

Image 36.8
This scanning electron micrograph (SEM) revealed the thickened, layered edge of severe acute respiratory syndrome–infected Vero E6 culture cells. The thickened edges of the infected cells were ruffled and appeared to comprise layers of folded plasma membranes. Note the layered cell edge (arrow) on SEM. Virus particles (arrowheads) are extruded from the layered surfaces. Courtesy of Centers for Disease Control and Prevention.

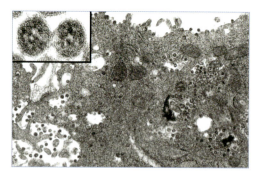

Image 36.9
Note the coronaviruses contained within cytoplasmic membrane–bound vacuoles and cisternae of the rough endoplasmic reticulum. This thin-section electron micrograph of an infected Vero E6 cell reveals coronavirus particles. Courtesy of Centers for Disease Control and Prevention.

CHAPTER 37
Cryptococcus neoformans and Cryptococcus gattii Infections
(Cryptococcosis)

CLINICAL MANIFESTATIONS

Primary pulmonary infection is acquired by inhalation of aerosolized *Cryptococcus* fungal propagules found in contaminated soil or organic material (eg, trees, rotting wood, and bird guano), and infection is often asymptomatic or mild. Pulmonary disease, when symptomatic, is characterized by cough, chest pain, and constitutional symptoms. Chest radiographs may reveal solitary or multiple masses; patchy, segmental, or lobar consolidation, which is often multifocal; or a nodular or reticulonodular pattern with interstitial changes. Pulmonary cryptococcosis may manifest as acute respiratory distress syndrome and can mimic *Pneumocystis* pneumonia. Hematogenous dissemination occurs particularly to the central nervous system, bones, skin, and other body sites and almost always occurs in children with defects in T-lymphocyte–mediated immunity, including children with leukemia or lymphoma, those taking corticosteroids, those with congenital immunodeficiency such as hyperimmunoglobulin M syndrome or severe combined immunodeficiency syndrome, those with AIDS, or those who have undergone solid organ transplant. Usually several sites are infected, but manifestations of involvement at one site predominate. Cryptococcal meningitis, the most common and serious form of cryptococcal disease, often follows an indolent course, but symptoms can be more acute in severely immunosuppressed patients. Symptoms are characteristic of meningitis, meningoencephalitis, or space-occupying lesions but sometimes manifest only as subtle, nonspecific findings such as fever, headache, or behavioral changes. Cryptococcal fungemia without apparent organ involvement occurs in patients with HIV infection but is rare in children.

ETIOLOGY

There are more than 30 species of *Cryptococcus*, but only 2, *Cryptococcus neoformans* (subspecies [subsp] *neoformans* and subsp *grubii*) and *Cryptococcus gattii*, are regarded as human pathogens.

EPIDEMIOLOGY

C neoformans subsp *neoformans* and *C neoformans* subsp *grubii* are isolated primarily from soil contaminated with pigeon or other bird droppings and cause most human infections, especially in immunocompromised hosts. *C neoformans* infects 5% to 10% of adults with AIDS, but cryptococcal disease is rare in HIV-infected and non–HIV-infected children. *C gattii* is associated with certain trees and the surrounding soil and has emerged as a pathogen producing a respiratory syndrome with or without neurological findings in individuals from British Columbia, Canada, the Pacific Northwest region of the United States, and, occasionally, other regions of the United States. A high frequency of disease has also been reported among Aboriginal people in Australia and in the central province of Papua New Guinea. *C gattii* causes disease in both immunocompetent and immunocompromised individuals, and cases have been reported in children. Person-to-person transmission does not generally occur.

The **incubation period** for *C neoformans* is unknown; dissemination often represents reactivation of latent disease acquired previously. The **incubation period** for *C gattii* is estimated at 8 weeks to 13 months.

DIAGNOSTIC TESTS

The cerebrospinal fluid (CSF) profile of cryptococcal meningoencephalitis is characterized by low cell counts, low glucose level, and elevated protein level. Opening pressure may be markedly elevated, especially in HIV-infected individuals. Laboratory diagnosis of cryptococcal infection is best performed by using cryptococcal antigen (CRAG) detection methods or by culture. The latex agglutination test, lateral flow immunoassay, and enzyme immunoassay for detection of cryptococcal capsular polysaccharide antigen (galactoxylomannan) in serum or CSF specimens are excellent rapid diagnostic tests for those with suspected meningitis. CRAG is detected in CSF or serum specimens from more than 95% of patients with cryptococcal meningitis. Antigen test results can be falsely negative when antigen concentrations are very high (prozone effect), which can be addressed by dilution of samples. A lateral flow immunoassay, which shows good agreement with standard CRAG testing, is a common test in both resource-available and resource-limited settings.

Definitive diagnosis requires isolation of the yeast from body fluid or tissue specimens. Encapsulated yeast cells can be visualized by using India ink or other stains of CSF and bronchoalveolar lavage specimens, but this method has limited sensitivity and is not recommended as a stand-alone rapid test. Sabouraud dextrose agar is useful for isolation of *Cryptococcus* organisms from sputum, bronchopulmonary lavage, tissue, or CSF specimens. Differentiation between *C neoformans* and *C gattii* can be made by use of the selective medium L-canavanine, glycine, bromothymol blue agar. A MALDI-TOF (matrix-assisted laser desorption/ionization–time-of-flight) mass spectrometer can be used to identify yeasts to species level accurately and rapidly. Polymerase chain multiplex reaction assays are available (BioFire) but may miss low burden infections with yeasts. Focal pulmonary or skin lesions can be biopsied for fungal staining and culture.

TREATMENT

No trials dedicated to children have been performed, so optimal dosing and duration of therapy for children with cryptococcal infection is unknown. Amphotericin B deoxycholate (1 mg/kg/day), liposomal amphotericin B (5–7.5 mg/kg/day), or amphotericin B lipid complex (5 mg/kg/day) is indicated in combination with oral flucytosine (25 mg/kg/dose, 4 times/day when renal function is normal) as first-line induction therapy for pediatric patients with meningeal and/or other serious cryptococcal infections. Frequent monitoring of blood counts and/or serum peak flucytosine concentrations (with a target of 40–60 μg/mL 2 hours after the dose) are recommended to prevent neutropenia. Patients with meningitis should receive induction combination therapy for at least 2 weeks and until a repeated CSF culture is negative, followed by consolidation therapy with fluconazole (10–12 mg/kg/day, in 2 divided daily doses; maximum 800 mg/day) for a minimum of 8 weeks. If flucytosine cannot be administered, amphotericin B alone has been successfully used in pediatric cryptococcosis, or amphotericin B can be combined with fluconazole for the induction phase of therapy. A lumbar puncture should be performed after 2 weeks of therapy to document microbiological clearance. The 20% to 40% of patients whose culture is positive after 2 weeks of therapy will require a more prolonged induction treatment course. For any relapse, induction antifungal therapy should be restarted for 4 to 10 weeks, CSF cultures should be repeated every 2 weeks until sterile, and antifungal susceptibility of the relapse isolate should be determined and compared to that of the original isolate. Monitoring of serum CRAG is not useful to determine response to therapy in patients with cryptococcal meningitis.

Increased intracranial pressure occurs frequently despite microbiological response and is often associated with clinical deterioration. Significant elevation of intracranial pressure is a major source of morbidity and should be managed with frequent repeated lumbar punctures or placement of a lumbar drain in those with high intracranial pressures and symptoms. Immune reconstitution inflammatory syndrome is described in children. In antiretroviral-naive HIV patients with newly diagnosed cryptococcal meningitis or disseminated disease, delay in potent antiretroviral therapy (ART) may be prudent until the end of the first 2 weeks of induction therapy.

Children with HIV infection who have completed initial therapy for cryptococcosis should receive long-term suppressive/maintenance therapy with fluconazole (6 mg/kg daily; maximum dose 400 mg). Discontinuing suppressive/maintenance therapy for cryptococcosis (after receiving secondary prophylaxis for at least 1 year) can be considered for asymptomatic children 6 years and older, with an increase in their $CD4^+$ T-lymphocyte counts to $100/\mu$L or greater and an undetectable viral load after receiving ART for 3 months or longer. Suppressive/maintenance therapy should be reinitiated if the $CD4^+$ T-lymphocyte count decreases to less than $100/\mu$L. Most experts would not discontinue secondary prophylaxis for patients younger than 6 years.

Patients with less severe nonmeningeal disease (pulmonary disease) can be treated with fluconazole alone, but data on use of fluconazole for children with *C neoformans* infection are limited; itraconazole is a potential alternative. Another potential treatment option for patients in whom amphotericin B treatment is not possible is the combination therapy with fluconazole and flucytosine. Echinocandins are not active against cryptococcal infections and should not be used.

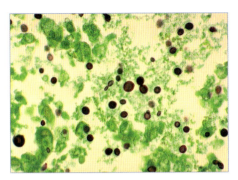

Image 37.1
Cryptococcosis of lung in a patient with AIDS (methenamine silver stain). Histopathologic features of lung show numerous extracellular yeasts of *Cryptococcus neoformans* within an alveolar space. Yeasts show narrow-base budding and characteristic variation in size. Courtesy of Centers for Disease Control and Prevention.

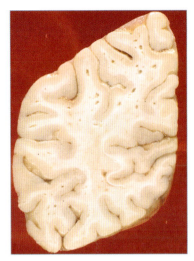

Image 37.2
Cryptococcus meningitis. Cystic lesions resulting from accumulation of organisms in perivascular spaces. Courtesy of Dimitris P. Agamanolis, MD.

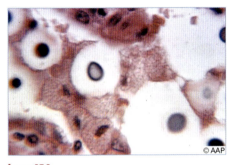

Image 37.3
Cryptococcosis of the liver (original magnification ×810) in a patient with immunodeficiency and disseminated disease. The mucinous capsules are prominent. Courtesy of Edgar O. Ledbetter, MD, FAAP.

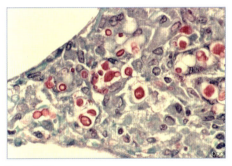

Image 37.4
Cryptococcosis of lung in a patient with AIDS (mucicarmine stain). Histopathologic features of lung show widened alveolar septum containing a few inflammatory cells and numerous yeasts of *Cryptococcus neoformans*. The inner layer of the yeast capsule stains red. Courtesy of Centers for Disease Control and Prevention/Edwin P. Ewing Jr, MD.

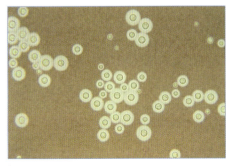

Image 37.5
This photomicrograph depicts *Cryptococcus neoformans* observable with a light India ink staining preparation. Courtesy of Centers for Disease Control and Prevention.

CHAPTER 38
Cryptosporidiosis

CLINICAL MANIFESTATIONS

Cryptosporidiosis commonly manifests with frequent, nonbloody, watery diarrhea, although infection can be asymptomatic. Other symptoms include abdominal cramps, fatigue, fever, vomiting, anorexia, and weight loss. In an immunocompetent person, symptomatic cryptosporidiosis is self-limited, usually resolving within 2 to 3 weeks.

In an immunocompromised person, such as a child who has received a solid organ transplant or has advanced HIV disease, cryptosporidiosis can result in profuse diarrhea lasting weeks to months, leading to severe dehydration, malnutrition, wasting, and death. The diagnosis of cryptosporidiosis should be considered in any immunocompromised person with diarrhea. Extraintestinal (eg, pulmonary or biliary tract) cryptosporidiosis has been reported in immunocompromised people and is associated with $CD4^+$ T-lymphocyte counts less than 50/µL.

ETIOLOGY

Cryptosporidia are oocyst-forming coccidian protozoa. Oocysts are excreted in feces of an infected host. Approximately 20 *Cryptosporidium* species or genotypes have been reported to infect humans, but *Cryptosporidium hominis* and *Cryptosporidium parvum* cause more than 90% of cases of human cryptosporidiosis. The organism is highly infectious, with 10 or fewer oocysts causing infection. *Cryptosporidium* oocysts can tolerate extreme environmental conditions and can survive in water and soil for several months. Even in properly chlorinated pools, *Cryptosporidium* oocysts can survive for more than 7 days.

EPIDEMIOLOGY

Cryptosporidium organisms can be transmitted between humans and to humans via contaminated water and food and from animals. Extensive waterborne disease outbreaks have been associated with contamination of drinking water and recreational water (eg, pools, lakes, and water playgrounds). *Cryptosporidium* infection has become the leading cause of outbreaks associated with treated recreational water venues (eg, swimming pools), responsible for 212 (58%) of 363 such outbreaks during 2000–2014 for which an infectious cause was identified.

Among children, the incidence of cryptosporidiosis is greatest during summer and early fall, corresponding to the outdoor swimming season. Cases are reported most frequently in children 1 through 4 years of age, followed by those 5 through 9 years.

Foodborne transmission can occur; *Cryptosporidium* organisms have been detected in raw produce and in raw or unpasteurized apple cider and milk. People can acquire infections from pets, from livestock, and from animals found in petting zoos, particularly preweaned bovine calves, lambs, and goat kids. *Cryptosporidium* organisms can spread by person-to-person transmission and result in outbreaks in child care settings and are a cause of travelers diarrhea.

The **incubation period** of *Cryptosporidium* species is usually 2 to 10 days. Recurrence of symptoms has been reported frequently. In immunocompetent people, oocyst shedding usually ceases within 2 weeks after symptoms abate. In immunocompromised people, the period of oocyst shedding can continue for months.

DIAGNOSTIC TESTS

Routine laboratory examination of stool for ova and parasites might not include testing for *Cryptosporidium* species, so testing for the organism should be requested specifically. The direct fluorescent antibody method for microscopic detection of oocysts in stool and multiwell plate enzyme immunoassays (EIAs) targeting cryptosporidial antigens are widely available and are recommended for laboratory diagnosis of cryptosporidiosis. Some EIAs target *Cryptosporidium* species and *Giardia duodenalis* in a single test format. The detection of oocysts on microscopic examination of stool specimens can be accomplished by direct wet mount if concentration of the oocysts is high. Alternatively, the formalin–ethyl acetate stool concentration method can be used, followed by staining of the stool specimen with a modified Kinyoun acid-fast stain. Oocysts are generally small (4–6 µm in diameter) and can be missed in a rapid scan of a slide.

Because shedding can be intermittent, at least 3 stool specimens collected on separate days should be examined before considering test results to be negative. Organisms can also be identified in intestinal biopsy tissue or sampling of intestinal fluid. Molecular methods are being used increasingly for diagnosis of cryptosporidiosis, particularly nucleic acid amplification tests that target multiple gastrointestinal tract pathogens in a single assay.

TREATMENT

Immunocompetent people might not need specific therapy. If treatment of diarrhea associated with cryptosporidiosis is indicated, a 3-day course of nitazoxanide oral suspension has been approved by the US Food and Drug Administration for non–HIV-infected immunocompetent people 1 year or older. Longer courses of nitazoxanide (up to ≥14 days) are recommended for immunocompromised children for treatment of diarrhea caused by *Cryptosporidium*, although efficacy is questionable. Disease in immunocompromised children, especially those with solid organ transplant or those with HIV infection, can be refractory to treatment with nitazoxanide.

In HIV-infected people, improvement in $CD4^+$ T-lymphocyte count associated with antiretroviral therapy (ART) can lead to resolution of symptoms and cessation of oocyst shedding. For this reason, administration of combination ART is the primary treatment of cryptosporidiosis in patients with HIV infection. Given the seriousness of cryptosporidiosis in immunocompromised people, use of nitazoxanide can be considered in immunocompromised HIV-infected children in conjunction with immune restoration with ART. Paromomycin or azithromycin is an alternative for children who do not respond to nitazoxanide.

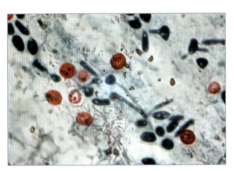

Image 38.1
This micrograph of a direct fecal smear is stained to detect *Cryptosporidium* species, an intracellular protozoan parasite. With a modified cold Kinyoun acid-fast staining technique and under an oil immersion lens, *Cryptosporidium* species oocysts, which are acid fast, stain red, and yeast cells, which are not acid fast, stain green. Courtesy of Centers for Disease Control and Prevention.

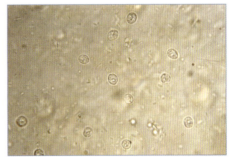

Image 38.2
This micrograph of a stool smear reveals *Cryptosporidium parvum* as the cause of this patient's cryptosporidiosis. *Cryptosporidium* is a microscopic parasite that can live in the intestines of humans and animals. The parasite is protected by an outer shell that allows it to survive outside the body for long periods and makes it resistant to chlorine disinfection. Courtesy of Centers for Disease Control and Prevention.

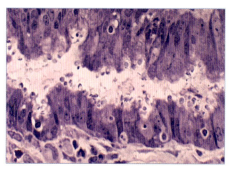

Image 38.3
Histopathologic features of cryptosporidiosis, intestine. Plastic-embedded, toluidine blue–stained section shows numerous *Cryptosporidium* organisms at luminal surfaces of epithelial cells. Courtesy of Centers for Disease Control and Prevention.

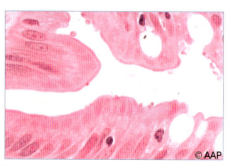

Image 38.4
Cryptosporidium, a spore-forming coccidian protozoan, can be seen on the brush border of intestinal mucosa. *Cryptosporidium* does not invade below the epithelial layer of the mucosa, so fecal leukocytes are absent.

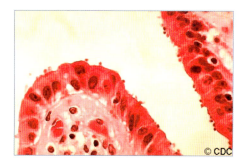

Image 38.5
Cryptosporidiosis of gallbladder in a patient with AIDS. Histopathologic features of gallbladder epithelium include numerous *Cryptosporidium* organisms along luminal surfaces of epithelial cells. Courtesy of Centers for Disease Control and Prevention.

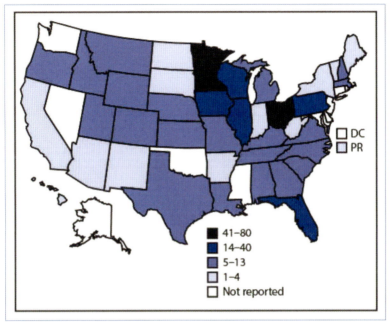

Image 38.6
Reported cryptosporidiosis outbreaks (N = 444), by exposure jurisdiction—United States, 2009–2017. Exposure districts are states, DC, and PR. These numbers largely depend on public health capacity and reporting requirements, which vary across jurisdictions and do not necessarily indicate the actual occurrence of cryptosporidiosis outbreaks in a given jurisdiction. Courtesy of *Morbidity and Mortality Weekly Report*.

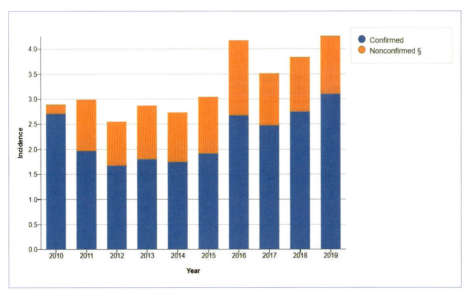

Image 38.7
Incidence* of reported cryptosporidiosis cases, by year and case classification—National Notifiable Diseases Surveillance System, United States, 2010–2019 (N = 105,211). * Cases per 100,000 population per year. § Probable, suspected, or unknown cases. Courtesy of Centers for Disease Control and Prevention.

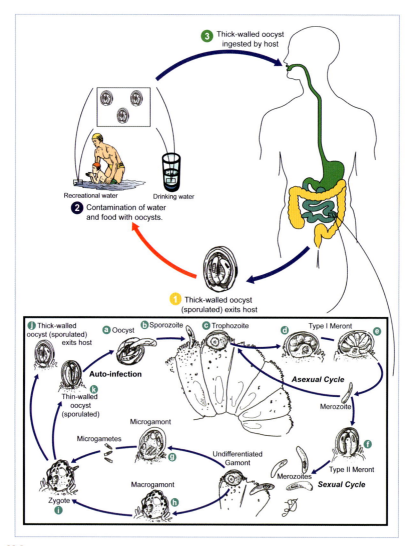

Image 38.8

Life cycle of *Cryptosporidium*. Sporulated oocysts, containing 4 sporozoites, are excreted by the infected host through feces and, possibly, other routes, such as respiratory secretions (1). Transmission of *Cryptosporidium parvum* occurs mainly through contact with contaminated water (eg, drinking or recreational water). Occasionally, food sources, such as chicken salad, may serve as vehicles for transmission. Many outbreaks in the United States have occurred in water parks, community swimming pools, and child care centers. Zoonotic transmission of *C parvum* occurs through exposure to infected animals or exposure to water contaminated by feces of infected animals (2). Following ingestion (and, possibly, inhalation) by a suitable host (3), excystation (a) occurs. The sporozoites are released and parasitize epithelial cells (b, c) of the gastrointestinal tract or other tissues. In these cells, the parasites undergo asexual multiplication (schizogony or merogony) (d–f) and then sexual multiplication (gametogony), producing microgamonts (male) (g) and macrogamonts (female) (h). On fertilization of the macrogamonts by the microgametes (i), oocysts (j, k) develop that sporulate in the infected host. Two different types of oocysts are produced: the thick-walled, which is commonly excreted from the host (j), and the thin-walled (k), which is primarily involved in autoinfection. Oocysts are infective on excretion, thus permitting direct and immediate fecal-oral transmission. Note that oocysts of *Cyclospora cayetanensis*, another important coccidian parasite, are unsporulated at excretion and do not become infective until sporulation is completed. Refer to the life cycle of *C cayetanensis* for further details. Courtesy of Centers for Disease Control and Prevention.

CHAPTER 39
Cutaneous Larva Migrans

CLINICAL MANIFESTATIONS

Cutaneous larva migrans is a clinical diagnosis based on advancing serpiginous tracks in the skin with associated intense pruritus. Certain nematode larvae may penetrate intact skin and produce pruritic reddish papules at the site of skin entry. Signs and symptoms typically develop several days after larval penetration of the skin, but in rare cases, onset of disease may be delayed for weeks to months. As the larvae migrate through skin, advancing up to 20 mm per day, intensely pruritic serpiginous tracks are formed, a condition also referred to as *creeping eruption*. Bullae may develop later as a complication of the larval migration. Larval activity can continue for several weeks, but the infection is self-limiting. Rarely, in infections with certain species of parasites, larvae may penetrate deeper tissues and cause pneumonitis (Löffler syndrome), which can be severe. Occasionally, the larvae of *Ancylostoma caninum* can reach the intestine and may cause eosinophilic enteritis.

ETIOLOGY

Infective larvae of cat and dog hookworms (most often *Ancylostoma braziliense;* also *A caninum, Ancylostoma ceylanicum*, and *Uncinaria stenocephala*) cause cutaneous larva migrans. Other skin-penetrating nematodes are occasional causes of similar clinical manifestations (eg, larva currens caused by *Strongyloides*).

EPIDEMIOLOGY

Cutaneous larva migrans is a disease of children, utility workers, gardeners, sunbathers, and others who come in contact with soil contaminated with cat and dog feces. Locally acquired cases in the United States are mostly in the Southeast. Most identified cases are not acquired locally but occur in travelers to tropical and subtropical regions, particularly those who have walked barefoot or have unprotected skin contact on beaches.

The **incubation period** is typically short, with signs and symptoms developing several days after larval penetration of the skin.

DIAGNOSTIC TESTS

The diagnosis is made clinically, and biopsies are not indicated. Biopsy specimens typically demonstrate an eosinophilic inflammatory infiltrate, but the migrating parasite is not visualized. Eosinophilia and increased immunoglobulin E serum concentrations occur in some cases. Larvae have been detected in sputum and gastric washings in patients with the rare complication of pneumonitis. Enzyme immunoassay or Western blot analysis by using antigens of *A caninum* have been developed in research laboratories, but these assays are not available for routine diagnostic use.

TREATMENT

The disease is usually self-limited, with spontaneous cure after several weeks; treatment may hasten resolution of symptoms. Orally administered ivermectin or albendazole is the recommended therapy. The safety of ivermectin in children weighing less than 15 kg and in pregnant women has not been established. Ingestion of ivermectin with a meal increases its bioavailability.

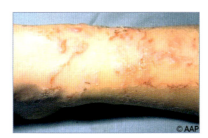

Image 39.1
Cutaneous larva migrans lesions on the leg (caused by hookworm larvae of *Ancylostoma braziliense* and *Ancylostoma caninum*).

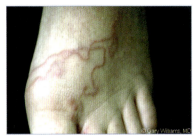

Image 39.2
Cutaneous larva migrans lesions of the foot of a 10-year-old girl. In the United States, this dog and cat hookworm infection is most commonly encountered in the Southeast. These raised, serpiginous, pruritic, migrating eruptions may extend rapidly. Copyright Gary Williams, MD.

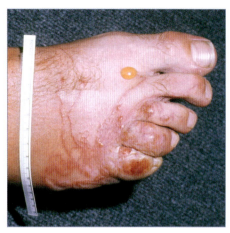

Image 39.3
Cutaneous larva migrans infection of the foot in an adolescent boy. Courtesy of George Nankervis, MD.

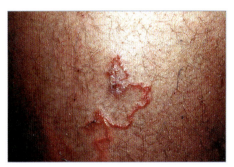

Image 39.4
Adult who noted a migrating skin lesion on the left thigh for 2 weeks. Copyright Larry I. Corman.

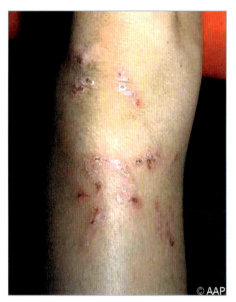

Image 39.5
Cutaneous larva migrans 48 hours after treatment. Orally administered albendazole or ivermectin is the recommended therapy.

CHAPTER 40
Cyclosporiasis

CLINICAL MANIFESTATIONS

Watery diarrhea is the most common symptom of cyclosporiasis and can be profuse and protracted. Anorexia, nausea, vomiting, substantial weight loss, flatulence, abdominal cramping, myalgia, and prolonged fatigue can occur. Low-grade fever occurs in approximately 50% of patients. Biliary tract disease has been reported. Infection is usually self-limited, but untreated people may have remitting, relapsing symptoms for weeks to months. Asymptomatic infection has been documented most commonly in settings where cyclosporiasis is endemic.

ETIOLOGY

Cyclospora cayetanensis is a coccidian protozoan; oocysts (rather than cysts) are passed in stools. These oocysts must then sporulate at temperatures between 22 and 32 °C (72 and 90 °F) for days to weeks before they are infectious.

EPIDEMIOLOGY

C cayetanensis is endemic in many resource-limited countries and has been reported as a cause of travelers diarrhea. Foodborne and waterborne outbreaks have been reported. Most outbreaks in the United States and Canada for which a food vehicle and its source have been identified have been associated with consumption of imported fresh produce (eg, basil, cilantro, raspberries, sugar snap peas, lettuce).

Humans are the only known hosts for *C cayetanensis*. Direct person-to-person transmission is unlikely, because excreted oocysts take days to weeks under favorable environmental conditions to sporulate and become infective. Oocysts are resistant to most disinfectants used in food and water processing and can remain viable for prolonged periods in cool, moist environments.

The **incubation period** is typically 1 week but can range from 2 days to 2 weeks or more.

DIAGNOSTIC TESTS

Diagnosis is made by identification of oocysts (8–10 μm in diameter) in stool, intestinal fluid/aspirates, or intestinal biopsy specimens. Oocysts may be shed at low levels, even by people with profuse diarrhea. This constraint underscores the utility of repeated stool examinations, sensitive recovery methods (eg, concentration procedures including formalin–ethyl acetate sedimentation or sucrose centrifugal flotation), and detection methods that highlight the organism. Oocysts are autofluorescent and are variably acid fast after modified acid-fast staining of stool specimens. Molecular diagnostic assays (eg, polymerase chain reaction) are available commercially as part of a multiplex gastrointestinal panel and at the Centers for Disease Control and Prevention.

TREATMENT

Trimethoprim-sulfamethoxazole, typically for 7 to 10 days, is the drug of choice; immunocompromised patients may need longer courses of therapy. No highly effective alternatives have been identified for people who cannot tolerate trimethoprim-sulfamethoxazole.

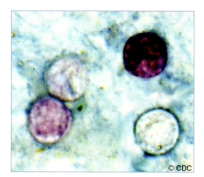

Image 40.1
Four *Cyclospora* oocysts from fresh stool fixed in 10% formalin (acid-fast stain). Compared with the oocysts of wet mounts, the oocysts from fixation are less perfectly round and have a wrinkled appearance. Most important, the staining is variable among the 4 oocysts. Courtesy of Centers for Disease Control and Prevention.

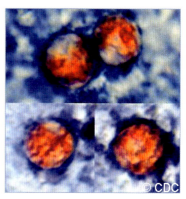

Image 40.2
Four *Cyclospora* oocysts from fresh stool fixed in 10% formalin and stained with safranin, showing the uniform staining of oocysts by this method. Courtesy of Centers for Disease Control and Prevention.

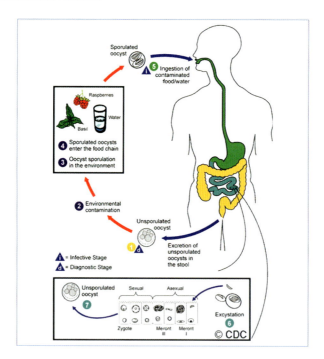

Image 40.3
Cyclospora cayetanensis. When freshly passed in stools, the oocyst is noninfective (1) (thus, direct fecal-oral transmission cannot occur; this differentiates *Cyclospora* from another important coccidian parasite, *Cryptosporidium*). In the environment (2), sporulation occurs after days or weeks at temperatures between 22 and 32 °C (71.6 and 89.6 °F), resulting in division of the sporont into 2 sporocysts, each containing 2 elongate sporozoites (3). Fresh produce and water can serve as vehicles for transmission (4), and the sporulated oocysts are ingested (in contaminated food or water) (5). The oocysts excyst in the gastrointestinal tract, freeing the sporozoites, which invade the epithelial cells of the small intestine (6). Inside the cells, they undergo asexual multiplication and sexual development to mature into oocysts, which will be shed in stools (7). The potential mechanisms of contamination of food and water are still under investigation. Some of elements of this figure were created on the basis of an illustration by Ortega et al. Courtesy of Centers for Disease Control and Prevention.

CHAPTER 41
Cystoisosporiasis (formerly Isosporiasis)

CLINICAL MANIFESTATIONS

Watery diarrhea is the most common symptom of cystoisosporiasis and can be profuse and protracted, even in immunocompetent people. Manifestations are similar to those caused by other enteric protozoa (eg, *Cryptosporidium* and *Cyclospora* species) and can include abdominal pain, cramping, anorexia, nausea, vomiting, weight loss, and low-grade fever. The proportion of infected people who are asymptomatic is unknown. Severity of infection ranges from self-limiting in immunocompetent hosts to chronic, debilitating, sometimes life-threatening diarrheal infection with wasting in immunocompromised patients, particularly people infected with HIV. Infections of the biliary tract and reactive arthritis have also been reported. Peripheral eosinophilia may occur.

ETIOLOGY

Cystoisospora belli (formerly *Isospora belli*) is a coccidian protozoan; oocysts (rather than cysts) are passed in stools.

EPIDEMIOLOGY

Infection occurs predominantly in tropical and subtropical regions of the world and results from ingestion of sporulated oocysts (eg, in food or water contaminated with human feces). Humans are the only known host for *C belli* and shed noninfective oocysts in feces. These oocysts must mature (sporulate) outside the host in the environment to become infective. Under favorable conditions, sporulation can be completed in 1 to 2 days and perhaps more quickly in some settings. Oocysts are probably resistant to most disinfectants and can remain viable for prolonged periods in a cool, moist environment.

The **incubation period** averages 1 week but may range from several days to 2 or more weeks.

DIAGNOSTIC TESTS

Identification of oocysts in feces or in duodenal aspirates or finding of developmental stages of the parasite in biopsy specimens (eg, of the small intestine) is diagnostic. Oocysts in stool are elongate and ellipsoidal (length, 25–35 μm). Oocysts can be shed in low numbers, even by people with profuse diarrhea. This underscores the utility of repeated stool examinations and sensitive recovery methods (eg, concentration methods) and the need for detection methods that highlight the organism (eg, oocysts stain bright red with modified acid-fast staining techniques and autofluoresce when viewed with UV fluorescence microscopy). Like *Cryptosporidium* and *Cyclospora* species, *Cystoisospora* organisms are not usually detected by routine stool ova and parasite examination. Therefore, the laboratory should be notified specifically when any coccidian parasite is suspected on clinical grounds so any special microscopic methods are used in addition to traditional ova and parasite examination.

TREATMENT

In the immunocompetent host, treatment may be unnecessary, because symptoms are usually self-limited. If symptoms do not start to resolve by 5 to 7 days, and in immunocompromised patients, trimethoprim-sulfamethoxazole, typically for 7 to 10 days, is the drug of choice. Immunocompromised patients may need higher doses and longer therapy. Pyrimethamine (plus leucovorin, to prevent myelosuppression) is an alternative for people who cannot tolerate (or whose infection does not respond to) trimethoprim-sulfamethoxazole. Nitazoxanide has been reported to be effective, but data are limited. In adolescents and adults coinfected with HIV with $CD4^+$ T-lymphocyte counts of less than 200/μL, maintenance therapy is recommended to prevent recurrent disease. In adults, secondary prophylaxis may be discontinued once the $CD4^+$ T-lymphocyte count is greater than 200/μL for longer than 6 months because of antiretroviral therapy (ART). In children, a reasonable time to discontinue secondary prophylaxis would be after sustained improvement (for >6 months) in $CD4^+$ T-lymphocyte count or $CD4^+$ T-lymphocyte percentage from Centers for Disease Control and Prevention immunologic category 3 to 1 or 2, in response to ART. These individuals should be monitored closely for recurrent symptoms. Supportive treatment of dehydration and/or malnutrition associated with severe diarrheal illness may be required.

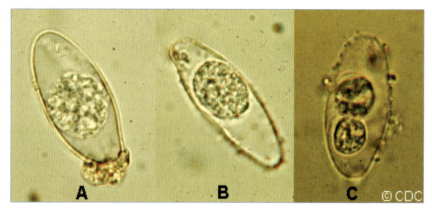

Image 41.1
Oocysts of *Cystoisospora belli* (iodine stain). The oocysts are large (25–30 μm) and have a typical ellipsoidal shape. When excreted, they are immature and contain 1 sporoblast (A, B). The oocyst matures after excretion; the single sporoblast divides into 2 sporoblasts (C), which develop cyst walls, becoming sporocysts, which eventually contain 4 sporozoites each. Courtesy of Centers for Disease Control and Prevention.

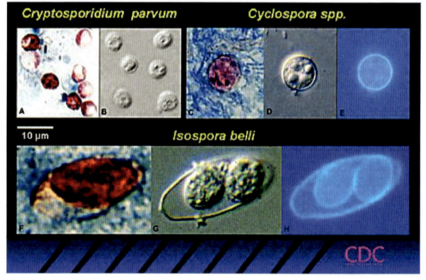

Image 41.2
Oocysts of *Cystoisospora belli* can also be stained with acid-fast stain and visualized by epifluorescence on wet mounts, as illustrated. Three coccidian parasites that most commonly infect humans, observed in acid-fast stained smears (A, C, F), bright-field differential interference contrast (B, D, G), and epifluorescence (E, H, C; *Cryptosporidium parvum* oocysts do not autofluoresce). Courtesy of Centers for Disease Control and Prevention.

CYSTOISOSPORIASIS (FORMERLY ISOSPORIASIS)

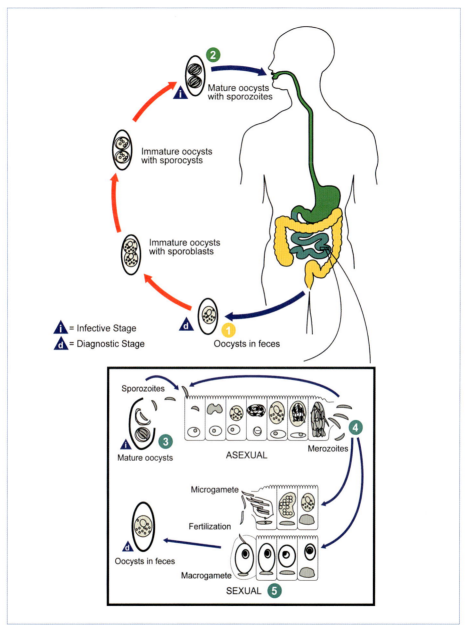

Image 41.3
At excretion, the immature oocyst usually contains 1 sporoblast (more rarely, 2) (1). In further maturation after excretion, the sporoblast divides into 2 (the oocyst now contains 2 sporoblasts); the sporoblasts secrete a cyst wall, thus becoming sporocysts; and the sporocysts divide twice to produce 4 sporozoites each (2). Infection occurs by ingestion of sporocyst-containing oocysts. The sporocysts excyst in the small intestine and release their sporozoites, which invade the epithelial cells and initiate schizogony (3). On rupture of the schizonts, the merozoites are released, invade new epithelial cells, and continue the cycle of asexual multiplication (4). Trophozoites develop into schizonts that contain multiple merozoites. After a minimum of 1 week, the sexual stage begins with the development of male and female gametocytes (5). Fertilization results in the development of oocysts that are excreted in the stool (1). *Cystoisospora belli* infects humans and animals. Courtesy of Centers for Disease Control and Prevention.

CHAPTER 42
Cytomegalovirus Infection

CLINICAL MANIFESTATIONS

Manifestations of acquired human cytomegalovirus (CMV) infection vary with the age and immunocompetence of the host. Asymptomatic infections are the most common, particularly in children. An infectious mononucleosis-like syndrome with prolonged fever and mild hepatitis, occurring in the absence of heterophile antibody production ("monospot negative"), may occur in adolescents and adults. End-organ disease, including pneumonia, colitis, retinitis, meningoencephalitis, or transverse myelitis, or a CMV syndrome characterized by fever, thrombocytopenia, leukopenia, and mild hepatitis may occur in immunocompromised hosts, including people receiving treatment of malignant neoplasms, people infected with HIV, and people receiving immunosuppressive therapy for solid organ or hematopoietic stem cell transplant. Less commonly, patients treated with biologic response modifiers can exhibit CMV end-organ disease, such as retinitis and hepatitis.

Congenital CMV infection has a spectrum of clinical manifestations but is not usually evident at birth (asymptomatic congenital CMV infection). Approximately 10% of infants with congenital CMV infection exhibit clinical findings that are evident at birth (symptomatic congenital CMV disease), with manifestations including jaundice attributable to direct hyperbilirubinemia, petechiae attributable to thrombocytopenia, purpura, hepatosplenomegaly, microcephaly, intracerebral (typically periventricular) calcifications, and retinitis; developmental delays can occur in affected infants in later infancy and early childhood. Death attributable to congenital CMV is estimated to occur in 3% to 10% of infants with symptomatic disease or 0.3% to 1.0% of all infants with congenital CMV infection.

Congenital CMV infection is the leading nongenetic cause of sensorineural hearing loss (SNHL) in children in the United States. Approximately 20% of all hearing loss at birth and 25% of all hearing loss at 4 years of age is attributable to congenital CMV infection. SNHL is the most common sequela following congenital CMV infection, with SNHL occurring in up to 50% of children with congenital infections that are symptomatic at birth and up to 15% of those with asymptomatic infections. Approximately 40% of infected children who ultimately develop SNHL will not have hearing loss detectable within the first month after birth, illustrating the risk of late-onset SNHL in these populations. Approximately 50% of children with CMV-associated SNHL continue to have further deterioration (progression) of their hearing loss over time.

Infection acquired during the intrapartum period from maternal cervical secretions or in the postpartum period from human milk is not usually associated with clinical illness in full-term infants. In preterm infants, however, postpartum infection resulting from human milk or from transfusion from CMV-seropositive donors has been associated with hepatitis, interstitial pneumonia, hematologic abnormalities including thrombocytopenia and leukopenia, and a viral sepsis syndrome.

ETIOLOGY

Human CMV, also known as human herpesvirus 5, is a member of the herpesvirus family (*Herpesviridae*), the beta-herpesvirus subfamily (*Betaherpesvirinae*), and the *Cytomegalovirus* genus. The viral genome contains double-stranded DNA that ranges in size from 196,000 to 240,000 base pairs encoding at least 166 proteins and is the largest of the human herpesvirus genomes.

EPIDEMIOLOGY

CMV is highly species specific, and only human CMV has been shown to infect and cause disease in humans. The virus is ubiquitous, and CMV strains exhibit extensive genetic diversity. Transmission occurs horizontally (by direct person-to-person contact with virus-containing secretions), vertically (from mother to infant before, during, or after birth), and via transfusions of blood, platelets, and white blood cells from infected donors. CMV can also be transmitted with solid organ or hematopoietic stem cell transplant. Infections have no seasonal predilection. CMV persists in leukocytes and tissue cells after a primary infection, with intermittent virus shedding; symptomatic infection can occur throughout the lifetime of the infected person, particularly under conditions of immunosuppression. Reinfection with other strains of CMV can occur in seropositive hosts, including pregnant women. In the United States, there appears to be 3 periods in life when there is an increased incidence of CMV acquisition: early childhood, adolescence, and the childbearing years.

Horizontal transmission probably results from exposure to saliva, urine, or genital secretions from infected individuals. Spread of CMV in households and child care centers is well-documented. Excretion rates from urine or saliva in children 1 to 3 years of age who attend child care centers usually range from 30% to 40% but can be as high as 70%. In addition, children who attend child care frequently excrete large quantities of virus for prolonged periods. Young children can transmit CMV to their parents, including mothers who may be pregnant, and other caregivers, including child care staff. In adolescents and adults, sexual transmission occurs, as evidenced by detection of virus in seminal and cervical fluids. As such, CMV is considered a sexually transmitted infection.

CMV-seropositive healthy people have latent CMV in their leukocytes and tissues; hence, blood transfusions and organ transplant can result in transmission. Severe CMV disease following transfusion or solid organ transplant is more likely to occur if the recipient is CMV seronegative before transplant. In contrast, among nonautologous hematopoietic stem cell transplant recipients, CMV-seropositive individuals who receive transplants from seronegative donors have greatest risk for disease when exposed to CMV after transplant, likely because of the failure of the transplanted graft to provide immunity to the recipient. Latent CMV may reactivate in immunosuppressed individuals and result in disease if immunosuppression is severe (eg, in patients with AIDS or with solid organ or hematopoietic stem cell transplant).

Vertical transmission of CMV to an infant occurs in one of the following periods: (1) in utero, by transplacental passage of maternal bloodborne virus; or (2) at birth, by passage through an infected maternal genital tract. Postnatal acquisition occurs via ingestion of CMV-positive human milk. Approximately 5 per 1,000 live-born infants are infected in utero and excrete CMV at birth, making this the most common congenital viral infection in the United States. Significant racial and ethnic differences exist in the prevalence of congenital CMV, with the highest prevalence of CMV among Black newborns (9.5 per 1,000 live births) and lower prevalence in non-Hispanic white infants (2.7 per 1,000 live births) and Hispanic white infants (3.0 per 1,000 live births). In utero fetal infection can occur in women with no preexisting CMV immunity (maternal primary infection) or in women with preexisting antibody to CMV (maternal nonprimary infection) by acquisition of a different viral strain during pregnancy or by reactivation of an existing maternal infection. Congenital infection and associated sequelae can occur irrespective of the trimester of pregnancy when the mother is infected, but severe sequelae are associated more commonly with maternal infection acquired during the first trimester. Damaging fetal infections and sequelae can occur following both primary and nonprimary maternal infections. It is estimated that more than three-quarters of infants with congenital CMV infection in the United States are born to women with nonprimary infection, and in populations with higher maternal CMV seroprevalence than that of the United States, most damaging congenital CMV infections occur in infants born to women with nonprimary infection.

Among infants who acquire infection from maternal cervical secretions or human milk, preterm infants born before 32 weeks' gestation and with a birth weight less than 1,500 g have greater risk for developing CMV disease than do full-term infants. Most infants who acquire CMV from ingestion of human milk from CMV-seropositive mothers do not develop clinical illness or sequelae, likely because of the presence of passively transferred maternal antibody.

The **incubation period** for horizontally transmitted CMV infections is highly variable. Infection usually manifests 3 to 12 weeks after blood transfusions and 1 to 4 months after organ transplant. For vertical transmission through human milk in preterm infants, the median time to onset of CMV viruria is 7 weeks (range, 3–24 weeks).

DIAGNOSTIC TESTS

The diagnosis of CMV disease is confounded by the ubiquity of the virus, the high rate of asymptomatic excretion, the frequency of reactivated infections, reinfection with different strains of CMV, the development of serum immunoglobulin M (IgM) CMV-specific antibody in some episodes of reactivation and reinfection, and concurrent infection with other pathogens.

Viral DNA can be detected by polymerase chain reaction (PCR) and other nucleic acid amplification assays in tissues and some fluids, including cerebrospinal fluid (CSF), amniotic fluid, human milk, aqueous and vitreous humor fluids, urine, saliva and other respiratory secretions, and peripheral blood. Detection of CMV DNA by PCR assay in blood does not necessarily indicate acute infection or disease, especially in immunocompetent people. Several quantitative PCR assays for detection of CMV have been cleared by the US Food and Drug Administration (FDA). These assays are sensitive, provide more rapid results than culture, and are generally the preferred method for detecting viremia. The same specimen type should always be used when testing any given patient over time. Antigenemia assays have also been cleared by the FDA, but they are labor intensive and require timely processing of specimens to obtain accurate results.

CMV can be isolated in conventional cell culture from urine, saliva, peripheral blood leukocytes, human milk, semen, cervical secretions, and other tissues and body fluids. Recovery of virus from a target organ provides strong evidence that the disease is caused by CMV infection. Standard viral cultures must be maintained for more than 28 days before considering such cultures negative.

Various serological assays, including immunofluorescence assays, latex agglutination assays, and enzyme immunoassays, are available for detecting both immunoglobulin G (IgG) and IgM CMV-specific antibodies. Single serum specimens for IgG antibody testing are useful in screening for past infection in individuals with risk for CMV reactivation or for screening potential organ transplant donors and recipients. For diagnosis of suspected recent infection, testing for CMV IgG in paired sera obtained at least 2 weeks apart and testing for IgM in a single serum specimen may be useful.

Fetal CMV infection can be diagnosed by detection of CMV DNA in amniotic fluid. Congenital infection with CMV requires detection of CMV or CMV DNA in urine, saliva, blood, or CSF obtained within 3 weeks of birth; detection beyond this initial period after birth could reflect postnatal acquisition of virus. PCR testing of saliva swab specimens from neonates has been shown to be more than 95% sensitive for the identification of congenital CMV infection. Positive saliva swab specimen test results may require confirmation with testing of urine because of potential contamination of saliva with CMV in human milk. The analytical sensitivity of CMV PCR of dried blood spots is low, limiting use of this type of specimen for widespread screening for congenital CMV infection. A positive PCR assay result from a neonatal dried blood spot confirms congenital infection, but a negative result does not rule out congenital infection. Differentiation between congenital and perinatal infection is difficult at later than 2 to 4 weeks of age unless clinical manifestations of the former, such as chorioretinitis or intracranial calcifications, are present.

TREATMENT

Intravenous ganciclovir is approved for induction and maintenance treatment of retinitis caused by acquired or recurrent CMV infection in immunocompromised adult patients, including HIV-infected patients, and for prophylaxis and treatment of CMV disease in adult transplant recipients. Valganciclovir, the oral prodrug of ganciclovir, is approved for treatment (induction and maintenance) of CMV retinitis in immunocompromised adult patients, including HIV-infected patients, and for prevention of CMV disease in kidney, kidney-pancreas, or heart transplant recipients with high risk for CMV disease. Valganciclovir is also approved for prevention of CMV disease in pediatric kidney transplant patients 4 months and older and for pediatric heart transplant patients 1 month and older. Ganciclovir and valganciclovir are used to treat CMV infections of other sites (ie, esophagus, colon, lungs) and for preemptive treatment of immunosuppressed adults with CMV antigenemia or viremia. Valganciclovir is available in both tablet and powder for oral solution formulations.

Neonates with symptomatic congenital CMV disease with or without central nervous system involvement have improved audiological and neurodevelopmental outcomes at 2 years of age when treated with oral valganciclovir for 6 months. Therapy can be accomplished by using oral valganciclovir for the entire treatment course, because drug exposure following appropriate dosing of valganciclovir is the same as that achieved with intravenous ganciclovir. If an infant is unable to absorb medications reliably from the gastrointestinal tract (eg, because of necrotizing enterocolitis or other bowel disorders), intravenous ganciclovir can be used initially. Significant neutropenia occurs in one-fifth of infants treated with oral valganciclovir and in two-thirds of infants treated with parenteral ganciclovir. Absolute neutrophil counts should be performed weekly for 6 weeks, then at 8 weeks, then monthly for the duration of antiviral treatment; serum alanine aminotransferase concentration should be measured monthly during treatment. Antiviral therapy should be limited to patients with moderate to severe symptomatic congenital CMV disease who are able to start treatment within the first month after birth. Infants with asymptomatic congenital CMV infection should not receive antiviral treatment. Neonates with mild symptomatic disease or with isolated SNHL and no other disease manifestations should not routinely receive antiviral treatment, because of a lack of data suggesting benefit in this less severely affected population.

Patients with symptomatic or asymptomatic congenital CMV infection should undergo serial audiological assessments throughout childhood.

Preterm infants with perinatally acquired CMV infection can have symptomatic, end-organ disease (eg, pneumonitis, hepatitis, thrombocytopenia). Antiviral treatment has not been studied in this population. If such patients are treated with parenteral ganciclovir, a reasonable approach is to treat for 2 weeks and then reassess responsiveness to therapy. If clinical data suggest benefit of treatment, an additional 1 to 2 weeks of parenteral ganciclovir can be considered if symptoms and signs have not resolved.

In hematopoietic stem cell transplant recipients, the combination of immune globulin intravenous (IGIV) or CMV IGIV and intravenous ganciclovir has been reported to be synergistic in treatment of CMV pneumonia. Valganciclovir and foscarnet have been approved for treatment of and maintenance therapy for CMV retinitis in adults with AIDS, and letermovir has been approved for prophylaxis of CMV infection and disease in adult CMV-seropositive recipients of an allogeneic hematopoietic stem cell transplant. Foscarnet is more toxic (with high rates of limiting nephrotoxicity) but may be advantageous for some patients with HIV infection, including people with disease caused by ganciclovir-resistant virus or people who are unable to tolerate ganciclovir. Cidofovir is efficacious for CMV retinitis in adults with AIDS but is associated with significant nephrotoxicity.

CMV establishes lifelong persistent infection; as such, it is not eliminated from the body with antiviral treatment of CMV disease. Until immune reconstitution is achieved with antiretroviral therapy, chronic suppressive therapy should be administered to HIV-infected patients with a history of CMV end-organ disease (eg, retinitis, colitis, pneumonitis) to prevent recurrence. Discontinuing prophylaxis may be considered for pediatric patients 6 years and older with $CD4^+$ T-lymphocyte counts of greater than $100/\mu L$ for more than 6 consecutive months and for children younger than 6 years with $CD4^+$ T-lymphocyte percentages of greater than 15% for more than 6 consecutive months. All patients whose anti-CMV maintenance therapy has been discontinued should continue to undergo regular ophthalmologic monitoring at 3- to 6-month intervals for early detection of CMV relapse as well as immune reconstitution uveitis.

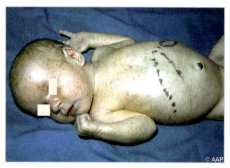

Image 42.1
A 3-week-old with congenital cytomegalovirus infection with purpuric skin lesions and hepatosplenomegaly. Courtesy of Edgar O. Ledbetter, MD, FAAP.

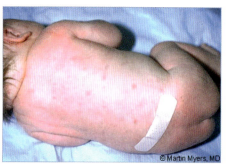

Image 42.2
A newborn with cytomegalovirus infection and hemorrhagic skin lesions on the back.

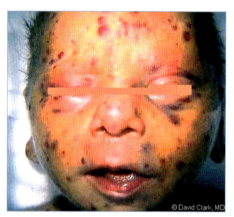

Image 42.3
Cytomegalovirus infection, congenital, with characteristic "blueberry muffin" lesions. Copyright David Clark, MD.

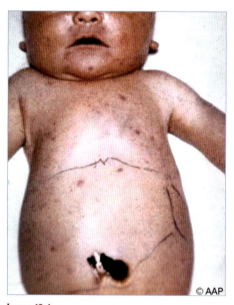

Image 42.4
Infant with lethal congenital cytomegalovirus disease with purpuric skin lesions and striking hepatosplenomegaly. Courtesy of Edgar O. Ledbetter, MD, FAAP.

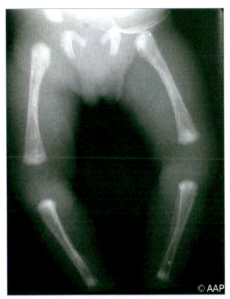

Image 42.5
Infant in Image 42.4, with lethal cytomegalovirus disease, with radiographic changes in long bones of osteitis characterized by fine vertical metaphyseal striations. Courtesy of Edgar O. Ledbetter, MD, FAAP.

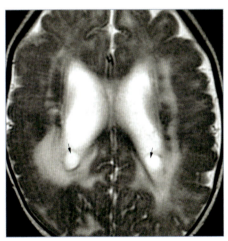

Image 42.8
Axial T2-weighted magnetic resonance image demonstrates periventricular germinolytic cysts (arrows). Also notable are the periventricular white matter hyperintensities that represent demyelination and gliosis.

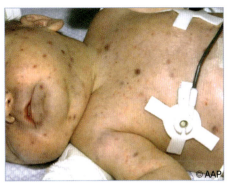

Image 42.6
Neonate with congenital cytomegalovirus infection with purpuric skin lesions.

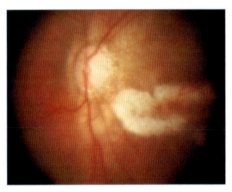

Image 42.7
Characteristic white perivascular infiltrates in the retina of an infant with congenital cytomegalovirus infection. Courtesy of George Nankervis, MD.

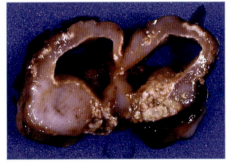

Image 42.9
Congenital cytomegalovirus encephalitis. Microcephaly and cerebral calcification. Courtesy of Dimitris P. Agamanolis, MD.

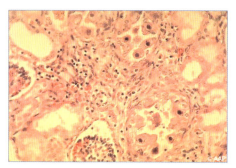

Image 42.10
Cytomegalovirus inclusion cells within renal glomeruli. Courtesy of Edgar O. Ledbetter, MD, FAAP.

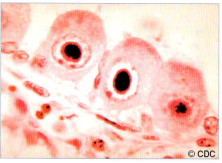

Image 42.11
Histopathologic features of cytomegalovirus infection of the kidney. Intranuclear inclusions are surrounded by a halo and the nuclear membrane, giving an owl-eye appearance. Courtesy of Centers for Disease Control and Prevention.

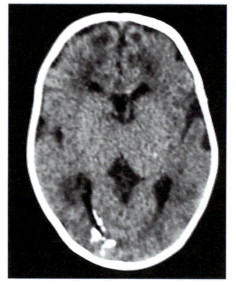

Image 42.12
Cytomegalovirus infection with periventricular calcification. Courtesy of Benjamin Estrada, MD.

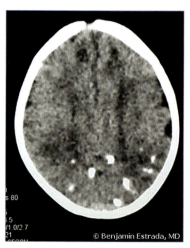

Image 42.13
Cytomegalovirus infection with periventricular calcification. Courtesy of Benjamin Estrada, MD.

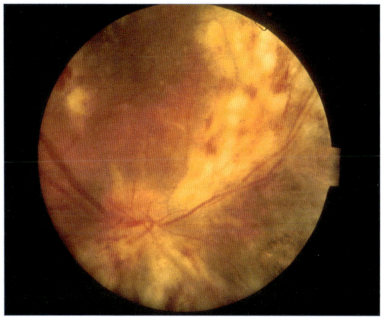

Image 42.14
Widespread "brushfire retinitis" in an infant with congenital cytomegalovirus infection. The perivascular infiltrates and diffuse hemorrhage may result in complete blindness whenever macular involvement occurs. Courtesy of George Nankervis, MD.

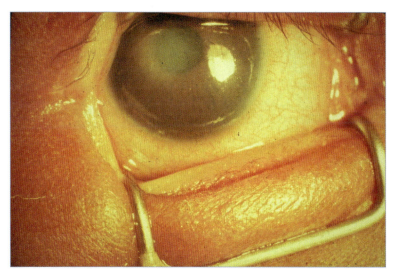

Image 42.15
A neonate with congenital cytomegalovirus infection with Peters anomaly, which was later treated by corneal transplant. *Peters anomaly* is the term most frequently used when the mesodermal dysgenesis of the anterior ocular segment includes a central stromal opacity with a defect in the posterior stroma and the Descemet membrane. Courtesy of Larry Frenkel, MD.

CHAPTER 43
Dengue

CLINICAL MANIFESTATIONS

Dengue infection may be asymptomatic or, if symptomatic, may have a wide range of clinical manifestations. The 2009 World Health Organization classification for dengue severity is divided into (1) **Dengue without warning signs:** fever plus 2 of the following criteria: nausea/vomiting, rash, aches and pains, leukopenia, or positive tourniquet test; (2) **Dengue with warning signs:** dengue as defined above plus any of the following criteria: abdominal pain or tenderness, persistent vomiting, clinical fluid accumulation (ie, ascites, pleural effusion), mucosal bleeding, lethargy, restlessness, or liver enlargement greater than 2 cm; and (3) **Severe dengue:** dengue with at least one of the following criteria: severe plasma leakage leading to shock or fluid accumulation with respiratory distress, severe bleeding as evaluated by a clinician, or severe organ involvement (eg, aspartate aminotransferase or alanine aminotransferase ≥1,000 IU/L, impaired consciousness, failure of heart and other organs). Less common clinical syndromes include myocarditis, pancreatitis, hepatitis, hemophagocytic lymphohistiocytosis, and neurological disease, including acute meningoencephalitis and post-dengue acute disseminated encephalomyelitis.

Dengue begins abruptly with a nonspecific, acute febrile illness lasting 2 to 7 days (**febrile phase**), often accompanied by muscle, joint, and/or bone pain; headache; retro-orbital pain; facial erythema; injected oropharynx; macular or maculopapular rash; leukopenia; and petechiae or other minor bleeding manifestations. During defervescence, usually on days 3 through 7 of illness, an increase in vascular permeability in parallel with increasing hematocrit (hemoconcentration) may occur. The period of clinically significant plasma leakage usually lasts 24 to 48 hours (**critical phase**), followed by a **convalescent phase** with gradual improvement and stabilization of the hemodynamic status. Warning signs and symptoms of progression to severe dengue occur in the late febrile phase and include persistent vomiting, severe abdominal pain, mucosal bleeding, difficulty breathing, early signs of shock, and a rapid decline in platelet count with an increase in hematocrit. Patients with nonsevere disease begin to improve during the critical phase, but people with clinically significant plasma leakage attributable to increased vascular permeability develop severe disease that may include pleural effusions, ascites, hypovolemic shock, and hemorrhage.

ETIOLOGY

Four related RNA viruses of the genus *Flavivirus*, dengue viruses 1, 2, 3, and 4, cause symptomatic (approximately 25%) and asymptomatic (approximately 75%) infections. Infection with one dengue virus serotype most often produces lifelong immunity against that serotype, and a period of cross-protection (often lasting 1–3 years) against infection with the other 3 serotypes can be observed. After this period of cross-protection, infection with a different serotype may predispose to more severe disease. A person has a lifetime risk of up to 4 dengue virus infections.

EPIDEMIOLOGY

Dengue virus is primarily transmitted to humans through the bite of infected *Aedes aegypti* (and, less commonly, *Aedes albopictus* or *Aedes polynesiensis*) mosquitoes. Humans are the main amplifying host of dengue virus and the main source of virus for *Aedes* mosquitoes. A sylvatic nonhuman primate dengue virus transmission cycle exists in parts of Africa and Southeast Asia but rarely crosses to humans. Other forms of transmission are relatively rare and include vertical transmission; transmission via breastfeeding, blood, or organ donation; and health care–associated transmission via needlestick or mucocutaneous exposure. The rate of vertical transmission is approximately 20% and is even higher when maternal dengue occurs late in pregnancy near delivery. Sexual transmission is also possible but is considered a rare route of infection.

Dengue is a major public health problem in the tropics and subtropics; approximately 3.9 billion people in 128 countries have risk for infection with dengue viruses. Approximately 390 million dengue infections occur annually worldwide, of which 96 million have clinical manifestations, including 500,000 hospitalizations and 20,000 deaths every year. Dengue is endemic in the United States territories of Puerto Rico, the US Virgin Islands, and American Samoa. Puerto Rico has the highest incidence of dengue among all US territories (3,000–27,000 cases per year). Incidence rates are highest from July to September and vary significantly by geographic locale, affected by factors such as population density, elevation, and mosquito breeding and water supply patterns. Outbreaks with local dengue virus transmission have occurred in Texas, Hawaii, and Florida and in Mexican cities bordering Yuma, Arizona (ie, San Luis Río Colorado, Sonora), and Calexico, CA (ie, Mexicali, Baja California). Although up to 28 states now have *A aegypti* and 40 states have *A albopictus* mosquitoes, local dengue virus transmission is uncommon because of infrequent contact between people and infected mosquitoes. Millions of US travelers, including children, have risk; dengue is the leading cause of febrile illness in travelers returning from the Caribbean, Latin America, and South Asia. Dengue occurs in people of all ages but occurs at higher rates among healthy adolescents and young adults and is most likely to cause severe disease in infants, pregnant women, and patients with chronic diseases (eg, asthma, sickle cell anemia, and diabetes mellitus). Severe dengue disease is most likely to occur with second heterologous dengue serotype infections, and although less likely, it can occur with a third or fourth heterologous dengue serotype infections.

The **incubation period** for dengue virus replication in mosquitoes is 8 to 12 days (extrinsic incubation); mosquitoes remain infectious for the remainder of their life cycle. In humans, the **incubation period** is 3 to 14 days before symptom onset (intrinsic incubation). Infected people, both symptomatic and asymptomatic, can transmit dengue virus to mosquitoes 1 to 2 days before symptoms develop and throughout the approximately 7-day viremic period.

DIAGNOSTIC TESTS

Laboratory confirmation of the clinical diagnosis of dengue can be made on a single serum specimen obtained during the febrile phase of the illness by testing both virologically (by detection of dengue virus RNA by reverse transcriptase–polymerase chain reaction [RT-PCR] assay or by detection of dengue virus nonstructural protein 1 [NS-1] antigen by immunoassay) and serologically (anti-dengue virus immunoglobulin M [IgM] antibodies by enzyme immunoassay [EIA]). Dengue virus is detectable by RT-PCR or NS-1 antigen EIAs from the beginning of the febrile phase until day 7 to 10 after illness onset. Anti-dengue virus IgM antibodies are detectable beginning 3 to 5 days after illness onset; 99% of patients have IgM antibodies by day 10. IgM levels peak after 2 weeks and then often decline to undetectable levels over 2 to 3 months but can cross-react with IgM antibodies against Zika virus and other closely related flaviviruses. Testing for NS-1 antigen and anti-dengue IgM in a single serum specimen collected during the first 10 days of illness accurately identifies 90% or more of dengue primary and secondary cases. Anti-dengue virus immunoglobulin G (IgG) antibody titer remains elevated for life after dengue virus infection. Anti-dengue virus IgG antibody may be falsely positive in people with previous infection with or immunization against other flaviviruses (eg, West Nile, Japanese encephalitis, yellow fever, or Zika virus). A 4-fold or greater increase in anti-dengue virus IgG antibody titers between the acute ($\leq$5 days after onset of symptoms) and convalescent ($>$15 days after onset of symptoms) samples confirms recent infection. Dengue diagnostic testing is available through commercial reference laboratories and some state public health laboratories; reference testing is available from the Dengue Branch of the Centers for Disease Control and Prevention (**www.cdc.gov/dengue**).

TREATMENT

No specific antiviral therapy exists for dengue. During the febrile phase, patients should stay well hydrated and avoid use of aspirin (acetylsalicylic acid), salicylate-containing drugs, and other nonsteroidal anti-inflammatory drugs (eg, ibuprofen) to minimize potential for bleeding. Additional supportive care is required if the patient becomes dehydrated or develops warning signs of severe disease at or around the time of defervescence.

Early recognition of shock and intensive supportive therapy can reduce risk of death from severe dengue from approximately 5% to 10% to less than 1%. During the critical phase, maintenance of fluid volume and hemodynamic status is crucial to management of severe cases. Patients should be monitored for early signs of shock, occult bleeding, and plasma leak to avoid prolonged shock, end-organ damage, and fluid overload. It is important to watch for signs of fluid overload, which may manifest as a decrease in the patient's hematocrit level as a result of the dilutional effect of reabsorbed fluid.

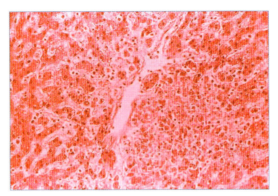

Image 43.1
Cytoarchitectural changes found in a liver tissue specimen extracted from a patient with dengue hemorrhagic fever in Thailand (hematoxylin-eosin stain, magnification ×70). This particular view reveals "mid-lobular necrosis, with accompanying acidophilic degeneration, and moderate hypertrophy of Kupffer cells." Courtesy of Dr Yves Robin and Dr Jean Renaudet, Arbovirus Laboratory at the Pasteur Institute in Dakar, Senegal; World Health Organization.

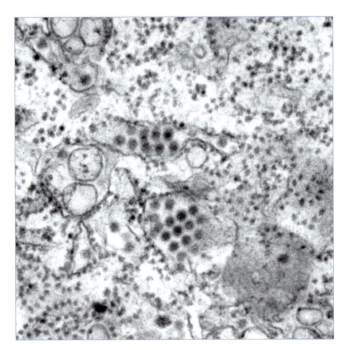

Image 43.2
This transmission electron micrograph depicts a number of round dengue virus particles that were revealed in this tissue specimen. Courtesy of Centers for Disease Control and Prevention.

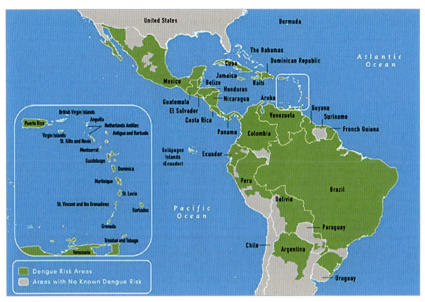

Image 43.3
Distribution of dengue, Western hemisphere. Courtesy of Centers for Disease Control and Prevention.

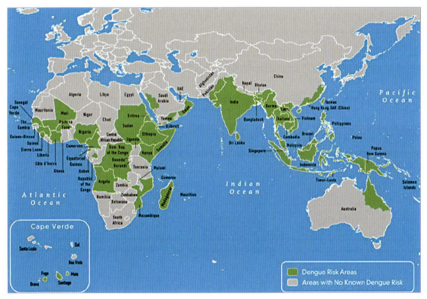

Image 43.4
Distribution of dengue, Eastern hemisphere. Courtesy of Centers for Disease Control and Prevention.

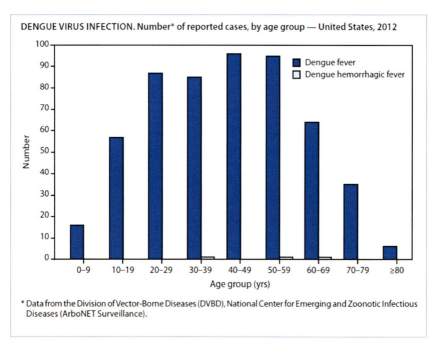

Image 43.5
Dengue virus infection. Number of reported cases, by age-group—United States, 2012. Courtesy of *Morbidity and Mortality Weekly Report.*

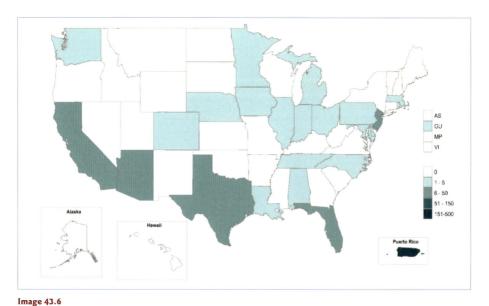

Image 43.6
States and territories reporting dengue cases—United States, 2021 (as of December 1, 2021). Courtesy of Centers for Disease Control and Prevention.

CHAPTER 44
Diphtheria

CLINICAL MANIFESTATIONS

Respiratory tract diphtheria usually manifests as membranous nasopharyngitis, obstructive laryngotracheitis, or bloody nasal discharge. Local infections are associated with low-grade fever and gradual onset of manifestations over 1 to 2 days. Less commonly, diphtheria manifests as cutaneous, vaginal, conjunctival, or otic infection. Cutaneous diphtheria is more common in tropical areas and with urban homelessness. Extensive neck swelling with cervical lymphadenitis (bull neck) is a sign of severe disease. Life-threatening complications of respiratory diphtheria include upper airway obstruction caused by membrane formation; myocarditis, with heart block; and cranial and peripheral neuropathies. Palatal palsy, noted by nasal speech, frequently occurs in pharyngeal diphtheria. Case-fatality rates are 5% to 10%, and up to 50% in untreated people.

ETIOLOGY

Diphtheria is caused by toxigenic strains of *Corynebacterium diphtheriae*. Toxigenic strains of *Corynebacterium ulcerans* have also emerged as an important cause of diphtheria-like illness. *C diphtheriae* is an irregularly staining, gram-positive, non–spore-forming, nonmotile, pleomorphic bacillus with 4 biotypes (*mitis, intermedius, gravis,* and *belfanti*). All biotypes of *C diphtheriae* may be toxigenic or nontoxigenic. Bacteria remain confined to superficial layers of skin or mucosal surfaces, inducing a local inflammatory reaction. Within several days of respiratory tract infection, a dense pseudomembrane forms, becoming adherent to tissue. Toxigenic strains produce an exotoxin that consists of an enzymatically active A domain and a binding B domain, which promotes the entry of A into the cell. The toxin, an ADP-ribosylase toxin, inhibits protein synthesis in all cells, including myocardial, renal, and peripheral nerve cells, resulting in myocarditis, acute tubular necrosis, and delayed peripheral nerve conduction. Nontoxigenic strains of *C diphtheriae* can cause sore throat and, rarely, other invasive infections, including endocarditis and infections related to foreign bodies.

EPIDEMIOLOGY

Humans are the sole reservoir of *C diphtheriae*. Infection is spread by respiratory tract droplets and by contact with discharges from skin lesions. In untreated people, organisms can be present in discharges from the nose and throat and from eye and skin lesions for 2 to 6 weeks after infection. Patients treated with an appropriate antimicrobial agent are not usually infectious 48 hours after treatment is initiated. Transmission results from close contact with patients or carriers. People traveling to areas with endemic diphtheria or people coming into contact with infected travelers from such areas have increased risk for being infected; rarely, fomites or milk products can serve as vehicles of transmission. Severe disease occurs more often in people who are unimmunized or inadequately immunized. Fully immunized people may be asymptomatic carriers or have mild sore throat.

Before 2019, respiratory disease caused by *C diphtheriae*, regardless of toxigenicity status, was nationally notifiable. Beginning in 2019, national notifications were restricted to disease caused by toxigenic *C diphtheriae* but could originate from respiratory or nonrespiratory sites. From 2000 through 2018, 6 cases of respiratory diphtheria were reported in the United States; however, the last bacteriologically confirmed case caused by toxigenic *C diphtheriae* occurred in 1997. There has been increasing recognition of cutaneous diphtheria; 4 toxigenic cases were identified from 2015 to 2018 in travelers to areas with endemic diphtheria. The incidence of respiratory diphtheria is greatest during fall and winter, but summer epidemics may occur in warm climates where skin infections are prevalent. Globally, endemic diphtheria occurs in Africa, Latin American, Asia, the Middle East, and parts of Europe where immunization coverage with diphtheria toxoid–containing vaccines is suboptimal. Since 2011, large outbreaks have been reported in Indonesia, Laos, Haiti, Venezuela, Yemen, and Bangladesh. In 2017, the World Health Organization reported 8,819 global cases of diphtheria.

The **incubation period** is usually 2 to 5 days (range, 1–10 days).

DIAGNOSTIC TESTS

Laboratory personnel should be notified that *C diphtheriae* is suspected. Specimens for culture should be obtained from the nares and throat or any mucosal or cutaneous lesion. Obtaining multiple samples from respiratory sites increases yield of culture. Material should be obtained for culture from beneath the membrane (if present) or a portion of the membrane. Specimens collected for culture can be placed into any transport medium or into a sterile container and transported at 4 °C (39 °F). All isolates of *C diphtheriae* should be sent through the state health department to the Centers for Disease Control and Prevention (CDC) to verify toxigenicity status.

TREATMENT

Antitoxin

Because patients can deteriorate rapidly, a single dose of diphtheria (equine) antitoxin (DAT) should be administered on the basis of clinical manifestation, history of travel, and vaccination status before culture results are available. DAT, its indications for use, suggested dosage, and instructions for administration are available through the CDC (CDC Emergency Operations Center [telephone: 770/488-7100] or **www.cdc.gov/diphtheria/dat.html**). DAT is not available from any commercial source. To neutralize toxin as rapidly as possible, intravenous administration of antitoxin is preferred. Before intravenous administration of antitoxin, tests for sensitivity to horse serum should be performed according to instructions provided with the material. Allergic reactions to horse serum varying from anaphylaxis to rash can be expected in 5% to 20% of patients. The dose of antitoxin depends on the site and size of the membrane, duration of illness, and degree of toxic effects, and specific recommendations are available from the CDC.

Antimicrobial Therapy

Erythromycin administered orally or parenterally for 14 days, aqueous penicillin G administered intravenously for 14 days, or penicillin G procaine administered intramuscularly for 14 days constitutes acceptable therapy. Antimicrobial therapy is required to stop toxin production, eradicate *C diphtheriae* organism, and prevent transmission but is not a substitute for antitoxin. Elimination of the organisms should be documented 24 hours after completion of treatment by 2 consecutive negative cultures from specimens taken 24 hours apart.

Immunization

Active immunization against diphtheria should be undertaken during convalescence from diphtheria, because disease does not necessarily confer immunity.

Cutaneous Diphtheria

Thorough cleansing of the lesion with soap and water and administration of an appropriate antimicrobial agent for 10 days are recommended.

Carriers (Regardless of Toxigenic Strain or Not)

If unimmunized, carriers should receive active immunization promptly and measures should be taken to ensure completion of the immunization schedule. If a carrier has been immunized previously but has not received a booster of diphtheria toxoid within 5 years, a booster dose of age-appropriate vaccine containing diphtheria toxoid (DTaP, Tdap, DT, or Td) should be administered. Carriers should receive oral erythromycin for 10 to 14 days or a single intramuscular dose of penicillin G benzathine (600,000 U for children weighing <30 kg and 1.2 million U for children weighing ≥30 kg or adults). Two follow-up cultures should be performed after completing antimicrobial treatment to detect persistence of carriage, which occurs following erythromycin treatment in some cases. The first culture should be performed 24 hours after completing treatment. If results of cultures are positive, an additional 10-day course of oral erythromycin should be administered, and follow-up cultures should be performed again.

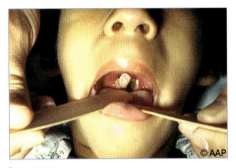

Image 44.1
Pharyngeal diphtheria with membranes covering the tonsils and uvula in a 15-year-old girl. Tonsillar and pharyngeal diphtheria may need to be differentiated from group A streptococcal pharyngitis, infectious mononucleosis, Vincent angina, acute toxoplasmosis, thrush, and leukemia, as well as other, less common entities, including tularemia and acute cytomegalovirus infection.

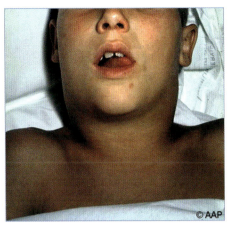

Image 44.2
Bull neck appearance of diphtheritic cervical lymphadenopathy in a 13-year-old boy.

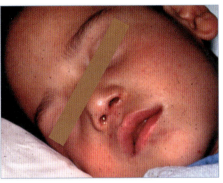

Image 44.3
A 5-year old boy with nasal diphtheria. Courtesy of Paul Wehrle, MD.

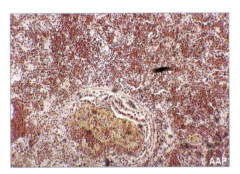

Image 44.4
Diphtheria pneumonia (hemorrhagic) with bronchiolar membranes (hematoxylin-eosin stain). Courtesy of Edgar O. Ledbetter, MD, FAAP.

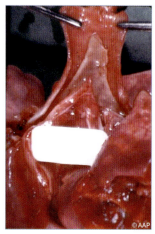

Image 44.5
Diphtheritic tracheobronchial membranes at autopsy of the patient in Image 44.4. Courtesy of Edgar O. Ledbetter, MD, FAAP.

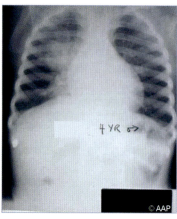

Image 44.6
A 4-year-old boy with fatal sub-laryngeal tracheal diphtheria and hemorrhagic diphtheria pneumonia. Courtesy of Edgar O. Ledbetter, MD, FAAP.

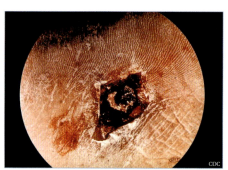

Image 44.7
This is a close-up of a diphtheria skin lesion caused by the organism *Corynebacterium diphtheriae*. Courtesy of Centers for Disease Control and Prevention/Brodsky, MD.

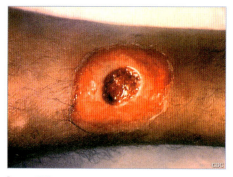

Image 44.8
A diphtheria skin lesion on the leg. *Corynebacterium diphtheriae* can not only affect the respiratory, cardiovascular, renal, and neurological systems but the cutaneous system as well, where it sometimes manifests as an open, isolated wound. Courtesy of Centers for Disease Control and Prevention.

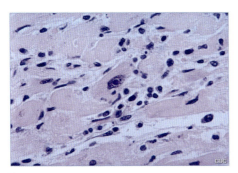

Image 44.9
This micrograph reveals an intranuclear inclusion body in a heart section from a patient with diphtheria-related myocarditis. Courtesy of Centers for Disease Control and Prevention/Martin Hicklin, MD.

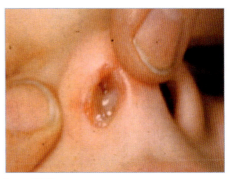

Image 44.10
Nasal membrane of diphtheria in a preschool-aged boy. Courtesy of George Nankervis, MD.

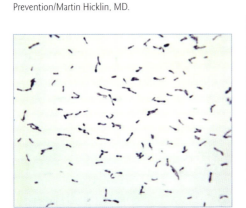

Image 44.11
This photomicrograph depicts numerous gram-positive, rod-shaped *Corynebacterium diphtheriae* bacteria. Courtesy of Centers for Disease Control and Prevention/ Graham Heid.

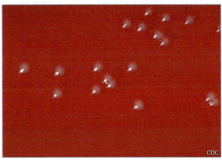

Image 44.12
Blood agar plate culture of *Corynebacterium diphtheriae* mitis. Courtesy of Centers for Disease Control and Prevention/W. A. Clark, MD.

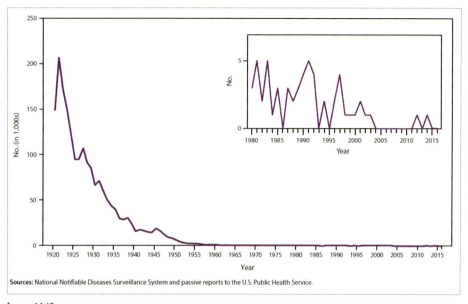

Image 44.13
Number of reported diphtheria cases—United States, 1920–2016. Courtesy of Centers for Disease Control and Prevention.

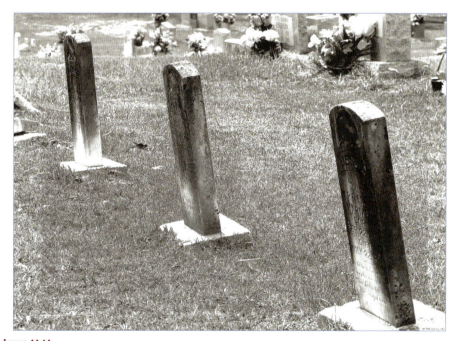

Image 44.14
Baby graves dating from the 1890s in a central Mississippi family cemetery. Diphtheria was a common cause of these infant deaths before the introduction of a toxoid vaccine around 1921. In the preantibiotic era, treatment was limited to comfort care or tracheotomy. Vaccination of children and adults has reduced the number of diphtheria cases in the United States. However, reluctance to immunize children sets the stage for another generation of rows of tiny memories. Courtesy of Will Sorey, MD.

CHAPTER 45

Ehrlichia, Anaplasma, and Related Infections

(Human Ehrlichiosis, Anaplasmosis, and Related Infections Attributable to Bacteria in the Family *Anaplasmataceae*)

CLINICAL MANIFESTATIONS

Early signs and symptoms of infections by members of the bacterial family *Anaplasmataceae* (genera *Anaplasma*, *Ehrlichia*, and *Neorickettsia* and the proposed genus *Candidatus* Neoehrlichia) can be nonspecific. All are acute febrile illnesses with common systemic manifestations including fever, headache, chills, rigors, malaise, myalgia, and nausea. More variable symptoms include arthralgia, vomiting, diarrhea, anorexia, cough, and confusion. Severe manifestations of these diseases can include acute respiratory distress syndrome, encephalopathy, meningitis, disseminated intravascular coagulation, toxic shock–like or septic shock–like syndromes, spontaneous hemorrhage, hepatic failure, and renal failure. Symptoms typically last 1 to 2 weeks, but prompt treatment with doxycycline shortens duration of illness and reduces risk of serious manifestations and sequelae. Fatigue can last several weeks, and neurological sequelae have been reported in some children after severe disease, more commonly with *Ehrlichia* infections.

A maculopapular rash is observed in up to 60% of **Ehrlichia chaffeensis infections** in children but in less than 30% of adults. The rash typically begins 5 days after symptom onset (notably fever). In adults, skin rash is reported more often for *Ehrlichia* infections than for *Anaplasma* infections. Severe disease and fatal outcome are more common in *E chaffeensis* infections (approximately 1%–3% case fatality) than with *Anaplasma phagocytophilum* infection (approximately <1% case fatality).

Coinfections of **Anaplasma** with other tickborne diseases, including babesiosis and Lyme disease, can cause illness that is more severe or of longer duration than a single infection.

Significant laboratory findings in **both Anaplasma and Ehrlichia infections** may include leukopenia with neutropenia (anaplasmosis) or lymphopenia (ehrlichiosis), thrombocytopenia, hyponatremia, and elevated serum hepatic aminotransferase concentrations. Cerebrospinal fluid abnormalities (eg, pleocytosis with a predominance of lymphocytes and increased total protein concentration) are common. People with underlying immunosuppression have greater risk for severe disease.

Because of the nonspecific manifesting symptoms, Rocky Mountain spotted fever should be considered in the differential diagnosis in the United States. Heartland virus infection also manifests with similar clinical features and should be considered in patients without a more likely explanation who have tested negative for *Ehrlichia* and *Anaplasma* infections or have not responded to doxycycline therapy.

ETIOLOGY

Ehrlichia and *Anaplasma* species are obligate intracellular bacteria, which appear as gram-negative cocci that measure 0.5 to 1.5 μm in diameter. Although genetically different, *Anaplasma* and *Ehrlichia* infections are often grouped with rickettsia because of overlapping clinical manifestation and their vectorborne spread (Table 45.1). Ehrlichiosis is the manifestation of (predominantly) *E chaffeensis*, although *Ehrlichia ewingii* and

Table 45.1
Taxonomy of *Rickettsiales*

Order	Rickettsiales			
Family	Rickettsiaceae		Anaplasmataceae	
Genera	Rickettsiae		Anaplasma	Ehrlichia
Species	Spotted fever group: Rocky Mountain spotted fever, Mediterranean spotted fever, Japanese spotted fever, etc	Typhus group: endemic, epidemic	Anaplasma phagocytophilum	Ehrlichia chaffeensis, Ehrlichia ewingii, Ehrlichia muris eauclairensis

Ehrlichia muris eauclairensis are also found in the United States (Table 45.2). Anaplasmosis is predominately caused by *A phagocytophilum* in the United States.

EPIDEMIOLOGY

Reported and suspected cases of ehrlichiosis and anaplasmosis are confined to geographic regions where their vectors are prevalent. Increased incidence is observed with heightened tick activity (mostly warm summer months) as well as with human activities with high levels of exposure to ticks. As with other tickborne diseases, patients often have no memory of being bitten by a tick.

The reported incidence of **E chaffeensis infection** in the United States in 2017 was 5.2 cases per million population. Reported incidence of *E ewingii* infection in 2017 was 0.1 cases per million population, but the incidence is believed to be underreported because of nonspecific illness like *E chaffeensis* infections. Ehrlichiosis caused by *E chaffeensis* and *E ewingii* is reported most commonly from the south-central and southeastern United States, from the East Coast extending westward to Texas. *E chaffeensis* and *E ewingii* are transmitted by the bite of the lone star tick (*Amblyomma americanum*) and are reported from states within its geographic range. Cases attributable to *E muris eauclairensis* have been reported only from Minnesota and Wisconsin and are transmitted by the black-legged tick (*Ixodes scapularis*). Cases of ehrlichiosis have occurred after blood transfusion or solid organ donation from asymptomatic donors.

The reported incidence of **Anaplasma infections** in the United States in 2017 was 18.3 cases per million population. Cases of human anaplasmosis are reported most frequently from the northeastern and upper midwestern United States. Cases of anaplasmosis have also been reported in northern California. In most of the United States, *A phagocytophilum* is transmitted by *I scapularis*, which is also the vector for ehrlichiosis caused by *E muris eauclairensis*, Lyme disease (*Borrelia burgdorferi*), Powassan virus infection, and babesiosis (*Babesia microti*). In the western United States, the western black-legged tick (*Ixodes pacificus*) is the main vector for *A phagocytophilum*. Cases of Anaplasmataceae infections have occurred after blood transfusion or solid organ donation from asymptomatic donors.

The **incubation period** is usually 5 to 14 days for both *E chaffeensis* and *A phagocytophilum*.

Table 45.2
Human Ehrlichiosis, Anaplasmosis, and Related Infections in the United States

Disease	Causal Agent	Major Target Cell	Tick Vector	Geographic Distribution
Ehrlichiosis caused by *Ehrlichia chaffeensis*	*E chaffeensis*	Usually monocytes	Lone star tick (United States) (*Amblyomma americanum*)	Predominantly southeastern, south-central, from the East Coast extending westward to Texas; has been reported outside the United States
Anaplasmosis	*Anaplasma phagocytophilum*	Usually granulocytes	Black-legged tick (*Ixodes scapularis*) or Western black-legged tick (*Ixodes pacificus*) (United States)	Northeastern and upper midwestern states, northern California; Europe, Asia
Ehrlichiosis caused by *Ehrlichia ewingii*	*E ewingii*	Usually granulocytes	Lone star tick (United States) (*A americanum*)	Southeastern, south-central, and midwestern states; Africa, Asia
Ehrlichiosis caused by *Ehrlichia muris eauclairensis*	*E muris eauclairensis*	Unknown, suspected in monocytes	Black-legged tick (*I scapularis*)	Minnesota, Wisconsin

DIAGNOSTIC TESTS

Treatment of ehrlichiosis or anaplasmosis with doxycycline should not be delayed while awaiting confirmation of the diagnosis. Polymerase chain reaction (PCR) testing of whole blood for the organism is most sensitive for anaplasmosis and ehrlichiosis. Sensitivity of PCR testing decreases rapidly following administration of doxycycline, and a negative result does not rule out the diagnosis.

Serological testing may be used to demonstrate a 4-fold change in immunoglobulin G (IgG)–specific antibody titer by indirect immunofluorescent antibody assay between paired acute and convalescent specimens taken 2 to 4 weeks apart. A single mildly elevated IgG titer may not be diagnostic, particularly in regions with high prevalence. Immunoglobulin M (IgM) serological assays are prone to false-positive reactions, and IgM level can remain elevated for lengthy periods, reducing its diagnostic utility. Specific antigens are available for serological testing of *E chaffeensis* and *A phagocytophilum* infections, although cross-reactivity between species can make interpretation difficult in areas where geographic distributions overlap.

Occasionally, *Anaplasmataceae* and *Ehrlichia* bacteria can be identified in Giemsa- or Wright-stained peripheral blood smears or buffy-coat leukocyte preparations in the first week of illness. These morulae can be seen within granulocytes (targeted by *Anaplasma*) or monocytes (targeted by *Ehrlichia*). Culture for isolation of these pathogens is not performed routinely.

TREATMENT

Doxycycline is the treatment of choice for all tickborne rickettsial diseases, including ehrlichiosis and anaplasmosis, and all other tickborne rickettsial diseases. Early initiation of therapy can minimize complications and should not be delayed while awaiting laboratory confirmation. Treatment with doxycycline is recommended in patients of all ages, including children younger than 8 years, when rickettsial diseases are being considered. After doxycycline is initiated, fever generally subsides within 24 to 48 hours.

Patients with suspected **ehrlichiosis** should be treated with doxycycline until at least 3 days after defervescence and until evidence of clinical improvement, typically 5 to 7 days. Patients with suspected **anaplasmosis** should be treated with doxycycline for 10 to 14 days to provide appropriate length of therapy for possible concurrent *B burgdorferi* (Lyme disease) infection.

Rifampin may provide an alternative to doxycycline in patients with anaplasmosis who demonstrate hypersensitivity to doxycycline. Small numbers of children younger than 8 years have also been treated successfully for anaplasmosis with rifampin for a 7- to 10-day course.

Treatment with trimethoprim-sulfamethoxazole has been linked to more severe outcomes and is contraindicated.

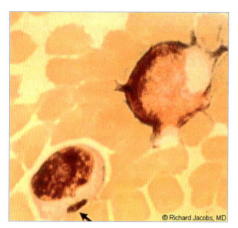

Image 45.1
The intracytoplasmic inclusion, or morula, of human monocytic ehrlichiosis in a cytocentrifuge preparation of cerebrospinal fluid from a patient with central nervous system involvement. Copyright Richard Jacobs, MD.

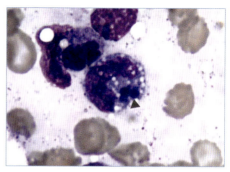

Image 45.2
Bone marrow examination (Wright stain, magnification ×1,000). Intraleukocytic morulae of *Ehrlichia* can be observed (arrow) within monocytoid cells. Courtesy of *Emerging Infectious Diseases*.

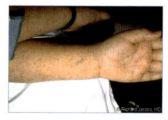

Image 45.4
The petechial and vasculitic rash of human monocytic ehrlichiosis in the patient in Image 45.3. Copyright Richard Jacobs, MD.

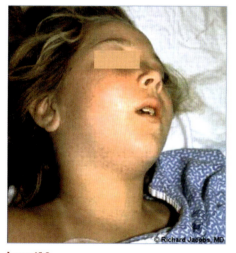

Image 45.3
Human monocytic ehrlichiosis (HME). A semicomatose 16-year-old girl with leukopenia, lymphopenia, thrombocytopenia, and elevated transaminase levels. The HME polymerase chain reaction and serological test results were positive for HME. Copyright Richard Jacobs, MD.

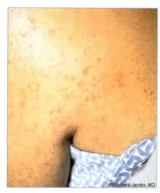

Image 45.5
The same characteristic rash of human monocytic ehrlichiosis in the patient in images 45.3 and 45.4. The differential diagnosis of this rash includes Rocky Mountain spotted fever, meningococcemia, and Stevens-Johnson syndrome. Other tickborne diseases, such as Lyme disease, babesiosis, Colorado tick fever, relapsing fever, and tularemia, may need to be considered. Kawasaki disease has also caused some diagnostic confusion. Copyright Richard Jacobs, MD.

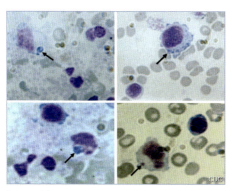

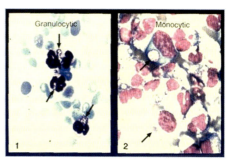

Image 45.6
Peripheral blood smears (buffy-coat preparation) showing variable-sized basophilic inclusions (arrows) in mononuclear cells from a 9-year-old boy with human monocytic ehrlichiosis in Carabobo, Venezuela (Dip Quick [Jorgensen Laboratories Inc, Loveland, CO] staining, magnification ×1,000). Courtesy of Centers for Disease Control and Prevention/*Emerging Infectious Diseases* and Maria C. Martinez.

Image 45.7
Etiologic agents of ehrlichiosis. Photomicrographs of human white blood cells infected with the agent of human granulocytic ehrlichiosis (1, *Anaplasma phagocytophilum*) and the agent of human monocytic ehrlichiosis (2, *Ehrlichia chaffeensis*). Courtesy of Centers for Disease Control and Prevention.

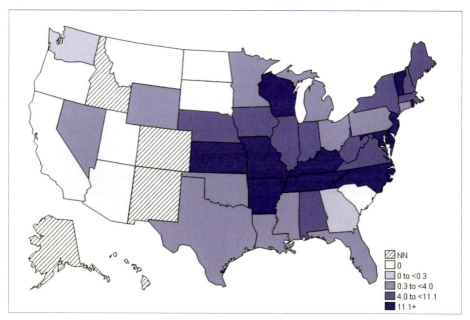

Image 45.8
Annual incidence (per million population) of reported *Ehrlichia chaffeensis* ehrlichiosis—United States, 2019. Courtesy of Centers for Disease Control and Prevention.

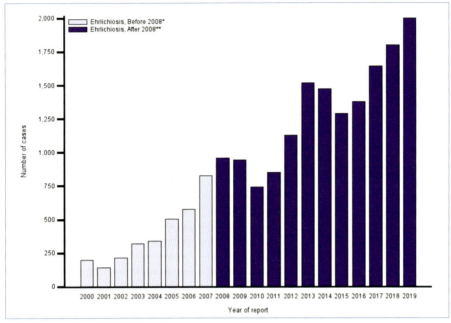

Image 45.9
Number of reported cases of *Ehrlichia chaffeensis* ehrlichiosis—United States, 2000–2019. Courtesy of Centers for Disease Control and Prevention.

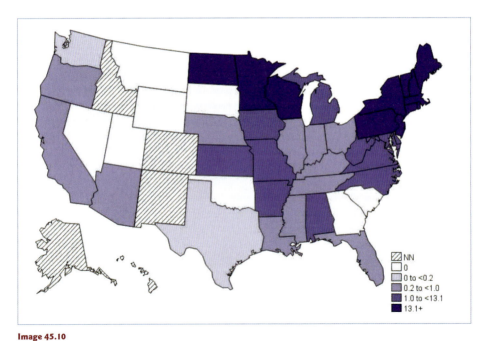

Image 45.10
Annual incidence (per million population) of reported anaplasmosis—United States, 2019. NN indicates not notifiable. Courtesy of Centers for Disease Control and Prevention.

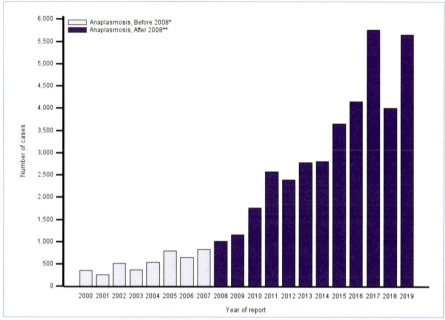

Image 45.11
Number of reported cases of anaplasmosis—United States, 2000–2019. Courtesy of Centers for Disease Control and Prevention.

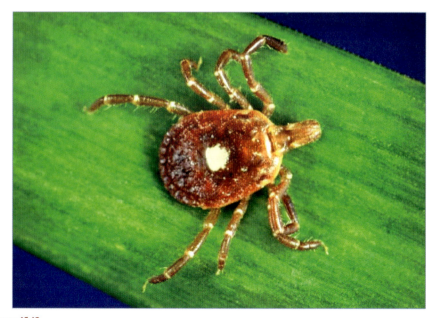

Image 45.12
This is a female lone star tick, *Amblyomma americanum*, and is found in the southeastern and mid-Atlantic United States. This tick is a vector of several zoonotic diseases, including human monocytic ehrlichiosis, southern tick–associated rash illness, tularemia, and Rocky Mountain spotted fever. Courtesy of Centers for Disease Control and Prevention.

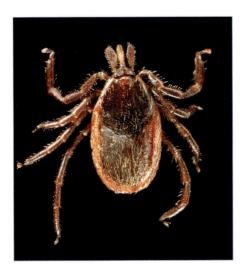

Image 45.13
Dorsal view of an adult female western black-legged tick, *Ixodes pacificus*, which has been shown to transmit *Borrelia burgdorferi*, the agent of Lyme disease, and *Anaplasma phagocytophilum*, the agent of human granulocytic anaplasmosis (previously known as human granulocytic ehrlichiosis), in the western United States. The small scutum, or tough, chitinous dorsal abdominal plate, does not cover its entire abdomen, thereby allowing the abdomen to expand many times when this tick ingests its blood meal (and helping identify this specimen as a female). The 4 pairs of jointed legs place these ticks in the phylum *Arthropoda* and the class *Arachnida*. Courtesy of Centers for Disease Control and Prevention/Amanda Loftis, MD; William Nicholson, MD; Will Reeves, MD; and Chris Paddock, MD.

CHAPTER 46

Serious Neonatal Bacterial Infections Caused by *Enterobacteriaceae*

(Including Septicemia and Meningitis)

CLINICAL MANIFESTATIONS

Neonatal septicemia or meningitis caused by *Escherichia coli* and other gram-negative bacilli cannot be differentiated clinically from septicemia or meningitis caused by other organisms. The early signs of sepsis can be subtle and similar to signs observed in noninfectious processes. Signs of septicemia include fever, temperature instability, heart rate abnormalities, grunting respirations, apnea, cyanosis, lethargy, irritability, anorexia, vomiting, jaundice, abdominal distention, cellulitis, and diarrhea. Meningitis, especially early in the course, can occur without overt signs suggesting central nervous system involvement. Some gram-negative bacilli, such as *Citrobacter koseri*, *Cronobacter* (formerly *Enterobacter*) *sakazakii*, *Serratia marcescens*, and *Salmonella* species, are associated with increased risk for brain abscesses in infants with meningitis caused by these organisms.

ETIOLOGY

Enterobacteriaceae are a large family of gram-negative, facultatively anaerobic, rod-shaped bacteria that include *Escherichia* species, *Klebsiella* species, *Enterobacter* species, *Proteus* species, *Providencia* species, and *Serratia* species, among many others. *E coli* strains, often those with the K1 capsular polysaccharide antigen, are the most common cause of septicemia and meningitis in neonates. Other important gram-negative bacilli causing neonatal septicemia include *Klebsiella* species, *Enterobacter* species, *Proteus* species, *Citrobacter* species, *Salmonella* species, and *Serratia* species. Nonencapsulated strains of *Haemophilus influenzae* and anaerobic gram-negative bacilli are rare causes. *Elizabethkingia meningoseptica* has been associated with outbreaks of neonatal meningitis, with infections in immunocompromised people or with other health care–associated outbreaks related to environmental contamination. *Elizabethkingia anophelis* has been reported as a recent cause of health care–associated infection in adults older than 65 years, with rare cases reported in neonates.

EPIDEMIOLOGY

The source of *E coli* and other *Enterobacteriaceae* in neonatal infections during the first days after birth is typically the maternal genital tract. Reservoirs for gram-negative bacilli can be present within the health care environment. Acquisition of gram-negative organisms can occur through person-to-person transmission from hospital nursery personnel as well as from nursery environmental sites such as sinks, countertops, powdered infant formula, and respiratory therapy equipment, especially by very preterm infants who require prolonged neonatal intensive care management. Predisposing factors in neonatal gram-negative bacterial infections include maternal intrapartum infection, gestation less than 37 weeks, low birth weight, and prolonged rupture of membranes. Metabolic abnormalities (eg, galactosemia), fetal hypoxia, and acidosis have been implicated as predisposing factors. Neonates with defects in the integrity of skin or mucosa (eg, myelomeningocele) or abnormalities of gastrointestinal or genitourinary tracts have increased risk for gram-negative bacterial infections. In neonatal intensive care units, systems for respiratory and metabolic support, invasive or surgical procedures, and indwelling vascular catheters are risk factors for infection. Frequent use of broad-spectrum antimicrobial agents enables selection and proliferation of strains of gram-negative bacilli that may be resistant to multiple antimicrobial agents.

Multiple mechanisms of resistance in gram-negative bacilli can be present simultaneously. Resistance resulting from production of chromosomally encoded or plasmid-derived **AmpC β-lactamases** or from plasmid-mediated **extended-spectrum β-lactamases (ESBLs)** occurs primarily in *E coli, Klebsiella* species, and *Enterobacter* species but has been reported in many other gram-negative species. Resistant gram-negative infections have been associated with nursery outbreaks, especially among very low birth weight infants. Additional risk factors for neonatal infection with ESBL-producing organisms include prolonged mechanical ventilation, extended hospital stay, use of invasive devices, and use of antimicrobial agents. Infants born to mothers colonized with ESBL-producing *E coli* are themselves at an increased risk of becoming colonized with ESBL-producing *E coli* compared with infants born to noncolonized mothers. Organisms that produce ESBLs are typically resistant to penicillins, cephalosporins, and monobactams and can be resistant to aminoglycosides. **Carbapenemase-producing Enterobacteriaceae** have also emerged, especially *Klebsiella pneumoniae*, *E coli*, and *Enterobacter cloacae*. ESBL- and carbapenemase-producing bacteria often carry additional plasmid-borne genes that encode for high-level resistance to aminoglycosides, fluoroquinolones, and trimethoprim-sulfamethoxazole.

The **incubation period** is variable; time of onset of infection ranges from birth to several weeks after birth or longer in very low birth weight, preterm infants with prolonged hospitalizations.

DIAGNOSTIC TESTS

Diagnosis is established by growth of *E coli* or other gram-negative bacilli from blood, cerebrospinal fluid (CSF), or other usually sterile sites. Isolates may be identified by traditional biochemical tests, commercially available biochemical test systems, mass spectrometry of bacterial cell components, or molecular methods. Multiplexed molecular tests capable of rapidly helping identify a variety of gram-negative rods, including *E coli*, directly in positive blood culture bottles have been cleared by the US Food and Drug Administration. Molecular diagnostics are being used increasingly for identification of pathogens; specimens should be saved for resistance testing.

TREATMENT

- Initial empirical treatment of suspected early-onset gram-negative sepsis in neonates should be based on local and regional antimicrobial susceptibility data. The proportion of *E coli* bloodstream infections with onset within 72 hours after birth that are resistant to ampicillin is high (approximately two-thirds) among very low birth weight infants. These *E coli* infections are almost invariably susceptible to gentamicin, although monotherapy with an aminoglycoside is not recommended.

- Ampicillin and an aminoglycoside may be first-line therapy for neonatal sepsis in areas with low ampicillin resistance. An alternative regimen of ampicillin and an extended-spectrum cephalosporin (such as cefotaxime or, if that is unavailable, ceftazidime or cefepime) can be used, but rapid emergence of cephalosporin-resistant organisms, especially *Enterobacter* species, *Klebsiella* species, and *Serratia* species, and increased risk of colonization or infection with ESBL-producing *Enterobacteriaceae* can occur when cephalosporin use is routine in a neonatal unit. The empirical addition of broader-spectrum antibiotic therapy may be considered until culture results are available if the patient is a severely ill preterm infant with the highest risk for early-onset gram-negative sepsis (such as infants with very low birth weight born after prolonged premature rupture of membranes and infants with exposure to prolonged courses of antepartum antibiotic therapy) or a full-term neonate with critical illness. When there is a concern for gram-negative meningitis, an extended-spectrum cephalosporin (eg, cefotaxime or, if that is unavailable, ceftazidime or cefepime) should be used unless local resistance profiles increase the likelihood of a multidrug-resistant gram-negative organism, in which case a carbapenem is the preferred choice for empirical therapy.

- Once the causative agent and its in vitro antimicrobial susceptibility pattern are known, non-meningeal infections should be treated with ampicillin, an appropriate aminoglycoside, or an extended-spectrum cephalosporin (such as cefotaxime) on the basis of the susceptibility results. Some experts treat nonmeningeal infections caused by *Enterobacter* species, *Serratia* species, and some other less commonly occurring gram-negative bacilli with a β-lactam antimicrobial agent and an aminoglycoside.

- For ampicillin-susceptible CSF isolates of *E coli*, meningitis can be treated with ampicillin or cefotaxime; meningitis caused by an ampicillin-resistant, cefotaxime-susceptible isolate can be treated with cefotaxime. Combination therapy of ampicillin or cefotaxime with an aminoglycoside is used until CSF is sterile. Expert advice from an infectious disease specialist is helpful for management of meningitis.

- A carbapenem is the drug of choice for treatment of *Enterobacteriaceae* infections caused by ESBL-producing organisms, especially certain *K pneumoniae* isolates. Of the aminoglycosides, amikacin retains the most activity against ESBL-producing strains. An aminoglycoside or cefepime can be used if the organism is susceptible, because cefepime does not induce chromosomal AmpC enzymes.

- *E meningoseptica* is intrinsically resistant to most β-lactams, including carbapenems, and has variable susceptibility to trimethoprim-sulfamethoxazole and fluoroquinolones; most are susceptible to piperacillin-tazobactam and rifampin. Expert advice from an infectious disease specialist is helpful in management of multidrug-resistant infection (eg, *E meningoseptica*) and ESBL-producing gram-negative infections in neonates.

- The treatment of infections caused by carbapenemase-producing gram-negative organisms is guided by the susceptibility profile, which depends in part on the carbapenemase type. Treatment can include an aminoglycoside, especially amikacin; trimethoprim-sulfamethoxazole; or colistin. Isolates are often susceptible to tigecycline, fluoroquinolones, and polymyxin B, for which experience in neonates is limited. Ceftazidime-avibactam may be effective in some cases and is approved for children and teens 3 months to 18 years of age for the treatment of complicated urinary tract infection or complicated intrabdominal infection (in the latter case, additional therapy such as metronidazole is needed for anaerobic coverage). Some carbapenemase-producing isolates may retain susceptibility to aztreonam. Combination therapy is often used. Expert advice from an infectious disease specialist is helpful in management of carbapenemase-producing gram-negative infections.

- All neonates with gram-negative meningitis should undergo repeated lumbar puncture to ensure sterility of the CSF after 24 to 48 hours of therapy. If CSF remains culture positive, choice and doses of antimicrobial agents should be reevaluated, and another lumbar puncture should be performed after another 48 to 72 hours.

- Duration of therapy is based on clinical and bacteriologic response of the patient and the site(s) of infection; the usual duration of therapy for uncomplicated bacteremia is 10 to 14 days, and for meningitis, minimum duration is 21 days.

- All infants with gram-negative meningitis should undergo careful follow-up examinations, including testing for hearing loss, neurological abnormalities, and developmental delay.

- Immune globulin intravenous therapy for newborns receiving antimicrobial agents for suspected or proven serious infection has been shown to have no effect on outcomes measured and is not recommended.

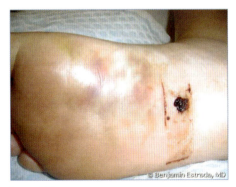

Image 46.1
Aeromonas cellulitis in an 11-year-old boy who previously sustained an injury to the plantar surface of his right foot. Courtesy of Benjamin Estrada, MD.

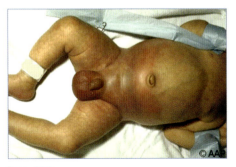

Image 46.2
Icteric preterm neonate with septicemia and perineal and abdominal wall cellulitis caused by *Escherichia coli*.

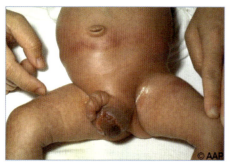

Image 46.3
Neonate in Image 46.2 with *Escherichia coli* septicemia and perineal cellulitis, scrotal necrosis, and abdominal wall abscesses below the navel that required surgical drainage and antibiotics.

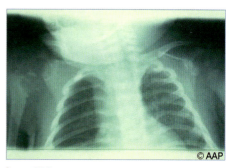

Image 46.4
Infant with osteomyelitis of the proximal right humerus caused by *Escherichia coli*.

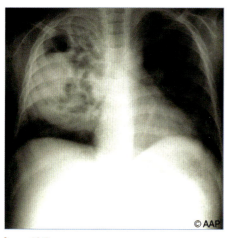

Image 46.5
Pneumonia caused by *Klebsiella pneumoniae* with pulmonary necrosis and downward "bulging" of the pleural fissure secondary to accumulation of tenacious secretions.

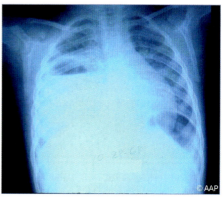

Image 46.6
Lung abscess, anteroposterior view, with air-fluid level. *Klebsiella pneumoniae* was cultured from bronchoscopy secretions. Courtesy of Edgar O. Ledbetter, MD, FAAP.

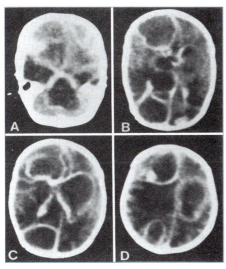

Image 46.7
A–D, Computed tomographic scan of the head of a neonate 3 weeks after therapy for *Escherichia coli* meningitis demonstrating widespread destruction of cerebral cortex secondary to vascular thrombosis. The neonate was blind, deaf, and globally intellectually disabled and had diabetes insipidus. Courtesy of Carol J. Baker, MD, FAAP.

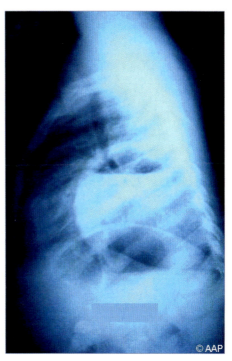

Image 46.8
Lateral view of the patient in Image 46.6, with *Klebsiella pneumoniae* pneumonia, demonstrating large lung abscess with air-fluid level. Repeated bronchoscopy was necessary for adequate drainage. Courtesy of Edgar O. Ledbetter, MD, FAAP.

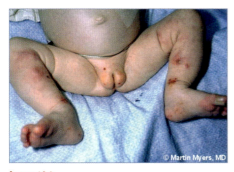

Image 46.9
A 5-week-old girl with *Klebsiella pneumoniae* sepsis and meningitis with bilateral saphenous vein thrombophlebitis (illness began with diarrhea). Copyright Martin G. Myers, MD.

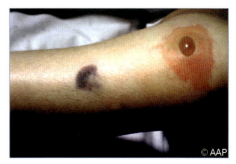

Image 46.10
Skin lesions caused by *Pseudomonas aeruginosa* in a child with neutropenia and septicemia.

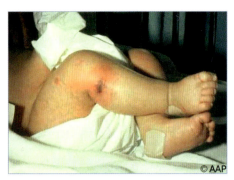

Image 46.11
Sepsis caused by *Pseudomonas aeruginosa* with early ecthyma gangrenosum.

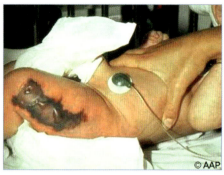

Image 46.12
Sepsis caused by *Pseudomonas aeruginosa* with rapidly progressing ecthyma gangrenosum. This is the same patient as in Image 46.11.

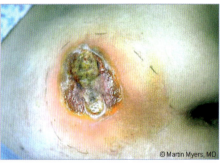

Image 46.13
A preschool-aged boy with acute lymphoblastic leukemia and necrotizing *Pseudomonas* skin lesions called *ecthyma gangrenosum*. Copyright Martin G. Myers, MD.

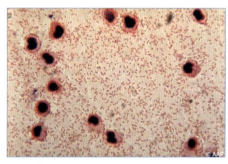

Image 46.14
Gram stain of *Escherichia coli* in the cerebrospinal fluid of a neonate with meningitis.

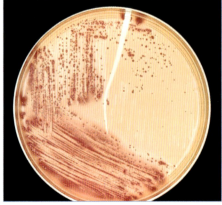

Image 46.15
After 24 hours, this inoculated MacConkey agar culture plate cultivated colonial growth of gram-negative *Escherichia coli* bacteria. Courtesy of Centers for Disease Control and Prevention.

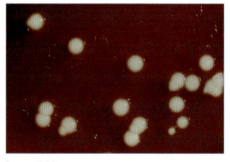

Image 46.16
This blood agar plate grew colonies of gram-negative, small rod-shaped, and facultatively anaerobic *Klebsiella pneumoniae* bacteria. Courtesy of Centers for Disease Control and Prevention.

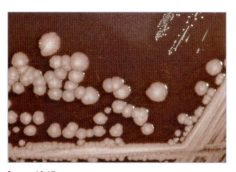

Image 46.17
This photograph depicts the colonies of *Proteus mirabilis* bacteria grown on a xylose-lysine-deoxycholate agar plate. Courtesy of Centers for Disease Control and Prevention.

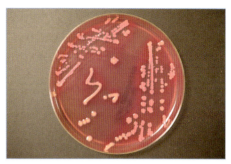

Image 46.18
Citrobacter freundii on MacConkey agar plate. Colonies appear dark pink on this type of medium, indicating lactose fermentation. Courtesy of Julia Rosebush, DO; Robert Jerris, PhD; and Theresa Stanley, M(ASCP).

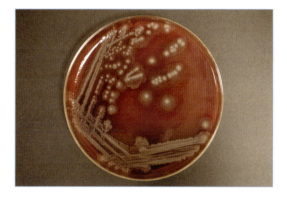

Image 46.19
Proteus vulgaris on blood agar plate. Because of its motility, *Proteus* species often appear to be swarming on chocolate and blood agar plates, as in this photograph. They may sometimes have the odor of chocolate cake. Courtesy of Julia Rosebush, DO; Robert Jerris, PhD; and Theresa Stanley, M(ASCP).

CHAPTER 47
Enterovirus (Nonpoliovirus)
(Group A and B Coxsackieviruses, Echoviruses, Numbered Enteroviruses)

CLINICAL MANIFESTATIONS

Nonpolio enteroviruses are responsible for significant and frequent illnesses in infants and children and result in protean clinical manifestations. The most common manifestation is nonspecific febrile illness, which in young infants may lead to evaluation for bacterial sepsis. Other manifestations can include (1) respiratory: coryza, pharyngitis, herpangina, stomatitis, parotitis, croup, bronchiolitis, pneumonia, pleurodynia, and bronchospasm; (2) skin: hand-foot-and-mouth disease, onychomadesis (shedding of nails), and nonspecific exanthems (particularly associated with echoviruses); (3) neurological: aseptic meningitis, encephalitis, and motor paralysis (acute flaccid myelitis [AFM]); (4) gastrointestinal/genitourinary: vomiting, diarrhea, abdominal pain, hepatitis, pancreatitis, and orchitis; (5) eye: acute hemorrhagic conjunctivitis and uveitis; (6) heart: myopericarditis; and (7) muscle: pleurodynia and other skeletal myositis. Neonates, especially those who acquire infection in the absence of type-specific maternal antibody, have risk for severe and life-threatening disease, including viral sepsis, meningoencephalitis, myocarditis, hepatitis, coagulopathy, and pneumonitis. Acute flaccid myelitis is a rare but serious neurological illness that manifests with acute onset of limb weakness, most often accompanied by cerebrospinal fluid (CSF) pleocytosis and nonenhancing lesions localized to the gray matter of the spinal cord on magnetic resonance imaging. Multiple viruses are known to cause this condition, including enteroviruses.

Infection with enterovirus A71 is associated with hand-foot-and-mouth disease, herpangina, and, in a small proportion of cases, severe neurological disease, including brainstem encephalomyelitis and AFM; secondary pulmonary edema/hemorrhage and cardiopulmonary collapse can occur, resulting in fatalities and sequelae among survivors.

Other noteworthy but not exclusive clinical associations include coxsackieviruses A6, A10, and A16 with hand-foot-and-mouth disease (including severe hand-foot-and-mouth disease, "eczema coxsackium," and atypical cutaneous involvement with coxsackievirus A6); coxsackievirus A24 variant and enterovirus D70 with acute hemorrhagic conjunctivitis; and coxsackieviruses B1 through B5 with pleurodynia and myopericarditis. Enterovirus D68 (EV-D68) is associated with mild to severe respiratory illness in infants, children, and teenagers and has been responsible for localized and large multinational outbreaks of respiratory disease. Disease is usually characterized by exacerbation of preexisting asthma or new-onset wheezing in children without history of asthma, often requiring hospitalization and, in some patients, intensive supportive care. EV-D68 has also been epidemiologically linked to biennial outbreaks of AFM beginning in 2014, although this pattern was disrupted during the COVID-19 pandemic year 2020.

Patients with humoral and combined immunodeficiencies can develop persistent central nervous system infections, a dermatomyositis-like syndrome, arthritis, hepatitis, and/or disseminated infection. Severe and/or chronic neurological or multisystem disease is reported in hematopoietic stem cell and solid organ transplant recipients, children with malignancies, and patients treated with anti-CD20 monoclonal antibody (eg, rituximab).

ETIOLOGY

The enteroviruses, along with the rhinoviruses, comprise a genus of small, nonenveloped, single-stranded, positive-sense RNA viruses in the *Picornaviridae* family. The nonpolio enteroviruses include more than 110 distinct types formerly subclassified as group A coxsackieviruses, group B coxsackieviruses, echoviruses, and newer numbered enteroviruses. A more recent classification system groups the enteroviruses into 4 species (enteroviruses A, B, C, and D) on the basis of genetic similarity, although traditional serotype names are retained for some individual types. Echovirus 22 has been reclassified as parechovirus 1; echovirus 23, as parechovirus 2.

EPIDEMIOLOGY

Humans are the principal reservoir for enteroviruses, although some primates can become infected. Enterovirus infections are common and are distributed worldwide; most infections are asymptomatic. Enteroviruses are spread by fecal-oral and respiratory routes and from mother to infant in the prenatal period, in the peripartum period, and, rarely, via breastfeeding. EV-D68 is believed to be spread primarily by respiratory transmission. Enteroviruses may survive on environmental surfaces for periods long enough to allow transmission from fomites, and transmission via contaminated water and food can occur. Hospital nursery and other institutional outbreaks may occur. Infection incidence, clinical attack rates, and disease severity are typically greatest among infants and young children, and infections occur more frequently in tropical areas and where poor sanitation, poor hygiene, and high population density are present. Most enterovirus infections in temperate climates occur in the summer and fall (June through October in the Northern hemisphere), but seasonal patterns are less evident in the tropics. Fecal shedding of most enteroviruses can persist for several weeks or months after onset of infection, but respiratory tract shedding is usually limited to 1 to 3 weeks or less. Fecal shedding is uncommon with EV-D68 infection. Enterovirus infection and viral transmission can occur without signs of clinical illness.

The usual **incubation period** for enterovirus infections is 3 to 6 days, except for acute hemorrhagic conjunctivitis, for which the **incubation period** is 24 to 72 hours.

DIAGNOSTIC TESTS

Enteroviruses can generally be detected by qualitative reverse transcriptase–polymerase chain reaction (RT-PCR) assay and culture from a variety of specimens, including stool, rectal swab specimens, throat swab specimens, nasopharyngeal aspirates, conjunctival swab specimens, tracheal aspirates, vesicle fluid, blood, urine, tissue biopsy specimens, and CSF. RT-PCR assay is rapid and more sensitive than isolation of enteroviruses in cell culture and can detect all enteroviruses, including types that are difficult to cultivate in cell cultures. RT-PCR assays for detection of enterovirus RNA are available at many reference and commercial laboratories for CSF, blood, and other specimens.

Patients with enterovirus A71 neurological disease often have negative results of RT-PCR assay and culture of CSF (even in the presence of CSF pleocytosis) and blood; RT-PCR assay and culture of throat or rectal swab and/or vesicle fluid specimens (in cases of hand-foot-and-mouth disease) are more frequently positive.

EV-D68 is demonstrated primarily in respiratory tract specimens and can be detected with multiplex respiratory RT-PCR assays, but these assays do not distinguish enteroviruses from rhinoviruses. Definitive identification of EV-D68 requires partial genomic sequencing or amplification with an EV-D68–specific RT-PCR assay.

Sensitivity of culture ranges from 0% to 80% depending on type and cell lines used. Many group A coxsackieviruses grow poorly or not at all in vitro. Culture usually requires 3 to 8 days to detect growth. The type of enterovirus may be identified by genomic sequencing and may be indicated in cases of special clinical interest or for epidemiological purposes (eg, for investigation of disease clusters or outbreaks). Acute infection with a known enterovirus type can be determined at reference laboratories by demonstration of a change in neutralizing antibody titer between acute and convalescent serum specimens or by detection of type-specific immunoglobulin M, but serological assays are relatively insensitive, may lack specificity, and are rarely used for diagnosis of acute infection.

TREATMENT

No specific therapy is available for enterovirus infections. Immune globulin intravenous (IGIV), administered intravenously or via intraventricular administration, may be beneficial for chronic enterovirus meningoencephalitis in immunodeficient patients. IGIV has also been used for life-threatening neonatal enterovirus infections (maternal convalescent plasma has also been used); severe enterovirus infections in transplant recipients and people with malignancies; suspected viral myocarditis; enterovirus A71 neurological disease; and AFM, but proof of efficacy for these uses is lacking. Interferons have occasionally been used for treatment of enterovirus-associated myocarditis and chronic enterovirus meningoencephalitis, without definitive proof of efficacy.

The antiviral drug pleconaril has activity against many enteroviruses but is not commercially available. Pocapavir is another antiviral drug that is being developed primarily for the treatment of chronic poliovirus infection in patients with a primary immunodeficiency and has some activity in vitro against some nonpolio enteroviruses. Like pleconaril, pocapavir is not commercially available.

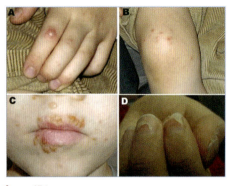

Image 47.1
Vesicular eruptions in the hand (A), foot (B), and mouth (C) of a 6-year-old boy with coxsackievirus A6 infection. Several of his fingernails shed (D) 2 months after the pictures were taken. Courtesy of Centers for Disease Control and Prevention/*Emerging Infectious Diseases*.

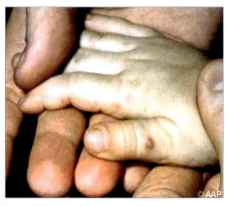

Image 47.2
Enterovirus infection in a preschool-aged girl. Hand-foot-and-mouth disease lesions are caused by coxsackievirus A16 and enterovirus 71.

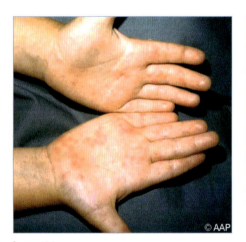

Image 47.3
Enterovirus infection (hand-foot-and-mouth disease) affecting the hands.

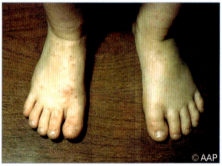

Image 47.4
Enterovirus infection (hand-foot-and-mouth disease) affecting the feet.

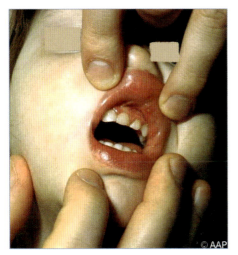

Image 47.5
Enterovirus infection (hand-foot-and-mouth disease) affecting the anterior buccal mucosa. These lesions are generally less painful than herpes simplex lesions.

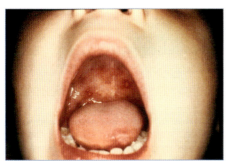

Image 47.7
Characteristic papulovesicular lesions of hand-foot-and-mouth disease in a 2-year-old boy. Courtesy of George Nankervis, MD.

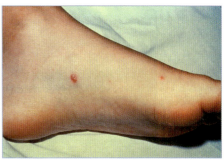

Image 47.6
A papulovesicular lesion on the medial aspect of the foot of a 6-year-old boy with hand-foot-and-mouth disease. Courtesy of George Nankervis, MD.

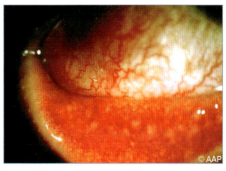

Image 47.8
Enterovirus 71 acute hemorrhagic conjunctivitis, on the second or third day. No neurological sequelae were present. Courtesy of Jerri Ann Jenista, MD.

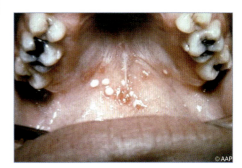

Image 47.9
Herpangina (coxsackievirus) lesions on the posterior palate of a male young adult. Coxsackievirus lesions are usually found in the posterior aspect of the oropharynx and may progress rapidly to painful ulceration.

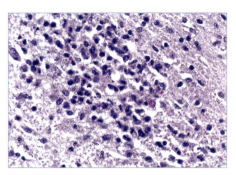

Image 47.10
Enterovirus encephalitis. Microglial nodule. Courtesy of Dimitris P. Agamanolis, MD.

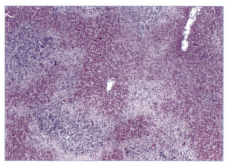

Image 47.11
Extensive hepatic necrosis caused by an enterovirus infection. Courtesy of Dimitris P. Agamanolis, MD.

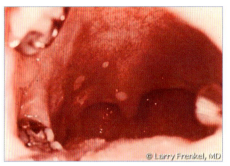

Image 47.12
A 4-year-old girl with pharyngeal inflammation and palatal lesions of hand-foot-and-mouth disease, a coxsackievirus A infection. Courtesy of Larry Frenkel, MD.

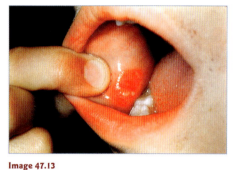

Image 47.13
This 7-year-old girl presented with low-grade fever, malaise, sore throat, and these interesting, slightly raised oral lesions opposite the first molar. She also had approximately 10 maculopapular lesions on each buttock and a few on each foot. She had classic hand-foot-and-mouth disease. Coxsackievirus A16 was grown from throat and rectal swabs. Courtesy of Neal Halsey, MD.

CHAPTER 48
Epstein-Barr Virus Infections
(Infectious Mononucleosis)

CLINICAL MANIFESTATIONS

Infectious mononucleosis is the most common manifestation of primary symptomatic Epstein-Barr virus (EBV) infection. It manifests typically as fever, pharyngitis with or without petechiae, exudative pharyngitis, lymphadenopathy, hepatosplenomegaly, and atypical lymphocytosis. The spectrum of disease is wide, ranging from asymptomatic to fatal infection. Infections are unrecognized or nonspecific in infants and young children. Rash can occur in up to 20% of patients and is more common in patients treated with antibiotics, most commonly with ampicillin or amoxicillin as well as with other penicillins. Central nervous system (CNS) manifestations include aseptic meningitis, encephalitis, myelitis, optic neuritis, cranial nerve palsies, transverse myelitis, Alice in Wonderland syndrome, and Guillain-Barré syndrome. Hematologic complications include splenic rupture, thrombocytopenia, agranulocytosis, hemolytic anemia, and hemophagocytic lymphohistiocytosis (HLH, or hemophagocytic syndrome). Pneumonia, orchitis, and myocarditis are observed infrequently. Early in the course of primary infection, 1% to 10% of circulating B lymphocytes are infected with EBV, and EBV-specific cytotoxic/suppressor T lymphocytes account for up to 50% of the $CD8^+$ T lymphocytes in the blood. Replication of EBV in B lymphocytes results in T-lymphocyte proliferation and inhibition of B-lymphocyte proliferation by T-lymphocyte cytotoxic responses, natural killer (NK) cell activation, and the production of neutralizing antibodies. Fatal disseminated infection or B-lymphocyte, T-lymphocyte, or NK-cell lymphomas rarely occur in children with no detectable immunologic abnormality as well as in children with congenital or acquired cellular immunodeficiencies.

EBV is associated with several other distinct disorders, including X-linked lymphoproliferative syndrome, posttransplant lymphoproliferative disorder (PTLD), Burkitt lymphoma, nasopharyngeal carcinoma, undifferentiated B- or T-lymphocyte lymphomas, and leiomyosarcoma. X-linked lymphoproliferative syndrome occurs most often in people with an inherited, maternally derived, recessive genetic defect in the SH2D1A or XIAP/BIRC4 gene, which is important in several lymphocyte signaling pathways. The syndrome is characterized by several phenotypic expressions, including occurrence of fatal infectious mononucleosis early in life in boys; HLH; nodular B-lymphocyte lymphomas, often with CNS involvement; and profound pancytopenia. Similarly, X-linked immunodeficiency with magnesium defect, EBV infection, and neoplasia disease is characterized by loss-of-function mutations in the gene encoding magnesium transporter 1 (MAGT1), chronic high-level EBV DNAemia with increased EBV-infected B cells, and heightened susceptibility to EBV-associated lymphomas. Several other genetic mutations associated with the failure to control EBV infection because of changes in T lymphocyte and NK cell function have also been described.

EBV-associated lymphoproliferative disorders can also occur in patients who are immunocompromised, such as transplant recipients or people infected with HIV. The highest incidence of these disorders occurs among small-intestine transplant recipients, with moderate risk in liver, pancreas, lung, and heart transplant recipients. Proliferative states range from benign lymph node hypertrophy to monoclonal lymphomas. Other EBV-associated lymphoproliferative syndromes are of greater importance outside the United States, such as Burkitt lymphoma, which can be endemic or sporadic. EBV is present in virtually 100% of endemic Burkitt lymphoma (a B-lymphocyte tumor predominantly found in head and neck lymph nodes primarily in Central Africa) versus 20% in sporadic Burkitt lymphoma (a B-lymphocyte tumor of abdominal lymphoid tissue predominantly in North America and Europe). EBV is found in nearly 100% of nasopharyngeal carcinoma in Southeast Asia and the Inuit populations. EBV has also been associated with Hodgkin disease (a B-lymphocyte tumor), non-Hodgkin lymphomas (both B- and T-lymphocyte types), gastric carcinoma "lymphoepitheliomas," and a variety of other epithelial malignancies.

Chronic fatigue syndrome is not directly caused by EBV infection; however, fatigue lasting 6 months or more may follow approximately 10% of cases of classic infectious mononucleosis.

ETIOLOGY

EBV (also known as human herpesvirus 4) is a gamma herpesvirus of the *Lymphocryptovirus* genus and is the most common cause of infectious mononucleosis (>90% of cases).

EPIDEMIOLOGY

Humans are the only known reservoir of EBV, and approximately 90% of US adults have been infected. Close personal contact is usually required for transmission. The virus is viable in saliva for several hours outside the body; the role of fomites in transmission is unknown. EBV may be transmitted by blood transfusion or transplant. Infection is commonly contracted early in life, particularly by members of lower-income groups, where crowding and intrafamilial spread is common. Endemic infectious mononucleosis is common in group settings of adolescents, such as educational or military institutions. No seasonal pattern has been clearly documented. Intermittent excretion in saliva is lifelong after infection and likely explains viral spread and persistence in the population.

The **incubation period** of infectious mononucleosis is estimated to be 30 to 50 days.

DIAGNOSTIC TESTS

Routine diagnosis depends on serological testing. Nonspecific tests for heterophile antibody, including the Paul-Bunnell test and slide agglutination reaction test, are available most commonly and are approximately 90% sensitive and specific. The heterophile antibody response is primarily immunoglobulin M (IgM), which appears during the first 2 weeks of illness and usually disappears over 6 months. The results of heterophile antibody tests are often negative in children younger than 4 years with EBV infection, but heterophile antibody tests help identify at least 85% of cases of classic infectious mononucleosis in older children and adults during the second week of illness. An absolute increase in atypical lymphocytes during the second week of illness with infectious mononucleosis is another characteristic but nonspecific finding.

Multiple specific serological antibody tests for EBV infection are available (Table 48.1 and Figure 48.1). The most commonly performed test is for antibody against the viral capsid antigen (VCA) of EBV. Because immunoglobulin G (IgG) antibodies against VCA occur in high titer early in infection and persist for life at modest levels, testing of acute and convalescent serum specimens for IgG anti-VCA alone is not useful for establishing the presence of active infection. In contrast, testing for the presence of IgM anti-VCA antibody and the absence or very low titers of antibodies to Epstein-Barr nuclear antigen (EBNA) is useful for identifying active and recent infections. Because serum antibody against EBNA is not present until several weeks to months after onset of infection and rises with convalescence, a very elevated anti-EBNA antibody concentration typically excludes active primary infection. Testing for antibodies against early antigen is not usually required to assess EBV-associated mononucleosis. Typical patterns of antibody responses to EBV infection are illustrated in Table 48.1 and Figure 48.1.

Serological testing for EBV is useful, particularly for evaluating patients who have heterophile-negative infectious mononucleosis, who are younger than 4 years, or in whom the infectious mononucleosis syndrome is not classic. Testing

Table 48.1
Serum Epstein-Barr Virus (EBV) Antibodies in EBV Infection

Infection	VCA IgG	VCA IgM	EA (D)	EBNA
No previous infection	−	−	−	−
Acute infection	+	+	±	−
Recent infection	+	±	±	±
Past infection	+	−	±	+

EA (D) indicates early antigen diffuse staining; EBNA, Epstein-Barr nuclear antigen; VCA IgG, immunoglobulin G class antibody to viral capsid antigen; and VCA IgM, immunoglobulin M class antibody to viral capsid antigen.

Figure 48.1
Schematic Representation of the Evolution of Antibodies to Various Epstein-Barr Virus Antigens in Patients With Infectious Mononucleosis

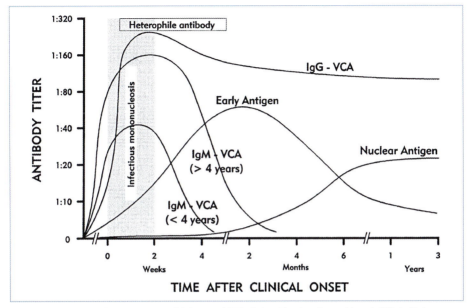

IgG indicates immunoglobulin G; IgM, immunoglobulin M; and VCA, viral capsid antigen. Source: *Manual of Clinical Laboratory Immunology*. American Society for Microbiology; 1997:636. © 1997 American Society for Microbiology. Used with permission. No further reproduction or distribution is permitted without the prior written permission of American Society for Microbiology.

for other agents, especially cytomegalovirus, *Toxoplasma*, human herpesvirus 6, adenovirus, and HIV (in those with HIV risk factors), may be indicated for some patients. Diagnosis of the entire range of EBV-associated illness requires use of additional molecular and antibody techniques, particularly for patients with immunodeficiencies.

Polymerase chain reaction (PCR) assay for detection of EBV DNA in serum, plasma, and tissue and reverse transcriptase–PCR assay for detection of EBV RNA in lymphoid cells, tissue, and/or body fluids are available and can be useful in evaluation of immunocompromised patients and in complex clinical situations.

TREATMENT

Currently, there is no antiviral treatment approved for EBV infection. Patients suspected to have infectious mononucleosis should not receive ampicillin or amoxicillin, which may cause nonallergic morbilliform rashes in a proportion of patients with active EBV infection. Although therapy with short-course corticosteroids may have a beneficial effect on some acute symptoms, because of potential adverse effects, its use is usually considered only for patients with marked tonsillar inflammation with impending airway obstruction, massive splenomegaly, myocarditis, hemolytic anemia, or HLH. The dosage of prednisone is usually 1 mg/kg/day, orally (maximum 60 mg/day), for 5 to 7 days, in some cases with tapering. Life-threatening HLH has been treated with cytotoxic agents and immunomodulators, including etoposide, cyclosporine, and/or corticosteroids. Decreasing immunosuppressive therapy is often beneficial for patients with EBV-induced PTLD. Rituximab, a monoclonal antibody directed against $CD20^+$ B lymphocytes, is also used both preemptively in hematopoietic stem cell transplant patients and for treatment of PTLD in solid organ transplant patients.

Strenuous activity and contact sports should be avoided for at least 21 days after onset of symptoms of infectious mononucleosis. After 21 days, limited noncontact aerobic activity can be allowed if there are no symptoms and there is no overt splenomegaly. Clearance to participate in contact sports is appropriate after 4 to 7 weeks following the onset of symptoms if the athlete is asymptomatic and has no overt splenomegaly. Repeated mononucleosis spot or EBV serological testing is not useful in most clinical situations. It may take 3 to 6 months or longer following mononucleosis for an athlete to return to preillness fitness.

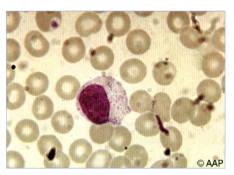

Image 48.1
Atypical lymphocyte in a peripheral blood smear of a patient with infectious mononucleosis. This lymphocyte is larger than normal-sized lymphocytes, with a higher ratio of cytoplasm to nucleus. The cytoplasm is vacuolated and basophilic. This may also be present in cytomegalovirus infections.

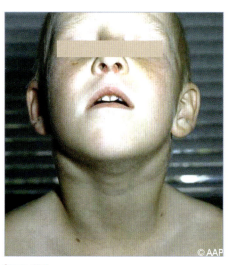

Image 48.2
Bilateral cervical lymphadenopathy in an 8-year-old boy with Epstein-Barr virus disease who remained relatively asymptomatic. Courtesy of Edgar O. Ledbetter, MD, FAAP.

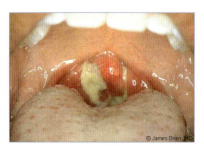

Image 48.3
Epstein-Barr virus disease with pharyngeal and tonsillar exudate. Copyright James Brien.

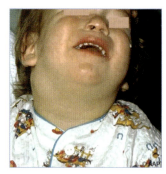

Image 48.4
Cervical lymphadenopathy in a 2-year-old girl with infectious mononucleosis.

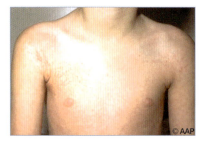

Image 48.5
Rash in a 9-year-old girl with infectious mononucleosis who was prescribed ampicillin.

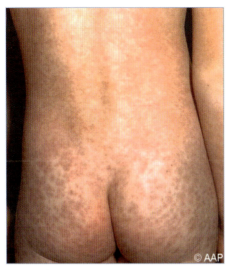

Image 48.6
Rash in the same patient as in Image 48.5, with infectious mononucleosis who was prescribed ampicillin. These morbilliform rashes are considered nonallergic.

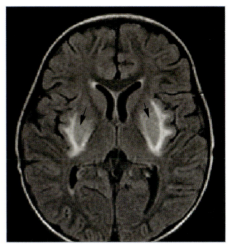

Image 48.7
Epstein-Barr virus encephalitis. Axial fluid–attenuated inversion-recovery magnetic resonance image shows basal ganglia hyperintensity (arrows).

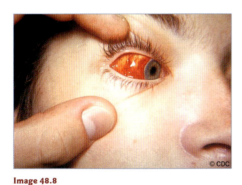

Image 48.8
A conjunctival hemorrhage of the right eye of a patient with infectious mononucleosis. At times, noninfectious conjunctivitis, as well as other corneal abnormalities, may manifest itself because of the body's systemic response to viral infections such as infectious mononucleosis. Courtesy of Centers for Disease Control and Prevention.

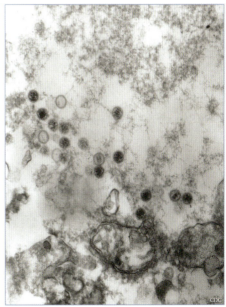

Image 48.9
This negatively stained transmission electron micrograph revealed the presence of numerous Epstein-Barr virus virions, members of the *Herpesviridae* virus family. Epstein-Barr virus is also known as human herpesvirus 4. At the core of its proteinaceous capsid, the Epstein-Barr virus contains a double-stranded DNA linear genome. Courtesy of Centers for Disease Control and Prevention/ Fred Murphy, MD.

CHAPTER 49
Escherichia coli Diarrhea
(Including Hemolytic-Uremic Syndrome)

CLINICAL MANIFESTATIONS

Escherichia coli is a common bacterial cause of diarrheal illness. At least 5 pathotypes of diarrhea-producing *E coli* strains have been identified. Clinical features of disease caused by each pathotype are summarized as follows (see also Table 49.1):

- **Shiga toxin–producing *E coli* (STEC)** organisms are associated with diarrhea, hemorrhagic colitis, and hemolytic-uremic syndrome (HUS). STEC O157:H7 is the serotype most often implicated in outbreaks and is consistently a virulent STEC serotype, but other serotypes can also cause illness. STEC illness typically begins with nonbloody diarrhea. Stools usually become bloody after 2 or 3 days, representing the onset of hemorrhagic colitis. Severe abdominal pain is typically short-lived, and low-grade fever is present in approximately one-third of cases. Diseases caused by *E coli* O157:H7 and other STEC organisms should be considered in people with presumptive diagnoses of intussusception, appendicitis, inflammatory bowel disease, or ischemic colitis. There are 2 types of Shiga toxin (Stx), Stx1 and Stx2; several variants of each type exist. In general, STEC strains that produce Stx2, especially variants Stx2a, Stx2c, and Stx2d, are more virulent than strains that produce only Stx1.

- Diarrhea caused by **enteropathogenic *E coli* (EPEC)** is watery. Illness occurs almost exclusively in children younger than 2 years and predominantly in resource-limited countries, either sporadically or epidemically, or in travelers to those settings. Although usually mild, diarrhea can result in dehydration and even death, particularly in resource-limited countries. EPEC diarrhea can be persistent and can result in wasting or growth restriction. EPEC infection is uncommon in breastfed infants. EPEC can also cause travelers diarrhea.

- Diarrhea caused by **enterotoxigenic *E coli* (ETEC)** is a 1- to 5-day, self-limited illness of moderate severity, typically with watery stools and abdominal cramps. ETEC is common in infants in resource-limited countries and in travelers to those countries. With increasing use of culture-independent tests, ETEC infections may be detected more frequently, especially in late summer into fall.

Table 49.1
Classification of *Escherichia coli* Associated With Diarrhea

Pathotype	Epidemiology	Type of Diarrhea	Mechanism of Pathogenesis
Shiga toxin–producing *Escherichia coli* (STEC)	Hemorrhagic colitis and hemolytic-uremic syndrome in all ages	Bloody or nonbloody	Shiga toxin production, large bowel adherence, coagulopathy
Enteropathogenic *Escherichia coli* (EPEC)	Acute and chronic endemic and epidemic diarrhea in infants in resource-limited countries; certain atypical strains in industrialized countries may cause disease.	Watery	Small-bowel adherence and effacement
Enterotoxigenic *Escherichia coli* (ETEC)	Infant diarrhea in resource-limited countries, travelers diarrhea in all ages, and some cases in nontravelers	Watery	Small-bowel adherence, heat-stable and/or heat-labile enterotoxin production
Enteroinvasive *Escherichia coli* (EIEC)	Diarrhea with fever in all ages	Bloody or nonbloody; dysentery	Mucosal invasion and inflammation of large bowel
Enteroaggregative *Escherichia coli* (EAEC)	Acute and chronic diarrhea in all ages	Watery, occasionally bloody	Small- and large-bowel adherence, enterotoxin and cytotoxin production

- Diarrhea caused by **enteroinvasive *E coli* (EIEC)** is similar clinically to diarrhea caused by *Shigella* species. Although dysentery can occur, diarrhea is usually watery without blood or mucus. Patients are often febrile, and stools can contain leukocytes.

- **Enteroaggregative *E coli* (EAEC)** organisms cause watery diarrhea and are common in people of all ages in industrialized as well as resource-limited countries. EAEC is a common cause of childhood diarrhea in developing countries, acute diarrhea in travelers, and persistent diarrhea in children or HIV-infected patients. EAEC has been associated with prolonged diarrhea (≥14 days). Asymptomatic infection can be accompanied by subclinical inflammatory enteritis, which can cause linear growth faltering.

Sequelae of STEC Infection

HUS is a serious sequela of STEC enteric infection. STEC O157:H7, particularly strains producing Stx2, are most commonly associated with HUS, which is defined by the triad of microangiopathic hemolytic anemia, thrombocytopenia, and acute renal dysfunction. HUS occurs in approximately 15% of children younger than 5 years (children 1–4 years of age have higher risk than infants) with laboratory-confirmed *E coli* O157 infection, as compared with approximately 6% among people of all ages. HUS occurs in approximately 1% of patients of all ages with laboratory confirmed non-O157 STEC infection. HUS typically develops 7 days (up to 2 weeks and rarely 2–3 weeks) after onset of diarrhea. More than 50% of children with HUS require dialysis, and 3% to 5% die. Patients with HUS can develop neurological complications (eg, seizures, coma, cerebral vessel thrombosis). Children presenting with an increased white blood cell count ($>20 \times 10^9$/mL) or oliguria or anuria have higher risk for poor outcome, as do, seemingly paradoxically, children with hematocrit close to normal rather than low. Most patients who survive have a very good prognosis, which can be predicted by normal creatinine clearance and no proteinuria or hypertension 1 year or more after HUS.

ETIOLOGY

The 5 pathotypes of diarrhea-producing *E coli* have been distinguished by genetic, pathogenic, and clinical characteristics. Each pathotype is defined by the presence of virulence-related genes, and each comprises characteristic serotypes, indicated by somatic (O) and flagellar (H) antigens. Diarrhea is caused by the direct effects of the pathogens in the intestine.

EPIDEMIOLOGY

Transmission of most diarrhea-associated *E coli* strains is from food or water contaminated with human or animal feces or from infected symptomatic people. STEC is shed in feces of cattle and, to a lesser extent, sheep, deer, and other ruminants. Human infection is acquired via contaminated food or water or via contact with an infected person, a fomite, or a carrier animal or its environment. Many foods have caused *E coli* O157 outbreaks, including raw leafy vegetables, undercooked ground beef, and unpasteurized milk and juice. Outbreak investigations have implicated petting zoos, drinking water, and ingestion of recreational water. The infectious dose is low; thus, person-to-person transmission is common in households and child care centers. Less is known about the epidemiology of STEC strains other than O157. The non-O157 STEC serogroups most commonly linked to illness in the United States are O26, O111, O103, O121, O45, and O145. Outbreaks from these serogroups are uncommon and are generally attributable to contaminated food or person-to-person transmission (often in a child care setting). A severe outbreak of bloody diarrhea and HUS occurred in Europe in 2011; the outbreak was attributed to an EAEC strain of serotype O104:H4 that had acquired the Stx2a-encoding phage. This experience highlights the importance of considering serogroups other than O157 in outbreaks and cases of HUS.

With the exception of EAEC, non-STEC pathotypes are most commonly associated with disease in resource-limited countries, where food and water supplies are commonly contaminated and facilities and supplies for hand hygiene are suboptimal. For young children in resource-limited countries, transmission of ETEC, EPEC, and other diarrheal pathogens via contaminated weaning foods (sometimes by use of untreated drinking water in the foods) is common. ETEC diarrhea occurs in people of all ages but is especially frequent and severe in infants in resource-limited countries. Breastfeeding is protective in such settings. ETEC is a major cause of travelers diarrhea.

The **incubation period** for most diarrhea-associated E coli strains is 10 hours to 6 days; for E coli O157:H7, the **incubation period** is usually 3 to 4 days (range, 1–10 days).

DIAGNOSTIC TESTS

Several US Food and Drug Administration (FDA)–cleared multiplex polymerase chain reaction assays (usually offered as diagnostic panels) can detect a variety of enteric pathogens, including EAEC, EPEC, ETEC, and STEC, the last by detection of the genes encoding Stx1 and Stx2. In most children, EAEC, EPEC, and ETEC are codetected with at least 1 other pathogen, raising questions about the clinical significance of these codetections on multiplex panels.

Several commercially available, sensitive, specific, and rapid immunologic assays for Shiga toxins in stool or broth culture of stool, including enzyme immunoassays (EIAs) and immunochromatographic assays, have been approved by the FDA. The Shiga toxin assays performed on broth-enriched stool specimens (usually incubated for 18–24 hours) are generally more sensitive than those testing stool directly.

Ideally, all stool specimens submitted for routine diagnosis of acute community-acquired diarrhea (regardless of patient age, season, or presence or absence of blood in the stool) should be simultaneously cultured for E coli O157 and tested for non-O157 Shiga toxins or the genes encoding these toxins.

Rapid diagnosis facilitates patient treatment and prompt institution of fluid rehydration. Hydration is the cornerstone of management for all diarrhea cases and may be particularly protective against the development of nephropathy associated with HUS. Most E coli O157 isolates can be identified presumptively when grown on sorbitol-containing selective media because they cannot ferment sorbitol within 24 hours. All presumptive E coli O157 isolates and all Shiga toxin–positive stool specimens that did not yield a presumptive E coli O157 isolate should be sent to a public health laboratory for further characterization.

STEC should be sought in stool specimens from all patients diagnosed with postdiarrheal HUS. However, the absence of STEC does not preclude the diagnosis of probable STEC-associated HUS, because HUS is typically diagnosed a week or more after onset of diarrhea, when the organism may not be detectable by conventional bacteriologic methods. In this setting, the selective enrichment of stool samples followed by immunomagnetic separation can markedly enhance the isolation of E coli O157 and other STEC for which immunomagnetic reagents are available. The test is available at some state public health laboratories and, through requests to state health departments, at the Centers for Disease Control and Prevention (CDC). Serological diagnosis by using EIA to detect serum antibodies to E coli O157 and O111 lipopolysaccharides is available at the CDC for outbreak investigations and for patients with HUS; the testing can be arranged through state health departments.

TREATMENT

Treatment is primarily supportive for all diarrhea-producing E coli. Orally administered electrolyte-containing solutions are usually adequate to prevent or treat dehydration and electrolyte abnormalities. Antimotility agents should not be administered to children with inflammatory or bloody diarrhea. Patients with proven or suspected STEC infection should be rehydrated fully but prudently as soon as clinically feasible. Many experts advocate intravenous volume expansion during the first 4 days of proven STEC infection to maintain renal perfusion and reduce the risk of renal injury. Careful monitoring of patients with hemorrhagic colitis (including complete blood cell count with smear, serum urea nitrogen, and creatinine concentrations) is recommended to detect changes suggestive of HUS. If patients have no laboratory evidence of hemolysis, thrombocytopenia, or nephropathy 3 days after resolution of diarrhea, their risk of developing HUS is low.

In resource-limited countries, nutritional rehabilitation, including supplemental zinc and vitamin A, should be provided as part of case management algorithms for diarrhea where feasible. Feeding, including breastfeeding, should be continued for young children with E coli enteric infection.

Bismuth subsalicylate has been approved by the FDA for use in children 12 years and older and may be used in mild cases of travelers diarrhea. It contains salicylate and should not be used if a viral infection, such as varicella or influenza, is also suspected.

Antimicrobial Therapy

Antimicrobial therapy in patients with STEC infection remains controversial because of its association with an increased risk of developing HUS in some studies. Most experts advise not prescribing antimicrobial therapy for children with *E coli* O157 enteritis or a clinical or epidemiological picture strongly suggestive of STEC infection.

Empirical self-treatment of diarrhea for travelers to a resource-limited country can slightly reduce duration of diarrhea; however, the prevalence of antimicrobial-resistant enteric pathogens in resource-limited settings is increasing. Azithromycin or a fluoroquinolone has been the most reliable agent for therapy; the choice of therapy depends on the pathogen and local antibiotic resistance patterns. Rifaximin may be used for people 12 years and older.

Patients with domestically acquired atypical EPEC (ie, that detected only by homology with the *eae* gene on molecular panel), EAEC, or ETEC generally have self-limited diarrhea that does not require antimicrobial therapy. For patients with moderate or severe illness with persistent (>14 days) diarrhea attributable to diarrheagenic *E coli* and no other pathogen detected, a treatment regimen similar to that used for travelers diarrhea (azithromycin, a fluoroquinolone, or rifaximin) may be used.

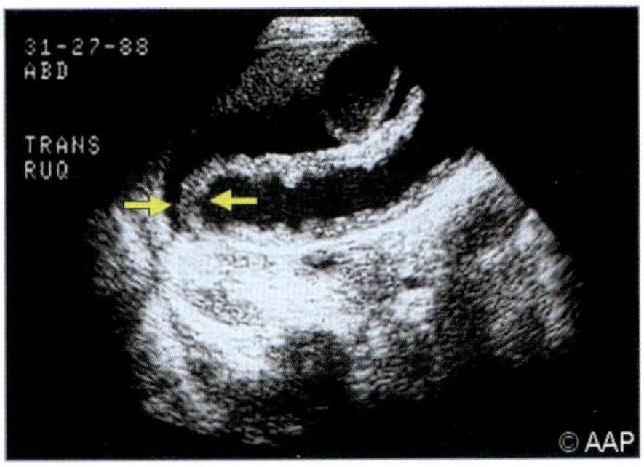

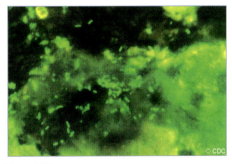

Image 49.1
Ultrasound of a 6-year-old boy with hemorrhagic colitis from *Escherichia coli* O157:H7 who developed hemolytic-uremic syndrome. Note the bowel wall edema (arrows).

Image 49.2
Escherichia coli in the intestine of an 8-month-old experiencing chronic diarrhea (fluorescent antibody stain). In a small number of individuals (mostly children <5 years of age and elderly people), *E coli* can cause hemolytic-uremic syndrome, in which the red blood cells are destroyed and the kidneys fail. Courtesy of Centers for Disease Control and Prevention.

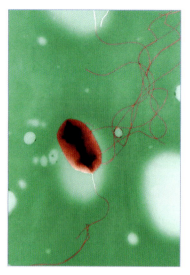

Image 49.3
Transmission electron micrograph of *Escherichia coli* O157:H7. Courtesy of Centers for Disease Control and Prevention/Peggy S. Hayes.

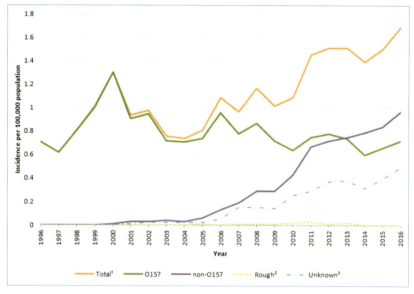

Image 49.4
Incidence of human Shiga toxin–producing *Escherichia coli* (STEC) infection reported to Laboratory-based Enteric Disease Surveillance (LEDS), by reporting partner, United States, 2016 (n = 7,015). The "Total" category includes culture-confirmed infections of serogroup O157, non-O157 serogroups, and rough isolates. [2] The "Rough" category includes isolates with an O antigen that could not be determined because the strain autoagglutinated (agglutinated in all antisera and diluent). Strains behaving in this manner are often blocked in one or more steps of O antigen synthesis and typically appear flat with irregular edges when grown on solid media. These isolates could be O157 or non-O157 STEC. [3] The "Unknown" category includes STEC infections detected exclusively with culture-independent diagnostic tests and culture-confirmed STEC infections reported to LEDS without serogroup information. LEDS does not currently collect information on test type and cannot differentiate between these 2 types of reports. Courtesy of Centers for Disease Control and Prevention.

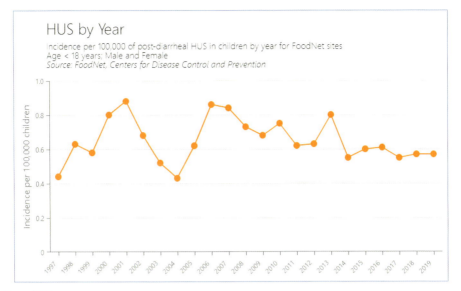

Image 49.5
Hemolytic-uremic syndrome (HUS) by year. Incidence per 100,000 of postdiarrheal HUS in children by year for Foodborne Diseases Active Surveillance Network (FoodNet) sites. Courtesy of Centers for Disease Control and Prevention.

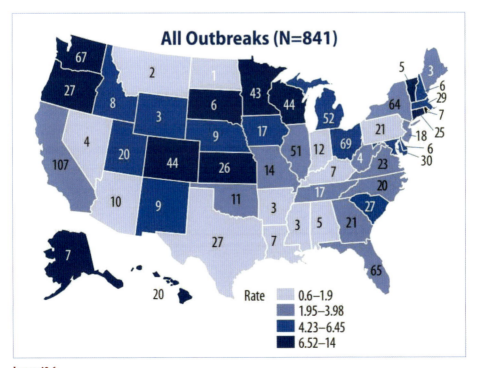

Image 49.6
Rate of reported foodborne disease outbreaks per 1 million population and number of outbreaks, by state and confirmed and suspected etiologic agent—Foodborne Disease Outbreak Surveillance System, United States, 2017. Courtesy of Centers for Disease Control and Prevention.

CHAPTER 50

Other Fungal Diseases

Uncommonly encountered fungi can cause infection in infants and children with immunosuppression or other underlying conditions. Fungi can cause invasive mold infections, such as mucormycosis, fusariosis, scedosporiosis, and the phaeohyphomycoses (black molds), as well as invasive yeast infections with organisms such as *Malazzesia, Trichosporon, Rhodotorula,* and many more (more common mycoses, including aspergillosis, blastomycosis, candidiasis, coccidioidomycosis, cryptococcosis, histoplasmosis, paracoccidioidomycosis, and sporotrichosis, are discussed in individual chapters). Children can acquire infection from these fungi through inhalation via the respiratory tract or direct inoculation after traumatic disruption of cutaneous barriers. A list of some of these fungi and the pertinent underlying host conditions, reservoirs or routes of entry, clinical manifestations, diagnostic laboratory tests, and treatments can be found in Table 50.1. Taken as a group, few in vitro antifungal susceptibility data are available on which to base treatment recommendations for these uncommon invasive fungal infections, especially in children. Physicians should consider consultation with a pediatric infectious disease specialist experienced in the diagnosis and treatment of invasive fungal infections when treating a child infected with one of these mycoses.

Table 50.1
Additional Fungal Diseases

Disease and Agent	Underlying Host Condition(s)	Reservoir(s) or Route(s) of Entry	Common Clinical Manifestation(s)	Diagnostic Laboratory Test(s)	Treatment
Hyalohyphomycosis					
Fusarium species	Granulocytopenia; hematopoietic stem cell transplant; severe immunocompromise; severe neutropenia and/or T-lymphocyte immunodeficiency	Respiratory tract; sinuses; skin; ingestion	Pulmonary infiltrates; cutaneous lesions (eg, ecthyma); sinusitis; disseminated infection	Culture of blood or tissue specimen, histopathologic examination of tissue	Voriconazole, posaconazole,[a,b] isavuconazole,[a,b] or amphotericin B deoxycholate[c]
Pseudallescheria boydii/ Scedosporium apiospermum complex	None or trauma or immunosuppression; cystic fibrosis; chronic granulomatous disease; chronic glucocorticoid use; hematologic malignancy	Environment; respiratory tract; direct inoculation (eg, skin puncture)	Pneumonia; localized pulmonary process or disseminated infection; osteomyelitis or septic arthritis; mycetoma (immunocompetent patients): endocarditis; keratitis and endophthalmitis; brain abscesses; lesions of the skin, soft tissue, or bone	Culture and histopathologic examination of tissue	Voriconazole or isavuconazole[b]
Lomentospora (formerly *Scedosporium*) *prolificans*					Voriconazole; consider addition of an echinocandin or terbinafine.
Talaromycosis					
Talaromyces (*Penicillium*) *marneffei*	HIV infection and exposure to Southeast Asia	Respiratory tract	Pneumonitis; invasive dermatitis; disseminated infection	Culture of blood, bone marrow, or tissue; histopathological examination of tissue	Amphotericin B; alternative, itraconazole[b]
Phaeohyphomycosis					
Alternaria species	None or trauma or immunosuppression	Respiratory tract; skin	Sinusitis; cutaneous lesions	Culture and histopathologic examination of tissue	Voriconazole[b] or amphotericin B deoxycholate[c]
Bipolaris species	None or trauma, immunosuppression, or chronic sinusitis	Environment	Sinusitis; cerebral and disseminated infection	Culture and histopathologic examination of tissue	Voriconazole,[b] posaconazole,[b] itraconazole,[d] or amphotericin B deoxycholate[c]; surgical excision

(continues)

Table 50.1 (continued)

Disease and Agent	Underlying Host Condition(s)	Reservoir(s) or Route(s) of Entry	Common Clinical Manifestation(s)	Diagnostic Laboratory Test(s)	Treatment
Phaeohyphomycosis (continued)					
Cladophialophora species	None or trauma or immunosuppression	Environment	Cerebral infection	Culture and histopathologic examination of tissue	Voriconazole,[b] posaconazole,[b] itraconazole,[d] or amphotericin B deoxycholate[c]; surgical excision
Curvularia species	Immunosuppression; altered skin integrity; asthma or nasal polyps; chronic sinusitis	Environment	Allergic fungal sinusitis; invasive dermatitis; disseminated infection	Culture and histopathologic examination of tissue	Allergic fungal sinusitis: surgery and corticosteroids
Invasive disease: voriconazole,[b] itraconazole,[b,d] or amphotericin B deoxycholate[c]					
Exophiala species, *Exserohilum* species	None or trauma or immunosuppression	Environment	Sinusitis; cutaneous lesions; disseminated infection; meningitis associated with contaminated steroid for epidural use	Culture and histopathologic examination of tissue	Voriconazole,[b,e] itraconazole,[b,d] amphotericin B deoxycholate, or surgical excision
Invasive Yeasts					
Trichosporon species	Immunosuppression: central venous catheter; hematologic malignancy, often with neutropenia; AIDS; extensive burns; glucocorticoid treatment; heart valve surgery; exposure to tropical environments	Environment; normal flora of gastrointestinal tract	Bloodstream infection; superficial skin lesions endocarditis; peritonitis; pneumonitis; disseminated infection	Blood culture; histopathologic examination of tissue or nodules; urine, sputum, and cerebrospinal fluid cultures; bronchoscopy with alveolar lavage cultures	For invasive infections, voriconazole or amphotericin B deoxycholate[b] For superficial infections, shaving of the hair and application of a topical azole antifungal to the affected areas

OTHER FUNGAL DISEASES

Organism	Risk Factors	Site	Diagnosis	Treatment
Malassezia species	Immunosuppression; preterm birth; exposure to parenteral nutrition that includes fat emulsions	Skin	Pityriasis versicolor, seborrheic dermatitis, central catheter–associated bloodstream infection; interstitial pneumonitis; urinary tract infection; meningitis	Culture of blood, catheter tip, or tissue specimen (requires special laboratory handling)	Removal of catheters and temporary cessation of lipid infusion; amphotericin B deoxycholate, azole therapy

Mucormycosis (formerly Zygomycosis)

Organism	Risk Factors	Site	Diagnosis	Treatment
Rhizopus; Mucor; Lichtheimia (formerly *Absidia*) species; *Rhizomucor* species; *Cunninghamella* species	Immunosuppression; hematologic malignant neoplasm; renal failure; diabetes mellitus; iron overload syndromes	Respiratory tract; skin	Rhinocerebral infection; pulmonary infection; disseminated infection; skin (traumatic wounds) and gastrointestinal tract (less commonly)	Histopathologic examination of tissue and culture	Amphotericin B deoxycholate for initial therapy and consider posaconazole[a] for maintenance therapy, with surgical excision and debridement, as feasible; isavuconazole (voriconazole has no activity); echinocandins (eg, caspofungin) may have clinical utility when combined with amphotericin B.

If the patient is intolerant of or refractory to amphotericin B deoxycholate, liposomal amphotericin B can be substituted.

[a] Demonstrates activity in vitro, but few clinical data are available for children.
[b] No US Food and Drug Administration approval for this indication.
[c] Consider use of a lipid-based formulation of amphotericin B.
[d] Itraconazole has been shown to be effective for cutaneous disease in adults, but safety and efficacy have not been established in children <18 years of age.
[e] Voriconazole demonstrates activity in vitro, but no clinical data are available.

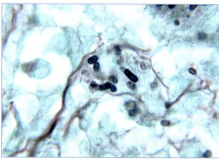

Image 50.1
Note the histopathologic changes observable in a mouse testicle and indicative of penicilliosis caused by *Penicillium marneffei*. With methenamine silver stain, the histopathologic changes indicative of penicilliosis, caused specifically by *P marneffei*, include the presence of globe-shaped yeast cells undergoing multiplication through fission. Courtesy of Centers for Disease Control and Prevention.

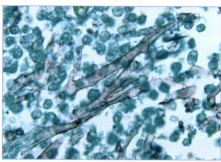

Image 50.2
This slide shows the histopathologic changes observable in a heart valve and resultant from zygomycosis caused by *Rhizomucor pusillus*. With methenamine silver stain, one can detect the presence of fungal elements associated with zygomycosis, including sparsely septate hyphae, among a mostly acute inflammatory process with some island of chronic granulomatous inflammation. Courtesy of Centers for Disease Control and Prevention.

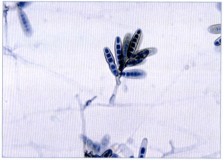

Image 50.3
This micrograph reveals a conidia-laden conidiophore of the fungus *Bipolaris hawaiiensis*. *Bipolaris* species are known to be one of the causative agents of the fungal illness phaeohyphomycosis, which can be superficially confined to the skin or systemically disseminated and can involve the brain, lungs, and bones. Courtesy of Centers for Disease Control and Prevention.

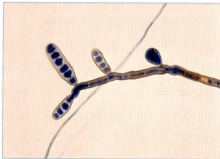

Image 50.4
Note the fine branching tubes of the fungus *Exserohilum rostratum*, which is the cause of phaeohyphomycosis. Phaeohyphomycosis is a fungal infection characterized by superficial and deep tissue involvement caused by dematiaceous, dark-walled fungi that form pigmented hyphae, or fine branching tubes, and yeastlike cells in the infected tissues. Courtesy of Centers for Disease Control and Prevention.

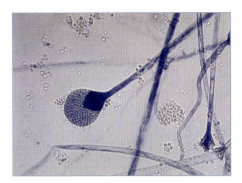

Image 50.5
This photomicrograph reveals a mature sporangium of a *Mucor* species fungus. *Mucor* is a common indoor mold and is among the fungi that cause the group of infections known as zygomycosis. The infection typically involves the rhino-facial-cranial area, lungs, gastrointestinal tract, or skin or less commonly involves other organ systems. Courtesy of Centers for Disease Control and Prevention.

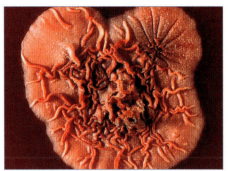

Image 50.6
The surface of a *Penicillium marneffei* colony. *P marneffei* is endemic to Southeast Asia, where it is one of the more common HIV-related opportunistic infections. Courtesy of Centers for Disease Control and Prevention.

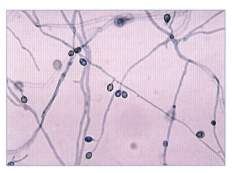

Image 50.8
This micrograph depicts a number of mycelia with attached conidia of the fungal organism *Pseudallescheria boydii*. The opportunistic pathogen *P boydii* is responsible for the infection known as pseudallescheriasis, which normally affects those who are immunocompromised, and is also known to be a cause of white grain mycetoma. Courtesy of Centers for Disease Control and Prevention.

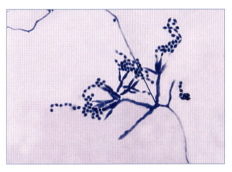

Image 50.7
This micrograph depicts multiple conidia-laden conidiophores and phialides of a *Penicillium marneffei* fungal organism. *Penicillium* species are known to cause penicilliosis, which usually affects individuals with immunocompromise, such as those with AIDS or undergoing chemotherapy. *P marneffei* is normally acquired though inhalation of airborne spores. Courtesy of Centers for Disease Control and Prevention.

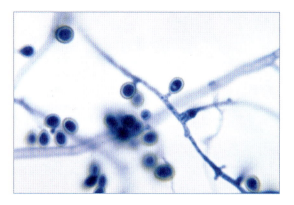

Image 50.9
This photomicrograph reveals the conidiophores with conidia of the fungus *Pseudallescheria boydii* from a slide culture. *P boydii* is pathogenic in humans, especially those who are immunocompromised, causing infections in almost all body regions, and is classified under the broad heading of pseudallescheriasis. Courtesy of Centers for Disease Control and Prevention.

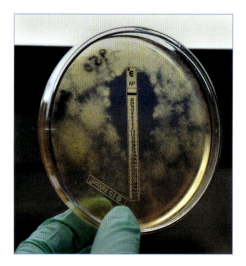

Image 50.10
This culture plate revealed the results of a susceptibility test to the antifungal drug amphotericin B. The drug inhibited growth of the fungal organism *Exserohilum* in the clear area where the amphotericin B had diffused into the medium, whereas the *Exserohilum* organisms were growing elsewhere on the plate, where the drug had not diffused into the medium.

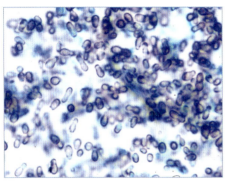

Image 50.11
Malassezia furfur pneumonitis. Organisms observable with a tissue stain for fungi. Courtesy of Dimitris P. Agamanolis, MD.

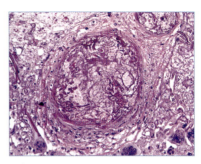

Image 50.12
Cerebral mucormycosis. Fungal organism invaded the vessel wall. The vessel is thrombosed. Courtesy of Dimitris P. Agamanolis, MD.

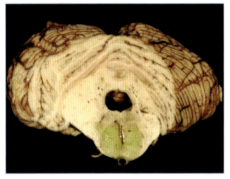

Image 50.13
Cerebral mucormycosis in a patient with acute lymphoblastic leukemia. Occlusion of the basilar artery and infarct of the pons. The patient had jaundice. Courtesy of Dimitris P. Agamanolis, MD.

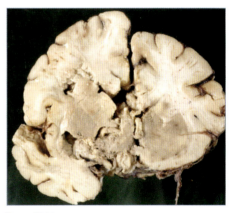

Image 50.14
Extensive cerebral necrosis in a patient with mucormycosis. Courtesy of Dimitris P. Agamanolis, MD.

CHAPTER 51

Fusobacterium Infections
(Including Lemierre Syndrome)

CLINICAL MANIFESTATIONS

Fusobacterium species, including *Fusobacterium necrophorum* and *Fusobacterium nucleatum*, can be isolated from oropharyngeal specimens in healthy people and are frequent components of human dental plaque with the potential to lead to periodontal disease. Invasive disease attributable to *Fusobacterium* species has been associated with otitis media, tonsillitis, gingivitis, and oropharyngeal trauma including dental and oropharyngeal surgery such as tonsillectomy. Ten percent of cases of invasive *Fusobacterium* infections are associated with concomitant Epstein-Barr virus infection.

Preceding oropharyngeal infection is the most frequent primary source for invasive infection. Invasive infections can be characterized by peritonsillar abscess, deep neck space infection, mastoiditis, and sinusitis that can be complicated by meningitis, cerebral abscess, and dural sinus venous thrombosis. Otogenic sources of infection have also been reported.

Invasive infection following tonsillitis was described early in the 20th century and was referred to as **postanginal sepsis** or **Lemierre syndrome**. The classic syndrome starts with sore throat symptoms, which may improve or may continue to worsen. Fever and sore throat are followed by severe neck pain (anginal pain) that can be accompanied by unilateral neck swelling, trismus, dysphagia, and rigors associated with development of suppurative jugular venous thrombosis (JVT). Patients with classic Lemierre syndrome have a sepsis syndrome with multiple organ dysfunction. Metastatic complications from septic embolic phenomena associated with JVT are common and may manifest as multiple pleural septic emboli, pleural empyema, pyogenic arthritis, osteomyelitis, or disseminated intravascular coagulation. Laboratory abnormalities associated with Lemierre syndrome can include significantly elevated inflammatory marker levels, thrombocytopenia, elevated aminotransferase levels, hyperbilirubinemia, and elevated creatinine level. Persistent headache or other neurological signs may indicate the presence of cerebral venous sinus thrombosis (eg, cavernous sinus thrombosis), meningitis, or brain abscess. *Fusobacterium* species (most commonly *F necrophorum*) are often isolated from blood or other normally sterile sites and account for at least 80% of Lemierre syndrome cases. Lemierre-like syndromes have also been reported following infection with *Arcanobacterium haemolyticum*, *Bacteroides* species, anaerobic *Streptococcus* species, other anaerobic bacteria, and methicillin-susceptible and methicillin-resistant strains of *Staphylococcus aureus*.

JVT can be completely vaso-occlusive. Some children with JVT associated with Lemierre syndrome have evidence of thrombophilia at diagnosis. These findings often resolve over several months and can indicate response to the inflammatory, prothrombotic process associated with infection rather than an underlying hypercoagulable state.

Fusobacterium species have also been associated with intra-abdominal and pelvic infections including acute appendicitis, suppurative portomesenteric vein thrombosis, and suppurative thrombosis of the pelvic vasculature.

ETIOLOGY

Fusobacterium species are filamentous, anaerobic, non–spore-forming, gram-negative bacilli. Human infection usually results from *F necrophorum* subspecies *funduliforme*, but infections with other species including *F nucleatum*, *Fusobacterium gonidiaformans*, *Fusobacterium naviforme*, *Fusobacterium mortiferum*, and *Fusobacterium varium* have been reported. Infection with *Fusobacterium* species, alone or in combination with other oral anaerobic bacteria, may result in Lemierre syndrome, but unlike with other anaerobic infections, *Fusobacterium* species are frequently the only organisms identified in these infections.

EPIDEMIOLOGY

Fusobacterium species are commonly found in soil and in the respiratory tracts of animals, including cattle, dogs, fowl, goats, sheep, and horses, and can be isolated from the oropharynx of healthy people. *Fusobacterium* infections are most common in adolescents and young adults, but infections, including fatal cases of Lemierre syndrome, have been reported in infants and young children.

DIAGNOSTIC TESTS

Fusobacterium species can be isolated by using conventional liquid anaerobic blood culture media. However, the organism grows best on semisolid media for fastidious anaerobic organisms or blood agar supplemented with vitamin K, hemin, menadione, and a reducing agent. Colonies are generally cream to yellow colored, smooth, and round and may show a narrow zone of alpha or beta hemolysis on blood agar, depending on the species of blood used in the medium; however, *F nucleatum* may appear as bread crumb-like colonies. Many strains fluoresce chartreuse green under UV light. Most *Fusobacterium* organisms are indole positive. On Gram stain, *F nucleatum* usually exhibits spindle-shaped cells with tapered ends, whereas *F necrophorum* and other species may be highly pleomorphic with swollen areas. The accurate identification of anaerobes to the species level has become important with the increasing incidence of microorganisms that are resistant to multiple drugs. Conventional and commercial culture-based biochemical test systems are reasonably accurate, at least to the genus level. Sequencing of the 16S ribosomal RNA gene, and phylogenetic analysis or the use of mass spectrometry of bacterial cell components, can accurately identify *Fusobacterium* species to the species level.

One should consider Lemierre syndrome in ill-appearing febrile children and especially in adolescents having a sore throat with exquisite neck pain and swelling over the angle of the jaw, accompanied by rigors. Aerobic and anaerobic blood cultures should be performed to detect invasive *Fusobacterium* species and other possible pathogens. Imaging studies of the internal jugular veins should be performed, but it is important to note that a significant proportion of patients with a diagnosis of Lemierre syndrome do not have a thrombus detected by imaging. Computed tomography and magnetic resonance imaging are more sensitive than ultrasonography to document thrombosis and thrombophlebitis of the internal jugular vein early in the course of illness and to better identify thrombus extension beyond the areas visible by ultrasonography, including under the mandible and clavicle.

TREATMENT

Aggressive and prompt antimicrobial therapy is the mainstay of treatment. *Fusobacterium* species are generally susceptible to metronidazole, clindamycin, chloramphenicol, penicillin with β-lactamase inhibitor combinations (ampicillin-sulbactam or piperacillin-tazobactam), carbapenem, cefoxitin, and ceftriaxone. Antimicrobial resistance has increased in anaerobic bacteria; therefore, susceptibility testing is indicated for all clinically significant anaerobic isolates, including *Fusobacterium* species. Combination therapy with metronidazole or clindamycin, in addition to a β-lactam agent active against aerobic oral and respiratory tract pathogens (cefotaxime, ceftriaxone, or cefuroxime), is recommended for patients with invasive infection caused by *Fusobacterium* species. Alternatively, some experts recommend monotherapy with a penicillin–β-lactamase inhibitor combination (ampicillin-sulbactam or piperacillin-tazobactam) or a carbapenem (meropenem, imipenem, or ertapenem). Up to 50% of *F nucleatum* and 20% of *F necrophorum* isolates produce β-lactamases, rendering them resistant to penicillin, ampicillin, and some cephalosporins. *Fusobacterium* species are intrinsically resistant to gentamicin, fluoroquinolone agents, and, typically, macrolides.

The duration of antimicrobial therapy depends on the anatomical location and severity of infection but is usually several weeks. Surgical intervention involving debridement or incision and drainage of abscesses may be necessary. Anticoagulation therapy has been used in both adults and children with JVT and cavernous sinus thrombosis. However, evidence for the role of anticoagulation in thrombosis outcome is lacking.

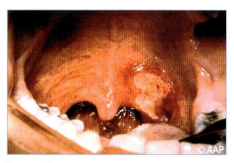

Image 51.1
Vincent stomatitis has been confused with diphtheria, although this infection is usually a mixed infection, including fusiform and spirochetal anaerobic bacteria such as *Fusobacterium*, and is associated with severe pain and halitosis. Note ulceration of the soft palate with surrounding erythema. Courtesy of Edgar O. Ledbetter, MD, FAAP.

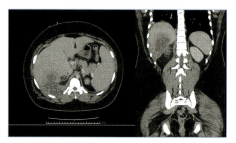

Image 51.2
This 15-year-old with obesity had a dental cleaning 7 days before presentation. The patient was found to have monomicrobial liver abscess with *Fusobacterium nucleatum*. The patient responded well to combined therapy with percutaneous drainage and antimicrobials for 6 weeks. Copyright Shom Dasgupta-Tsinikas, MD, FAAP.

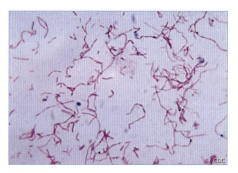

Image 51.3
This photomicrograph shows *Fusobacterium nucleatum* after being cultured in a thioglycolate medium for 48 hours. Courtesy of Centers for Disease Control and Prevention.

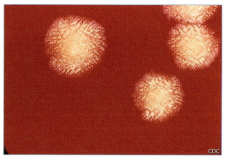

Image 51.4
This photograph demonstrates the morphological features of 4 colonies of *Fusobacterium fusiforme* bacteria that were grown on blood agar medium for 48 hours. *F fusiforme* is a spindle-shaped, gram-negative bacteria that colonizes the gingival sulcus of the human oral cavity and has also been isolated from infections of the upper respiratory tract. Courtesy of Centers for Disease Control and Prevention/V. R. Dowell Jr, MD.

CHAPTER 52
Giardia duodenalis (formerly Giardia lamblia and Giardia intestinalis) Infections
(Giardiasis)

CLINICAL MANIFESTATIONS

Symptoms of *Giardia* infection are attributable to dysfunction of the small bowel caused by residing trophozoites and range from asymptomatic carriage to fulminant diarrhea and dehydration. Most infections are asymptomatic, but children are more often symptomatic than adults. Symptomatic patients are mildly to moderately ill and frequently report intermittent abdominal cramping and bloating, and almost intolerable foul-smelling flatus and stools. Chronic infection, often with weight loss, is common. A more fulminant manifestation with acute and chronic diarrhea, malabsorption, failure to thrive, and weight loss may occur, but systemic symptoms, other than malaise, are uncommon.

Symptoms are also caused by lactose intolerance and malabsorption, which result in voluminous diarrhea often described as "greasy or fatty" and foul smelling. Sometimes atypical upper gastrointestinal symptoms of belching, nausea, and vomiting predominate, causing a delay in diagnosis. Fever, mucus, and blood in stool are distinctly atypical and suggest infection with another agent(s). Chronic symptoms similar to those of irritable bowel may be confused with giardiasis and are also sequelae of giardiasis. The natural history of acquired untreated infections is not well-documented, but duration of infection is typically prolonged, can be abnormally long-standing in young people, and can last years in immunosuppressed individuals. In children, development of immunity is poor and repeated infections are common. Patients with cystic fibrosis have an increased prevalence of *Giardia duodenalis* infection. Extraintestinal involvement is unusual. Giardiasis is not associated with eosinophilia.

ETIOLOGY

G duodenalis (syn *Giardia lamblia* and *Giardia intestinalis*) is a flagellate protozoan that exists in trophozoite and cyst forms; the infective form is the cyst. Infection is limited to the small intestine and biliary tract. *Giardia* cysts are infectious immediately after being excreted in feces and remain viable for 3 months in water at 4 °C (39 °F).

EPIDEMIOLOGY

Giardiasis has a worldwide distribution and is the most common intestinal parasitic infection of humans identified in the United States and the world. Highest incidence in the United States is reported among children 1 through 9 years of age, adults 25 to 29 years of age, and adults 55 through 59 years of age and residents of northern states. Peak illness onset occurs from early summer through early fall. As few as 10 to 100 cysts are able to initiate infection. Transmission of *G duodenalis* is most likely to occur when exposure to infected feces is likely, including (1) child care centers; (2) areas of the world with endemic disease; (3) close contact, including sexual contact, with infected people; (4) swallowing of contaminated drinking or recreational water; and (5) consumption of unfiltered or untreated water such as during outdoor activities (eg, camping or backpacking). Although less common, outbreaks associated with food or food handlers have been reported. Surveys conducted in the United States have helped identify overall prevalence rates of *Giardia* organisms in stool specimens that range from 5% to 7%, with variations depending on age, geographic location, and seasonality. Duration of cyst excretion is variable but can range from weeks to months. Giardiasis is communicable for as long as the infected person excretes cysts.

The **incubation period** is usually 1 to 3 weeks.

DIAGNOSTIC TESTS

Giardia cysts or trophozoites are not consistently found in the stools of infected patients. Diagnostic sensitivity can be increased by examining up to 3 stool specimens over several days. New molecular enteric panel assays generally include *Giardia* as a target pathogen. Diagnostic techniques include direct fluorescence antibody (considered the gold standard), rapid immunochromatographic cartridge assays, enzyme immunoassay kits, microscopy with trichrome staining, and molecular assays. If there is a suspicion of false-negative results, repeated testing should be performed and use of a different methodology considered. Molecular testing (such as polymerase chain reaction testing) can be used to identify the genotypes and subtypes of *Giardia*, but this is not helpful clinically. Retesting is recommended only if symptoms persist after treatment.

TREATMENT

Some infections are self-limited, and treatment may not be required. Tinidazole, metronidazole, and nitazoxanide are the drugs of choice. A 5- to 7-day course of metronidazole has an efficacy of 80% to 100% in pediatric patients. A single dose of tinidazole, a nitroimidazole for children 3 years and older, has a median efficacy of 91% in pediatric patients (range, 80%–100%) and has fewer adverse effects than metronidazole. A 3-day course of nitazoxanide oral suspension has efficacy similar to metronidazole and has the advantage(s) of treating other intestinal parasites and of being approved for use in children 1 year and older. If treatment is needed during pregnancy, paromomycin, a poorly absorbed aminoglycoside, is 50% to 70% effective and is the recommended treatment.

Symptom recurrence after completing antimicrobial treatment can be attributable to reinfection or recurrence, post-*Giardia* irritable bowel, residual lactose intolerance (occurs in 20%–40% of patients), or symptoms attributable to another process or infection. Recurrences are associated with immunosuppression or poor immunity, insufficient treatment, drug resistance, or reexposure.

Because new or residual symptoms are nonspecific, repeated testing should be performed. There is no clear best course for re-treatment, but options include treatment with an alternative drug of a different class, a longer course of the first failed drug, or a combined drug regimen consisting of 2 different drug types.

Patients who are immunocompromised because of hypogammaglobulinemia or lymphoproliferative disease have higher risk for giardiasis, and a cure is more difficult for these patients. Among HIV-infected children and adults without AIDS, effective combination antiretroviral therapy and antiparasitic therapy are the major initial treatments of these infections. Patients with AIDS often respond to standard therapy, but in some cases, additional treatment is required. If giardiasis is refractory to standard treatment of HIV-infected patients with AIDS, longer treatment duration or combination antiparasitic therapy (eg, tinidazole, nitazoxanide, or metronidazole plus one of the following drugs: paromomycin, albendazole, or quinacrine) may be appropriate.

Treatment of asymptomatic carriers is controversial but recommended in the United States and other areas of low prevalence to prevent infection within families or of other children. Treatment of children likely to be reinfected, such as those residing in areas of high prevalence, is not recommended unless medically indicated.

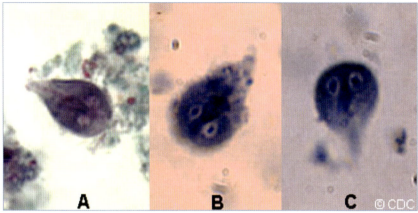

Image 52.1
Three trophozoites of *Giardia intestinalis* (A, trichrome stain; B and C, iron hematoxylin stain). Each cell has 2 nuclei with a large, central karyosome. Cell length is 9–21 μm. Trophozoites are usually found in fresh diarrheal stool or in duodenal mucus. Courtesy of Centers for Disease Control and Prevention.

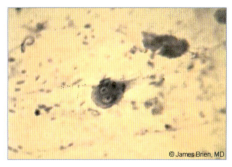

Image 52.2
Giardia intestinalis cyst in a stool preparation. Giardiasis is the most common protozoal infection in the United States. Copyright James Brien.

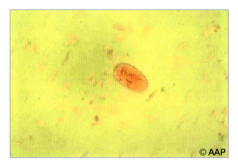

Image 52.3
Giardia intestinalis cyst in a stool preparation. The ingested cyst produces trophozoites in the proximal small intestine. As the trophozoites pass through the intestinal tract, they form cysts that are passed in the stool and are the infective form of *G intestinalis*.

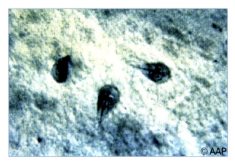

Image 52.4
Giardia intestinalis cysts (trichrome stain). Person-to-person transmission is the most common mode of transmission of giardiasis.

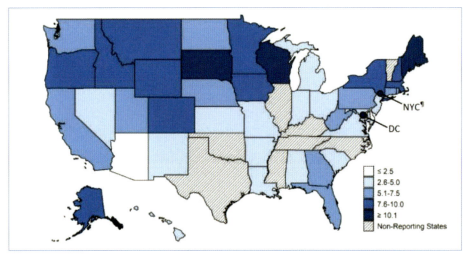

Image 52.5
Incidence of giardiasis cases (per 100,000 population), by reporting jurisdiction—National Notifiable Diseases Surveillance System, United States, 2018 (n = 15,579). Giardiasis is geographically widespread across the United States. Although incidence rates appear to be consistently higher in the northern states, differences in incidence might reflect differences in risk factors or modes of transmission of *Giardia*, the magnitude of outbreaks, or the capacity or requirements to detect, investigate, and report cases. Non-reporting states included Illinois, Kentucky, Mississippi, North Carolina, Oklahoma, Tennessee, Texas, and Vermont. New York State and New York City data are mutually exclusive. Courtesy of Centers for Disease Control and Prevention.

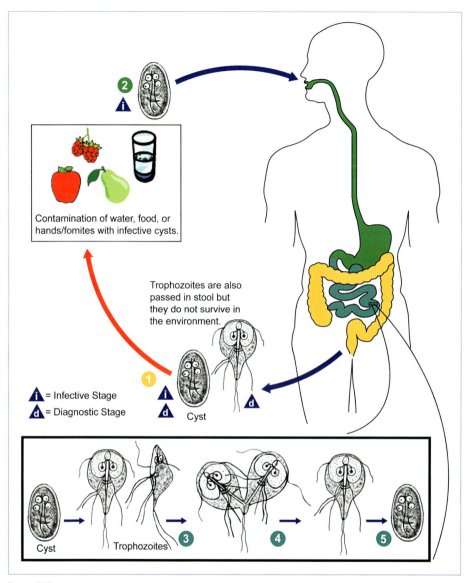

Image 52.6

Cysts are resistant forms and are responsible for transmission of giardiasis. Cysts and trophozoites can be found in the feces (diagnostic stages) (1). The cysts are hardy and can survive several months in cold water. Infection occurs by the ingestion of cysts in contaminated water or food or by the fecal-oral route (hands or fomites) (2). In the small intestine, excystation releases trophozoites (each cyst produces 2 trophozoites) (3). Trophozoites multiply by longitudinal binary fission, remaining in the lumen of the proximal small bowel, where they can be free or attached to the mucosa by a ventral sucking disk (4). Encystation occurs as the parasites transit toward the colon. The cyst is the stage found most commonly in nondiarrheal feces (5). Because the cysts are infectious when passed in the stool or shortly afterward, person-to-person transmission is possible. While animals are infected with *Giardia*, their importance as a reservoir is unclear. Courtesy of Centers for Disease Control and Prevention.

CHAPTER 53

Gonococcal Infections

CLINICAL MANIFESTATIONS

Gonococcal infections demonstrate a spectrum of clinical manifestations, ranging from asymptomatic carriage, to characteristic localized infections (usually mucosal), to disseminated disease, and should be considered in 3 distinct age-groups: newborns, prepubertal children, and postpubertal sexually active adolescents and young adults. Multiple sites of infection can occur simultaneously in one individual.

- **Asymptomatic carriage** has been detected in the oropharynx of child sexual abuse survivors and in the urogenital tract of sexually active females (up to 80% are asymptomatic) and males (around 10% can be asymptomatic). In all age-groups, most pharyngeal infections are asymptomatic. Likewise, most rectal infections are asymptomatic; rectal carriage can accompany 20% to 70% of female urogenital infections.

- **Localized disease** manifests at the site of inoculation and includes (1) scalp abscess, which can be associated with fetal scalp monitoring during labor if the mother has an undiagnosed gonococcal infection; (2) either ophthalmia neonatorum in newborns following exposure to an infected birth canal or conjunctivitis in any age-group following eye inoculation with infected secretions (eg, through hand transfer from the urogenital tract); (3) acute tonsillopharyngitis, accompanied by cervical adenopathy; (4) urethritis (with mucopurulent discharge, dysuria, and/or suprapubic pain) in any age-group or sex; (5) genital disease such as vulvitis and/or vaginitis in prepubertal females (with vaginal discharge and/or dysuria), bartholinitis and/or cervicitis in postpubertal females (with mucopurulent discharge, intermenstrual bleeding, and/or dyspareunia), and penile abscess; and (6) proctitis (symptoms range from painless mucopurulent discharge and scant rectal bleeding to overt proctitis with associated rectal pain and tenesmus). Extension to the upper genital tract and beyond (less common in prepubertal children) can result in pelvic inflammatory disease (endometritis and/or salpingitis) and perihepatitis (Fitz-Hugh–Curtis syndrome) in females and epididymitis, prostatitis, and/or seminal vesiculitis in males, with resultant scarring, ectopic pregnancy, impairment of fertility, and chronic pelvic pain, particularly in females.

- Disseminated gonococcal infection (DGI) occurs in up to 3% of untreated people with mucosal gonorrhea. DGI can manifest as petechial or pustular skin lesions and as asymmetrical polyarthralgia, tenosynovitis, or oligoarticular septic arthritis (arthritis-dermatitis syndrome). In neonates, DGI can manifest as sepsis, arthritis, or meningitis. Bacteremia can result in a maculopapular rash with necrosis, tenosynovitis, and migratory arthritis. Arthritis may be reactive (sterile) or septic in nature. Meningitis and endocarditis occur rarely.

ETIOLOGY

Neisseria gonorrhoeae is a gram-negative, oxidase-positive diplococcus.

EPIDEMIOLOGY

Gonococcal infections occur only in humans. The source of the organism is exudate and secretions from infected mucosal surfaces; *N gonorrhoeae* is communicable as long as a person harbors the organism. Transmission results from intimate contact, such as sexual acts and parturition. Sexual abuse is the most frequent cause of gonococcal infection in prepubertal children beyond the newborn period.

N gonorrhoeae infection is the second most commonly reported sexually transmitted infection (STI) in the United States, following *Chlamydia trachomatis* infection. As of October 2019, a total of 583,405 cases of gonorrhea (179 cases per 100,000 population) were reported in the United States for 2018 according to Centers for Disease Control and Prevention (CDC) surveillance reports. Reported gonorrhea cases continued to be highest among adolescents and young adults. In 2018, the highest rates for females were observed among those aged 20 through 24 years (702.6 cases per 100,000 females) and 15 through 19 years (548.1 cases per 100,000 females). For males, the rate was highest among those aged 20 through 24 years (720.9 cases per 100,000 males) and 25 through 29 years

(674.0 cases per 100,000 males). Rates of reported gonorrhea are highest in the southern United States and have significant racial and ethnic disparities. In 2018, the rate of reported gonorrhea cases remained highest among Black people (548.9 cases per 100,000 population), a rate 7.7 times the rate among white people (71.1 cases per 100,000 population). Comparable differences in gonorrhea rates were also observed among other racial and ethnic groups versus white people: 4.6 times higher among American Indian/Alaska Native people, 2.6 times higher among Native Hawaiian/Other Pacific Islander populations, 1.6 times higher among Hispanic people, and 1.3 times higher among multiracial people. However, the rate among Asian people (35.1 cases per 100,000 population) was half the rate among white people. Disparities in gonorrhea rates are also observed by sexual behavior. Surveillance networks that monitor trends in STI prevalence among men who have sex with men (MSM) have found very high proportions of positive gonorrhea pharyngeal, urethral, and rectal test results as well as coinfection with other STIs. Populations with greater risk for DGI include asymptomatic carriers; neonates; menstruating, pregnant, and postpartum females; MSM; and individuals with complement deficiency.

Diagnosis of genitourinary tract gonorrhea infection should also prompt investigation for other STIs, including chlamydia, trichomoniasis, syphilis, and HIV infection. Concurrent infection with *C trachomatis* is common.

The **incubation period** is usually 2 to 7 days.

DIAGNOSTIC TESTS

Microscopic examination of Gram-stained smears of exudate from the conjunctivae, male urethra, skin lesions, synovial fluid, and, when clinically warranted, cerebrospinal fluid (CSF) may be useful in the initial evaluation. Identification of gram-negative intracellular diplococci in these smears can be helpful, particularly if the organism is not recovered in culture. However, because of low sensitivity, a negative smear result should not be considered sufficient for ruling out infection. Intracellular gram-negative diplococci identified on Gram stain of conjunctival exudate justify presumptive treatment of gonorrhea after appropriate cultures for *N gonorrhoeae* are performed.

N gonorrhoeae can be isolated from normally sterile sites, such as blood, CSF, or synovial fluid, by using nonselective chocolate agar with incubation in 5% to 10% carbon dioxide. Selective media that inhibit normal flora and nonpathogenic *Neisseria* organisms are used for cultures from nonsterile sites, such as the cervix, vagina, rectum, urethra, and pharynx. Specimens for *N gonorrhoeae* culture from mucosal sites should be inoculated immediately onto appropriate agar, because the organism is extremely sensitive to drying and temperature changes.

A nucleic acid amplification test (NAAT) is far superior in overall performance than other *N gonorrhoeae* culture and nonculture diagnostic methods to test genital and extragenital specimens. Most commercially available products are now cleared by the US Food and Drug Administration (FDA) for testing male urethral swab specimens, female endocervical or vaginal swab specimens (provider or patient collected), male or female urine specimens, oropharynx or rectal swab specimens, or liquid cytology specimens. Although NAATs are not FDA cleared for *N gonorrhoeae* testing on conjunctival swab specimens, they have been shown to be more sensitive than *N gonorrhoeae* culture. For urogenital infections, the CDC recommends that optimal specimen types for gonorrhea screening via NAATs include first-void urine from men and vaginal swab specimens from women. Patient-collected samples can be used in place of provider-collected samples in clinical settings when testing by NAAT for urine (men and women) vaginal, rectal, and oropharyngeal swab specimens. Certain NAAT platforms also permit combined testing of specimens for *N gonorrhoeae, C trachomatis,* and *Trichomonas vaginalis.*

Infants and Children

Culture can be used to test urogenital and extragenital sites in girls and boys. NAAT can be used to test for *N gonorrhoeae* from vaginal and urine specimens of girls and urine of boys. Although data on NAAT from extragenital sites in children are more limited and performance is test dependent, no evidence suggests that performance of NAAT for detection of *N gonorrhoeae* in children would differ from that in adults. Consultation with an expert is necessary before using NAAT in this context, both to minimize the possibility of cross-reaction with nongonococcal *Neisseria* species and other commensals. Gram stains are inadequate for evaluating prepubertal children for gonorrhea and should not be used to diagnose or exclude gonorrhea. If evidence of DGI exists, gonorrhea culture and antimicrobial susceptibility testing should be performed on specimens from relevant clinical sites.

TREATMENT

A single dose of intramuscular ceftriaxone is the recommended treatment of uncomplicated gonorrhea infections of the cervix, urethra, and rectum. If chlamydial infection has not been excluded, treatment of *C trachomatis* with oral doxycycline for 7 days should also be provided. A single 500-mg dose of intramuscular ceftriaxone is also recommended for the treatment of uncomplicated gonococcal infections of the pharynx. Gonococcal infections of the pharynx are more difficult to eradicate than are infections at urogenital and anorectal sites.

Resistance to penicillin and tetracycline is widespread, and as of 2007, the CDC no longer recommends the use of fluoroquinolones for gonorrhea because of the increased prevalence of quinolone-resistant *N gonorrhoeae* in the United States. Over the past decade, the minimum inhibitory concentrations for cefixime against *N gonorrhoeae* strains circulating in the United States and other countries has increased and treatment failure following the use of cefixime has been described. As of 2012, the CDC no longer recommends the use of cefixime as a first-line treatment of gonococcal infection. Only ceftriaxone is recommended currently for treatment of gonorrhea in the United States.

To maximize adherence with recommended therapies and reduce complications and transmission, medication for gonococcal infection should be provided on-site and directly observed. If medications are unavailable when treatment is indicated, linkage to an STI treatment facility should be provided for same-day treatment. To minimize disease transmission, people treated for gonorrhea should be instructed to abstain from sexual activity for 7 days after treatment and until all sexual partners are adequately treated (7 days after receiving treatment and resolution of symptoms, if present).

Neonatal Infection

Infants with clinical evidence of ophthalmia neonatorum or scalp abscess attributable to *N gonorrhoeae* should be hospitalized, treated in consultation with an infectious disease specialist, and evaluated for disseminated infection (ie, sepsis, arthritis, meningitis).

One dose of ceftriaxone (25–50 mg/kg, intravenously or intramuscularly, not to exceed 250 mg) is adequate therapy for gonococcal ophthalmia. Cefotaxime, 100 mg/kg, intravenously or intramuscularly as a single dose, can be administered for neonates who are unable to receive ceftriaxone because of simultaneous administration of intravenous calcium. Topical antibiotic therapy alone is inadequate and unnecessary if systemic treatment is administered.

For gonococcal scalp abscesses and DGIs in neonates, treatment is with ceftriaxone (25–50 mg/kg/day, intravenously, in a single daily dose) or cefotaxime (50 mg/kg/day in 2 divided daily doses, intravenously or intramuscularly) for 7 days, with a duration of 10 to 14 days if meningitis is documented.

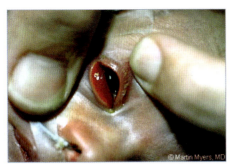

Image 53.1
An infant with gonococcal ophthalmia. In-hospital evaluation and treatment are recommended for infants with gonococcal ophthalmia. Copyright Martin G. Myers, MD.

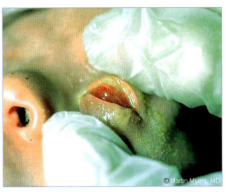

Image 53.2
An 8-day-old with gonococcal ophthalmia. Copyright Martin G. Myers, MD.

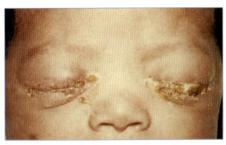

Image 53.3
This newborn has gonococcal ophthalmia neonatorum caused by a maternally transmitted gonococcal infection. Unless preventive measures are taken, it is estimated that gonococcal ophthalmia neonatorum will develop in 28% of neonates born to women with gonorrhea. It affects the corneal epithelium, causing microbial keratitis, ulceration, and perforation. Courtesy of Centers for Disease Control and Prevention.

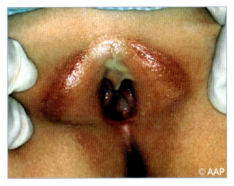

Image 53.4
Profuse, purulent vaginal discharge in an 18-month-old girl who has gonococcal vulvovaginitis. In preadolescent children, this infection is almost always associated with sexual abuse. Identification of the species of cultured gonococci is imperative in suspected cases of sexual abuse.

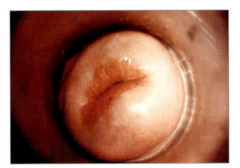

Image 53.5
This colposcopic view of this patient's cervix revealed an eroded ostium caused by *Neisseria gonorrhoeae* infection. A chronic *N gonorrhoeae* infection can lead to complications that can be apparent, such as this cervical inflammation, and some can be quite insipid, giving the impression that the infection has subsided although treatment is still needed. Courtesy of Centers for Disease Control and Prevention.

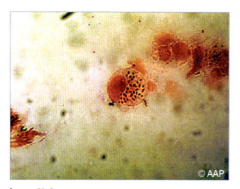

Image 53.6
Gram stain of cervical discharge in an adolescent who has gonococcal cervicitis. Note multiple intracellular diplococci. In children with suspected abuse, it is imperative that the gonococcus be cultured and identified to distinguish pathogens from normal flora.

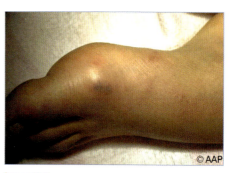

Image 53.7
Gonococcemia with maculopapular and petechial skin lesions, most commonly observed on the hands and feet.

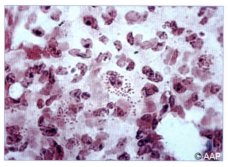

Image 53.8
Intracellular gram-negative diplococci (*Neisseria gonorrhoeae*) isolated on culture of a petechial skin lesion.

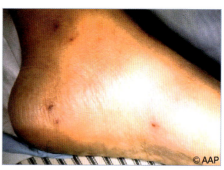

Image 53.9
Adolescent with septic arthritis of the left ankle with petechial and necrotic skin lesions on the feet. Blood cultures were positive for *Neisseria gonorrhoeae*.

GONOCOCCAL INFECTIONS

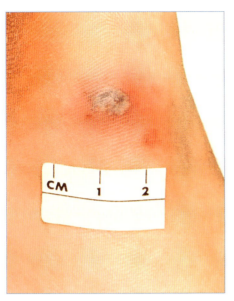

Image 53.10
This patient presented with a cutaneous gonococcal lesion caused by a disseminated *Neisseria gonorrhoeae* bacterial infection. Although gonorrhea is a sexually transmitted infection, if a gonococcal infection is allowed to go untreated, *N gonorrhoeae* bacteria can disseminate throughout the body, forming lesions in extragenital locations. Courtesy of Centers for Disease Control and Prevention.

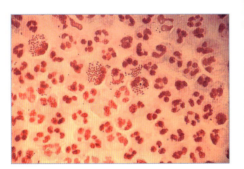

Image 53.12
This photomicrograph reveals the histopathologic features in an acute case of gonococcal urethritis (Gram stain). This image demonstrates the nonrandom distribution of gonococci among polymorphonuclear neutrophils. Note that there are intracellular and extracellular bacteria in the field of view. Courtesy of Centers for Disease Control and Prevention.

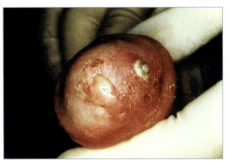

Image 53.11
This male presented with purulent penile discharge caused by gonorrhea with an overlying penile pyoderma lesion. Pyoderma involves the formation of a purulent skin lesion, as in this case, located on the glans penis and overlying the sexually transmitted gonorrhea. Courtesy of Centers for Disease Control and Prevention.

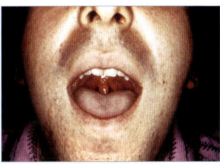

Image 53.13
This patient presented with symptoms later diagnosed as caused by gonococcal pharyngitis. Gonococcal pharyngitis is a sexually transmitted infection acquired through oral sex with an infected partner. Most patients with throat infections caused by gonococci have no symptoms, but some with the infection can experience mild to severe sore throat. Courtesy of Centers for Disease Control and Prevention.

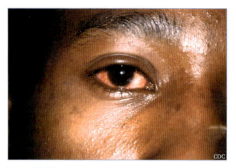

Image 53.14
This patient presented with gonococcal urethritis and gonococcal conjunctivitis of the right eye. If untreated, *Neisseria gonorrhoeae* may spread to the bloodstream and throughout the body. Courtesy of Centers for Disease Control and Prevention/Joe Miller.

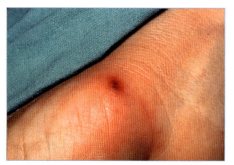

Image 53.15
Disseminated gonococcal infection. Courtesy of Gary Overturf, MD.

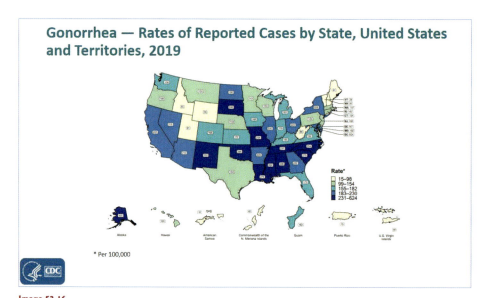

Image 53.16
Rates of reported gonorrhea cases by state, United States and territories, 2019. Courtesy of Centers for Disease Control and Prevention.

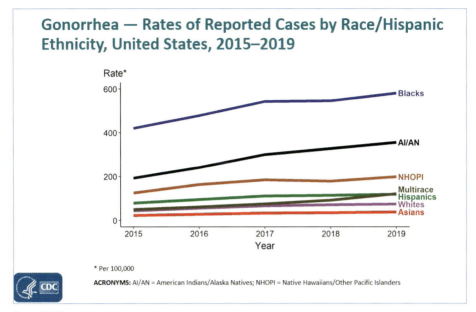

Image 53.17
Rates of reported gonorrhea cases by race/Hispanic ethnicity, United States, 2015–2019. Courtesy of Centers for Disease Control and Prevention.

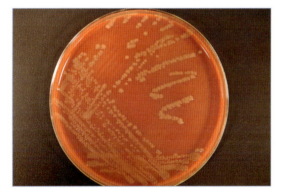

Image 53.18
Neisseria gonorrhoeae on chocolate agar. Colonies appear off-white with no discoloration of the agar. Courtesy of Julia Rosebush, DO; Robert Jerris, PhD; and Theresa Stanley, M(ASCP).

CHAPTER 54

Granuloma Inguinale
(Donovanosis)

CLINICAL MANIFESTATIONS

Initial lesions of this sexually transmitted genital ulcerative disease are single or multiple painless subcutaneous nodules that gradually ulcerate. These nontender, granulomatous ulcers have raised, rolled margins; are beefy red and highly vascular; and bleed readily on contact. "Kissing" lesions may occur from autoinoculation on adjacent skin. Lesions usually involve the genitalia or perineum without regional adenopathy; however, lesions at both the genitalia and inguinal regions occur in 5% to 10% of patients. Subcutaneous granulomas extending into the inguinal area can mimic inguinal adenopathy (ie, "pseudobubo"). Extragenital lesions (eg, face, mouth) account for 6% of cases. Dissemination to intra-abdominal organs and bone is rare.

ETIOLOGY

The disease, donovanosis, is caused by *Klebsiella granulomatis* (formerly known as *Calymmatobacterium granulomatis*), an intracellular, gram-negative bacillus.

EPIDEMIOLOGY

Indigenous granuloma inguinale occurs very rarely in the United States and most industrialized nations. The disease is endemic in some tropical and developing areas, including India, Papua New Guinea, the Caribbean, and southern Africa. The incidence of infection seems to correlate with sustained high temperatures and high relative humidity. Infection is usually acquired by sexual contact, most commonly with a person with active infection. Young children and others, however, can, less commonly, acquire infection by contact with infected secretions. The period of communicability extends throughout the duration of active lesions.

The **incubation period** is uncertain; a range of 1 to 360 days has been reported.

DIAGNOSTIC TESTS

The causative organism is difficult to culture, and diagnosis requires microscopic demonstration of dark-staining intracytoplasmic Donovan bodies on Wright, Leishman, or Giemsa staining of a crush preparation from subsurface scrapings of a lesion or tissue. The microorganism can also be detected by histological examination of biopsy specimens. Culture of *K granulomatis* is difficult to perform and is not available routinely. Diagnosis by polymerase chain reaction assay and serological testing is available only in research laboratories.

TREATMENT

The recommended treatment regimen is azithromycin for at least 3 weeks and until all lesions have completely healed. Treatment has been shown to halt progression of lesions. Partial healing is usually noted within 7 days of initiation of therapy and typically proceeds inward from the ulcer margins. Prolonged therapy is usually required to permit granulation and reepithelialization of the ulcers. Relapse can occur, especially if the antimicrobial agent is stopped before the primary lesion has healed completely. In addition, relapse can occur 6 to 18 months after apparently effective therapy.

Patients should be evaluated for other sexually transmitted infections, including chlamydia, trichomoniasis, syphilis, and HIV infection.

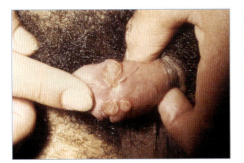

Image 54.1
This patient's penile lesions were caused by gram-negative *Klebsiella granulomatis*, formerly known as *Calymmatobacterium granulomatis*. *K granulomatis* causes granuloma inguinale, or donovanosis, a sexually transmitted infection that is a slowly progressive, ulcerative condition of the skin and lymphatics of the genital and perianal area. A definitive diagnosis is achieved when a tissue smear is positive for *K granulomatis* (Donovan bodies). Courtesy of Centers for Disease Control and Prevention.

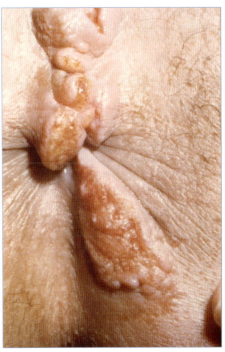

Image 54.2
This 19-year-old young woman presented with a perianal granuloma inguinale lesion of about 8 months' duration. A genital ulcerative disease caused by the intracellular gram-negative bacterium *Klebsiella granulomatis* (formerly known as *Calymmatobacterium granulomatis*), granuloma inguinale, also known as donovanosis, occurs rarely in the United States. Courtesy of Centers for Disease Control and Prevention.

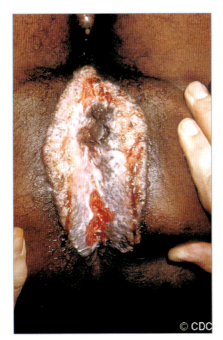

Image 54.3
Granuloma inguinale accompanied by perianal skin ulceration caused by the bacterium *Klebsiella granulomatis*, formerly known as *Calymmatobacterium granulomatis*. The ulcerations are, for the most part, painless and granulomatous (ie, chronic inflammation). Courtesy of Centers for Disease Control and Prevention/ Dr Thomas F. Sellers/Emory University.

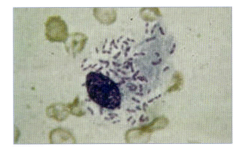

Image 54.4
Giemsa-stained *Klebsiella granulomatis* (Donovan bodies, formerly known as *Calymmatobacterium granulomatis*) of granuloma inguinale. Courtesy of Robert Jerris, PhD.

CHAPTER 55
Haemophilus influenzae Infections

CLINICAL MANIFESTATIONS

Haemophilus influenzae type b (Hib) causes pneumonia, bacteremia, meningitis, epiglottitis, septic arthritis, cellulitis, otitis media, purulent pericarditis, and, less commonly, endocarditis, endophthalmitis, osteomyelitis, peritonitis, and gangrene. Infections caused by encapsulated but non–type b H influenzae manifest similarly to type b infections. Nonencapsulated strains more commonly cause infections of the respiratory tract (eg, otitis media, sinusitis, pneumonia, conjunctivitis), but cases of bacteremia, meningitis, chorioamnionitis, and neonatal septicemia are well described.

ETIOLOGY

H influenzae is a pleomorphic, gram-negative coccobacillus. Encapsulated strains express 1 of 6 antigenically distinct capsular polysaccharides (a–f); nonencapsulated strains lack complete capsule genes and are designated nontypeable.

EPIDEMIOLOGY

The mode of transmission is person to person by inhalation of respiratory tract droplets or by direct contact with respiratory tract secretions. In neonates, infection is acquired intrapartum by aspiration of amniotic fluid or by contact with genital tract secretions containing the organism. Pharyngeal colonization by H influenzae is relatively common, especially with nontypeable strains. In the pre-Hib vaccine era, the major reservoir of Hib was young infants and toddlers, who may asymptomatically carry the organism in their upper respiratory tracts.

Before introduction of effective Hib conjugate vaccines, Hib was the most common cause of bacterial meningitis in young children in the United States. The peak incidence of invasive Hib infections occurred between 6 and 18 months of age. In contrast, the peak age for Hib epiglottitis was 2 to 4 years of age.

Unimmunized children younger than 5 years have increased risk for invasive Hib disease. Other factors that predispose to invasive disease include sickle cell disease, asplenia, HIV infection, certain immunodeficiency syndromes, and chemotherapy for malignant neoplasms. Historically, invasive Hib infection was more common in Black and American Indian/Alaska Native children, boys, child care attendees, children living in crowded conditions, and children who were not breastfed.

Since introduction of Hib conjugate vaccines in the United States, the incidence of invasive Hib disease has decreased by more than 99% in children younger than 5 years. In 2017, 33 cases of invasive type b disease were reported in children younger than 5 years (0.17 cases per 100,000). In the United States, invasive Hib disease occurs primarily in underimmunized children and in infants too young to have completed the primary immunization series. Hib remains an important pathogen in many resource-limited countries where Hib vaccine coverage is suboptimal.

The epidemiology of invasive H influenzae disease in the United States has shifted in the post-Hib vaccination era. Nontypeable H influenzae is now the most common cause of invasive H influenzae disease in all age-groups. In 2017, the annual incidence of invasive nontypeable H influenzae disease was 1.7 per 100,000 among children younger than 5 years, and the rate was highest among children younger than 1 year (5.4 per 100,000). Among the cases in children younger than 1 year, more than half were diagnosed within the first 2 weeks after birth; many were preterm neonates who had a positive culture on the day of birth. In addition to invasive disease, nontypeable H influenzae causes approximately 50% of episodes of acute otitis media and sinusitis in children and commonly causes recurrent otitis media.

H influenzae type a (Hia) has emerged as the most common encapsulated serotype causing invasive disease, with a clinical manifestation similar to Hib. In some North American Indigenous populations (eg, Alaska Native children, northern Canadian Indigenous children), the rate of invasive Hia infection has been increasing and there is evidence of secondary cases having occurred. Although the incidence of invasive Hia is lower among the general population of US children, it has also been increasing in recent years, with a nearly 300% increase over the past 10 years among children younger than 1 year. Invasive disease may also be caused by other encapsulated non–type b strains c, d, e, and f.

The **incubation period** is unknown.

DIAGNOSTIC TESTS

The diagnosis of invasive disease is established by growth on appropriate media of H influenzae from cerebrospinal fluid (CSF), blood, synovial fluid, pleural fluid, or pericardial fluid. Because occult meningitis is known to occur in young children with invasive Hib disease, a lumbar puncture should be strongly considered in the presence of invasive disease, even in the absence of central nervous system signs and symptoms. Gram stain of an infected body fluid specimen can facilitate presumptive diagnosis. Antigen detection methods, which have historically been used on CSF, blood, and urine specimens, are not recommended because they lack sensitivity and specificity. Nucleic acid amplification tests available in multiplexed assays to detect H influenzae DNA directly in blood or CSF may be particularly useful in patients whose specimens are obtained after the initiation of antibiotics. Most of these assays do not determine the capsular polysaccharide type.

The capsular polysaccharide of H influenzae isolates associated with invasive infection should be determined. Serotyping by slide agglutination with polyclonal antisera can have suboptimal sensitivity and specificity depending on reagents used and the experience of the technologist. Capsule typing by molecular methods, such as polymerase chain reaction assay of genes in the cap locus are preferred methods for capsule typing. If serotyping or capsule typing by molecular methods are not available locally, isolates should be submitted to the state health department or to a reference laboratory for testing.

TREATMENT

- Initial therapy for children with H influenzae meningitis is cefotaxime or ceftriaxone. Intravenous ampicillin may be substituted if the isolate is found to be susceptible. Treatment of other invasive H influenzae infections is similar. Therapy is continued for 7 days by the intravenous route and longer in complicated infections.

- Dexamethasone is beneficial for treatment of infants and children with Hib meningitis to diminish the risk of hearing loss, if administered before or concurrently with the first dose of antimicrobial agent(s).

- Epiglottitis is a medical emergency. An airway must be established promptly via controlled intubation.

- Infected pleural or pericardial fluid should be drained.

- For acute suppurative otitis media (AOM), amoxicillin (80–90 mg/kg/day) is recommended for infants younger than 6 months, for those 6 through 23 months of age with bilateral disease, and for those older than 6 months with severe signs and symptoms. A watch-and-wait option can be considered for older children and those with nonsevere disease. Optimal duration of therapy is uncertain. For younger children and children with severe disease at any age, a 10-day course is recommended; for children 6 years and older with mild or moderate disease, a duration of 5 to 7 days is appropriate. Otalgia should be treated symptomatically. Patients whose initial management fails should be reassessed at 48 to 72 hours to confirm the diagnosis of AOM and exclude other causes of illness. If AOM is confirmed in the patient treated initially with observation, amoxicillin should be administered. If the initial antibacterial therapy fails, a change in antibacterial agent is indicated. Suitable alternative agents should be active against penicillin-nonsusceptible pneumococci as well as β-lactamase–producing H influenzae (in the United States, approximately 30%–40% of H influenzae isolates produce β-lactamase) and Moraxella catarrhalis. Such agents include high-dose oral amoxicillin-clavulanate; oral cefdinir, cefpodoxime, or cefuroxime; or 3 daily doses of intramuscular ceftriaxone. Patients whose therapy with one of the aforementioned oral agents continues to fail should be treated with a 3-day course of parenteral ceftriaxone. Macrolide resistance among Streptococcus pneumoniae is high, so clarithromycin and azithromycin are not considered appropriate alternatives for initial therapy even in patients with a type I (immediate, anaphylactic) reaction to a β-lactam agent. In such cases, treatment with clindamycin (if susceptibility is known) or levofloxacin is preferred. For patients with a history of non–type I allergic reaction to penicillin, agents such as cefdinir, cefuroxime, or cefpodoxime can be used orally.

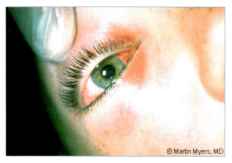

Image 55.1
A 12-year-old boy with periorbital cellulitis, conjunctivitis, and ethmoid sinusitis caused by *Haemophilus influenzae* type b. Copyright Martin G. Myers, MD.

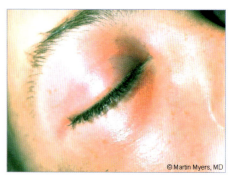

Image 55.2
A 12-year-old boy with periorbital cellulitis and ethmoid sinusitis caused by *Haemophilus influenzae* type b. This is the same patient as in Image 55.1. Copyright Martin G. Myers, MD.

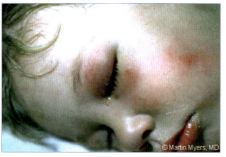

Image 55.3
A 16-month-old girl with periorbital and facial cellulitis caused by *Haemophilus influenzae* type b. The patient had no history of trauma. Copyright Martin G. Myers, MD.

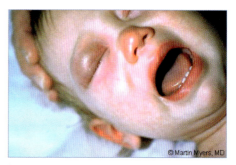

Image 55.4
A 10-month-old boy with periorbital cellulitis caused by *Haemophilus influenzae* type b. Copyright Martin G. Myers, MD.

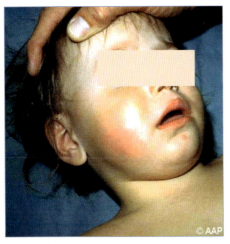

Image 55.5
Haemophilus influenzae type b cellulitis of the face proven by positive results from subcutaneous aspirate cultures and blood cultures. The result from cerebrospinal fluid culture was negative. (This is the first of 3 preschool boys from the same child care center who were examined within a period of 72 hours.)

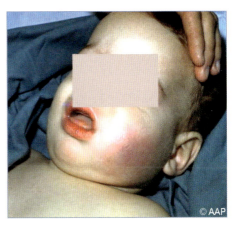

Image 55.6
The second of 3 preschool-aged boys with *Haemophilus influenzae* type b cellulitis of the face proved by positive results from subcutaneous aspirate cultures and blood cultures.

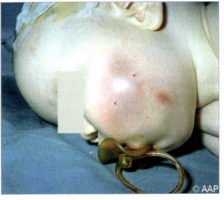

Image 55.7
The third of 3 preschool-aged boys with *Haemophilus influenzae* type b (Hib) cellulitis of the face proved by positive results from subcutaneous aspirate cultures and blood cultures. The routine administration of the Hib vaccine prevents most of these invasive infections.

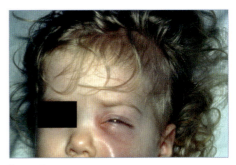

Image 55.8
A classic manifestation of *Haemophilus influenzae* type b (Hib) facial cellulitis in a 10-month-old girl. This once-common infection has been nearly eliminated in children who have been immunized with the Hib vaccine. Courtesy of George Nankervis, MD.

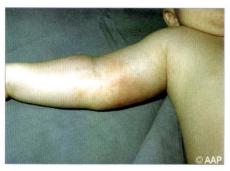

Image 55.9
Haemophilus influenzae type b cellulitis of the arm proved by positive results from blood culture.

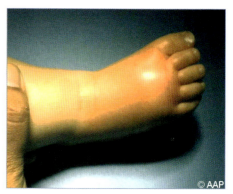

Image 55.10
Haemophilus influenzae type b cellulitis of the foot proved by positive results from blood culture.

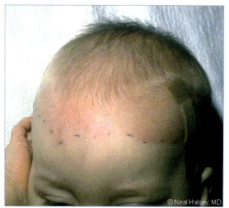

Image 55.11
Haemophilus influenzae type b cellulitis of the forehead proved by positive results from blood culture. Courtesy of Neal Halsey, MD.

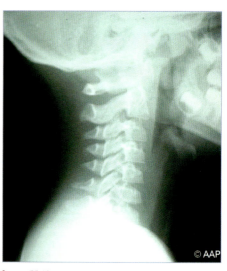

Image 55.12
Acute epiglottitis caused by *Haemophilus influenzae* type b proved by blood culture. The swollen inflamed epiglottis looks like the shadow of a thumb on the lateral neck radiograph.

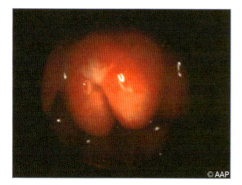

Image 55.13
Acute *Haemophilus influenzae* type b epiglottitis with striking erythema and swelling of the epiglottis. Courtesy of Edgar O. Ledbetter, MD, FAAP.

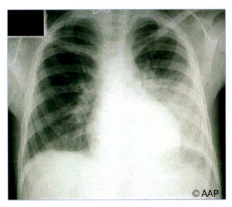

Image 55.14
Haemophilus influenzae type b pneumonia, bilateral, in a patient with acute epiglottitis (proved by blood culture). This is the same patient as in Image 55.13.

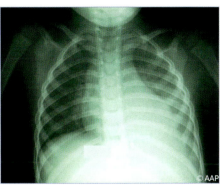

Image 55.15
Haemophilus influenzae type b (Hib) pneumonia with left pleural effusion. Pleural fluid culture and blood culture were positive for Hib. Courtesy of Edgar O. Ledbetter, MD, FAAP.

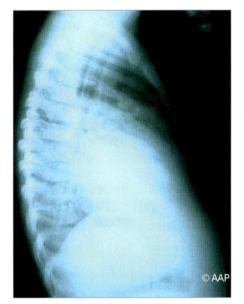

Image 55.16
Lateral radiograph of the patient shown in Image 55.15, with fulminant *Haemophilus influenzae* type b pneumonia. Courtesy of Edgar O. Ledbetter, MD, FAAP.

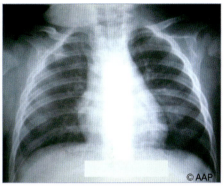

Image 55.17
Retrocardiac *Haemophilus influenzae* type b pneumonia proved by blood culture. Note the air bronchogram.

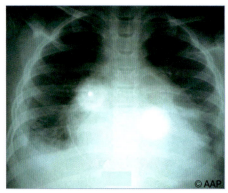

Image 55.18
Haemophilus influenzae type b bilateral pneumonia, empyema, and purulent pericarditis. Pericardiostomy drainage is important in prevention of cardiac restriction.

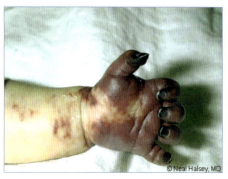

Image 55.19
Haemophilus influenzae type b sepsis with peripheral gangrene. Courtesy of Neal Halsey, MD.

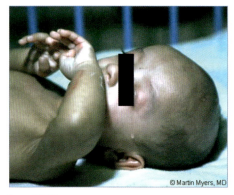

Image 55.20
A 2-year-old boy with *Haemophilus influenzae* type b meningitis and subdural empyema. Note the prominent anterior fontanelle secondary to increased intracranial pressure. Copyright Martin G. Myers, MD.

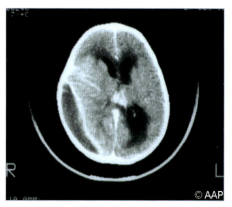

Image 55.21
Magnetic resonance image showing subdural empyema that developed in a patient with *Haemophilus influenzae* type b meningitis.

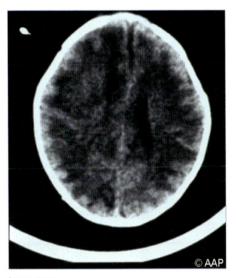

Image 55.22
Magnetic resonance image showing cerebral infarction in a patient with *Haemophilus influenzae* type b meningitis.

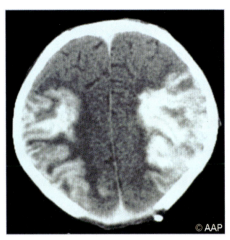

Image 55.23
Magnetic resonance image showing cerebral infarction in a patient who had *Haemophilus influenzae* type b (Hib) meningitis. The routine administration of Hib vaccine has virtually eliminated this type of devastating illness in the United States.

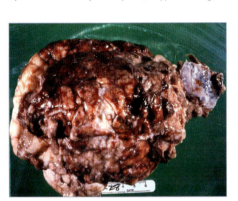

Image 55.24
Haemophilus influenzae meningitis in a 4-month-old who was evaluated in the morning for a health supervision visit and normal clinical findings. By afternoon, the child had necrosis of the hands and feet and died 12 hours later. This is the brain of the infant 24 hours after the health supervision visit. No immunologic deficit was diagnosed. Copyright Jerri Ann Jenista, MD.

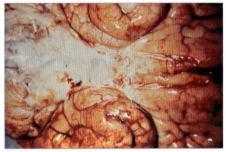

Image 55.25
This is an inferior view of a brain from a child who died of *Haemophilus influenzae* bacteremia and meningitis. Courtesy of Centers for Disease Control and Prevention.

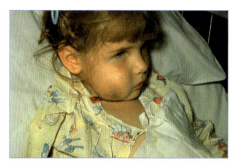

Image 55.26
This girl was hospitalized with *Haemophilus influenzae* type b infection involving deep tissue of her face. *H influenzae* disease can also lead to brain damage, seizures, paralysis, hearing loss, and death. Courtesy of the Immunization Action Coalition.

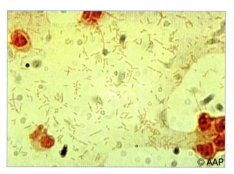

Image 55.27
Gram stain of cerebrospinal fluid (culture positive for *Haemophilus influenzae* type b).

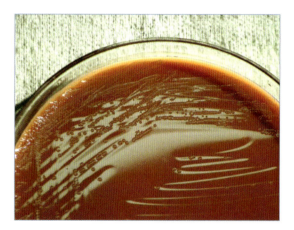

Image 55.28
This photograph depicts the colonial morphological features displayed by gram-negative *Haemophilus influenzae* bacteria, which was grown on a medium of chocolate agar for a 24-hour period at a temperature of 37 °C (98.6 °F). Invasive disease caused by *H influenzae* type b can affect many organ systems. The most common types of invasive disease are pneumonia, occult febrile bacteremia, meningitis, epiglottitis, septic arthritis, cellulitis, otitis media, purulent pericarditis, and other, less common infections such as endocarditis and osteomyelitis. Courtesy of Centers for Disease Control and Prevention.

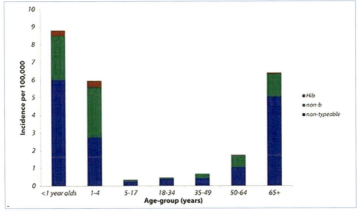

Image 55.29
Estimated US incidence of *Haemophilus influenzae* type b (Hib) by age-group and serotype, 2009–2014. Courtesy of Centers for Disease Control and Prevention.

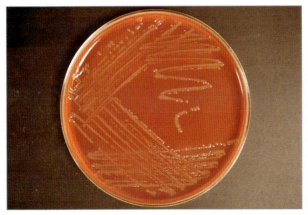

Image 55.30
Haemophilus influenzae on chocolate agar. This organism thrives on chocolate agar because of the supplication of factors X and V required for its growth. Individual colonies appear gray and sometimes mucoid or glistening. Courtesy of Julia Rosebush, DO; Robert Jerris, PhD; and Theresa Stanley, M(ASCP).

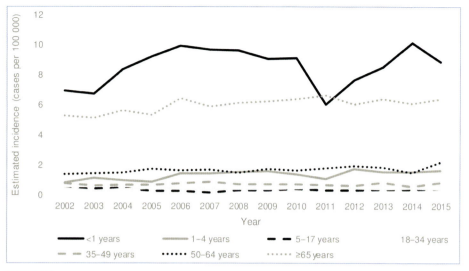

Image 55.31
Trends in estimated incidence of invasive *Haemophilus influenzae* disease, by age-group—United States, 2002–2015. Soeters HM, Blain A, Pondo T, et al. Current epidemiology and trends in invasive *Haemophilus influenzae* disease—United States, 2009–2015. *Clin Infect Dis.* 2018;67(6):881–889.

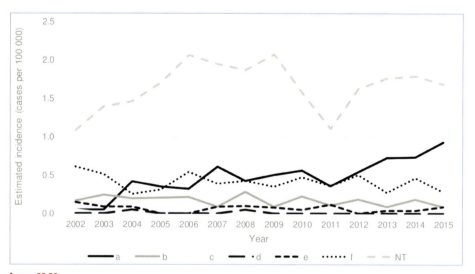

Image 55.32
Trends in estimated incidence of invasive *Haemophilus influenzae* disease among children aged <5 years, by serotype—United States, 2002–2015. Soeters HM, Blain A, Pondo T, et al. Current epidemiology and trends in invasive *Haemophilus influenzae* disease—United States, 2009–2015. *Clin Infect Dis.* 2018;67(6):881–889.

CHAPTER 56
Hantavirus Pulmonary Syndrome

CLINICAL MANIFESTATIONS

Hantaviruses cause 2 distinct clinical syndromes: (1) hantavirus pulmonary syndrome (HPS), also known as hantavirus cardiopulmonary syndrome, characterized by noncardiogenic pulmonary edema, which is observed in the Americas; and (2) hemorrhagic fever with renal syndrome, which occurs worldwide. After an incubation period of 1 to 6 weeks, the prodromal illness of HPS lasts 3 to 7 days and is characterized by fever, chills, headache, myalgia, nausea, vomiting, diarrhea, dizziness, and, sometimes, cough. Respiratory tract symptoms or signs do not usually occur during the first 3 to 7 days, but then pulmonary edema and severe hypoxemia appear abruptly and manifest as cough and dyspnea. The disease then progresses over hours. In severe cases, myocardial dysfunction causes hypotension, which is why the syndrome is sometimes called *hantavirus cardiopulmonary syndrome.*

Extensive bilateral interstitial and alveolar pulmonary edema with pleural effusions are attributable to diffuse pulmonary capillary leak. Intubation and assisted ventilation are usually required for only 2 to 4 days, with resolution heralded by onset of diuresis and rapid clinical improvement.

The severe myocardial depression is different from that of septic shock, with low cardiac indices and stroke volume index, normal pulmonary wedge pressure, and increased systemic vascular resistance. Poor prognostic indicators include persistent hypotension, marked hemoconcentration, a cardiac index of less than 2, and abrupt onset of lactic acidosis with a serum lactate concentration of greater than 4 mmol/L (36 mg/dL).

The mortality rate for patients with HPS is between 30% and 40%; death usually occurs in the first 1 or 2 days of hospitalization. A disproportionate number of cases occur in American Indian/Alaska Native populations, and case-fatality rates for these populations (46%) are higher than for non-Native populations. Milder forms of disease have been reported. Limited information suggests that clinical manifestations and prognosis are similar in adults and children. Serious sequelae are uncommon.

ETIOLOGY

Hantaviruses are RNA viruses of the *Hantaviridae* family. Sin Nombre virus (SNV) is the major cause of HPS in the western and central regions of the United States. Bayou virus, Black Creek Canal virus, Monongahela virus, and New York virus are responsible for sporadic cases in Louisiana, Texas, Florida, New York, and other areas of the eastern United States. Andes virus, Oran virus, Laguna Negra virus, and Choclo virus are responsible for cases in South and Central America. There are typically 20 to 40 cases of HPS reported annually in the United States, with the majority (>95%) of cases occurring west of the Mississippi River. Cases in children younger than 10 years are exceedingly rare. Children may be less likely to become infected than adults.

EPIDEMIOLOGY

Rodents are natural hosts for hantaviruses and acquire lifelong, asymptomatic, chronic infection with prolonged viruria and virus in saliva and feces. Humans acquire infection through direct contact with infected rodents, rodent droppings, or rodent nests or through the inhalation of aerosolized virus particles from rodent urine, droppings, or saliva. Rarely, infection may be acquired from rodent bites or contamination of broken skin with excreta. At-risk activities include handling or trapping rodents, cleaning or entering closed or rarely used rodent-infested structures, cleaning feed storage or animal shelter areas, hand plowing, and living in a home with an increased density of mice. For backpackers or campers, sleeping in a structure inhabited by rodents has been associated with HPS, with a notable outbreak occurring in 2012 in Yosemite National Park secondary to rodent-infested cabins. Exceptionally heavy rainfall improves rodent food supplies, resulting in an increase in the rodent population with more frequent contact between humans and infected rodents, resulting in more human disease. Most cases occur during the spring and summer, with the geographic location determined by the habitat of the rodent carrier.

SNV is transmitted by the deer mouse, *Peromyscus maniculatus;* Black Creek Canal virus is transmitted by the cotton rat, *Sigmodon hispidus;* Bayou virus is transmitted by the rice rat, *Oryzomys palustris;* and the New York and Monongahela viruses are transmitted by the white-footed mouse, *Peromyscus leucopus.*

Andes virus is transmitted by the long-tailed rice rat (*Oligoryzomys longicaudatus*), endemic to most of Argentina and Chile. Unlike all other hantaviruses, Andes virus can also be transmitted person to person.

DIAGNOSTIC TESTS

HPS should be considered when thrombocytopenia occurs with severe pneumonia clinically resembling acute respiratory distress syndrome in the proper epidemiological setting. Other characteristic laboratory findings include neutrophilic leukocytosis with immature granulocytes, including more than 10% immunoblasts (basophilic cytoplasm, prominent nucleoli, and an increased nuclear-to-cytoplasmic ratio) and increased hematocrit.

Molecular detection of virus has been described in peripheral blood mononuclear cells and other clinical specimens from the early phase of the disease but not usually in bronchoalveolar lavage fluids. Viral culture is not useful. Hantavirus-specific immunoglobulin M and immunoglobulin G (IgG) antibodies are often present at the onset of clinical disease, and serological testing remains the method of choice for diagnosis. IgG may be negative in rapidly fatal cases.

Immunohistochemical staining of tissues (capillary endothelial cells of the lungs and almost every organ in the body) can establish the diagnosis at autopsy.

TREATMENT

Patients with suspected HPS should be transferred immediately to a tertiary care facility where supportive management of pulmonary edema, severe hypoxemia, and hypotension can occur during the first critical 24 to 48 hours.

In severe forms, early mechanical ventilation and inotropic and pressor support are necessary. Extracorporeal membrane oxygenation should be considered when pulmonary wedge pressure and cardiac indices have deteriorated, and it may provide short-term support for the severe capillary leak syndrome in the lungs.

Ribavirin is active in vitro against hantaviruses, including SNV. However, 2 clinical studies of intravenous ribavirin (1 open-label study and 1 randomized, placebo-controlled, double-blind study) failed to show benefit in treatment of HPS in the cardiopulmonary stage.

Cytokine-blocking agents for HPS may theoretically have a role, but these agents have not been evaluated in a systematic fashion. Antibacterial agents are unlikely to offer benefit.

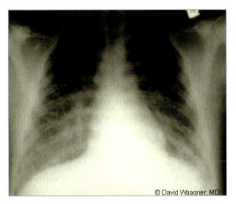

Image 56.1
Hantavirus pulmonary syndrome in a 16-year-old boy with a 36-hour history of fever, myalgia, and shortness of breath. Diffuse interstitial infiltrates with Kerley B lines. Diffuse nodular confluent alveolar opacities with some consolidation consistent with adult respiratory distress syndrome. Hantavirus serological reaction confirmatory by immunoglobulin M at 1:6,400. Patient recovered with supportive care including inhaled nitric oxide. Copyright David Waagner, MD.

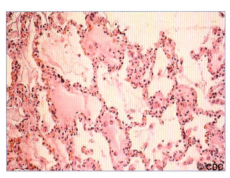

Image 56.2
Histopathologic features of lung in hantavirus pulmonary syndrome include interstitial pneumonitis and intra-alveolar edema. Courtesy of Centers for Disease Control and Prevention.

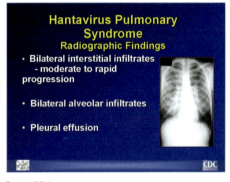

Image 56.4
Radiographic findings of hantavirus pulmonary syndrome (HPS). Findings usually include interstitial edema, Kerley B lines, hilar indistinctness, and peribronchial cuffing with normal cardiothoracic ratios. HPS begins with minimal changes of interstitial pulmonary edema and rapidly progresses to alveolar edema with severe bilateral involvement. Pleural effusions are common and are often large enough to be evident radiographically. Courtesy of Centers for Disease Control and Prevention.

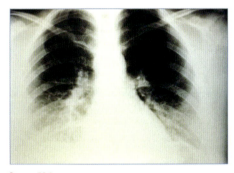

Image 56.3
This anterolateral chest radiograph reveals the early stages of bilateral pulmonary effusion caused by hantavirus pulmonary syndrome (HPS). The radiological evolution of HPS begins with minimal changes of interstitial pulmonary edema and progresses to alveolar edema with severe bilateral involvement. Pleural effusions are common and are often large enough to be evident radiographically. Courtesy of Centers for Disease Control and Prevention.

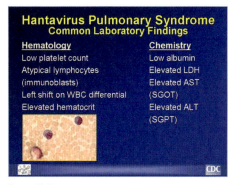

Image 56.5
Common laboratory findings. Notable hematologic findings include low platelet count, immunoblasts, left shift on white blood cell count (WBC) differential, elevated WBC, and elevated hematocrit. The large atypical lymphocyte shown is an example of one of the laboratory findings that, when combined with a bandemia and dropping platelet count, are characteristic of hantavirus pulmonary syndrome. Notable blood chemistry findings include low albumin, elevated lactate dehydrogenase (LDH), elevated aspartate aminotransferase (AST), and elevated alanine aminotransferase (ALT; previously serum glutamic-pyruvic transaminase). Courtesy of Centers for Disease Control and Prevention.

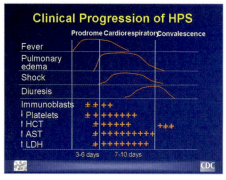

Image 56.6
Clinical progression of hantavirus pulmonary syndrome (HPS) starts with a febrile prodrome that may ultimately lead to hypotension and end-organ failure. The onset of the immune response precedes severe organ failure, which is thought to be immunopathologic in nature. Hypotension does not result in shock until the onset of respiratory failure, but this may reflect the severe physiological effect of lung edema. AST indicates aminotransferase; HCT, hematocrit; and LDH, lactate dehydrogenase. Courtesy of Centers for Disease Control and Prevention.

CHAPTER 57
Helicobacter pylori Infections

CLINICAL MANIFESTATIONS

Most *Helicobacter pylori* infections in children are believed to be asymptomatic. *H pylori* may cause chronic active gastritis and may result in duodenal and, to a lesser extent, gastric ulcers. Persistent infection with *H pylori* also increases risk for the development of gastric cancers including mucosal-associated lymphoid tissue (MALT) lymphoma and adenocarcinoma in adults; however, this is an infrequent complication in children. In children, acute *H pylori* infection can result in gastroduodenal inflammation that manifests as epigastric pain, nausea, vomiting, hematemesis, and guaiac-positive stools; these symptoms are usually self-limited. There is no clear association between infection and recurrent abdominal pain in the absence of peptic ulcer disease. The presence of nighttime wakening can distinguish children with peptic ulcer disease from those with chronic gastritis attributable to *H pylori* infection (for whom nighttime wakening rarely occurs). Endoscopic findings of *H pylori* infection include nodular gastritis, chronic gastritis, and, rarely, the presence of gastric or duodenal erosions or ulcers. In children, extraintestinal conditions that have been associated with *H pylori* infection include treatment-refractory iron-deficiency anemia and chronic immune thrombocytopenia purpura (cITP).

ETIOLOGY

H pylori is a gram-negative, spiral, curved, or U-shaped microaerobic bacillus that has single or multiple flagella at one end. The organism is positive for catalase, oxidase, and urease activity. The 2 main virulence factors associated with more severe disease include the cytotoxin-associated gene A and the vacuolating cytotoxin A.

EPIDEMIOLOGY

H pylori organisms have been isolated from humans and other primates. An animal reservoir for human transmission has not been demonstrated. Organisms are thought to be transmitted from infected humans by the fecal-oral, gastro-oral, and oral-oral routes.

H pylori is estimated to have infected 70% of people living in resource-limited countries and 30% to 40% of people living in industrialized countries. Infection rates in children are low in resource-rich, industrialized countries, except in children from lower-income groups, immigrants from resource-limited countries, and those living in poor hygienic conditions. Most infections are acquired in the first 8 years after birth. The organism can persist in the stomach for years or for life.

Although all infected people have gastritis, over a lifetime, approximately 10% to 15% will develop peptic ulcer disease and less than 1% will develop gastric cancer.

The **incubation period** is unknown.

DIAGNOSTIC TESTS

H pylori infection can be diagnosed by culture of gastric biopsy tissue on nonselective media (eg, chocolate agar, brucella agar, brain-heart infusion agar) or selective media (eg, Skirrow agar) at 37 °C (99 °F) under microaerophilic conditions (decreased oxygen, increased carbon dioxide, and increased hydrogen concentrations) for 3 to 10 days. Colonies are small, smooth, and translucent and are positive for catalase, oxidase, and urease activity. Antimicrobial susceptibility testing of cultured isolates should be performed to guide therapy. Organisms can be visualized on histological sections with Warthin-Starry silver, Steiner, Giemsa, or Genta staining. Presence of *H pylori* can be confirmed but not excluded on the basis of hematoxylin-eosin stains. Immunohistological staining with specific *H pylori* antibodies may improve specificity. Because of production of high levels of urease by these organisms, urease testing of a gastric biopsy specimen can be used to detect the presence of *H pylori*.

Noninvasive, commercially available tests include urea breath tests and stool antigen tests; these tests are designed for detection of active infection and have high sensitivity and specificity. Stool antigen tests by enzyme immunoassay monoclonal antibodies are available commercially and can be used for children of any age. Testing is appropriate to confirm eradication of infection following completion of treatment.

The European Society for Paediatric Gastroenterology, Hepatology and Nutrition and the North American Society for Pediatric Gastroenterology, Hepatology & Nutrition (ESPGHAN/NASPGHAN) joint guideline recommends against a "test and treat" strategy for *H pylori* infection in children. Instead, they make the following recommendations:

- The diagnosis of *H pylori* infection should be based on either (a) histopathology (*H pylori*–positive gastritis) plus at least 1 other positive biopsy-based test result or (b) positive culture.

- When testing for *H pylori*, wait at least 2 weeks after stopping a proton pump inhibitor (PPI) and 4 weeks after stopping antimicrobial agents.

- Testing for *H pylori* should be performed in children with gastric or duodenal ulcers. If *H pylori* infection is identified, treatment should be advised and eradication should be confirmed.

- Diagnostic testing for *H pylori* infection should not be performed as part of the initial investigation in children with iron-deficiency anemia. In children with refractory iron-deficiency anemia in which other causes have been ruled out, testing for *H pylori* during upper endoscopy may be considered.

TREATMENT

Treatment options are detailed in tables 57.1 and 57.2. Treatment is recommended for infected patients who have peptic ulcer disease, gastric MALT-type lymphoma, or early gastric cancer. Treatment of *H pylori* infection, if found, may be considered for children who have unexplained and

Table 57.1
Recommended Options for First-line Therapy for *Helicobacter pylori* Infections[a,b]

Helicobacter pylori Antimicrobial Susceptibilities	Suggested First-line Treatment
Susceptible to clarithromycin, susceptible to metronidazole	PPI + amoxicillin + clarithromycin for 14 days[c]
Resistant to clarithromycin, susceptible to metronidazole	PPI + amoxicillin + metronidazole for 14 days OR Bismuth-based therapy as detailed in "Susceptibilities unknown" row
Susceptible to clarithromycin, resistant to metronidazole	PPI + amoxicillin + clarithromycin for 14 days
Resistant to clarithromycin, resistant to metronidazole ("double resistant")	<8 years of age: PPI + amoxicillin + metronidazole + bismuth for 14 days ≥8 years of age: PPI + tetracycline + metronidazole + bismuth for 14 days
Susceptibilities unknown	<8 years of age: PPI + amoxicillin + metronidazole + bismuth for 14 days ≥8 years of age: PPI + tetracycline + metronidazole + bismuth for 14 days

ESPGHAN/NASPGHAN indicates European Society for Paediatric Gastroenterology, Hepatology and Nutrition and North American Society for Pediatric Gastroenterology, Hepatology & Nutrition; PPI, proton pump inhibitor.

[a] Adapted from Jones NL, Koletzko S, Goodman K, et al; ESPGHAN, NASPGHAN. Joint ESPGHAN/NASPGHAN guidelines for the management of *Helicobacter pylori* in children and adolescents (update 2016). *J Pediatr Gastroenterol Nutr.* 2017;64(6):991–1003.
[b] Refer to joint ESPGHAN/NASPGHAN guidelines for antibiotic dosing.
[c] Sequential therapy for 10 days (PPI + amoxicillin for 5 days, followed by PPI + clarithromycin + metronidazole for 5 days) is equally effective but has the disadvantage of exposing the child to 3 different antibiotics.

Table 57.2
Rescue Therapies in Pediatric Patients Whose Therapy Fails[a,b]

Initial Antibiotic Susceptibilities	Past Treatment Regimen	Suggested Rescue Treatment
Susceptible to clarithromycin, susceptible to metronidazole	PPI + amoxicillin + clarithromycin	PPI + amoxicillin + metronidazole
	PPI + amoxicillin + metronidazole	PPI + amoxicillin + clarithromycin
Susceptible to clarithromycin, susceptible to metronidazole	Sequential therapy (See footnote **c** in Table 57.1.)	Consider performing a second endoscopy and use a tailored treatment for 14 days OR Treat like "double resistant" in Table 57.1.
Resistant to clarithromycin	PPI + amoxicillin + metronidazole	Treat like "double resistant" in Table 57.1.
Resistant to metronidazole	PPI + amoxicillin + clarithromycin	Consider performing a second endoscopy and use a tailored treatment for 14 days OR Treat like "double resistant" in Table 57.1.
Susceptibilities unknown	PPI + amoxicillin + clarithromycin OR PPI + amoxicillin + metronidazole OR Sequential therapy (See footnote **c** in Table 57.1.)	Consider performing a second endoscopy to assess secondary antimicrobial susceptibility OR Treat like "double resistant" in Table 57.1.

[a] Adapted from Jones NL, Koletzko S, Goodman K, et al; ESPGHAN, NASPGHAN. Joint ESPGHAN/NASPGHAN guidelines for the management of *Helicobacter pylori* in children and adolescents (update 2016). *J Pediatr Gastroenterol Nutr*. 2017;64(6):991–1003.
[b] Refer to joint ESPGHAN/NASPGHAN guidelines for antibiotic dosing.

refractory iron-deficiency anemia. Additionally, both the ESPGHAN/NASPGHAN and American Society of Hematology guidelines recommend eradication if infection is associated with cITP. For patients with *H pylori* infection in the absence of clinical or endoscopic evidence of peptic ulcer disease, treatment is not recommended unless the patient is within a risk group or region with high incidence of gastric cancer. Adherence is critical to the success of eradication therapy.

The backbone of all recommended therapies includes a PPI and amoxicillin. Additions of metronidazole, clarithromycin, and/or bismuth are based on the patient's previous treatment experience or known susceptibilities to clarithromycin and metronidazole. Reports of increasing prevalence of antibiotic-resistant strains (particularly clarithromycin resistance) as well as increasing failures of triple therapies suggest the need for bismuth-based quadruple therapy regimens (meaning 3 antibiotics and bismuth) and longer durations (14 days) for eradication of *H pylori*. There is no current evidence to support the use of probiotics to reduce medication adverse effects or improve eradication of *H pylori*.

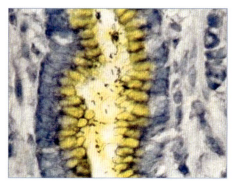

Image 57.1
Histological features of the gastric mucosa demonstrate the characteristic curved organisms in the gastric glands. Courtesy of H. Cody Meissner, MD, FAAP.

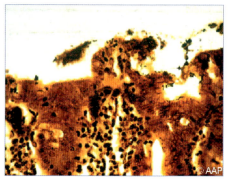

Image 57.2
Gastric mucosal biopsy demonstrating *Helicobacter pylori*. This organism has been isolated from humans and other primates.

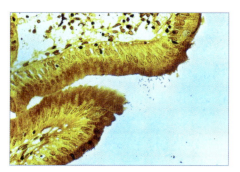

Image 57.3
A biopsy of gastric mucosa stained with Warthin-Starry silver stain showing *Helicobacter pylori* organisms. Courtesy of Brian Oliver, MD.

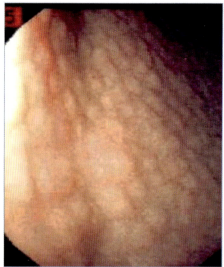

Image 57.4
Helicobacter pylori infection is a known risk factor for gastritis and duodenal ulcers in children and adults. Rarely, and primarily in older adulthood, *H pylori* is also associated with a gastric lymphoma of the mucosal-associated lymphoid tissue. The gold standard for the diagnosis of *H pylori* infection of the stomach is endoscopy with biopsy. Endoscopy may show a nodular gastritis of the antrum. Courtesy of H. Cody Meissner, MD, FAAP.

CHAPTER 58

Hemorrhagic Fevers Caused by Arenaviruses

CLINICAL MANIFESTATIONS

Arenaviruses are responsible for several hemorrhagic fever (HF) syndromes. Arenaviruses are divided into 2 groups: the New World or Tacaribe complex and the Old World or lymphocytic choriomeningitis virus (LCMV)–Lassa virus (LASV) complex. Disease associated with arenaviruses ranges from asymptomatic or mild, acute, febrile infections to severe illnesses in which vascular leak, shock, and multiorgan dysfunction are prominent features. Fever, weakness, malaise, headache, arthralgia, myalgia, conjunctival suffusion, retro-orbital pain, facial flushing, anorexia, vomiting, diarrhea, and abdominal pain are common early symptoms in all infections. Thrombocytopenia, leukopenia, petechiae, generalized lymphadenopathy, and encephalopathy are usually present in Argentine HF, Bolivian HF, and Venezuelan HF, and exudative pharyngitis often occurs in Lassa fever. Mucosal bleeding generally occurs in severe cases as a consequence of vascular damage, coagulopathy, thrombocytopenia, and platelet dysfunction. However, hemorrhagic manifestations occur in only one-third of patients with Lassa fever. Proteinuria is common, but renal failure is unusual. Increased serum concentrations of aspartate aminotransferase can portend a severe or possibly fatal outcome of Lassa fever. Shock develops 7 to 9 days after onset of illness in more severely ill patients with these infections. Upper and lower respiratory tract symptoms can develop in people with Lassa fever. Encephalopathic signs, such as tremor, alterations in consciousness, and seizures, can occur in South American HFs and in severe cases of Lassa fever. Transient or permanent deafness is reported in 30% of convalescents of Lassa fever. The overall mortality rate in Lassa fever is 1% to 20% of all infections, but it is highest among hospitalized patients (15%–50%); for South American HFs, the mortality rate is 10% to 35%, and for Lujo HF, the mortality rate is 80%. Pregnant women have substantially higher risk for mortality (approximately 80%) and spontaneous abortion, with 95% mortality in fetuses of infected mothers. Symptoms resolve 10 to 15 days after disease onset in surviving patients.

ETIOLOGY

Mammalian arenaviruses (mammarenaviruses) are enveloped, bisegmented, single-stranded RNA viruses. Old World arenaviruses include LCMV, which causes lymphocytic choriomeningitis, LASV (Lassa HF), and Lujo virus (Lujo HF) in western and southern Africa. New World arenaviruses include Junín virus (Argentine HF) Machupo virus (Bolivian HF), Sabiá virus (Brazilian HF), Guanarito virus (Venezuelan HF), and Chapare virus (Chapare HF). Whitewater Arroyo virus is a rare cause of human disease in North America. Antibodies to Tamiami viruses have been detected in people in North America, but clinical disease has not been confirmed. Several other arenaviruses are known only from their rodent reservoirs in the Old and New Worlds.

EPIDEMIOLOGY

Arenaviruses are maintained in nature by association with specific rodent hosts, in which they produce chronic viremia and viruria. The principal routes of infection are inhalation and direct contact of mucous membranes and skin (eg, through cuts, scratches, or abrasions) with urine and salivary secretions from these persistently infected rodents. Ingestion of food contaminated by rodent excrement may also cause disease transmission. All arenaviruses are infectious as aerosols, and human-to-human transmission may occur in community or hospital settings following unprotected contact or through droplets. Excretion of arenaviruses in urine and semen for several weeks after infection has been documented. Arenaviruses causing HF should be considered highly hazardous to people working with any of these viruses in the laboratory. Laboratory-acquired infections have been documented with Lassa, Machupo, Junín, and Sabiá viruses. The geographic distribution and habitats of the specific rodents that serve as reservoir hosts largely determine areas with endemic infection and populations with risk. Before a vaccine became available in Argentina, several hundred cases of Argentine HF occurred annually in agricultural workers and inhabitants of the Argentine pampas; the Argentine HF vaccine is not licensed in the United States. Epidemics of Bolivian HF occurred in small towns between 1962 and 1964; sporadic disease activity in the countryside has continued since then. Venezuelan HF was first identified in 1989 and occurs in rural north-central Venezuela. Lassa fever is endemic in most of western Africa, where rodent hosts live in proximity to humans, causing thousands of infections annually. Lassa fever has been reported in the United States and western Europe in people who have traveled to western Africa.

The **incubation periods** for these HF range from 6 to 21 days.

DIAGNOSTIC TESTS

Viral nucleic acid can be detected in acute disease by reverse transcriptase–polymerase chain reaction assay. These viruses may be isolated from blood of acutely ill patients as well as from various tissues obtained postmortem, but isolation should be attempted only under biosafety level–4 conditions. Virus antigen is detectable by enzyme immunoassay in acute specimens and postmortem tissues. Virus-specific immunoglobulin M antibodies are present in the serum during acute stages of illness by immunofluorescent antibody or enzyme-linked immunosorbent assays but may be undetectable in rapidly fatal cases. The immunoglobulin G antibody response is delayed. Diagnosis can be made retrospectively by immunohistochemical staining of formalin-fixed tissues obtained from autopsy.

TREATMENT

Intravenous ribavirin substantially decreases the mortality rate of patients with severe Lassa fever, particularly if they are treated early, during the first week of illness. For Argentine HF, transfusion of immune plasma in defined doses of neutralizing antibodies is the standard specific treatment when administered during the first 8 days from onset of symptoms and reduces mortality rate to 1% to 2%. Intravenous ribavirin has been used with success to abort a Sabiá laboratory infection and to treat Bolivian HF patients and the only known Lujo virus infection survivor. Ribavirin did not reduce mortality rate when initiated 8 days or more after onset of Argentine HF symptoms. Whether ribavirin treatment initiated early in the course of the disease has a role in the treatment of Argentine HF remains to be seen. Meticulous fluid and electrolyte balance is an important aspect of supportive care in each case of the HFs.

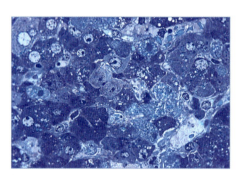

Image 58.1
This photomicrograph shows hepatitis caused by the Lassa virus (toluidine-blue–azure II stain). The Lassa virus, which can cause altered liver morphological features with hemorrhagic necrosis and inflammation, is a member of the family *Arenaviridae* and is a single-stranded RNA, zoonotic, or animalborne pathogen. Courtesy of Centers for Disease Control and Prevention.

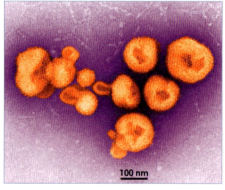

Image 58.2
This transmission electron micrograph depicts virions (viral particles) that are members of the genus *Arenavirus*. Arenaviruses include lymphocytic choriomeningitis virus and the agents of 5 hemorrhagic fevers, including West African Lassa fever virus and Bolivian hemorrhagic fever, also known as Machupo virus. Spread to humans occurs through inhalation of airborne particulates originating from rodent excrement, which can occur during the simple act of sweeping a floor. Courtesy of Centers for Disease Control and Prevention/Charles Humphrey.

CHAPTER 59

Hemorrhagic Fevers Caused by Bunyaviruses

CLINICAL MANIFESTATIONS

Bunyaviruses are arthropodborne or rodentborne infections that often result in severe febrile disease with multisystem involvement and may be associated with high rates of morbidity and mortality.

Hemorrhagic fever with renal syndrome (HFRS) is a complex, multiphasic disease characterized by vascular instability and varying degrees of renal insufficiency. Fever, flushing, conjunctival injection, headache, blurred vision, abdominal pain, and lumbar pain are followed by hypotension, oliguria, and, subsequently, polyuria. Petechiae are frequent, but more serious bleeding manifestations are rare. Shock and acute renal insufficiency may occur.

Crimean-Congo hemorrhagic fever (CCHF) is a multisystem disease characterized by hepatitis and hemorrhagic manifestations. Fever, headache, and myalgia are followed by signs of a diffuse capillary leak syndrome with facial suffusion, conjunctivitis, icteric hepatitis, proteinuria, and disseminated intravascular coagulation associated with petechiae and purpura on the skin and mucous membranes. A hypotensive crisis often occurs after the appearance of frank hemorrhage from the gastrointestinal tract, nose, mouth, or uterus.

Rift Valley fever (RVF), in most cases, is a self-limited undifferentiated febrile illness. In 8% to 10% of cases, however, hemorrhagic fever with shock and icteric hepatitis, encephalitis, or retinitis develops.

ETIOLOGY

The order *Bunyavirales* includes segmented, single-stranded RNA viruses with different geographic distributions depending on their vector or reservoir. Hemorrhagic fever syndromes are associated with viruses from 3 families: *Hantaviridae* (Old World hantaviruses), *Nairoviridae* (CCHF Virus), and *Phenuiviridae* (RVF virus). Old World hantaviruses (Hantaan, Seoul, Dobrava, and Puumala viruses) cause HFRS, and New World hantaviruses (Sin Nombre and related viruses) cause hantavirus pulmonary syndrome.

EPIDEMIOLOGY

The epidemiology of these diseases is a function of the distribution and behavior of their reservoirs and vectors. All families except *Hantaviridae* are associated with arthropod vectors. Hantavirus infections are transmitted via coming into contact with virus shed in rat urine, saliva, or droppings; inhaling virus in dust from contaminated nesting materials; or being bitten by an infected rat.

Classic HFRS occurs throughout much of Asia and Europe, with up to 100,000 cases per year. The most severe form of the disease is caused by the prototype Hantaan and Dobrava viruses in rural Asia and Europe, respectively; Puumala virus is associated with milder disease (nephropathia epidemica) in western Europe. Seoul virus is distributed worldwide in association with brown Norway rats (*Rattus* species) and can cause a disease of variable severity. Cases have been reported in the United States in rat fanciers. Person-to-person transmission has never been reported with HFRS. Fatal outcome occurs in 1% to 15% of cases, depending on the species of virus and the level of care.

CCHF occurs in much of sub-Saharan Africa, the Middle East, northwestern China, part of the Indian subcontinent, Ukraine, Russia, Georgia, Armenia, central Asia, and Southeast Europe. CCHF virus is transmitted by hard ticks and occasionally by contact with viremic livestock and wild animals at slaughter. Health care–associated transmission of CCHF is a frequent and serious hazard. Fatal outcome occurs in 9% to 50% of hospitalized patients.

RVF occurs throughout sub-Saharan Africa, Egypt, Saudi Arabia, and Yemen. The virus is mosquitoborne and can also be directly transmitted from domestic livestock to humans via contact with infected aborted tissues or freshly slaughtered infected animal carcasses. Person-to-person transmission has not been reported, but laboratory-acquired cases are well-documented. Overall fatal outcome occurs in 1% to 2% of cases but has been reported to be up to 30% in hospitalized patients.

The **incubation periods** for CCHF and RVF range from 2 to 10 days; for HFRS, the **incubation period** is usually longer, ranging from 7 to 42 days.

DIAGNOSTIC TESTS

Viral culture of blood and/or tissue, acute-phase reverse transcriptase–quantitative polymerase chain reaction (RT-qPCR), and serological testing may facilitate diagnosis (Table 59.1). Immunoglobulin M (IgM) antibodies or increasing immunoglobulin G (IgG) titers in paired serum specimens, as demonstrated by enzyme immunoassay, are diagnostic; neutralizing antibody tests provide greater virus-strain specificity but are rarely used. Serum IgM and IgG virus-specific antibodies typically develop early in convalescence in CCHF and RVF but can be absent in rapidly fatal cases of CCHF. In HFRS, IgM and IgG antibodies are usually detectable at illness onset or within 48 hours, when it is too late for virus isolation and RT-qPCR assay. Diagnosis can be made retrospectively by immunohistochemical staining of formalin-fixed tissues.

TREATMENT

Ribavirin, administered intravenously to patients with HFRS within the first 4 days of illness, may be effective in decreasing renal dysfunction, vascular instability, and mortality. However, intravenous ribavirin is not available commercially in the United States and is available only from the manufacturer through an investigational new drug protocol. Health care professionals who need to obtain intravenous ribavirin should contact the US Food and Drug Administration. Supportive therapy for HFRS should include (1) treatment of shock; (2) monitoring of fluid balance; (3) dialysis for complications of renal failure; (4) control of hypertension during the oliguric phase; and (5) early recognition of possible myocardial failure with appropriate therapy.

Oral and intravenous ribavirin, when administered early in the course of CCHF, has been associated with milder disease, although no controlled studies have been performed. Ribavirin may also be efficacious as postexposure prophylaxis of CCHF. Ribavirin should be avoided in RVF owing to an increased risk for development of encephalitis in patients receiving ribavirin.

Table 59.1
Diagnostic Tests to Be Performed for Hemorrhagic Fevers Caused by Bunyaviruses

Diagnostic Testing	HFRS	CCHF	RVF
Virus culture of blood or tissue	No (not usually detected at time of illness)	Yes (in BSL-4 conditions)	Yes (in BSL-4 conditions)
Acute-phase virus RT-qPCR	Yes, but not routinely done	Yes	Yes
IgM and IgG serology	Yes (at illness onset or within 48 hours)	Yes (detectable in early convalescence, but could be absent in fatal cases)	Yes (detectable in early convalescence)

BSL indicates biosafety level; CCHF, Crimean-Congo hemorrhagic fever; HFRS, hemorrhagic fever with renal syndrome; RVF, Rift Valley fever; and RT-qPCR, reverse transcriptase–quantitative polymerase chain reaction.

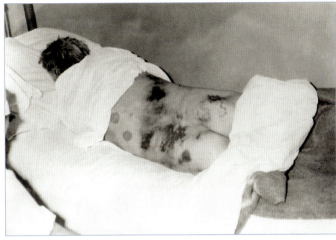

Image 59.1
Isolated male patient diagnosed with Crimean-Congo hemorrhagic fever, a tickborne hemorrhagic fever with documented person-to-person transmission and a case-fatality rate of approximately 30%. This widespread virus has been found in Africa, Asia, the Middle East, and eastern Europe. Courtesy of Centers for Disease Control and Prevention.

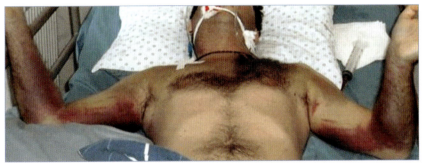

Image 59.2
Intubated patient with Crimean-Congo hemorrhagic fever, Republic of Georgia, 2009, showing massive ecchymoses on the upper extremities that extend to the chest. Courtesy of *Emerging Infectious Diseases*.

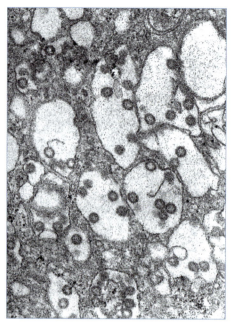

Image 59.3
Electron micrograph of the Rift Valley fever virus, which is a member of the genus *Phlebovirus* in the family *Bunyaviridae*, first reported in livestock in Kenya around 1900. Courtesy of Centers for Disease Control and Prevention.

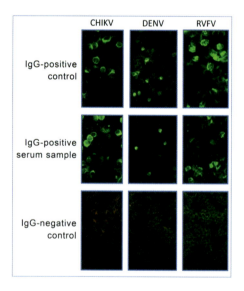

Image 59.4
Images from immunofluorescence assays in Vero E6 cells for immunoglobulin G (IgG) against chikungunya virus (CHIKV), dengue virus (DENV), and Rift Valley fever virus (RVFV) (original magnification ×100 and ×200). Courtesy of *Emerging Infectious Diseases*.

CHAPTER 60

Hemorrhagic Fevers Caused by Filoviruses: Ebola and Marburg

CLINICAL MANIFESTATIONS

Data on Ebola and Marburg virus infections are primarily derived from adult populations. More is known about Ebola virus disease (EVD) than Marburg virus disease, although the same principles apply generally to the 2 filoviruses known to cause human disease. Historically, the overall incidence of EVD infections is lower in children than in adults. However, pediatric mortality is high, with the youngest children having the highest case-fatality rates. Symptomatic disease ranges from mild to severe; case-fatality rates for severely affected people range from 25% to 90%. After a typical incubation period of 8 to 10 days (range, 2–21 days), disease in children and adults begins with nonspecific signs and symptoms including fever, severe headache, myalgia, fatigue, abdominal pain, and weakness, followed several days later by vomiting, diarrhea, and, sometimes, unexplained bleeding or bruising. Data from the 2014–2016 Ebola outbreak in West Africa, the largest since the virus was identified in 1976, indicate that children may have shorter incubation periods than adults. Respiratory symptoms are more common, and central nervous system (CNS) manifestations are less common, in children than in adults. A fleeting maculopapular rash on the torso or face after approximately 4 to 5 days of illness may occur. Conjunctival injection or subconjunctival hemorrhage may be present. Leukopenia, frequently with lymphopenia, is followed later by elevated neutrophil counts, a left shift, and thrombocytopenia. Hepatic dysfunction, with elevations in aspartate aminotransferase at markedly higher concentrations than alanine aminotransferase, and metabolic derangements, including hypokalemia, hyponatremia, hypocalcemia, and hypomagnesemia, are common. In the most severe cases, microvascular instability ensues around the end of the first week of disease. Although hemostasis is impaired, hemorrhagic manifestations develop in a minority of patients. The most common hemorrhagic manifestations consist of bleeding from the gastrointestinal tract, sometimes with oozing from the mucous membranes or venipuncture sites in late stages. Twenty percent of infected children have no fever at presentation.

CNS manifestations and renal failure are frequent in end-stage disease. In fatal cases, death typically occurs around 10 to 12 days after symptom onset, usually resulting from viral- or bacterial-induced septic shock and multiorgan system failure. Factors associated with pediatric Ebola deaths in the 2014–2016 outbreak were age younger than 5 years, bleeding at any time during hospitalization, and high viral load.

Approximately 30% of pregnant women with EVD present with spontaneous abortion and vaginal bleeding. Maternal mortality approaches 90% when infection occurs during the third trimester. Ebola virus can cross the placenta, and pregnant women infected with the virus will likely transmit the virus to the fetus. In infants born to infected mothers, Ebola virus RNA has been detected in amniotic fluid, fetal meconium, umbilical cord, and buccal swab specimens. There has been only 1 report of survival of a neonate born to a mother with active EVD. The neonate was treated with monoclonal antibodies, a buffy-coat transfusion from an Ebola survivor, and the antiviral drug remdesivir shortly after birth. The exact mechanism of neonatal deaths is unknown, but high viral loads of Ebola virus have been documented in amniotic fluid, placental tissue, and fetal tissues of stillborn neonates. EVD survivors have risk for reactivation of disease in immune-privileged sites, such as the eye or the CNS, because of persistence of Ebola virus. However, disease reactivation is currently thought to be a rare event. Long-term shedding of virus in semen has been implicated in the origin of several clusters of EVD in West Africa.

ETIOLOGY

Filoviruses (from the Latin *filo*, meaning "thread," referring to their filamentous shape) are single-stranded, negative-sense RNA viruses. There are 6 genera in the family *Filoviridae*, but only 2, *Marburgvirus* and *Ebolavirus*, cause disease in humans. This includes 4 of the 6 viruses within the genus *Ebolavirus* and both known viruses within the genus *Marburgvirus*. These filoviruses are endemic only in Africa.

EPIDEMIOLOGY

Fruit bats are believed to be the animal reservoir for most filoviruses. Human infection is believed to occur from inadvertent exposure to infected bat excreta or saliva following entry into roosting areas in caves, mines, and forests. Nonhuman primates, especially gorillas and chimpanzees, and other wild animals (eg, rodents, small antelopes) may become infected from bat contact and serve as intermediate hosts that transmit filoviruses to humans through contact with their blood and bodily fluids, usually associated with hunting and butchering. For unclear reasons, filovirus outbreaks tend to occur after prolonged dry seasons.

Molecular epidemiological evidence shows that most outbreaks result from a single point introduction (or very few) into humans from wild animals, followed by human-to-human transmission, almost invariably fueled by health care–associated transmission in areas with inadequate infection-control equipment and resources. Filoviruses are the most transmissible of all hemorrhagic fever viruses. The secondary attack rate in households is generally between 10% and 20% in African communities. Risk to household contacts is associated with direct physical contact, with little to no transmission observed otherwise. Human-to-human transmission usually occurs through oral, mucous membrane, or nonintact skin exposure to blood or bodily fluids of a symptomatic person with filovirus disease or by exposure to objects contaminated with infected blood or bodily fluids, most often in providing care to a sick family or community member (community transmission) or patient (health care–associated transmission). Funeral rituals that entail the touching of the corpse have also been implicated. Sexual transmission has been documented and implicated in several clusters of disease. Ebola virus has been detected in human milk. Respiratory spread of virus does not occur. Infection through fomites cannot be excluded. Health care–associated transmission is highly unlikely if rigorous infection-control practices are in place in health care facilities. Filoviruses are not spread through the air, by water, or in general by food (except for bushmeat).

Children may be less likely to become infected from interfamilial spread than adults when a primary case occurs in a household, possibly because they are not typically primary caregivers of sick individuals and are less likely to take part in funeral rituals that involve touching and washing of the deceased person's body.

The degree of viremia correlates with the clinical state. People are most infectious late in the course of severe disease, especially when copious vomiting, diarrhea, and/or bleeding is present. Disease transmission does not occur during the incubation period, when the person is asymptomatic. Virus may persist in a few sites for several weeks to months after clinical recovery, including in testicles/semen, vaginal fluid, placenta, amniotic fluid, human milk, saliva, the CNS (particularly cerebrospinal fluid), joints, conjunctivae, and the chambers of the eye (resulting in transient uveitis and other ocular problems). Because of the proven risk of sexual transmission, abstinence or use of condoms is recommended for at least 12 months after recovery and possibly longer.

Updated information on identification, current treatment of people traveling from areas of transmission or having contact with a person with Ebola virus infection, and communicating with children about Ebola can be found on the Centers for Disease Control and Prevention (CDC) website (**www.cdc.gov/vhf/ebola** and **www.cdc.gov/vhf/ebola/pdf/how-talk-children-about-ebola.pdf**) and HealthyChildren.org, the official American Academy of Pediatrics website for parents (**www.healthychildren.org/English/health-issues/conditions/infections/Pages/Ebola.aspx**).

The **incubation period** for EVD is 8 to 10 days (range, 2–21 days).

DIAGNOSTIC TESTS

The diagnosis of filovirus infection should be considered in a person who develops a fever within 21 days of travel to an area with endemic infection. Because initial clinical manifestations are difficult to distinguish from those of more common febrile diseases, prompt laboratory testing is imperative in a suspected case. Malaria, measles, typhoid fever, Lassa fever, dengue, and influenza should be included in the differential diagnosis of a symptomatic person returning from Africa within 21 days and are much more likely than a filovirus to be the cause of fever. Filovirus disease can be diagnosed by testing of blood by reverse transcriptase–polymerase chain reaction (RT-PCR) assay, enzyme-linked immunosorbent assay for viral antigens or immunoglobulin M (IgM), and virus isolation early in the disease course, with the latter being attempted only under biosafety level–4 conditions. Viral RNA is generally detectable by RT-PCR assay within 3 days after the onset of symptoms. IgM and immunoglobulin G antibodies may be used later in disease course or after recovery. Postmortem diagnosis can be made via immunohistochemical staining of skin or liver or spleen tissue. Testing is generally not performed routinely in clinical laboratories. Local and state public health department officials must be contacted and can facilitate testing at a regional certified laboratory or at the CDC.

In October 2019, the US Food and Drug Administration (FDA) allowed marketing of the OraQuick Ebola Rapid Antigen Test, a rapid diagnostic test (RDT) for detecting Ebola virus in both symptomatic patients and recently deceased people. The RDT should be used only when more sensitive molecular testing is unavailable. All OraQuick Ebola Rapid Antigen Test results are presumptive; all test results (positive and negative) must be verified through real-time RT-PCR testing at a Laboratory Response Network laboratory located in 49 states and at the CDC.

TREATMENT

People suspected of having filovirus infection should be placed in isolation immediately, and public health officials should be notified. Treatment of patients with filovirus disease is primarily supportive, including oral or intravenous fluids with electrolyte repletion, vasopressors, blood products, oxygen, total parenteral nutrition, analgesics, antipyretics, and antimalarial and antimicrobial medications when coinfections are suspected or confirmed. Volume losses can be enormous (10 L/day in adults), and some centers in the United States report better results with repletion by using lactated Ringer solution rather than normal saline solution in treatment of adult patients. When antimicrobial agents are used to treat sepsis, the medications should have coverage for intestinal microbiota based on limited evidence of translocation of gut bacteria into the blood of patients with filovirus disease.

On October 14, 2020, the FDA approved the first treatment of Zaire ebolavirus infection in adult and pediatric patients. Under the brand name Inmazeb, it consists of a mixture of 3 monoclonal antibodies: atoltivimab, maftivimab, and odesivimab-ebgn. On December 21, 2020, a second monoclonal antibody therapy, ansuvimab-zykl, which goes by the brand name Ebanga, received FDA approval, also for use in adult and pediatric patients. There currently are no specific therapies approved by the FDA for other filovirus infections.

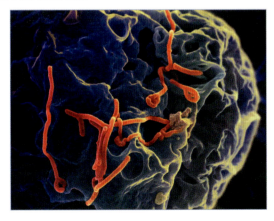

Image 60.1
Under very high magnification, this digitally colorized scanning electron micrograph depicts a number of filamentous Ebola virus particles (red) that had budded from the surface of a Vero cell (blue-gray) of the African green monkey kidney epithelial cell line. Courtesy of National Institute of Allergy and Infectious Diseases.

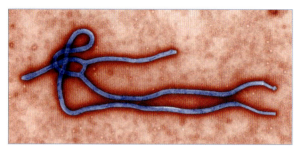

Image 60.2
Created by Centers for Disease Control and Prevention microbiologist Cynthia Goldsmith, this colorized transmission electron micrograph reveals some of the ultrastructural morphological features displayed by an Ebola virus virion. Courtesy of Centers for Disease Control and Prevention/Cynthia Goldsmith.

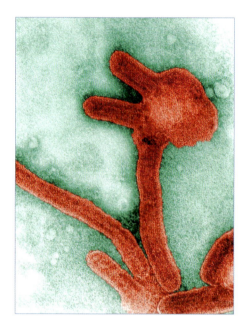

Image 60.3
This colorized, negative-stained transmission electron micrograph, captured by F.A. Murphy in 1968, depicts a number of Marburg virus virions, which had been grown in an environment of tissue culture cells. Marburg hemorrhagic fever is a rare, severe type of hemorrhagic fever that affects humans and nonhuman primates. Caused by a genetically unique zoonotic (ie, animalborne) RNA virus of the *Filovirus* family, its recognition led to the creation of this virus family. The 4 species of Ebola virus are the only other known members of the *Filovirus* family. After an incubation period of 5–10 days, onset of the disease is sudden and is marked by fever, chills, headache, and myalgia. Around the fifth day after the onset of symptoms, a maculopapular rash, most prominent on the trunk (ie, chest, back, stomach), may occur. Nausea, vomiting, chest pain, a sore throat, abdominal pain, and diarrhea may then develop. Symptoms become increasingly severe and may include jaundice, inflammation of the pancreas, severe weight loss, delirium, shock, liver failure, and multiorgan dysfunction. Because many of the signs and symptoms of Marburg hemorrhagic fever are like those of other infectious diseases, such as malaria or typhoid fever, diagnosis of the disease can be difficult, especially if only a single case is involved. Courtesy of Centers for Disease Control and Prevention/F.A. Murphy.

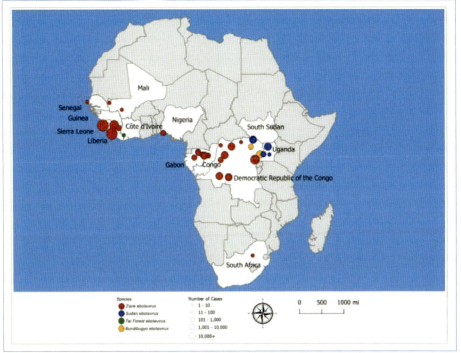

Image 60.4
Ebola virus outbreaks by species and size, since 1976. Courtesy of Centers for Disease Control and Prevention.

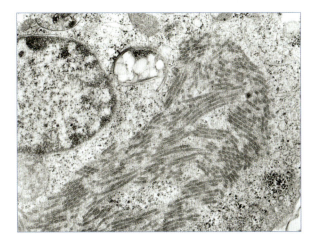

Image 60.5
This electron micrograph shows a thin section containing the Ebola virus, the causative agent of African hemorrhagic fever. The image shows an intracytoplasmic inclusion of Ebola virus nucleocapsids. Courtesy of Centers for Disease Control and Prevention.

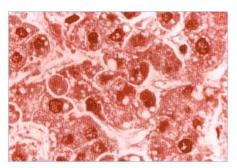

Image 60.6
Under a high magnification of ×400, this hematoxylin-eosin–stained photomicrograph depicts the cytoarchitectural changes found in a liver tissue specimen extracted from a patient with Ebola virus infection in the Democratic Republic of the Congo. This particular view reveals an acidophilic necrosis leading to the formation of a Councilman body and cytoplasmic inclusions. A steatotic (fatty change) vesicle was caught in the process of formation. Courtesy of Centers for Disease Control and Prevention.

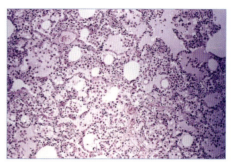

Image 60.7
This photomicrograph reveals the cytoarchitectural histopathologic changes detected in a lung biopsy tissue section from a patient with Marburg virus infection who was treated in Johannesburg, South Africa. Note the necrotic changes indicated by the breakdown of the alveolar walls resulting in pulmonary edema. There is also the presence of numerous alveolar macrophages caused by the *Filovirus* infiltrate. Courtesy of Centers for Disease Control and Prevention.

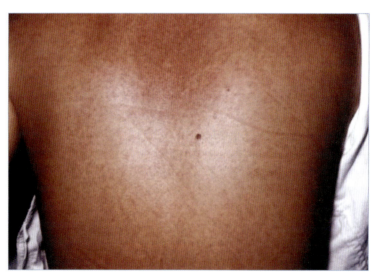

Image 60.8
This patient with Marburg virus infection presented with a measles-like rash located on her back and was hospitalized in Johannesburg, South Africa. This type of maculopapular rash, which can appear on patients with Marburg virus infection around the fifth day after the onset of symptoms, may usually be found on the patient's chest, back, and stomach. This patient's skin blanched under pressure, which is a common characteristic of a Marburg virus rash. Courtesy of Centers for Disease Control and Prevention.

CHAPTER 61
Hepatitis A

CLINICAL MANIFESTATIONS

Hepatitis A is an acute, self-limited illness associated with fever, malaise, jaundice, anorexia, and nausea that typically lasts less than 2 months, although 10% to 15% of symptomatic people have prolonged or relapsing disease that lasts as long as 6 months. Symptomatic hepatitis A virus (HAV) infection occurs in approximately 30% of infected children younger than 6 years, but few of these children will have jaundice. In older children and adults, infection is usually symptomatic, with jaundice occurring in 70% or more of cases. Fulminant hepatitis is rare but is more common in people with underlying liver disease. Chronic infection does not occur.

ETIOLOGY

HAV is a small, nonenveloped, positive-sense RNA virus with an icosahedral capsid and is classified as a member of the family *Picornaviridae*, genus *Hepatovirus*.

EPIDEMIOLOGY

The most common mode of transmission is person to person, resulting from fecal contamination and oral ingestion (ie, the fecal-oral route). In resource-limited countries where infection is endemic, most people are infected during the first decade after birth. In the United States, rates of HAV infection decreased by 95% from 1996 to 2011 following implementation of universal infant vaccination in 2006. Recently, HAV incidence has increased from a historic low of 1,239 cases reported in 2014 to more than 11,000 cases reported in 2018, primarily related to outbreaks associated with contaminated food, men who have sex with men, and people who use drugs or experience homelessness. Hepatitis A vaccination coverage (≥1 dose) for children 19 to 35 months of age was 86% in 2017. Significant decreases in anti-HAV seroprevalence in adults 40 years and older have occurred because of reduced exposure to HAV earlier in life since the introduction of universal infant vaccination, resulting in an increased proportion of adults in the United States being susceptible to HAV infection. Most HAV infection cases are now in adults 20 years and older.

Recognized risk groups for HAV infection include people who have close personal contact with a person infected with HAV, people with chronic liver disease, people with clotting factor disorders, people with HIV infection, men who have sex with men, people who use injection and noninjection drugs, people who experience homelessness, people traveling to or working in countries that have highly or intermediately endemic HAV, people who anticipate close contact with an adoptee from a country of high or intermediate endemic HAV during the first 60 days following arrival, and people who work with HAV-infected primates or with HAV in a research laboratory setting. Although HAV infections and outbreaks have been associated with food-service establishments and food handlers, health care institutions, institutions for people with developmental disabilities, schools, and child care facilities, they typically reflect transmission in the community.

Outbreaks have been associated with consumption of raw produce (eg, green onions) and fruits (eg, strawberries) and oysters and mussels. Waterborne outbreaks are rare and are typically associated with sewage-contaminated or inadequately treated water.

People with HAV infection are most infectious during the 1 to 2 weeks before onset of jaundice or elevation of liver enzyme levels, when concentration of virus in the stool is highest. Risk of transmission subsequently diminishes and is minimal by 1 week after onset of jaundice. HAV can be detected in stool for longer periods, especially in neonates and young children.

The **incubation period** is 15 to 50 days, with an average of 28 days.

DIAGNOSTIC TESTS

Serological tests for HAV-specific total antibody (ie, immunoglobulin G [IgG] plus immunoglobulin M [IgM]), IgG-only anti-HAV, and IgM-only anti-HAV are available commercially, primarily in enzyme immunoassay format. A single total or IgG anti-HAV test does not have diagnostic value for acute infection. The presence of serum IgM anti-HAV indicates current or recent infection, although false-positive results may occur, particularly if the person is asymptomatic. IgM anti-HAV is generally included in most acute hepatitis serological test panels offered by hospital or reference laboratories. IgM anti-HAV is detectable in up to 20% of hepatitis A vaccine recipients when measured 2 weeks after vaccination. In most people with HAV infection, serum IgM anti-HAV becomes detectable 5 to 10 days before onset of symptoms and declines to undetectable concentrations within 6 months after infection. People who have positive test results for IgM anti-HAV more than 1 year after infection have been reported. IgG anti-HAV is detectable shortly after appearance of IgM. A positive IgG anti-HAV or total anti-HAV (IgM and IgG) test result with a negative IgM anti-HAV test result indicates immunity from past infection or vaccination. Polymerase chain reaction assays for hepatitis A are available and may be considered to detect very early infections and to assist with interpretation of questionable IgM anti-HAV results.

TREATMENT

Supportive care, and management of complications.

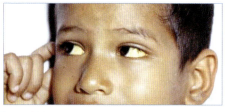

Image 61.1
Acute hepatitis A virus infection with scleral icterus in a 10-year-old boy. Courtesy of Edgar O. Ledbetter, MD, FAAP.

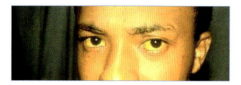

Image 61.2
Hepatitis A virus infection has caused this man's skin and the whites of his eyes to turn yellow. Other symptoms of hepatitis A virus infection can include loss of appetite, abdominal pain, nausea or vomiting, fever, headaches, and dark urine.

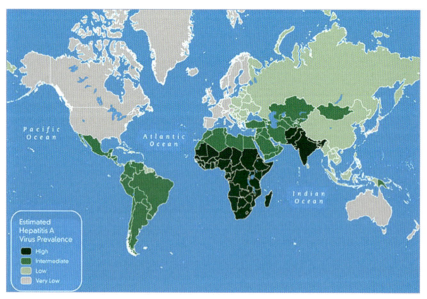

Image 61.3
Estimated prevalence of hepatitis A virus. Courtesy of Centers for Disease Control and Prevention.

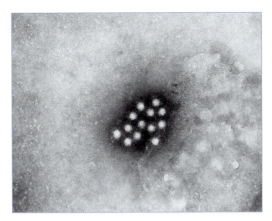

Image 61.4
An electron micrograph of the hepatitis A virus, an RNA virus classified as a member of the picornavirus group. Courtesy of Centers for Disease Control and Prevention.

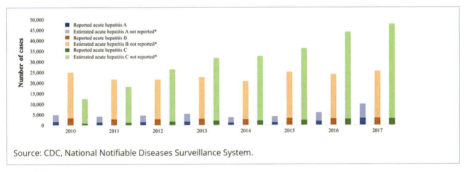

Image 61.5
Actual number of acute viral hepatitis cases submitted to the Centers for Disease Control and Prevention (CDC) by states and estimated number of acute viral hepatitis cases—United States, 2010–2017. * The number of estimated viral hepatitis cases was determined by multiplying the number of reported cases by a factor that adjusted for under-ascertainment and underreporting. Courtesy of Centers for Disease Control and Prevention.

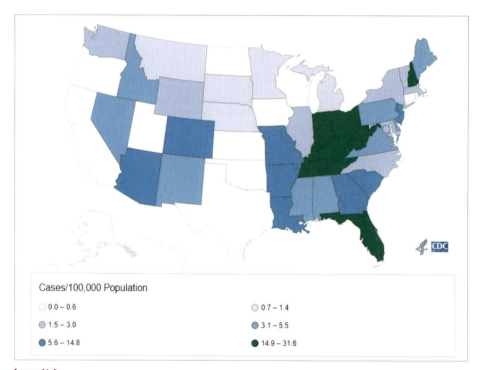

Image 61.6
Rates of reported hepatitis A virus infection, by state or jurisdiction—United States, 2019. Courtesy of Centers for Disease Control and Prevention.

CHAPTER 62
Hepatitis B

CLINICAL MANIFESTATIONS

People acutely infected with hepatitis B virus (HBV) may be asymptomatic or symptomatic. The likelihood of developing symptoms of acute hepatitis is age dependent: less than 1% of infants younger than 1 year, 5% to 15% of children 1 through 5 years of age, and 30% to 50% of people 6 through 30 years of age are symptomatic. Few data are available for adults older than 30 years. The spectrum of signs and symptoms is varied and includes subacute illness with nonspecific symptoms (eg, anorexia, nausea, or malaise), clinical hepatitis with jaundice, or fulminant hepatitis. Gianotti-Crosti syndrome (papular acrodermatitis), urticaria, macular rash, or purpuric lesions may be observed in acute HBV infection. Extrahepatic manifestations associated with circulating immune complexes that have been reported in HBV-infected children include arthralgias, arthritis, polyarteritis nodosa, thrombocytopenia, and glomerulonephritis. Acute HBV infection cannot be distinguished from other forms of acute viral hepatitis on the basis of clinical signs and symptoms or nonspecific laboratory findings.

Chronic HBV infection is defined as persistence in serum for at least 6 months of any one of the following substances: hepatitis B surface antigen (HBsAg), HBV DNA, or hepatitis B e antigen (HBeAg). Chronic HBV infection is likely in the presence of HBsAg, HBV DNA, or HBeAg in serum from a person who tests negative for antibody of the immunoglobulin M subclass to hepatitis B core antigen (IgM anti-HBc).

Age at the time of infection is the primary determinant of risk of progressing to chronic infection. Up to 90% of infants infected in the perinatal period or in the first year after birth will develop chronic HBV infection. Between 25% and 50% of children infected between 1 and 5 years of age become chronically infected, whereas 5% to 10% of infected older children and adults develop chronic HBV infection. Patients who become infected with HBV while immunosuppressed or with an underlying chronic illness (eg, end-stage renal disease) have an increased risk for developing chronic infection. In the absence of treatment, up to 25% of infants and children who acquire chronic HBV infection will die prematurely of HBV-related hepatocellular carcinoma (HCC) or cirrhosis.

The clinical course of untreated chronic HBV infection varies according to the population studied, reflecting differences in age at acquisition, rate of loss of HBeAg, and possibly HBV genotype. Most children have asymptomatic infection. For years to decades after initial infection, perinatally infected children are in an "immune tolerant" phase with normal or minimally elevated alanine aminotransferase (ALT) concentrations and minimal or mild liver histological abnormalities, detectable HBeAg, and high HBV DNA concentrations ($\geq$20,000 IU/mL). Some children with chronic HBV may exhibit growth impairment. Chronic HBV infection acquired during later childhood or adolescence is usually accompanied by more active liver disease and increased serum aminotransferase concentrations. Patients with detectable HBeAg (*HBeAg-positive chronic hepatitis B*) usually have high concentrations of HBV DNA and HBsAg in serum and are more likely to transmit infection. Over time (years to decades), HBeAg becomes undetectable in many chronically infected people. This transition is often accompanied by development of antibody to HBeAg (anti-HBe) and decreases in serum HBV DNA and serum aminotransferase concentrations and may be preceded by a temporary exacerbation of liver disease. These patients have **inactive chronic infection** but may still have exacerbations of hepatitis. Serological reversion (reappearance of HBeAg) is more common if loss of HBeAg is not accompanied by development of anti-HBe; reversion with loss of anti-HBe can also occur. Because HBV-associated liver injury is thought to be immune-mediated, in people coinfected with HIV and HBV, the return of immunocompetence with antiretroviral treatment of HIV infection may lead to a reactivation of HBV-related liver inflammation and damage.

Some patients who lose HBeAg may continue to have ongoing histological evidence of liver damage and moderate to high concentrations of HBV DNA (*HBeAg-negative chronic hepatitis B*). Patients with histological evidence of chronic HBV infection, regardless of HBeAg status, continue to have higher risk for death attributable to liver failure than HBV-infected people with no histological evidence of liver inflammation and fibrosis.

Resolved hepatitis B is defined as clearance of HBsAg, normalization of serum aminotransferase concentrations, and development of antibody to HBsAg (anti-HBs). Chronically infected adults clear HBsAg and develop anti-HBs at the rate of 1% annually; during childhood, the annual clearance rate is less than 1%. Reactivation of resolved chronic infection in HBsAg-positive patients is possible if these patients become immunosuppressed, as well as receive antitumor necrosis factor agents or disease-modifying antirheumatic drugs (12% of such patients), and has been reported in patients with chronic HCV infection being treated with direct-acting antiviral agents (21%).

ETIOLOGY

HBV is a partially double-stranded DNA–containing 42-nm–diameter enveloped virus in the family *Hepadnaviridae*. Important components of the viral particle include an outer lipoprotein envelope containing HBsAg and an inner nucleocapsid consisting of hepatitis B core antigen.

EPIDEMIOLOGY

HBV is transmitted through infected blood or body fluids. Although HBsAg has been detected in multiple body fluids including human milk, saliva, and tears, the most potentially infectious fluids include blood, serum, semen, vaginal secretions, and cerebrospinal, synovial, pleural, pericardial, peritoneal, and amniotic fluids. People with chronic HBV infection are the primary reservoirs for infection. Common modes of transmission include percutaneous and permucosal exposure to infectious body fluids; sharing or using nonsterilized needles, syringes, or glucose monitoring equipment or devices; sexual contact with an infected person; perinatal exposure to an infected mother; and household exposure to a person with chronic HBV infection. The risks of HBV acquisition when a susceptible child bites a child who has chronic HBV infection or when a susceptible child is bitten by a child with chronic HBV infection are unknown. A theoretical risk exists if HBsAg-positive blood enters the oral cavity of the biter, but transmission by this route has not been reported. Transmission by transfusion of contaminated blood or blood products is rare in the United States because of routine screening of blood donors and viral inactivation of certain blood products before administration.

Perinatal transmission of HBV is highly efficient and usually occurs from blood exposures during labor and delivery. In utero transmission accounts for less than 2% of all vertically transmitted HBV infections in most studies. Without postexposure prophylaxis, the risk of an infant acquiring HBV from an infected mother by perinatal exposure is 70% to 90% for infants born to mothers who are HBsAg and HBeAg positive; the risk is 5% to 20% for infants born to HBsAg-positive but HBeAg-negative mothers. Infants born to mothers with very high HBV DNA levels (>200,000 IU/mL) have high risk for breakthrough infection despite receipt of recommended prophylaxis.

Prevalence of HBV infection and patterns of transmission vary markedly throughout the world (Figure 62.1). Approximately 80% of people worldwide live in regions of intermediate to high HBV endemicity, defined as prevalence of chronic HBV infection of 2% or greater. Historically, most new HBV infections occurred because of perinatal or early childhood infections in regions of high HBV endemicity, where the prevalence of HBV infection is 8% or greater. Infant immunization programs in some of these countries have, in recent years, greatly reduced seroprevalence of HBsAg, but many countries with endemic HBV have yet to implement widespread routine birth-dose and/or childhood hepatitis B immunization programs. In regions of intermediate HBV endemicity (prevalence of HBV infection 2%–7%), multiple modes of transmission (ie, perinatal, household, sexual, injection drug use, and health care–associated) contribute to the burden of infection. In countries with low endemicity (chronic HBV infection prevalence <2%) and where routine immunization has been adopted, new infections occur most often in age-groups in which routine immunization is not conducted.

In regions of the world with high prevalence of chronic HBV infection, transmission between children in household settings may account for a substantial amount of transmission. Precise mechanisms of transmission from child to child are unknown, but frequent interpersonal contact

Figure 62.1
Map of Hepatitis B Prevalence Globally

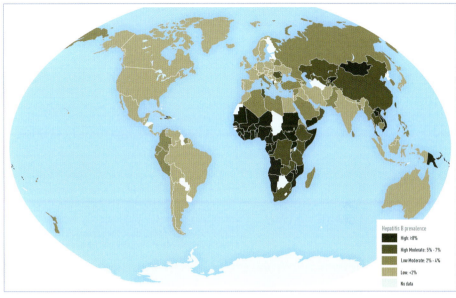

Reproduced from Centers for Disease Control and Prevention. *CDC Yellow Book 2020: Health Information for National Travel.* Oxford University Press; 2019. Accessed June 23, 2022. https://www.cdc.gov/travel-static/yellowbook/2020/map_4-04.pdf.

of nonintact skin or mucous membranes with blood-containing secretions, open skin lesions, or blood-containing saliva are potential means of transmission. Transmission from sharing inanimate objects, such as razors or toothbrushes, may also occur. HBV can survive in the environment for 7 or more days but is inactivated by commonly used disinfectants, including household bleach diluted 1:10 with water. HBV is not transmitted by the fecal-oral route.

The **incubation period** for acute HBV infection is 45 to 160 days, with an average of 90 days.

DIAGNOSTIC TESTS

Serological protein antigen tests are available commercially to detect HBsAg and HBeAg. Serological antibody assays are also available for detection of anti-HBs, total anti-HBc, IgM anti-HBc, and anti-HBe (Table 62.1, Figure 62.2, and Figure 62.3). Most laboratories now use real-time polymerase chain reaction assays for analysis of HBV DNA.

HBsAg is detectable during acute and chronic infection. If HBV infection is self-limited, HBsAg disappears in most patients within a few weeks to several months after infection, followed by appearance of anti-HBs. The time between disappearance of HBsAg and appearance of anti-HBs is termed the *window period* of infection. During the window period, the only marker of acute infection is IgM anti-HBc. IgM anti-HBc is not usually present in infants infected perinatally. People with chronic HBV infection have circulating HBsAg and circulating total anti-HBc (Figure 62.3); in a minority of chronically infected individuals, anti-HBs is also present. Both anti-HBs and total anti-HBc are present in people with resolved infection, whereas anti-HBs alone is present in people immunized with hepatitis B vaccine. The presence of HBeAg in serum correlates with higher concentrations of HBV DNA and greater infectivity. Tests for HBeAg and HBV DNA are useful in selection of candidates to receive antiviral therapy and to monitor response to therapy.

Transient presence of HBsAg can occur following receipt of hepatitis B vaccine, with HBsAg being detected as early as 24 hours after and up to 3 weeks following administration of the vaccine.

Table 62.1
Diagnostic Tests for Hepatitis B Virus (HBV) Antigens and Antibodies

Factors to Be Tested	HBV Antigen or Antibody	Use
HBsAg	Hepatitis B surface antigen	Detection of acutely or chronically infected people; antigen used in hepatitis B vaccine; can rarely be detected for up to 3 weeks after a dose of hepatitis B vaccine
Anti-HBs	Antibody to HBsAg	Identification of people who have resolved infections with HBV; determination of immunity after immunization
HBeAg	Hepatitis B e antigen	Identification of infected people with increased risk for transmitting HBV
Anti-HBe	Antibody to HBeAg	Identification of infected people with lower risk for transmitting HBV
Anti-HBc (total)	Antibody to HBcAg[a]	Identification of people with acute, resolved, or chronic HBV infection (not present after immunization); passively transferred maternal anti-HBc is detectable for as long as 24 months in infants born to HBsAg-positive women
IgM anti-HBc	IgM antibody to HBcAg	Identification of people with acute or recent HBV infection (including HBsAg-negative people during the *window period* of infection; unreliable for detecting perinatal HBV infection)

HBcAg indicates hepatitis B core antigen; IgM, immunoglobulin M.
[a] No test is available commercially to measure HBcAg.

Figure 62.2
Typical Serological Course of Acute Hepatitis B Virus Infection With Recovery

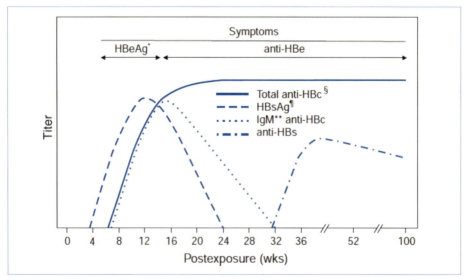

* Hepatitis B e antigen.
§ Antibody to hepatitis B core antigen.
¶ Hepatitis B surface antigen.
** Immunoglobulin M.
From Centers for Disease Control and Prevention. Recommendations for identification and public health management of persons with chronic hepatitis B virus infection. *MMWR Recomm Rep.* 2008;57(RR-8):1–20.

Figure 62.3
Typical Serological Course of Acute Hepatitis B Virus (HBV) Infection With Progression to Chronic HBV Infection

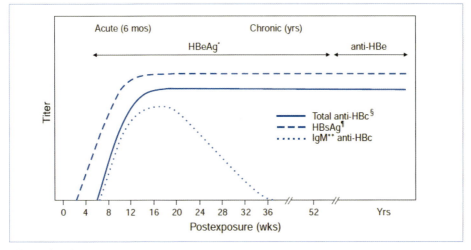

* Hepatitis B e antigen.
§ Antibody to hepatitis B core antigen.
¶ Hepatitis B surface antigen.
** Immunoglobulin M.
From Centers for Disease Control and Prevention. Recommendations for identification and public health management of persons with chronic hepatitis B virus infection. *MMWR Recomm Rep.* 2008;57(RR-8):1–20.

TREATMENT

No therapy for uncomplicated *acute* HBV infection is recommended. Treatment with a nucleoside or nucleotide analogue is indicated if there is concern for severe infection with acute liver failure. Acute HBV infection may be difficult to distinguish from reactivation of HBV. If reactivation is a possibility, referral to a hepatitis specialist would be warranted. Hepatitis B immune globulin and corticosteroids are not effective treatment of acute or chronic disease.

The goal of treatment in chronic HBV infection is to prevent progression to cirrhosis, hepatic failure, and HCC, with anti-HBe seroconversion as the surrogate end point. Current indications for treatment of chronic HBV infection include evidence of ongoing HBV viral replication, as indicated by the longer-than-6-months presence of serum HBV DNA greater than 20,000 IU/mL with HBeAg positivity or greater than 2,000 IU/mL without HBeAg positivity, AND elevated serum ALT concentrations for longer than 6 months or evidence of chronic hepatitis on liver biopsy. Children without necroinflammatory liver disease and children in the immunotolerant phase (ie, normal ALT concentrations despite the presence of HBV DNA) do not warrant antiviral therapy. Treatment response is measured by biochemical, virological, and histological response. It is recommended that women with viral loads greater than 200,000 IU/mL be offered antiviral therapy to prevent transmission to their child.

The US Food and Drug Administration (FDA) has approved 3 nucleoside analogues (entecavir, lamivudine, and telbivudine), 3 nucleotide analogues (tenofovir disoproxil fumarate, tenofovir alafenamide fumarate, and adefovir), and 2 interferon-alfa drugs (interferon alfa-2b and pegylated interferon alfa-2a) for treatment of chronic HBV infection in adults. Tenofovir disoproxil fumarate, tenofovir alafenamide fumarate, entecavir, and pegylated interferon alfa-2a are preferred in adults as first-line therapy because of the lower likelihood of developing antiviral resistance mutations over long-term therapy. FDA licensure in the pediatric population is as follows: interferon alfa-2b, 1 year and older; entecavir, 2 years and older; tenofovir disoproxil fumarate, 2 years and older; and telbivudine, 16 years and older. Pegylated interferon alfa-2a is not approved for treatment of children with chronic hepatitis B but is approved for children 5 years and older to treat chronic hepatitis C infection.

Consultation with health care professionals with expertise in treating chronic hepatitis B in children is recommended.

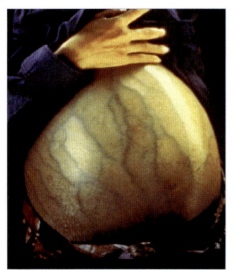

Image 62.1
This female Cambodian patient presented with a distended abdomen caused by a hepatoma resulting from chronic hepatitis B virus infection. Courtesy of Centers for Disease Control and Prevention.

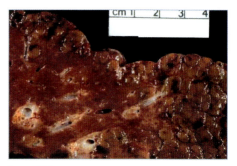

Image 62.2
Section of liver damaged by hepatitis B virus infection. Note the enlarged cells and blistering capsular surface. Courtesy of Immunization Action Coalition.

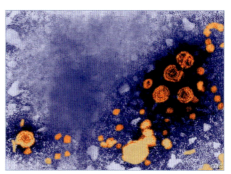

Image 62.4
This transmission electron micrograph reveals the presence of hepatitis B virions. Courtesy of Centers for Disease Control and Prevention/Erskine Palmer, MD.

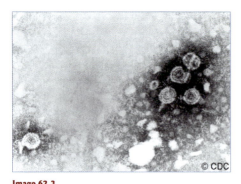

Image 62.3
Transmission electron micrograph of hepatitis B virions, also known as Dane particles. Courtesy of Centers for Disease Control and Prevention.

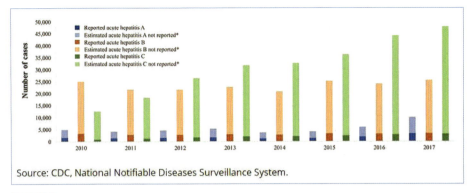

Source: CDC, National Notifiable Diseases Surveillance System.

Image 62.5
Actual number of acute viral hepatitis cases submitted to the Centers for Disease Control and Prevention (CDC) by states and estimated number of acute viral hepatitis cases—United States, 2010–2017. * The number of estimated viral hepatitis cases was determined by multiplying the number of reported cases by a factor that adjusted for under-ascertainment and underreporting. Courtesy of Centers for Disease Control and Prevention.

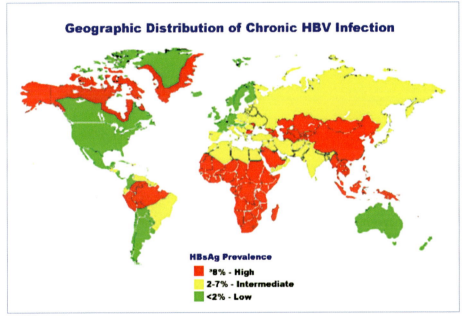

Image 62.6
World map for hepatitis B virus (HBV) infection endemicity. HBsAg indicates hepatitis B surface antigen. Courtesy of Centers for Disease Control and Prevention.

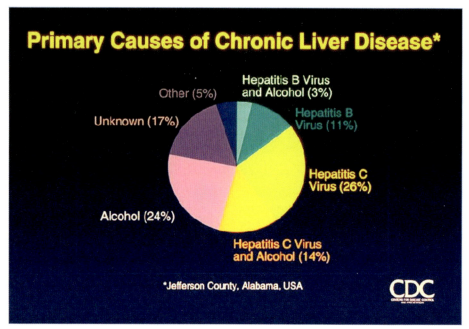

Image 62.7
Pie chart showing causes of chronic liver disease in residents of Jefferson County, Alabama. Hepatitis B and C viruses contributed to most cases of chronic liver disease in this population. Courtesy of Centers for Disease Control and Prevention.

Hepatitis C

CLINICAL MANIFESTATIONS

Signs and symptoms of hepatitis C virus (HCV) infection are indistinguishable from those of hepatitis A or hepatitis B virus infections. Acute disease tends to be mild and insidious in onset, and most infections are asymptomatic. Jaundice occurs in less than 20% of patients with HCV infection, and abnormalities in serum alanine aminotransferase concentrations are generally less pronounced than in patients with hepatitis B virus infection. Persistent infection with HCV occurs in up to 80% of infected children, even in the absence of biochemical evidence of liver disease. In general, higher rates of spontaneous viral clearance have been observed in children with perinatal infection, with roughly 20% clearing virus by 2 years of age. Most children with chronic infection are asymptomatic. Liver failure secondary to HCV infection is one of the leading indications for liver transplant among adults in the United States. Limited data indicate that cirrhosis and hepatocellular carcinoma occur less commonly in children than in adults.

ETIOLOGY

HCV is a small, single-stranded, positive-sense RNA virus and is a member of the family *Flaviviridae* in the genus *Hepacivirus*. At least 7 HCV genotypes exist, with more than 50 subtypes. Distribution of genotypes and subtypes varies by geographic location, with genotype 1a being the most common in the United States.

EPIDEMIOLOGY

Prevalence of HCV infection in the general population of the United States is estimated at 1.0%, equating to an estimated 2.7 (2.0–2.8) million people in the United States with chronic HCV infection. Incidence of HCV infection decreased markedly in the United States in all age-groups from the 1990s to reach its lowest incidence in 2006–2010. After 2010, there was an increase in reported cases of acute HCV infection in the United States, largely related to injection drug use, with the highest incidence among people 20 through 29 years of age. Worldwide, the prevalence of chronic HCV infection is highest in eastern Europe, central Asia, northern Africa, and the Middle East.

HCV is transmitted primarily through percutaneous (parenteral) exposures to infectious blood that can result from injection drug use, needlestick injuries, and inadequate infection control in health care settings. The most common risk factors for adults are injection drug use and male-to-male sexual contact. The most common route of infection for children is maternal-fetal transmission. The current risk of HCV infection after blood transfusion in the United States is estimated to be less than 1 per 2 million units transfused because of exclusion of high-risk donors and of HCV-positive units after antibody testing as well as screening of pools of blood units by nucleic acid amplification tests (NAATs). All intravenous and intramuscular immune globulin and plasma products now available commercially in the United States undergo an inactivation procedure for HCV or are documented to be HCV RNA negative before release.

Approximately 60% of acute HCV infections reported to public health authorities are in people who acknowledge that they inject drugs and that they have shared needles or injection paraphernalia. Data from recent multicenter, population-based cohort studies indicate that approximately one-third of people who inject drugs and are 18 to 30 years of age are infected with HCV. People with sporadic percutaneous exposures, such as health care professionals, may be infected; per-exposure risk of HCV transmission from needlestick is estimated at 0.1%. Health care–associated outbreaks have been documented, especially among nonhospital settings with inadequate infection control and injection safety procedures. Prevalence of HCV is higher among people with frequent direct percutaneous exposures, such as patients receiving hemodialysis (7%).

Sexual transmission of HCV between monogamous heterosexual partners is extremely rare. Transmission can occur in male-to-male sexual contact, especially in association with sexual practices that result in mucosal trauma, presence of concurrent anogenital ulcerative disease, HIV-positive serostatus, or sex while using methamphetamines. HCV has been identified in semen, rectal fluids, and the genital tracts of women, especially in those coinfected with HCV and HIV.

Transmission among family contacts could occur from direct or inapparent percutaneous or mucosal exposure to blood, but this is extremely uncommon.

Seroprevalence among pregnant women in the United States is estimated at 1% to 2% but is higher in some areas. Risk of perinatal transmission averages 5% to 6%, and transmission is associated with presence of HCV viremia at or near the time of delivery. The exact timing of HCV transmission from mother to infant is not established. It is recommended that all pregnant women be tested for HCV with each pregnancy. Factors that increase risk of perinatal transmission include internal fetal monitoring, vaginal lacerations, and prolonged rupture of membranes (>6 hours). Method of delivery has no effect on perinatal infection risk. Antibody to HCV (anti-HCV) and HCV RNA have been detected in colostrum, but risk of HCV transmission is similar in breastfed and formula-fed infants. Maternal coinfection with HIV is associated with increased risk of perinatal transmission of HCV (2-fold greater). Early and sustained control of HIV viremia with antiretroviral therapy may reduce risk of HCV transmission to infants.

All people with HCV RNA in their blood are considered to be infectious.

The **incubation period** for HCV infection averages 6 to 7 weeks, with a range of 2 weeks to 6 months. The time from exposure to development of viremia is generally 2 to 3 weeks.

DIAGNOSTIC TESTS

Diagnostic assays for the detection of anti-HCV antibody are available in various formats, which include enzyme immunoassays, chemiluminescent immunoassays, and immunochromatographic or rapid tests. NAATs for both qualitative and quantitative detection of HCV RNA are used to detect current HCV infection and to monitor response to antiviral therapy. Screening for HCV infection is usually accomplished by serological testing for anti-HCV with reflex testing of positive or equivocal HCV antibody test results, with NAAT testing to diagnose current infection. Third-generation anti-HCV assays cleared by the US Food and Drug Administration (FDA) are at least 97% sensitive and more than 99% specific. Anti-HCV antibodies can be detected approximately 8 to 11 weeks after exposure. Within 15 weeks after exposure and within 5 to 6 weeks after onset of hepatitis, 80% of patients will have positive test results for anti-HCV antibody. In infants born to anti-HCV–positive mothers, passively acquired maternal antibody may persist for up to 18 months. In clinical settings where exposure to HCV is considered likely, testing for HCV RNA by NAAT should be performed regardless of the anti-HCV result.

NAATs for detection of HCV RNA are available commercially and recommended as reflex testing for patients with anti-HCV positive test results. HCV RNA can be detected in serum or plasma within 1 to 2 weeks after exposure to the virus and weeks before onset of liver enzyme abnormalities or appearance of anti-HCV antibody. Assays for detection of HCV RNA are used commonly in clinical practice to (1) detect HCV infection after needlestick or transfusion and before seroconversion; (2) identify active infection in anti-HCV–positive patients; (3) identify infection in infants early in life (ie, perinatal transmission) when maternal antibody interferes with ability to detect antibody produced by the infant; (4) identify HCV infection in severely immunocompromised or hemodialysis patients in whom antibody test results may be falsely negative; and (5) monitor patients receiving antiviral therapy. False-positive and false-negative results of NAATs can occur from improper handling, storage, and contamination of test specimens. Highly sensitive quantitative assays for measuring the concentration of HCV RNA have largely replaced qualitative assays. HCV genotyping is still needed for determining which direct-acting antiviral (DAA) agents should be used in individual patients.

Because infants exposed to HCV perinatally have a low risk for HCV acquisition, because they do not usually exhibit symptoms for years, and because there are no antiviral therapies available in the first 3 years after birth, testing for HCV infection usually relies on serological testing at 18 months of age. Liver enzyme testing can be performed at approximately 6-month intervals to detect the rare perinatally HCV-infected infant who has significant liver injury before 18 months of age. When there is concern about follow-up of a perinatally HCV-exposed infant until 18 months of age, NAAT for HCV RNA detection can be performed between 2 and 6 months of age. Regardless of the NAAT test result, serological testing should also be performed at 18 months of age for more definitive diagnosis.

TREATMENT

Children with a diagnosis of HCV infection should be referred to a pediatric infectious diseases specialist or gastroenterologist for clinical monitoring and consideration for treatment. A number of highly effective interferon-free DAA drug regimens have been approved by the FDA, an increasing number of which are now approved in children as young as 3 years. All HCV-infected children 3 years or older should be treated with FDA age-approved antiviral medications.

Management of Chronic HCV Infection

Because of the very high rate of severe hepatitis in patients with HCV-associated chronic liver disease, all patients with chronic HCV infection should be immunized against hepatitis A and hepatitis B. Risk of liver-related morbidity and mortality, including cirrhosis and primary hepatocellular carcinoma, increases with advancing age in individuals with chronic HCV infection. In children, progression of liver disease appears to be accelerated when comorbid conditions, including HIV, childhood cancer, iron overload, or thalassemia, are present. Pediatricians should be alert for conditions that may worsen liver disease in patients with HCV infection, such as concomitant infections, alcohol use, and concomitant use of prescription and nonprescription drugs, such as acetaminophen, some antiretroviral agents, and herbal medications. Children with chronic infection should be followed up closely, including sequential monitoring of serum alanine aminotransferase concentrations, because of the potential for chronic liver disease.

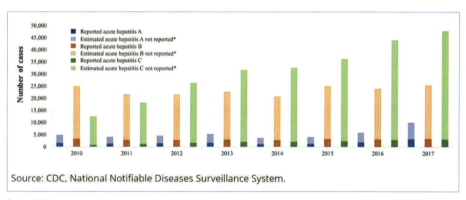

Source: CDC, National Notifiable Diseases Surveillance System.

Image 63.1
Actual number of acute viral hepatitis cases submitted to the Centers for Disease Control and Prevention (CDC) by states and estimated number of acute viral hepatitis cases—United States, 2010–2017. * The number of estimated viral hepatitis cases was determined by multiplying the number of reported cases by a factor that adjusted for underascertainment and underreporting. Courtesy of Centers for Disease Control and Prevention.

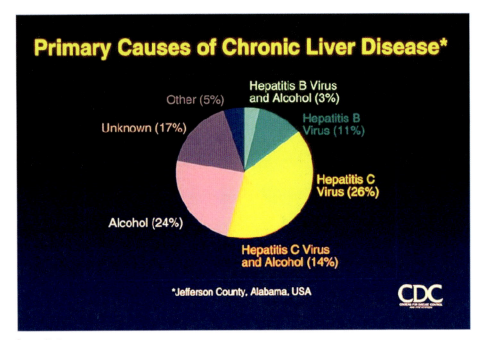

Image 63.2
Pie chart showing causes of chronic liver disease in residents of Jefferson County, Alabama. Hepatitis B and C viruses contributed to most cases of chronic liver disease in this population. Courtesy of Centers for Disease Control and Prevention.

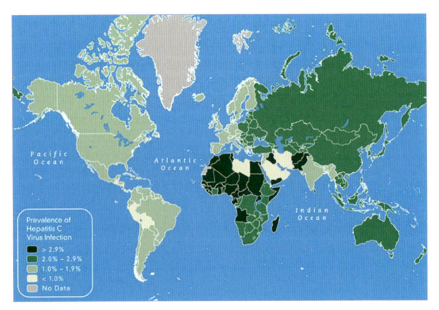

Image 63.3
Prevalence of chronic hepatitis C virus infection. Courtesy of Centers for Disease Control and Prevention.

CHAPTER 64
Hepatitis D

CLINICAL MANIFESTATIONS

Hepatitis D virus (HDV) causes infection only in people with acute or chronic hepatitis B virus (HBV) infection. HDV requires hepatitis B surface antigen (HbsAg) for virion assembly and secretion. The importance of HDV infection lies in its ability to convert an asymptomatic or mild chronic HBV infection into more severe or rapidly progressive disease. HDV infection can be acquired either simultaneously with HBV infection (coinfection) or subsequently to HBV infection in people already positive for HbsAg (superinfection). Coinfection is indistinguishable from acute hepatitis B and is usually transient and self-limited, whereas superinfection often results in chronic illness. Acute infection with HDV usually causes an illness indistinguishable from other viral hepatitis infections, except that the likelihood of fulminant hepatitis can be as high as 5%.

ETIOLOGY

Hepatitis delta virus is the only species in the *Deltavirus*. HDV has a circular, negative-sense single-stranded RNA genome and approximately 70 copies of hepatitis delta antigen, all of which is coated with HbsAg.

EPIDEMIOLOGY

HDV infection is present worldwide, in all age-groups. Over the past 20 years, HDV prevalence has varied geographically, with decreases in some regions attributable to long-standing hepatitis B vaccination. HDV remains a significant health problem in resource-limited countries. At least 8 genotypes of HDV have been described, each with a typical geographic pattern, with genotype 1 being found worldwide. Acquisition of HDV is by parenteral transmission from infected blood or body fluids such as through injection drug use or sexual contact. Transmission from mother to newborn is uncommon. Intrafamilial spread can occur among people with chronic HBV infection. High-prevalence areas include parts of eastern Europe, South America, Africa, central Asia, and the Middle East. HDV infection is found in the United States most commonly in people who use injection drugs and people who have emigrated from areas with endemic HDV infection.

The **incubation period** for HDV superinfection is approximately 2 to 8 weeks. When HBV and HDV infect simultaneously, the incubation period is similar to that of HBV (45–160 days; average, 90 days).

DIAGNOSTIC TESTS

People with chronic HBV infection have risk for HDV superinfection. Because of the dependence of HDV on HBV, the diagnosis of hepatitis D cannot be made in the absence of markers of HBV infection. Testing should be considered for patients with unusually severe or protracted hepatitis and for HbsAg-positive patients with specific risk factors, such as emigration from a region with endemic infection (such as eastern European countries, Mediterranean countries, and countries in Central America), injection drug use, men who have sex with men, coinfection with hepatitis C virus or HIV, or high-risk sexual practices. Anti-HDV becomes detectable several weeks after illness onset. In a person with anti-HDV, absence of immunoglobulin M hepatitis B core antibody, which is indicative of chronic HBV infection, suggests that the person has both chronic HBV infection and superinfection with HDV. Because immunoglobulin G anti-HDV is detectable during acute, chronic, and resolved phases of infection, testing for HDV RNA is required for diagnosing current HDV infection and for monitoring antiviral therapy. Patients with circulating HDV RNA should be staged for severity of liver disease, have surveillance for development of hepatocellular carcinoma, and be considered for treatment.

TREATMENT

HDV has proven difficult to treat, and there are no approved therapies. Data suggest pegylated interferon alfa may result in up to 40% of patients having a sustained response to treatment. Clinical trials suggest that at least a year of therapy may be associated with sustained responses, and longer courses may be warranted if the patient is able to tolerate therapy. Novel therapies under investigation in adults include viral entry inhibitors, assembly inhibitors, and HbsAg secretion inhibitors.

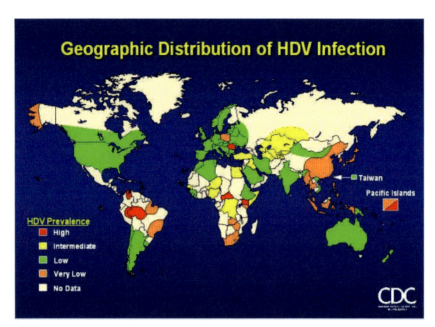

Image 64.1
Hepatitis D virus (HDV) infections are found worldwide, but the prevalence varies in different geographic areas. Anti-HDV antibodies are found in 20%–40% of hepatitis B surface antigen (HBsAg) carriers in Africa, the Middle East, and southern Italy. HDV infection in the United States is relatively uncommon, except in people who use drugs and people who have hemophilia, who exhibit prevalence rates of 1%–10%. Both gay men and health care workers have high risk for contracting hepatitis B virus infection but have surprisingly low risk for HDV infection for unclear reasons. Additionally, HDV infection is uncommon in the large population of HBsAG carriers in Southeast Asia and China. Additional groups with high risk for contracting HDV include patients undergoing hemodialysis, sex contacts of infected individuals, and infants born to infected mothers (rare). Worldwide, >10 million people are infected with HDV. Courtesy of Centers for Disease Control and Prevention.

CHAPTER 65
Hepatitis E

CLINICAL MANIFESTATIONS

Hepatitis E virus (HEV) infection can be asymptomatic or can cause an acute illness with symptoms including jaundice, malaise, anorexia, fever, abdominal pain, and arthralgia. Disease is more common in young adults than in children and is more severe in pregnant women, whose mortality rates can reach 10% to 25% if infection occurs during the third trimester. Chronic HEV infection is rare and, to date, has been reported only in more developed countries, mostly in organ transplant recipients with immunosuppression. Approximately 60% of recipients of solid organ transplants fail to clear the virus and develop chronic hepatitis, and 10% will develop cirrhosis.

ETIOLOGY

HEV is a spherical, nonenveloped, positive-sense, single-stranded RNA virus. HEV is classified in the genus *Orthohepevirus* of the family *Hepeviridae*. *Orthohepevirus* A comprises 8 genotypes (based on phylogenetic analyses); these may infect humans (HEV-1, -2, -3, -4, and -7), pigs (HEV-3 and -4), rabbits (HEV-3), wild boars (HEV-3, -4, -5, and -6), mongooses (HEV-3), deer (HEV-3), yaks (HEV-4), and camels (HEV-7 and -8). There is also a report of human infection caused by *Orthohepevirus* C, which is usually found in rats and ferrets.

EPIDEMIOLOGY

An estimated 20 million HEV infections occur each year worldwide, resulting in 3.4 million cases of acute hepatitis and 44,000 deaths. Almost all HEV infections occur in resource-limited countries, where ingestion of fecally contaminated water is the most common route of HEV transmission, and large waterborne outbreaks occur frequently. HEV infection has been reported throughout the world, including Africa and Asia. Foodborne infection has occurred sporadically in developed countries following consumption of uncooked or undercooked pork or deer meat or sausage as well as from shellfish. Person-to-person transmission appears to be much less efficient than with hepatitis A virus but occurs sporadically and in outbreak settings. Mother-to-infant transmission of HEV, mainly HEV-1, occurs frequently and accounts for substantial fetal loss and perinatal mortality. It is unclear whether breastfeeding is a potential route of HEV transmission; there is sufficient concern to discourage breastfeeding by confirmed HEV-infected mothers.

HEV is also transmitted through blood and blood product transfusion. Transfusion-transmitted hepatitis E occurs primarily in countries with endemic disease and is also reported in areas without endemic infection. Serological studies have demonstrated that approximately 6% of the population of the United States has immunoglobulin G (IgG) antibodies against HEV, but symptomatic HEV infection in the United States is uncommon and generally occurs in people who acquire HEV-1 infection while traveling in countries with endemic HEV infection. A number of people without a travel history have been diagnosed with acute hepatitis E, and evidence for the infection should be sought in patients with acute hepatitis of unknown etiology. Hepatitis E may masquerade as drug-induced liver injury.

The **incubation period** is 2 to 10 weeks.

DIAGNOSTIC TESTS

HEV infection should be considered in any person with symptoms of viral hepatitis who has traveled to or from a region with endemic hepatitis E or from a region where an outbreak has been identified and who tests negative for serological markers of hepatitis A, B, and C, and other hepatotropic, viruses. Testing for anti-HEV immunoglobulin M and IgG is available through some research and commercial reference laboratories. Because anti-HEV assays are not approved by the US Food and Drug Administration and their performance characteristics are not well-defined, results should be interpreted with caution, particularly in cases lacking a discrete onset of illness associated with jaundice or with no recent history of travel to a country with endemic HEV transmission. Definitive diagnosis can be made by demonstrating viral RNA in serum or stool samples by means of reverse transcriptase–polymerase chain reaction assay, which is available at a limited number of commercial laboratories and with prior approval through the Centers for Disease Control and Prevention. Because virus circulates in the body for a relatively short period, the inability to detect HEV in serum or stool does not eliminate the possibility that the person was infected with HEV.

TREATMENT

Management is supportive.

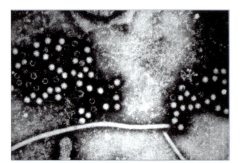

Image 65.1
This electron micrograph depicts hepatitis E viruses (HEVs). HEV was classified as a member of the *Caliciviridae* family but has been reclassified in the genus *Hepevirus* of the family *Hepeviridae*. There are 4 major recognized genotypes with a single known serotype. HEV, the major etiologic agent of enterically transmitted non-A, non-B hepatitis worldwide, is a spherical, nonenveloped, single-stranded RNA virus that is approximately 32–34 nm in diameter. Courtesy of Centers for Disease Control and Prevention.

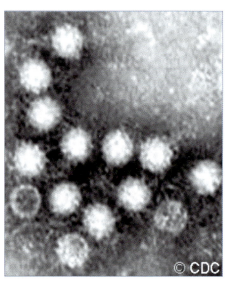

Image 65.2
Electron micrograph of nonhuman primate (marmoset)–passaged hepatitis E virus (HEV) (Nepal isolate). Virus is aggregated with convalescent antisera to HEV and negatively stained in phosphotungstic acid. Particle size ranges from 27–30 nm. Courtesy of Centers for Disease Control and Prevention.

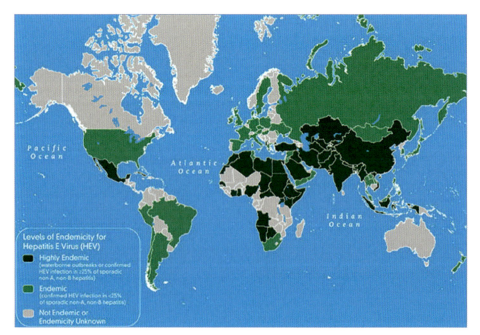

Image 65.3
Distribution of hepatitis E virus infection, 2010. Courtesy of Centers for Disease Control and Prevention.

CHAPTER 66
Herpes Simplex

CLINICAL MANIFESTATIONS

Neonatal

In newborns, herpes simplex virus (HSV) infection can manifest as (1) *disseminated disease* involving multiple organs, most prominently liver and lungs, and, in 60% to 75% of cases, also involving the central nervous system (CNS); (2) *localized CNS disease*, with or without skin, eye, or mouth involvement (CNS disease); or (3) *disease localized to the skin, eyes, and/or mouth* (SEM disease). Approximately 25% of cases of neonatal HSV manifest as disseminated disease, 30% manifest as CNS disease, and 45% manifest as SEM disease. Both HSV type 1 (HSV-1) and type 2 (HSV-2) can cause any of these manifestations of neonatal HSV disease. In the absence of skin lesions, the diagnosis of neonatal HSV infection is challenging. More than 80% of neonates with SEM disease have skin vesicles; those without vesicles have infection limited to the eyes and/or oral mucosa. Approximately two-thirds of neonates with disseminated or CNS disease have skin lesions, but these lesions may not be present at the onset of symptoms. Disseminated infection should be considered in neonates with sepsis syndrome with negative bacteriologic culture results, severe liver dysfunction, consumptive coagulopathy, or suspected viral pneumonia, especially hemorrhagic pneumonia. HSV should be considered as a causative agent in neonates with fever (especially within the first 3 weeks after birth), a vesicular rash, or abnormal cerebrospinal fluid (CSF) findings (especially in the presence of seizures or during a time of year when enteroviruses are not circulating in the community). Although asymptomatic HSV infection is common in older children, it rarely, if ever, occurs in neonates. Recurrent skin lesions are common in surviving infants, occurring in approximately 50% of survivors, often within 1 to 2 weeks of completing the initial treatment course of parenteral acyclovir.

Initial signs of HSV infection can occur anytime between birth and approximately 6 weeks of age, although almost all infected infants develop clinical disease within the first month after birth. Infants with disseminated disease and SEM disease have an earlier age of onset, typically presenting between the first and second weeks after birth; infants with CNS disease usually present with illness between the second and third weeks after birth.

Children Beyond the Neonatal Period and Adolescents

Most primary HSV childhood infections beyond the neonatal period are asymptomatic. Gingivostomatitis, which is the most common clinical manifestation of HSV during childhood, is almost exclusively caused by HSV-1 and is characterized by fever, irritability, tender submandibular adenopathy, and an ulcerative enanthem involving the gingiva and mucous membranes of the mouth, often with perioral vesicular lesions.

Genital herpes is characterized by vesicular or ulcerative lesions of the male or female genitalia, perineum, or perianal areas. Until the past 2 decades, genital herpes was most often caused by HSV-2, but, likely because of an increase in oral sexual practices by adolescents and young adults, HSV-1 now accounts for more than half of all cases in the United States. Most cases of primary genital herpes infection in males and females are asymptomatic, so they are not recognized by the infected person or diagnosed by a health care professional.

In immunocompromised patients, severe local lesions and, less commonly, disseminated HSV infection with generalized vesicular skin lesions and visceral involvement can occur.

After primary infection, HSV persists for life in a latent form. Reactivation of latent virus is most commonly asymptomatic. When symptomatic, recurrent HSV-1 herpes labialis manifests as single or grouped vesicles in the perioral region, usually on the vermilion border of the lips (typically called "cold sores" or "fever blisters"). Symptomatic recurrent genital herpes manifests as vesicular lesions on the penis, scrotum, vulva, cervix, buttocks, perianal areas, thighs, or back. In immunocompromised patients, genital HSV-2 recurrences are more frequent and of longer duration. Recurrences may be heralded by a prodrome of burning or itching at the site of an incipient recurrence, identification of which can be useful in instituting early antiviral therapy.

Ocular manifestations of HSV include conjunctivitis and keratitis that can result from primary or recurrent HSV infection. In addition, HSV can cause acute retinal necrosis and uveitis.

Eczema herpeticum can develop in patients with atopic dermatitis who are infected with HSV and can be difficult to distinguish from poorly controlled atopic dermatitis. Examination may reveal skin with punched-out erosions, hemorrhagic crusts, and/or vesicular lesions. Pustular lesions attributable to bacterial superinfection may also occur. Herpetic whitlow consists of single or multiple vesicular lesions on the distal parts of fingers. Wrestlers can develop herpes gladiatorum if they become infected with HSV-1. HSV infection can be a precipitating factor of other cutaneous manifestations, such as erythema multiforme. Recurrent erythema multiforme is often caused by symptomatic or asymptomatic HSV recurrences.

HSV encephalitis (HSE) occurs in children beyond the neonatal period, in adolescents, and in adults, and it can result from primary or recurrent HSV-1 infection. One fifth of HSE cases occur in the pediatric age-group. Symptoms and signs usually include fever, alterations in the state of consciousness, personality changes, seizures, and focal neurological findings. Encephalitis commonly has an acute onset with a fulminant course, leading to coma and death in untreated patients. HSE usually involves the temporal lobe, and magnetic resonance imaging is the most sensitive imaging modality to detect this. CSF pleocytosis with a predominance of lymphocytes is typical. Historically, erythrocytes in the CSF were considered suggestive of HSE, but with earlier diagnosis (before development of a hemorrhagic encephalitis), this finding is rare today.

HSV infection can also manifest as mild, self-limited aseptic meningitis, usually associated with genital HSV-2 infection. Unusual CNS manifestations of HSV include Bell palsy, atypical pain syndromes, trigeminal neuralgia, ascending myelitis, transverse myelitis, postinfectious encephalomyelitis, and recurrent (Mollaret) meningitis.

ETIOLOGY

HSVs are large, enveloped, double-stranded DNA viruses. They are members of the family *Herpesviridae* and, along with varicella-zoster virus (human herpesvirus 3), the subfamily *Alphaherpesviridae*. Two distinct HSV types exist: HSV-1 and HSV-2. Infections with HSV-1 traditionally involve the face and skin above the waist; however, an increasing number of genital herpes cases are attributable to HSV-1. Infections with HSV-2 usually involve the genitalia and skin below the waist in sexually active adolescents and adults. Both HSV-1 and HSV-2 cause herpetic disease in neonates. HSV-1 and HSV-2 establish latency following primary infection, with periodic reactivation to cause recurrent symptomatic disease or asymptomatic viral shedding. Genital HSV-2 infection is more likely to recur than is genital HSV-1 infection.

EPIDEMIOLOGY

HSV infections can be transmitted from people who are symptomatic or asymptomatic with primary or recurrent infections.

Neonatal

The incidence of neonatal HSV infection in the United States has increased over the past 2 decades to approximately 1 in 2,000 live births. HSV is transmitted to a neonate most often during birth through an infected maternal genital tract but can be caused by an ascending infection through ruptured or apparently intact amniotic membranes. Other less common sources of neonatal infection include postnatal transmission from a parent, a sibling, or other caregivers, most often from a nongenital infection (eg, mouth or hands), transmission from the mouth of a religious circumciser (mohel) to the infant penis during ritual Jewish circumcisions that include direct orogenital suction (metzitzah b'peh), and intrauterine infection causing congenital malformations.

The risk of transmission to a neonate born to a mother who acquires primary genital HSV infection near the time of delivery is estimated to be 25% to 60%. In contrast, the risk to a neonate born to a mother shedding HSV because of reactivation of infection acquired during the first half of pregnancy or earlier is less than 2%. More than three-quarters of infants who contract HSV infection are born to women with no history or clinical findings suggestive of genital HSV infection during or preceding pregnancy. Therefore, a lack of history of maternal genital HSV infection does not preclude a diagnosis of neonatal HSV disease.

Children Beyond the Neonatal Period and Adolescents

Patients with primary gingivostomatitis or genital herpes usually shed virus for at least 1 week and occasionally shed it for several weeks. Patients with symptomatic recurrences shed virus for a shorter period, typically 3 to 4 days. Intermittent asymptomatic reactivation of oral and genital herpes is common and likely occurs throughout the remainder of a person's life. The greatest concentration of virus is shed during symptomatic primary infections; the lowest, during asymptomatic reactivation.

Several single gene defects have been reported that predispose to HSE. These are mainly involved in the toll-like receptor 3 (*TLR3*) pathway, including deficiencies of *TLR3* itself or in downstream signal transduction pathways (ie, *UNC93B1, TRIF/ TICAM1, TRAF, TBK1*) or deficiencies in innate/ type 1 interferon (IFN) pathways (ie, IFN-α/ IFN-β, IFN-λ, *STAT1, IRF3*).

The **incubation period** for HSV infection occurring beyond the neonatal period ranges from 2 days to 2 weeks.

DIAGNOSTIC TESTS

HSV grows readily in traditional cell culture. Cytopathogenic effects typical of HSV infection are usually observed 1 to 3 days after inoculation. Methods of culture confirmation include fluorescent antibody staining, enzyme immunoassays (EIAs), and monolayer culture with typing. Cultures that remain negative by day 5 will likely remain negative.

Polymerase chain reaction (PCR) assay can usually detect HSV DNA in CSF from neonates with CNS infection (neonatal HSV CNS disease) and from older children and adults with HSE and is the diagnostic method of choice for CNS HSV involvement. PCR assay of CSF can yield negative results in HSE, especially early in the disease course. In difficult cases in which HSV CNS disease is expected but repeated CSF PCR assay results are negative, histological examination and viral culture of a brain tissue biopsy specimen is the most definitive method of confirming the diagnosis of HSE. Detection of intrathecal antibody against HSV can also assist in the diagnosis. Viral cultures of CSF from a patient with HSE are usually negative.

For diagnosis of neonatal HSV infection, all the following specimens should be obtained for each patient: (1) swab specimens from the conjunctivae, mouth, nasopharynx, and anus ("surface specimens") for HSV culture (if available) or PCR assay (can use a separate swab for each site, or a single swab starting with the conjunctivae); (2) specimens of skin vesicles for HSV culture (if available) or PCR assay; (3) CSF sample for HSV PCR assay; (4) whole blood sample for HSV PCR assay; and (5) whole blood sample for measuring alanine aminotransferase. Positive cultures obtained from any of the surface sites more than 12 to 24 hours after birth indicate viral replication and suggest infant infection, and risk of progression to neonatal HSV disease, rather than mere contamination after intrapartum exposure. As with any PCR assay, false-negative and false-positive results can occur. Any of the 3 manifestations of neonatal HSV disease (ie, disseminated, CNS, SEM) can have associated viremia, so a positive whole blood PCR assay result does not define an infant as having disseminated HSV and, therefore, should not be used to determine extent of disease and duration of treatment. Likewise, no data exist to support use of serial blood PCR assays to monitor response to therapy. Rapid diagnostic techniques are available, such as direct fluorescent antibody staining of vesicle scrapings or EIA detection of HSV antigens. These techniques are as specific but less sensitive than culture.

HSV PCR assay and cell culture are the preferred tests for detecting HSV in genital lesions. The sensitivity of viral culture is low, especially for recurrent lesions, and declines rapidly as lesions begin to heal. PCR assays for HSV DNA are more sensitive and are increasingly used in many settings. Failure to detect HSV in genital lesions by culture or PCR assay does not rule out HSV infection, because viral shedding is intermittent.

Type-specific antibodies to HSV develop during the first several weeks after infection and persist indefinitely. Approximately 20% of HSV-2 first episode patients seroconvert by 10 days, and the median time to seroconversion is 21 days with a type-specific enzyme-linked immunosorbent assay; more than 95% of people seroconvert by 12 weeks following infection. Although type-specific HSV-2 antibody usually indicates previous anogenital infection, the presence of HSV-1 antibody does not distinguish anogenital from orolabial infection reliably because a substantial proportion of initial genital infections and virtually all initial orolabial infections are caused by HSV-1. Serological testing is not useful in neonates.

TREATMENT

Neonatal

Parenteral acyclovir is the treatment of neonatal HSV infections. The dosage of acyclovir is 60 mg/kg per day in 3 divided doses (20 mg/kg/dose), administered intravenously for 14 days in SEM disease and for a minimum of 21 days in CNS disease or disseminated disease. All infants with CNS involvement should undergo a repeated lumbar puncture performed near the end of therapy to document that the CSF is negative for HSV DNA on PCR assay; in the unlikely event that the PCR result remains positive near the end of a 21-day treatment course, intravenous acyclovir should be administered for another week, with repeated CSF PCR assay performed near the end of the extended treatment period and another week of parenteral therapy if the result remains positive. Parenteral antiviral therapy should not be stopped until the CSF PCR result for HSV DNA is negative. Consultation with a pediatric infectious diseases specialist is warranted in these cases.

Infants surviving neonatal HSV disease of any classification (disseminated, CNS, or SEM) should receive oral acyclovir suppression at 300 mg/m^2/dose, administered 3 times daily for 6 months after the completion of parenteral therapy for acute disease; the dose should be adjusted monthly to account for growth. Absolute neutrophil counts should be assessed at 2 and 4 weeks after initiating suppressive acyclovir therapy and then monthly during the treatment period. Longer durations or higher doses of antiviral suppression do not further improve neurodevelopmental outcomes. Valacyclovir has not been studied for longer than 5 days in young infants, so it should not be used routinely for antiviral suppression in this age-group.

All infants with neonatal HSV disease, regardless of disease classification, should undergo an ophthalmologic examination and neuroimaging to establish baseline brain anatomy. Magnetic resonance imaging is the most sensitive imaging modality; acceptable alternatives are computed tomography or ultrasonography of the head. Topical ophthalmic drug (1% trifluridine or 0.15% ganciclovir), in addition to parenteral antiviral therapy, may be indicated in infants with ocular involvement attributable to HSV infection, and an ophthalmologist should be involved in the management and treatment of acute neonatal ocular HSV disease.

Genital Infection

Primary

Oral acyclovir therapy shortens the duration of illness and viral shedding. Valacyclovir and famciclovir are not more effective than acyclovir but offer the advantage of less frequent dosing. Intravenous acyclovir is indicated for patients with a severe or complicated primary infection that requires hospitalization. Treatment of primary herpetic lesions does not affect the subsequent frequency or severity of recurrences.

Recurrent

Antiviral therapy for recurrent genital herpes can be administered either episodically to ameliorate or shorten the duration of lesions or continuously as suppressive therapy to decrease the frequency of recurrences. Many patients benefit from antiviral therapy, and treatment options should be discussed with patients with recurrent disease. Acyclovir, valacyclovir, and famciclovir have been approved for suppression of genital herpes in immunocompetent adults. Acyclovir and valacyclovir are most commonly used in pregnant women with first-episode genital herpes or severe recurrent herpes, and acyclovir should be administered intravenously to pregnant women with severe HSV infection.

Mucocutaneous

Immunocompromised Hosts

Intravenous acyclovir is effective for treatment of mucocutaneous HSV infections. Acyclovir-resistant strains of HSV have been isolated from immunocompromised people receiving prolonged treatment with acyclovir. Foscarnet is the drug of choice for acyclovir-resistant HSV isolates.

Immunocompetent Hosts

Limited data are available on effects of acyclovir on the course of primary or recurrent nongenital mucocutaneous HSV infections in immunocompetent hosts. Therapeutic benefit has been noted in a limited number of children with primary gingivostomatitis treated with oral acyclovir. A small therapeutic benefit of oral acyclovir therapy has been demonstrated among adults with recurrent herpes labialis. Famciclovir or valacyclovir can also be considered.

Other HSV Infections

Central Nervous System

Patients with HSE should be treated for 21 days with intravenous acyclovir. Use of concomitant corticosteroids is not routinely recommended.

Ocular

Treatment of eye lesions should be undertaken in consultation with an ophthalmologist. Several topical drugs, such as 1% trifluridine and 0.15% ganciclovir, have proven efficacy for superficial keratitis. Topical corticosteroids administered without concomitant antiviral therapy are contraindicated in suspected HSV conjunctivitis; however, ophthalmologists may choose to use corticosteroids in conjunction with antiviral drugs to treat locally invasive infections. For children with recurrent ocular lesions, oral suppressive therapy with acyclovir may be of benefit and may be indicated for months or even years.

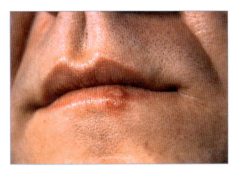

Image 66.1
This is a close-up of a herpes simplex lesion on the lower lip on the second day after onset. Also known as a "cold sore," this lesion is caused by the contagious herpes simplex virus type 1 and should not be confused with a canker sore, which is not contagious. Courtesy of Centers for Disease Control and Prevention.

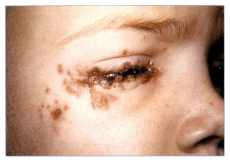

Image 66.2
This 7-year-old with a history of recurrent herpes labialis presented with periocular herpes simplex. Courtesy of Centers for Disease Control and Prevention.

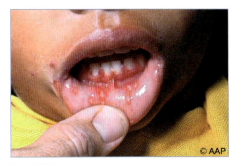

Image 66.3
Herpes simplex stomatitis, primary infection of the anterior oral mucous membranes. Tongue lesions are also common with primary herpes simplex.

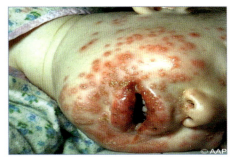

Image 66.4
Herpes simplex stomatitis, primary infection with extension to the face.

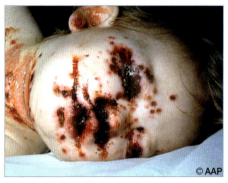

Image 66.5
Herpes simplex in a child with eczema with Kaposi varicelliform eruption and Stevens-Johnson syndrome.

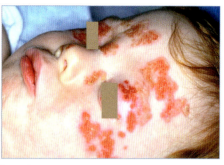

Image 66.6
Eczema herpeticum on the face of a boy with eczema and primary herpetic gingivostomatitis, day 3–4 of the onset. The herpetic lesions spread over 2–3 days to extensive covering of the skin, and systemic therapy with acyclovir was provided. The patient recovered after a prolonged hospital stay for secondary nosocomial bacterial infections. Copyright Jerri Ann Jenista, MD.

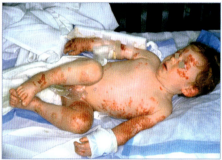

Image 66.7
Patient in Image 66.6, with generalized eczema and primary herpetic gingivostomatitis with extensive eczema herpeticum. Copyright Jerri Ann Jenista, MD.

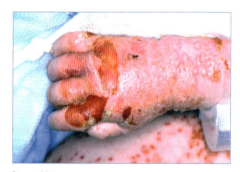

Image 66.8
Hand of the patient in images 66.6 and 66.7, with eczema and primary herpetic gingivostomatitis that spread over 2–3 days to extensively cover the skin. Copyright Jerri Ann Jenista, MD.

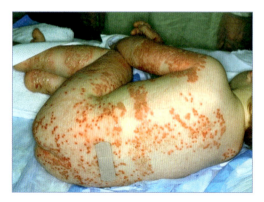

Image 66.9
The patient shown in images 66.6, 66.7, and 66.8, with extensive eczema herpeticum and primary herpetic gingivostomatitis. Copyright Jerri Ann Jenista, MD.

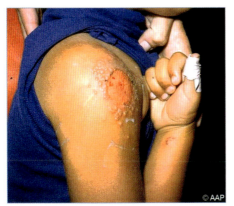

Image 66.10
Herpes simplex virus infection at a diphtheria, tetanus, and pertussis vaccine injection site reflecting self-inoculation. Courtesy of Edgar O. Ledbetter, MD, FAAP.

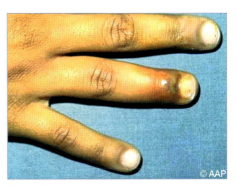

Image 66.11
Herpetic whitlow in a 10-year-old boy with recurrent herpes simplex infection.

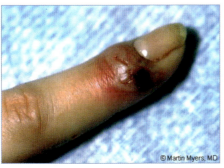

Image 66.12
An adolescent girl with herpetic whitlow secondary to orolabial lesions with self-inoculation. Copyright Martin G. Myers, MD.

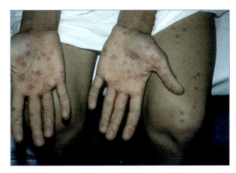

Image 66.13
Disseminated herpes simplex infection in a 17-year-old boy with Hodgkin disease. Courtesy of George Nankervis, MD.

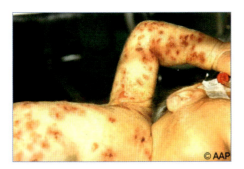

Image 66.14
Neonatal herpes simplex infection with disseminated vesicular lesions.

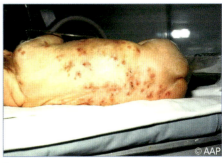

Image 66.15
Neonatal herpes simplex infection. This is the same patient as in Image 66.14.

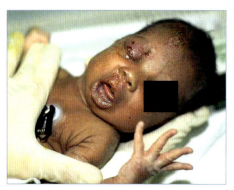

Image 66.16
Neonatal herpes skin lesions of the face. A preterm 14-day-old developed vesicular lesions over the right eye and face on days 11–14 after birth. Herpes simplex virus type 2 was recovered from viral culture of the vesicular fluid. Keratoconjunctivitis was diagnosed by ophthalmologic examination, and the neonate was treated with topical antiviral eye drops in addition to intravenous acyclovir. The neonate was born via a spontaneous vaginal delivery with a vertex presentation. Membranes had ruptured 8 hours before delivery. There was no history of genital herpes or fever blisters in either parent. The lesions were concentrated on the face and head, the presenting body parts in delivery. Copyright Barbara Jantausch, MD, FAAP.

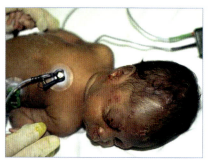

Image 66.17
Neonatal herpes skin lesions of the head and face. This is the same patient as shown in Image 66.16. Copyright Barbara Jantausch, MD, FAAP.

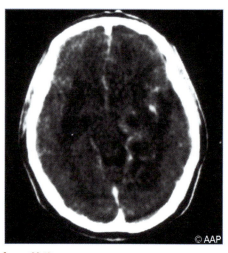

Image 66.18
Computed tomographic scan of a patient with herpes simplex encephalitis with temporal lobe changes.

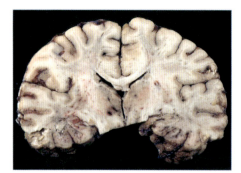

Image 66.19
Postneonatal herpes simplex encephalitis. Hemorrhagic necrosis of the temporal lobes. Courtesy of Dimitris P. Agamanolis, MD.

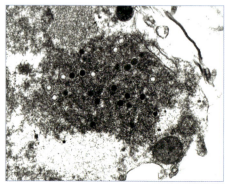

Image 66.20
Herpes simplex encephalitis. Viral particles in an intranuclear inclusion. Courtesy of Dimitris P. Agamanolis, MD.

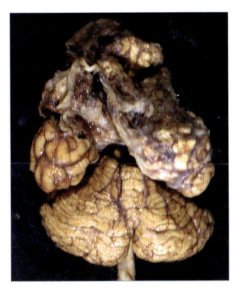

Image 66.21
Burned-out neonatal herpes simplex encephalitis. Severe atrophy and distortion of the cerebral hemispheres. Courtesy of Dimitris P. Agamanolis, MD.

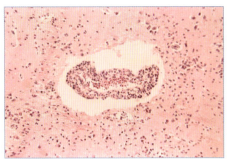

Image 66.22
Histopathologic changes observable in brain tissue, caused by herpes simplex encephalitis (hematoxylin-eosin stain, magnification ×125). Herpes simplex encephalitis is characterized by headaches, fever, and altered mental state caused by inflammation of the brain. Herpes simplex virus, the cause of herpes simplex encephalitis, is one of the main causes of non-epidemic, sporadic encephalitis. Courtesy of Centers for Disease Control and Prevention.

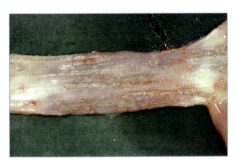

Image 66.23
Herpes simplex esophagitis. Courtesy of Dimitris P. Agamanolis, MD.

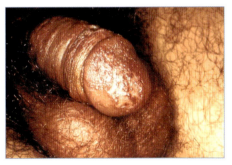

Image 66.24
This male presented with primary vesiculopapular herpes genitalis lesions on his glans penis and penile shaft. When signs of herpes genitalis occur, they typically appear as ≥1 blisters on or around the genitals or rectum. The blisters break, leaving tender ulcers (sores) that may take 2–4 weeks to heal the first time they occur. Courtesy of Centers for Disease Control and Prevention.

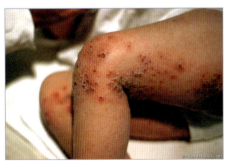

Image 66.25
Herpes simplex infection in a 4-year-old boy with eczema (Kaposi varicelliform eruption). Courtesy of Ed Fajardo, MD.

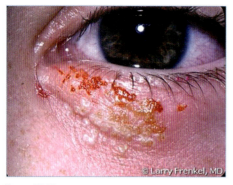

Image 66.26
A 15-year-old girl with recurrent facial and ocular herpes simplex infection. Courtesy of Larry Frenkel, MD.

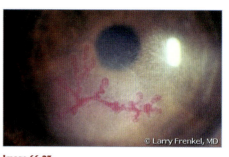

Image 66.27
A 15-year-old girl with recurrent facial and ocular herpes simplex infection. This is the same patient as in Image 66.26. Courtesy of Larry Frenkel, MD.

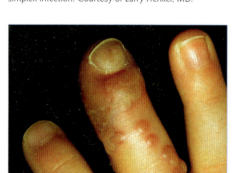

Image 66.28
A 2-year-old boy with herpes simplex infection of the index finger. Courtesy of Larry Frenkel, MD.

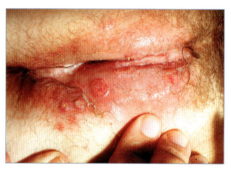

Image 66.29
A 15-year-old girl with primary herpes simplex infection of the genital area. Courtesy of Larry Frenkel, MD.

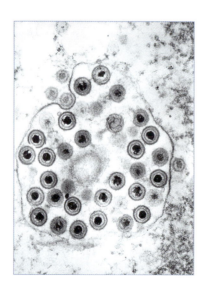

Image 66.30
This negatively stained transmission electron micrograph reveals the presence of numerous herpesvirus virions, members of the *Herpesviridae* virus family. Courtesy of Centers for Disease Control and Prevention.

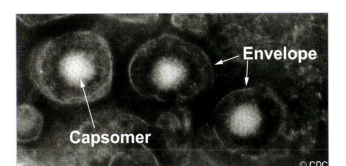

Image 66.31
Electron micrograph image of herpesvirus (negative stain). A viral envelope surrounds the nucleocapsid, which measures approximately 100 nm and is composed of an icosahedron formed by hollow capsomers. Courtesy of Centers for Disease Control and Prevention.

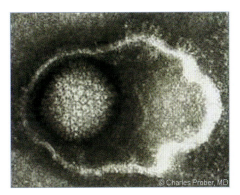

Image 66.32
Herpesvirus, electron micrograph. Copyright Charles Prober, MD.

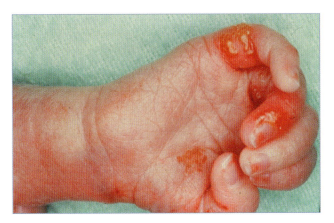

Image 66.33
A full-term 3-week-old who presented with fever and poor feeding. A blood culture grew group B *Streptococcus*. On day 2 of antibiotic therapy, these vesicular lesions on the hand were noted and lesion fluid grew herpes simplex virus type 2. Courtesy of Carol J. Baker, MD.

CHAPTER 67
Histoplasmosis

CLINICAL MANIFESTATIONS

Histoplasma capsulatum causes symptoms in less than 5% of infected people. Clinical manifestations are classified according to site (pulmonary or disseminated), duration (acute, subacute, or chronic), and pattern (primary or reactivated) of infection. Most symptomatic patients have acute pulmonary histoplasmosis, a brief, self-limited illness characterized by fever, chills, nonproductive cough, and malaise. Radiographic findings may consist of hilar or mediastinal adenopathy, or diffuse interstitial or reticulonodular pulmonary infiltrates. Most patients recover without treatment 2 to 3 weeks after onset of symptoms.

Exposure to a large inoculum of conidia can cause severe pulmonary infection associated with high fevers, hypoxemia, diffuse reticulonodular infiltrates, and acute respiratory distress syndrome. Mediastinal involvement, a rare complication of pulmonary histoplasmosis, includes mediastinal lymphadenitis, which can cause airway encroachment in young children. Inflammatory syndromes (pericarditis and rheumatologic syndromes) can develop; erythema nodosum can occur in adolescents and adults. Primary cutaneous infections after trauma are rare, and chronic cavitary pulmonary histoplasmosis is extremely rare in children.

Progressive disseminated histoplasmosis (PDH) may occur in otherwise healthy infants and children younger than 2 years or in older children with primary or acquired cellular immune dysfunction. It can be a rapidly progressive illness following acute infection or can be a more chronic, slowly progressive disease. Early manifestations of PDH in children include prolonged fever, failure to thrive, and hepatosplenomegaly; if untreated, malnutrition, diffuse adenopathy, pneumonitis, mucosal ulceration, pancytopenia, disseminated intravascular coagulopathy, and gastrointestinal tract bleeding can ensue. PDH in adults occurs most often in people with underlying immunodeficiency (eg, HIV/AIDS, solid organ transplant, hematologic malignancy, and biologic response modifiers including tumor necrosis factor antagonists). Central nervous system (CNS) involvement occurs in 5% to 25% of patients with chronic progressive disease. Chronic PDH generally occurs in adults with immunosuppression and is characterized by prolonged fever, night sweats, weight loss, and fatigue; signs include hepatosplenomegaly, mucosal ulcerations, adrenal insufficiency, and pancytopenia. Clinicians should be alert to the risk of disseminated endemic mycoses in patients receiving tumor necrosis factor–α antagonists and disease-modifying antirheumatic drugs.

ETIOLOGY

Histoplasma strains, which may be classified into at least 7 distinct clades, are thermally dimorphic, endemic fungi that grow in the environment as a spore-bearing mold but convert to the yeast phase at 37 °C (99 °F).

EPIDEMIOLOGY

H capsulatum is encountered in most parts of the world (including Africa, the Americas, Asia, and Europe) and is highly endemic in the central and eastern United States, particularly the Mississippi, Ohio, and Missouri River valleys; Central America; the northernmost part of South America; and Argentina. *H capsulatum* subspecies *duboisii* is found only in central and western Africa.

Infection is acquired following inhalation of conidia that are aerosolized by disturbance of soil, especially when contaminated with bat guano or bird droppings. Infections occur sporadically or rarely in point-source epidemics after exposure to activities that disturb contaminated sites. In regions with endemic disease, recreational activities, such as playing in hollow trees and caving, and occupational activities, such as construction, excavation, demolition, farming, and cleaning of contaminated buildings, have been associated with outbreaks. Person-to-person transmission may occur via transplant of infected organs, through vertical transmission, or through exposure to cutaneous lesions. Prior infection confers partial immunity; reinfection can occur but may require a larger inoculum.

The **incubation period** is variable but is usually 1 to 3 weeks.

DIAGNOSTIC TESTS

Detection of *H capsulatum* polysaccharide antigen in serum, urine, bronchoalveolar lavage (BAL) fluid, or cerebrospinal fluid by using a quantitative enzyme immunoassay is the preferred method of testing. Antigen detection is most sensitive for progressive disseminated infections. Combining both urine and serum antigen testing increases the likelihood of antigen detection. Results are often transiently positive early in the course of acute, self-limited pulmonary infections. A negative test result does not exclude infection. If the result is initially positive, the antigen test is also useful for monitoring treatment response and, thereafter, identifying relapse or reinfection. Cross-reactions may occur in patients with dimorphic fungal diseases (eg, blastomycosis, coccidioidomycosis, paracoccidioidomycosis, sporotrichosis, *Emergomyces africanus* disease, and talaromycosis [formerly penicilliosis]); clinical and epidemiological distinctions aid in differentiating these entities.

Antibody detection testing is available and is most useful in patients with subacute or chronic pulmonary disease and CNS involvement. Complement fixation and immunodiffusion are available. A 4-fold increase in mycelial-phase complement fixation titers or a single titer of 1:32 or greater in either test is strong presumptive evidence of active or recent infection in patients exposed to or residing within endemic regions. Cross-reacting antibodies can result most commonly from *Blastomyces* and *Coccidioides* species. The immunodiffusion test is a qualitative method that is more specific, but slightly less sensitive, than the complement fixation test. It detects the H and M glycoproteins of *H capsulatum* found in histoplasmin. The M band develops with acute infection, generally by 6 weeks after infection; is often present in chronic forms of histoplasmosis; and persists for months to years after the infection has resolved. The H band is much less common; is rarely, if ever, found without an M band; and is indicative of chronic or severe acute forms of histoplasmosis. The immunodiffusion assay is approximately 80% sensitive but is more specific than the complement fixation assay. It is commonly used in conjunction with the complement fixation test.

Culture is the definitive method of diagnosis. *H capsulatum* organisms from bone marrow, blood, sputum, and tissue specimens grow in the mycelia (mold) phase on standard mycological media, including Sabouraud dextrose or potato dextrose agar incubated at 25 to 30 °C (77–86 °F) in 1 to 6 weeks. The yeast phase of the organism can be recovered on primary culture by using enriched media, such as brain-heart infusion agar with blood (BHIB) incubated at 35 to 37 °C (95–99 °F). Mycelial-phase organisms in culture can be confirmed as *H capsulatum* by conversion to yeast-phase organisms by repeated passage on BHIB at 35 to 37 °C (95–99 °F). The lysis-centrifugation method is preferred for blood and bone marrow cultures. A DNA probe for *H capsulatum* permits rapid identification of cultured isolates. Care should be taken in working with the organism in the laboratory, because mold-phase growth may release large numbers of infectious microconidia into the air.

Demonstration of typical intracellular yeast forms by examination with Wright or Giemsa stains of blood, bone marrow, or BAL specimens strongly supports the diagnosis of histoplasmosis when clinical, epidemiological, and other laboratory studies are compatible.

TREATMENT

Immunocompetent children with uncomplicated or mild to moderate acute pulmonary histoplasmosis may not require antifungal therapy, because infection is usually self-limited. If the patient does not improve within 4 weeks, itraconazole should be given for 6 to 12 weeks.

Treatment is imperative for all forms of disseminated histoplasmosis, which can be either acute (rapid onset and progression, usually in an immunocompromised patient) or chronic (slower evolution, usually in an immunocompetent patient) illness. Treatment with a lipid formulation of amphotericin B is recommended for severe acute pulmonary infection. Methylprednisolone during the first 1 to 2 weeks of therapy may be considered if severe respiratory complications develop but should be used only in conjunction with antifungals.

After clinical improvement occurs in 1 to 2 weeks, itraconazole is recommended for an additional 12 weeks. Itraconazole is preferred over other mold-active azoles by most experts; when used in adults, itraconazole is more effective, has fewer adverse effects, and is less likely to induce resistance than is fluconazole. Serum trough concentrations of itraconazole should be 1 to 2 μg/mL.

Concentrations should be checked after several days of therapy to ensure adequate drug exposure. When measured by high-pressure liquid chromatography, both itraconazole and its bioactive hydroxy-itraconazole metabolite are reported, the sum of which should be considered in assessing drug levels.

All patients with chronic pulmonary histoplasmosis (eg, progressive cavitation of the lungs) should be treated. Mild to moderate cases should be treated with itraconazole for 1 to 2 years. Severe cases should be treated initially with a lipid formulation amphotericin B followed by itraconazole for the same duration.

Mediastinal and inflammatory manifestations of infection do not generally need to be treated with antifungal agents. Mediastinal adenitis that causes obstruction of a bronchus, the esophagus, or another mediastinal structure may improve with a brief course of corticosteroids. In these instances, itraconazole should be used concurrently and continued for 6 to 12 weeks thereafter. Dense fibrosis of mediastinal structures without an associated granulomatous inflammatory component does not respond to antifungal therapy, and surgical intervention may be necessary for severe cases. Pericarditis and rheumatologic syndromes may respond to treatment with nonsteroidal anti-inflammatory agents (indomethacin).

For treatment of moderately severe to severe PDH in an infant or a child, a lipid formulation of amphotericin B is the drug of choice and is usually given for a minimum of 2 weeks. When the child has demonstrated substantial clinical improvement and a decline in the serum concentration of *Histoplasma* antigen, oral itraconazole is administered for a total of at least 12 months. Lifelong suppressive therapy with itraconazole may be required for patients with primary immunodeficiency syndromes, acquired immunodeficiency that cannot be reversed, or relapse despite appropriate therapy. For those with mild to moderate PDH, itraconazole for at least 12 months is recommended. After completion of treatment of PDH, urine antigen concentrations should be monitored for 12 months. Stable, low, and decreasing concentrations that are unaccompanied by signs of active infection may not necessarily require prolongation or resumption of treatment.

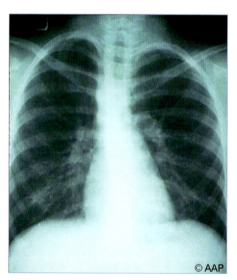

Image 67.1
Acute, primary histoplasmosis in a 13-year-old girl. Progressive disseminated histoplasmosis is unusual in otherwise healthy children.

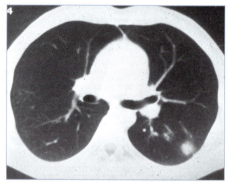

Image 67.2
Computed tomographic scan showing a single pulmonary nodule of histoplasmosis. Courtesy of Centers for Disease Control and Prevention.

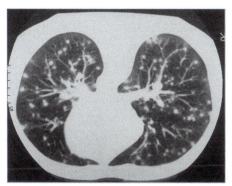

Image 67.3
Computed tomographic scan of lungs showing classic snowstorm appearance of acute histoplasmosis. Courtesy of Centers for Disease Control and Prevention.

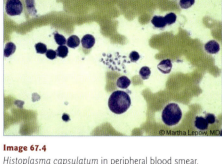

Image 67.4
Histoplasma capsulatum in peripheral blood smear. Copyright Martha Lepow, MD.

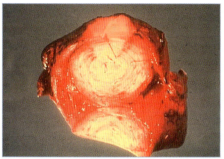

Image 67.5
Gross pathological specimen of lung showing cut surface of fibrocaseous nodule caused by *Histoplasma capsulatum*. Courtesy of Centers for Disease Control and Prevention.

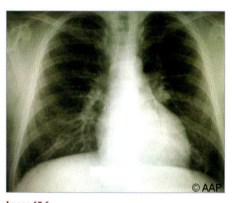

Image 67.6
A preadolescent with left bilateral calcified hilar lymph nodes secondary to histoplasmosis.

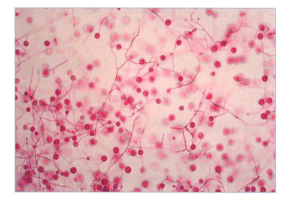

Image 67.7
This photomicrograph shows the smooth macroconidia of the Jamaican isolate of *Histoplasma capsulatum*. *H capsulatum* is a dimorphic fungus (ie, it morphologically grows in 2 different forms). It takes a mycelial form when grown at a lower temperature (ie, 25 °C [77 °F]), creating macroconidia, and a yeast form when grown at 35 °C (95 °F), on enriched media. Courtesy of Centers for Disease Control and Prevention.

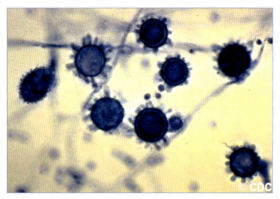

Image 67.8
Asexual spores (conidia). Tuberculate macroconidia of *Histoplasma capsulatum* (toluidine blue stain). Microconidia are also present. Courtesy of Centers for Disease Control and Prevention.

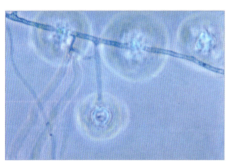

Image 67.9
This photomicrograph reveals a conidiophore of the fungus *Histoplasma capsulatum*. *H capsulatum* grows in soil and material contaminated with bat or bird droppings. Spores become airborne when contaminated soil is disturbed. Breathing the spores causes pulmonary histoplasmosis. Courtesy of Centers for Disease Control and Prevention.

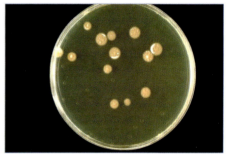

Image 67.10
Pictured is a Sabhi agar plate culture of the fungus *Histoplasma capsulatum* grown at 20 °C (68 °F). Positive results from a histoplasmin skin test occur in as many as 80% of the people living in areas where *H capsulatum* is common, such as the eastern and central United States. Courtesy of Centers for Disease Control and Prevention.

CHAPTER 68
Hookworm Infections
(*Ancylostoma duodenale* and *Necator americanus*)

CLINICAL MANIFESTATIONS

Patients with hookworm infection are often asymptomatic. The most common clinical manifestation is iron deficiency resulting from direct blood loss at the site where adult worms attach to the mucosa of the small intestine. Chronic hookworm infection is a common cause of moderate and severe hypochromic, microcytic anemia in people living in resource-limited tropical countries, and heavy infection can cause hypoproteinemia with edema. Chronic hookworm infection in children may lead to physical growth delay, deficits in cognition, and developmental delay. Transmission occurs when larvae in contaminated soil penetrate the skin, frequently through the feet. A stinging or burning sensation may occur, followed by pruritus and a papulovesicular rash ("ground itch"), persisting for 1 to 2 weeks. Pneumonitis associated with migrating larvae (Löffler-like syndrome) is uncommon and usually mild, except in heavy infections. Colicky abdominal pain, nausea, diarrhea, and marked eosinophilia may develop 4 to 6 weeks after exposure. Blood loss secondary to hookworm infection develops 10 to 12 weeks after initial infection, and symptoms related to serious iron-deficiency anemia can develop in long-standing moderate or heavy hookworm infections. Pharyngeal itching, hoarseness, nausea, and vomiting may also develop after ingestion of infectious *Ancylostoma duodenale* larvae.

ETIOLOGY

Necator americanus is the major cause of hookworm infection worldwide, although *A duodenale* is also an important hookworm in some regions. *Ancylostoma ceylanicum*, a zoonotic (eg, dogs and cats) hookworm, is increasingly being identified as a major cause of hookworm infections in humans, particularly in Asia. Mixed infections can occur. Each of these roundworms (nematodes) has a similar life cycle, except for *A ceylanicum*. Other animal hookworm species (ie, *Ancylostoma braziliense*, *Ancylostoma caninum*, *Uncinaria stenocephala*) cause cutaneous larva migrans when filariform larvae penetrate the skin and migrate in the upper dermis, causing an intensely pruritic track, although they do not usually develop further or cause systemic infection (an exception is *A caninum*, which may rarely migrate to the intestine and cause eosinophilic enteritis).

EPIDEMIOLOGY

Hookworm is the second most common human helminthic infection following ascariasis. It has worldwide distribution but is most prominent in rural, tropical, and subtropical areas where soil is conducive to organism development and where contamination with human feces is common. *N americanus* is predominant in the Western hemisphere, sub-Saharan Africa, Southeast Asia, and a number of Pacific Islands. *A duodenale* is the predominant species in the Mediterranean region, northern Asia, and selected foci of South America. *A ceylanicum* is found in Asia, Australia, some Pacific Islands, South Africa, and Madagascar. Larvae and eggs survive in loose, sandy, moist, shady, well-aerated, warm soil (optimal temperature 23–33 °C [73–91 °F]). Hookworm eggs from stool hatch in soil in 1 to 2 days as rhabditiform larvae. These larvae develop into infective filariform larvae in soil within 5 to 7 days and can survive for 3 to 4 weeks. Percutaneous infection occurs after exposure to infectious larvae. *A duodenale* transmission can occur by ingestion and, possibly, through human milk. Untreated infected patients can harbor worms for 5 years or longer.

The **incubation period** from exposure to development of noncutaneous symptoms is 4 to 12 weeks. Eggs appear in feces approximately 5 to 8 weeks from the time of infection.

DIAGNOSTIC TESTS

Microscopic demonstration of hookworm eggs in feces is diagnostic. A direct stool smear with saline solution or potassium iodide saturated with iodine is adequate for diagnosis of heavy hookworm infection; light infections require concentration techniques. Quantification techniques (eg, Kato-Katz, Beaver direct smear, or Stoll egg-counting techniques) to determine the clinical significance of infection and the response to treatment may be available from state or reference laboratories. Stool microscopy is not very sensitive, and multiple samples may be needed to detect infection; some experts recommend examining at least 3 consecutive samples by using concentration techniques when index of suspicion of infection is high. Cutaneous larva migrans attributable to transient cutaneous infection with dog or cat hookworms is diagnosed clinically.

TREATMENT

Albendazole and mebendazole are recommended in the treatment of hookworm infection, and pyrantel pamoate is an effective alternative. Albendazole should be taken with food; a fatty meal increases oral bioavailability. Pyrantel pamoate suspension can be mixed with milk or fruit juice. Studies in children as young as 1 year of age suggest that albendazole can be administered safely to this population. Re-treatment is indicated for persistent or recurrent infection. Nutritional supplementation, including iron, is important when addressing associated iron-deficiency anemia. Severely affected children may require blood transfusion.

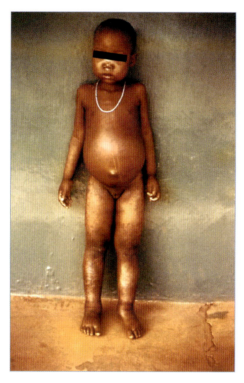

Image 68.1
This child with hookworm shows visible signs of edema and was diagnosed with anemia as well. Courtesy of Centers for Disease Control and Prevention.

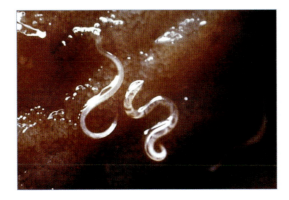

Image 68.2
This enlargement shows hookworms, *Ancylostoma caninum*, attached to the intestinal mucosa. Barely visible larvae penetrate the skin (often through bare feet), are carried to the lungs, go through the respiratory tract to the mouth, are swallowed, and eventually reach the small intestine. This journey takes about 1 week. Courtesy of Centers for Disease Control and Prevention.

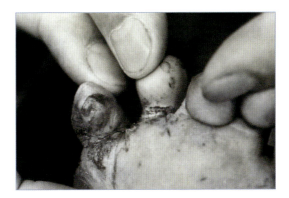

Image 68.3
This patient presented with a hookworm infection involving the toes of the right foot, which is also known as "ground itch." Usually the first sign of infection is itching and a rash at the site where skin touched contaminated soil or sand, which occurs when the larvae penetrate the skin, followed by anemia, abdominal pain, diarrhea, loss of appetite, and weight loss. Courtesy of Centers for Disease Control and Prevention.

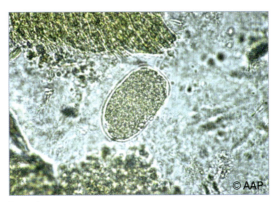

Image 68.4
Hookworm (*Necator americanus*) ova in stool preparation.

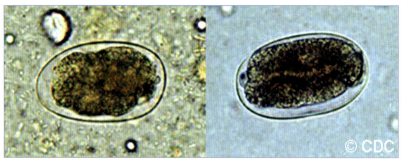

Image 68.5
Hookworm eggs examined on wet mount (eggs of *Ancylostoma duodenale* and *Necator americanus* cannot be morphologically distinguished). Diagnostic characteristics: 57–76 μm × 35–47 μm, oval or ellipsoidal, thin shell. The embryo (right) has begun cellular division and is at an early developmental stage (gastrula). Courtesy of Centers for Disease Control and Prevention.

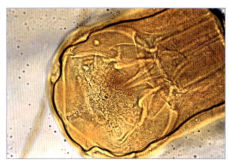

Image 68.6
This micrograph reveals the head of the hookworm *Necator americanus* and its mouth's cutting plates (magnification ×400). The hookworm uses these sharp cutting teeth to grasp firmly to the intestinal wall and, while remaining fastened in place, ingests the host's blood, obtaining its nutrients in this fashion. Courtesy of Centers for Disease Control and Prevention.

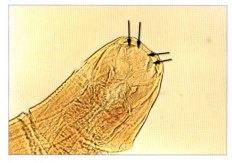

Image 68.7
This unstained micrograph reveals the *Ancylostoma duodenale* hookworm's mouth parts (magnification ×125). Courtesy of Centers for Disease Control and Prevention.

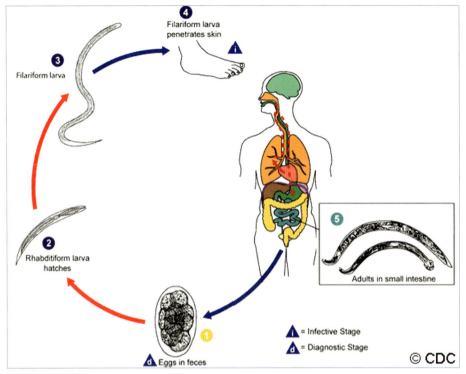

Image 68.8
Eggs are passed in the stool (1), and under favorable conditions (ie, moisture, warmth, shade), larvae hatch in 1-2 days. The released rhabditiform larvae grow in the feces and/or the soil (2), and after 5-10 days (and 2 molts), they become filariform (third-stage) larvae that are infective (3). These infective larvae can survive 3-4 weeks in favorable environmental conditions. On contact with the human host, the larvae penetrate the skin and are carried through the veins to the heart and then to the lungs. They penetrate into the pulmonary alveoli, ascend the bronchial tree to the pharynx, and are swallowed (4). The larvae reach the small intestine, where they reside and mature into adults. Adult worms live in the lumen of the small intestine, where they attach to the intestinal wall with resultant blood loss by the host (5). Most adult worms are eliminated in 1-2 years, but longevity records can reach several years. Some *Ancylostoma duodenale* larvae, following penetration of the host skin, can become dormant (in the intestine or muscle). In addition, infection by *A duodenale* may also occur by the oral and transmammary route. *Necator americanus*, however, requires a transpulmonary migration phase. Courtesy of Centers for Disease Control and Prevention.

CHAPTER 69

Human Herpesviruses 6 (Including Roseola) and 7

CLINICAL MANIFESTATIONS

Human herpesviruses 6 and 7 comprise 3 distinct viral species, *Human herpesvirus 6B*, *Human herpesvirus 6A*, and *Human herpesvirus 7*. Although many infections are asymptomatic, clinical manifestations of primary infection with human herpesvirus 6B (HHV-6B) include roseola (exanthem subitum) in approximately 20% of infected children as well as a nonspecific febrile illness without rash or localizing signs. Acute HHV-6B infection may be accompanied by cervical and characteristic postoccipital lymphadenopathy, gastrointestinal tract or respiratory tract signs, and inflamed tympanic membranes. Fever may be high (temperature >39.5 °C [103.0 °F]) and persist for 3 to 7 days. Approximately 20% of all emergency department visits for febrile children 6 through 12 months of age are attributable to HHV-6B. Roseola is distinguished by an erythematous maculopapular rash that typically appears once fever resolves and can last hours to days. Febrile seizures, sometimes leading to status epilepticus, are the most common complication and reason for hospitalization of children with primary HHV-6B infection. Approximately 10% to 15% of children with primary HHV-6B infection develop febrile seizures, predominantly between the ages of 6 and 18 months. Other reported neurological manifestations include a bulging fontanelle and encephalopathy or encephalitis, the latter more commonly noted in infants in Japan than in the United States or Europe. Hepatitis has been reported as a rare manifestation of primary HHV-6B infection. Congenital infection with HHV-6B and human herpesvirus 6A (HHV-6A), which occurs in approximately 1% of newborns, has not been linked to any clinical disease. In contrast to HHV-6B, primary infection with HHV-6A has not been associated with any recognized disease.

The clinical manifestations occurring with human herpesvirus 7 (HHV-7) infection are less clear than with HHV-6B. Most primary infections with HHV-7 are presumably asymptomatic or mild and not distinctive. Some initial infections can manifest as typical roseola and may account for second or recurrent cases of roseola. Febrile illnesses associated with seizures have also been documented to occur during primary HHV-7 infection.

Following infection, HHV-6B, HHV-6A, and HHV-7 remain in a latent state and may reactivate. The clinical circumstances and manifestations of reactivation in healthy people are unclear. Illness associated with HHV-6B reactivation has been described primarily in recipients of solid organ and hematopoietic stem cell transplants. Clinical findings associated with HHV-6B reactivation in solid organ and hematopoietic stem cell transplants include fever, rash, hepatitis, bone marrow suppression, acute graft-versus-host disease, graft rejection, pneumonia, delirium, and encephalitis. The best characterized of these is posttransplant acute limbic encephalitis, a specific syndrome associated with HHV-6B reactivation in the central nervous system (CNS) characterized by anterograde amnesia, seizures, insomnia, confusion, and the syndrome of inappropriate antidiuretic hormone secretion. Patients undergoing cord blood transplant have an increased risk for developing posttransplant acute limbic encephalitis, with significant morbidity and mortality attributed to this complication. A few cases of CNS symptoms have been reported in association with HHV-7 reactivation in immunocompromised hosts, but clinical findings have generally been reported much less frequently with HHV-7 than with HHV-6B reactivation.

ETIOLOGY

HHV-6B, HHV-6A, and HHV-7 are lymphotropic viruses that are closely related members of the *Herpesviridae* family, subfamily *Betaherpesvirinae*. As betaherpesviruses, HHV-6B, HHV-6A, and HHV-7 are most closely related to cytomegalovirus. As with all human herpesviruses, they establish lifelong latency after initial acquisition. In 2012, *Human herpesvirus 6A* and *Human herpesvirus 6B* were recognized as distinct species rather than as variants of the same species. This recognition increased the number of known human herpesviruses to 9.

EPIDEMIOLOGY

HHV-6B and HHV-7 cause ubiquitous infections in children worldwide. Humans are the only known natural host. Nearly all children acquire

HHV-6B infection within the first 2 years after birth, probably resulting from asymptomatic shedding of infectious virus in upper respiratory tract secretions of a healthy family member or other close contact. Virus-specific maternal antibody, which is present uniformly in the sera of infants at birth, provides transient partial protection. As maternal antibody concentration decreases during the first year after birth, the infection rate increases rapidly, peaking between 6 and 24 months of age. During the acute phase of primary infection, HHV-6B and HHV-7 can be isolated from peripheral blood mononuclear cells; HHV-7, from saliva of some children. Viral DNA may subsequently be detected throughout life by polymerase chain reaction (PCR) assay in multiple body sites, including blood mononuclear cells, salivary glands, lung, skin, and the CNS. Infections occur throughout the year without a seasonal pattern. Occasional outbreaks of roseola have been reported.

Several genetic mutations have been associated with severe CNS disease during primary HHV-6B infection. These include *RANBP2*, *POLG*, and carnitine palmitoyl-transferase 2 gene mutations.

Congenital infection occurs in approximately 1% of newborns, as determined by the presence of HHV-6A or HHV-6B DNA in cord blood. Most congenital infections appear to result from the germline passage of maternal or paternal chromosomally integrated HHV-6 (ciHHV-6), a unique mechanism of transmission of human viral congenital infection. Transplacental HHV-6 infection may also occur from reinfection or reactivation of maternal HHV-6 infection or possibly from reactivated maternal ciHHV-6. HHV-6 has not been identified in human milk. Congenital infection is typically asymptomatic, and the clinical implications of ciHHV-6 are not fully known. However, reactivation of ciHHV-6 in severely immunocompromised hosts is possible and can be associated with disease.

HHV-7 infection usually occurs later in childhood than HHV-6B infection. By adulthood, the seroprevalence of HHV-7 is approximately 85%. Infectious HHV-7 is present in more than 75% of saliva specimens obtained from healthy adults. Acquisition of virus via infected respiratory tract secretions of healthy contacts is the probable mode of transmission of HHV-7 to young children.

HHV-7 DNA has been detected in human milk, peripheral blood mononuclear cells, cervical secretions, and other body sites. Congenital HHV-7 infection has not been demonstrated.

The mean **incubation period** for HHV-6B is 9 to 10 days. For HHV-7, the **incubation period** is unknown.

DIAGNOSTIC TESTS

Multiple assays for detection of HHV-6 and HHV-7 have been developed; some are available commercially, but because laboratory diagnosis of HHV-6 or HHV-7 does not usually influence clinical management (infections in severely immunocompromised patients are an exception), these tests have limited utility in clinical practice.

Reference laboratories offer diagnostic testing for HHV-6B, HHV-6A, and HHV-7 infections by detection of viral DNA in blood, cerebrospinal fluid (CSF), other body fluids, or tissue specimens. However, detection of HHV-6A, HHV-6B, or HHV-7 DNA by PCR assay might not differentiate between new infection, persistence of virus from past infection, or chromosomal integration of HHV-6. At least one multiplexed PCR diagnostic panel designed to detect agents of meningitis and encephalitis in CSF cleared by the US Food and Drug Administration contains HHV-6 as one of its target pathogens; however, given the prevalence of ciHHV-6 (1%), which would yield a positive CSF PCR result, a positive test result should be interpreted with caution if there are no other findings to suggest encephalitis. Quantitative PCR assay has been used for monitoring the effectiveness of antiviral treatment in immunocompromised patients with viral reactivation.

Chromosomal integration of HHV-6 is supported by consistently positive PCR test results for HHV-6 DNA in whole blood, tissue, or other fluids, often with high viral loads (eg, 1×10^6 copies in whole blood, which, with a normal white blood cell count, is approximately 1 copy of HHV-6 DNA per cell). Droplet digital PCR or quantitative comparison of viral DNA copies to human cell number copies in whole blood samples may also be used to identify ciHHV-6.

Serological tests including immunofluorescent antibody assay, virus neutralization, immunoblot, and enzyme immunoassay are often difficult to interpret. A 4-fold increase in serum antibody concentration alone does not necessarily indicate new infection, because an increase in titer may occur with reactivation and in association with other infections, especially other betaherpesvirus infections. However, documented seroconversion is considered evidence of recent primary infection in infants and young children, and serological tests may be useful for epidemiological studies. Detection of specific immunoglobulin M (IgM) antibody is not reliable for diagnosing new infection, because IgM antibodies to HHV-6 and HHV-7 are not always detectable in children with primary infection and may also be present in asymptomatic previously infected people. These antibody assays do not differentiate HHV-6A from HHV-6B infections. In addition, the diagnosis of primary HHV-7 infection in children with previous HHV-6B infection is confounded by concurrent increase in HHV-6 antibody titer from antigenic cross-reactivity or from reactivation of HHV-6B by a new HHV-7 infection. Detection of low-avidity HHV-6 or HHV-7 antibody with subsequent maturation to high-avidity antibody has been used in these situations to identify recent primary infection.

TREATMENT

Management is supportive. The use of ganciclovir (and, therefore, valganciclovir) or foscarnet may be beneficial for immunocompromised patients with HHV-6 or HHV-7 disease and is recommended for treatment of HHV-6 encephalitis in hematopoietic stem cell and solid organ transplant patients. Antiviral resistance may occur. Routine monitoring of HHV-6 and HHV-7 DNA levels in blood during transplant is not recommended.

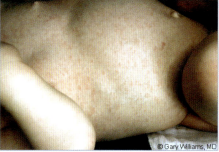

Image 69.2
Roseola rash in a 10-month-old. Seizures are somewhat common during the febrile phase of primary infections. Copyright Gary Williams, MD.

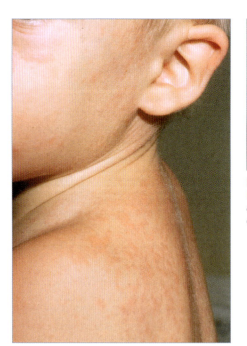

Image 69.1
A 13-month-old boy developed high fever that persisted for 4 days without recognized cause. The child appeared relatively well, and the fever subsided to be followed by a maculopapular rash that began on the trunk and spread to involve the face and extremities. The course was typical for roseola infantum. Courtesy of George Nankervis, MD.

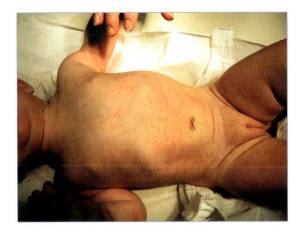

Image 69.3
An 8-month-old with a temperature between 38.3 and 39.4 °C (101 and 103 °F) for 3 consecutive days. The child appeared well, with no additional symptoms aside from mild irritability and decreased appetite. After cessation of the fever, the patient developed a maculopapular rash heavy on the trunk, but, aside from this, the patient still appeared well. The rash resolved in the next 48 hours. The clinical course and rash are compatible with roseola. Copyright Stan Block, MD, FAAP.

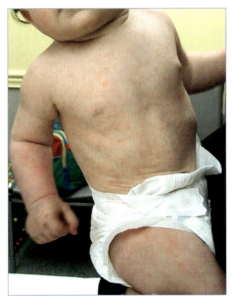

Image 69.4
Clinical course and rash compatible with roseola. This is the same patient as in Image 69.3. Copyright Stan Block, MD, FAAP.

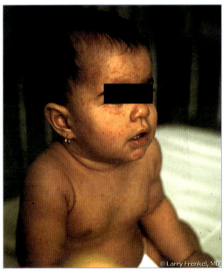

Image 69.5
A female toddler with the exanthem of roseola following several days of high fever. Courtesy of Larry Frenkel, MD.

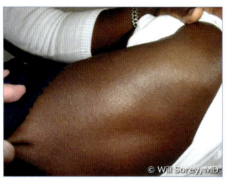

Image 69.6
A 3-year-old with 2 days of bounding fever to 39.4 °C (103 °F). Although the child was febrile, he had still been active between fever spikes. He had a brief tonic-clonic seizure, but anticonvulsants were not started because of his well appearance at the emergency department. He was diagnosed with a febrile seizure. The fever resolved, but the child was restricted from child care because of a fine rash all over. He was asymptomatic at the time his rash developed and was diagnosed with roseola. Despite reassurance, school admission was refused until the rash faded. Courtesy of Will Sorey, MD.

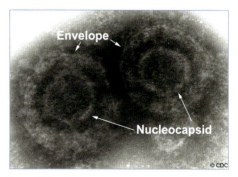

Image 69.7
Thin-section electron micrograph image of human herpesvirus 7, which, like human herpesvirus 6, can cause roseola. Virions consist of a darkly staining core within the capsid that is surrounded by a proteinaceous tegument layer and enclosed within the viral envelope. Courtesy of Centers for Disease Control and Prevention.

CHAPTER 70

Human Herpesvirus 8

CLINICAL MANIFESTATIONS

Human herpesvirus 8 (HHV-8), also known as Kaposi sarcoma–associated herpesvirus, causes Kaposi sarcoma (KS), primary effusion lymphoma, multicentric Castleman disease (MCD), and the Kaposi sarcoma herpesvirus-associated inflammatory cytokine syndrome (KICS). HHV-8 also potentially triggers hemophagocytic lymphohistiocytosis. In regions with endemic HHV-8, a nonspecific primary infection syndrome in immunocompetent children consists of fever and a maculopapular rash, often accompanied by upper respiratory tract symptoms. Primary infection in immunocompromised people tends to lead to more severe manifestations including pancytopenia, fever, rash, lymphadenopathy, splenomegaly, diarrhea, arthralgia, disseminated disease, and/or KS. In parts of Africa where HHV-8 is endemic, KS is a frequent, aggressive malignancy in children both with and without HIV infection. Clinical manifestations can vary, but younger children most often present with prominent (>2 cm), firm, nontender lymphadenopathy; with associated cytopenias (significant anemia and thrombocytopenia); and frequently without the characteristic cutaneous lesions or "woody" edema more commonly found in adults. In the United States, KS is rare in children and occurs primarily in adults with poorly controlled HIV infection. Immune reconstitution inflammatory syndrome–KS can occur, most notably in HIV-positive children adopted from HHV-8–endemic countries. Among solid organ and, less often, bone marrow transplant recipients, KS is an important cause of cancer-related deaths. Primary effusion lymphoma is rare in children. MCD has been described in immunosuppressed and immunocompetent children, but the proportion of cases attributable to infection with HHV-8 is unknown.

ETIOLOGY

HHV-8 is a member of the family *Herpesviridae*, the subfamily *Gammaherpesvirinae*, and the *Rhadinovirus* genus and is a DNA virus closely related to Epstein-Barr virus and to *Herpesvirus saimiri* of monkeys.

EPIDEMIOLOGY

In areas of Africa, the Amazon basin, the Mediterranean, and the Middle East with endemic HHV-8, seroprevalence ranges from approximately 30% to 80%. Low rates of seroprevalence, generally less than 5%, have been reported in the United States, Northern and central Europe, and most areas of Asia. Higher rates, however, occur in specific geographic regions, among adolescents and adults with or with high risk of acquiring HIV infection, people using injection drugs, and children adopted from endemic regions including some eastern European countries.

Acquisition of HHV-8 in areas with endemic infection frequently occurs before puberty, likely by exposure to saliva of close contacts, especially mothers and siblings. Virus is shed frequently in saliva of infected people and becomes latent for life in peripheral blood mononuclear cells and lymphoid tissue. In areas where infection is not endemic, sexual transmission appears to be the major route of infection, especially among men who have sex with men. Studies from areas with endemic infection have suggested that transmission may occur by blood transfusion, but in the United States, evidence for this is lacking. Transplant of infected donor organs has been documented to result in HHV-8 infection in the recipient. HHV-8 DNA has been detected in blood drawn at birth from infants born to HHV-8–seropositive mothers, but vertical transmission seems rare. Viral DNA has also been detected in human milk, but transmission via human milk is yet to be proven.

The **incubation period** of HHV-8 is unknown.

DIAGNOSTIC TESTS

Nucleic acid amplification testing and serological assays for HHV-8 are available. Polymerase chain reaction (PCR) tests may be used on peripheral blood, fluid from body cavity effusions, and tissue biopsy specimens. When KS is suspected, biopsy with histological confirmation is the gold standard. Detection of HHV-8 in peripheral blood specimens by PCR assay has also been used to identify exacerbations of other HHV-8–associated diseases, primarily MCD and KICS (especially at high copy number in these 2 diseases); however, HHV-8 DNA can be detected in the peripheral blood of asymptomatically infected people, and, conversely, HHV-8 infected people may not have active viremia.

Currently available serological assays measuring antibodies to HHV-8 include immunofluorescent antibody assay, enzyme immunoassays, and Western blot assays with recombinant HHV-8 proteins. These serological assays detect both latent and lytic infection, but each poses challenges with accuracy or convenience, with resulting limitations on their use in the diagnosis and management of acute clinical disease.

TREATMENT

Epidemic KS (KS in HIV-positive children) should be treated with both HIV antiretroviral therapy plus chemotherapy based on clinical staging. For clinically significant disease with tissue or fluid (primary effusion lymphoma) burden, the most widely used treatment modality is chemotherapy. Treatment of transplant KS may benefit from reduction in immunosuppressive therapy and use of sirolimus in lieu of tacrolimus as the suppressive agent.

Several antiviral agents have in vitro activity against HHV-8. Case reports document an effect of ganciclovir, valganciclovir, ganciclovir combined with zidovudine, cidofovir, and foscarnet. Antiviral therapy may play a more significant role in the treatment of diseases associated with active, lytic HHV-8 replication, specifically MCD and KICS.

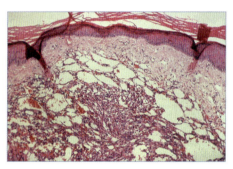

Image 70.1
This photomicrograph of a human skin biopsy specimen reveals histopathologic changes observed in what was diagnosed as a Kaposi sarcoma (KS) lesion. Of importance is the appearance of the dermal layer, which contains a cellular infiltrate, and a proliferation of vascular elements. KS is a malignant tumor of the lymphatic endothelium caused by the human herpesvirus 8, also known as Kaposi sarcoma–associated herpesvirus, and arises from a cancer of the lymphatic endothelial lining. It is characterized by bluish-red cutaneous nodules. Kaposi sarcoma is thought of as an opportunistic infection, affecting patients whose immune systems have been compromised, as in patients with HIV/AIDS. Courtesy of Centers for Disease Control and Prevention.

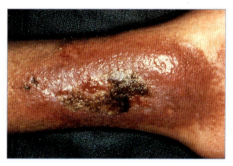

Image 70.2
This image depicts a medial view of a patient's distal left leg and ankle, where a Kaposi sarcoma (KS) cutaneous lesion can be observed. KS is a malignant tumor of the lymphatic endothelium caused by the human herpesvirus 8, also known as Kaposi sarcoma–associated herpesvirus, and arises from a cancer of the lymphatic endothelial lining. It is characterized by bluish-red cutaneous nodules. Kaposi sarcoma is thought of as an opportunistic infection, affecting patients whose immune systems have been compromised, as in patients with HIV/AIDS. Courtesy of Centers for Disease Control and Prevention.

CHAPTER 71
Human Immunodeficiency Virus Infection

CLINICAL MANIFESTATIONS

HIV infection results in a wide array of clinical manifestations. HIV type 1 (HIV-1) is much more common in the United States than HIV type 2 (HIV-2). Unless otherwise specified, this chapter addresses HIV-1 infection. AIDS is the name given to an advanced stage of HIV infection based on specific criteria for children, adolescents, and adults established by the Centers for Disease Control and Prevention (CDC).

Acute retroviral syndrome develops in 50% to 90% of adolescents and adults within the first few weeks after they become infected with HIV and is characterized by nonspecific mononucleosis-like symptoms, including fever, malaise, lymphadenopathy, and skin rash.

Clinical manifestations of untreated pediatric HIV infection include unexplained fevers, generalized lymphadenopathy, hepatomegaly, splenomegaly, failure to thrive, persistent oral and diaper candidiasis, recurrent diarrhea, parotitis, hepatitis, central nervous system (CNS) disease (eg, encephalopathy, hyperreflexia, hypertonia, floppiness, developmental delay), lymphoid interstitial pneumonia, recurrent invasive bacterial infections, and opportunistic infections (OIs) (eg, viral, parasitic, and fungal).

In the era of antiretroviral therapy (ART), there has been a substantial decrease in frequency of all OIs. In the pre-ART era, the most common OIs observed in children in the United States were infections caused by invasive encapsulated bacteria, *Pneumocystis jirovecii* (previously called *Pneumocystis carinii*, hence the still-used acronym PCP for *P carinii* pneumonia), varicella-zoster virus, cytomegalovirus, herpes simplex virus, *Mycobacterium avium* complex, *Cryptococcus neoformans*, and *Candida* species. Less commonly observed opportunistic pathogens included Epstein-Barr virus, *Mycobacterium tuberculosis*, *Cryptosporidium* species, *Cystoisospora* (formerly *Isospora*) species, other enteric pathogens, *Aspergillus* species, and *Toxoplasma gondii*.

Immune reconstitution inflammatory syndrome (IRIS) is a paradoxical clinical deterioration often encountered in severely immunosuppressed individuals that occurs shortly after the initiation of ART. Local and/or systemic symptoms develop secondary to an inflammatory response as cell-mediated immunity is restored. IRIS is observed in patients with previous infections with mycobacteria (including *M tuberculosis*), BCG vaccine, herpesviruses, and fungi (including *Cryptococcus* species).

Malignant neoplasms in children with HIV infection are relatively uncommon, but leiomyosarcomas and non-Hodgkin B-cell lymphomas of the Burkitt type (including those in the CNS) occur more commonly in children with HIV infection than in immunocompetent children. Kaposi sarcoma, caused by human herpesvirus 8, is rare in children in the United States but has been documented in HIV-infected children who have emigrated from sub-Saharan African countries. The incidence of malignant neoplasms among HIV-infected children has decreased during the ART era.

ETIOLOGY

HIV-1 and HIV-2 are cytopathic lentiviruses (genus *Lentivirus*) belonging to the family *Retroviridae*. Three distinct genetic groups of HIV exist: M (major), O (outlier), and N (new). Group M viruses are the most prevalent worldwide and comprise 8 genetic subtypes, or clades, known as A through K, each of which has a distinct geographic distribution.

HIV-2, the second AIDS-causing virus, is found predominantly in West Africa. HIV-2 has a milder disease course with a longer time to development of AIDS than that of HIV-1. Accurate diagnosis of HIV-2 is important clinically, because HIV-2 is intrinsically resistant to nonnucleoside reverse transcriptase inhibitors and the fusion inhibitor enfuvirtide.

EPIDEMIOLOGY

Humans are the only known reservoir for HIV-1 and HIV-2. Latent virus persists in peripheral blood mononuclear cells and in cells of the brain, bone marrow, and genital tract even when plasma viral load is undetectable. Only blood, semen, cervicovaginal secretions, and human milk have been implicated in transmission of infection.

Established modes of HIV transmission include (1) sexual contact (vaginal, anal, or orogenital); (2) percutaneous blood exposure (from contaminated needles or other sharp materials); (3) mucous membrane exposure to contaminated blood or other body fluids; (4) mother-to-child transmission (MTCT) during prepartum, intrapartum, and postpartum periods, including breastfeeding postnatally; and (5) transfusion with contaminated blood products. Cases of HIV transmission from HIV-infected caregivers to children through feeding blood-tinged premasticated food and from contact of nonintact skin with blood-containing body fluids have been reported in the United States. Because of highly effective screening assays and protocols, transfusion of blood, blood components, and clotting factors has virtually been eliminated as a cause of HIV transmission in the United States since 1985. Since the mid-1990s, the number of reported pediatric AIDS cases has decreased significantly, primarily because of prevention of MTCT of HIV and the widespread availability of ART for children with HIV.

In the absence of breastfeeding, the risk of HIV infection for infants born to untreated women living with HIV (WLHIV) in the United States is approximately 25%, with most transmission occurring near the time of delivery. Maternal viral load is the critical determinant affecting the likelihood of MTCT of HIV, although transmission has been observed across the entire range of maternal viral loads. Current US guidelines recommend cesarean delivery before labor and before rupture of membranes at 38 completed weeks of gestation for WLHIV with a viral load of 1,000 copies/mL or greater (irrespective of antiretroviral [ARV] use in pregnancy) and for women with unknown viral load near the time of delivery.

The rate of acquisition of HIV infection among infants has decreased significantly in the United States. The overall rate of new HIV infections among adolescents and young adults aged 13 to 24 years is also decreasing but is increasing for young men who have sex with men in this age-group. HIV infection in adolescents occurs disproportionately in youth of minority race or ethnicity and is attributable primarily to sexual exposure.

INCUBATION PERIOD

The usual age of onset of symptoms is approximately 12 to 18 months for untreated infants and children in the United States who acquire HIV infection through MTCT. However, some HIV-infected children become ill in the first few months after birth, whereas others remain relatively asymptomatic for more than 5 years and, rarely, until early adolescence.

Acute retroviral syndrome occurring in adolescents and adults following HIV acquisition occurs 7 to 14 days following viral acquisition and lasts for 5 to 7 days. Only a minority of patients are ill enough to seek medical care with acute retroviral syndrome.

DIAGNOSTIC TESTS

Serological Assays

Immunoassays are used widely as the initial test for serum HIV antibody or for p24 antigen and HIV antibody. Serological assays that are cleared by the US Food and Drug Administration (FDA) for the diagnosis of HIV include

- Antigen/antibody combination immunoassays (fourth-generation tests) that detect HIV-1/HIV-2 antibodies as well as HIV-1 p24 antigen: recommended for initial testing

- HIV-1/HIV-2 immunoassays that detect immunoglobulin M (third-generation antibody tests): alternative for initial testing

- HIV-1/HIV-2 antibody differentiation immunoassay that differentiates HIV-1 antibodies from HIV-2 antibodies (HIV-1/HIV-2 test): recommended for supplemental confirmatory testing

- HIV-1 Western blot and HIV-1 indirect immunofluorescent antibody assays (first-generation tests): alternative for supplemental confirmatory testing

- HIV-1 and HIV-2 antibodies (separate results for each) as well as p24 antigen (fifth-generation test): FDA cleared for initial HIV screening but not as a confirmatory test

The 2018 CDC HIV laboratory testing algorithm recommends an initial FDA-approved HIV-1/HIV-2 antigen/antibody combination immunoassay (fourth-generation assay). Specimens with a reactive antigen/antibody immunoassay result should be tested with an FDA-approved HIV-1/HIV-2 antibody differentiation immunoassay. Specimens that are reactive on the initial antigen/antibody immunoassay and nonreactive or indeterminate on the HIV-1/HIV-2 antibody differentiation immunoassay should be tested with an FDA-approved HIV-1 nucleic acid amplification test (NAAT). If acute HIV infection or end-stage AIDS is suspected, virological testing may be indicated because of false-negative antibody assay results in these populations.

Nucleic Acid Amplification Tests

Plasma HIV DNA or RNA assays have been used to diagnose HIV infection. The DNA polymerase chain reaction (PCR) assays can detect 1 to 10 DNA copies of proviral DNA in peripheral blood mononuclear cells and are used qualitatively to diagnose HIV infection. An RNA qualitative assay that can detect 100 RNA copies/mL is also cleared by the FDA for diagnosis, by using transcription-mediated amplification. Quantitative RNA PCR (viral load) assays cleared by the FDA provide results that serve as a predictor of disease progression and are useful in monitoring changes in viral load during treatment with ART.

HIV-2 Detection

Most HIV immunoassays currently approved by the FDA detect but do not routinely differentiate between HIV-1 and HIV-2 antibodies. It is important to notify the laboratory when ordering serological tests for a patient in whom HIV-2 infection is a possibility so FDA-approved HIV-1/HIV-2 antibody differentiation immunoassays can be used. NAATs approved by the FDA for detection and quantitation of viral load are specific to HIV-1 and do not detect HIV-2.

Diagnosis of Perinatally and Postnatally Acquired Infection

Because children born to HIV-infected mothers passively acquire maternal antibodies, antibody assays are not informative for the diagnosis of infection in children younger than 18 months unless assay results are negative. Therefore, laboratory diagnosis of HIV infection during the first 18 months after birth is based on HIV NAATs (Table 71.1). In children 18 to 24 months and older, HIV antibody assays can be used for diagnosis. Despite a median age of "seroreversion" of 13.9 months, 14% of infants remain seropositive after 18 months, 4.3% remain seropositive after 21 months, and 1.2% remain seropositive after 24 months.

HIV-1 RNA or DNA NAATs for diagnosis of infection in infants are equally recommended in current diagnostic guidelines (figures 71.1 and 71.2). Because DNA PCR detects proviral DNA in cells while HIV RNA tests measure viral RNA in plasma, there is the potential for DNA testing to be more sensitive in infants with very low viral loads. However, studies have shown that RNA and DNA NAATs for the diagnosis of HIV-1 infection in infants produce comparable results, leading to the current recommendation that either assay can be used in this setting. HIV-1 RNA assays help identify 25% to 58% of infected infants in the

Table 71.1
Laboratory Diagnosis of HIV Infection[a]

Test	Comment
HIV DNA PCR or RNA PCR	Preferred tests to diagnose HIV infection in infants and children <18–24 months; highly sensitive and specific by 2 weeks of age and available; DNA test performed on peripheral blood mononuclear cells; RNA test performed on plasma
HIV p24 Ag	Less sensitive, false-positive results during first month after birth, variable results; not recommended
ICD p24 Ag	Negative test result does not rule out infection; not recommended
HIV culture	Expensive, not readily available, requires up to 4 weeks for results; not recommended

Ag indicates antigen; ICD, immune complex dissociated; and PCR, polymerase chain reaction.

[a] Adapted from Read JS; American Academy of Pediatrics Committee on Pediatric AIDS. Diagnosis of HIV-1 infection in children younger than 18 months in the United States. *Pediatrics.* 2007;120(6):e1547–e1562. Reaffirmed June 2015. Accessed June 23, 2022. https://publications.aap.org/pediatrics/article/120/6/e1547/70580/Diagnosis-of-HIV-1-Infection-in-Children-Younger.

Figure 71.1
Newborn Testing and Prophylaxis Recommendations Following Low-risk Perinatal HIV Exposure

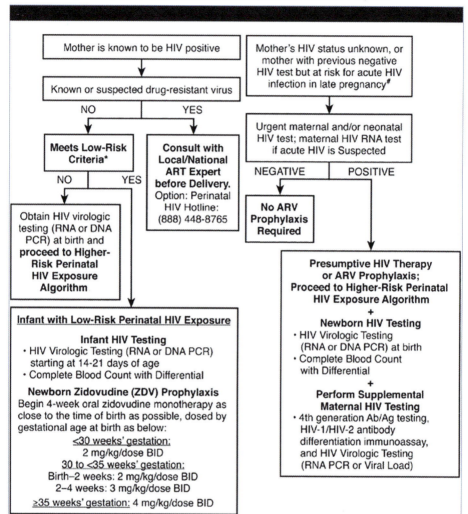

Figure 71.2
Newborn Testing and Prophylaxis Recommendations Following Higher-risk Perinatal HIV Exposure

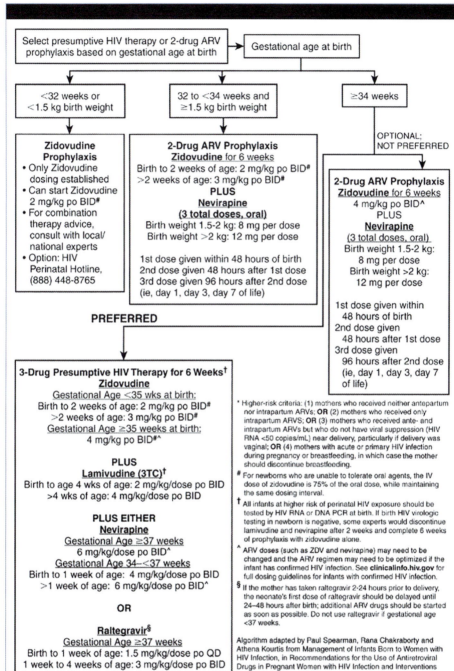

first week after birth; 89%, by 1 month of age; and 90% to 100%, by 2 to 3 months of age. An HIV RNA assay result with only a low-level viral copy number in an HIV-exposed infant may indicate a false-positive result.

In HIV-exposed infants, diagnostic testing with HIV DNA or RNA assays is recommended at 14 to 21 days of age and, if results are negative, again at 1 to 2 months of age and at 4 to 6 months of age (Figure 71.3). An infant is considered infected if 2 samples from 2 different time points produce positive test results by DNA or RNA NAAT. For infants with higher risk for perinatal HIV transmission, additional virological diagnostic testing is recommended at birth and at 8 to 10 weeks after birth (which is 2–4 weeks after cessation of ARV prophylaxis) (Figure 71.3). If testing is performed shortly after birth, umbilical cord blood should not be used because of possible contamination with maternal blood. HIV-infected infants should promptly be transitioned from neonatal ARV prophylaxis to ART treatment.

In HIV-exposed children with 2 negative HIV DNA or RNA assay results, many clinicians confirm the absence of antibody (ie, loss of passively acquired maternal antibody, or seroreversion) to HIV on testing at 18 through 24 months of age. Some clinicians have a slightly more stringent requirement that the 2 separate antibody-negative blood samples obtained after 6 months of age be drawn at least 1 month apart for a child to be considered HIV uninfected.

Adolescents and HIV Testing

The American Academy of Pediatrics recommends that routine HIV screening be offered to all youth 15 years or older, at least once in health care settings. Following initial screening, youth with increased risk, including those who are sexually active, should be rescreened at least annually, potentially as frequently as every 3 to 6 months if they have very high risk (males reporting male sexual contact; youth actively using injection drugs; transgender youth; youth with sexual partners who have HIV infection, vary in gender, or use injection drugs; youth exchanging sex for drugs or money; or those who have had a diagnosis of or request testing for other sexually transmitted infections [STIs]). Use of any FDA-cleared HIV antibody test is appropriate. For any positive test result, immediate referral to an HIV specialist is appropriate to confirm diagnosis and initiate management. HIV testing is recommended and should be routine for all patients in STI clinics and those seeking treatment of STIs in other clinical settings.

Figure 71.3
Recommended Virologic Testing Schedules for Infants Exposed to HIV by Perinatal HIV Transmission Risk

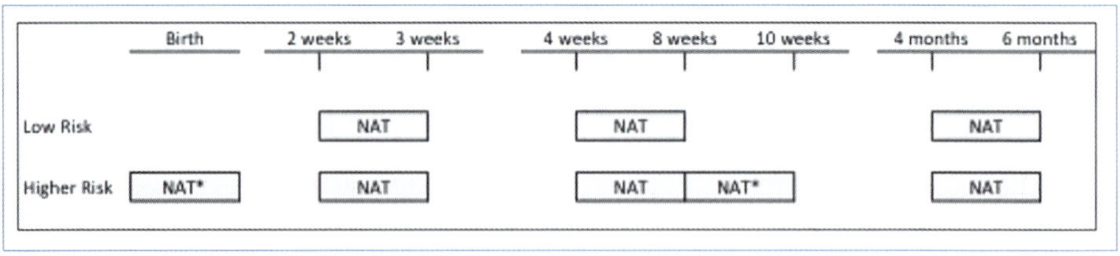

NAT indicates nucleic acid amplification test (referred to as NAAT in this chapter).

Low Risk: Infants born to mothers who received standard antiretroviral therapy (ART) during pregnancy with sustained viral suppression (usually defined as confirmed HIV RNA level below the lower limits of detection of an ultrasensitive assay) and no concerns related to maternal adherence.

Higher Risk: Infants born to women living with HIV infection who did not receive prenatal care, did not receive antepartum or intrapartum antiretrovirals (ARVs), received intrapartum ARV drugs only, initiated ART late in pregnancy (late second or third trimester), were diagnosed with acute HIV infection during pregnancy, or had detectable HIV viral loads close to the time of delivery, including those who received combination ARV drugs and did not have sustained viral suppression.

* For higher-risk infants, additional virologic diagnostic testing should be considered at birth and 2 to 4 weeks after cessation of ARV prophylaxis (ie, at 8–10 weeks of life).

Reproduced with permission from Spach DH. Preventing perinatal HIV transmission. National HIV Curriculum, Infectious Diseases Education and Assessment, University of Washington. Updated January 24, 2022. Accessed June 23, 2022. https://www.hiv.uw.edu/go/prevention/preventing-perinatal-transmission/core-concept/all.

Suspicion of acute retroviral syndrome should prompt urgent assessment with an antigen/antibody immunoassay or HIV RNA NAAT in conjunction with an antibody test. If the immunoassay result is negative or indeterminate, testing for HIV RNA by using a NAAT should follow. Clinicians should not assume that a laboratory report of a negative HIV antibody test result indicates that the necessary RNA screening for acute HIV infection has been conducted. HIV home-testing kits detect only HIV antibodies and, therefore, will not detect acute HIV infection.

TREATMENT

Antiretroviral Therapy

Consultation with an expert in pediatric HIV infection is recommended in the care of HIV-infected infants, children, and adolescents. Whenever possible, enrollment of HIV-infected infants, children, and adolescents in clinical trials should be encouraged.

ART is indicated for HIV-infected pediatric patients and should be initiated as soon as possible after diagnosis of HIV infection is established. Initiation of treatment of adolescents generally follows guidelines for adults and is recommended strongly for all HIV-infected adolescents or adults regardless of $CD4^+$ T-lymphocyte count, as long as medication readiness is apparent. In general, ART with at least 3 active drugs is recommended for all HIV-infected individuals requiring ARV therapy. ARV resistance testing (viral genotyping) is recommended before starting treatment. Sustained suppression of virus to undetectable levels is the desired goal. A change in ARV therapy should be considered if there is evidence of disease progression (virological, immunologic, or clinical), toxicity of or intolerance to drugs, development of drug resistance, or availability of data suggesting the possibility of a superior regimen.

Opportunistic Infections

Guidelines for prevention and treatment of OIs in children and adolescents and adults provide indications for administration of drugs for infection with *P jirovecii*, *M avium* complex, cytomegalovirus, *T gondii*, and other organisms.

Immunization Recommendations

All recommended childhood vaccinations should be administered to HIV-exposed infants. If HIV infection is confirmed, guidelines for the HIV-infected child should be followed. Children and adolescents with HIV infection should undergo immunization as soon as is age appropriate with all inactivated vaccines. Inactivated influenza vaccine should be administered annually according to the most current recommendations. The 3-dose series of human papillomavirus vaccine; tetanus toxoid, reduced diphtheria toxoid, and acellular pertussis vaccine; and meningococcal conjugate vaccine are all indicated in HIV-infected adolescents.

The live-virus measles-mumps-rubella (MMR) vaccine and monovalent varicella vaccine can be administered to asymptomatic HIV-infected children and adolescents without severe immunosuppression (ie, can be administered to children 1–13 years of age with a $CD4^+$ T-lymphocyte percentage $\geq$15% and to adolescents $\geq$14 years with a $CD4^+$ T-lymphocyte count $\geq$200/μL). Severely immunocompromised HIV-infected infants, children, adolescents, and young adults (eg, children 1–13 years of age with a $CD4^+$ T-lymphocyte percentage <15% and adolescents $\geq$14 years with a $CD4^+$ T-lymphocyte count <200/μL) should not receive measles virus–containing vaccine, because vaccine-related pneumonia has been reported. The quadrivalent measles-mumps-rubella-varicella vaccine should not be administered to any HIV-infected infant, regardless of degree of immunosuppression, because of lack of safety data in this population.

Rotavirus vaccine should be administered to HIV-exposed and HIV-infected infants irrespective of $CD4^+$ T-lymphocyte percentage or count.

All HIV-infected children should receive a dose of 23-valent polysaccharide pneumococcal vaccine after turning 24 months of age, with a minimal interval of 8 weeks since the last pneumococcal conjugate vaccine.

HIV-infected children who are 5 years and older and have not received *Haemophilus influenzae* type b (Hib) vaccine should receive 1 dose of Hib vaccine.

Infants and children who have HIV infection and are 2 months or older should receive an age-appropriate series of the meningococcal ACWY conjugate vaccine (MenACWY). The same vaccine product should be used for all doses. However, if the product used for previous doses is unknown or unavailable, the vaccination series may be completed with any age- and formulation-appropriate MenACWY. Although no data on interchangeability of meningococcal conjugate vaccines in HIV-infected people are available, limited data from a postlicensure study in healthy adolescents suggests that safety and immunogenicity of MenACWY-CRM are not adversely affected by prior immunization with MenACWY-D. For HIV-infected children 2 through 23 months of age, only MenACWY-CRM (Menveo) should be used, because interference with the immune response to pneumococcal conjugate vaccine occurs with MenACWY-D (Menactra), and MenACWY-TT (MenQuadfi) is not licensed for use in children younger than 2 years.

Children Who Are HIV Uninfected Residing in the Household of an HIV-Infected Person

Members of households in which an adult or a child has HIV infection can receive MMR vaccine, because these vaccine viruses are not transmitted from person to person. To decrease the risk of transmission of influenza to patients with symptomatic HIV infection, all household members 6 months or older should receive yearly influenza immunization. Immunization with varicella vaccine of siblings and susceptible adult caregivers of patients with HIV infection is encouraged to prevent acquisition of wild-type varicella-zoster virus infection, which can cause severe disease in immunocompromised hosts. Transmission of varicella vaccine virus from an immunocompetent host to a household contact is very uncommon.

Postexposure Passive Immunization of HIV-Infected Children

Measles

HIV-infected children who are exposed to measles require prophylaxis on the basis of immune status and measles vaccine history. HIV-infected children who have serological evidence of immunity or who received 2 doses of measles vaccine after initiation of ART with no to moderate immunosuppression should be considered immune and do not require any additional measures to prevent measles. Asymptomatic mildly or moderately immunocompromised HIV-infected people without evidence of immunity to measles should receive immune globulin intramuscular at a dose of 0.5 mL/kg (maximum 15 mL), regardless of immunization status. Severely immunocompromised patients (eg, HIV-infected people with $CD4^+$ T-lymphocyte percentages <15% [all ages] or $CD4^+$ T-lymphocyte counts <200/µL [age >5 years], regardless of immunization status, and those who have not received MMR vaccine since receiving ART) who are exposed to measles should receive immune globulin intravenous (IGIV) prophylaxis, 400 mg/kg, after exposure to measles, because they may not be protected by the vaccine. Some experts would include all HIV-infected people, regardless of immunologic status or MMR vaccine history, as needing IGIV prophylaxis. HIV-infected children who have received IGIV within 3 weeks of exposure do not require additional passive immunization.

Tetanus

HIV-infected children with severe immunosuppression who sustain wounds classified as tetanus prone should receive tetanus immune globulin regardless of immunization status.

Varicella

HIV-infected children without a history of previous varicella or without evidence of immunity to varicella should receive varicella-zoster immune globulin, if available, ideally within 96 hours but potentially beneficial up to 10 days, after close contact with a person who has chickenpox or shingles. An alternative to varicella-zoster immune globulin for passive immunization is IGIV, 400 mg/kg, administered once within 10 days after exposure. Children who have received IGIV for other reasons within 3 weeks of exposure do not require additional passive immunization.

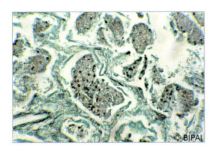

Image 71.1
Pneumocystis jirovecii (formerly *Pneumocystis carinii*) pneumonia lung biopsy specimen from a child with HIV infection and pneumonia. Numerous dark-staining cysts of *P jirovecii* (Grocott-Gomori methenamine–silver nitrate stain). Copyright Baylor International Pediatric AIDS Initiative/Mark Kline, MD, FAAP.

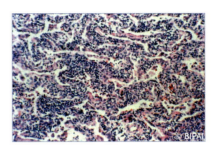

Image 71.2
Lung biopsy specimen showing mononuclear interstitial infiltration in a child with HIV infection and lymphoid interstitial pneumonitis/pulmonary lymphoid hyperplasia (LIP/PLH). The pathogenesis of LIP/PLH is poorly understood, but Epstein-Barr virus has been implicated as a cofactor in its development. Copyright Baylor International Pediatric AIDS Initiative/Mark Kline, MD, FAAP.

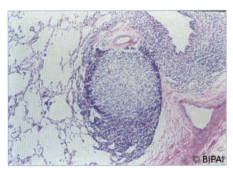

Image 71.3
Biopsy specimen showing a nodular aggregate of mononuclear cells in the lung of a child with HIV infection and lymphoid interstitial pneumonitis/pulmonary lymphoid hyperplasia. Copyright Baylor International Pediatric AIDS Initiative/Mark Kline, MD, FAAP.

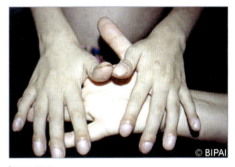

Image 71.4
Digital clubbing in a child with HIV infection and lymphoid interstitial pneumonitis/pulmonary lymphoid hyperplasia (LIP/PLH). Marked lymphadenopathy, hepatosplenomegaly, and salivary gland enlargement are also observed in many children with LIP/PLH. The clinical course of LIP/PLH is variable. Exacerbation of respiratory distress and hypoxemia can occur in association with intercurrent viral respiratory illnesses. Spontaneous clinical remission is sometimes observed. Copyright Baylor International Pediatric AIDS Initiative/Mark Kline, MD, FAAP.

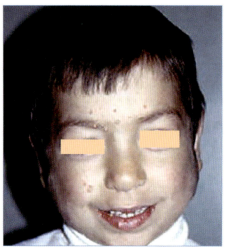

Image 71.5
Bilateral parotid gland enlargement in a male child with HIV infection and lymphoid interstitial pneumonitis/pulmonary lymphoid hyperplasia. Note the presence of multiple lesions of molluscum contagiosum, which are commonly found in patients with HIV infection, particularly those with a low CD4 lymphocyte count. (See also Molluscum Contagiosum.) Copyright Baylor International Pediatric AIDS Initiative/Mark Kline, MD, FAAP.

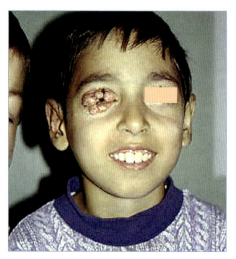

Image 71.6
Severe molluscum contagiosum in a boy with HIV infection. Some HIV-infected children develop molluscum contagiosum lesions that are unusually large or widespread. They are often seated more deeply in the epidermis. (See also Molluscum Contagiosum.) Copyright Baylor International Pediatric AIDS Initiative/Mark Kline, MD, FAAP.

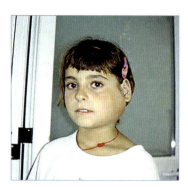

Image 71.7
Suppurative parotitis in a girl with HIV infection. Note the marked swelling and redness overlying the left parotid gland. On palpation of the gland, pus could be observed exuding from the Stensen duct. Copyright Baylor International Pediatric AIDS Initiative/Mark Kline, MD, FAAP.

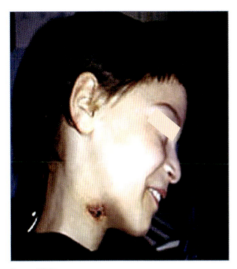

Image 71.8
An 8-year-old boy with HIV and tuberculous lymphadenitis (scrofula). Copious amounts of pus spontaneously drained from this lesion. In a child with immunocompromise, other causes of lymphadenitis include infections with gram-positive bacteria, atypical mycobacterium, and *Bartonella henselae* (cat-scratch disease); malignant neoplasms such as lymphoma; masses such as branchial cleft cysts or cystic hygromas masquerading as lymph nodes; and adenitis caused by HIV itself. (See also Nontuberculous Mycobacteria.) Copyright Baylor International Pediatric AIDS Initiative/ Mark Kline, MD, FAAP.

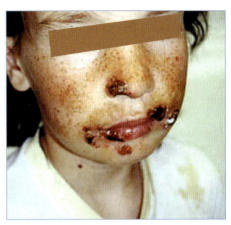

Image 71.9
Herpes simplex infection in a girl with HIV infection. Chronic or progressive herpetic skin lesions are observed occasionally in HIV-infected children, although unlike varicella-zoster virus infections in these patients, herpes simplex infections much less commonly cause disseminated disease. (See also Herpes Simplex.) Copyright Baylor International Pediatric AIDS Initiative/ Mark Kline, MD, FAAP.

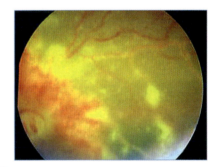

Image 71.11
Funduscopic examination of a 16-year-old girl with HIV infection and cytomegalovirus retinitis. There are extensive areas of hemorrhage, with white retinal exudates. Children with cytomegalovirus retinitis usually present with painless visual impairment. (See also Cytomegalovirus Infection.) Copyright Baylor International Pediatric AIDS Initiative/Mark Kline, MD, FAAP.

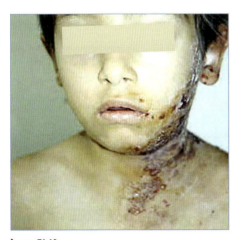

Image 71.10
Herpes zoster (shingles) in a boy with HIV infection. These cases can be complicated by chronicity or dissemination. (See also Varicella-Zoster Virus Infections.) Copyright Baylor International Pediatric AIDS Initiative/ Mark Kline, MD, FAAP.

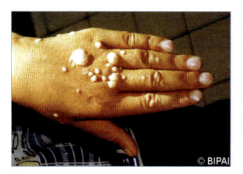

Image 71.12
Severe cutaneous warts (human papillomavirus infection) in a boy with HIV infection. Copyright Baylor International Pediatric AIDS Initiative/Mark Kline, MD, FAAP.

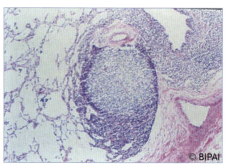

Image 71.13
Pseudomembranous candidiasis in a person with HIV infection. (See also Candidiasis.) Copyright Baylor International Pediatric AIDS Initiative/Mark Kline, MD, FAAP.

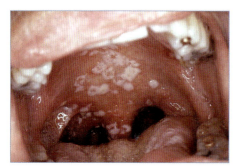

Image 71.14
This patient with HIV/AIDS presented with secondary oral pseudomembranous candidiasis. The immune system weakens when HIV therapy undergoes a dramatic reduction in its effectiveness, resulting in the greater possibility of secondary infections, as in this patient. This infection responded to fluconazole, 100 mg daily, for 1 week. Courtesy of Centers for Disease Control and Prevention.

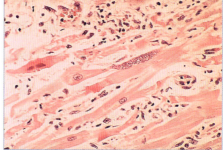

Image 71.15
Histopathologic features of toxoplasmosis of the heart in a fatal case of AIDS. Courtesy of Centers for Disease Control and Prevention.

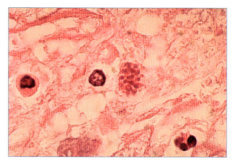

Image 71.17
Histopathologic features of toxoplasmosis of the brain in a fatal case of AIDS. Courtesy of Centers for Disease Control and Prevention.

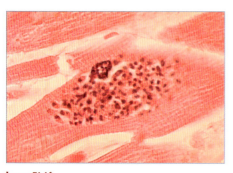

Image 71.16
Toxoplasmosis of the heart in a patient with AIDS. Courtesy of Centers for Disease Control and Prevention.

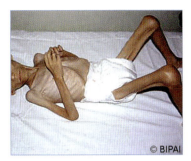

Image 71.18
Severe wasting in a patient with HIV infection. Copyright Baylor International Pediatric AIDS Initiative/Mark Kline, MD, FAAP.

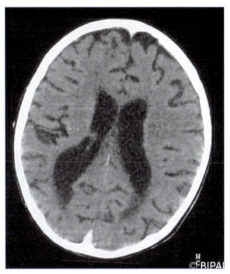

Image 71.19
Computed tomographic scan of the brain of an 8-year-old boy with HIV infection and generalized brain atrophy Cerebral atrophy is observed commonly in children with HIV-associated encephalopathy, but it may also be observed in children with typical neurological function and development. Copyright Baylor International Pediatric AIDS Initiative/Mark Kline, MD, FAAP.

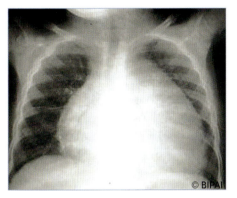

Image 71.20
Chest radiograph showing cardiomegaly in a 5-year-old girl with HIV infection, cardiomyopathy, and congestive heart failure. Many children with HIV infection with congestive heart failure respond well to medical management. Copyright Baylor International Pediatric AIDS Initiative/Mark Kline, MD, FAAP.

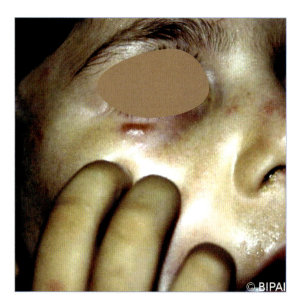

Image 71.21
A 7-year-old girl with HIV infection and a Kaposi sarcoma lesion. This tumor is rarely diagnosed in US children, with the occasional exceptions of children of Haitian descent with vertical HIV infection or older adolescents. Kaposi sarcoma is observed more commonly in HIV-infected children in some other geographic locales, including parts of Africa (eg, Zambia, Uganda) and Romania. Kaposi sarcoma has been linked to infection with a novel herpesvirus, now known as human herpesvirus 8 or Kaposi sarcoma–associated virus. Copyright Baylor International Pediatric AIDS Initiative/Mark Kline, MD, FAAP.

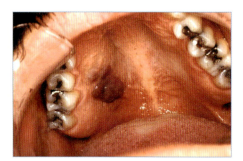

Image 71.22
This patient with HIV infection presented with intraoral Kaposi sarcoma of the hard palate secondary to his AIDS infection. Approximately 7.5%–10% of patients with AIDS display signs of oral Kaposi sarcoma, which can range in appearance from small asymptomatic growths that are flat purple-red to larger nodular growths. Courtesy of Centers for Disease Control and Prevention.

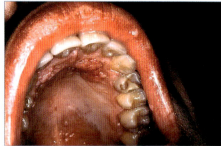

Image 71.23
This HIV-positive patient was exhibiting signs of a secondary condyloma acuminata infection (ie, venereal warts). This intraoral eruption of condyloma acuminata, or venereal warts, was caused by human papillomavirus (HPV). Although oral HPV is a rare occurrence, HIV reduces the body's immune response; therefore, such secondary infections can manifest themselves. Courtesy of Centers for Disease Control and Prevention.

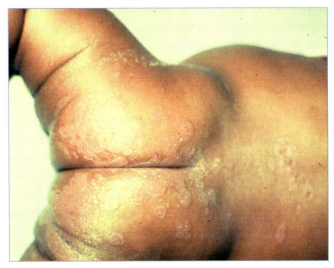

Image 71.24
A 12-month-old boy with HIV infection with a chronic *Trichophyton* infection (tinea corporis) mostly marked over the buttocks and lower extremities. Courtesy of Larry Frenkel, MD.

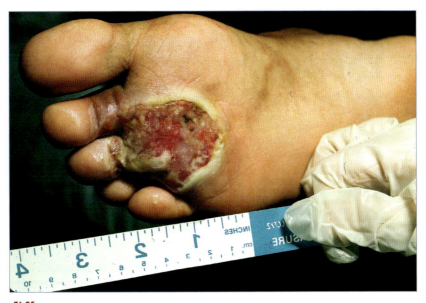

Image 71.25
A 17-year-old boy with HIV infection with an ulcerative lesion on the plantar surface of the left foot of several months' duration. A viral culture result was positive for human herpesvirus, which led to the diagnosis of HIV. Courtesy of Larry Frenkel, MD.

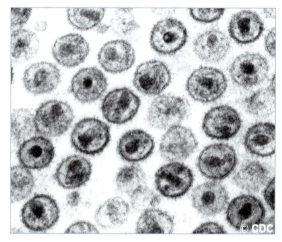

Image 71.26
HIV type 1 transmission electron micrograph. Cone-shaped cores are sectioned in various orientations. Viral genomic RNA is located in the electron-dense wide end of core. Courtesy of Centers for Disease Control and Prevention.

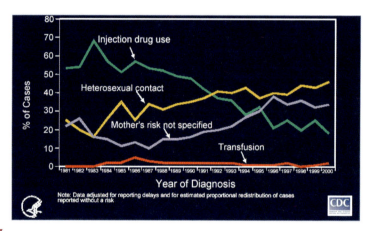

Image 71.27
Mothers' exposure category, by year of diagnosis for perinatally acquired AIDS, 1981–2000, United States. Changes have occurred in the distribution of exposure categories for the mothers of children who were infected perinatally and in whom AIDS developed. In the 1980s, most of the women who transmitted HIV vertically were exposed to HIV through injection drug use, and a smaller proportion through heterosexual contact. In the 1990s, a smaller proportion of women who transmitted HIV vertically were exposed to HIV through injection drug use; a larger proportion, through heterosexual contact. Courtesy of Centers for Disease Control and Prevention.

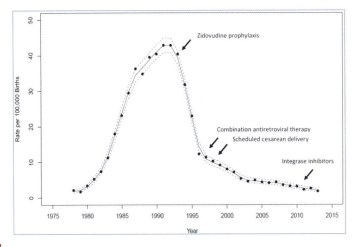

Image 71.28
The estimated incidence of perinatally acquired HIV infections per 100,000 live births (points) with a smoothed curve (solid line) and 95% confidence bands (dashed lines). The timing of important advances in recommendations for prevention of maternal-to-child transmission of HIV is noted on the figure. The arrows indicate the year in which the interventions (eg, "Zidovudine prophylaxis") occurred. From Nesheim SR, Wiener J, Fitz Harris LF, et al. Brief report: estimated incidence of perinatally acquired HIV infection in the United States, 1978–2013. *JAIDS J Acquir Immune Defic Syndr.* 2017;76(5):461–464.

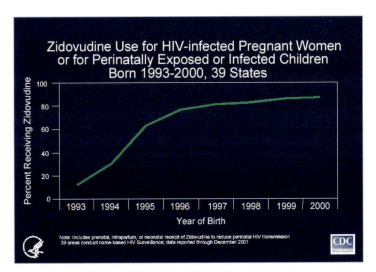

Image 71.29
Zidovudine (ZDV) use for pregnant women with HIV infection or for children who were born from 1993–2000 and perinatally exposed or infected, 39 states. In April 1994, the US Public Health Service released guidelines for the use of ZDV to reduce perinatal HIV transmission; in 1995, recommendations for HIV counseling and voluntary testing for pregnant women were published; and in 2002, recommendations on the use of antiretroviral drugs in pregnant women with HIV infection were updated. Since then, the proportion of children who were perinatally exposed to or infected with HIV who received ZDV has increased markedly. This increase in ZDV use, including receipt by the mother during the prenatal or intrapartum period and receipt by the neonate, has been accompanied by a decrease in the number of children perinatally infected with HIV and is responsible for the dramatic decline in cases of AIDS acquired perinatally. The data presented are from the 30 states with name-based HIV infection surveillance and may not represent all states in the United States. Courtesy of Centers for Disease Control and Prevention.

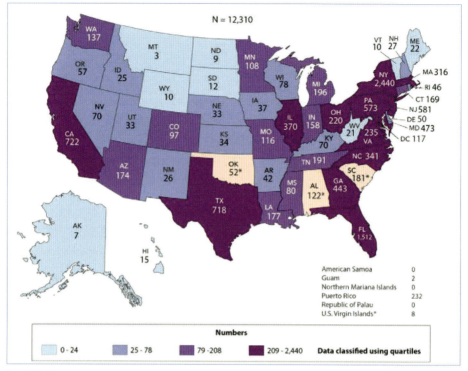

Image 71.30
People living with diagnosed perinatally acquired HIV infection, year-end 2018—United States and 6 dependent areas. Data for the year 2018 are preliminary and based on deaths reported to the Centers for Disease Control and Prevention through December 2019. Data are based on address of residence as of December 31, 2018 (ie, most recent known address). * indicates incomplete reporting.

CHAPTER 72
Human Papillomaviruses

CLINICAL MANIFESTATIONS

Most human papillomavirus (HPV) infections are subclinical, and 90% resolve spontaneously within 2 years. However, persistent HPV infection can cause benign epithelial proliferation (warts) of the skin and mucous membranes as well as cancers of the lower anogenital tract and the oropharynx. HPVs can be grouped into cutaneous and mucosal types. The cutaneous types cause common skin warts, plantar warts, flat warts, and threadlike (filiform) warts. These cutaneous warts are benign. Certain mucosal types (low risk) are associated with warts or papillomas of mucous membranes, including the upper respiratory tract and anogenital, oral, nasal, and conjunctival areas. Other mucosal types (high risk) can cause precancers and cancers, including cervical, anogenital, and oropharyngeal cancers.

Warts are common, benign lesions, although they may be associated with significant clinical problems. Common **skin warts** are dome shaped with conical projections that give the surface a rough appearance. Skin warts are usually painless and multiple, occurring commonly on the hands and around or under the nails. When small dermal vessels become thrombosed, black dots appear in the warts.

Plantar warts on the foot are often larger than warts at other sites and may not project through much of the skin surface. They can be painful when walking and are characterized by marked hyperkeratosis, sometimes with black dots.

Flat warts ("juvenile warts") are commonly found on the face and extremities of children and adolescents. Flat warts are usually small, multiple, and flat topped; seldom exhibit papillomatosis; and rarely cause pain. **Filiform warts** occur on the face and neck.

Anogenital warts, also called **condylomata acuminata,** are skin-colored warts with a papular, flat, or cauliflower-like surface that range in size from a few millimeters to several centimeters; these warts often occur in groups. In males, these warts may be found on the penis, scrotum, anal, or perianal area. In females, these lesions may occur on the vulvar, anal, or perianal areas and, less commonly, in the vagina or on the cervix. Warts are usually painless, although they may cause itching, burning, local pain, or bleeding.

Invasive cancers attributable to HPV include those of the cervix, vagina, vulva, penis, anus, and oropharynx (back of throat, base of tongue, and tonsils). Cervical cancer is the most common HPV-attributable cancer in females, and oropharyngeal cancer is the most common HPV-attributable cancer in males. Anogenital low-grade squamous intraepithelial lesions (LSILs) can result from persistent infection with low-risk or high-risk HPV types, whereas high-grade squamous intraepithelial lesions (HSILs) can result from persistent infection with high-risk HPV types. In the cervix, HSILs include cervical intraepithelial neoplasia (CIN) grades 2 or 3, and adenocarcinoma in situ (AIS), which are precancerous lesions. Intraepithelial lesions are detected through routine screening with cytological testing (Papanicolaou [Pap] test); tissue biopsy is required to diagnose CIN.

Recurrent respiratory papillomatosis (RRP) is a rare condition characterized by recurring papillomas in the larynx or other areas of the upper or lower respiratory tract. Age of onset can be in childhood or adulthood. RRP is referred to as *juvenile-onset RRP* (JORRP) when it occurs before 12 years of age and as *adult-onset RRP* (AORRP) in those 12 years and older. JORRP is believed to result most frequently from vertical transmission of HPV from a mother to her infant at the time of delivery. JORRP is diagnosed most commonly in children between 2 and 5 years of age, with manifestations of voice change (eg, hoarseness, abnormal cry), stridor, or respiratory distress. Respiratory papillomas can cause respiratory tract obstruction in young children, and repeated surgeries are often needed. Most cases of JORRP are caused by HPV type 6 or 11.

Epidermodysplasia verruciformis is a rare inherited disorder believed to be a consequence of a deficiency of cell-mediated immunity, resulting in an abnormal susceptibility to certain HPV types and manifesting as chronic cutaneous lesions and skin cancers. Lesions may resemble flat warts or pigmented plaques covering the torso and upper extremities. Most appear during the first decade after birth, but malignant transformation, which occurs in 30% to 60% of affected people, is usually delayed until adulthood.

ETIOLOGY

HPVs are small, nonenveloped, double-stranded DNA viruses of the *Papillomaviridae* family, which can be grouped into a number of types based on DNA sequence variation. Different types display different specific tissue tropism. Types 6 and 11 cause anogenital warts (condylomata acuminata), RRP, and conjunctival papillomas but are rarely found in cancer. High-risk HPV types can be detected in almost all cervical precancers and invasive cervical cancers. Approximately 50% of cervical cancers worldwide are attributable to HPV type 16; 70% are attributable to type 16 or 18. Most other HPV-related cancers—anogenital cancers (ie, vulvar, vaginal, penile, anal) and oropharyngeal cancers—are also attributable to HPV type 16. Infection with a high-risk HPV type is considered necessary but insufficient to cause cancer. Most people with an HPV infection will not develop cancer. Risk of developing cancer precursors or cancers is greater for people with certain immunocompromising conditions, such as HIV infection or cellular immunodeficiencies.

EPIDEMIOLOGY

Virtually all adults will be infected with some type of HPV during their lives. In the United States, HPV infection prevalence is 79 million, and annual incidence is 14 million infections.

Nongenital hand and foot warts occur commonly in school-aged children. Acquisition can occur through casual contact and is facilitated by minor skin trauma. Autoinoculation can result in spread of lesions. The intense and often widespread appearance of cutaneous warts in people with compromised cellular immunity (particularly those who have undergone transplant or who have HIV infection) suggests that alterations in T-lymphocyte immunity may impair clearance of infection.

Genital HPV infections are transmitted by intimate skin-to-skin contact (eg, through sexual intercourse or other close genital contact). In US females, the highest prevalence of infection is among 20- to 24-year-olds. Most infections are subclinical and clear spontaneously within 1 or 2 years. Cancer is an uncommon outcome of infection that generally requires decades of persistent infection with high-risk HPV types. There are more than 33,000 cases of HPV-attributable cancers annually in the United States. HPV-attributable cervical cancer accounts for approximately one-third of new HPV-attributable cancer cases and 4,000 deaths annually in the United States. HPV-attributable oropharyngeal cancer accounts for more than one-third of new HPV-attributable cancer cases per year. HPV is the cause of at least 90% of all cervical cancers, 70% of oropharyngeal cancers, and most vulvar, vaginal, penile, and anal cancers.

Rarely, HPV infection is transmitted to a child through the birth canal during delivery or transmitted from nongenital sites postnatally. When anogenital warts are diagnosed in a child, the possibility of sexual abuse must be considered, while noting the possibility of vertical transmission to neonates.

The **incubation period** for symptoms of HPV infection is estimated to range from 3 months to several years, but most infections are asymptomatic. The period from infection to neoplastic changes is usually years to decades.

DIAGNOSTIC TESTS

Most cutaneous and anogenital warts can be diagnosed through clinical inspection. Routine cervical cancer screening guidelines direct the age of initiation and interval at which screening with cytology (Pap testing) and/or HPV nucleic acid testing (primary screening or "cotesting") should be added and when colposcopic evaluation and biopsy should be performed. Vulvar, vaginal, penile, and anal lesions may be identified by using visual inspection, sometimes by using magnification; in some cases, cytological screening is used and suspicious lesions are biopsied, but there is no routine screening recommended for cancers at these sites. For all anogenital, oropharyngeal, and respiratory tract precancers and cancers, diagnosis is made on the basis of histological findings.

Although cytological and histological changes can be suggestive of HPV, these findings are nondiagnostic of HPV. Documentation of HPV infection is based on detection of viral nucleic acid (DNA or RNA). Nucleic acid tests for high-risk HPV types may be used as a primary screening for cervical cancer in women starting at age 25 years, in combination with Pap testing in women 30 years or older and for triage of equivocal Pap test abnormalities (atypical squamous cells of undetermined significance) in women 21 years or older. The benefit of HPV nucleic acid testing is that a negative test result for high-risk HPV types allows longer intervals (eg, 3–5 years) between routine screening.

A number of HPV DNA or messenger RNA detection and genotyping assays have been cleared for use in the United States by the US Food and Drug Administration (FDA). Liquid-based cytology collection and transport kits permit performance of Pap smear cytology and HPV detection and genotyping on the same specimen. There are differences in the appropriate clinical applications for each of these assays, including whether they can be used as an initial stand-alone test (ie, without cervical cytology) or in a primary screening algorithm; none is recommended for use in women younger than 21 years or for men.

TREATMENT

There is no FDA approved treatment of HPV infection. Treatment may be directed toward lesions caused by HPV.

Regression of **nongenital and genital warts** occurs in approximately 30% of cases within 6 months, even without treatment. Most methods of treatment of cutaneous warts use chemical or physical destruction of the infected epithelium, including cryotherapy with liquid nitrogen, laser or surgical removal of warts, application of salicylic acid products, or application of topical immune-modulating agents.

Daily treatment with tretinoin has been useful for widespread flat warts in children. Systemic treatments, including cimetidine, have been used for refractory warts with variable success. Treatments for genital warts are characterized as patient applied or provider administered. Interventions include ablational/excisional treatments, topical antiproliferative medications, or immune-modulating medications. Oral warts can be removed through cryotherapy, electrocautery, or surgical excision. Although most forms of therapy are successful for initial removal of warts, treatment may not eradicate HPV infection from the surrounding tissue. Recurrences are common and may be attributable to reactivation rather than reinfection.

Cancer precursor lesions that are identified in the cervix (eg, HSILs, AIS) or elsewhere in the genital tract may require excision or destruction. Treatment of cervical lesions can cause substantial economic, emotional, and reproductive adverse effects, including higher risk of preterm birth and perinatal mortality. Management of invasive cervical and other anogenital and oropharyngeal cancers requires a specialist and should be conducted according to current guidelines.

Respiratory papillomatosis is difficult to treat and is best managed by an experienced otolaryngologist. Local recurrence is common, and repeated surgical debulking procedures are often necessary to relieve airway obstruction. Extension or dissemination of respiratory papillomas from the larynx into the trachea, bronchi, or lung parenchyma happens rarely but results in increased morbidity and mortality; malignant transformation occurs rarely.

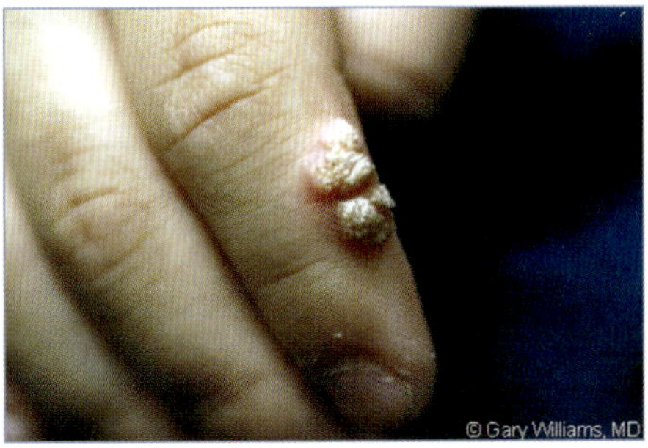

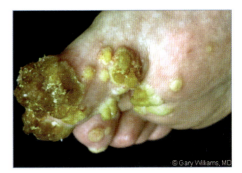

Image 72.1
Digitate human papillomavirus wart with fingerlike projections on a child's index finger. Copyright Gary Williams, MD.

Image 72.2
Human papillomavirus warts on the foot of a 14-year-old boy with immunocompromise. Copyright Gary Williams, MD.

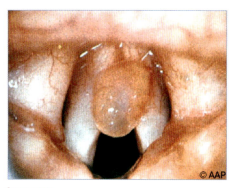

Image 72.3
Laryngeal papillomas may cause hoarseness. Although rare, they can occur in infants of mothers infected with human papillomavirus.

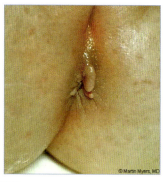

Image 72.4
A 13-month-old girl with condyloma acuminata around the anus from sexual abuse (sodomy). Copyright Martin G. Myers, MD.

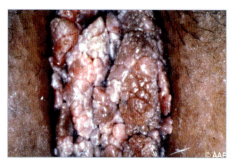

Image 72.5
Massive condyloma acuminata (genital warts) in a 10-year-old girl who had been sexually abused. These genital warts are commonly caused by human papillomavirus, especially types 6 and 11.

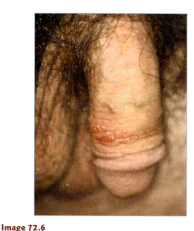

Image 72.6
This patient with condylomata acuminata presented with soft, wartlike growths on the penis (12 hours postpodophyllin application). *Condylomata acuminata* refers to an epidermal manifestation caused by epidermotropic human papillomavirus. The most commonly affected areas are the penis, vulva, vagina, cervix, perineum, and perianal area. Courtesy of Centers for Disease Control and Prevention.

CHAPTER 73
Influenza

CLINICAL MANIFESTATIONS

Influenza illness typically begins with sudden onset of fever, often accompanied by nonproductive cough, chills or rigors, diffuse myalgia, headache, and malaise. Subsequently, respiratory tract symptoms, including sore throat, nasal congestion, rhinitis, and cough, become more prominent. Less commonly, abdominal pain, nausea, vomiting, and diarrhea are associated with influenza illness. In some children, influenza can appear as an upper respiratory tract illness or as a febrile illness with few respiratory tract symptoms. In infants, influenza can produce a nonspecific sepsis-like illness picture, and in infants and young children, influenza can cause otitis media, croup, pertussis-like illness, bronchiolitis, or pneumonia. Acute myositis secondary to influenza can manifest with calf tenderness and refusal to walk.

Although most children with influenza recover fully after 3 to 7 days of illness, complications may occur, even in previously healthy children. Neurological complications associated with influenza range from febrile seizures to severe encephalopathy and encephalitis with status epilepticus, resulting in neurological sequelae or death. Reye syndrome, now a very rare condition, has been associated with influenza and the use of aspirin therapy during the illness. Children with influenza or suspected influenza should not be given aspirin, and children with diseases that necessitate long-term aspirin therapy or salicylate-containing medication, including juvenile idiopathic arthritis or Kawasaki disease, should be recognized as having increased risk for complications from influenza. Death from influenza-associated myocarditis has been reported. Invasive secondary infections or coinfections with *Staphylococcus aureus* (including methicillin-resistant *S aureus*), *Streptococcus pneumoniae*, group A streptococcus, or other bacterial pathogens can result in severe disease and death.

ETIOLOGY

Influenza viruses are orthomyxoviruses of 3 genera or types (A, B, and C). Annual epidemics are caused by influenza virus types A and B, and both influenza A and B virus antigens are included in seasonal influenza vaccines. Type C influenza viruses can cause sporadic mild influenzalike illness in children. Type C antigens are not included in influenza vaccines. Influenza A viruses are subclassified into subtypes based on their surface antigens, hemagglutinin (HA) and neuraminidase (NA). Examples of these virus subtypes include H1N1 and H3N2 influenza A viruses. Specific antibodies to these various antigens, especially to HA, are important determinants of immunity.

A minor antigenic variation that leads to changes in the HA or NA surface proteins of influenza A or B viruses is termed *antigenic drift*. Antigenic drift occurs continuously and results in new strains of influenza A and B viruses, resulting in seasonal epidemics.

A major antigenic variation that leads to new subtypes containing a unique HA and/or NA is termed *antigenic shift*. When the new virus subtype can infect humans and be transmitted efficiently from person to person in a sustained manner, this can lead to a pandemic because the human population has little or no preexisting immunity to the newly emerged influenza strain. Antigenic shift occurs only among influenza A viruses and has produced 4 influenza pandemics in the 20th and 21st centuries, the most recent in 2009. As with previous antigenic shifts, the 2009 pandemic influenza A (H1N1) viral strain subsequently replaced the previously circulating seasonal influenza A (H1N1) strain in the ensuing influenza seasons.

Humans of all ages may sporadically be infected with emerging influenza A viruses of swine or avian origin. Most notable among avian influenza viruses are A (H5N1), which emerged in 1997 in Hong Kong, and A (H7N9), first detected in 2013 in China, both of which have been associated with severe disease and high case-fatality rates. Since 2017, A (H7N9) is considered the influenza virus with the highest potential pandemic risk. Infection with a novel influenza A virus is a nationally notifiable disease and should be reported to the Centers for Disease Control and Prevention (CDC) through state health departments.

EPIDEMIOLOGY

Influenza is spread person to person, primarily through large-particle respiratory droplet transmission (eg, coughing, sneezing), which requires close proximity between the person who is the source and the person who is the recipient because droplets generally travel only short distances. Another mode of transmission comes from contact with influenza virus from droplet-contaminated hands or surfaces, where it can remain for up to 24 hours, with transfer from hands to mucosal surfaces of the face. Airborne transmission via small-particle aerosols in the vicinity of the infectious individual may also occur. Influenza is highly contagious, and patients may be infectious 24 hours before onset of symptoms. Viral shedding in nasal secretions usually peaks during the first 3 days of illness and ceases within 7 days but can be prolonged ($\geq$10 days) in young children and immunodeficient patients.

Influenza activity in the United States can occur anytime from October to May but most commonly peaks between December and February. Seasonal epidemics can last 8 to 12 weeks or longer. Circulation of 2 or 3 influenza virus strains in a community may be associated with a prolonged influenza season and may produce bimodal peaks in activity.

Seasonal influenza epidemics are associated with an estimated 9.3 to 45 million illnesses, 140,000 to 810,000 hospitalizations, and 12,000 to 61,000 respiratory and circulatory deaths annually in the United States. The CDC estimates that on average, 8% (range, 3%–11%) of the US population develops symptomatic influenza illness each season, depending on the circulating strains. During community outbreaks of influenza, the highest influenza incidence occurs among children, ranging from 10% to 40%, particularly school-aged children. Secondary spread to adults and other children within a family is common.

Hospitalization rates among children younger than 5 years are high and are like hospitalization rates among people 65 years and older. Although rates vary across studies (190–480 per 100,000 population) because of differences in methodology and severity of influenza seasons, children younger than 2 years consistently have a substantially higher risk for hospitalization than do older children. Rates of hospitalization and morbidity attributable to complications, such as bronchitis and pneumonia, are greater among children with high-risk conditions, including chronic pulmonary diseases such as asthma, neurological and neurodevelopmental disorders, hemodynamically significant cardiac disease, obesity, immunosuppression, metabolic diseases such as diabetes mellitus, and hemoglobinopathies such as sickle cell disease. However, 40% to 50% of all children hospitalized with influenza have no known underlying conditions, and almost half of children who die of influenza do not have an underlying high-risk condition. The number of reported annual influenza-related deaths of both chronically ill and previously healthy children usually ranges from 35 to 188, with higher numbers reported in some seasons. All influenza-associated pediatric deaths are nationally notifiable and must be reported to the CDC through state health departments.

The **incubation period** is usually 1 to 4 days, with a mean of 2 days.

DIAGNOSTIC TESTS

Influenza testing should be performed when the results are anticipated to influence clinical management (eg, to inform the decision to initiate antiviral therapy or antibiotic agents, to pursue other diagnostic testing, or to implement infection prevention and control measures). The decision to test is related to the level of local influenza activity, clinical suspicion for influenza, and the sensitivity and specificity of commercially available influenza tests (Table 73.1). These include rapid molecular assays for influenza RNA or nucleic acid detection, reverse transcriptase–polymerase chain reaction (RT-PCR) single-plex or multiplex assays, real-time or other RNA-based assays, immunofluorescence assays (direct or indirect fluorescent antibody staining) for antigen detection, rapid influenza diagnostic tests based on antigen detection, rapid cell culture (shell vial culture), and viral tissue cell culture (conventional) for virus isolation. The optimal choice of influenza test depends on the clinical setting.

The sensitivity and specificity of any influenza test varies by type of test used, time from illness onset to specimen collection, quality of specimen collected, source of specimen, and handling and processing of specimen, including time from

Table 73.1
Summary of Influenza Diagnostic Tests

Influenza Diagnostic Test	Method	Availability	Typical Processing Time	Sensitivity, %	Types Detected
Rapid influenza diagnostic tests[a]	Antigen detection	Wide	<15 min	10–70	A and B
Rapid molecular assays[b]	RNA or nucleic acid detection	Wide	15–30 min	86–100	A and B
Nucleic acid amplification (RT-PCR and other molecular assays)[c]	RNA or nucleic acid detection	Limited	1–8 h	86–100	A and B
Direct and indirect immunofluorescent antibody assays[c]	Antigen detection	Wide	1–4 h	70–100	A and B
Rapid cell culture (shell vials and cell mixtures)[c]	Virus isolation	Limited	1–3 days	100	A and B
Tissue cell culture[c]	Virus isolation	Limited	3–10 days	100	A and B

CLIA indicates Clinical Laboratory Improvement Amendments; RT-PCR, reverse transcriptase–polymerase chain reaction. May be single-plex or multiplex, real-time, and other RNA-based assays.

[a] Most rapid influenza diagnostic tests are CLIA waived.
[b] Some rapid influenza molecular assays are CLIA waived, depending on the specimen.
[c] Not CLIA waived. Requires laboratory expertise.

Adapted from Influenza (flu). Information for clinicians on influenza virus testing. Centers for Disease Control and Prevention. Accessed June 23, 2022. https://www.cdc.gov/flu/professionals/diagnosis/index.htm.

specimen collection to testing. To diagnose influenza in the outpatient or inpatient setting, testing should occur as soon after illness onset as possible, because the quantity of virus shed decreases rapidly as illness progresses. Nasopharyngeal swab specimens have the highest yield of upper respiratory tract specimens for detection of influenza viruses. Mid-turbinate nasal swab or wash specimens are also acceptable. Testing with combined nasal and throat swab specimens may increase the detection of influenza viruses over single specimens from either site (particularly over throat swab specimens alone). Using flocked swabs improves influenza virus detection over nonflocked swabs. For patients with respiratory failure receiving mechanical ventilation, including patients with negative influenza testing results on upper respiratory tract specimens, endotracheal aspirate or bronchoalveolar lavage fluid specimens should be obtained. Nonrespiratory specimens such as blood, plasma, serum, cerebrospinal fluid, urine, and stool should not be used for routine diagnosis of influenza. Results of influenza testing should be properly interpreted in the context of clinical findings and local community influenza activity, because the prevalence of circulating influenza viruses influences the positive and negative predictive values of these influenza screening tests. False-positive results are more likely to occur during periods of low influenza activity; false-negative results are more likely to occur during periods of peak influenza activity.

TREATMENT

In the United States, 3 classes of antiviral medications with different mechanisms of action are currently approved for treatment or prophylaxis of influenza. Two of these classes are used in clinical management of influenza disease: 3 drugs in the NA inhibitor class (oral oseltamivir, inhaled zanamivir, and intravenous peramivir) and 1 drug in the cap-dependent endonuclease inhibitor class (oral baloxavir marboxil). Guidance for use of these antiviral agents is summarized in Table 73.2.

Oseltamivir remains the antiviral drug of choice for treatment of influenza A and B. The US Food and Drug Administration has approved oseltamivir for influenza treatment in children as young as 2 weeks of age. Given available pharmacokinetic data and safety data, though, oseltamivir can be used to treat influenza in both full-term and preterm infants from birth, because benefits of therapy are likely to outweigh possible risks of treatment.

Table 73.2
Antiviral Drugs for Influenza[a]

Drug (Trade Name)	Virus	Administration	Treatment Indications	Chemoprophylaxis Indications	Adverse Effects
Oseltamivir (Tamiflu)	A and B	Oral twice daily for 5 days	Birth or older[b]	3 months or older	Nausea, vomiting, headache; skin reactions
Zanamivir (Relenza)	A and B	Inhalation twice daily for 5 days	7 years or older	5 years or older	Bronchospasm, skin reactions
Peramivir (Rapivab)	A and B[c]	Intravenous as a single dose	2 years or older	Not recommended	Diarrhea, skin reactions
Baloxavir marboxil (Xofluza)[d]	A and B	Oral as a single dose	12 years or older and weight ≥40 kg	Not recommended	Nausea, vomiting, diarrhea

[a] For current recommendations about treatment and chemoprophylaxis of influenza, including specific dosing information, see www.aapredbook.org/flu and www.cdc.gov/flu/professionals/antivirals/index.htm. Antiviral susceptibilities of viral strains are reported weekly at www.cdc.gov/flu/weekly/fluactivitysurv.htm.
[b] Approved by the US Food and Drug Administration for children as young as 2 weeks. Given available pharmacokinetic data and limited safety data, the American Academy of Pediatrics believes that oseltamivir can be used to treat influenza in both full-term and preterm infants from birth because benefits of therapy are likely to outweigh possible risks of treatment.
[c] Peramivir efficacy is based on clinical trials in which the predominant influenza virus type was influenza A; a limited number of participants infected with influenza B virus were enrolled.
[d] Long-acting endonuclease inhibitor with different mechanism of action than that of neuraminidase inhibitors. Greater activity on influenza B reported compared with oseltamivir.

Inhaled zanamivir is an acceptable alternative for older children. Intravenous peramivir is approved for use in people 2 years and older. Oral baloxavir is approved for people 12 years and older.

Resistance to oseltamivir and zanamivir has been documented in less than 1% of the tested influenza viral samples during the past seasons. Decreased susceptibility to baloxavir has been reported in Japan, where use has been more common, and surveillance for resistance among circulating influenza viruses is ongoing in the United States.

Regardless of influenza vaccination status and duration of symptoms, antiviral treatment should be offered as early as possible to any hospitalized child with suspected or confirmed influenza disease; any child, inpatient or outpatient, with severe, complicated, or progressive influenza illness; and children with influenza virus infection of any severity who have high risk for complications of influenza.

Antiviral treatment may be considered for any otherwise healthy child clinically presumed to have influenza disease if treatment can be initiated within 48 hours of illness onset and for those whose siblings or household contacts are younger than 6 months or have a high-risk condition that predisposes them to complications of influenza.

Children with severe influenza should be evaluated carefully for possible coinfection with bacterial pathogens (eg, *S aureus* or *S pneumoniae*) that might require antimicrobial therapy.

The most common adverse effects of oseltamivir are nausea and vomiting. Postmarketing reports, almost exclusively from Japan, have noted self-injury and delirium with use of oseltamivir in pediatric patients, but other data suggest that these occurrences may have been related to influenza disease itself rather than antiviral therapy. Zanamivir use has been associated with bronchospasm in some people and is not recommended for use in patients with underlying reactive airway disease. The most common adverse effects of baloxavir are nausea, vomiting, and diarrhea.

Control of fever with acetaminophen or another appropriate nonsalicylate-containing antipyretic agent may be important in some children, because fever and other symptoms of influenza could exacerbate underlying chronic conditions. Children and adolescents with influenza should not receive aspirin or any salicylate-containing products because of the potential risk of developing Reye syndrome.

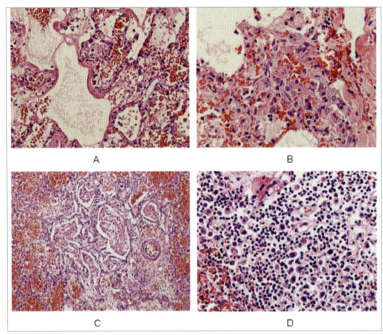

Image 73.1
Pathological findings from a patient with confirmed influenza A (H5N1) infection (hematoxylin-eosin stain, magnification ×40). A, Hyaline membrane formation lining the alveolar spaces of the lung and vascular congestion with a few infiltrating lymphocytes in the interstitial areas. Reactive fibroblasts are also present. B, An area of lung with proliferating reactive fibroblasts within the interstitial areas. Few lymphocytes are visible, and no viral intranuclear inclusions are visible. C, Fibrinous exudates filling the alveolar spaces, with organizing formation and few hyaline membranes. The surrounding alveolar spaces contain hemorrhage. D, A section of spleen showing numerous atypical lymphoid cells scattered around the white pulp. No viral intranuclear inclusions are visible. Courtesy of Centers for Disease Control and Prevention.

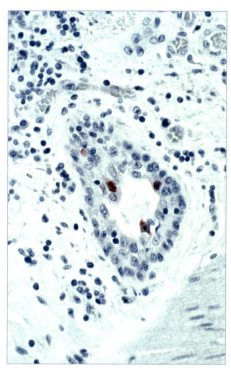

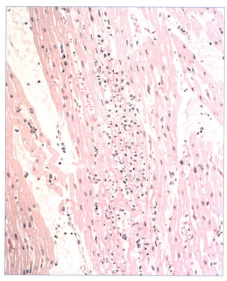

Image 73.3
Focal myocarditis observed in a patient with influenza B infection. Note myocardial necrosis associated with areas of mostly mononuclear inflammation. Courtesy of Centers for Disease Control and Prevention.

Image 73.2
Influenza viral antigens in bronchial epithelial lining cells as visualized with immunohistochemistry. Courtesy of Centers for Disease Control and Prevention.

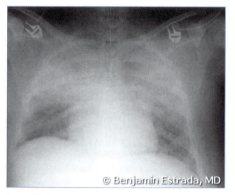

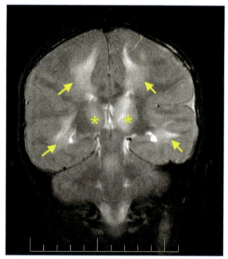

Image 73.4
Influenza pneumonia in a 12-year-old boy with respiratory failure. Courtesy of Benjamin Estrada, MD.

Image 73.5
Coronal T2-weighted magnetic resonance image of a 5-year-old with influenza-associated encephalopathy demonstrating bilateral confluent signal hyperintensity in the white matter (arrows) and thalami (asterisks). Courtesy of James Sejvar, MD.

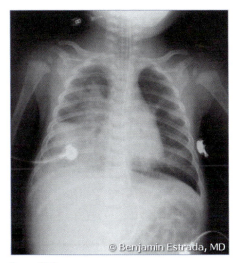

Image 73.6
Influenza A with *Staphylococcus aureus* pneumonia with empyema in a preschool-aged child. Courtesy of Benjamin Estrada, MD.

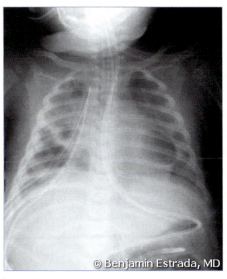

Image 73.7
Influenza A with *Staphylococcus aureus* superinfection in a 6-year-old. Note the presence of bilateral pneumatoceles. Courtesy of Benjamin Estrada, MD.

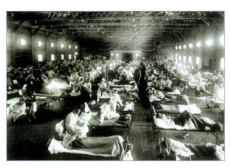

Image 73.8
Emergency hospital during 1918 influenza epidemic, Camp Funston, KS. Source: National Museum of Health and Medicine, Armed Forces Institute of Pathology, Washington, DC, Image NCP 1603. Courtesy of Immunization Action Coalition.

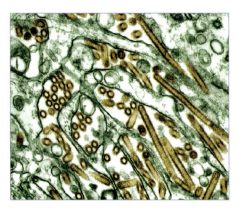

Image 73.9
Colorized transmission electron micrograph of avian influenza A (H5N1) viruses (gold) grown in Madin-Darby canine kidney epithelial cells (green). Avian influenza A viruses do not usually infect humans; however, several instances of human infections and outbreaks have been reported since 1997. When such infections occur, public health authorities monitor these situations closely. Courtesy of Centers for Disease Control and Prevention.

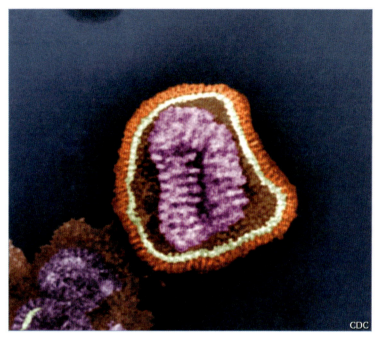

Image 73.10
This negative-stained transmission electron micrograph depicts the ultrastructural details of an influenza virus particle, or virion. Courtesy of Centers for Disease Control and Prevention/Erskine L. Palmer, MD/M. L. Martin, MD.

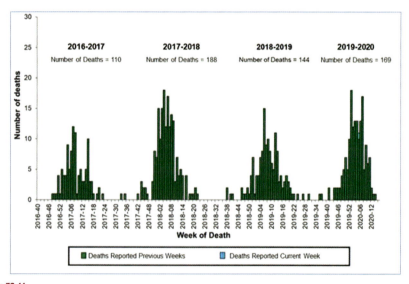

Image 73.11
Influenza-associated pediatric deaths by week of death, 2016–2017 season to 2019–2020 season. Courtesy of Centers for Disease Control and Prevention.

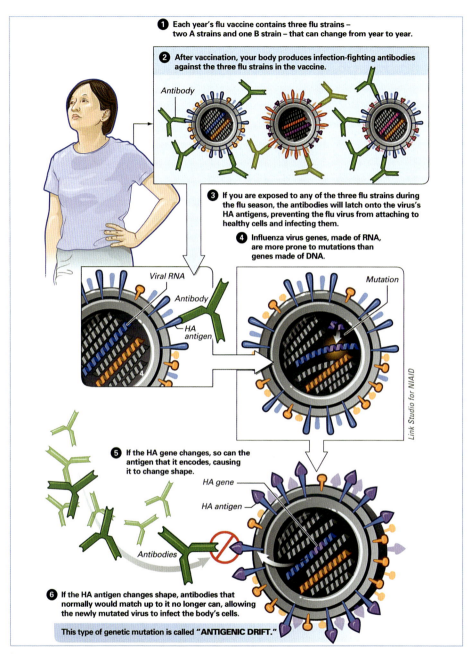

Image 73.12

Antigenic drift. Each year's flu vaccine contains 3 flu strains—2 A strains and 1 B strain—that can change from year to year. After vaccination, the body produces infection-fighting antibodies against the 3 flu strains in the vaccine. If a vaccinated individual is exposed to any of the 3 flu strains during the flu season, the antibodies will latch on to the virus hemagglutinin (HA) antigens, preventing the flu virus from attaching to healthy cells and infecting them. Influenza virus genes, made of RNA, are more prone to mutations than genes made of DNA. If the HA gene changes, so can the antigen that it encodes, causing it to change shape. If the HA antigen changes shape, antibodies that would normally match up to it no longer can, allowing the newly mutated virus to infect the body's cells. This type of genetic mutation is called *antigenic drift*. Courtesy of National Institute of Allergy and Infectious Diseases.

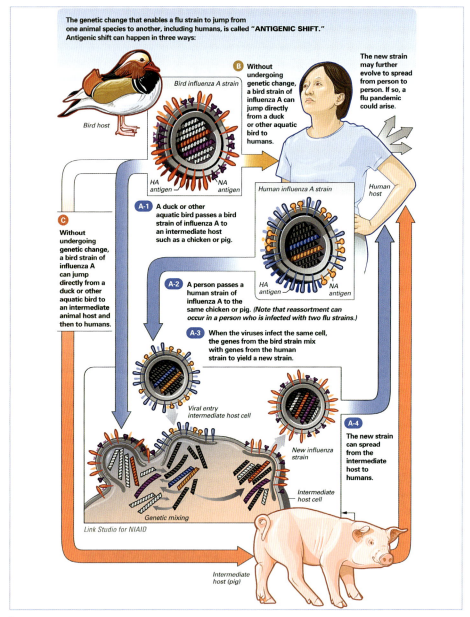

Image 73.13

Antigenic shift. The genetic change that enables a flu strain to jump from one animal species to another, including humans, is called *antigenic shift*. Antigenic shift can happen in 3 ways. Antigenic shift 1: A duck or other aquatic birds pass a bird strain of influenza A to an intermediate host, such as a chicken or pig. A person passes a human strain of influenza A to the same chicken or pig. When the viruses infect the same cell, genes from the bird strain mix with genes from the human strain to yield a new strain. The new strain can spread from the intermediate host to humans. Antigenic shift 2: Without undergoing genetic change, a bird strain of influenza A can jump directly from a duck or other aquatic birds to humans. Antigenic shift 3: Without undergoing genetic change, a bird strain of influenza A can jump directly from a duck or other aquatic birds to an intermediate animal host and then to humans. The new strain may further evolve to spread from person to person. If so, a flu pandemic could arise. HA indicates hemagglutinin; NA, neuraminidase. Courtesy of National Institute of Allergy and Infectious Diseases.

CHAPTER 74
Kawasaki Disease

CLINICAL MANIFESTATIONS

Kawasaki disease is a vasculitis of medium-sized arteries, the diagnosis of which is made in patients with fever in addition to the presence of the following clinical criteria:

1. Bilateral injection of the bulbar conjunctivae with limbic sparing and without exudate
2. Erythematous mouth and pharynx, strawberry tongue, and red, cracked lips
3. A polymorphous, generalized, erythematous rash, often with accentuation in the groin, which can be morbilliform, maculopapular, scarlatiniform, or erythema multiforme–like
4. Changes in the peripheral extremities consisting of erythema of the palms and soles and firm, sometimes painful, induration of the hands and feet, often with periungual desquamation usually beginning 10 to 14 days after fever onset
5. Acute, nonsuppurative, usually unilateral, anterior cervical lymphadenopathy with at least 1 node 1.5 cm or greater in diameter

The diagnosis of classic (or complete) Kawasaki disease is based on the presence of 5 or more days of fever and 4 or more of the 5 principal features described. Clinicians should consider Kawasaki disease in their differential diagnosis before the fifth day of fever if several of the principal features are present without alternative explanation. Individual clinical manifestations may appear and self-resolve rather than be present simultaneously. It is important to question about previous presence of relevant manifestations when a patient seeks medical attention for persistent fever.

The correct diagnosis is sometimes delayed in patients who seek medical attention because of fever and unilateral neck swelling, which are mistakenly thought to be attributable to bacterial lymph node or parapharyngeal or retropharyngeal infection. A distinguishing clinical and imaging feature in these cases is that suppuration is generally not observed in Kawasaki disease. Concurrent viral upper respiratory tract infection is sometimes present in a patient with Kawasaki disease and, even if confirmed by virus detection, should not delay treatment of Kawasaki disease. (An exception is the patient with fever, exudative conjunctivitis, and exudative pharyngitis, in whom adenovirus is detected. In such cases, Kawasaki disease is considered extremely unlikely.)

The following mucocutaneous or laboratory findings should prompt a search for an alternative diagnosis to Kawasaki disease: bullous, vesicular, or petechial rash; oral ulcers; pharyngeal or conjunctival exudates; generalized lymphadenopathy or splenomegaly; or leukopenia or relative lymphocyte predominance. Prior infection with SARS-CoV-2, the virus that causes COVID-19 and has caused the worldwide pandemic that began in early 2020, increases the likelihood of multisystem inflammatory syndrome in children (MIS-C) as the cause in a child presenting with symptoms suggestive of Kawasaki disease. Although features of MIS-C overlap with those of Kawasaki disease, MIS-C has a wider spectrum of symptoms. Patients with MIS-C are typically older than 7 years, are of African or Hispanic origin, and show greater elevation of inflammatory marker levels. More than 80% of patients with MIS-C also present with an unusual cardiac injury shown by high concentrations of troponin and brain natriuretic peptide, whereas others develop arrhythmia, left ventricle dysfunction, and unusual coronary dilatation or aneurysms.

The diagnosis of incomplete Kawasaki disease should be considered in children with unexplained fever who lack all 5 of the principal clinical criteria. Supportive laboratory and echocardiography data are also sought when considering the diagnosis of incomplete Kawasaki disease. In 2017, the American Heart Association (AHA) published updated guidelines for the diagnosis, treatment, and long-term management of Kawasaki disease. An algorithm for diagnosis and treatment of suspected incomplete Kawasaki disease is provided in Figure 74.1. A high index of suspicion for Kawasaki disease should be maintained for infants, particularly those younger than 6 months, because compared with older children, infants have heightened risk for incomplete manifestations, delayed diagnosis, and development of coronary artery aneurysms. Kawasaki disease should be considered in infants younger than

Figure 74.1
Evaluation of Suspected Incomplete Kawasaki Disease[a]

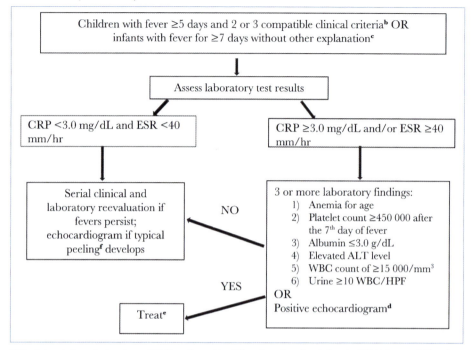

ALT indicates alanine aminotransferase; CRP, C-reactive protein; ESR, erythrocyte sedimentation rate; HPF, high-power field; and WBC, white blood cell.

[a] In the absence of a gold standard for diagnosis, this algorithm cannot be evidence based but rather represents the informed opinion of the expert committee. Consultation with an expert should be sought anytime assistance is needed.
[b] See text for clinical findings of Kawasaki disease.
[c] Infants ≤6 months of age are the most likely to develop prolonged fever without other clinical criteria for Kawasaki disease; these infants are at particularly high risk of developing coronary artery abnormalities.
[d] Echocardiography is considered positive for purposes of this algorithm if any of 3 conditions are met: z score of left anterior descending coronary artery or right coronary artery ≥2.5; coronary artery aneurysm is observed; or ≥3 other suggestive features exist, including decreased left ventricular function, mitral regurgitation, pericardial effusion, or z scores in left anterior descending coronary artery or right coronary artery of 2–2.5.
[e] Treatment should be given within 10 days of fever onset. See text for indications for treatment after the tenth day of fever.
[f] Typical peeling begins under the nail beds of fingers and toes.

Source: McCrindle BW, Rowley AH, Newburger JW, et al; American Heart Association Rheumatic Fever, Endocarditis, and Kawasaki Disease Committee of the Council on Cardiovascular Disease in the Young; Council on Cardiovascular and Stroke Nursing; Council on Cardiovascular Surgery and Anesthesia; and Council on Epidemiology and Prevention. Diagnosis, treatment, and long-term management of Kawasaki disease: a scientific statement for health professionals from the American Heart Association. *Circulation.* 2017;135(17):e927–e999. Accessed June 23, 2022. https://www.ahajournals.org/doi/full/10.1161/CIR.0000000000000484.

12 months with prolonged unexplained fever, with or without aseptic meningitis, with evidence of systemic inflammation, even with fewer than 2 of the characteristic features of Kawasaki disease. Other manifestations of Kawasaki disease include infants and children with a shock-like syndrome in whom an inciting infection is not confirmed and those with presumed bacterial cervical lymphadenitis or parapharyngeal or retropharyngeal phlegmon that fails to respond to appropriate antibiotic therapy.

If coronary artery aneurysm or ectasia is evident (z score ≥2.5) in any patient evaluated for fever, a presumptive diagnosis of Kawasaki disease should be made. A normal early echocardiographic study is typical and does not exclude the diagnosis but may be useful in evaluation of patients with suspected incomplete Kawasaki disease. In one study, 80% of patients with Kawasaki disease who ultimately developed coronary artery disease had abnormalities (z score ≥2.5) on an echocardiogram obtained during the first 10 days of illness.

Other clinical features of Kawasaki disease include irritability, abdominal pain, diarrhea, and vomiting. Other examination and laboratory findings include urethritis with sterile pyuria (70% of cases), mild anterior uveitis (80%), mild elevation of serum hepatic aminotransferase concentrations (50%), arthralgia or arthritis (10%–20%), marked irritability with cerebrospinal fluid pleocytosis (40%), hydrops of the gallbladder (<10%), pericardial effusion of at least 1 mm (<5%), myocarditis manifesting as congestive heart failure (<5%), and cranial nerve palsy (<1%). Persistent resting tachycardia and a hyperdynamic precordium are common findings, and an S_3 gallop can be present. Fine desquamation in the groin area can occur in the acute phase of disease (Fink sign). Inflammation or ulceration may be observed at the inoculation scar of previous BCG immunization. Rarely, Kawasaki disease can manifest with acute shock; these children often have significant thrombocytopenia attributable to consumption coagulopathy, which also causes a low erythrocyte sedimentation rate (ESR). Group A streptococcal or *Staphylococcus aureus* toxic shock syndrome should be excluded in such cases.

The average duration of fever in untreated Kawasaki disease is 10 days; however, fever can last 2 weeks or longer. After fever resolves, patients can remain anorexic and/or irritable with decreased energy for 2 to 3 weeks. During this phase, branny desquamation of fingers, toes, hands, and feet may occur. Transverse lines across the nails (Beau lines) are sometimes noted month(s) later. Recurrent disease develops in approximately 1% to 2% of patients in the United States at a median of 1.5 years after the index episode. The recurrence rate is 3.5% in Asian and Pacific Islander populations.

Coronary artery abnormalities are serious sequelae of Kawasaki disease, occurring in 20% to 25% of untreated children. Increased risk of developing coronary artery abnormalities is associated with male sex; age younger than 12 months or older than 8 years; fever for more than 10 days; white blood cell count greater than 15,000/μL; high relative neutrophil (>80%) and band count; low hemoglobin concentration (<10 g/dL); hypoalbuminemia, hyponatremia, or thrombocytopenia; and fever persisting or recurring more than 36 hours after completion of immune globulin intravenous (IGIV) administration. Aneurysms of the coronary arteries most typically occur between 1 and 4 weeks after onset of illness; onset later than 6 weeks is extremely uncommon. Giant coronary artery aneurysms (internal diameter ≥8 mm) are highly predictive of long-term complications. Aneurysms occurring in other medium-sized arteries (eg, iliac, femoral, renal, and axillary vessels) are uncommon and do not generally occur in the absence of significant coronary abnormalities. In addition to coronary artery disease, carditis can involve the pericardium, myocardium, or endocardium, and mitral or aortic regurgitation or both can develop. Carditis generally resolves when fever resolves.

In children with only mild coronary artery dilation, coronary artery dimensions often return to baseline within 6 to 8 weeks after onset of disease. Approximately 50% of coronary aneurysms (but only a small proportion of giant aneurysms) regress by echocardiography to normal luminal size within 1 to 2 years, although this process can result in luminal stenosis or a poorly compliant, fibrotic vessel wall or both.

The current case-fatality rate for Kawasaki disease in the United States and Japan is less than 0.2%. The principal cause of death is myocardial infarction resulting from coronary artery occlusion attributable to thrombosis or progressive stenosis. The relative risk of mortality is highest within 6 weeks of onset of acute symptoms, but myocardial infarction and sudden death can occur months to years after the acute episode. There is no current evidence that the vasculitis of Kawasaki disease predisposes to premature atherosclerotic coronary artery disease.

ETIOLOGY

The etiology is unknown. Epidemiological and clinical features suggest an infectious and/or an environmental cause or trigger in genetically susceptible individuals.

EPIDEMIOLOGY

Peak age of occurrence in the United States is 6 to 24 months. Fifty percent of patients are younger than 2 years, and 80% are younger than 5 years; cases are uncommon in children older than 8 years, but rare cases have occurred even in adults. The prevalence of coronary artery abnormalities is higher if treatment (IGIV) is delayed beyond the 10th day of illness. The male-to-female ratio is approximately 1.5:1. In the United States, 4,000 to 5,500 cases are estimated to occur each year; the incidence is highest among children of Asian ancestry. Kawasaki disease was first described in Japan, where a pattern of endemic occurrence with superimposed epidemic outbreaks was recognized. More cases, including clusters, occur during winter and spring. Little evidence indicates person-to-person or common-source spread, although the incidence is 10-fold higher among siblings of children with the disease than among the general population, and more than 50% of sibling cases occur within 10 days of the index case.

The **incubation period** is unknown.

DIAGNOSTIC TESTS

No specific diagnostic test is available. The diagnosis is established by fulfillment of the clinical criteria after consideration of other possible illnesses, such as staphylococcal or streptococcal toxin-mediated disease; drug reactions (eg, Stevens-Johnson syndrome); MIS-C; measles, adenovirus, Epstein-Barr virus, parvovirus B19, or enterovirus infections; rickettsial exanthems; leptospirosis; systemic-onset juvenile idiopathic arthritis; and reactive arthritis. The identification of a respiratory virus by molecular testing does not exclude the diagnosis of Kawasaki disease in infants and children whose condition has otherwise met diagnostic criteria. A markedly increased ESR and/or serum C-reactive protein (CRP) concentration during the first 2 weeks of illness and an increased platelet count (>450,000/μL) on days 10 to 21 of illness are almost universal laboratory features. ESR and platelet count are usually normal within 6 to 8 weeks; CRP concentration returns to normal much sooner.

TREATMENT

Management during the acute phase is directed at decreasing inflammation of the myocardium and coronary artery wall and providing supportive care. Therapy should be initiated as soon as the diagnosis is established or strongly suspected. Once the acute phase has subsided, therapy is directed at prevention of coronary artery thrombosis.

Primary Treatment

Immune Globulin Intravenous

A single dose of IGIV, 2 g/kg, administered over 10 to 12 hours, results in rapid resolution of fever and other clinical and laboratory indicators of acute inflammation in approximately 85% of patients and has been proven to reduce the risk of coronary artery aneurysms from 17% to 4% in children with a normal first echocardiogram. IGIV plus aspirin is the treatment of choice and should be initiated as soon as the diagnosis is established or strongly suspected and alternative diagnoses are unlikely, whether or not coronary artery abnormalities are detected. Despite prompt treatment with IGIV and aspirin, approximately 2% to 4% of patients develop coronary artery aneurysms even when treatment is initiated before the onset of coronary artery abnormalities.

Efficacy of therapy initiated later than the 10th day of illness or after detection of aneurysms has not been evaluated fully. However, therapy with IGIV and aspirin should be provided for patients whose diagnosis is made more than 10 days after the onset of fever (ie, the diagnosis was not made earlier) and who have manifestations of continuing inflammation (ie, elevated ESR or CRP level ≥3.0 mg/dL) plus either fever or coronary artery luminal dimension z score greater than 2.5.

IGIV infusion reactions (ie, fever, chills, hypotension) are somewhat common. Occasionally, Coombs-positive hemolytic anemia can complicate IGIV therapy, especially in individuals with AB blood type, and usually occurs within 5 to 10 days of infusion. Aseptic meningitis can result from IGIV therapy and resolves quickly without neurological sequelae. IGIV infusion results in elevation of the ESR; therefore, ESR is not a useful test to monitor disease activity after infusion. CRP is not affected by IGIV administration and can be used.

Aspirin

Aspirin is used for its anti-inflammatory (high-dose) and antithrombotic (low-dose) activity, although aspirin alone does not decrease the risk of coronary artery abnormalities. Guidelines vary with regard to dose, with Japanese and western European clinicians frequently using 30 to 50 mg/kg/day and US clinicians using 80 to 100 mg/kg/day in 4 divided doses when the diagnosis is made and concurrently with IGIV administration. Children with acute Kawasaki disease have decreased aspirin absorption and increased clearance and rarely achieve therapeutic serum concentrations. It is generally unnecessary to monitor salicylate concentrations. High-dose aspirin therapy is usually given until the patient has been afebrile for 48 to 72 hours. Low-dose aspirin (3–5 mg/kg/day, in a single daily dose; maximum 81–325 mg/day) is then given until a follow-up echocardiogram at 6 to 8 weeks after onset of illness is normal in findings or is continued indefinitely for children in whom coronary artery abnormalities are present. In general, ibuprofen should be avoided in children who have coronary aneurysms and are taking aspirin, because ibuprofen and other nonsteroidal anti-inflammatory drugs with known or potential effects on the cyclooxygenase pathway interfere with the antiplatelet effect of acetylsalicylic acid to prevent thrombosis. The child and all household contacts older than 6 months should receive influenza vaccine according to seasonal recommendations. The inactivated injectable influenza vaccine (not live attenuated vaccine) should be used in the child receiving aspirin. Family members can receive either inactivated or live attenuated influenza vaccine.

Adjunctive Therapies for Primary Treatment

The following are 2017 consensus recommendations of the AHA: (1) single-dose pulse methylprednisolone should not be administered with IGIV as routine primary therapy for patients with Kawasaki disease and (2) administration of a longer course of corticosteroids (eg, prednisolone, 2 mg/kg/day intravenously, divided every 8 hours until afebrile, then an oral corticosteroid until CRP level normalizes, with subsequent tapering over 2–3 weeks) together with IGIV and aspirin may be considered for treatment of high-risk patients with acute Kawasaki disease, when such risk can be identified before initiation of treatment.

Management of IGIV Resistance and Re-treatment

Approximately 30% of patients who receive IGIV, 2 g/kg, plus aspirin have fever within the first 36 hours after completing the IGIV infusion, which does not indicate therapeutic failure. However, 10% to 20% of treated patients have recrudescent or persistent fever beyond 36 hours after completion of their IGIV infusion and are termed *IGIV resistant*. In these situations, the diagnosis of Kawasaki disease should be reevaluated. If Kawasaki disease is still considered to be most likely, re-treatment with IGIV, 2 g/kg, is usually given and high-dose aspirin is continued. Several small series and observational studies have described children with IGIV-resistant Kawasaki disease in whom administration of a single dose of infliximab or a variety of regimens of corticosteroids were associated with an improvement of symptoms, without adverse events.

Treatment of patients with Kawasaki disease refractory to a second dose of IGIV, infliximab, or a course of corticosteroids has included use of cyclosporine, other immune-modulating therapies, or plasma exchange but should be undertaken in consultation with an expert in Kawasaki disease.

Cardiac Care

Echocardiography should be performed at the time of suspected diagnosis and repeated at 2 weeks and 6 to 8 weeks after diagnosis in children with normal coronary arteries on initial evaluation. Coronary abnormalities warrant closer follow-up with echocardiography. Children with higher risk (eg, children with persistent or recrudescent fever after initial IGIV, children with baseline coronary artery abnormalities, very young patients) may require more frequent echocardiography to guide the need for additional therapies. Children should be assessed during this time for arrhythmias, congestive heart failure, and valvular regurgitation. The care of patients with significant cardiac abnormalities should involve a pediatric cardiologist experienced in treating patients with Kawasaki disease and in assessing echocardiographic studies of coronary arteries in children.

Long-term management of Kawasaki disease should be based on the extent of coronary artery involvement. In patients with persistent moderately large coronary artery aneurysms that are not large enough to warrant anticoagulation, clopidogrel (0.2–1 mg/kg/day) to antagonize adenosine diphosphate–mediated platelet activation in combination with prolonged low-dose aspirin is recommended.

Development of giant coronary artery aneurysms (luminal diameter ≥8 mm in a child, but smaller diameter in an infant on the basis of relative body surface area, z score ≥10) usually requires addition of anticoagulant therapy, such as warfarin or low-molecular-weight heparin, to prevent thrombosis. The AHA has provided recommendations regarding criteria for systemic anticoagulation and frequency of echocardiography in those with coronary aneurysms.

Subsequent Immunization

Measles- and varicella-containing vaccines should be deferred until 11 months after receipt of IGIV, 2 g/kg, for treatment of Kawasaki disease because of possible interference with development of an adequate immune response. If the child's risk of exposure to measles or varicella within this period is high, the child should be immunized and then reimmunized at least 11 months after administration of IGIV. Live attenuated varicella-containing vaccines should be avoided during aspirin therapy because of a theoretical concern of Reye syndrome. The schedule for administration of inactivated childhood vaccines should not be interrupted.

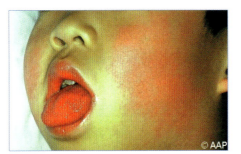

Image 74.1
A child with Kawasaki disease with striking facial rash and erythema of the oral mucous membrane.

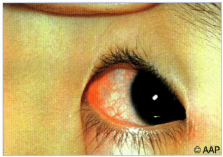

Image 74.2
A child with Kawasaki disease with conjunctivitis. Note the absence of conjunctival discharge.

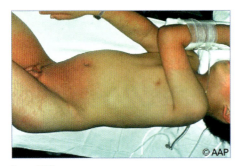

Image 74.3
Characteristic distribution of erythroderma of Kawasaki disease. The rash is accentuated in the perineal area in approximately two-thirds of patients.

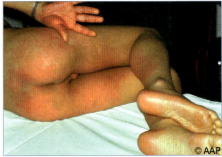

Image 74.4
Generalized erythema and early perianal and palmar desquamation. This is the same patient as in Image 74.3.

KAWASAKI DISEASE

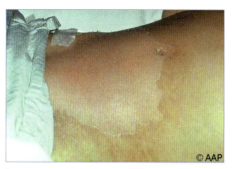

Image 74.5
Characteristic desquamation of the skin over the abdomen in a patient with Kawasaki disease. This is the same patient as in images 74.3 and 74.4.

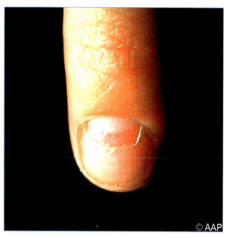

Image 74.6
Periungual desquamation of a patient with Kawasaki disease. This is the same patient as in images 74.3–74.5.

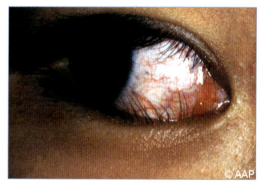

Image 74.7
Bulbar conjunctivitis in a patient is generally absent.

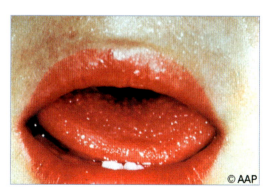

Image 74.8
Erythematous lips and injection of the oropharyngeal membranes in a patient with Kawasaki disease. Scarlet fever, toxic shock syndrome, staphylococcal scalded skin syndrome, and measles may be confused with this disease.

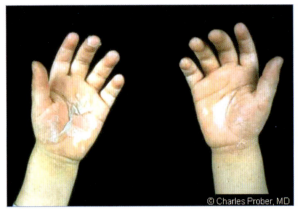

Image 74.9
A child with the characteristic desquamation of the hands in a later stage of Kawasaki disease. Copyright Charles Prober, MD.

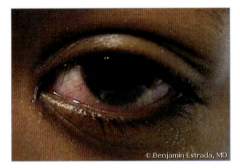

Image 74.10
Bulbar conjunctivitis in a 3-year-old boy with Kawasaki disease. Courtesy of Benjamin Estrada, MD.

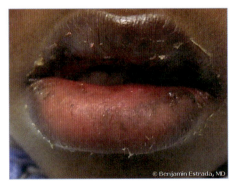

Image 74.11
Mucositis in a 3-year-old boy with Kawasaki disease. Courtesy of Benjamin Estrada, MD.

CHAPTER 75
Kingella kingae Infections

CLINICAL MANIFESTATIONS

The most common infections attributable to *Kingella kingae* are pyogenic arthritis, osteomyelitis, and bacteremia. Other infections caused by *K kingae* include diskitis, endocarditis (*K kingae* belongs to the HACEK group of organisms), meningitis, ocular infections, and pneumonia. The vast majority of *K kingae* infections affect children between 6 and 48 months of age, with most cases occurring in children younger than 2 years.

K kingae is a primary cause of skeletal infections in the first 4 years after birth. *K kingae* pyogenic arthritis is generally monoarticular and most commonly involves the knee, hip, or ankle. *K kingae* osteomyelitis most often involves the femur or tibia. The organism also shows an unusual predilection for the small joints of the hand and foot. Compared with the clinical manifestations of pyogenic arthritis and osteomyelitis in immunocompetent children caused by other pathogens, skeletal infections caused by *K kingae* can be milder and evolution can be more insidious, resulting in a more subacute manifestation in many cases. Evolution to chronicity or long-term sequelae are rare; however, Brodie abscesses of bone that are attributable to *K kingae* have been reported.

K kingae bacteremia can occur in children with previous health and in children with preexisting chronic medical problems. Children with *K kingae* bacteremia present with fever and frequently have concurrent symptoms of respiratory or gastrointestinal tract disease.

ETIOLOGY

K kingae is a gram-negative, encapsulated organism that belongs to the *Neisseriaceae* family. It is a fastidious, facultative anaerobic, β-hemolytic coccobacillus that appears as pairs or short chains with tapered ends. It often resists decolorization, sometimes resulting in misidentification as a gram-positive organism.

EPIDEMIOLOGY

The usual habitat of *K kingae* is the human posterior pharynx. The organism colonizes young children more frequently than older children or adults and can be transmitted among children in child care centers, occasionally causing clusters of cases. Infection may be associated with preceding or concomitant viral infections that cause hand-foot-and-mouth disease, herpetic gingivostomatitis, or nonspecific upper respiratory tract infections.

The **incubation period** relative to acquisition of colonization is not well-defined.

DIAGNOSTIC TESTS

K kingae can be isolated from blood, synovial fluid, bone, cerebrospinal fluid, respiratory tract secretions, and other fluid or tissues. Patients with pyogenic arthritis or osteomyelitis attributable to *K kingae* often have negative blood cultures. Organisms grow best in aerobic conditions with enhanced carbon dioxide. *K kingae* is difficult to isolate on routinely used solid media. Therefore, synovial fluid and bone aspirates from patients with suspected *K kingae* infection should be inoculated on both solid media and into an aerobic blood culture vial and held for 5 to 7 days to maximize recovery. Once the organism is recovered in culture, standard biochemical tests readily identify it; alternatively, mass spectrometry of bacterial cellular components may be used for rapid identification. When available, conventional and real-time polymerase chain reaction methods markedly improve detection of *K kingae* in young children with culture-negative skeletal infections. Such methods are available only in specialty laboratories.

TREATMENT

K kingae is usually highly susceptible to penicillins and cephalosporins, but in vitro susceptibility to oxacillin is relatively reduced. Nearly all isolates are susceptible to aminoglycosides, macrolides, tetracyclines, and fluoroquinolones. Between 40% and 100% of isolates are resistant to clindamycin, and virtually all isolates are resistant to glycopeptide antibiotics (eg, vancomycin) and trimethoprim (although most strains are susceptible to trimethoprim-sulfamethoxazole). Occasional isolates in parts of the United States and other countries have demonstrated TEM-I β-lactamase production resulting in low-level resistance to penicillin and ampicillin. The TEM-I β-lactamase is susceptible to β-lactamase inhibitors and lacks activity against second- and third-generation cephalosporins.

Ampicillin-sulbactam or a first- or second-generation cephalosporin is recommended for children with osteoarticular infections suspected to be attributable to *K kingae* (definitive therapy can be determined after β-lactamase production of the isolate is known). For more invasive or severe infections (eg, endocarditis), treatment with a third-generation cephalosporin or, if β-lactamase production has been ruled out, ampicillin plus an aminoglycoside should be considered.

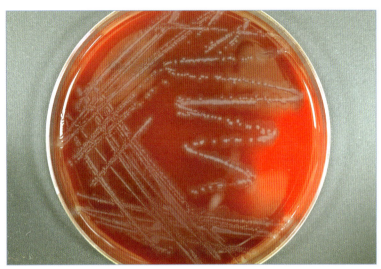

Image 75.1
Kingella kingae on blood agar. Smooth, gray colonies may pit the agar and are surrounded by a small but distinct zone of beta hemolysis on blood agar. Courtesy of Julia Rosebush, DO; Robert Jerris, PhD; and Theresa Stanley, M(ASCP).

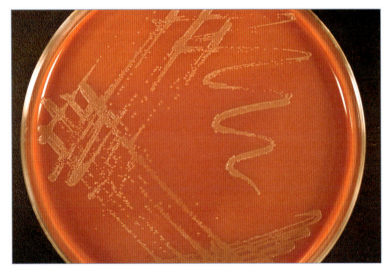

Image 75.2
Kingella kingae on chocolate agar. Colonies appear after 2–4 days of incubation on blood and chocolate agar. This species demonstrates beta hemolysis on blood agar. Courtesy of Julia Rosebush, DO; Robert Jerris, PhD; and Theresa Stanley, M(ASCP).

CHAPTER 76
Legionella pneumophila Infections

CLINICAL MANIFESTATIONS

Legionellosis is associated primarily with 2 clinically and epidemiologically distinct illnesses: legionnaires' disease and Pontiac fever. **Legionnaires' disease** manifests as pneumonia characterized by fever, cough with or without chest pain, and progressive respiratory distress. Legionnaires' disease can be associated with chills and rigors, headache, myalgia, and gastrointestinal tract, central nervous system, and renal manifestations. Overall (including adults) case-fatality rate is approximately 10%. **Pontiac fever** is a milder febrile illness, without pneumonia, that is characterized by an abrupt onset of a self-limited, influenzalike illness (ie, fever, myalgia, headache, weakness) resulting from the host inflammatory response to the bacterium. Cervical lymphadenitis caused by *Legionella* species has been reported and may produce a syndrome clinically similar to nontuberculous mycobacterial infection. Other extrapulmonary infections including endocarditis, graft infections, joint infections, and wound infections have also been reported.

ETIOLOGY

Legionella species are fastidious, small, gram-negative, aerobic bacilli that grow on buffered charcoal–yeast extract (BCYE) media. They constitute a single genus in the family *Legionellaceae*. At least 20 of the more than 60 known species have been implicated in human disease, but the most common species causing infections in the United States is *Legionella pneumophila*, with most isolates belonging to serogroup 1. Multiplication of *Legionella* organisms in water sources occurs optimally in temperatures between 25 °C (77 °F) and 42 °C (108 °F), although *Legionella* organisms have been recovered from water outside this temperature range.

EPIDEMIOLOGY

Legionnaires' disease is usually acquired through inhalation of aerosolized water containing *Legionella* species. Less frequently, transmission can occur via aspiration of *Legionella*-containing water. Only one case of possible person-to-person transmission has been reported. Outbreaks are commonly associated with buildings or structures that have complex water systems, like hotels and resorts, long-term care facilities, hospitals, and cruise ships. The most likely sources of infection include *Legionella*-containing water aerosolized from showerheads, cooling towers (parts of centralized air-conditioning systems for large buildings), hot tubs, decorative fountains, and humidifiers. Health care–associated infections can be related to contamination of the hot water supply. Legionnaires' disease should be considered in the differential diagnosis of patients who develop pneumonia during or after their hospitalization. Most cases of legionnaires' disease are sporadic, although they may be connected with unrecognized outbreaks or clusters. Legionnaires' disease is more common in older individuals (≥50 years), males, smokers, and individuals with weakened immune systems, malignancy, or chronic disease. Infection in children is rare, with 1% or less cases of pneumonia caused by *Legionella* infection, and may be asymptomatic or mild and unrecognized. Severe disease has occurred in children with malignancy, severe combined immunodeficiency, chronic granulomatous disease, organ transplant, end-stage renal disease, and underlying pulmonary disease and those treated with systemic corticosteroids or other immunosuppression. Health care–associated cases of *Legionella* infection in newborns, including severe and sometimes fatal cases, have been associated with a *Legionella*-containing water source (eg, humidifiers). Severe and fatal infections in neonates have occurred after birth in water (eg, using a birthing pool or hot tub).

The **incubation period** for legionnaires' disease is most commonly 2 to 10 days, with an average of 5 to 6 days, but can rarely occur up to 26 days. For Pontiac fever, the **incubation period** is generally 1 to 3 days but can be as short as 4 hours.

DIAGNOSTIC TESTS

When a patient is suspected of having legionnaires' disease, testing should include both culture of a lower respiratory tract specimen and testing for antigen in urine. Recovery of *Legionella* organisms from lower respiratory tract secretions, lung tissue, pleural fluid, or other normally sterile fluid specimens by using supplemented BCYE media provides definitive evidence of infection, but the sensitivity of culture is laboratory dependent.

Detection of *Legionella* lipopolysaccharide antigen in urine by commercially available immunoassays is highly specific. This test detects only *L pneumophila* serogroup 1; thus, other testing methods are needed to detect other *L pneumophila* serogroups and other *Legionella* species. Urinary antigen test sensitivity depends on the assay method used and on the severity of disease.

Genus-specific polymerase chain reaction (PCR)–based assays have been developed that detect *Legionella* DNA in lower respiratory tract specimens and blood. There is a commercially available PCR assay, present in a multiplexed nucleic acid format for detection of *L pneumophila* in lower respiratory tract specimens.

Detection of serum immunoglobulin M antibodies is not useful for diagnosis, and the positive predictive value of a single immunoglobulin G (IgG) titer of 1:256 or greater is low. A 4-fold increase in *L pneumophila*–specific IgG antibody titer, as measured by indirect immunofluorescent antibody (IFA), confirms a recent infection. This serological result is not useful for treatment decisions, however, because convalescent titers take 3 to 4 weeks to increase (and the increase may be delayed for 8–12 weeks). Antibodies to several gram-negative organisms, including *Pseudomonas* species, *Bacteroides fragilis*, and *Campylobacter jejuni*, can cause false-positive IFA test results.

TREATMENT

Patients with legionnaires' disease should receive antimicrobial agents. Intravenously administered azithromycin or levofloxacin (or another respiratory fluoroquinolone) is recommended. Once the patient's condition is improved clinically, oral therapy can be substituted. Doxycycline is an alternative agent; however, *Legionella longbeachae* is often resistant (this species is common in some geographic areas such as Australia and New Zealand). Duration of therapy is 5 to 10 days for azithromycin and 14 to 21 days for other drugs, with the longer courses of therapy for patients who are immunocompromised or who have severe disease.

Antimicrobial treatment for patients with Pontiac fever is not recommended.

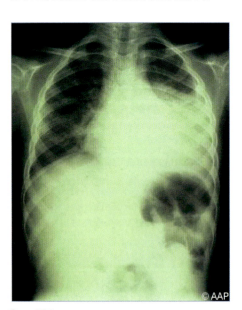

Image 76.1
An adult with pneumonia caused by *Legionella pneumophila*. *Legionella* infections are rare in otherwise healthy children. Although nosocomial infections and hospital outbreaks are reported, this infection is not transmitted from person to person.

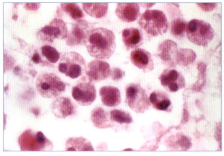

Image 76.2
This hematoxylin-eosin–stained micrograph of lung tissue biopsied from a patient with legionnaires' diseases revealed the presence of an intra-alveolar exudate consisting of macrophages and polymorphonuclear leucocytes. The *Legionella pneumophila* bacteria are not stained in this preparation (magnification ×500).
Courtesy of Centers for Disease Control and Prevention.

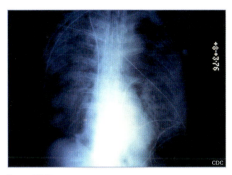

Image 76.3
This anteroposterior radiograph revealed bilateral pulmonary infiltrates in a patient with legionnaires' disease. Legionnaires' disease is an acute and sometimes fatal respiratory illness caused by *Legionella pneumophila* bacteria, whereby headache, high fever, cough, and flulike symptoms accompany the condition. Courtesy of Centers for Disease Control and Prevention.

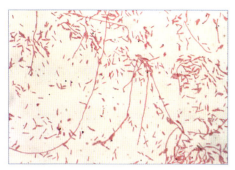

Image 76.4
This Gram-stained micrograph reveals chains and solitary gram-negative *Legionella pneumophila* bacteria found within a sample taken from an individual in the 1976 legionnaires' disease outbreak in Philadelphia, PA. Legionnaires' disease is the more severe form of legionellosis and is characterized by pneumonia, commencing 2–10 days after exposure. Pontiac fever is an acute-onset, flulike, non-pneumonic illness, occurring within 1–2 days of exposure. Courtesy of Centers for Disease Control and Prevention.

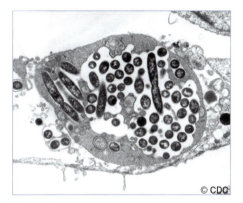

Image 76.5
Legionella pneumophila multiplying inside a cultured human lung fibroblast. Courtesy of Centers for Disease Control and Prevention.

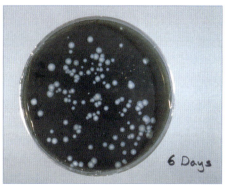

Image 76.6
Charcoal–yeast extract agar plate culture of *Legionella pneumophila*. Courtesy of Centers for Disease Control and Prevention.

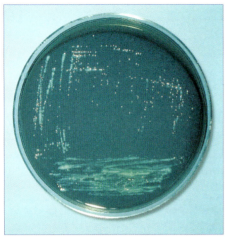

Image 76.7
Charcoal–yeast extract agar plate culture of *Legionella pneumophila*. Courtesy of Centers for Disease Control and Prevention.

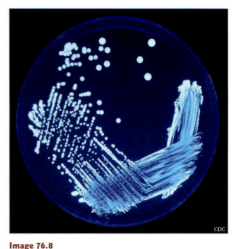

Image 76.8
This photograph shows numbers of *Legionella* species colonies, which had been cultivated on an agar-cultured plate and illuminated with UV light. At least 46 *Legionella* species and 70 serogroups have been identified. *Legionella pneumophila*, a ubiquitous aquatic bacterial organism that thrives in warm environments, primarily at temperatures ranging from 32–45 °C (89.6–113.0 °F), causes >90% of cases of legionnaires' disease in the United States. Courtesy of Centers for Disease Control and Prevention.

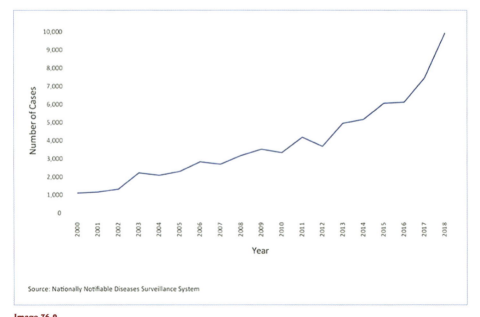

Image 76.9
Legionnaires' disease is on the rise in the United States, 2000–2018. Courtesy of Centers for Disease Control and Prevention.

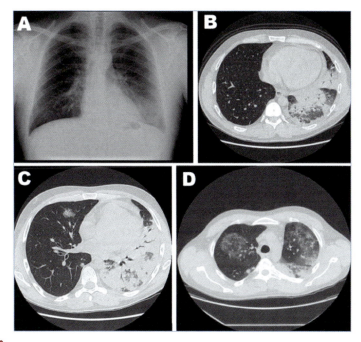

Image 76.10

Imaging studies of a 42-year-old man with severe pneumonia caused by *Legionella pneumophila* serogroup 11, showing lobar consolidation of the left lower lung lobe, with an air bronchogram within the homogeneous airspace consolidation. Consensual mild pleural effusion was documented by a chest radiograph (A) and high-resolution computed tomographic scan (B). A week after hospital admission, repeated high-resolution computed tomography of the chest showed extensive and homogeneous consolidation of left upper and lower lobes, accompanied by bilateral ground-glass opacities (C, D). Courtesy of *Emerging Infectious Diseases*.

CHAPTER 77
Leishmaniasis

CLINICAL MANIFESTATIONS

Cutaneous Leishmaniasis

After inoculation by the bite of an infected female phlebotomine sand fly (approximately 2–3 mm long), parasites proliferate locally in mononuclear phagocytes, leading to an erythematous papule, which typically enlarges slowly to become a nodule and then an ulcerative lesion with raised, indurated borders. Ulcerative lesions may become dry and crusted or may develop a moist granulating base with overlying exudate. Lesions can, however, persist as nodules, papules, or plaques and may be single or multiple. Lesions commonly appear on exposed areas of the body (eg, face and extremities) and may be accompanied by satellite lesions, sporotrichoid-like nodules, and regional adenopathy. Spontaneous resolution of lesions may take weeks to years—depending, in part, on the *Leishmania* species/strain—and usually results in a flat, atrophic scar.

Mucosal Leishmaniasis (Espundia)

Mucosal leishmaniasis traditionally refers to a metastatic sequela of New World cutaneous infection resulting from dissemination of the parasite from the skin to the naso-oropharyngeal/laryngeal mucosa. This form of leishmaniasis is typically caused by species in the *Viannia* subgenus. (Mucosal involvement attributable to local extension of cutaneous facial lesions has a different pathophysiology.) Mucosal disease usually becomes clinically evident months to years after the original cutaneous lesions have healed, although mucosal and cutaneous lesions may be noted simultaneously, and some affected people have had subclinical cutaneous infection. Untreated mucosal leishmaniasis can progress to cause ulcerative destruction of the mucosa (eg, perforation of the nasal septum) and facial disfigurement.

Visceral Leishmaniasis (Kala-Azar)

After cutaneous inoculation by an infected sand fly, the parasite spreads throughout the reticuloendothelial system (ie, within macrophages in spleen, liver, and bone marrow), leaving no or a minimal skin lesion at the bite site. Clinical manifestations include fever, weight loss, hepatosplenomegaly, pancytopenia (anemia, leukopenia, and thrombocytopenia), hypoalbuminemia, and hypergammaglobulinemia. Hemophagocytic lymphohistiocytosis has been reported as a complication of visceral leishmaniasis. Peripheral lymphadenopathy is common in East Africa (eg, South Sudan). Some patients in South Asia (the Indian subcontinent) develop grayish discoloration of their skin; this manifestation gave rise to the Hindi term *kala-azar* ("black sickness"). Untreated, advanced cases of visceral leishmaniasis are almost always fatal, either directly from the disease or from complications, such as secondary bacterial infections or hemorrhage. Visceral infection can, alternatively, be asymptomatic or have few symptoms. Latent visceral infection can reactivate years to decades after exposure in people who become immunocompromised (eg, because of coinfection with HIV or immunosuppressive/immunomodulatory therapy). Some patients develop post–kala-azar dermal leishmaniasis (PKDL) during or after treatment of visceral leishmaniasis.

Post–Kala-Azar Dermal Leishmaniasis

PKDL is a dermatosis that generally develops as a sequela after apparent successful cure from visceral leishmaniasis. In the Indian subcontinent variant, polymorphic lesions (coexistence of macules/patches along with papulonodules) are prevalent, whereas the Sudanese variant has papular or nodular lesions.

ETIOLOGY

In the human host, *Leishmania* species are obligate intracellular protozoan parasites of mononuclear phagocytes. Together with *Trypanosoma* species, they constitute the family *Trypanosomatidae*. Approximately 20 *Leishmania* species (in the *Leishmania* and *Viannia* subgenera) are known to infect humans. Cutaneous leishmaniasis is typically caused by Old World species *Leishmania tropica*, *Leishmania major*, and *Leishmania aethiopica* and by New World species *Leishmania mexicana*, *Leishmania amazonensis*, *Leishmania (Viannia) braziliensis*, *Leishmania (V) panamensis*, *Leishmania (V) guyanensis*, and *Leishmania (V) peruviana*. Mucosal leishmaniasis is typically caused by species in the *Viannia* subgenus (especially *L [V] braziliensis* but also *L [V] panamensis* and *L [V] guyanensis*). Most cases of visceral leishmaniasis are caused by *Leishmania donovani* or *Leishmania infantum* (*Leishmania chagasi* is synonymous). *L donovani* and *L infantum* can also cause cutaneous and mucosal leishmaniasis, although people with typical cutaneous leishmaniasis caused by these organisms rarely develop visceral leishmaniasis. Recently, emerging foci of both cutaneous and visceral infection with *Leishmania enriettii* complex have been reported from the Caribbean, Ghana, and Thailand. PKDL has been reported to be caused primarily by *L donovani*, in both the Indian subcontinent and Sudan.

EPIDEMIOLOGY

In most settings, leishmaniasis is a zoonosis, with mammalian reservoir hosts, such as rodents or dogs. Some transmission cycles are anthroponotic: infected humans are the primary or only reservoir hosts of *L donovani* in South Asia (potentially also in East Africa) and of *L tropica*. Congenital and parenteral (ie, shared needles, blood transfusion) transmission have also been reported.

Leishmaniasis has been endemic in more than 90 countries in the tropics, the subtropics, and southern Europe. Visceral leishmaniasis (50,000–90,000 new cases annually) is found in focal areas in the Old World; in parts of Asia (particularly in South, Southwest, and central Asia), Africa (particularly in East Africa), the Middle East, and southern Europe; and in the New World, particularly in Brazil. Most (>95%) of the world's cases of visceral leishmaniasis occur in 10 countries: Bangladesh, Brazil, China, Ethiopia, India, Kenya, Nepal, Somalia, South Sudan, and Sudan.

Cutaneous leishmaniasis is more common (0.6 million–1.0 million new cases annually). Approximately 90% of cutaneous leishmaniasis cases occur in the Americas, the Mediterranean basin, parts of the Middle East, and central Asia. In 2017, 7 countries (Afghanistan, Algeria, Brazil, Colombia, Iran, Iraq, and Syria) accounted for 95% of new cases. Cutaneous leishmaniasis has been acquired in Texas and occasionally in Oklahoma. In general, the geographic distribution of leishmaniasis cases identified in the United States reflects immigration from and travel patterns to regions with endemic disease.

PKDL is confined mainly to 2 regions with endemic kala-azar: the Indian subcontinent (India, Nepal, Sri Lanka, and Bangladesh) and East Africa, mainly Sudan, although case reports have emanated from China, Iraq, and Iran. In the Indian subcontinent, transmission of visceral leishmaniasis is anthroponotic, whereas in Sudan it is zoonotic and anthroponotic; therefore, patients with PKDL are the proposed disease reservoir of visceral leishmaniasis in the Indian subcontinent. Young adults are more affected in the Indian subcontinent, and children are more affected in Sudan.

Incubation periods for the various forms of leishmaniasis range from weeks to years. The primary skin lesions of cutaneous leishmaniasis typically appear within several weeks of exposure. The **incubation period** of visceral infection usually ranges from approximately 2 to 6 months. PKDL in Sudan develops within 6 months of treatment but in India can develop decades after cure of visceral leishmaniasis.

DIAGNOSTIC TESTS

Definitive diagnosis is made by detecting the parasite (amastigote stages) in infected tissue (eg, of aspirates, scrapings, touch preparations, or histological sections) by light-microscopic examination of slides stained with Giemsa, hematoxylin, and eosin or other stains; by in vitro culture (available at reference laboratories); or increasingly by molecular methods (detection of parasite DNA by polymerase chain reaction [PCR] testing). The molecular methods are reported to be more sensitive than microscopy or culture. The SMART-Leish PCR used by the US military leishmaniasis diagnostic laboratory is cleared by the US Food and Drug Administration (FDA) for use. In cutaneous and mucosal disease, tissue can be obtained by a 3-mm punch biopsy, lesion scrapings, or needle aspiration of the raised nonnecrotic edge (biopsy) or the ulcer base of the lesion. In visceral leishmaniasis, although the sensitivity is highest (approximately 95%) for splenic aspiration, the procedure can be associated with life-threatening hemorrhage; bone marrow aspiration is safer and generally preferred. Other potential sources of specimens include liver, lymph node, and, in some patients (eg, those coinfected with HIV), whole blood or buffy coat. Identification of *Leishmania* species (eg, via isoenzyme analysis of cultured parasites or molecular approaches) may affect prognosis and influence treatment decisions. The Centers for Disease Control and Prevention (CDC) (**www.cdc.gov/parasites/leishmaniasis**) can assist in all aspects of diagnostic testing. Serological testing is not usually helpful in the evaluation of potential cases of cutaneous leishmaniasis but can provide supportive evidence for the diagnosis of visceral or mucosal leishmaniasis, particularly if the patient is immunocompetent. The rK39 immunochromatographic assay is FDA cleared for the presumptive diagnosis of visceral leishmaniasis and is commercially available.

TREATMENT

Guidelines published in 2016 from the Infectious Diseases Society of America and the American Society of Tropical Medicine and Hygiene provide a detailed approach to diagnosis and treatment. Systemic antileishmanial treatment is always indicated for patients with visceral or mucosal leishmaniasis, whereas not all patients with cutaneous leishmaniasis need to be treated or require systemic therapy. Consultation with infectious disease or tropical medicine specialists and with staff of the CDC Division of Parasitic Diseases and Malaria is recommended. The relative merits of the various treatment approaches/regimens for an individual patient should be considered, taking into account that the therapeutic response may vary, not only for different *Leishmania* species but also for the same species in different geographic regions. Special considerations apply in the United States regarding the availability of particular medications. For example, the pentavalent antimonial compound, sodium stibogluconate, is not commercially available but can be obtained by US-licensed physicians through the CDC Drug Service (404/639-3670), under an investigational new drug protocol, for parenteral (intravenous or, less commonly, intramuscular) treatment of leishmaniasis. Liposomal amphotericin B is approved by the FDA for treatment of visceral leishmaniasis. The oral agent miltefosine is approved for treatment of cutaneous, mucosal, and visceral leishmaniasis; the FDA-approved indications are limited to infection caused by particular *Leishmania* species and to patients who are at least 12 years of age, weigh at least 30 kg (66 lb), and are not pregnant or breastfeeding during and for 5 months after the treatment course.

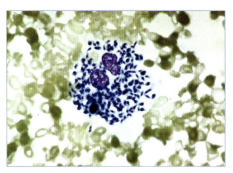

Image 77.1
Leishmania organisms in a peripheral blood smear from a young man with HIV infection who had visited a jungle in Central America. (See also Human Immunodeficiency Virus Infection.)

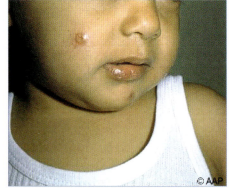

Image 77.2
Cutaneous leishmaniasis, as in this boy from India, seldom disseminates in people with immunocompetence. Multiple organisms can usually be found on biopsy of the border of a lesion.

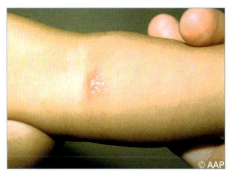

Image 77.3
Cutaneous leishmaniasis. Infected sand fly inoculation site with satellite lesions. The organism may be demonstrated by punch biopsy of the margin of a cutaneous lesion. This is the same child as in Image 77.2.

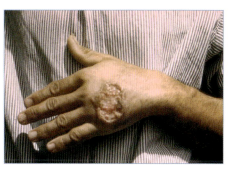

Image 77.4
Skin ulcer caused by leishmaniasis; hand of Central American adult. Courtesy of Centers for Disease Control and Prevention.

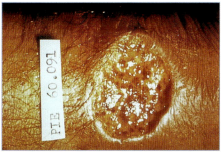

Image 77.5
Crater lesion of leishmaniasis, skin. Courtesy of Centers for Disease Control and Prevention.

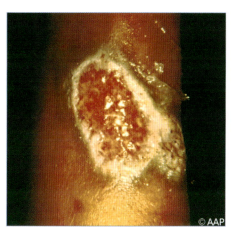

Image 77.6
Leishmaniasis of the forearm with severe cutaneous involvement. Courtesy of Hugh Moffet, MD.

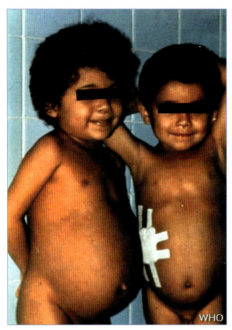

Image 77.7
Two young boys experiencing visceral leishmaniasis, with distended abdomens caused by hepatosplenomegaly. Courtesy of World Health Organization/TDR/Lainson/Wellcome Trust.

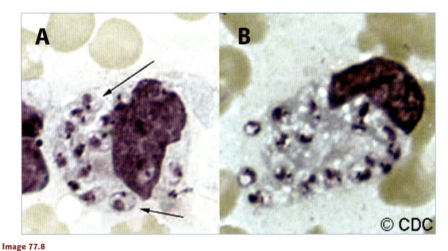

Image 77.8
Leishmania tropica amastigotes from a skin touch preparation. A, Still intact macrophage is practically filled with amastigotes, several of which have a clearly visible nucleus and a kinetoplast (arrows). B, Amastigotes are being freed from a rupturing macrophage. The patient has a history of travel to Egypt, Africa, and the Middle East. Culture in Novy-MacNeal-Nicolle medium followed by isoenzyme analysis helped identify the species as *L tropica* minor. Courtesy of Centers for Disease Control and Prevention.

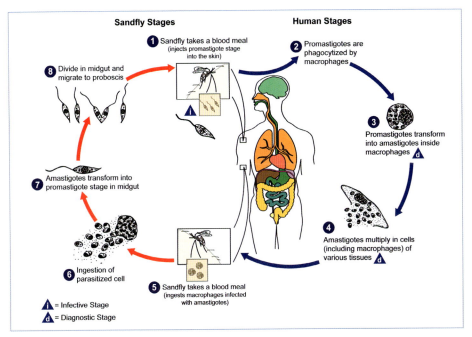

Image 77.9
Leishmaniasis is transmitted by the bite of female *Phlebotomine* species sand flies. The sand flies inject the infective stage, promastigotes, during blood meals (1). Promastigotes that reach the puncture wound are phagocytized by macrophages (2) and transform into amastigotes (3). Amastigotes multiply in infected cells and affect different tissues, depending, in part, on the *Leishmania* species (4). This originates the clinical manifestations of leishmaniasis. Sand flies become infected during blood meals on an infected host when they ingest macrophages infected with amastigotes (5, 6). In the sand fly's midgut, the parasites differentiate into promastigotes (7), which multiply and migrate to the proboscis (8). Courtesy of Centers for Disease Control and Prevention.

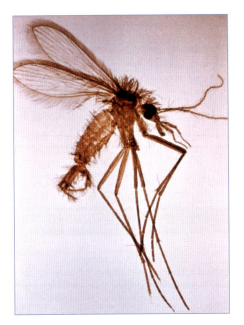

Image 77.10
This image depicts a mounted male *Phlebotomus* species fly, which, because of its resemblance, may be mistaken for a mosquito. *Phlebotomus* species sand flies are bloodsucking insects that are very small and sometimes act as the vectors for various diseases, such as leishmaniasis and bartonellosis (also known as Carrión disease). Courtesy of Centers for Disease Control and Prevention.

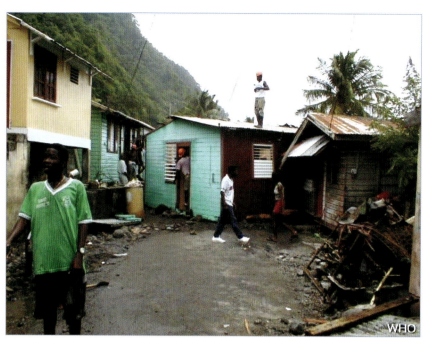

Image 77.11
A shantytown, another environment where *Leishmania* infection proliferates because of inadequate housing and lack of sanitation. Courtesy of World Health Organization.

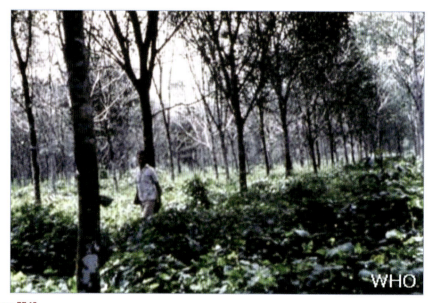

Image 77.12
Natural uncut forests are transmission sites for leishmaniasis. People who collect rubber or clear these areas for agriculture are prone to infection. Courtesy of World Health Organization/TDR/Lainson/Wellcome Trust.

CHAPTER 78

Leprosy

CLINICAL MANIFESTATIONS

Leprosy (Hansen disease) is a curable infection primarily involving skin, peripheral nerves, and mucosa of the upper respiratory tract. The clinical forms of leprosy reflect the cellular immune response to *Mycobacterium leprae* and, in turn, the number, size, structure, and bacillary content of the lesions. The organism has unique tropism for peripheral nerves, and all forms of leprosy exhibit nerve involvement. Leprosy skin lesions are quite varied and may manifest as macular hypopigmented or erythematous anesthetic lesions, discolored patches, scaly plaques, sharply defined macules with central clearing, painless ulcers, or nodules. Leprosy lesions do not usually itch or hurt. They lack sensation to heat, touch, and pain but otherwise may be difficult to distinguish from other common maladies. There may be madarosis (loss of eyelashes or eyebrows). Although the nerve injury caused by leprosy is irreversible, early diagnosis and drug therapy can prevent those sequelae.

Leprosy manifests over a broad clinical and histopathologic spectrum. In the United States, the Ridley-Jopling scale is used to classify patients according to the histopathologic features of their lesions and organization of the underlying granuloma. The scale is as follows: (1) tuberculoid; (2) borderline tuberculoid; (3) mid-borderline; (4) borderline lepromatous; and (5) lepromatous. When pathological examination and diagnosis are unavailable, a simplified scheme introduced by the World Health Organization (WHO) can be used. It is based purely on clinical skin examination. This scheme classifies leprosy by the number of skin patches as either paucibacillary (1–5 lesions, usually tuberculoid or borderline tuberculoid) or multibacillary (>5 lesions, usually mid-borderline, borderline lepromatous, or lepromatous). Patients in the tuberculoid spectrum have active cell-mediated immunity with low antibody responses to *M leprae* and few well-defined lesions containing few bacilli. Lepromatous spectrum cases have high antibody responses with little cell-mediated immunity to *M leprae* and several somewhat diffuse lesions usually containing numerous bacilli.

Serious consequences of leprosy occur from immune reactions and nerve involvement with resulting anesthesia, which can lead to repeated unrecognized trauma, ulcerations, fractures, and even bone resorption. Leprosy is a leading cause of permanent physical disability from communicable diseases worldwide. Eye involvement can occur, especially corneal scarring, and patients should be examined by an ophthalmologist. A diagnosis of leprosy should be considered in any patient with a hypoesthetic or anesthetic skin rash or skin patches who has a history of residence in areas with endemic leprosy or who has had contact with armadillos.

Leprosy Reactions

Acute clinical exacerbations reflect abrupt changes in the immunologic balance. These reactions are especially common during initial years of treatment but can occur in the absence of therapy. Two major types of leprosy reactions (LRs) are observed. Type 1 (reversal reaction [LR-1]) is observed predominantly in borderline tuberculoid and borderline lepromatous leprosy and is resultant from a sudden increase in effective cell-mediated immunity. Acute tenderness and swelling at the site of cutaneous and neural lesions with development of new lesions are major manifestations. Ulcerations can occur, but polymorphonuclear leukocytes are absent from the LR-1 lesion. Fever and systemic toxicity are uncommon. Type 2 (erythema nodosum leprosum [LR-2]) occurs in borderline and lepromatous forms as a systemic inflammatory response. Tender red subcutaneous papules or nodules resembling erythema nodosum can occur along with high fever, migrating polyarthralgia, painful swelling of lymph nodes and spleen, iridocyclitis, and, rarely, nephritis.

ETIOLOGY

Leprosy is caused by *M leprae,* an obligate intracellular rod-shaped bacterium that can have variable findings on Gram stain and is weakly acid fast on standard Ziehl-Neelsen staining but is best visualized by using the Fite stain. *M leprae* has not been cultured successfully in vitro. *M leprae* is the only bacterium known to infect Schwann cells of peripheral nerves, and demonstration of acid-fast bacilli in peripheral nerves is pathognomonic for leprosy. A newly described genomic variant, *Mycobacterium lepromatosis,* has also been implicated to cause leprosy, but the organism is not yet well characterized.

EPIDEMIOLOGY

Leprosy is considered a neglected tropical disease and is most prevalent in tropical and subtropical zones. It is not highly infectious. Several human genes have been identified that are associated with susceptibility to *M leprae*, and a minority of people appear to be genetically susceptible to the infection. Accordingly, spouses of leprosy patients are not likely to develop leprosy, but biological parents, children, and siblings who are household contacts of untreated patients with leprosy have some increased risk.

Transmission is believed to be most effective through long-term close contact with an infected individual and likely occurs through respiratory shedding of organisms. The 9-banded armadillo (*Dasypus novemcinctus*) is a recognized nonhuman reservoir of *M leprae*, and zoonotic transmission is reported in the southern United States. There are reports of *M leprae* infection in 9-banded armadillos as well as the 6-banded armadillo (*Euphractus sexcinctus*) in both Central and South America, mainly Argentina and Brazil. In addition, red squirrels (*Sciurus vulgaris*) in the British Isles may harbor *M leprae* and *M lepromatosis*. People living with HIV infection do not appear to have increased risk for becoming infected with *M leprae*. However, concomitant HIV infection and leprosy can lead to worsening of leprosy symptoms during HIV treatment and result in immune reconstitution inflammatory syndrome. Like many other chronic infectious diseases, onset of leprosy is associated increasingly with use of anti-inflammatory autoimmune therapies and immunologic senescence in elderly patients.

A total of 14,029 leprosy cases have been documented in the United States since 1894. There are approximately 6,500 people with leprosy currently living in the United States, with 3,500 under active medical management. Most leprosy cases reported in the United States occurred in residents of Texas, California, and Hawaii or in immigrants and other people who lived or worked in countries with endemic leprosy. More than 65% of the world's leprosy patients reside in South and Southeast Asia, primarily India. Other areas of high endemicity include Angola, Brazil, the Central African Republic, the Democratic Republic of Congo, Madagascar, Mozambique, the Republic of the Marshall Islands, South Sudan, the Federated States of Micronesia, and the United Republic of Tanzania.

The **incubation period** is usually 3 to 5 years but may range from 1 to 20 years.

DIAGNOSTIC TESTS

There are no diagnostic tests or methods to detect subclinical leprosy. Histopathologic examination of a skin biopsy by an experienced pathologist is the best method of establishing the diagnosis and establishing classification of the disease. Formalin-fixed or paraffin-embedded biopsies can be sent to the National Hansen's Disease (Leprosy) Program (NHDP [800/642-2477; **www.hrsa.gov/hansens-disease/diagnosis/biopsy.html**]). Acid-fast bacilli may be found in slit smears or biopsy specimens of skin lesions from patients with lepromatous (multibacillary) forms of the disease but are rarely visualized from patients with the paucibacillary tuberculoid and indeterminate (first lesion with slightly diminished sensation) forms of disease. A polymerase chain reaction test for *M leprae* and *M lepromatosis* is also available at the NHDP, as are molecular tests for genetic mutations associated with drug resistance, and strain typing based on single nucleotide polymorphisms and other genomic elements.

TREATMENT

Leprosy is curable. Therapy for patients with leprosy should be undertaken in consultation with an expert in leprosy. The NHDP (800/642-2477) consults on clinical and pathological issues and information about local Hansen disease clinics and clinicians who have experience with the disease. Prevention of permanent nerve damage and disability is an important goal of treatment and care and requires education and self-awareness of the patient. Combination antimicrobial multidrug therapy can be obtained free of charge from the NHDP in the United States and from the WHO in other countries (**www.hrsa.gov/hansensdisease/diagnosis/recommendedtreatment.html**).

The infectivity of leprosy patients to others ceases within only a few days of initiating standard multidrug therapy. It is important to treat *M leprae* infections with more than one antimicrobial agent to minimize development of antimicrobial-resistant organisms. Adults are treated with dapsone, rifampin, and clofazimine. Regimens and doses for children are available and should be chosen with assistance from the NHDP. Resistance to all 3 drugs has been documented but is extremely rare. Before beginning antimicrobial therapy, patients should be tested for glucose-6-phosphate dehydrogenase deficiency, have baseline complete blood cell count and serum aminotransferase results documented, and be evaluated for any evidence of tuberculosis infection, especially if infected with HIV. This consideration is important to avoid monotherapy of active tuberculosis with rifampin while treating active leprosy.

Management of leprosy reactions is complex, and expert guidance should be sought. Reactions should be treated aggressively to prevent peripheral nerve damage. Treatment with prednisone (1 mg/kg/day, orally) can be initiated for short-term management and rescue situations. Long-term use of prednisone should incorporate a sparing agent such as methotrexate. LR-2 may be treated with thalidomide (100–400 mg/day for 4 days). Thalidomide is used under strict supervision and is available through Celgene (**www.thalomidrems.com** or 888/423-5436). Thalidomide is not approved for use in children younger than 12 years. Rehabilitative measures, including surgery and physical therapy, may be necessary for some patients.

All patients with leprosy should be educated about signs and symptoms of neuritis and cautioned to report them immediately so corticosteroid therapy can be instituted. Patients should receive counseling because of the social and psychological effects of this disease.

Relapse of disease after completing multidrug therapy is rare (0.01%–0.14%); the manifestation of new skin patches is usually attributable to a late type 1 reaction (LR-1). When it does occur, relapse is usually attributable to reactivation of drug-susceptible organisms. People with relapses of disease require another course of multidrug therapy.

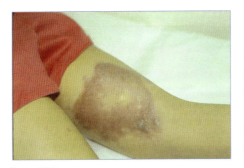

Image 78.1
Hansen disease. A young Vietnamese boy who spent 2 years in a refugee camp in the Philippines presented with the nodular violaceous skin lesion shown. The results of a biopsy of the lesion showed acid-fast organisms surrounding blood vessels. A diagnosis of lepromatous leprosy was made, and the child was treated with a multidrug regimen. Copyright Barbara Jantausch, MD, FAAP.

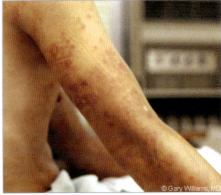

Image 78.2
Erythema nodosum leprosum in a 29-year-old man. Copyright Gary Williams, MD.

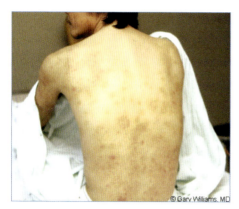

Image 78.3
Erythema nodosum leprosum in the same patient as in Image 78.2. Copyright Gary Williams, MD.

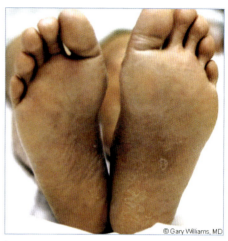

Image 78.4
Erythema nodosum leprosum in the same patient as in images 78.2 and 78.3. Copyright Gary Williams, MD.

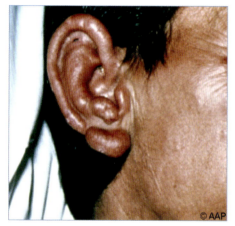

Image 78.5
Lepromatous leprosy in a man. Newly diagnosed cases are considered contagious until treatment is established and should be reported to local and state public health departments. Courtesy of Hugh Moffet, MD.

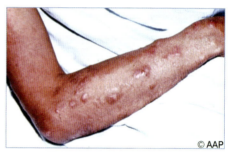

Image 78.6
A male adult with lepromatous leprosy. Courtesy of Hugh Moffet, MD.

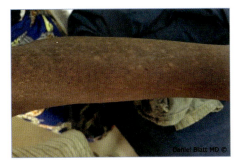

Image 78.7
Hypopigmented skin lesions in the arm of an 18-month-old boy with multibacillary leprosy. This patient experienced lack of sensation during a pinprick test performed on the lesions. Courtesy of Daniel Blatt, MD.

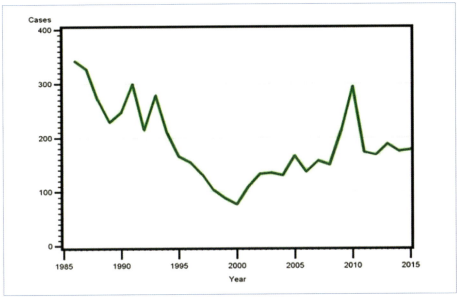

Image 78.8
US-reported Hansen disease cases by year, 1985–2015. Courtesy of Health Resources & Services Administration.

CHAPTER 79
Leptospirosis

CLINICAL MANIFESTATIONS

Leptospirosis is an acute febrile disease with varied manifestations. The severity of disease ranges from asymptomatic or subclinical to a self-limited systemic febrile illness (approximately 90% of patients) to a life-threatening illness that can include jaundice, renal failure (oliguric or nonoliguric), myocarditis, hemorrhage (particularly pulmonary), aseptic meningitis, or refractory shock. Clinical manifestation may be monophasic or biphasic. Classically described biphasic leptospirosis has an acute septicemia phase usually lasting up to 1 week, during which *Leptospira* organisms are present in blood, followed by a second immune-mediated phase that is less likely to respond to antimicrobial therapy. Regardless of its severity, the acute phase is characterized by nonspecific symptoms, including fever, chills, headache, myalgia, nausea, vomiting, or rash. Distinct clinical findings include notable conjunctival suffusion without purulent discharge (28%–99% of cases) and myalgia of the calf and lumbar regions (40%–97% of cases). Manifestations of the immune phase are more variable and milder than those of the initial illness. The hallmark of the immune phase is aseptic meningitis; uveitis is a late finding (4–8 months after the illness has begun). Supportive therapies are appropriate during this phase. Severe manifestations include jaundice and renal dysfunction (Weil syndrome), pulmonary hemorrhage, cardiac arrhythmias, and circulatory collapse. Abnormal potassium (high or low) and/or magnesium (low) levels may require aggressive management. The estimated case-fatality rate is 5% to 15% with severe illness, although it can increase to greater than 50% in patients with pulmonary hemorrhage syndrome.

ETIOLOGY

Leptospirosis is caused by pathogenic spirochetes of the genus *Leptospira*. Leptospires are classified by species and subdivided into more than 300 antigenically defined serovars and grouped into serogroups on the basis of antigenic relatedness. Currently, the molecular classification divides the genus into 23 named pathogenic (n = 10), intermediate (n = 5) and saprophytic (nonpathogenic; n = 8) genomospecies as determined by DNA-DNA hybridization, 16S ribosomal gene phylogenetic clustering, and whole genome sequencing. This newer nomenclature supersedes the former division of these organisms into 2 species: *Leptospira interrogans*, comprising all pathogenic strains, and *Leptospira biflexa*, comprising all saprophytic stains found in the environment. All leptospires are tightly coiled spirochetes, obligate aerobic, with an optimum growth temperature of 28 to 30 °C (82–86 °F).

EPIDEMIOLOGY

Leptospirosis is among the most important zoonoses globally, affecting people in resource-rich and resource-limited countries in both urban and rural contexts. It has been estimated that more than 1 million people worldwide are infected annually (95% CI, 434,000–1,750,000), with approximately 58,900 deaths (95% CI, 23,800–95,900) occurring each year. The reservoirs for *Leptospira* species include a wide range of wild and domestic animals, including rodents, dogs, livestock (ie, cattle, pigs), and horses that may shed organisms asymptomatically for years. *Leptospira* organisms excreted in animal urine may remain viable in moist soil or water for weeks to months in warm climates. Humans usually become infected via entry of leptospires through contact of mucosal surfaces (especially conjunctivae) or abraded skin with urine-contaminated environmental sources such as soil and water. Infection may also be acquired through direct contact with infected animals or their tissues, urine, or other body fluids. Epidemics are associated with seasonal flooding and natural disasters, including hurricanes and monsoons. Populations in regions of high endemicity in the tropics and subtropics likely encounter *Leptospira* organisms during routine activities of daily living. People predisposed by occupation include abattoir and sewer workers, miners, veterinarians, farmers, and military personnel. Recreational exposures and clusters of disease have been associated with adventure travel, sporting events including triathlons, and wading, swimming, or boating in contaminated water, particularly during flooding or following heavy rainfall. Common history includes head submersion in or swallowing water during such activities. Person-to-person transmission is not described convincingly.

The **incubation period** is usually 5 to 14 days (range, 2–30 days).

DIAGNOSTIC TESTS

Leptospira organisms can be isolated from blood during the early septicemic phase (first week) of illness, from urine specimens starting approximately 1 week after symptom onset, and from cerebrospinal fluid (CSF) when clinical signs of meningitis are present. Specialized culture media are required but are not available routinely in most clinical laboratories. *Leptospira* organisms can be subcultured to specific *Leptospira* semisolid medium (ie, EMJH [Ellinghausen-McCullough-Johnson-Harris]) from blood culture bottles used in automated systems within 1 week of inoculation. Isolation of the organism may be difficult, requiring incubation for up to 16 weeks. Sensitivity of culture for diagnosis is low. Isolated leptospires are identified by serological methods with agglutinating antisera or, more recently, by molecular methods.

Serum specimens should always be obtained to facilitate diagnosis, and paired acute and convalescent sera are recommended, ideally collected 10 to 14 days apart. Antibodies develop by 5 to 7 days after onset of illness, but increases in antibody titer may not be detected until more than 10 days after onset, especially if antimicrobial therapy is initiated early. Antibodies can be measured by commercially available immunoassays, most of which are based on sonicates of the saprophyte *L biflexa*. These assays have variable sensitivity according to regional differences of the various *Leptospira* species. In populations with high endemicity, background reactivity requires establishing regionally relevant diagnostic criteria and establishing diagnostic versus background titers. Antibody increases can be transient, delayed, or absent in some patients, which may be related to antibiotic use, bacterial virulence, immunogenetics of the individual, or other unknown factors. Microscopic agglutination, the gold standard serological test, is performed only in reference laboratories, and seroconversion demonstrated between acute and convalescent specimens is diagnostic.

Immunohistochemical and immunofluorescent techniques can detect leptospiral antigens in infected tissues. Polymerase chain reaction assays for detection of *Leptospira* DNA in clinical specimens are available but are sensitive only in acute specimens and, sometimes, convalescent urine. *Leptospira* DNA can be detected in whole blood during the first 7 days of illness, with highest sensitivity between days 1 and 4; *Leptospira* DNA can be found after 7 days of illness in urine and may be detectable for weeks to months in the absence of antimicrobial treatment. *Leptospira* DNA can also be detected in CSF from symptomatic patients with clinical signs of meningitis.

TREATMENT

Antimicrobial therapy should be initiated as soon as possible after symptom onset. Intravenous penicillin is the drug of choice for patients with severe infection requiring hospitalization; penicillin has been shown to be effective in shortening duration of fever when given as late as 7 days into the course of illness. Penicillin G decreases the duration of systemic symptoms and persistence of associated laboratory abnormalities and may prevent development of leptospiruria. A Jarisch-Herxheimer reaction (an acute febrile reaction accompanied by headache, myalgia, and an aggravated clinical picture lasting <24 hours) can develop after initiation of penicillin therapy, as with other spirochetal infections. Parenteral cefotaxime, ceftriaxone, and doxycycline have been demonstrated in randomized clinical trials to be equal in efficacy to penicillin G for treatment of severe leptospirosis. For patients with mild disease, oral doxycycline has been shown to shorten the course of illness and decrease the occurrence of leptospiruria; doxycycline can be used for short durations (ie, ≤21 days) without regard to patient age. Ampicillin or amoxicillin can also be used to treat mild disease. Azithromycin has been demonstrated in a clinical trial to be as effective as doxycycline. Severe cases require appropriate supportive care, including fluid and electrolyte replacement. Patients with oliguric renal insufficiency require prompt dialysis, and those with pulmonary hemorrhage may require mechanical ventilation to improve clinical outcome.

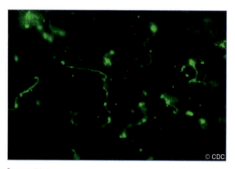

Image 79.1
Leptospira bacteria in liver impression smear (fluorescent antibody stain). Patient died of leptospirosis. Courtesy of Centers for Disease Control and Prevention.

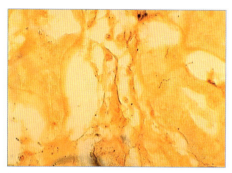

Image 79.2
Histopathologic features of leptospirosis, kidney. *Leptospira* bacteria are visible at the right (Dieterle stain). Courtesy of Centers for Disease Control and Prevention.

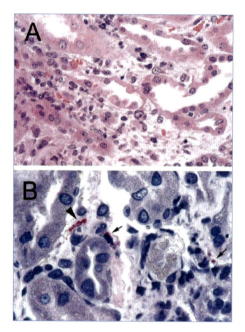

Image 79.3
A, Renal biopsy shows inflammatory cell infiltrate in the interstitium and focal denudation of tubular epithelial cells (hematoxylin-eosin, original magnification ×100). B, Immunostaining of fragmented leptospire (arrowhead) and granular form of bacterial antigens (arrows) (original magnification ×158). Courtesy of *Emerging Infectious Diseases*.

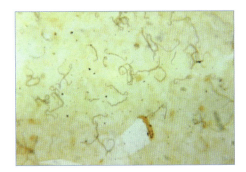

Image 79.4
A photomicrograph of a liver smear, by use of a silver staining technique, taken from a patient with a fatal case of leptospirosis. Humans become infected by swallowing water contaminated by infected animals or through skin contact, especially with mucosal surfaces, such as the eyes or nose, or with broken skin. The disease is not known to be spread from person to person. Courtesy of Centers for Disease Control and Prevention.

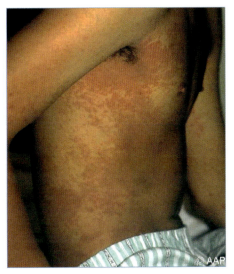

Image 79.5
Leptospirosis rash in an adolescent boy that shows the generalized vasculitis caused by this infection.

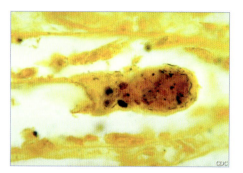

Image 79.6
Photomicrograph of kidney tissue, by use of a silver staining technique, revealing the presence of *Leptospira* bacteria. Courtesy of Centers for Disease Control and Prevention/Martin Hicklin, MD.

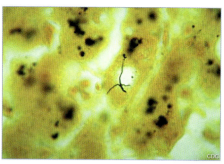

Image 79.7
Photomicrograph of liver tissue revealing the presence of *Leptospira* bacteria. Humans become infected by swallowing water contaminated by infected animals or through skin contact, especially with mucosal surfaces, such as the eyes or nose, or with broken skin. The disease is not known to be spread from person to person. Courtesy of Centers for Disease Control and Prevention/Martin Hicklin, MD.

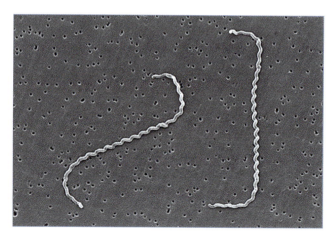

Image 79.8
Scanning electron micrograph of *Leptospira interrogans* strain RGA. Courtesy of Centers for Disease Control and Prevention.

CHAPTER 80
Listeria monocytogenes Infections
(Listeriosis)

CLINICAL MANIFESTATIONS

Listeriosis is a relatively uncommon but often severe invasive infection caused by *Listeria monocytogenes*. Transmission is predominantly foodborne, and illness, especially with severe manifestations, occurs most frequently in pregnant women and their fetuses or newborns, older adults, and people with impaired cell-mediated immunity resulting from underlying illness or treatment (eg, organ transplant, hematologic malignancy, immunosuppression resulting from therapy with corticosteroid or antitumor necrosis factor agents, or AIDS). Infections during pregnancy can result in spontaneous abortion, fetal death, preterm delivery, and neonatal illness or death. In pregnant women, infections can be asymptomatic or associated with a nonspecific febrile illness with myalgia, back pain, and, occasionally, gastrointestinal tract symptoms. Fetal infection generally results from transplacental transmission following maternal bacteremia. Additional mechanisms of infection in neonates with listeriosis are thought to include inhalation of infected amniotic fluid and infection ascending from maternal vaginal colonization. Approximately 65% of pregnant women with *Listeria* infection experience a prodromal illness before the diagnosis of listeriosis in their newborns. Amnionitis during labor, brown staining of amniotic fluid, or asymptomatic perinatal infection can occur.

Neonates can present with early- or late-onset disease. Preterm birth, pneumonia, and septicemia are common in early-onset disease (within the first week), with fatality rates of 14% to 56%. An erythematous rash with small, pale papules characterized histologically by granulomas, termed *granulomatosis infantisepticum*, can occur in severe newborn infection. Late-onset infections occur at 8 to 30 days following full-term deliveries and usually result in meningitis with fatality rates of approximately 25%. Late-onset infection may result from acquisition of the organism during passage through the birth canal or, rarely, from environmental sources. Health care–associated nursery outbreaks have been reported.

Clinical features characteristic of invasive listeriosis outside the neonatal period or pregnancy are bacteremia and meningitis, with or without parenchymal brain involvement, and, less commonly, brain abscess or endocarditis. *L monocytogenes* can also cause rhombencephalitis (brainstem encephalitis) in otherwise healthy adolescents and young adults. Outbreaks of febrile gastroenteritis caused by food contaminated with a very large inoculum of *L monocytogenes* have been reported.

ETIOLOGY

L monocytogenes is a facultatively anaerobic, nonspore-forming, nonbranching, motile, gram-positive rod that multiplies intracellularly. It has been assigned to the family *Listeriaceae* along with 5 other traditional and several newly named species. The organism grows readily on blood agar and produces incomplete hemolysis. *L monocytogenes* serotypes 1/2a, 4b, and 1/2b grow well at refrigerator temperatures (4–10 °C [39–50 °F]).

EPIDEMIOLOGY

L monocytogenes causes approximately 1,000 cases of invasive disease annually in the United States, and approximately 15% of cases are associated with pregnancy. Pregnant women are 10 times more likely to be infected than other people. The mortality rate is 15% to 20%, with higher rates among older adults and immunocompromised people, including neonates. The saprophytic organism is distributed widely in the environment and is an important cause of illness in ruminants. Foodborne transmission causes outbreaks and sporadic infections in humans. Commonly incriminated foods include deli-style, ready-to-eat meats, particularly poultry; unpasteurized milk; and soft cheeses, including Mexican-style cheese. Approximately 25% of global outbreaks are attributable to foods not traditionally associated as sources of *L monocytogenes*, such as ice cream and fresh and frozen fruits and vegetables. Listeriosis is a relatively rare foodborne illness (<1% of pathogens causing reported foodborne illness in the United States) but has the highest case-fatality rate among all foodborne pathogens and causes 20% of foodborne disease–related deaths. The incidence of listeriosis decreased substantially in the United States during the 1990s, when regulatory agencies began enforcing rigorous screening guidelines for

L monocytogenes in processed foods and better detection methods became available to identify contaminated foods. The prevalence of stool carriage of *L monocytogenes* among healthy, asymptomatic adults is estimated to be 1% to 5%.

The **incubation period** for invasive disease is longer for pregnancy-associated cases (2–4 weeks or occasionally longer) than for nonpregnancy-associated cases (1–14 days). The **incubation period** for self-limiting, febrile gastroenteritis following ingestion of a large inoculum is 24 hours; illness typically lasts 2 to 3 days.

DIAGNOSTIC TESTS

L monocytogenes can be recovered readily on blood agar from cultures of blood, cerebrospinal fluid (CSF), meconium, placental or fetal tissue specimens, amniotic fluid, and other infected tissue specimens, including joint, pleural, or peritoneal fluid. Gram stain of meconium, placental tissue, biopsy specimens of the rash of early-onset infection, or CSF from an infected patient may demonstrate the organism. The organisms can be gram variable and can resemble diphtheroids, cocci, or diplococci. Laboratory misidentification is somewhat common, and the isolation of a diphtheroid from blood or CSF should always alert one to the possibility that the organism is *L monocytogenes*.

A number of laboratory-derived polymerase chain reaction (PCR) assays have been described for detection of *L monocytogenes* in blood and CSF. At least 1 multiplexed PCR diagnostic panel designed to detect agents of meningitis and encephalitis in CSF cleared by the US Food and Drug Administration contains *L monocytogenes* as one of its target organisms; however, there are limited clinical data with the use of PCR for this purpose, and parallel culture of CSF should also be performed to allow for susceptibility testing and molecular characterization, especially for outbreak detection.

TREATMENT

No controlled trials have established the drug(s) of choice or duration of therapy for listeriosis. Combination therapy with ampicillin and a second agent in doses appropriate for meningitis is recommended for severe infections. An aminoglycoside, typically gentamicin, is usually used as the second agent in combination therapy. Use of an alternative second agent that is active intracellularly (eg, trimethoprim-sulfamethoxazole [contraindicated in infants <2 months], fluoroquinolones, linezolid, or rifampin) is supported by case reports in adults. In the penicillin-allergic patient, options include either penicillin desensitization or use of either trimethoprim-sulfamethoxazole or a fluoroquinolone, both of which have been used successfully as monotherapy for *Listeria* meningitis and in the setting of brain abscess. Treatment failures with vancomycin have been reported. Cephalosporins are not active against *L monocytogenes*.

For bacteremia without associated central nervous system infection, 14 days of treatment is recommended. For *L monocytogenes* meningitis, most experts recommend 3 to 4 weeks of treatment. Longer courses are necessary for patients with endocarditis or parenchymal brain infection (ie, cerebritis, rhombencephalitis, brain abscess). Diagnostic imaging of the brain near the end of the anticipated duration of therapy allows determination of parenchymal involvement of the brain and the need for prolonged therapy in neonates with complicated courses and in immunocompromised patients.

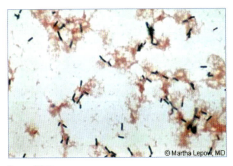

Image 80.1
Cerebrospinal fluid showing characteristic gram-positive rods (Gram stain). Listeriosis is a severe but relatively uncommon infection. Listeriosis occurs most frequently in pregnant women and their fetuses or newborns, people of advanced age, or people with immunocompromise. Copyright Martha Lepow, MD.

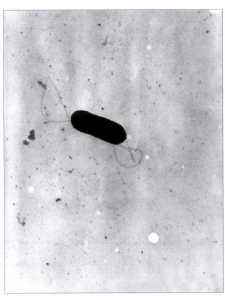

Image 80.2
Electron micrograph of a flagellated *Listeria monocytogenes* bacterium (magnification ×41,250). Courtesy of Centers for Disease Control and Prevention.

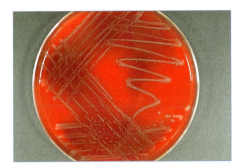

Image 80.3
Listeria monocytogenes on blood agar. Courtesy of Julia Rosebush, DO; Robert Jerris, PhD; and Theresa Stanley, M(ASCP).

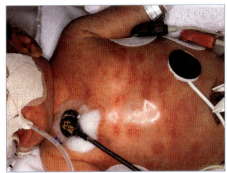

Image 80.4
Skin lesions present at birth in a neonate with congenital pneumonia. *Listeria monocytogenes* was isolated from blood and skin lesion cultures.

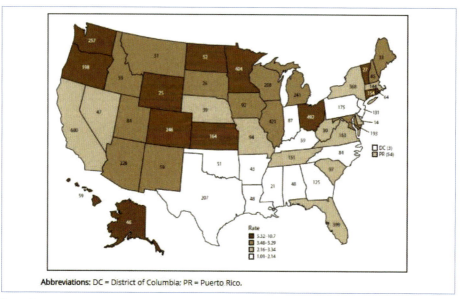

Image 80.5
Number* and rate[†] of reported foodborne disease outbreaks—Foodborne Disease Outbreak Surveillance System, United States and Puerto Rico 2009–2015. *Total number of reported outbreaks in each area (N = 5,760), includes 177 multistate outbreaks (ie, outbreaks in which exposure occurred in more than one state) assigned as an outbreak to each state involved. Multistate outbreaks involved a median of seven states (range, 2–45). [†]Per 1 million population using U.S. Census Bureau estimates of the mid-year populations for 2009–2015. Source: US Census Bureau. Population and housing unit estimates. US Dept of Commerce; 2016.

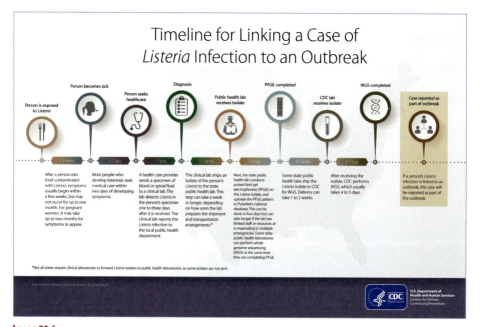

Image 80.6
The timeline for linking a case of *Listeria* infection to an outbreak. CDC indicates Centers for Disease Control and Prevention. Courtesy of Centers for Disease Control and Prevention.

CHAPTER 81
Lyme Disease
(Lyme Borreliosis, *Borrelia burgdorferi* sensu lato Infection)

CLINICAL MANIFESTATIONS

Clinical manifestations of Lyme disease are divided into 3 stages: early localized, early disseminated, and late manifestations. Early localized disease is characterized by a distinctive lesion, erythema migrans (EM), at the site of a recent tick bite. EM is by far the most common manifestation of Lyme disease in children. EM appears days to weeks after a tick bite and begins as a red macule or papule that usually expands to form a large (often ≥5 cm in diameter) annular, erythematous lesion, sometimes with partial central clearing. The lesion is typically painless and nonpruritic. Localized EM can vary greatly in size and shape and can be confused with cellulitis; lesions may have a purplish discoloration or central vesicular or necrotic areas. A classic bull's-eye appearance with concentric rings appears in a minority of cases. Factors that distinguish EM from local allergic reaction to a tick bite include larger size, gradual expansion, less pruritus, and slower onset of EM. Constitutional symptoms, such as malaise, headache, mild neck stiffness, myalgia, and arthralgia, but not joint swelling or effusion, often accompany EM. Fever may be present but is not universal and is generally mild.

In early disseminated disease, multiple EM lesions may appear several weeks after an infective tick bite and consist of secondary annular, erythematous lesions like the primary lesion but usually smaller. Other manifestations of early disseminated illness (which may occur with or without a skin lesion) are palsies of the cranial nerves (most commonly cranial nerve VII), lymphocytic meningitis (often associated with cranial neuropathy or papilledema), and radiculitis. Carditis usually manifests as various degrees of atrioventricular block and can be life threatening. Systemic symptoms, such as low-grade fever, arthralgia, myalgia, headache, and fatigue, may be present during the early disseminated stage.

Patients with early Lyme disease can be infected simultaneously with *Borrelia miyamotoi* and agents of babesiosis and anaplasmosis. These diagnoses should be suspected in patients who manifest high fever, have hematologic abnormalities consistent with these infections, or do not respond as expected to therapy prescribed for Lyme disease, such as fever persisting for more than 1 day after starting treatment. Patients who contract Lyme disease may be coinfected with Powassan virus (deer tick virus) if bitten in the United States or with tickborne encephalitis virus if infection was acquired in Europe.

Late Lyme disease occurs in patients who are not treated at an earlier stage of illness and manifests in children most commonly as arthritis. Lyme arthritis is characterized by inflammatory arthritis that is usually monoarticular or oligoarticular and affects large joints, particularly the knees. Although arthralgia can be present at any stage of Lyme disease, Lyme arthritis has objective evidence of joint swelling and white blood cells in synovial fluid specimens. Most cases of arthritis occur without a history of earlier stages of illness (including EM) or prior treatment. Compared with pyogenic arthritis, Lyme arthritis tends to manifest with joint swelling/effusion out of proportion to pain or disability and with lower peripheral blood neutrophilia and erythrocyte sedimentation rate. The effusion may be episodic, lasting weeks at a time, and then resolve with later occurrence. Polyneuropathy, encephalopathy, and encephalitis are rare late manifestations. Children treated with antimicrobial agents in the early stage of disease rarely develop late manifestations.

Other rare clinical manifestations include ophthalmic conditions such as conjunctivitis, optic neuritis, keratitis, and uveitis.

Lyme disease is not thought to produce a congenital infection syndrome. No causal relationship between maternal Lyme disease and abnormalities of pregnancy or congenital disease caused by *Borrelia burgdorferi* sensu lato has been documented. No evidence exists that Lyme disease can be transmitted via human milk.

ETIOLOGY

In the United States, Lyme disease is caused by the spirochete *B burgdorferi* sensu stricto (hereafter referred to as *B burgdorferi*) and rarely by the recently discovered *Borrelia mayonii*. In Eurasia, *B burgdorferi*, *Borrelia afzelii*, and *Borrelia garinii* cause borreliosis. *Borrelia* species are members of the family *Spirochaetaceae*, which also includes *Treponema* species.

EPIDEMIOLOGY

In 2017, 29,513 confirmed cases of Lyme disease were reported in the United States, although the actual number of cases may be up to 10-fold greater because of underreporting. Lyme disease occurs primarily in 2 distinct geographic regions of the United States, with more than 80% of cases occurring in New England and the eastern Mid-Atlantic States, as far south as Virginia. The disease also occurs, but with lower frequency, in the upper Midwest, especially Wisconsin and Minnesota. The geographic range is not static and has expanded considerably in the eastern and Midwestern states since 2000. Transmission also occurs at a low level on the West Coast, especially in northern California. The occurrence of cases in the United States correlates with distribution and frequency of infected tick vectors—*Ixodes scapularis* in the east and Midwest and *Ixodes pacificus* in the west. In southern states, *I scapularis* ticks are rarer than in the Northeast; the ticks that are present do not feed commonly on competent reservoir mammals and are less likely to bite humans because of different questing habits. Cases reported from states without known endemic transmission may have been imported from endemic states or may be misdiagnoses resulting from false-positive serological test results or results that are misinterpreted as positive. Late manifestations, such as arthritis, can occur months after exposure, highlighting the importance of eliciting a travel history to areas with endemic transmission.

Most cases of early localized and early disseminated Lyme disease occur between April and October; approximately 50% occur during June and July. People of all ages can be affected, but incidence in the United States is highest among children 5 through 9 years of age and adults 55 through 69 years of age.

With lesion(s) like EM, southern tick–associated rash illness (STARI) has been reported mainly in south-central and southeastern states without endemic *B burgdorferi* infection. The etiology is unknown. STARI results from the bite of the lone star tick, *Amblyomma americanum*, which is abundant in southern states and is biologically incapable of transmitting *B burgdorferi*. Patients with STARI may present with constitutional symptoms in addition to EM, but STARI has not been associated with any of the disseminated complications of Lyme disease. Appropriate treatment of STARI is unknown.

B mayonii is a newly described species identified in a small number of patients from the upper Midwest with symptoms like those of Lyme disease. Patients with *B mayonii* infection can be expected to test positive for Lyme disease via the 2-tiered serological testing described later in this chapter, and therapy used for Lyme disease is effective against *B mayonii*.

Lyme disease is also endemic in eastern Canada, Europe, states of the former Soviet Union, China, Mongolia, and Japan. The primary tick vector in Europe is *Ixodes ricinus*, and the primary tick vector in Asia is *Ixodes persulcatus*. Clinical manifestations vary somewhat from those seen in the United States. European Lyme disease can cause the skin lesions borrelial lymphocytoma and acrodermatitis chronica atrophicans and is more likely to produce neurological disease, whereas arthritis is uncommon. These differences are attributable to the different genospecies of *Borrelia* responsible for European Lyme disease.

The **incubation period** for US Lyme disease from tick bite to appearance of single or multiple EM lesions ranges from 3 to 32 days, with a median time of 11 days. Late manifestations such as arthritis can occur months after the tick bite in people who do not receive antimicrobial therapy.

DIAGNOSTIC TESTS

Diagnosis of Lyme disease rests first and foremost on the recognition of a consistent clinical illness in people who have had plausible geographic exposure. Early Lyme disease in patients with EM is diagnosed clinically on the basis of the characteristic appearance of this skin lesion. Although EM is not pathognomonic for Lyme disease, it is highly distinctive and characteristic. In areas with endemic Lyme disease, it is expected that the vast majority of EM occurring in the appropriate season is attributable to *B burgdorferi* infection. Sensitivity of serological testing is low during early infection, and less than half of children with solitary EM lesions will be seropositive. Patients who seek medical attention with 1 or more lesions of EM and without extracutaneous manifestations should be treated on the basis of a clinical diagnosis of Lyme disease without serological testing.

There is a broad differential diagnosis for extracutaneous manifestations of Lyme disease. Diagnosis of extracutaneous Lyme disease, including late-stage disease, requires a typical clinical illness, plausible geographic exposure, and a positive serological test result.

The standard testing method for Lyme disease is a 2-tiered serological algorithm. The initial screening test can be used to identify antibodies to a whole-cell sonicate, to peptide antigen, or to recombinant antigens of *B burgdorferi* via an enzyme-linked immunosorbent assay (ELISA) or enzyme immunoassay (EIA) or an immunofluorescent antibody (IFA) test. It should be noted that clinical laboratories vary somewhat in their description of this test. It may be described as "Lyme ELISA," "Lyme antibody screen," "total Lyme antibody," or "Lyme IgG/IgM." Many commercial laboratories offer EIA/IFA with reflex to Western immunoblot if the first-tier assay result is positive or equivocal. Although the initial EIA or IFA test result may be reported quantitatively, its sole importance is to categorize the result as negative, equivocal, or positive.

If the first-tier EIA result is negative, the patient is considered seronegative and no further testing is indicated. If the result is equivocal or positive, a second-tier test is required to confirm the result. There are 2 options for second-tier testing: (1) a Western immunoblot, which is the standard 2-tiered testing algorithm or (2) an EIA test that has been specifically cleared by the US Food and Drug Administration (FDA) for use as a second-tier confirmatory test, which is the modified 2-tiered testing algorithm (**www.cdc.gov/ mmwr/volumes/68/wr/mm6832a4.htm?s_ cid=mm6832a4_w**). Some assays marketed in the United States have reduced sensitivity for European strains of *B burgdorferi*.

Two-tiered serological testing increases test specificity. False-positive results are partly explained by antigenic components of *B burgdorferi* that are nonspecific to this species. Antibodies produced in response to other spirochetal infections, spirochetes in normal oral flora, other acute infections, and certain autoimmune diseases may be cross-reactive. In areas with endemic infection, previous subclinical infection with seroconversion may occur, and a seropositive patient's symptoms may be coincidental. Patients with active Lyme disease almost always have objective signs of infection (eg, EM, facial nerve palsy, arthritis). Nonspecific symptoms commonly accompany these specific signs but are almost never the only evidence of Lyme disease. Serological testing for Lyme disease should not be performed in children without symptoms or signs suggestive of Lyme disease and plausible geographic exposure.

Western immunoblot testing should not be performed if the initial EIA or IFA test result is negative or without a prior EIA or IFA test, because specificity of immunoblot diminishes if the test is performed alone. The immunoblot assay tests for presence of antibodies to specific *B burgdorferi* antigens, including immunoglobulin M (IgM) antibodies to 3 spirochetal antigens (the 23/24, 39, and 41 kDa polypeptides) and immunoglobulin G (IgG) antibodies to 10 spirochetal antigens (the 18, 23/24, 28, 30, 39, 41, 45, 60, 66, and 93 kDa polypeptides). Although some clinical laboratories report presence of antibody to each of 13 bands, describing each band as positive or negative, a positive immunoblot result is defined as presence of at least 2 IgM bands or 5 IgG bands. Physicians must be careful not to misinterpret a positive band as a positive test result or interpret a result as positive despite presence of 4 or fewer IgG bands. It is noteworthy that IgG antibodies to flagella protein, the p41 band, are present in 30% to 50% of healthy people.

A positive IgM immunoblot result can be falsely positive. The IgM assay is useful only for patients in the first 4 weeks after symptom onset. The IgM immunoblot result should be disregarded (or, if possible, not ordered) in patients who have had symptoms for longer than 4 weeks, or symptoms consistent with late Lyme disease, because false-positive IgM assay results are common and most untreated patients with disseminated Lyme disease will have a positive IgG result by week 4 of symptoms.

Lyme disease test results for *B burgdorferi* in patients treated for syphilis or other spirochete diseases are difficult to interpret. Consultation with an infectious diseases specialist is recommended. Although immunodeficiency could theoretically affect serological testing results, reports have described infected patients who produced anti–*B burgdorferi* antibodies and had positive test results despite various immunocompromising conditions.

Polymerase chain reaction (PCR) testing of joint fluid from a patient with Lyme arthritis often yields positive results and can be informative in establishing a diagnosis of Lyme arthritis. The role of a PCR assay on blood is not well established; test results are usually negative in early and late Lyme disease, so PCR assay is not recommended routinely. Yield of PCR testing on cerebrospinal fluid samples from patients with neuroborreliosis is too low to be useful in excluding this diagnosis.

Some patients treated with antimicrobial agents for early Lyme disease never develop detectable antibodies against *B burgdorferi*; they are cured and do not have risk for late disease. Development of antibodies in patients treated for early Lyme disease does not indicate lack of cure or presence of persistent infection. Ongoing infection without development of antibodies ("seronegative Lyme") has not been demonstrated. Most patients with early disseminated disease and virtually all patients with late disease have antibodies against *B burgdorferi*. Once such antibodies develop, they may persist for many years. Tests for antibodies should not be repeated or used to assess success of treatment.

A number of tests for Lyme disease have been found to be invalid on the basis of independent testing or to be too nonspecific to exclude false-positive results. These include urine tests for *B burgdorferi*, CD57 assay, novel culture techniques, and antibody panels that differ from those recommended as part of standardized 2-tier testing. Although these tests are commercially available from some clinical laboratories, they are not FDA cleared and are not appropriate diagnostic tests for Lyme disease.

Current evidence indicates that patients with *B mayonii* infection develop a serological response like that of patients infected with *B burgdorferi*. Standardized 2-tier testing can be expected to have positive results in patients with *B mayonii* infection.

TREATMENT

Consensus practice guidelines for assessment, treatment, and prevention of Lyme disease have been published by the Infectious Diseases Society of America. Care of children should follow recommendations in Table 81.1. Antimicrobial therapy for nonspecific symptoms or for asymptomatic seropositivity is not recommended. Antimicrobial agents administered for durations not specified in Table 81.1 are not recommended. Alternative diagnostic approaches or therapies without adequate validation studies and publication in peer-reviewed scientific literature are discouraged. Physicians have successfully treated patients with *B mayonii* infection with antimicrobial regimens used for Lyme disease.

Erythema Migrans (Single or Multiple)

Doxycycline, amoxicillin, or cefuroxime can be used to treat children of any age who present with EM. Azithromycin is generally regarded as a second-line antimicrobial agent for EM in the United States, but further research on the efficacy of this agent is warranted. Selection of an oral antimicrobial agent for treatment of EM should be based on the following considerations: presence of neurological disease (for which doxycycline is the drug of choice), drug allergy, adverse effects, frequency of administration (doxycycline and cefuroxime are administered twice a day, and amoxicillin is administered 3 times a day), ability to minimize sun exposure (photosensitivity may be associated with doxycycline use), likelihood of coinfection with *Anaplasma phagocytophilum* or *Ehrlichia muris*–like agent (neither is sensitive to β-lactam antimicrobial agents), and inability to easily distinguish *Staphylococcus aureus* cellulitis from EM (doxycycline is effective against most strains of methicillin-sensitive and methicillin-resistant *S aureus*). EM should be treated orally for 10 days if doxycycline is used and for 14 days if amoxicillin or cefuroxime is used. Because STARI may be indistinguishable from early Lyme disease and questions remain about appropriate treatment, some physicians treat STARI with the same antimicrobial agents orally as for Lyme disease.

Treatment of EM results in resolution of the skin lesion within several days of initiating therapy and almost always prevents development of later stages of Lyme disease.

Table 81.1
Recommended Treatment of Lyme Disease in Children

Disease Category	Drug(s) and Dose
Erythema migrans (single or multiple) (any age)	Doxycycline, 4.4 mg/kg/day, orally, divided into 2 doses (maximum 200 mg/day) for 10 days
	OR
	Amoxicillin, 50 mg/kg/day, orally, divided into 3 doses (maximum 1.5 g/day) for 14 days
	OR
	Cefuroxime, 30 mg/kg/day, orally, in 2 divided doses (maximum 1 g/day) for 14 days
	OR, for a patient unable to take a β-lactam or doxycycline,
	Azithromycin, 10 mg/kg/day, orally, once daily for 7 days
Isolated facial palsy	Doxycycline, 4.4 mg/kg/day, orally, divided into 2 doses (maximum 200 mg/day), for 14 days[a]
Arthritis	An oral agent as for early localized disease, for 28 days[b]
Persistent arthritis after first course of therapy	Re-treat by using an oral agent as for first-episode arthritis, for 28 days[b]
	OR
	Ceftriaxone sodium, 50–75 mg/kg, IV, once a day (maximum 2 g/day) for 14–28 days
Atrioventricular heart block or carditis	An oral agent as for early localized disease, for 14 days (range, 14–21 days)
	OR
	Ceftriaxone sodium, 50–75 mg/kg, IV, once a day (maximum 2 g/day) for 14 days (range, 14–21 days for a hospitalized patient); oral therapy (by using an agent as for early localized disease) can be substituted when the patient is stabilized or discharged, to complete the 14- to 21-day course.
Meningitis	Doxycycline, 4.4 mg/kg/day, orally, divided into 1 or 2 doses (maximum 200 mg/day) for 14 days
	OR
	Ceftriaxone sodium, 50–75 mg/kg, IV, once a day (maximum 2 g/day) for 14 days

IV indicates intravenously.

[a] Corticosteroids should not be given. Use of amoxicillin for facial palsy in children has not been studied. Treatment has no effect on the resolution of facial nerve palsy; its purpose is to prevent late disease.
[b] There are limited safety data on the use of doxycycline for >21 days in children <8 years of age.

Early Disseminated Disease

Oral antimicrobial agents are appropriate and effective for most manifestations of disseminated Lyme disease. Doxycycline is preferred therapy for facial nerve palsy caused by B burgdorferi in children of any age. The purpose of therapy for cranial nerve palsies is to reduce the risk of late disease; treatment has no effect on resolution of the facial palsy. Amoxicillin has not been studied sufficiently for treatment of facial nerve palsies in young children to make a recommendation. Amoxicillin is unlikely to reach therapeutic levels in the central nervous system.

A growing body of evidence suggests that oral doxycycline is effective for treatment of Lyme meningitis and may be used as an alternative to hospitalization and parenteral ceftriaxone therapy in children well enough to be treated as outpatients. Lumbar puncture is indicated for a child with a stiff neck and other symptoms of meningitis in whom the possibility of a bacterial (nonspirochetal) meningitis cannot be ruled out. Neurological disease is treated for 14 days.

Late Disseminated Disease

Children with Lyme arthritis are treated with oral antimicrobial agents for 28 days. Because of this duration, patients younger than 8 years should be treated with an oral agent other than doxycycline (eg, amoxicillin). For patients 8 years and older, any of the oral options, including doxycycline, may be used.

Treatment of patients with Lyme arthritis who have a partial response to therapy is uncertain. Consideration should be given to medication adherence, duration of symptoms before treatment, extent of synovial proliferation compared to joint swelling, cost, and patient preference. A second 28-day course of oral therapy is reasonable when synovial proliferation is more modest than joint swelling or when the patient prefers a trial of oral therapy before considering intravenous treatment. Patients who demonstrate no or minimal response or who experience worsening of their arthritis can be treated with ceftriaxone parenterally for 14 to 28 days.

Approximately 10% to 15% of patients treated for Lyme arthritis will develop persistent synovitis that can last for months to years. Theories of pathophysiology include delayed resolution of inflammation because of slow clearance of nonviable bacteria following treatment versus an autoimmune mechanism. Misdiagnosis should also be considered (ie, Lyme antibodies in serum present from a previous infection or cross-reacting because of another disorder). Persisting synovitis following Lyme disease, termed *antibiotic-refractory Lyme arthritis*, is a strongly HLA-associated phenomenon. Patients with persistent synovitis despite repeated treatment should initially be treated with nonsteroidal anti-inflammatory drugs. More severe cases should be referred to a rheumatologist who may treat the inflammation with an intra-articular steroid injection. Methotrexate has been used successfully in some cases. Arthroscopic synovectomy is required rarely for disabling or refractory cases.

Persistent Posttreatment Symptoms

Some patients have prolonged, persistent symptoms following standard treatment of Lyme disease. It is unclear whether this phenomenon is unique to Lyme disease or it is a more general occurrence during convalescence from other systemic illnesses. Persistent, treatment-refractory infection with *B burgdorferi* (chronic Lyme disease) has not been substantiated scientifically. Patients with persistent symptoms following Lyme disease usually respond to symptomatic treatment and recover gradually.

Several double-blinded, randomized, placebo-controlled trials have shown that re-treatment with additional antimicrobial agents for subjective symptoms of patients with residual posttreatment Lyme disease may be associated with harm and does not offer benefit.[1-4] Administration of additional antimicrobial agents to a patient with posttreatment Lyme disease symptoms following standard treatment of Lyme disease is strongly discouraged.

Re-treatment is appropriate for subsequent acute infections caused by *B burgdorferi*.

Pregnancy

Tetracyclines are contraindicated in pregnancy. Doxycycline has not been studied adequately during pregnancy to make a recommendation regarding its use. Otherwise, therapy is the same as recommended for nonpregnant people.

---

[1] Feder HM, Johnson BJ, O'Connell S, et al; Ad Hoc International Lyme Disease Group. A critical appraisal of "chronic Lyme disease." *N Engl J Med.* 2007;357(14):1422–1430.

[2] Lantos PM, Rumbaugh J, Bockenstedt LK, et al. Clinical practice guidelines by the Infectious Diseases Society of America (IDSA), American Academy of Neurology (AAN), and American College of Rheumatology (ACR): 2020 guidelines for the prevention, diagnosis and treatment of Lyme disease. *Clin Infect Dis.* 2021;72(1):e1–e48. The full guideline is available at **www.idsociety.org/practice-guideline/lyme-disease**.

[3] Berende A, ter Hofstede HJ, Vos FJ, et al. Randomized trial of longer-term therapy for symptoms attributed to Lyme disease. *N Engl J Med.* 2016;374(13):1209–1220.

[4] Marzec NS, Nelson C, Waldron PR, et al. Serious bacterial infections acquired during treatment of patients given a diagnosis of chronic Lyme disease—United States. *MMWR Morb Mortal Wkly Rep.* 2017;66(23):607–609.

LYME DISEASE

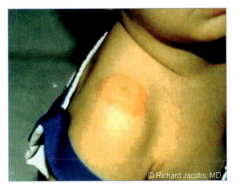

Image 81.1
Lyme disease. The rash of erythema migrans in a 4-year-old boy with infection caused by *Borrelia burgdorferi*. Copyright Richard Jacobs, MD.

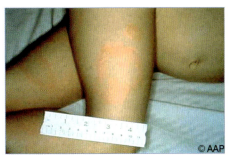

Image 81.2
Erythema migrans lesion at the site of a tick bite characteristic of early localized Lyme disease. It is annular with central clearing (ie, a target lesion), but in other cases, the initial lesion can be uniformly erythematous and can occasionally have a vesicular or necrotic center, as illustrated in Image 81.3. Systemic symptoms, such as fever, myalgia, headache, or malaise, can occur at this stage of infection.

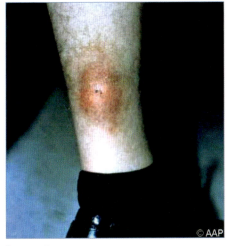

Image 81.3
The rash at the site of a tick bite on the lower leg indicates the variation in the initial rash of Lyme disease. Central clearing is incomplete, and a central necrotic area is apparent at the presumed site of the tick bite.

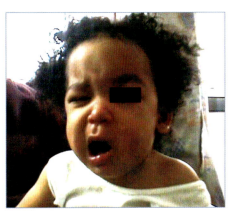

Image 81.4
A 15-month-old girl with left facial nerve palsy complicating Lyme disease. Copyright Michael Rajnik, MD, FAAP.

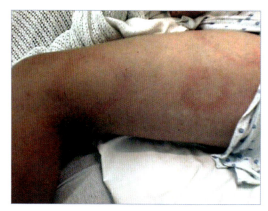

Image 81.5
Erythema migrans lesions in a 12-year-old boy who contracted Lyme disease in Maryland. Copyright Michael Rajnik, MD, FAAP.

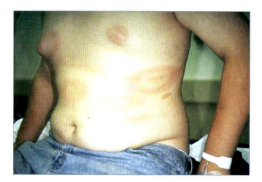

Image 81.6
A 14-year-old boy with multiple annular skin lesions and worsening headache associated with photophobia. Results from a lumbar puncture revealed a cerebrospinal fluid pleocytosis and aseptic meningitis. The characteristic erythema migrans skin lesions helped determine the diagnosis of Lyme disease. The patient was treated with intravenous ceftriaxone. Copyright Barbara Jantausch, MD, FAAP.

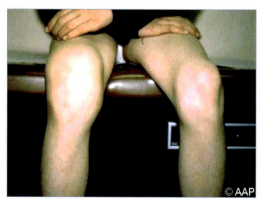

Image 81.7
Borrelia burgdorferi synovitis with marked swelling and only mild tenderness. Arthritis usually occurs within 1–2 months following the appearance of erythema migrans, and the knees are the most commonly affected joints.

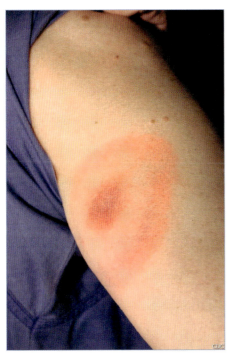

Image 81.8
This photograph depicts the pathognomonic erythematous rash in the pattern of a bull's-eye, which developed at the site of a tick bite on this Maryland woman's posterior right upper arm. Courtesy of Centers for Disease Control and Prevention/James Gathany.

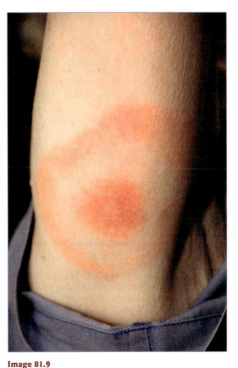

Image 81.9
This photograph depicts the pathognomonic erythematous rash (erythema migrans) in the pattern of a bull's-eye, which developed at the site of a tick bite on this Maryland woman's posterior right upper arm. The expanding rash reflects migration of the spirochetes after introduction of the organism during the tick bite. Courtesy of Centers for Disease Control and Prevention/James Gathany.

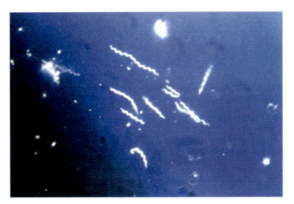

Image 81.10
Taken with darkfield microscopy technique, this photomicrograph reveals the presence of spirochetes, or corkscrew-shaped bacteria known as *Borrelia burgdorferi*, which are the pathogen responsible for causing Lyme disease (magnification ×400). *B burgdorferi* are helical-shaped bacteria and are about 10–25 μm long. These bacteria are transmitted to humans by the bite of an infected deer tick. Courtesy of Centers for Disease Control and Prevention.

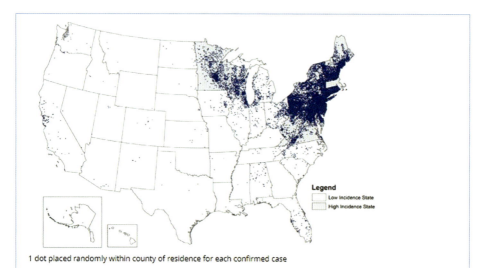

Image 81.11
Reported cases of Lyme disease—United States, 2019. One dot is placed randomly within county of residence for each confirmed case. Courtesy of Centers for Disease Control and Prevention.

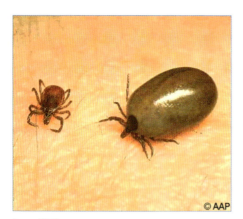

Image 81.12
Two deer ticks of the *Ixodes* genus that transmit *Borrelia burgdorferi* to humans. The engorged tick on the right demonstrates increased size from a blood meal. Both are magnified in this photograph.

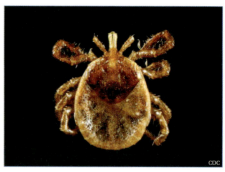

Image 81.13
This photograph depicts a dorsal view of an immature, or nymphal, lone star tick, *Amblyomma americanum*. Nymphal ticks are much smaller than adult ticks, and people might not notice a nymph until it has been feeding for a few days. Nymphs are therefore more likely than adult ticks to transmit diseases to people. Courtesy of Centers for Disease Control and Prevention/Amanda Loftis, MD; William Nicholson, MD; Will Reeves, MD; and Chris Paddock, MD.

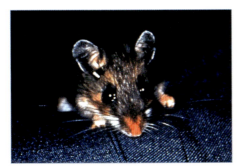

Image 81.14
This photograph depicts a white-footed mouse, *Peromyscus leucopus*, which is a wild rodent reservoir host of ticks, which are known to carry *Borrelia burgdorferi*, the bacteria responsible for Lyme disease. During their larval stage, *Ixodidae*, or hard ticks, feed on small mammals, particularly the white-footed mouse, which serves as the primary reservoir for *B burgdorferi*. Courtesy of Centers for Disease Control and Prevention.

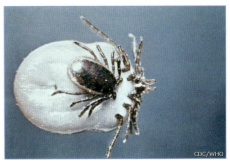

Image 81.15
This is a male *Ixodes ricinus* tick (smaller) shown copulating with a female tick (larger). *I ricinus*, the castor-bean tick, so called because of its resemblance to the castor bean, is a vector for the *Borrelia burgdorferi* spirochete, the cause of Lyme disease, and is commonly found on farm animals and deer. Courtesy of Centers for Disease Control and Prevention/World Health Organization.

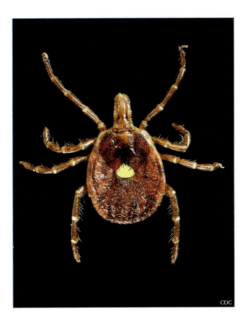

Image 81.16
This photograph depicts a dorsal view of a female lone star tick, *Amblyomma americanum*. Note the characteristic lone star marking located centrally on its dorsal surface, at the distal tip of its scutum. Courtesy of Centers for Disease Control and Prevention/Amanda Loftis, MD; William Nicholson, MD; Will Reeves, MD; and Chris Paddock, MD.

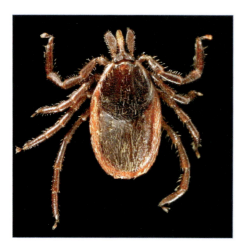

Image 81.17
This photograph depicts a dorsal view of an adult female western black-legged tick, *Ixodes pacificus*, which has been shown to transmit *Borrelia burgdorferi*, the agent of Lyme disease, and *Anaplasma phagocytophilum*, the agent of human granulocytic anaplasmosis (previously known as human granulocytic ehrlichiosis), in the western United States. The small scutum does not cover its entire abdomen, thereby allowing the abdomen to expand many times when this tick ingests its blood meal, and helps identify this specimen as a female. The 4 pairs of jointed legs place these ticks in the phylum *Arthropoda* and the class *Arachnida*. Courtesy of Centers for Disease Control and Prevention/Amanda Loftis, MD; William Nicholson, MD; Will Reeves, MD; and Chris Paddock, MD.

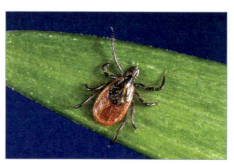

Image 81.18
This black-legged tick, *Ixodes scapularis*, is found on a wide range of hosts, including mammals, birds, and reptiles. *I scapularis* are known to transmit the agent of Lyme disease, *Borrelia burgdorferi*, to humans and animals during feeding when they insert their mouth parts into the skin of a host and slowly take in the nutrient-rich host blood. Courtesy of Centers for Disease Control and Prevention/Michael L. Levin, PhD.

CHAPTER 82

Lymphatic Filariasis
(Bancroftian, Malayan, and Timorian)

CLINICAL MANIFESTATIONS

Lymphatic filariasis (LF) is caused by infection with the filarial parasites *Wuchereria bancrofti, Brugia malayi,* or *Brugia timori.* Adult worms cause lymphatic dilatation and dysfunction, which result in abnormal lymph flow and may eventually lead to lymphedema in the legs, scrotal area (only for *W bancrofti*), and arms. Recurrent secondary bacterial infections hasten progression of lymphedema to the more severe form known as elephantiasis. Although the infection occurs commonly in young children living in areas with endemic LF, chronic manifestations of infection, such as hydrocele and lymphedema, occur infrequently in people younger than 20 years. Most filarial infections remain clinically asymptomatic, but even then, they commonly cause subclinical lymphatic dilatation and dysfunction. Lymphadenopathy, most frequently of the inguinal, crural, and axillary lymph nodes, is the most common clinical sign of LF in children. There can be an acute inflammatory response that progresses from the lymph node distally (retrograde) along the affected lymphatic vessel, usually in the limbs. Accompanying systemic symptoms, such as headache or fever, are generally mild. In postpubertal males, adult *W bancrofti* organisms are found most commonly in the intrascrotal lymphatic vessels; thus, inflammation around dead or dying adult worms may manifest as funiculitis (inflammation of the spermatic cord), epididymitis, or orchitis. A tender granulomatous nodule may be palpable at the site of dying or dead adult worms. Chyluria can occur as a manifestation of bancroftian filariasis. Tropical pulmonary eosinophilia, characterized by cough, fever, wheezing, marked eosinophilia, and high serum immunoglobulin E concentrations, is a rare manifestation of LF.

ETIOLOGY

Filariasis is caused by 3 filarial nematodes in the family *Filariidae: W bancrofti, B malayi,* and *B timori.*

EPIDEMIOLOGY

The parasite is transmitted by the bite of infected mosquitoes of various genera, including *Culex, Aedes, Anopheles,* and *Mansonia. W bancrofti,* the most prevalent cause of LF, is found in Haiti, the Dominican Republic, Guyana, northeast Brazil, sub-Saharan and North Africa, and Asia, extending from India through the Indonesian archipelago to the western Pacific Islands. Humans are the only definitive host for the parasite. *B malayi* is found mostly in Southeast Asia and parts of India. *B timori* is restricted to certain islands at the eastern end of the Indonesian archipelago. Live adult worms release microfilariae into the bloodstream. Adult worms live for an average of 5 to 8 years, and reinfection is common. Microfilariae that can infect mosquitoes may be present in a patient's blood for decades, although individual microfilariae have a life span between 3 and 12 months. The adult worm is not transmissible from person to person or by blood transfusion; microfilariae can be transmitted by transfusion, but they do not develop into adult worms.

The **incubation period** is not well established; the period from acquisition to the appearance of microfilariae in blood can be 3 to 12 months, depending on the species of parasite.

DIAGNOSTIC TESTS

Microfilariae can generally be detected microscopically on blood smears obtained at night (10:00 pm–4:00 am), although variations in the periodicity of microfilaremia have been described depending on the parasite strain and the geographic location. Adult worms or microfilariae can be identified on the basis of general morphology, size, and presence or absence of a sheath in Giemsa-stained fluid or tissue specimens obtained at biopsy. Serological enzyme immunoassays are available, but interpretation of results is affected by cross-reactions of filarial antibodies with antibodies against other helminths. Determination of serum antifilarial immunoglobulin G (IgG) and IgG4 is available through the Laboratory of Parasitic Diseases at the National Institutes of Health (301/496-5398) or for antifilarial IgG4 through the Centers for Disease Control and Prevention (CDC [404/718-4745; **parasites@cdc.gov**]). Assays for circulating filarial antigen of *W bancrofti* are available commercially but are not cleared for use by the

US Food and Drug Administration and are not available in the United States. Ultrasonography can be used to visualize adult worms. Patients with lymphedema may no longer have microfilariae or antifilarial antibody present.

TREATMENT

The main goal of treatment of an infected person is to kill the adult worm. Diethylcarbamazine citrate (DEC), which is both microfilaricidal and active against the adult worm, is the drug of choice for LF. DEC is no longer sold in the United States but can be obtained from the CDC (404/718-4745; **parasites@cdc.gov**; **www.cdc.gov/parasites/lymphaticfilariasis**). Treatment with DEC should be undertaken by a specialist with experience in treating LF, because DEC therapy has been associated with life-threatening adverse events, including encephalopathy and renal failure in people with circulating *Loa loa* microfilariae concentrations greater than 8,000/µL. Ivermectin is effective against the microfilariae of *W bancrofti* and the 2 *Brugia* species but has no effect on the adult parasite. Albendazole has also demonstrated macrofilaricidal activity. Studies in children as young as 1 year of age suggest that albendazole can be administered safely to this population. Two- or 3-drug combination therapies have been used in the Global Programme to Eliminate Lymphatic Filariasis. Doxycycline, a drug that targets *Wolbachia* species, an intracellular rickettsial-like bacterial endosymbiont in adult worms, has been shown to be macrofilaricidal and has been used in combination with DEC.

Antifilarial chemotherapy has been shown to have limited efficacy for reversing or stabilizing lymphedema in its early forms. Doxycycline, in limited studies, has been shown to decrease the severity of lymphedema. Complex decongestive physiotherapy can be effective for treating lymphedema and requires strict attention to hygiene in the affected anatomical areas. Prompt identification and treatment of bacterial superinfections, particularly streptococcal and staphylococcal infections, and careful treatment of intertriginous and ungual fungal infections are important aspects of therapy for lymphedema. Surgery may be indicated for management of hydrocele. Chyluria originating in the bladder responds to fulguration; chyluria originating in the kidney is difficult to correct.

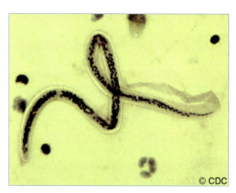

Image 82.1
Microfilaria of *Wuchereria bancrofti* from a patient in Haiti (thick blood smear; hematoxylin stain). The microfilaria is sheathed, its body is gently curved, and the tail is tapered to a point. The nuclear column (ie, the cells that constitute the body of the microfilaria) is loosely packed; the cells can be visualized individually and do not extend to the tip of the tail. The sheath is slightly stained by hematoxylin. Courtesy of Centers for Disease Control and Prevention.

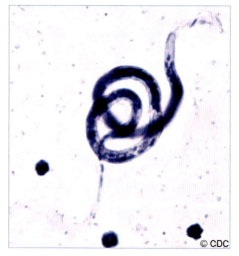

Image 82.2
Microfilaria of *Brugia malayi* (thick blood smear; hematoxylin stain). Like *Wuchereria bancrofti*, this species has a sheath (slightly stained in hematoxylin). In contrast with *W bancrofti*, the microfilariae in this species are more tightly coiled and the nuclear column is more tightly packed, preventing the visualization of individual cells. Courtesy of Centers for Disease Control and Prevention.

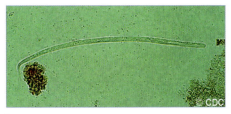

Image 82.4
Microfilaria of *Onchocerca volvulus* from skin snip from a patient in Guatemala (wet preparation). Some important characteristics of the microfilariae of this species are shown. No sheath is present, and the tail is tapered and is sharply angled at the end. Courtesy of Centers for Disease Control and Prevention.

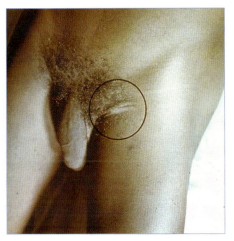

Image 82.3
Inguinal lymph nodes enlarged (circled) because of filariasis. Courtesy of Centers for Disease Control and Prevention.

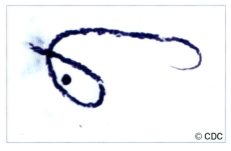

Image 82.6
Microfilaria of *Mansonella ozzardi* (thick blood smear; Giemsa stain). The microfilaria is typically small and unsheathed and has a slender, tapered tail that is hooked ("buttonhook"). The nuclei do not extend to the end of the tail. Courtesy of Centers for Disease Control and Prevention.

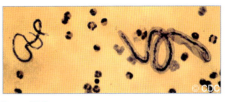

Image 82.5
Microfilariae of *Loa loa* (right) and *Mansonella perstans* (left) in a patient in Cameroon (thick blood smear; hematoxylin stain). *L loa* is sheathed, with a relatively dense nuclear column; its tail tapers and is frequently coiled, and nuclei extend to the end of the tail.
M perstans is smaller, has no sheath, and has a blunt tail with nuclei extending to the end of the tail. Courtesy of Centers for Disease Control and Prevention.

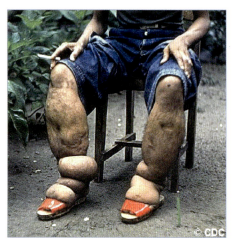

Image 82.7
Elephantiasis of both legs caused by filariasis. Luzon, Philippines. Courtesy of Centers for Disease Control and Prevention.

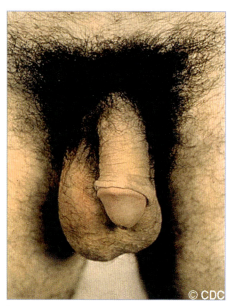

Image 82.8
Scrotal lymphangitis caused by filariasis. Courtesy of Centers for Disease Control and Prevention.

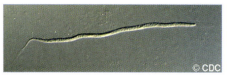

Image 82.9
Microfilaria of *Brugia malayi* collected by the Knott (centrifugation) concentration technique, in 2% formalin wet preparation. Note the erythrocyte ghosts (for size comparison) and the clearly visible sheath that extends beyond the anterior and posterior ends of the microfilaria. (There are 4 sheathed species: *Wuchereria bancrofti*, *B malayi*, *Brugia timori*, and *Loa loa*.) Courtesy of Centers for Disease Control and Prevention.

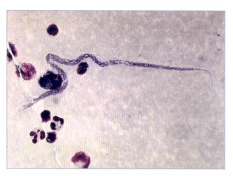

Image 82.10
Mansonella ozzardi, infectious agent of filariasis. Courtesy of Centers for Disease Control and Prevention.

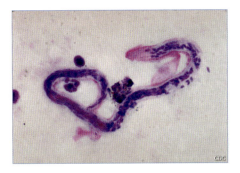

Image 82.11

This photomicrograph shows the inner body and cephalic space of a *Brugia malayi* microfilaria in a thick blood smear. *B malayi*, a nematode that can inhabit the lymphatics and subcutaneous tissues in humans, is one of the causative agents for lymphatic filariasis. The vectors for this parasite are mosquito species from the genera *Mansonia* and *Aedes*. Courtesy of Centers for Disease Control and Prevention/Mae Melvin, MD.

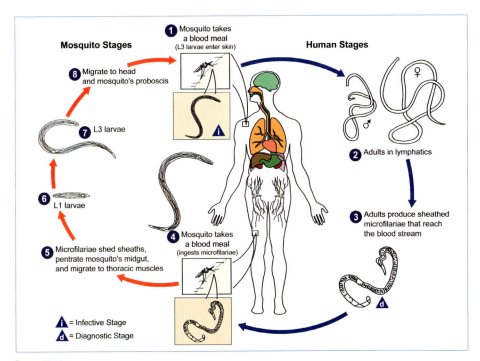

Image 82.12

The typical vector for *Brugia malayi* filariasis are mosquito species from the genera *Mansonia* and *Aedes*. During a blood meal, an infected mosquito introduces third-stage filarial larvae onto the skin of the human host, where they penetrate into the bite wound (1). They develop into adults that commonly reside in the lymphatics (2). The adult worms resemble those of *Wuchereria bancrofti* but are smaller. Female worms measure 43–55 mm in length × 130–170 μm in width, and males measure 13–23 mm in length × 70–80 μm in width. Adults produce microfilariae, measuring 177–230 μm in length and 5–7 μm in width, that are sheathed and have nocturnal periodicity. The microfilariae migrate into lymph and enter the bloodstream, reaching the peripheral blood (3). A mosquito ingests the microfilariae during a blood meal (1). After ingestion, the microfilariae lose their sheaths and work their way through the wall of the proventriculus and cardiac portion of the midgut to reach the thoracic muscles (5). There, the microfilariae develop into first-stage larvae (6) and, subsequently, into third-stage larvae (7). The third-stage larvae migrate through the hemocoel to the mosquito's proboscis (8) and can infect another human when the mosquito takes a blood meal (1). Courtesy of Centers for Disease Control and Prevention.

CHAPTER 83
Lymphocytic Choriomeningitis Virus

CLINICAL MANIFESTATIONS

Child and adult infections with lymphocytic choriomeningitis virus (LCMV) are asymptomatic in approximately one-third of cases. Symptomatic infection may result in a mild to severe illness, which can include fever, malaise, myalgia, retro-orbital headache, photophobia, anorexia, and nausea and vomiting. Sore throat, cough, arthralgia or arthritis, and orchitis may also occur. Initial symptoms may last from a few days to 3 weeks. Leukopenia, lymphopenia, thrombocytopenia, and elevation of lactate dehydrogenase and aspartate aminotransferase levels occur frequently. A biphasic febrile course is common; after a few days without symptoms, the second phase may occur in up to half of symptomatic patients, consisting of neurological manifestations that vary from aseptic meningitis to severe encephalitis. Transverse myelitis, eighth nerve deafness, Guillain-Barré syndrome, and hydrocephalus have also been reported, but a causal link remains to be established. Extraneural disease has included reports of myocarditis and dermatitis. Rarely, LCMV has caused a disease resembling viral hemorrhagic syndrome. Transmission of LCMV through organ transplant and infection in other immunocompromised populations can result in fatal disseminated infection with multiple organ failure.

Current prevalence and seasonality are unknown, because diagnostic testing is often not performed. Recovery without sequelae is the usual outcome, but convalescence may take several weeks, with asthenia, poor cognitive function, headaches, and arthralgia. LCMV infection should be suspected in presence of (1) aseptic meningitis or encephalitis, especially during periods of colder weather; (2) febrile illness, followed by brief remission, followed by onset of neurological illness; and (3) cerebrospinal fluid (CSF) findings of lymphocytosis and hypoglycorrhachia.

Infection during pregnancy has been associated with spontaneous abortion. Congenital infection may cause severe abnormalities, including hydrocephalus, chorioretinitis, intracranial calcifications, microcephaly, and intellectual disability. Congenital LCMV infection should be included in the differential diagnosis whenever intrauterine infections with toxoplasma, rubella, cytomegalovirus, herpes simplex virus, enterovirus, parechovirus, Zika virus, *Treponema pallidum*, or parvovirus B19 are being considered.

ETIOLOGY

LCMV is a single-stranded RNA virus that belongs to the family *Arenaviridae* (appearance on electron microscopy resembles grains of sand). Other members of this family included in the genus *Mammarenaviruses* are Lassa virus and the New World *Arenaviruses* Junin, Machupo, Guanarito, Sabiá, and Chapare.

EPIDEMIOLOGY

LCMV is a chronic infection of common house mice, which are often infected asymptomatically and which chronically shed virus in urine and other excretions. Congenital murine infection is common and results in a normal-appearing litter with chronic viremia and particularly high virus excretion. In addition, hamsters, laboratory mice, and guinea pigs can have chronic infection and can be sources of human infection. Humans are infected mostly by inhalation of aerosol generated by rodents shedding virus from the urine, feces, blood, or nasopharyngeal secretions. Other less likely routes of entry of infected secretions include conjunctival and other mucous membranes, ingestion, and cuts in the skin. The disease is observed more frequently in young adults. Human-to-human transmission has occurred during pregnancy from infected mothers to their fetus and through solid organ transplant from an infected organ donor. Several such clusters of cases have been described following transplant, and one case was traced to a pet hamster purchased by the donor. Laboratory-acquired LCMV infections have occurred, both through infected laboratory animals and contaminated tissue-culture stocks.

The **incubation period** is usually 6 to 13 days and is occasionally as long as 3 weeks.

DIAGNOSTIC TESTS

Patients with central nervous system disease have a mononuclear pleocytosis with 30 to 8,000 cells in CSF. Hypoglycorrhachia, as well as mild increase in protein level, may occur. LCMV can usually be isolated from CSF obtained during the acute phase of illness and, in severe disseminated infections, also from blood, urine, and nasopharyngeal secretion specimens. Reverse transcriptase–polymerase chain reaction assays available through reference or commercial laboratories can be used on serum during the acute stage and on CSF during the neurological phase. Serum specimens from the acute and convalescent phases of illness can be tested for increases in antibody titers by enzyme immunoassays and neutralization tests.

Demonstration of virus-specific immunoglobulin M antibodies in serum or CSF specimens is useful. In congenital infections, diagnosis is usually suspected when ocular or neurological signs develop, and diagnosis is usually made by serological testing. In immunosuppressed patients, seroconversion can take several weeks. Diagnosis can also be made by immunohistochemical assay of fixed tissues.

TREATMENT

Management is supportive.

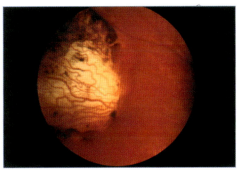

Image 83.1
Fundus photograph of a 9-month-old girl with congenital lymphocytic choriomeningitis virus infection. Extensive chorioretinal scarring is visible. Hydrocephalus and periventricular calcification were visible on computed tomographic and magnetic resonance images. Copyright Leslie L. Barton, MD, FAAP.

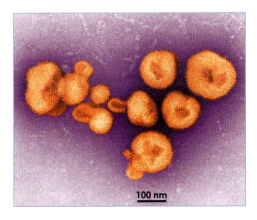

Image 83.2
This transmission electron micrograph depicts 8 virions (viral particles) of a newly discovered virus, which was determined to be a member of the genus *Arenavirus*. A cause of fatal hemorrhagic fever, it was confirmed that this virus was responsible for causing illness in 5 South Africans, 4 of whom died having succumbed to its devastating effects. Ultrastructurally, these round *Arenavirus* virions displayed the characteristic "sandy" or granular capsid (ie, outer skin), an appearance from which the Latin name, *arena*, was derived. Other members of the genus *Arenavirus* include the West African Lassa virus, lymphocytic choriomeningitis virus, and Bolivian hemorrhagic fever virus, also known as Machupo virus, all of which are spread to humans through their inhalation of airborne particulates originating from rodent excrement, which can occur during the simple act of sweeping a floor. Courtesy of Centers for Disease Control and Prevention/Charles Humphrey.

CHAPTER 84
Malaria

CLINICAL MANIFESTATIONS

The classic symptom of malaria, which may be paroxysmal, is high fever with chills, rigor, sweats, and headache. Other manifestations can include nausea, vomiting, diarrhea, cough, tachypnea, arthralgia, myalgia, and abdominal and back pain. Anemia and thrombocytopenia are common. Hepatosplenomegaly is frequently present in infected children in areas with endemic malaria and may be present in adults and in people previously not infected with malaria. Severe disease occurs more frequently in people without immunity acquired from previous infection; young children; pregnant women, especially primigravidae; or those who are immunocompromised.

Infection with *Plasmodium falciparum*, one of the 5 *Plasmodium* species that naturally infect humans, is potentially fatal and most commonly manifests as a nonspecific febrile illness often without localizing signs. Severe disease (which may occur with any of the infecting species but is most commonly caused by *P falciparum*) may manifest as one of the following clinical syndromes, all of which are medical emergencies and may be fatal unless treated:

- **Cerebral malaria,** characterized by altered mental status and manifesting with a range of neurological signs and symptoms, including generalized seizures, signs of increased intracranial pressure (confusion and progression to stupor or coma), and death.

- **Severe anemia** attributable to dyserythropoiesis, high parasitemia and hemolysis, sequestration of infected erythrocytes to capillaries, coagulopathy, and hemolysis of infected erythrocytes associated with hypersplenism; late-onset hemolytic anemia has been described following treatment of severe disease with artemisinin derivatives.

- **Hypoglycemia,** which can manifest with metabolic acidosis and hypotension associated with hyperparasitemia; it can also be a consequence of quinine or quinidine-induced hyperinsulinemia.

- **Renal failure** caused by acute tubular necrosis (rare in children <8 years).

- **Respiratory failure,** without pulmonary edema.

- **Abnormal bleeding,** which can include hemoglobinuria and is attributable to thrombocytopenia, an exaggerated hemolytic response, or disseminated coagulopathy.

- **Jaundice,** secondary to hemolysis of infected blood cells, coagulopathy, and/or hepatic dysfunction.

- **Metabolic acidosis,** usually attributed to lactic acidosis, hypovolemia, liver dysfunction, and impaired renal function.

- **Vascular collapse and shock** associated with hypothermia and adrenal insufficiency.

Syndromes primarily associated with *Plasmodium vivax* and *Plasmodium ovale* infection are as follows:

- **Anemia** attributable to acute parasitemia

- **Hypersplenism** with danger of splenic rupture

- **Thrombocytopenia,** which may be severe with *P vivax*

- **Relapse of infection,** for as long as 3 to 5 years after the primary infection, attributable to latent hepatic stages (hypnozoites)

- **Severe, and even fatal, infection** with *P vivax*

Syndromes associated with *Plasmodium malariae* infection include

- **Chronic asymptomatic parasitemia,** which persists at undetectable levels for as long as decades after the primary infection

- **Nephrotic syndrome** resulting from deposition of immune complexes in the kidney

Plasmodium knowlesi is a nonhuman primate malaria parasite that can also infect humans and has been misdiagnosed as *P malariae*, which causes more benign infection. Disease can be characterized by very rapid replication of the parasite and hyperparasitemia resulting in severe disease. *P knowlesi* infection should be treated aggressively, because hepatorenal failure and subsequent death have been documented.

Congenital malaria resulting from perinatal transmission occurs infrequently, with increased risk among primigravidae in areas with endemic infection. Most congenital cases have been caused by *P vivax* and *P falciparum; P malariae* and *P ovale* account for less than 20% of such cases. Manifestations can resemble those of neonatal sepsis, including fever and nonspecific symptoms of poor appetite, irritability, and lethargy.

ETIOLOGY

The genus *Plasmodium* includes species of intraerythrocytic parasites that infect a wide range of mammals, birds, and reptiles. The 5 species that infect humans are *P falciparum, P vivax, P ovale, P malariae,* and *P knowlesi.* Coinfection with multiple species has been documented.

EPIDEMIOLOGY

Malaria is endemic throughout the tropical areas of the world and is acquired primarily from the bite of the female *Anopheles* genus of mosquito. Half of the world's population lives in areas where transmission occurs. Worldwide, 219 million cases and 435,000 deaths were reported in 2017. Approximately 10% of these are cases of severe malaria, which have a significantly higher chance of death. Most deaths occur in children younger than 5 years. Infection by the malaria parasite poses substantial risks to pregnant women and their fetuses, especially primigravid women in areas with endemic infection, and may result in spontaneous abortion and stillbirth. Malaria also contributes to low birth weight in countries where *P falciparum* or *P vivax* is endemic.

Risk of malaria is highest, but variable, for travelers to sub-Saharan Africa, Papua New Guinea, the Solomon Islands, and Vanuatu; risk is intermediate on the Indian subcontinent and is low in most of Southeast Asia and Latin America. Potential for malaria reintroduction exists in areas where malaria has been eliminated. Climate change may also affect the geographic range of malaria. Health care professionals can check the Centers for Disease Control and Prevention (CDC) website for the most current information (**www.cdc.gov/ malaria**) to determine malaria endemicity when providing pretravel malaria advice or evaluating a febrile returned traveler. Transmission is possible in more temperate climates, including areas of the United States where *Anopheles* mosquitoes are present.

Nearly all the approximately 2,078 annual reported cases in the United States in 2016 resulted from infection acquired outside the United States. Uncommon modes of malaria transmission are congenital, through transfusions, or through the use of contaminated needles or syringes.

P vivax and *P falciparum* are the most prevalent species worldwide. *P vivax* malaria is prevalent on the Indian subcontinent and in Central America. *P falciparum* malaria is prevalent in Africa, in Papua New Guinea, and on the island of Hispaniola (Haiti and the Dominican Republic). *P vivax* and *P falciparum* are the most common malaria species in southern and Southeast Asia, Oceania, and South America. *P malariae,* although much less common, has a wide distribution. *P ovale* malaria occurs most frequently in West Africa but has been reported in other areas. Reported cases of human infections with *P knowlesi* have been from certain countries of Southeast Asia, specifically Borneo, Malaysia, Philippines, Thailand, Myanmar, Singapore, and Cambodia.

Relapses may occur in *P vivax* and *P ovale* infections because of a persistent hepatic (hypnozoite) stage of infection. Recrudescence of *P falciparum* and *P malariae* infection occurs when a persistent low-density parasitemia produces recurrence of symptoms of the disease, such as when incomplete treatment or drug resistance prevents elimination of the parasite. Asymptomatic parasitemia can occur in individuals with partial immunity.

Drug resistance in both *P falciparum* and *P vivax* has been evolving throughout areas with endemic malaria, generally proportional to the use of particular drugs in a population. The spread of chloroquine-resistant *P falciparum* strains throughout the world dates back to the 1960s. Chloroquine-resistant *P vivax* has been reported in Indonesia, Papua New Guinea, the Solomon Islands, Myanmar, India, and Guyana. *P falciparum* resistance to sulfadoxine-pyrimethamine is distributed throughout not only Africa but other endemic regions as well. Mefloquine resistance has been documented in Myanmar (Burma), Lao People's Democratic Republic (Laos), Thailand, Cambodia, and Vietnam. Resistance to artemisinin compounds has been reported across the same region.

The **incubation period** (time to onset of malaria symptoms) in most cases ranges from as soon as 7 days after being bitten by an infected mosquito to about 30 days and is shortest for *P falciparum* and longest for *P malariae*. Antimalarial drugs discontinued before completing the recommended course of prophylaxis for *P falciparum* may delay symptoms for weeks to months; relapses of *P vivax* and *P ovale* may occur months after initial infection.

DIAGNOSTIC TESTS

Definitive parasitological diagnosis has historically been based on identification of *Plasmodium* parasites microscopically on stained blood films. There is an increasing range of rapid diagnostic test methods available that detect specific malaria antigens in blood. Rapid diagnostic testing is recommended to be conducted in parallel with routine microscopy to provide further information needed for patient treatment, such as the percentage of erythrocytes harboring parasites. Both positive and negative rapid diagnostic test results should be confirmed by microscopic examination, because low-level parasitemia may not be detected (ie, false-negative result), false-positive results occur, and mixed infections may not be detected accurately. Both thick and thin blood films should be examined. The thick film allows for concentration of the blood to find parasites that may be present at low density, whereas the thin film is most useful for species identification and determination of the density of red blood cells infected with parasites. If initial blood smears test negative for *Plasmodium* species but malaria remains a possibility, the smear should be repeated every 12 to 24 hours during a 72-hour period, ideally with at least 3 smears.

Confirmation and identification of the species of malaria parasites on the blood smear are essential in guiding therapy. Serological testing is generally unhelpful, except in epidemiological surveys. Polymerase chain reaction (PCR) assay is available in reference laboratories and many state health departments. PCR is most useful to confirm species of malaria. Information about sensitivity of rapid diagnostic tests for the 3 less common species of malaria, *P ovale, P malariae*, and *P knowlesi*, is limited. Additional information is available (**www.cdc.gov/malaria/diagnosis_treatment/index.html**).

TREATMENT

Choice of malaria treatment is based on the infecting species, possible drug resistance, and severity of disease. Severe malaria (largely a consideration for *P falciparum* infections) is defined as one or more of the following signs: parasitemia greater than 5% of red blood cells infected, signs of central nervous system or other end-organ involvement, severe anemia requiring transfusion, shock, acidosis, abnormal bleeding, and/or hypoglycemia. Patients with severe malaria require intensive care and parenteral treatment with intravenous artesunate. Sequential blood smears to determine percentage of erythrocytes infected with parasites may be monitored to assess therapeutic efficacy. A recent review of available literature suggests that exchange transfusion for severe disease is not efficacious in patients with end-organ involvement.

For patients with severe malaria in the United States or patients with malaria who are unable to tolerate an oral medication despite attempts, intravenous artesunate is the treatment of choice. If commercially available intravenous artesunate is not available within 24 hours, intravenous artesunate is available through a CDC investigational new drug protocol. Assistance with management of malaria is available 24 hours a day through the CDC Emergency Operations Center (770/488-7100). Additional information on artesunate and guidelines for the treatment of malaria are available on the CDC website (**www.cdc.gov/malaria/diagnosis_treatment/artesunate.html** and **www.cdc.gov/malaria/resources/pdf/Malaria_Treatment_Table.pdf**).

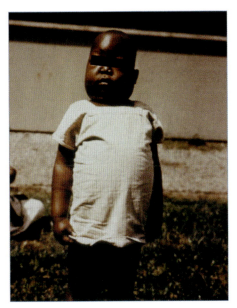

Image 84.1
The edema exhibited by this African child was brought on by nephrosis associated with malaria. Infection with one type of malaria, *Plasmodium falciparum*, if not promptly treated, may cause kidney failure. Swelling of the abdomen, eyes, feet, and/or hands is one of the symptoms of nephrosis brought on by the damaged kidneys. Courtesy of Centers for Disease Control and Prevention.

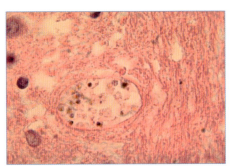

Image 84.2
Histopathologic features of malaria of the brain. Mature schizonts. Courtesy of Centers for Disease Control and Prevention.

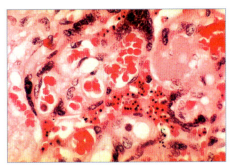

Image 84.3
A photomicrograph of placental tissue revealing the presence of the malarial parasite *Plasmodium falciparum*. Maternal or placental malaria predisposes the newborn to a low birth weight, preterm delivery, and increased mortality; the mother, to maternal anemia. Courtesy of Centers for Disease Control and Prevention.

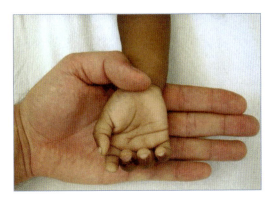

Image 84.4
Severe *Plasmodium vivax* malaria, Brazilian Amazon. Hand of a 2-year-old with severe anemia (hemoglobin level, 3.6 g/dL) showing intense pallor, compared with the hand of a healthy physician. Courtesy of *Emerging Infectious Diseases*.

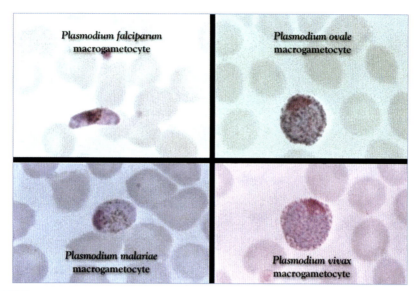

Image 84.5
This Giemsa-stained slide reveals a *Plasmodium falciparum*, *Plasmodium ovale*, *Plasmodium malariae*, and *Plasmodium vivax* gametocyte. The male (microgametocytes) and female (macrogametocytes) are ingested by an *Anopheles* mosquito during its blood meal. Known as the sporogonic cycle, while in the mosquito's stomach, the microgametes penetrate the macrogametes, generating zygotes. Courtesy of Centers for Disease Control and Prevention.

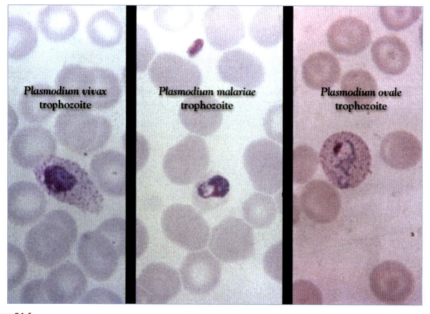

Image 84.6
This thin-film Giemsa-stained micrograph reveals growing *Plasmodium vivax*, *Plasmodium malariae*, and *Plasmodium ovale* trophozoites. As the parasite increases in size, the ring morphological features of the early trophozoite disappear and it becomes what is referred to as a *mature trophozoite*, which undergoes further transformation, maturing into a schizont. Courtesy of Centers for Disease Control and Prevention.

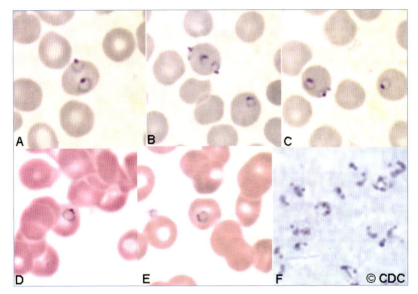

Image 84.7
Plasmodium falciparum ring-stage smears from patients. *P falciparum* rings have delicate cytoplasm and 1 or 2 small chromatin dots. Red blood cells (RBCs) that are infected are not enlarged; multiple infection of RBCs is more common in *P falciparum* than in other species. Occasional appliqué forms (rings appearing on the periphery of the RBC) can be present. A–C, Multiply infected RBCs with appliqué forms in thin blood smears. D, Signet ring form. E, Double chromatin dot. F, A thick blood smear showing many ring forms of *P falciparum*. Courtesy of Centers for Disease Control and Prevention.

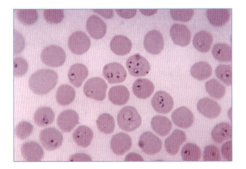

Image 84.8
Photomicrograph of a blood smear showing *Plasmodium falciparum* rings in erythrocytes. The term *ring* is derived from the morphological appearance of this stage, which includes chromatin (red) and cytoplasm (blue), often arranged in a ring shape around a central vacuole; biologically, the ring is a young trophozoite. Courtesy of Centers for Disease Control and Prevention.

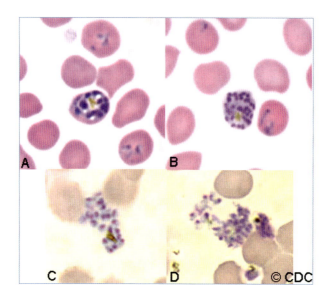

Image 84.9
Plasmodium falciparum schizont smears from patients. Schizonts are seldom observed in peripheral blood. Mature schizonts have 8–24 small merozoites with dark pigment and are clumped in one mass. A, Immature schizont in a thin blood smear. B, Mature schizont. C and D, Ruptured schizonts in a thin blood smear. Courtesy of Centers for Disease Control and Prevention.

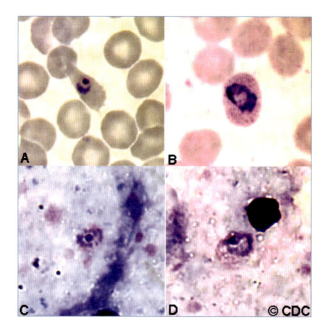

Image 84.10
Plasmodium ovale ring-stage parasites (smears from patients). *P ovale* rings have sturdy cytoplasm and large chromatin dots. Red blood cells (RBCs) are normal sized to slightly enlarged (×1.25), may be round to oval, and are sometimes fimbriated. Schüffner dots are visible under optimal conditions. A and B, *P ovale* rings in thin blood smears. A, Fimbriation of the infected RBC. B, Schüffner dots. C and D, Rings of *P ovale* in thick blood smears. Courtesy of Centers for Disease Control and Prevention.

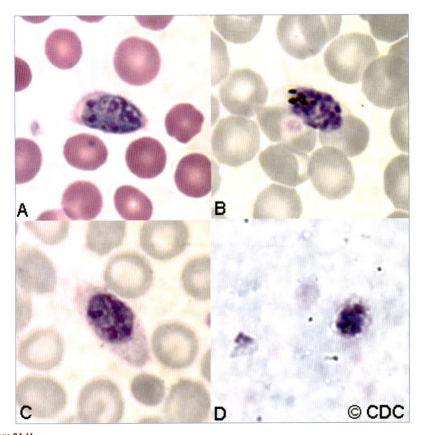

Image 84.11
Plasmodium ovale schizonts (smears from patients). *P ovale* schizonts have 6–14 merozoites with large nuclei, clustered around a mass of dark-brown pigment. Red blood cells are normal sized to slightly enlarged (×1.25), may be round to oval, and are sometimes fimbriated. Schüffner dots are visible under optimal conditions. A–C, Schizonts of *P ovale* in thin blood smears. All these infected blood cells are oval. A and C, Minor fimbriation. D, Schizont in a thick blood smear. Courtesy of Centers for Disease Control and Prevention.

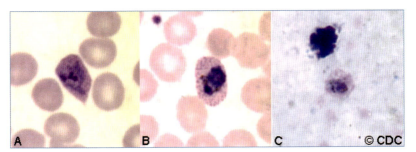

Image 84.12
Plasmodium ovale trophozoites (smears from patients). *P ovale* trophozoites have sturdy cytoplasm and large chromatin dots and can be compact to slightly amoeboid. Red blood cells are normal sized to slightly enlarged (×1.25), may be round to oval, and are sometimes fimbriated. Schüffner dots are visible under optimal conditions. A and B, Trophozoites of *P ovale* in thin blood smears. A, Slightly amoeboid. B, A more compact trophozoite and Schüffner dots. C, Trophozoite in a thick blood smear. Courtesy of Centers for Disease Control and Prevention.

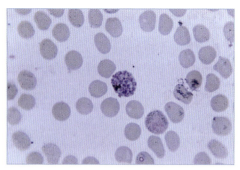

Image 84.13
This photomicrograph of a simian blood sample reveals the presence of a mature simian malarial schizont and gametocyte (magnification ×1,125). Courtesy of Centers for Disease Control and Prevention/W. A. Rogers Jr, MD.

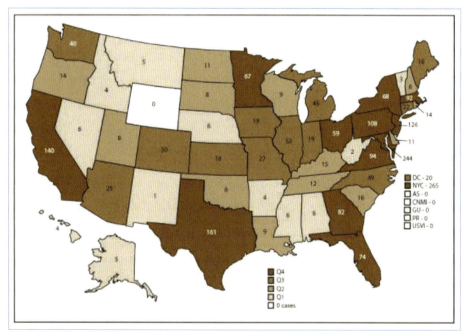

Image 84.14
Number of malaria cases, by state and quartile—United States, 2017. Courtesy of Centers for Disease Control and Prevention.

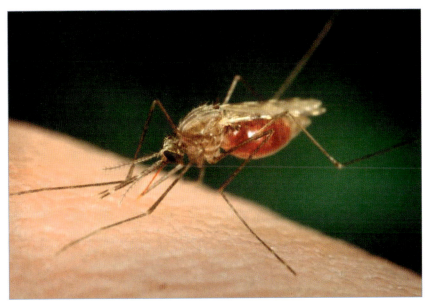

Image 84.15
This photograph depicts an *Anopheles funestus* mosquito partaking in a blood meal from its human host. Note the blood passing through the proboscis, which has penetrated the skin and entered a miniscule cutaneous blood vessel. The *A funestus* mosquito, along with *Anopheles gambiae*, is 1 of the 2 most important malaria vectors in Africa, where >80% of the world's malarial disease and deaths occurs. Courtesy of Centers for Disease Control and Prevention.

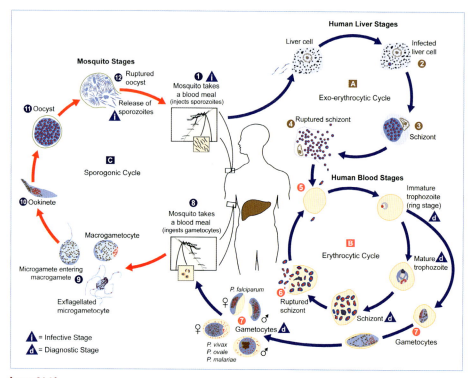

Image 84.16

The malaria parasite life cycle involves 2 hosts. During a blood meal, a malaria-infected female *Anopheles* species mosquito inoculates sporozoites into the human host (1). Sporozoites infect liver cells (2) and mature into schizonts (3), which rupture and release merozoites (4). (Of note, in *Plasmodium vivax* and *Plasmodium ovale*, a dormant stage [hypnozoites] can persist in the liver and cause relapses by invading the bloodstream weeks, or even years, later.) After this initial replication in the liver (exoerythrocytic schizogony) (A), the parasites undergo asexual multiplication in the erythrocytes (erythrocytic schizogony) (B). Merozoites infect red blood cells (5). The ring-stage trophozoites mature into schizonts, which rupture, releasing merozoites (6). Some parasites differentiate into sexual erythrocytic stages (gametocytes) (7). Blood stage parasites are responsible for the clinical manifestations of the disease. The gametocytes, male (microgametocytes) and female (macrogametocytes), are ingested by an *Anopheles* species mosquito during a blood meal (8). The parasite multiplication in the mosquito is known as the sporogonic cycle (C). While in the mosquito's stomach, the microgametes penetrate the macrogametes, generating zygotes (9). The zygotes, in turn, become motile and elongated (ookinetes) (10) and invade the midgut wall of the mosquito, where they develop into oocysts (11). The oocysts grow, rupture, and release sporozoites (12), which make their way to the mosquito's salivary glands. Inoculation of the sporozoites into a new human host perpetuates the malaria life cycle (1). Courtesy of Centers for Disease Control and Prevention.

CHAPTER 85
Measles

CLINICAL MANIFESTATIONS

Measles is an acute viral disease characterized by fever, cough, coryza, and conjunctivitis, followed by a maculopapular rash beginning on the face and spreading cephalocaudally and centrifugally. During the prodromal period, a pathognomonic enanthema (Koplik spots) may be present. Complications of measles, including otitis media, bronchopneumonia, laryngotracheobronchitis (croup), and diarrhea, occur commonly in young children and immunocompromised hosts. Acute encephalitis, which often results in permanent brain damage, occurs in approximately 1 of every 1,000 cases. In the postelimination era in the United States, death, predominantly resulting from respiratory and neurological complications, has occurred in 1 to 3 of every 1,000 cases reported. Case-fatality rates are increased among children younger than 5 years, pregnant women, and immunocompromised children, including children with leukemia, HIV infection, and severe malnutrition (including vitamin A deficiency). Sometimes the characteristic rash does not develop in immunocompromised patients.

Measles inclusion body encephalitis is a rare manifestation of measles infection in immunocompromised individuals usually manifesting within 1 year of measles infection. Disease onset is subacute with progressive neurological dysfunction occurring over weeks to months. Subacute sclerosing panencephalitis (SSPE) is a rare degenerative central nervous system disease characterized by behavioral and intellectual deterioration and seizures that occurs 7 to 11 years after wild-type measles virus infection, occurring at a rate of 4 to 11 per 100,000 measles cases. Rates of SSPE as high as approximately 1:1,000 measles cases have been seen in some recent studies, with the highest rates among children infected before 2 years of age.

Several recent studies have documented that children who have had measles have long-term blunted immune responses to other pathogens and increased mortality attributable to the known effects of measles virus on lymphocytes. This effect is another reason why measles prevention is so important.

ETIOLOGY

Measles virus is an enveloped RNA virus with 1 serotype, classified as a member of the genus *Morbillivirus* in the *Paramyxoviridae* family.

EPIDEMIOLOGY

The only natural host of measles virus is humans. Measles virus is transmitted by direct contact with infectious droplets or, less commonly, by airborne spread. Measles is one of the most highly communicable of all infectious diseases; the attack rate in a susceptible individual exposed to measles is 90% in close-contact settings. Population immunity as high as 95% or greater is often needed to stop ongoing transmission. In temperate areas, the peak incidence of infection usually occurs during late winter and spring. In the prevaccine era, most cases of measles in the United States occurred in preschool and young school-aged children, and few people remained susceptible by 20 years of age. Following implementation of routine childhood vaccination in the United States at age 12 to 15 months, measles occurred more often in infants younger than 1 year and in older adolescents and adults who had not been adequately vaccinated. Infant susceptibility occurs around the time when transplacentally acquired maternal antibodies are no longer present. The childhood and adolescent immunization program in the United States began with licensure of the measles vaccine in 1963 and has resulted in a greater than 99% decrease in the reported incidence of measles, with interruption of endemic disease transmission being declared in 2000.

From 1989 to 1991, the incidence of measles in the United States increased because of low immunization rates among preschool-aged children, especially in urban areas, and because of primary vaccine failures after 1 measles vaccine dose. Following improved coverage in preschool-aged children and implementation of a routine second dose of measles, mumps, and rubella vaccine for children, the incidence of measles declined to extremely low levels (<1 case per 1 million population). Unfortunately, increasing numbers of cases and outbreaks of measles have occurred over the past decade. Most of these cases are linked to importation of measles from countries where it is endemic, including countries in western Europe, and subsequent spread among unimmunized individuals, including intentionally unimmunized children.

Progress continues toward global control and regional measles elimination, with an 80% drop in measles deaths worldwide between 2000 and 2017. By the end of 2018, 89% of children globally had received 1 dose of measles vaccine by their second birthday. All World Health Organization (WHO) regions have established goals to eliminate measles, including the adoption of a second dose of a measles-containing vaccine for all children.

Inadequate response to vaccine (ie, primary vaccine failure) occurs in as many as 7% of people who received a single dose of vaccine at 12 months or older. Most cases of measles in previously immunized children seem to be attributable to primary vaccine failures, but waning immunity after immunization (ie, secondary vaccine failure) may be a factor in some cases. Primary vaccine failure was the main reason a 2-dose vaccine schedule was recommended routinely for children and for adults with high risk.

Patients infected with wild-type measles virus are contagious from 4 days before the rash through 4 days after appearance of the rash. Immunocompromised patients who may have prolonged excretion of the virus in respiratory tract secretions can be contagious for the duration of the illness. Patients with SSPE are not contagious.

The **incubation period** is generally 8 to 12 days from exposure to onset of prodromal symptoms. In family studies, the average interval between appearance of rash in the index case and subsequent cases is 14 days, with a range of 7 to 21 days. In SSPE, the mean **incubation period** of 84 cases reported between 1976 and 1983 was 10.8 years.

DIAGNOSTIC TESTS

Measles virus infection can be confirmed by (1) detection of measles viral RNA by reverse transcriptase–polymerase chain reaction (RT-PCR); (2) detection of measles virus–specific immunoglobulin M (IgM); (3) a 4-fold increase in measles immunoglobulin G antibody concentration in paired acute and convalescent serum specimens (collected at least 10 days apart); or (4) isolation of measles virus in cell culture. Detection of IgM in serum samples by enzyme immunoassay has been the preferred method for case confirmation; however, as the incidence of disease decreases, the positive predictive value of IgM detection decreases. For this reason, detection of viral RNA in blood; throat, nasal, and posterior nasopharyngeal swab specimens; bronchial lavage samples; or urine samples (respiratory samples are preferred specimens, and sampling >1 site may increase sensitivity) is playing an increasing role in case confirmation. A serum sample as well as a throat swab specimen should be obtained from any patient in whom measles is suspected. Additionally, it is ideal to obtain a urine sample because sampling from all 3 sites increases the likelihood of establishing a diagnosis. Many state public health laboratories and the Measles Virus Laboratory at the Centers for Disease Control and Prevention (CDC) can perform RT-PCR assays to detect measles RNA. Isolation of measles virus in cell culture is not recommended for routine case confirmation.

The sensitivity of measles IgM assays varies by timing of specimen collection, immunization status of the patient, and the assay method itself. Up to 20% of assays for IgM may produce a false-negative result in the first 72 hours after rash onset. If the measles IgM result is negative and the patient has a generalized rash lasting more than 72 hours, the measles IgM test should be repeated. Measles IgM is detectable for at least 1 month after rash onset in unimmunized people but might be absent or present only transiently in people immunized with 1 or 2 vaccine doses. Therefore, a negative IgM test result should not be used to rule out the diagnosis in immunized people.

Detection of viral RNA by RT-PCR provides a rapid and sensitive method for case confirmation. It is important to collect samples for RNA detection as soon as possible after rash onset, because viral shedding declines with time after rash.

In populations with high vaccine coverage, such as those in the United States, comprehensive serological and virological testing is generally not available locally and requires submitting specimens to state public health laboratories or the CDC. Individuals with a febrile rash illness who are seronegative for measles IgM and have negative RT-PCR assay results for measles should be tested for rubella via the same specimens.

TREATMENT

No specific antiviral therapy is available.

Vitamin A

The WHO currently recommends vitamin A for all children with measles, regardless of their country of residence, and many US experts concur for all children regardless of hospitalization status with measles in the United States. Vitamin A treatment of children with measles in resource-limited countries has been associated with decreased morbidity and mortality rates. Low serum concentrations of vitamin A have also been found in children in the United States, and children with more severe measles illness may have lower vitamin A concentrations. Vitamin A for treatment of measles is administered once daily for 2 days (ie, immediately on diagnosis and repeated the next day), at the following doses:

- 200,000 IU (60,000 μg retinol activity equivalent [RAE]) for children 12 months or older.
- 100,000 IU (30,000 μg RAE) for infants 6 through 11 months of age.
- 50,000 IU (15,000 μg RAE) for infants younger than 6 months.
- An additional (ie, a third) age-specific dose of vitamin A should be given 2 through 6 weeks later to children with clinical signs and symptoms of vitamin A deficiency.

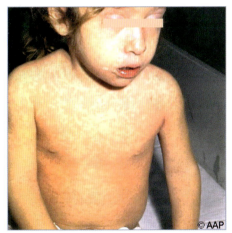

Image 85.1
Child with measles who exhibited an appearance of feeling miserable.

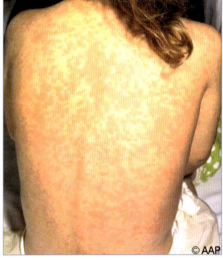

Image 85.2
Measles. This is the same patient as in Image 85.1.

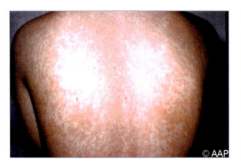

Image 85.3
Characteristic confluent measles rash over the back of this child.

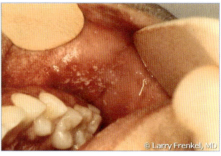

Image 85.4
Koplik spots of measles in a 7-year-old boy. Courtesy of Larry Frenkel, MD.

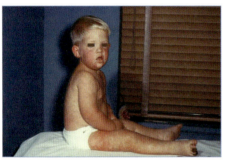

Image 85.5
This child with measles is displaying the characteristic red, blotchy pattern on his face and body during the third day of the rash. Courtesy of Centers for Disease Control and Prevention.

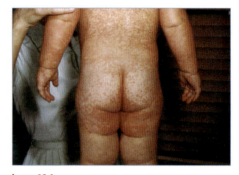

Image 85.6
This child with measles is showing the characteristic red, blotchy rash on his buttocks and back during the third day of the rash. Measles is an acute, highly communicable viral disease with prodromal fever, conjunctivitis, coryza, cough, and Koplik spots on the buccal mucosa. A red, blotchy rash appears around day 3 of the illness, first on the face and then becoming generalized. Courtesy of Centers for Disease Control and Prevention.

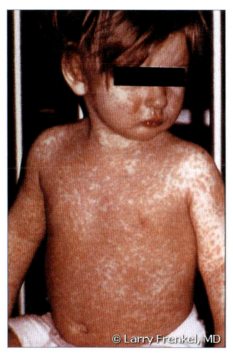

Image 85.7
A 2-year-old boy with the confluent rash of measles. Courtesy of Larry Frenkel, MD.

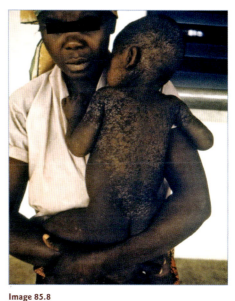

Image 85.8
This photograph shows a Nigerian mother and her child, who was recovering from measles. Note that the skin is sloughing on the child as he heals from his measles infection. Sloughing of the skin in recovering patients is often extensive and resembles that of a burn. Because of their weakened state, children such as the one shown need nursing care to avoid subsequent infections. Courtesy of Centers for Disease Control and Prevention.

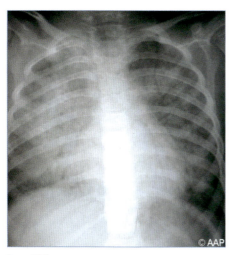

Image 85.9
Measles pneumonia in a 6-year-old with acute lymphoblastic leukemia. The child died of respiratory failure.

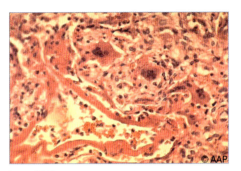

Image 85.10
Measles pneumonia with interstitial mononuclear cell infiltration, multinucleated giant cells, and hyaline membranes (hematoxylin-eosin stain, original magnification ×250). This is the same patient as in Image 85.9.

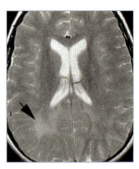

Image 85.11
This axial T2-weighted magnetic resonance image demonstrates an asymmetrical right peri-trigonal focus of white matter hyperintensity consistent with early demyelination in a patient with measles encephalitis.

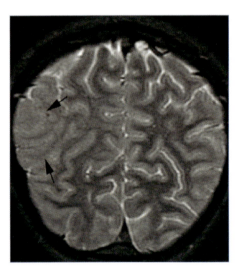

Image 85.12
This coronal T2-weighted magnetic resonance image shows swelling and hyperintensity of the right parietal occipital cortex (arrows) in a patient with measles encephalitis.

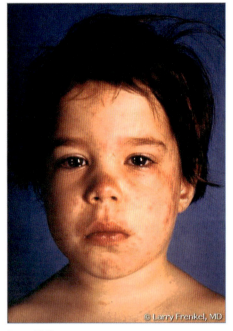

Image 85.13
A 6-year-old girl with the early facial rash and conjunctivitis of measles. Courtesy of Larry Frenkel, MD.

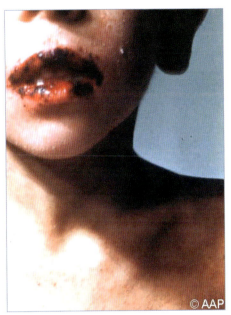

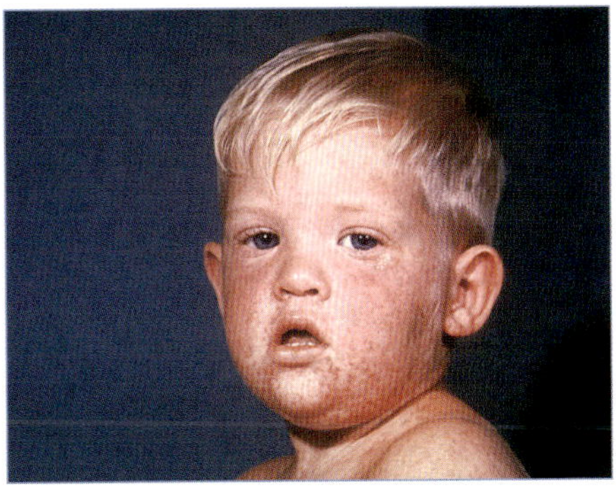

Image 85.15
The face of a boy with measles on the third day of the rash. Courtesy of Centers for Disease Control and Prevention.

Image 85.14
Hemorrhagic measles (black measles). Although uncommon, hemorrhagic measles may result in bleeding from the mouth, nose, and gastrointestinal tract. Courtesy of Edgar O. Ledbetter, MD, FAAP.

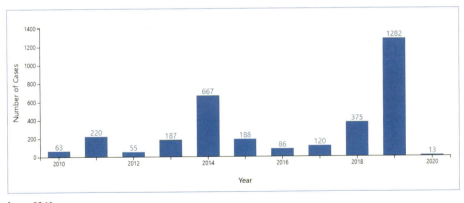

Image 85.16
Number of measles cases reported by year, 2010–2020 (as of December 31, 2020). Courtesy of Centers for Disease Control and Prevention.

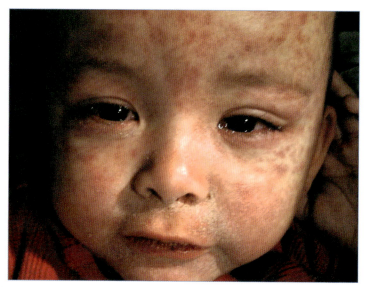

Image 85.17
This unvaccinated 11-month-old acquired measles while traveling to the Philippines to visit relatives. Note the bilateral conjunctivitis, crusting rhinorrhea, and morbilliform rash; he also had a prominent staccato cough. Courtesy of Carol J. Baker, MD.

CHAPTER 86
Meningococcal Infections

CLINICAL MANIFESTATIONS

Invasive meningococcal infection usually results in septicemia (35%–40% of cases), meningitis (approximately 50% of cases), or both. Bacteremic pneumonia is less common (10% of cases). Rarely, young children have occult bacteremia. Onset of invasive infections can be insidious and nonspecific, but onset of septicemia (meningococcemia) is typically abrupt, with fever, chills, malaise, myalgia, limb pain, prostration, and a rash that can initially be macular or maculopapular but typically becomes petechial or purpuric within hours. A similar rash can occur with viral infections or with severe sepsis attributable to other bacterial pathogens. In fulminant cases, purpura, limb ischemia, coagulopathy, pulmonary edema, shock, coma, and death can ensue within hours despite appropriate management. Signs and symptoms of meningococcal meningitis are indistinguishable from those associated with pneumococcal meningitis. In severe and fatal cases of meningococcal meningitis, raised intracranial pressure is a predominant manifesting feature. Invasive infections can be complicated by arthritis, myocarditis, pericarditis, and endophthalmitis. Noninvasive meningococcal infections, such as conjunctivitis and urethritis, also occur. The overall case-fatality rate for invasive meningococcal disease is 15% and is somewhat higher among late adolescents and among older adults. Clinical predictors of mortality include coma, hypotension, leukopenia, and thrombocytopenia. A self-limiting postinfectious inflammatory syndrome occurs in less than 10% of cases, begins a minimum of 4 days after onset of meningococcal infection, and most commonly manifests as fever and arthritis or vasculitis, with less common manifestations including iritis, scleritis, conjunctivitis, pericarditis, and polyserositis.

Sequelae associated with meningococcal disease occur in up to 19% of survivors and include hearing loss, neurological disability, digit or limb amputations, and skin scarring. In addition, patients may experience subtle long-term neurological deficits, such as impaired school performance, behavioral problems, and attention-deficit/hyperactivity disorder.

ETIOLOGY

Neisseria meningitidis is a gram-negative diplococcus with 12 confirmed serogroups based on capsular type.

EPIDEMIOLOGY

N meningitidis disease rates are highest among infants younger than 1 year, followed by children 1 year of age and adolescents and young adults 16 to 20 years of age. Household contacts of cases have 500 to 800 times the rate of disease for the general population. A predominance of US cases is observed in the winter, often noted 2 to 3 weeks following onset of influenza outbreaks, with peak of cases in January, February, and March. Patients with persistent complement-component deficiencies (eg, C3, C5–C9, properdin, or factor D or factor H deficiencies), with anatomical or functional asplenia or HIV, or treated with eculizumab have increased risk for invasive and recurrent meningococcal disease. Asymptomatic colonization of the upper respiratory tract is most common in older adolescents and young adults and is the reservoir from which the organism is spread. Transmission occurs from person to person through droplets from the respiratory tract and requires close contact. Patients should be considered capable of transmitting the organism for up to 24 hours after initiation of effective antimicrobial treatment.

Distribution of meningococcal serogroups in the United States has shifted in the past 2 decades. Serogroup B accounts for most cases currently, followed by serogroups C, W, and Y and nongroupable (nonencapsulated) meningococci. Serogroup distribution varies by age, location, and time. Greater than 85% of cases in adolescents and young adults are caused by serogroups B, C, Y, or W and, therefore, are potentially preventable with available vaccines. In infants and children younger than 60 months, approximately two-thirds of cases are caused by serogroup B.

Since the early 2000s, annual incidence rates for invasive meningococcal disease have decreased, and during 2017, a total of 350 cases occurred (incidence of 0.11 per 100,000 population) in the United States. The decrease in cases in the United States started before the 2005 introduction of meningococcal ACWY conjugate vaccine into the routine immunization schedule at age 11 through

12 years and the 2010 recommendation for a booster vaccine at age 16 years. Reasons for this decrease in incidence are postulated to be related to the increased use of influenza vaccine, reduction in the carriage rates, the use of meningococcal conjugate vaccines in preadolescents and adolescents, immunity of the population to circulating meningococcal strains unrelated to vaccination, and changes in behavioral risk factors (eg, decreases in smoking and exposure to secondhand smoke among adolescents and young adults).

Strains belonging to groups A, B, C, Y, W, and X are implicated most commonly in invasive disease worldwide. Serogroup A has historically been associated with epidemics outside the United States, primarily in sub-Saharan Africa. A serogroup A meningococcal conjugate vaccine was introduced in the "meningitis belt" of sub-Saharan Africa starting in December 2010, and its widespread use has been associated with a marked reduction in serogroup A disease rates; recent outbreaks in the meningitis belt have been associated with serogroups C, W, and X. In Europe, Australia, and South America, the incidence of meningococcal disease ranged from 0.3 to 2 cases per 100,000 population in recent years. Serogroups B, C, W, and Y are most commonly reported in these regions.

Most cases of meningococcal disease are sporadic, with less than 10% associated with outbreaks. Outbreaks occur in communities and institutions, including child care centers, schools, colleges, and military recruit camps. Multiple outbreaks of serogroup B meningococcal disease have occurred on college campuses, and outbreaks of serogroup C meningococcal disease have been reported among men who have sex with men and among people experiencing homelessness.

The **incubation period** for invasive disease is 1 to 10 days, usually less than 4 days.

DIAGNOSTIC TESTS

Cultures of blood and cerebrospinal fluid (CSF) are indicated for patients with suspected invasive meningococcal disease. Cultures of a petechial or purpuric lesion scraping, synovial fluid, and other usually sterile body fluid specimens are sometimes positive. Specimens for culture should be plated onto both sheep blood and chocolate agar and incubated at 35 to 37 °C (95–99 °F) with 5% carbon dioxide in a moist atmosphere. The organism is readily identified with standard biochemical tests as well as by the newer method of mass spectrometry of bacterial cell components. A Gram stain of a petechial or purpuric scraping, CSF, or buffy-coat smear of blood may reveal gram-negative diplococci. Because N meningitidis can be a component of the nasopharyngeal flora, isolation of N meningitidis from this site is not helpful diagnostically. A serogroup-specific polymerase chain reaction (PCR) test to detect N meningitidis from clinical specimens is useful, particularly in patients who receive antimicrobial therapy before cultures are obtained. In the United States, multiplex PCR assays have excellent sensitivity and specificity for detection of serogroups A, B, C, W, X, and Y.

Surveillance case definitions for invasive meningococcal disease are provided in Box 86.1. Serological typing and other characterization such as whole genome sequencing can be useful epidemiological tools during a suspected outbreak to detect concordance among invasive strains.

TREATMENT

The priority in management of meningococcal disease is treatment of shock in meningococcemia and of raised intracranial pressure in severe meningitis. Empirical therapy for suspected meningococcal disease should include cefotaxime or ceftriaxone. Once the microbiological diagnosis is established, treatment options include cefotaxime, ceftriaxone, penicillin G, or ampicillin. Five to 7 days of antimicrobial therapy is adequate. Because of recent detections of β-lactamase–producing organisms in the United States, meningococcal isolate susceptibility to penicillin should be determined before switching to penicillin or ampicillin. Ceftriaxone clears nasopharyngeal carriage effectively after 1 dose. For patients with a life-threatening penicillin allergy characterized by anaphylaxis, meropenem can be used with caution because the rate of cross-reactivity in penicillin-allergic adults is very low. In meningococcemia, early and rapid fluid resuscitation and early use of inotropic and ventilatory support may reduce mortality. The postinfectious inflammatory syndromes associated with meningococcal disease often respond to nonsteroidal anti-inflammatory drugs. Treating physicians should consider evaluating for conditions that increase risk of disease, such as underlying complement-component deficiencies.

Box 86.1
Surveillance Case Definitions for Invasive Meningococcal Disease

Confirmed case
A clinically compatible case and isolation of *Neisseria meningitidis* from a usually sterile site, such as

- Blood
- CSF
- Synovial fluid
- Pleural fluid
- Pericardial fluid
- Isolation from skin scraping of petechial or purpuric lesions

OR

Detection of *N meningitidis*–specific nucleic acid in a specimen obtained from a normally sterile body site (eg, blood, CSF), by using a validated PCR assay

Probable case
A clinically compatible case with EITHER a positive result of antigen test OR immunohistochemistry of formalin-fixed tissue

Suspected case
- A clinically compatible case and gram-negative diplococci in any sterile fluid, such as CSF, synovial fluid, or scraping from a petechial or purpuric lesion
- Clinical purpura fulminans without a positive culture

CSF indicates cerebrospinal fluid; PCR, polymerase chain reaction.

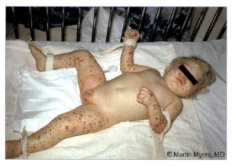

Image 86.1
Young boy with meningococcemia that demonstrates striking involvement of the extremities with sparing of the trunk. Copyright Martin G. Myers, MD.

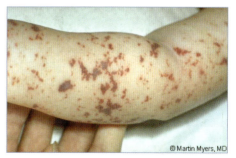

Image 86.2
The arm of the boy shown in Image 86.1, which demonstrates striking extremity involvement and characteristic angular lesions. Copyright Martin G. Myers, MD.

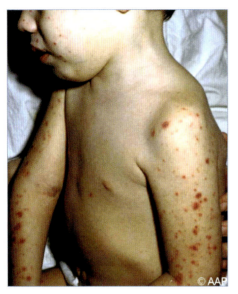

Image 86.3
Meningococcemia showing striking involvement of the extremities with relative sparing of the skin of the child's body surface.

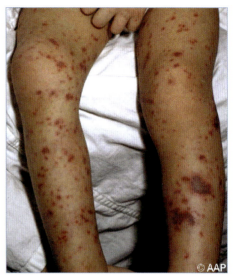

Image 86.4
Meningococcemia. This image shows the lower extremities of the patient in Image 86.3.

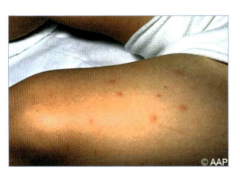

Image 86.5
Papular skin lesions of early meningococcemia.

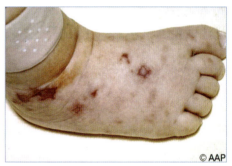

Image 86.6
Characteristic, angular, necrotic lesions on the foot of an infant boy with meningococcemia (after 2 days of intravenous penicillin treatment).

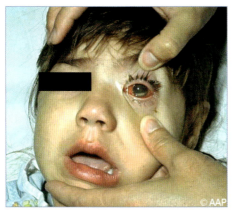

Image 86.7
Preschool-aged girl with meningococcal panophthalmitis. An infant sibling had meningococcal meningitis 1 week before the onset of this child's illness.

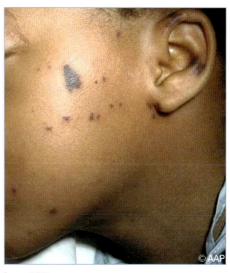

Image 86.8
Meningococcemia in an adolescent girl with disseminated intravascular coagulation.

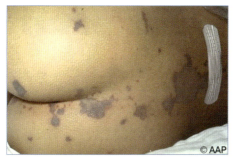

Image 86.9
Meningococcemia in the same patient as in Image 86.8.

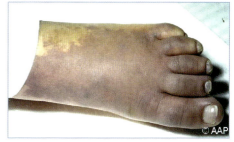

Image 86.10
Patient shown in images 86.8 and 86.9, with marked purpura of the left foot.

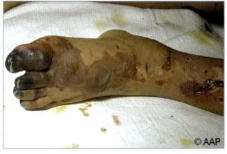

Image 86.11
Patient shown in images 86.8–86.10, with gangrene of the toes.

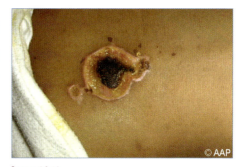

Image 86.12
Patient shown in images 86.8–86.11, with cutaneous necrosis.

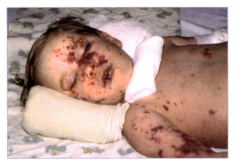

Image 86.13
A 2-year-old boy with acute meningococcemia with septic shock and purpura fulminans. Courtesy of George Nankervis, MD.

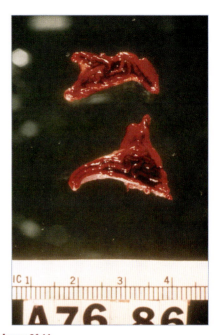

Image 86.14
Hemorrhagic adrenal glands from the 2-year-old child in Image 86.13, who had the characteristic histopathologic features of Waterhouse-Friderichsen syndrome at autopsy. Courtesy of George Nankervis, MD.

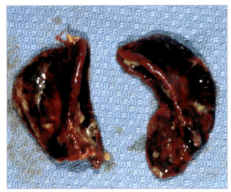

Image 86.15
Adrenal hemorrhage in a patient with gram-negative sepsis, a major complication of meningococcal disease with increased mortality. Courtesy of Dimitris P. Agamanolis, MD.

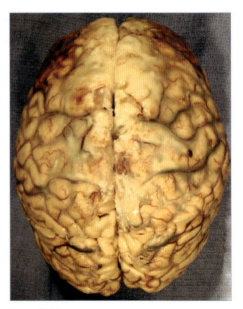

Image 86.16
Fatal meningococcal meningitis with purulent exudate in the subarachnoid space covering the cerebral convexities. Courtesy of Dimitris P. Agamanolis, MD.

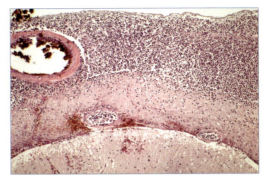

Image 86.17
Suppurative meningococcal meningitis. The subarachnoid space is filled with neutrophils. Courtesy of Dimitris P. Agamanolis, MD.

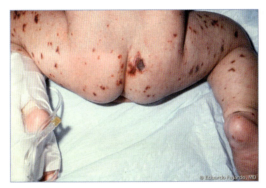

Image 86.18
Petechial rash with a necrotic lesion over the right buttock of an infant girl with *Neisseria meningitidis* septicemia and meningitis. Courtesy of Ed Fajardo, MD.

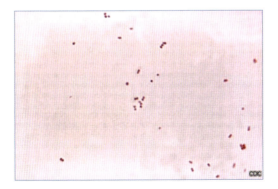

Image 86.19
This micrograph depicts the presence of aerobic gram-negative *Neisseria meningitidis* diplococcal bacteria (magnification ×1,150). Meningococcal disease is an infection caused by a bacterium called *N meningitidis* or meningococcus. Courtesy of Centers for Disease Control and Prevention.

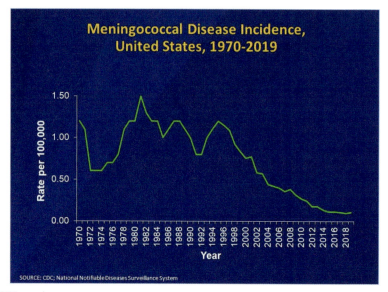

Image 86.20
Incidence rates (per 100,000 people) of meningococcal disease in the United States by year from 1970–2019. The incidence rate began declining in 1995 and has remained low in 2019. Courtesy of Centers for Disease Control and Prevention.

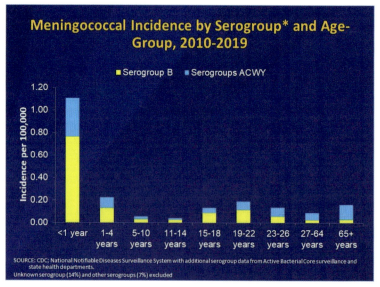

Image 86.21
The figure shows incidence rates (per 100,000 people) of meningococcal disease caused by serogroup B compared to those of serogroups A, C, W, and Y by age-group from 2010–2019. Serogroup B caused approximately 60% of cases among children <5 years old. Serogroups C, Y, or W, which are covered by meningococcal conjugate vaccines, caused approximately 2 in 3 cases of meningococcal disease among people ≥11 years old during this period. However, in 2019, serogroups C, Y, or W caused approximately 1 in 2 cases of meningococcal disease among people ≥11 years old. Courtesy of Centers for Disease Control and Prevention.

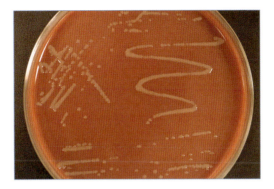

Image 86.22
Neisseria meningitidis on chocolate agar. Isolation of this species requires chocolate or Thayer-Martin agar. Colonies are gray-brown and can appear moist to mucoid or dry. *N meningitidis* can be distinguished from *Neisseria gonorrhoeae* by the fact that it ferments glucose and maltose. Courtesy of Julia Rosebush, DO; Robert Jerris, PhD; and Theresa Stanley, M(ASCP).

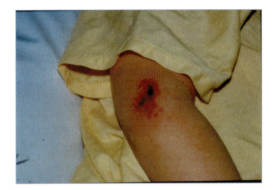

Image 86.23
Purpuric lesion on day 5 of therapy in a 6-year-old with group C *Neisseria meningitidis* sepsis and meningitis. Fever returned on day 6 with swelling of the left knee and mild discomfort. This represents the immune-mediated complication, which resolves with oral nonsteroidal medication. Courtesy of Carol J. Baker, MD.

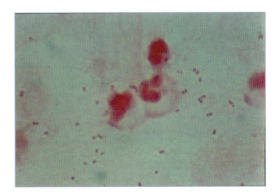

Image 86.24
Gram stain from the cerebrospinal fluid at admission from the patient in Image 86.23. Note the gram-negative cocci in pairs, typical of *Neisseria meningitides* morphological features. Courtesy of Carol J. Baker, MD.

CHAPTER 87

Human Metapneumovirus

CLINICAL MANIFESTATIONS

Human metapneumovirus (hMPV) causes acute respiratory tract illness in people of all ages and is one of the leading causes of bronchiolitis in infants. In children, hMPV also causes pneumonia, asthma exacerbations, croup, upper respiratory tract infections, and acute otitis media; these may be accompanied by fever. As with other respiratory viral infections, secondary bacterial pneumonia can occur. hMPV is associated with acute exacerbations of chronic obstructive pulmonary disease and pneumonia in adults. Otherwise healthy young children infected with hMPV usually have mild or moderate respiratory symptoms, but some young children have severe disease requiring hospitalization. hMPV infection in immunocompromised people can result in severe disease, and fatalities have been reported in hematopoietic stem cell or lung transplant recipients. Preterm birth and underlying cardiopulmonary disease are risk factors for severe disease and hospitalization. Recurrent infections occur throughout life and, in previously healthy people, are usually mild or asymptomatic.

ETIOLOGY

hMPV is an enveloped, single-stranded negative-sense RNA virus in the genus *Metapneumovirus* of the family *Pneumoviridae*. hMPV is divided into 2 major antigenic lineages further subdivided into 2 clades within each lineage (designated A1, A2, B1, and B2) based on sequence differences in the fusion (F) and attachment (G) surface glycoproteins. Viruses from these different clades cocirculate each year in varying proportions.

EPIDEMIOLOGY

Humans are the only source of infection. Spread occurs by direct or close contact with contaminated secretions. Health care–associated infections have been reported.

In temperate climates, hMPV circulation usually occurs during late winter and early spring, overlapping with parts of the respiratory syncytial virus (RSV) season, but typically peaks 1 to 2 months later than RSV. Sporadic infection may occur throughout the year. In otherwise healthy infants, the duration of viral shedding is 1 to 2 weeks. Prolonged shedding (weeks to months) has been reported in severely immunocompromised individuals.

Serological studies suggest that nearly all children are infected at least once by 5 years of age. The incidence of hospitalizations attributable to hMPV is lower than that attributable to RSV but comparable to that of both influenza and parainfluenza type 3 in children younger than 5 years. Large studies have shown that hMPV is detected in 5% to 15% of children with medically attended lower respiratory tract illnesses. Overall annual rates of hospitalization associated with hMPV infection are highest in the first year after birth but occur throughout childhood. In infants, the peak age of hospitalization is 6 to 12 months (compared to 2–3 months for RSV). Coinfection with other respiratory viruses occurs.

The **incubation period** is 3 to 7 days.

DIAGNOSTIC TESTS

Reverse transcriptase–polymerase chain reaction (RT-PCR) assays are the diagnostic method of choice for hMPV. Several RT-PCR assays for hMPV are available commercially. These include a test for hMPV alone and multiplexed tests for hMPV with other respiratory pathogens. hMPV is difficult to isolate in cell culture. Direct fluorescent antibody testing for hMPV detection in respiratory specimens is available in some reference laboratories, with reported sensitivity of 85%.

TREATMENT

Treatment is supportive. Antimicrobial agents are not indicated in the treatment of infants hospitalized with uncomplicated hMPV bronchiolitis or pneumonia unless evidence exists for the presence of a concurrent bacterial infection.

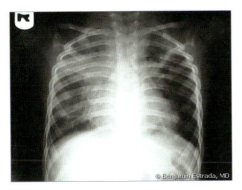

Image 87.1
Bilateral human metapneumovirus pneumonia in a 3-year-old boy. Courtesy of Benjamin Estrada, MD.

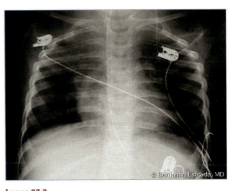

Image 87.2
Human metapneumovirus bronchiolitis in a 12-month-old boy. Courtesy of Benjamin Estrada, MD.

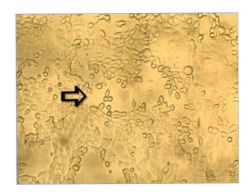

Image 87.3
Late cytopathic effect of human metapneumovirus in rhesus monkey kidney cell monolayers. Infected cells progressed slowly from focal rounding to detachment from cell monolayer (arrow) (magnification ×100). Courtesy of *Emerging Infectious Diseases*.

CHAPTER 88
Microsporidia Infections
(Microsporidiosis)

CLINICAL MANIFESTATIONS

Microsporidia infections can be asymptomatic; patients with symptomatic intestinal infection have watery, nonbloody diarrhea; nausea; and diffuse abdominal pain. Abdominal cramping can occur. Symptomatic intestinal infection, often protracted diarrhea, is most common in immunocompromised people, especially in recipients of organ transplants and people infected with HIV with low $CD4^+$ lymphocyte counts ($<100/\mu L$). Complications include malnutrition, progressive weight loss, and failure to thrive. Different infecting microsporidia species may result in different clinical manifestations, including ocular, biliary, cerebral, respiratory, muscle, and genitourinary involvement (Table 88.1). Chronic infection in immunocompetent people is rare.

ETIOLOGY

Microsporidia are obligate intracellular, spore-forming organisms classified as fungi. More than 1,400 species belonging to about 200 genera have been identified, with at least 15 reported in human infection (Table 88.1). *Enterocytozoon bieneusi* and *Encephalitozoon intestinalis* are the most commonly reported pathogens in humans and are most often associated with chronic diarrhea in HIV-infected people.

EPIDEMIOLOGY

Most microsporidia infections are transmitted by oral ingestion of spores. *Microsporidium* spores are commonly found in surface water, and strains responsible for human infection have been identified in municipal water supplies and groundwater. Spores can survive for extended periods in the environment. Several studies indicate that waterborne transmission occurs. Donor-derived infections in organ transplant recipients have been

Table 88.1
Clinical Manifestations of Microsporidia Infections

Microsporidia Species	Clinical Manifestation
Anncaliia algerae	Myositis, ocular infection, cellulitis myositis
Anncaliia connori	Disseminated disease
Anncaliia vesicularum	Myositis
Encephalitozoon cuniculi	Infection of the respiratory and genitourinary tracts, disseminated infection
Encephalitozoon hellem	Ocular infection
Encephalitozoon intestinalis	Infection of the gastrointestinal tract causing diarrhea, and dissemination to ocular, genitourinary, and respiratory tracts
Enterocytozoon bieneusi	Diarrhea, acalculous cholecystitis
Microsporidium species (*M africanum* and *M ceylonensis*)	Ocular infection
Nosema species (*N ocularum*)	Ocular infection
Pleistophora species	Myositis
Trachipleistophora anthropophthera	Disseminated infection, encephalitis, ocular infection
Trachipleistophora hominis	Myositis, sinusitis, encephalitis, ocular infection
Tubulinosema acridophagus	Disseminated infection, myositis
Vittaforma corneae	Ocular infection, urinary tract infection

Adapted from Han B, Weiss LM. Microsporidia: obligate intracellular pathogens within the fungal kingdom. *Microbiol Spectr.* 2017;5(2).

documented. Person-to-person spread by the fecal-oral route also occurs. Spores have also been detected in other body fluids, but their role in transmission is unknown. Data suggest the possibility of zoonotic transmission.

The **incubation period** is unknown.

DIAGNOSTIC TESTS

Infection with gastrointestinal tract microsporidia can be documented by microscopic identification of spores in stool or biopsy specimens. Microsporidia spores can be detected in formalin-fixed or unfixed stool, other fluid, or tissue specimens stained with a chromotrope-based stain (a modification of the trichrome stain) and examined by an experienced microscopist. Fluorescent techniques including calcofluor or Fungi-Fluor can also be used to detect organisms in stool or tissue sections. Identification and diagnostic confirmation of species requires transmission electron microscopy or molecular methods (polymerase chain reaction), which are available through the Centers for Disease Control and Prevention for some common species. The value of serological testing, when available, has not been substantiated.

TREATMENT

Restoration of immune function is critical for control of microsporidia infection. Effective antiretroviral therapy is the primary initial treatment of these infections in people infected with HIV. Albendazole is the drug of choice for infections caused by microsporidia other than *E bieneusi* and *Vittaforma corneae* infections, which may respond to fumagillin. Fumagillin for systemic use is not available in the United States; it is associated with bone marrow toxicity, and recurrence of diarrhea is common after therapy is discontinued. Limited data suggest that nitazoxanide may be effective for treatment of *E bieneusi* gastroenteritis. None of these therapies have been studied in children with microsporidia infection. Supportive care for malnutrition and dehydration may be necessary. Antimotility agents may be useful to control chronic diarrhea.

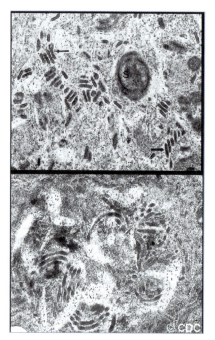

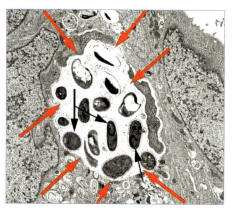

Image 88.2
Transmission electron micrograph showing developing forms of *Encephalitozoon intestinalis* inside a parasitophorous vacuole (red arrows) with mature spores (black arrows). Microsporidiosis, parasite. Courtesy of Centers for Disease Control and Prevention.

Image 88.1
Transmission electron micrographs showing developmental intracellular stages of microsporidia. Courtesy of Centers for Disease Control and Prevention.

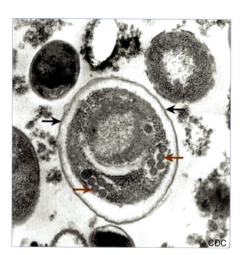

Image 88.3
Transmission electron micrograph of a mature microsporidian spore. Black arrows indicate the electron dense cell wall; red arrows, the coils of polar tubule. Although polymerase chain reaction assay can be used for diagnosis, serological tests are unreliable. Courtesy of Centers for Disease Control and Prevention.

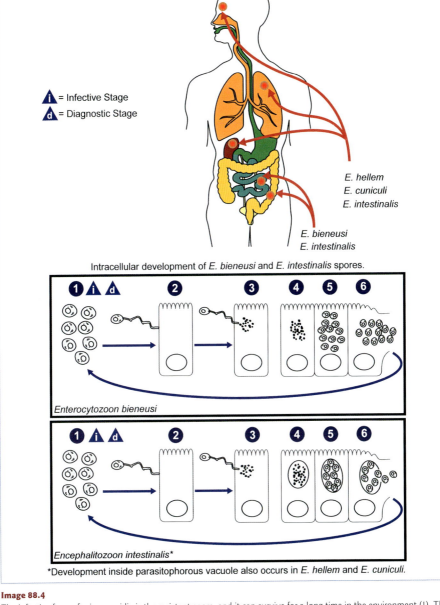

Image 88.4

The infective form of microsporidia is the resistant spore, and it can survive for a long time in the environment (1). The spore extrudes its polar tubule and infects the host cell (2). The spore injects the infective sporoplasm into the eukaryotic host cell through the polar tubule (3). Inside the cell, the sporoplasm undergoes extensive multiplication by either merogony (binary fission) (4) or schizogony (multiple fission). This development can occur either in direct contact with the host cell cytoplasm (eg, *Enterocytozoon bieneusi*) or inside a vacuole termed *parasitophorous vacuole* (eg, *Enterocytozoon intestinalis*). Free in the cytoplasm or inside a parasitophorous vacuole, microsporidia develop by sporogony to mature spores (5). During sporogony, a thick wall is formed around the spore that provides resistance to adverse environmental conditions. When the spores increase in number and completely fill the host cell cytoplasm, the cell membrane is disrupted and releases the spores to the surroundings (6). These free mature spores can infect new cells, thus continuing the cycle. Courtesy of Centers for Disease Control and Prevention.

CHAPTER 89

Molluscum Contagiosum

CLINICAL MANIFESTATIONS

Molluscum contagiosum is a benign viral infection of the skin with no systemic manifestations. It is usually characterized by 1 to 20 discrete 2- to 5-mm-diameter dome-shaped flesh-colored to translucent papules, some with central umbilication. Lesions commonly occur on the trunk, face, and extremities but are rarely generalized. Molluscum contagiosum is a self-limited epidermal infection with individual lesions often spontaneously resolving in 6 to 12 months but some taking as long as 3 to 4 years to disappear completely. An eczematous reaction (molluscum dermatitis) encircling the lesions is common. People with atopic dermatitis and immunocompromising conditions, including HIV infection and congenital *DOCK8* deficiency or *CARD11* mutations, tend to have more widespread and prolonged eruptions, which are often recalcitrant to therapy.

ETIOLOGY

Molluscum contagiosum virus is the sole member of the genus *Molluscipoxvirus*, family *Poxviridae*. Other poxviruses include the agents of smallpox, monkeypox, vaccinia, and cowpox.

EPIDEMIOLOGY

Humans are the only known source of the virus, which is spread by direct contact, scratching, shaving, sexual contact, or fomites. Vertical transmission has been linked with neonatal molluscum contagiosum. Lesions can be disseminated by autoinoculation. Infectivity is generally low, but occasional outbreaks may occur in facilities such as child care centers. The period of communicability is unknown.

The **incubation period** is generally between 2 and 7 weeks but may be as long as 6 months.

DIAGNOSTIC TESTS

The diagnosis can usually be made clinically from the characteristic appearance of umbilicated papules. Wright or Giemsa staining of cells expressed from the central core of a lesion reveals characteristic intracytoplasmic inclusions. Electron microscopic examination of these cells identifies typical poxvirus particles. If uncertainty persists in the differential diagnosis (eg, warts, trichoepithelioma, tuberous sclerosis), nucleic acid testing by polymerase chain reaction is available at certain reference centers. Genital molluscum contagiosum in adolescents and young adults should prompt a screening for other sexually transmitted infections.

TREATMENT

There is no consensus on management of molluscum contagiosum in children and adolescents. Genital lesions in older patients should be treated to prevent spread to sexual contacts. Treatment of nongenital lesions is sometimes provided for cosmetic reasons. Lesions in healthy people are typically self-limited, so treatment may be unnecessary. However, therapy may be warranted to (1) alleviate discomfort, including itching; (2) reduce autoinoculation; (3) limit transmission of the virus to close contacts; (4) reduce cosmetic concerns; and (5) prevent secondary infection.

Physical destruction of the lesions is the most rapid and effective means of curing molluscum contagiosum. Modalities available include curettage, CryoDestruction with liquid nitrogen, electrodesiccation, and chemical agents designed to initiate a local inflammatory response (podophyllin, tretinoin, cantharidin, 25%–50% trichloroacetic acid, liquefied phenol, silver nitrate, iodine tincture, or potassium hydroxide). When treatment is desired, the most support exists for cryotherapy, curettage, or cantharidin. These treatments require an experienced provider, because they can result in postprocedural pain, irritation, dyspigmentation, and scarring. Because physical destruction of the lesions is painful, appropriate local anesthesia may be required, particularly in young children.

Cidofovir is a cytosine nucleotide analogue with in vitro activity against molluscum contagiosum; successful intravenous treatment of immunocompromised adults with severe involvement has been reported. However, use of cidofovir should be reserved for extreme cases because of potential carcinogenicity and known toxicities (neutropenia and potentially permanent nephrotoxicity) associated with systemic administration of cidofovir. Successful treatment with compounded formulations of topical cidofovir has been reported in both adult and pediatric patients, most of whom were immunocompromised.

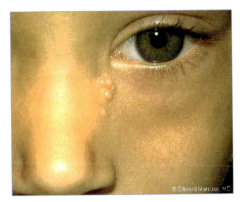

Image 89.1
Molluscum contagiosum lesions adjacent to the nasal bridge. Copyright Edgar K. Marcuse, MD.

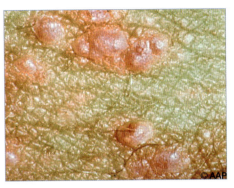

Image 89.2
A central dimple or umbilication is the hallmark of molluscum contagiosum. The lesions of molluscum contagiosum vary in size from 1–6 mm and, unlike venereal warts, are smooth and pearly and have an umbilicated center.

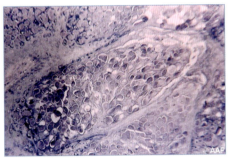

Image 89.3
Molluscum contagiosum lesions in a skin biopsy specimen (Giemsa stain, original magnification ×40). Courtesy of Edgar O. Ledbetter, MD, FAAP.

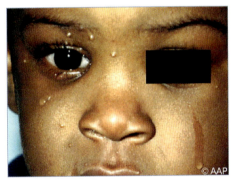

Image 89.4
Molluscum contagiosum is characterized by ≥1 translucent or white papules. Intracytoplasmic inclusions may be seen with Wright or Giemsa staining of material expressed from the core of a lesion.

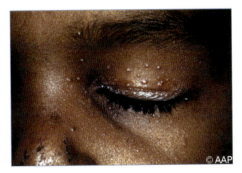

Image 89.5
Pearly papules on the forehead and eyelid in a child with molluscum contagiosum lesions, which commonly occur on the face.

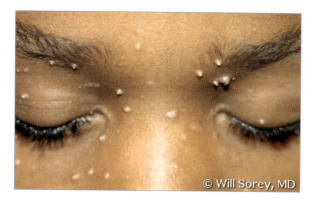

Image 89.6
This 10-year-old girl had multiple small bumps on the face for 1 month. These had started as a solitary papule on her eyebrow but spread over several weeks. They developed a small pointed core and embarrassed the child. School pictures were pending. The family strongly requested treatment. There was a family history of keloids. The family was counseled on the limited treatment options because of the potential for permanent scarring and keloid formation. Consultation with a dermatologist was arranged at the parents' request. Courtesy of Will Sorey, MD.

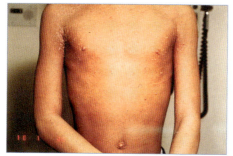

Image 89.7
A 15-year-old boy with HIV with numerous and widespread molluscum contagiosum lesions. Courtesy of Larry Frenkel, MD.

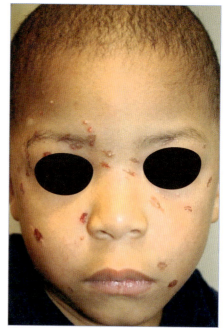

Image 89.8
This healthy 5-year-old boy with widespread molluscum was prescribed home treatment with a topical liquid salicylic acid preparation. He developed itchy crusted erosions around the treated lesions. Topical therapy was discontinued, and a topical antibiotic ointment was started, with rapid clearing of the irritant dermatitis. Courtesy of H. Cody Meissner, MD, FAAP.

CHAPTER 90
Moraxella catarrhalis Infections

CLINICAL MANIFESTATIONS

Moraxella catarrhalis is commonly implicated in acute otitis media (AOM), otitis media with effusion, and sinusitis. AOM caused by *M catarrhalis* occurs predominantly in younger infants and is frequently recovered from middle ear and sinuses as part of mixed infections. Since introduction of 13-valent pneumococcal conjugate vaccine, *M catarrhalis* appears to be recovered in a greater proportion of children undergoing tympanocentesis; however, it is unclear whether this represents an increase in cases attributable to *M catarrhalis* or a decrease in pneumococcal disease. *M catarrhalis* can cause pneumonia with or without bacteremia in immunocompetent infants and young children but is more common in children with chronic lung disease or impaired host defenses, such as leukemia with neutropenia or congenital immunodeficiency. In immunocompromised children, often no focus of infection is identified. Other clinical manifestations include hypotension with or without a rash indistinguishable from that observed in meningococcemia, neonatal meningitis, and focal infections, such as preseptal cellulitis, bacterial tracheitis, urethritis, osteomyelitis, or septic arthritis. Rare manifestations include endocarditis, peritonitis, shunt-associated ventriculitis, meningitis, and mastoiditis. Health care–acquired *M catarrhalis* bacteremia has been reported in hospitalized children with transnasal devices (nasogastric tube, elemental diet tube, or nasotracheal tube); foci of infection in these cases have included pneumonia or bronchitis.

ETIOLOGY

M catarrhalis is a gram-negative aerobic diplococcus.

EPIDEMIOLOGY

M catarrhalis is part of the normal microbiota of the upper respiratory tract of humans. At least two-thirds of children are colonized within the first year after birth. The mode of transmission is presumed to be direct contact with contaminated respiratory tract secretions or droplet spread. Infection is most common in infants and young children but also occurs in immunocompromised people at all ages. The duration of carriage by children with infection or colonization and the period of communicability are unknown. Recent studies suggest early colonization with *M catarrhalis* is associated with a stable microbiome and low risk for recurrent respiratory tract infection.

DIAGNOSTIC TESTS

The organism can be isolated on blood or chocolate agar culture media after incubation in air or with increased carbon dioxide. On Gram stain, *Moraxella* species are short and plump gram-negative cocci, usually occurring in pairs or short chains, and are mostly catalase and cytochrome oxidase positive. Polymerase chain reaction tests for *M catarrhalis* have been developed but are currently used only for research purposes.

TREATMENT

Almost all strains of *Moraxella* species produce β-lactamase and are resistant to amoxicillin, unlike other common pathogens causing acute otitis media. *M catarrhalis* are typically susceptible to ampicillin-sulbactam (and amoxicillin-clavulanate), second- or third-generation cephalosporins, trimethoprim-sulfamethoxazole, macrolides, and fluoroquinolones. The organism is resistant to clindamycin, vancomycin, and oxacillin.

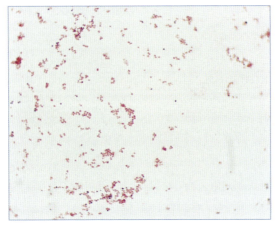

Image 90.1
Gram stain of *Moraxella catarrhalis* showing characteristic gram-negative diplococci morphological features (magnification ×100). Courtesy of Rita Yee, MT(ASCP)SM.

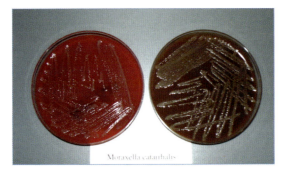

Image 90.2
Moraxella catarrhalis on blood and chocolate agar plates, both inoculated simultaneously. Courtesy of Rita Yee, MT(ASCP)SM.

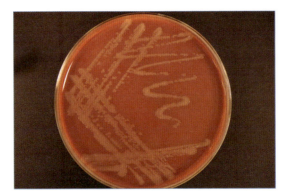

Image 90.3
Moraxella catarrhalis on chocolate agar. Courtesy of Julia Rosebush, DO; Robert Jerris, PhD; and Theresa Stanley, M(ASCP).

CHAPTER 91
Mumps

CLINICAL MANIFESTATIONS

Mumps is a systemic disease characterized by swelling of one or more of the salivary glands, usually the parotid glands. Approximately one-fifth of infections in unvaccinated people may be asymptomatic. The frequency of asymptomatic infection in vaccinated people is unknown, but mumps symptoms are usually milder and complications less common among vaccinated people. Orchitis is the most frequently reported complication and occurs in approximately 30% of unvaccinated and 6% of vaccinated postpubertal men. Approximately half of patients with mumps orchitis develop testicular atrophy of affected testicles. Greater than 50% of people with mumps have cerebrospinal fluid (CSF) pleocytosis, but less than 1% have symptoms of viral meningitis. Uncommon complications include oophoritis, pancreatitis, encephalitis, hearing loss (either transient or permanent), arthritis, thyroiditis, mastitis, glomerulonephritis, myocarditis, endocardial fibroelastosis, thrombocytopenia, cerebellar ataxia, and transverse myelitis. Emergence of contralateral parotitis within weeks to months after apparent recovery has been described. In the absence of an immunization program, mumps typically occurs during childhood. Infection in adults is more likely to result in complications. Although mumps virus can cross the placenta, no evidence exists that this transmission results in congenital malformation.

ETIOLOGY

Mumps is an enveloped RNA virus with 12 genotypes in the genus *Rubulavirus* in the family *Paramyxoviridae*. The genus also includes human parainfluenza virus types 2 and 4. Other common infectious causes of parotitis include Epstein-Barr virus, cytomegalovirus, parainfluenza virus types 1 and 3, influenza A virus, enteroviruses, lymphocytic choriomeningitis virus, HIV, nontuberculous mycobacterium, and gram-positive and gram-negative bacteria.

EPIDEMIOLOGY

Mumps occurs worldwide, and humans are the only known natural hosts. The virus is spread by contact with infectious respiratory tract secretions and saliva. Mumps virus is the only known cause of epidemic parotitis. Historically, the peak incidence of mumps was between January and May and among children younger than 10 years. Mumps vaccine was licensed in the United States in 1967 and recommended for routine childhood immunization in 1977. After implementation of the 2-dose measles-mumps-rubella (MMR) vaccine recommendation in 1989 for measles control in the United States, mumps further declined to extremely low levels, with an incidence of 0.1 per 100,000 by 1999. From 2000 to 2005, there were fewer than 300 reported cases per year. However, since then, there has been an increase in the number of reported mumps cases, with peak years in 2006, 2016–2017 (>6,000 cases each year), and 2019 (>3,000 cases). Most cases during these peak years were among college-aged young adults and people who previously received 2 doses of MMR vaccine.

The **incubation period** is usually 16 to 18 days, but cases may occur from 12 to 25 days after exposure. The period of maximum communicability begins several days before parotitis onset. The recommended isolation period is 5 days after onset of parotid swelling. However, virus has been detected in patients' saliva as early as 7 days before and until 9 days after onset of swelling. Mumps virus has been isolated from urine and seminal fluids up to 14 days after onset of parotitis.

DIAGNOSTIC TESTS

Unvaccinated and vaccinated people with parotitis, orchitis, or oophoritis without other apparent cause should undergo diagnostic testing to confirm mumps virus as the cause. Mumps can be confirmed by detection of mumps virus nucleic acid by reverse transcriptase–quantitative polymerase chain reaction (RT-qPCR) assay in buccal swab specimens (Stenson duct exudates), throat or oral swab specimens, urine, or CSF. The parotid should be massaged for 30 seconds before buccal swab specimen collection. The mumps RT-qPCR test developed by the Centers for Disease Control and Prevention (CDC) and available at the CDC, many state public health departments, and the Vaccine Preventable Disease Reference Centers is sensitive and specific. Other RT-PCR assays for mumps may be available at clinical or commercial laboratories, but the performance measures of these tests are unknown. Mumps virus may be isolated in cell culture with a variety of cell types, by using either standard or rapid isolation and identification techniques. However, RT-qPCR is the preferred test for confirmation of mumps infection.

Testing for mumps-specific immunoglobulin M (IgM) antibody, immunoglobulin G (IgG) seroconversion, or a significant increase between acute and convalescent IgG antibody titers can also aid in the diagnosis of mumps, but these serological assays do not confirm a diagnosis of mumps. In previously vaccinated patients who acquire mumps, IgM response may be transient, delayed, or not detected. Collection of serum 3 to 10 days after parotitis onset improves the ability to detect IgM. A negative IgM test result in a person with clinically compatible mumps symptoms does not rule out mumps as a diagnosis.

To distinguish wild-type mumps virus from vaccine virus in a person with clinically compatible mumps symptoms who was recently vaccinated, it is necessary to obtain a buccal/oral swab specimen for genotyping.

TREATMENT

Management is supportive.

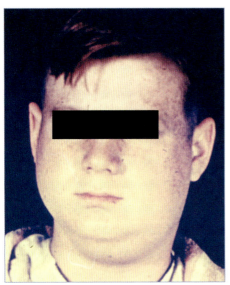

Image 91.1
A 10-year-old boy with bilateral mumps parotitis and submandibular edema. Courtesy of Paul Wehrle, MD.

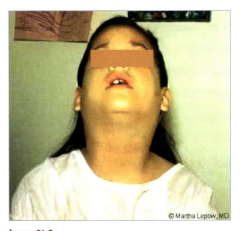

Image 91.2
Mumps with bilateral parotid and submandibular involvement. The differential diagnosis for acute infectious parotitis includes cytomegalovirus, parainfluenza viruses, lymphocytic choriomeningitis virus, coxsackieviruses and other enteroviruses, HIV, nontuberculous mycobacterium, and certain bacteria. Copyright Martha Lepow, MD.

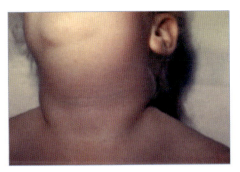

Image 91.3
This is a photograph of a patient with bilateral swelling in the submaxillary regions caused by mumps. Before vaccine licensure in 1967, 100,000–200,000 mumps cases were estimated to have occurred in the United States each year. Courtesy of Centers for Disease Control and Prevention.

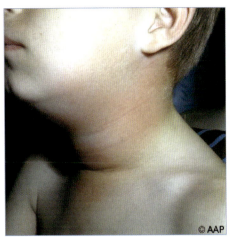

Image 91.4
Mumps parotitis with cervical and presternal edema and erythema that resolved spontaneously.

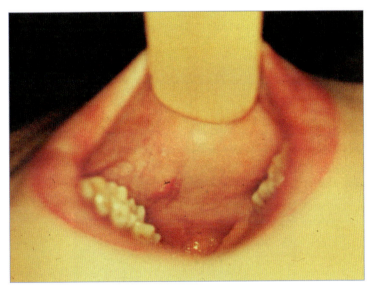

Image 91.5
Swelling and erythema of the Stensen duct in a 10-year-old boy with mumps parotitis. Courtesy of Paul Wehrle, MD.

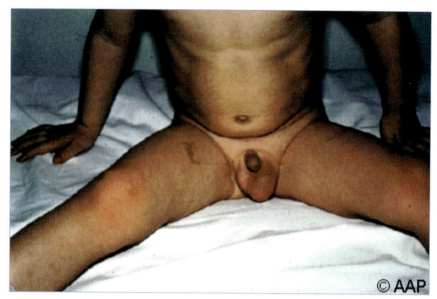

Image 91.6
Mumps orchitis in a 6-year-old boy. This complication is unusual in prepubertal boys. The highest risk for orchitis is in boys and men between 15 and 29 years of age.

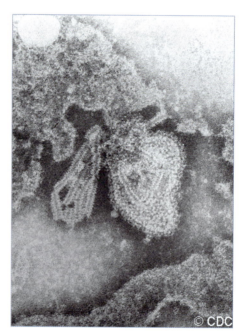

Image 91.7
Electron micrograph of the mumps virus. The mumps virus is a member of the *Paramyxoviridae* family and is enveloped by a helical ribonucleic-protein capsid, which has a Herring-body–like appearance. Courtesy of Centers for Disease Control and Prevention.

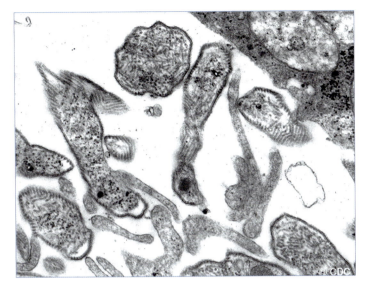

Image 91.8
Thin-section electron micrograph of mumps virus. Filamentous nucleocapsids can be observed within viral particles and juxtaposed along the viral envelope. Courtesy of Centers for Disease Control and Prevention.

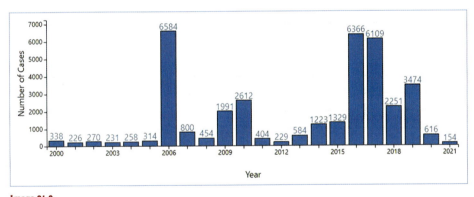

Image 91.9
Reported mumps cases by year, United States—2000-2021. Jurisdictions refer to any of the 50 states, New York City, and the District of Columbia. Courtesy of Centers for Disease Control and Prevention.

CHAPTER 92

Mycoplasma pneumoniae and Other Mycoplasma Species Infections

CLINICAL MANIFESTATIONS

Mycoplasma pneumoniae is a frequent cause of upper and lower respiratory tract infections in children, including pharyngitis, acute bronchitis, and pneumonia. Acute otitis media is uncommon. Bullous myringitis, once considered pathognomonic for mycoplasma, is now known to occur with other pathogens as well. Sinusitis and croup are rare. Symptoms are variable and include cough, malaise, fever, and, occasionally, headache. Acute bronchitis and upper respiratory tract illness caused by *M pneumoniae* are generally mild and self-limited. Approximately 25% of infected school-aged children develop pneumonia with cough and rales on physical examination within days after onset of constitutional symptoms. Cough, initially nonproductive, can become productive, persist for 3 to 4 weeks, and be accompanied by wheezing. Approximately 10% of children with *M pneumoniae* infection exhibit a rash, which is most often maculopapular. Radiographic abnormalities are variable; bilateral diffuse infiltrates or focal abnormalities, such as consolidation, effusion, or hilar adenopathy, can occur.

Unusual manifestations include nervous system disease (eg, aseptic meningitis, encephalitis, acute disseminated encephalomyelitis, cerebellar ataxia, transverse myelitis, and peripheral neuropathy) as well as myocarditis, pericarditis, arthritis (particularly in immunocompromised hosts), erythema nodosum, polymorphous mucocutaneous eruptions (eg, Stevens-Johnson syndrome or *Mycoplasma*-induced rash and mucositis syndrome), hemolytic anemia, thrombocytopenic purpura, and hemophagocytic syndromes. Severe pneumonia with pleural effusion can occur, particularly in patients with sickle cell disease, Down syndrome, immunodeficiencies, and chronic cardiorespiratory disease. Acute chest syndrome and pneumonia have been associated with *M pneumoniae* in patients with sickle cell disease. Infection has also been associated with exacerbations of asthma.

Several other *Mycoplasma* species colonize mucosal surfaces of humans and can produce disease in children. *Mycoplasma hominis* infection has been reported in neonates and children (both immunocompetent and immunocompromised). Intra-abdominal abscess, septic arthritis, endocarditis, pneumonia, meningoencephalitis, brain abscess, and surgical wound infection have been reported to be attributable to *M hominis*. *Mycoplasma genitalium* is now the second most common cause of nongonococcal urethritis in sexually active adolescents and adults, with a frequency only slightly lower than that of *Chlamydia trachomatis*.

ETIOLOGY

Mycoplasmas are pleomorphic bacteria that lack a cell wall. They are classified in the family Mycoplasmataceae, which includes the *Mycoplasma* and *Ureaplasma* genera.

EPIDEMIOLOGY

Mycoplasmas are ubiquitous in animals and plants, but *M pneumoniae* causes disease only in humans. *M pneumoniae* is transmissible by respiratory droplets during close contact with a symptomatic person. Outbreaks have been described in hospitals, military bases, colleges, and summer camps. Occasionally, *M pneumoniae* causes ventilator-associated pneumonia. *M pneumoniae* is a leading cause of pneumonia in school-aged children and young adults but is an infrequent cause of community-acquired pneumonia (CAP) in children younger than 5 years. In the United States, an estimated 2 million infections are caused by *M pneumoniae* each year. Overall, approximately 10% to 20% of cases of CAP in hospitalized patients are believed to be caused by *M pneumoniae*. Infections occur throughout the world, in any season, and in all geographic settings. In family studies, approximately 30% of household contacts develop pneumonia. Asymptomatic carriage after infection may occur for weeks to months. Immunity after infection is not long-lasting.

The **incubation period** is usually 2 to 3 weeks (range, 1–4 weeks), which can contribute to lengthy outbreaks.

DIAGNOSTIC TESTS

Nucleic acid amplification tests (NAATs), including polymerase chain reaction (PCR) tests for *M pneumoniae*, are available commercially and are increasingly replacing other tests, because PCR tests performed on respiratory tract specimens (nasal wash, nasopharyngeal swab, oropharyngeal swab, sputum, and bronchoalveolar lavage fluid) are rapid, have sensitivity and specificity between 80% and 100%, and yield positive results earlier in the course of illness. Identification of *M pneumoniae* by NAAT or culture in a patient with compatible clinical manifestations suggests causation. However, attributing a nonclassic clinical disorder to *M pneumoniae* is problematic, because the organism can colonize the respiratory tract for several weeks after acute infection (even after appropriate antimicrobial therapy) and has been detected by PCR in 17% to 25% of asymptomatic children 3 months to 16 years of age. PCR assay of body fluids for *M hominis* is available at reference laboratories and may be helpful diagnostically.

Serological tests by using immunofluorescent and enzyme immunoassays that detect *M pneumoniae*–specific immunoglobulin M (IgM), immunoglobulin A, and immunoglobulin G (IgG) antibodies are available commercially. IgM antibodies are generally not detectable within the first 7 days after onset of symptoms. Although the presence of IgM antibodies may indicate recent *M pneumoniae* infection, false-positive test results occur, and antibodies may persist in serum for several months or even years and, thus, may not indicate acute infection. IgM antibody titers may not be elevated in older children and adults who have had recurrent *M pneumoniae* infection. Serological diagnosis is best accomplished by demonstrating a 4-fold or greater increase in IgG antibody titer between acute and convalescent serum specimens. Complement-fixation assay results should be interpreted cautiously, because the assay is less sensitive and less specific than is immunofluorescent assay or enzyme immunoassay. Measurement of serum cold hemagglutinin titer has limited value.

The diagnosis of mycoplasma-associated central nervous system disease is challenging, because disease may not result from direct invasion and because there is no reliable single test for cerebrospinal fluid to establish a diagnosis.

TREATMENT

Evidence of benefit of antimicrobial therapy is limited for nonhospitalized children with lower respiratory tract disease attributable to *M pneumoniae*. Antimicrobial therapy is not recommended for preschool children with CAP, because viral pathogens are responsible for the great majority of cases. There is no evidence that treatment of other possible manifestations of *M pneumoniae* infection (eg, upper respiratory tract infection) with antimicrobial agents alters the course of illness.

Because mycoplasmas lack a cell wall, they are inherently resistant to β-lactam agents. Macrolides, including azithromycin, clarithromycin, and erythromycin, are the preferred antimicrobial agents for treatment of *Mycoplasma* pneumonia in school-aged children who have moderate to severe infection and those with underlying conditions, such as sickle cell disease. Fluoroquinolones and doxycycline are the other 2 classes of antibiotics to which *M pneumoniae* is sensitive. Macrolide-resistant strains are increasingly common in the United States (currently between 5% and 15%). The usual course of antimicrobial therapy for pneumonia is 7 to 10 days, except for azithromycin, for which it is usually 5 days.

M hominis is usually resistant to erythromycin and azithromycin but is variably susceptible to clindamycin, tetracyclines, and fluoroquinolones. Like *M pneumoniae*, to which it is closely related, *M genitalium* is susceptible in vitro to macrolides, tetracyclines, and fluoroquinolones. The new pleuromutilin antibiotic lefamulin has good in vitro activity against *M genitalium* but has not been studied in children.

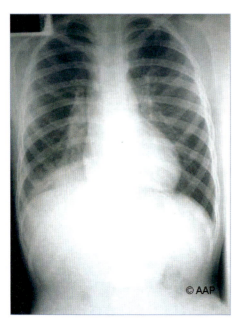

Image 92.1
A preadolescent boy with bilateral perihilar infiltration and right lower lobe pneumonia and pleural effusion caused by *Mycoplasma pneumoniae*. Courtesy of Edgar O. Ledbetter, MD, FAAP.

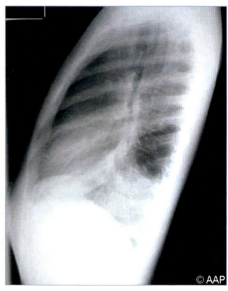

Image 92.2
Right lateral radiograph of the patient in Image 92.1, with pneumonia and pleural effusion. Pleural effusions associated with *Mycoplasma pneumoniae* infections generally resolve spontaneously without drainage. Courtesy of Edgar O. Ledbetter, MD, FAAP.

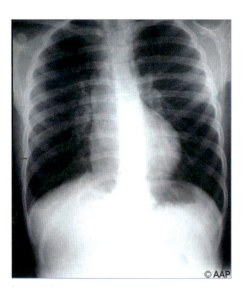

Image 92.3
Preadolescent boy with bilateral perihilar infiltrates caused by *Mycoplasma pneumoniae*.

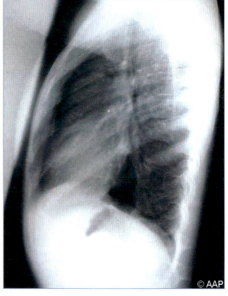

Image 92.4
Lateral radiograph of the patient in Image 92.3, with pneumonia caused by *Mycoplasma pneumoniae*.

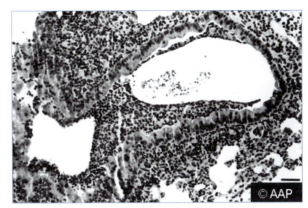

Image 92.5
Histopathologic study of *Mycoplasma pneumoniae*–infected lung tissue. The respiratory bronchiole is surrounded by an inflammatory mononuclear cell response. The intraluminal site is approximately 30% occluded by mucus and white blood cells. *M pneumoniae* is a common cause of pneumonia and tracheobronchitis in school-aged children and adolescents.

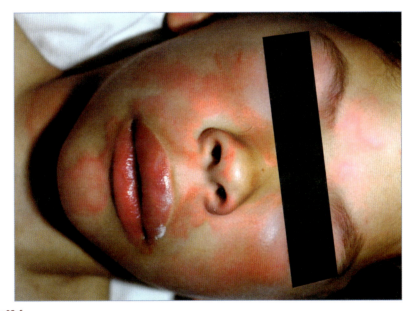

Image 92.6
Erythema multiforme associated with mycoplasma infection. This 10-year-old boy presented with fever and macular lesions on the face, chest, arms, and back, as well as facial swelling. He had a 4-day period of increasing cough and low-grade fever before the onset of the skin lesions and facial swelling. Chest radiograph revealed mild increased infiltrates in the right lung. Levels of cold agglutinins were markedly elevated, and he had a >4-fold rise in complement fixation antibody to *Mycoplasma pneumoniae*. Courtesy of Neal Halsey, MD.

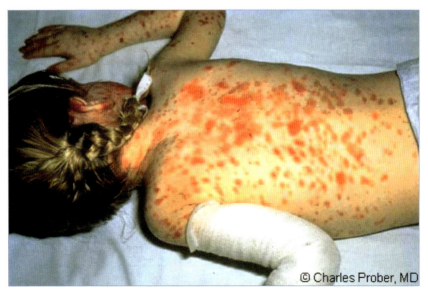

Image 92.7
Erythema multiforme rash (Stevens-Johnson syndrome) associated with *Mycoplasma pneumoniae* infection in a preadolescent girl. Copyright Charles Prober, MD.

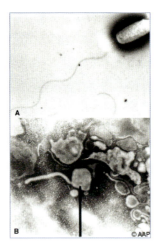

Image 92.8
A, Typical structure of a common gram-negative bacterium (*Pseudomonas aeruginosa*) and its flagellum, as observed on electron microscopy. B, Pleomorphic structure of *Mycoplasma pneumoniae*, as observed on electron microscopy. The bacterium is indicated by the black pointer. Mycoplasmas, including *M pneumoniae*, lack a cell wall.

CHAPTER 93

Nocardiosis

CLINICAL MANIFESTATIONS

Immunocompetent children typically develop cutaneous or lymphocutaneous disease with pustular or ulcerative lesions following soil contamination of a skin injury. Deep-seated tissue infection may follow traumatic soil-contaminated wounds. Immunocompromised people may develop invasive disease (pulmonary disease, which may disseminate). People with risk include those with chronic granulomatous disease, chronic obstructive pulmonary disease, HIV infection, disease requiring long-term systemic corticosteroid/immunosuppressive therapy, solid organ or bone marrow transplant, autoimmune disease, or receipt of tumor necrosis factor inhibitors. Pulmonary disease commonly manifests as rounded nodular infiltrates that can undergo cavitation; the infection may be acute, subacute, or chronic suppurative. The most common clinical symptoms include fever, cough, pleuritic chest pain, chills, and headache. Nocardia has a propensity to spread hematogenously to the brain (single or multiple abscesses) from the lungs. The organism may also spread to the skin (ie, pustules, pyoderma, abscesses, mycetoma) or occasionally to other organs. *Nocardia* organisms can be recovered from respiratory specimens of patients with cystic fibrosis, but the clinical significance of this pathogen in these patients is unclear.

ETIOLOGY

Nocardia are Gram-stain positive, aerobic, intracellular, nonmotile, filamentous bacteria in the order *Actinomycetales*. Cell walls of *Nocardia* organisms contain mycolic acid and, thus, may be described as *acid fast* or *partially acid fast* by using the modified Kinyoun or Fite-Faraco acid-fast staining and light microscopy.

EPIDEMIOLOGY

Nocardia species are ubiquitous environmental saprophytes, living in soil, organic matter, and fresh water or seawater. Infections caused by *Nocardia* species typically result from environmental exposure through inhalation of soil or dust particles or through traumatic inoculation with a soil-contaminated object. The most prevalent species reported from human clinical sources in the United States are *Nocardia nova* complex, *Nocardia farcinica*, *Nocardia cyriacigeorgica*, and *Nocardia abscessus* complex. Primary cutaneous infection and mycetoma are most often associated with *Nocardia brasiliensis*. Other less common pathogenic species include *Nocardia brevicatena-paucivorans* complex, *Nocardia otitidiscaviarum* complex, *Nocardia pseudobrasiliensis*, *Nocardia transvalensis* complex, and *Nocardia veterana*.

Health care–associated person-to-person transmission has rarely been reported. Animal-to-human transmission is not known to occur.

The **incubation period** is unknown.

DIAGNOSTIC TESTS

Isolation of *Nocardia* species from clinical specimens can require extended incubation periods because of their slow growth. Specimens from sterile sites can be inoculated directly onto enriched solid media such as trypticase soy agar supplemented with 5% sheep blood, chocolate, brain-heart infusion, Sabouraud dextrose agars, and buffered charcoal–yeast extract (BCYE) agar. Colonies look like white snowballs because of aerial hyphae. Specimens from nonsterile or contaminated sites, such as tissue or sputum, should be inoculated onto selective media, such as Thayer-Martin or BCYE agar supplemented with vancomycin, with a minimum incubation of 3 weeks. Recovery of *Nocardia* species from tissue can be improved if the laboratory is requested to observe cultures for up to 4 weeks in an appropriate liquid medium at optimal growth temperature (between 25 and 35 °C [77 and 95 °F] for most species). Smears of sputum, body fluids, or pus demonstrating beaded, branching rods that stain weakly gram positive and partially acid fast by the modified Kinyoun method suggest the diagnosis. The Brown-Brenn tissue Gram stain method and Grocott-Gomori methenamine–silver nitrate stains are recommended to demonstrate microorganisms in tissue specimens.

Accurate identification of *Nocardia* isolates paired with antimicrobial susceptibility testing greatly enhances selection of appropriate antimicrobial therapy, thereby increasing the likelihood of favorable patient care outcomes. Because of variability of phenotypic traits and difficulty growing organisms on commercial biochemical testing media, accurate identification is accomplished through molecular methods. MALDI-TOF (matrix-assisted laser desorption/ionization–time-of-flight) mass spectrometry has become an established method to identify the *Nocardia* isolate down to the species level. Other complementary methods include 16S ribosomal RNA gene sequence analysis of full-length or nearly full-length (approximately 1,440 base pair) sequences, and whole genome analysis. Serological tests for *Nocardia* species are not.

Some experts recommend cerebrospinal fluid examination and/or neuroimaging in patients with pulmonary disease, even with a nonfocal neurological examination, given the propensity of these organisms to infect the central nervous system (CNS).

TREATMENT

Rapid and accurate identification of *Nocardia* isolates and antimicrobial susceptibility testing are essential tools for successful treatment of nocardiosis. *Nocardia* species possess intrinsic resistance to multiple drugs.

Trimethoprim-sulfamethoxazole (TMP-SMX) or a sulfonamide alone (eg, sulfisoxazole, sulfamethoxazole) are the drugs of choice for mild infections. Certain *Nocardia* species including *N farcinica*, *N nova* complex, and *N otitidiscaviarum* complex may demonstrate intrinsic resistance to TMP-SMX. If infection does not respond to TMP-SMX, a fluoroquinolone or a carbapenem may be considered, although most *Nocardia* species are resistant to ertapenem. Linezolid has excellent activity against all *Nocardia* species. Other agents with specific *Nocardia* coverage include clarithromycin (*N nova* complex) and amoxicillin-clavulanate (*N brasiliensis* and *N abscessus* complex). Pediatric data are lacking for many of these agents in treatment of nocardiosis. Immunocompetent patients with lymphocutaneous disease usually respond after 6 to 12 weeks of monotherapy.

Combination drug therapy is recommended for patients with serious disease (ie, pulmonary infection, disseminated disease, CNS involvement) and for infection in immunocompromised hosts. Initial combination treatment should include TMP-SMX, amikacin, and a carbapenem-cilastatin (resistance noted for some strains of *N brasiliensis*) or linezolid until susceptibilities are available. Ceftriaxone or cefotaxime is an alternative agent, but resistance is noted for many strains of *N farcinica*, *N transvalensis* complex, and *N otitidiscaviarum* complex. Patients with immunocompromise and patients with serious disease should be treated for 6 to 12 months and for at least 3 months after apparent cure, because of the propensity for relapse. Patients living with HIV may need even longer therapy, and suppressive therapy should be considered for life. Patients with CNS disease should be monitored with serial neuroimaging studies.

Drainage of abscesses is beneficial, and removal of infected foreign bodies (eg, central venous catheters) is recommended.

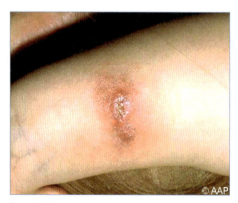

Image 93.1
Cutaneous nocardiosis of forearm in a preschool-aged boy with immunocompetence.

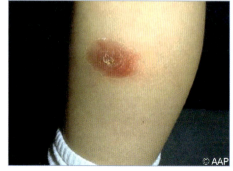

Image 93.2
Cutaneous nocardiosis of the leg of a preschool-aged girl with immunocompetence.

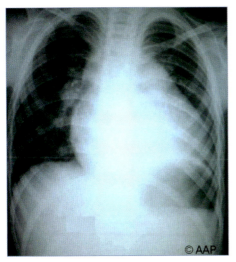

Image 93.3
Nocardia mediastinitis following surgical repair of ventricular septal defect (nosocomial infection). Courtesy of Edgar O. Ledbetter, MD, FAAP.

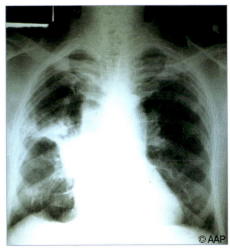

Image 93.4
Nocardia pneumonia, bilateral, in a child with immunocompromise. Invasive nocardiosis is unusual in children with immunocompetence.

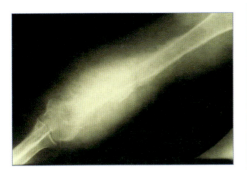

Image 93.5
This radiograph of a patient's right arm reveals the effects of actinomycotic mycetoma caused by *Nocardia asteroides*, which is among the most common actinomycetes that cause mycetoma worldwide. Mycetoma is a slowly progressive, destructive infection of the cutaneous and subcutaneous tissues and fascia, and, as shown, it affects bone as well. Courtesy of Centers for Disease Control and Prevention.

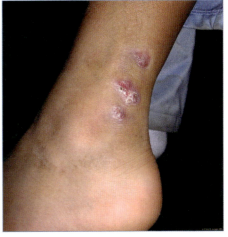

Image 93.6
A school-aged child with chronic rash on the lower left ankle. Histopathologic findings confirmed *Nocardia brasiliensis*. Courtesy of Preeti Jaggi, MD.

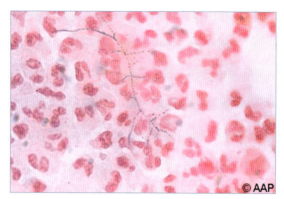

Image 93.7
Nocardia asteroides (Gram stain). Courtesy of Edgar O. Ledbetter, MD, FAAP.

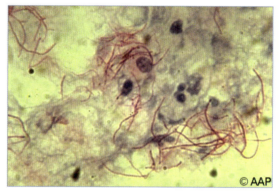

Image 93.8
Nocardia asteroides colony (tissue acid-fast stain).

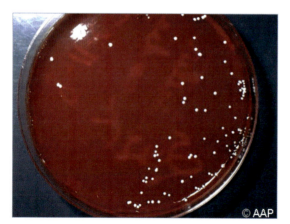

Image 93.9
Nocardia asteroides colonies (white, chalklike colonies on blood agar plate).

CHAPTER 94

Norovirus and Sapovirus Infections

CLINICAL MANIFESTATIONS

Abrupt onset of vomiting and/or watery diarrhea, accompanied by abdominal cramps and nausea, is characteristic of norovirus and sapovirus gastroenteritis. Symptoms typically last from 24 to 72 hours. However, more prolonged courses of illness can occur, particularly in elderly people, young children, and hospitalized patients. Norovirus illness is also recognized as one of the possible causes of chronic gastroenteritis in immunocompromised patients. Systemic manifestations, including fever, myalgia, malaise, anorexia, and headache, may accompany gastrointestinal tract symptoms.

ETIOLOGY

Norovirus and *Sapovirus* are genera in the family *Caliciviridae* and are 23- to 40-nm nonenveloped, single-stranded RNA viruses. Noroviruses are genetically diverse, with viruses from genogroup (G) I and GII causing most of the infections in humans. GII genotype 4 viruses have been causing greater than 50% of all outbreaks globally over the past 15 years. Sapovirus GI, GII, GIV, and GV cause acute gastroenteritis with symptoms indistinguishable to norovirus in humans. At least 17 different sapovirus genotypes have been recognized.

EPIDEMIOLOGY

Norovirus causes an estimated 1 in 15 US residents to become ill each year as well as 56,000 to 71,000 hospitalizations and 570 to 800 deaths annually, predominantly among young children and elderly people. Because of the success of rotavirus vaccines, noroviruses have become the predominant cause of medically attended acute gastroenteritis in the United States, causing both sporadic cases and outbreaks. Outbreaks of sapovirus infection are relatively rare, but its prevalence in children younger than 5 years ranges from 3% to 17%.

Outbreaks with high attack rates tend to occur among semiclosed populations, such as long-term care facilities, schools, child care centers, and cruise ships. Transmission is via the fecal-oral or vomitus-oral routes, either directly by person to person or indirectly by ingesting contaminated food or water or by touching surfaces contaminated with the virus and then touching the mouth. Common-source outbreaks have been described after ingestion of ice, shellfish, and a variety of ready-to-eat foods, including salads, berries, and bakery products, usually contaminated by infected food handlers. Transmission via vomitus has been documented, and exposure to contaminated surfaces and aerosolized vomitus has been implicated in some outbreaks. Asymptomatic shedding of norovirus is common across all age-groups, with the highest prevalence among children.

Most norovirus strains bind to histo-blood group antigens, which are expressed on intestinal epithelial cells and are genetically regulated by the fucosyltransferase 2 (*FUT2*) gene. Individuals with a functional *FUT2* gene are referred to as *secretors*, whereas nonsecretors have a single point mutation in *FUT2*, making them nonsusceptible to most norovirus infections.

The **incubation period** for both norovirus and sapovirus is 12 to 48 hours. Viral shedding may start before onset of symptoms, peaks several days after exposure, and, in some cases, may persist for 4 weeks or more. Prolonged shedding (>6 months) has been reported in immunocompromised hosts. Infection occurs year round but is more common during the colder months of the year.

DIAGNOSTIC TESTS

Molecular diagnostic methods, such as real-time reverse transcriptase–quantitative polymerase chain reaction (RT-qPCR), are the most sensitive assays to detect norovirus and sapovirus. Several multiplex nucleic acid–based assays for the detection of gastrointestinal pathogens are cleared by the US Food and Drug Administration, with most including norovirus testing and some including sapovirus testing. In children, interpretation of test results may be complicated by coinfection with other enteric pathogens.

State and local public health laboratories use RT-qPCR for detection of norovirus and sapovirus RNA in clinical specimens. Laboratory and epidemiological support for investigation of suspected viral gastroenteritis outbreaks in the United States is available through local and state health departments.

TREATMENT

Supportive therapy includes oral or intravenous rehydration solutions to replace and maintain fluid and electrolyte balance.

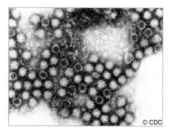

Image 94.1
Transmission electron micrograph of a feline calicivirus. Virions average 35–40 nm in diameter. Cuplike surface depressions sometimes manifest in a Star of David array. Courtesy of Centers for Disease Control and Prevention.

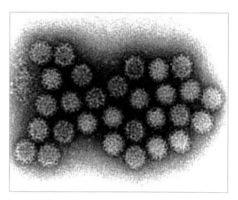

Image 94.2
This is a norovirus in a stool specimen from a patient with acute gastroenteritis, visualized by negative contrast staining and transmission electron microscopy. Particles frequently appear in clumps. Noroviruses are small, round-structured viruses (particle size, 28–32 nm) with a rough surface that contrasts with the smooth edge of astroviruses and picornaviruses, which can also be found in stool specimens. Copyright David O. Matson, MD, PhD, FAAP.

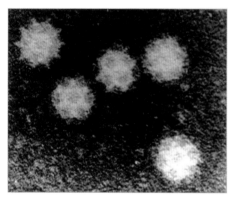

Image 94.3
Calicivirus from clinical specimens and after cryoelectronic image reconstruction. This is *Sapovirus* species in a stool specimen from a patient with acute gastroenteritis, visualized by negative contrast staining and transmission electron microscopy. *Sapovirus* species are typical caliciviruses because they manifest as a particle with 10 surface spikes (top left particle) or a Star of David (bottom left particle), depending on the particle orientation, as do many animal caliciviruses.

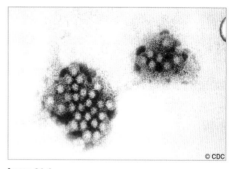

Image 94.4
An electron micrograph of a norovirus, with 27- to 32-nm viral particles. Noroviruses (and related caliciviruses) are important causes of nonbacterial gastroenteritis in the United States. An estimated 181,000 cases of this type of food poisoning occur annually.

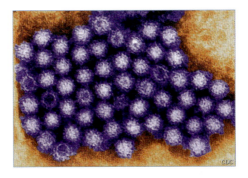

Image 94.5
This transmission electron micrograph revealed some of the ultrastructural morphological features displayed by norovirus virions (virus particles). Noroviruses belong to the genus *Norovirus* and the family *Caliciviridae*. They are a group of related nonenveloped, single-stranded RNA viruses that cause acute gastroenteritis in humans. Courtesy of Centers for Disease Control and Prevention/Charles D. Humphrey.

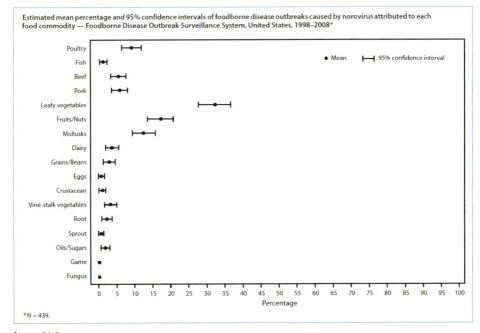

Image 94.6
Estimated mean percentage and 95% confidence intervals of foodborne disease outbreaks caused by norovirus attributed to each food commodity—Foodborne Disease Outbreak Surveillance System, United States, 1998–2008. Courtesy of *Morbidity and Mortality Weekly Report*.

CHAPTER 95

Onchocerciasis
(River Blindness, Filariasis)

CLINICAL MANIFESTATIONS

The disease involves skin, subcutaneous tissues, lymphatic vessels, and eyes. Subcutaneous, nontender nodules that can be up to several centimeters in diameter and contain male and female worms develop 6 to 12 months after initial infection. In patients in Africa, nodules tend to be found on the lower torso, pelvis, and lower extremities, whereas in patients in Central and South America, the nodules are more often located on the upper body (the head and trunk) but may also occur on the extremities. After the worms mature, fertilized female worms produce prelarval stages, called *microfilariae*, that migrate to the dermis and may cause a papular dermatitis. Pruritus is often highly intense, resulting in patient-inflicted excoriations over the affected areas. After a period of years, skin can become lichenified and hypopigmented or hyperpigmented. Microfilariae may invade ocular structures, leading to inflammation of the cornea, iris, ciliary body, retina, choroid, and optic nerve. Loss of visual acuity and blindness can result over time if the disease is left untreated. Infection with *Onchocerca volvulus* has been associated with development of epilepsy.

ETIOLOGY

O volvulus is a filarial nematode.

EPIDEMIOLOGY

O volvulus has no significant animal or environmental reservoir. Humans are infected when infectious larvae are transmitted through the bites of *Simulium* species flies (blackflies). Blackflies breed in fast-flowing streams and rivers (hence, the colloquial name for the disease, "river blindness"). The disease occurs primarily in equatorial Africa, but small foci are found in Venezuela, Brazil, and Yemen. Prevalence is greatest among people who live near vector breeding sites. The infection is not transmissible by person-to-person contact, blood transfusion, or breastfeeding; congenital transmission does not occur.

The **incubation period** from larval inoculation to microfilariae in the skin is usually 12 to 18 months but can be as long as 3 years.

DIAGNOSTIC TESTS

Direct microscopic examination of a 1- to 2-mm biopsy specimen of the epidermis and upper dermis (usually taken from the posterior iliac crest area), incubated in saline, can reveal emerging microfilariae. Microfilariae are not found in blood. Adult worms may be demonstrated in excised nodules that have been sectioned and stained. A slit-lamp examination of an involved eye may reveal motile microfilariae in the anterior chamber or "snowflake" corneal lesions. Eosinophilia is common. Specific serological tests and polymerase chain reaction techniques for detection of microfilariae in skin are available in the United States in research and public health laboratories, including those of the National Institutes of Health and Centers for Disease Control and Prevention.

TREATMENT

Ivermectin and moxidectin, microfilaricidal agents, are available for treatment of onchocerciasis. Moxidectin, approved by the US Food and Drug Administration in 2018 as a single oral dose for patients 12 years and older, showed superior efficacy to a single dose of ivermectin, but safety and efficacy of repeated doses have not been studied. Treatment decreases dermatitis and the risk of developing severe ocular disease but does not kill the adult worms (which can live for more than a decade) and, thus, is not curative. Oral ivermectin is given every 6 to 12 months until there are no symptoms. The safety of ivermectin in children weighing less than 15 kg and in pregnant women has not been established. Adverse reactions to treatment are caused by death of microfilariae and can include rash, edema, fever, myalgia, and, rarely, asthma exacerbation and hypotension. Such reactions are more common in people with higher skin loads of microfilaria and decrease with repeated treatment in the absence of reexposure. Precautions to ivermectin/moxidectin treatment include pregnancy (class C drug), central nervous system disorders, and coinfection with *Loa loa*. Treatment of patients with high levels of circulating *L loa* microfilaremia rarely result in fatal encephalopathy. Referral to a specialist familiar with treating these infections would be indicated for people coinfected with *O volvulus* and *L loa*. Ivermectin is usually compatible with breastfeeding. Because low levels of drug are found in human milk after maternal treatment, some experts recommend delaying maternal treatment until the neonate is 7 days of age, but risk versus benefit should be considered.

A 6-week course of doxycycline can be used to kill adult worms through depletion of the endosymbiotic rickettsial-like bacteria *Wolbachia*, which appear to be required for survival of *O volvulus*. Doxycycline can be used for short durations (ie, ≤21 days) without regard to patient age, but for the longer durations required for treatment of *O volvulus*, for whom the alternative treatment of ivermectin exists, doxycycline is not recommended for children younger than 8 years. Doxycycline may be used for children 8 years or older and nonpregnant adults to obviate the need for years of ivermectin treatment. Doxycycline treatment may be initiated 1 week after treatment with ivermectin-moxidectin; for patients without symptoms, a 6-week course of doxycycline may be given, followed by a dose of ivermectin-moxidectin.

The microfilaricide diethylcarbamazine is contraindicated for the treatment of onchocerciasis because it may cause adverse ocular reactions. Nodules can be removed surgically, but not all nodules may be clinically detectable or surgically accessible.

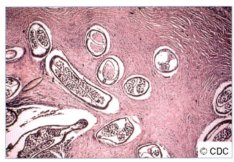

Image 95.1
Histopathologic features of *Onchocerca* nodule in onchocerciasis. Courtesy of Centers for Disease Control and Prevention.

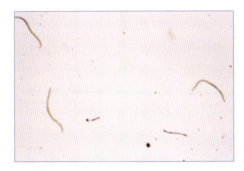

Image 95.2
This is a glycerin mount photomicrograph of the microfilarial pathogen *Onchocerca volvulus* in its larval form. Courtesy of Centers for Disease Control and Prevention.

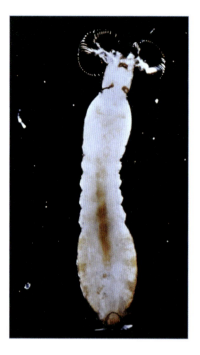

Image 95.3
As an adult, this *Simulium* species larva, or blackfly, is a vector of the disease onchocerciasis, or "river blindness." The blackfly larva is usually a filter feeder, feeding on nutrients extracted from passing currents. Before entering the pupal stage, a *Simulium* species larva passes through 6 larval stages and then encases itself in a silken, submerged cocoon. Courtesy of Centers for Disease Control and Prevention.

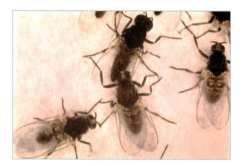

Image 95.4
These are *Simulium* species of flies, or blackflies, a vector of the disease onchocerciasis, or "river blindness." Courtesy of Centers for Disease Control and Prevention.

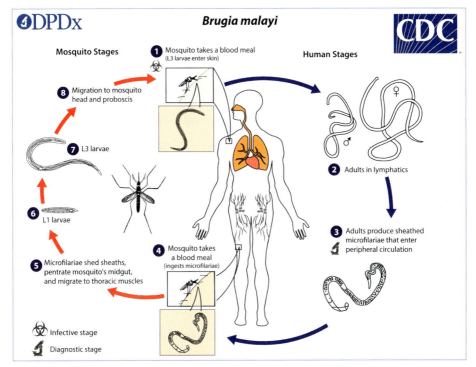

Image 95.5
During a blood meal, an infected mosquito (typically *Mansonia* species and *Aedes* species) introduces third-stage filarial larvae onto the skin of the human host, where they penetrate into the bite wound (1). They develop into adults that commonly reside in the lymphatics (2). The adult worms outwardly resemble those of *Wuchereria bancrofti* but are smaller. Female worms measure 43–55 mm in length × 130–170 μm in width, and males measure 13–23 mm in length × 70–80 μm in width. Adults produce microfilariae, measuring 177–230 μm in length and 5–7 μm in width, which are sheathed and have nocturnal periodicity (in some regions, *Brugia malayi* may be sub-periodic, and note that microfilariae are usually not produced in *Brugia pahangi* infections). The microfilariae migrate into lymph and enter the bloodstream, reaching the peripheral blood (3). A mosquito ingests the microfilariae during a blood meal (4). After ingestion, the microfilariae lose their sheaths and work their way through the wall of the proventriculus and cardiac portion of the midgut to reach the thoracic muscles (5). There the microfilariae develop into first-stage larvae (6) and subsequently into third-stage larvae (7). The third-stage larvae migrate through the hemocoel to the mosquito's proboscis (8) and can infect another human when the mosquito takes a blood meal (1). Courtesy of Centers for Disease Control and Prevention.

CHAPTER 96
Paracoccidioidomycosis
(Formerly Known as South American Blastomycosis)

CLINICAL MANIFESTATIONS

Most disease occurs in adults (90%–95% of cases), in whom the site of initial infection is the lungs. Clinical patterns include subclinical infection or progressive disease that can be either acute-subacute (juvenile type) or chronic (adult type). Constitutional symptoms, such as fever, malaise, anorexia, and weight loss, are common in both adult and juvenile forms.

In the juvenile form, the initial pulmonary infection is usually asymptomatic, and manifestations are related to dissemination of infection to the reticuloendothelial system, resulting in enlarged lymph nodes and involvement of liver, spleen, and bone marrow. Skin lesions are observed regularly and are located typically on the face, neck, and trunk. Involvement of bones, joints, and mucous membranes is less common. Enlarged lymph nodes occasionally coalesce and form abscesses or fistulas. The chronic form of the illness can be localized to the lungs or can disseminate. Oral mucosal lesions are observed in half the cases, and skin involvement is common but occurs in a smaller proportion than in patients with the acute-subacute form. Infection can be latent for years before causing illness.

ETIOLOGY

Paracoccidioides brasiliensis is a thermally dimorphic fungus with yeast and mycelia (mold) phases. *P brasiliensis* contains 4 different phylogenetic lineages (S1, PS2, PS3, and PS4). A new species, *Paracoccidioides lutzii*, also causes paracoccidioidomycosis.

EPIDEMIOLOGY

The infection occurs in Latin America, from Mexico to Argentina, with 80% of cases in Brazil. The natural reservoir is unknown, although soil is suspected, and most disease is associated with agricultural work. The mode of transmission is unknown, but transmission most likely occurs via inhalation of contaminated soil or dust; person-to-person transmission does not occur. The armadillo is a known reservoir of *P brasiliensis*.

The **incubation period** is highly variable, ranging from 1 month to decades. A history of prior residence in Latin America is critical.

DIAGNOSTIC TESTS

Diagnosis is confirmed by visualization of fungal elements. Round, multiple-budding yeast cells with a distinguishing pilot's wheel appearance can be observed in preparations of sputum, specimens of bronchoalveolar lavage, scrapings from ulcers, and material from lesions or in tissue biopsy specimens. Specimens can be prepared with several procedures, including wet or potassium hydroxide wet preparations, or histological staining with hematoxylin and eosin, silver, or periodic acid–Schiff reaction. The mycelia form of *P brasiliensis* can be cultured on most enriched media, including blood agar at 37 °C (99 °F) and Mycosel or Sabouraud dextrose agar at 25 to 30 °C (77–86 °F). Cultures should be held at least 6 weeks. Complement fixation and immunodiffusion are available for antibody detection; semiquantitative immunodiffusion is the preferred test and is the most widely available test in endemic regions.

TREATMENT

Oral therapy with itraconazole is the treatment of choice for less severe or localized infection; oral solution is preferred to capsules. Voriconazole may be as effective as itraconazole but has not been studied as extensively. Isavuconazole has been efficacious in adults, but there are no pediatric data for paracoccidioidomycosis. Prolonged therapy for 9 to 18 months is necessary to minimize the relapse rate, and children with severe disease can require a longer course.

Trimethoprim-sulfamethoxazole orally is an inferior alternative, and treatment must be continued for 2 years or longer to lessen risk of relapse, which occurs in 10% to 15% of optimally treated patients. Amphotericin B is generally given only for initial treatment of severe paracoccidioidomycosis for 2 to 4 weeks, with intravenous trimethoprim-sulfamethoxazole being another option. Children treated initially by the intravenous route can transition to orally administered therapy after clinical improvement has been observed, usually after 3 to 6 weeks.

Serial serological testing by complement fixation or semiquantitative immunodiffusion is useful for monitoring the response to therapy. The expected response is a progressive decline in titers after 1 to 3 months of treatment, with stabilization at a low titer for years or even for life.

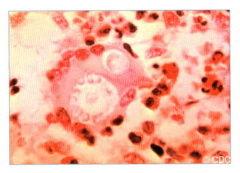

Image 96.1
Histopathologic features of paracoccidioidomycosis, skin. Budding cell of *Paracoccidioides brasiliensis* within multinucleated giant cell. Courtesy of Centers for Disease Control and Prevention.

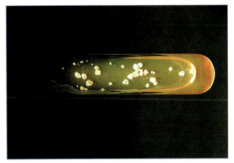

Image 96.2
Pictured is a Sabouraud dextrose agar slant culture of the fungus *Paracoccidioides brasiliensis* grown at 37 °C (98.6 °F). This is the only etiologic agent of the disease paracoccidioidomycosis. *P brasiliensis* is geographically restricted to areas of South and Central America. Courtesy of Centers for Disease Control and Prevention.

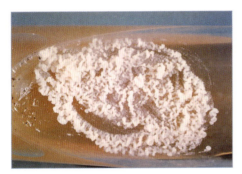

Image 96.3
This is a slant culture growing the fungus *Paracoccidioides brasiliensis* during its yeast phase. Inhalation of *P brasiliensis* conidia is presumably the route of acquisition. The primary infection is asymptomatic in most cases and can remain dormant for years within lymph nodes, reappearing later, usually because of some type of immunodeficiency. Courtesy of Centers for Disease Control and Prevention.

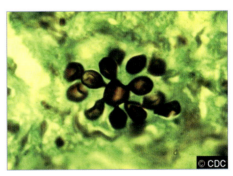

Image 96.4
Histopathologic features of paracoccidioidomycosis. Budding cell of *Paracoccidioides brasiliensis* (methenamine silver stain). Courtesy of Centers for Disease Control and Prevention.

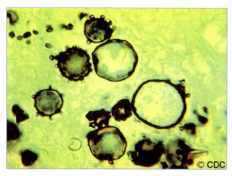

Image 96.5
Histopathologic features of paracoccidioidomycosis, liver. Minute buds on several cells of *Paracoccidioides brasiliensis* (methenamine silver stain). Courtesy of Centers for Disease Control and Prevention.

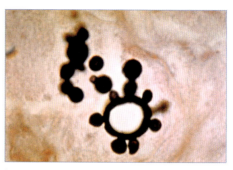

Image 96.6
Histopathologic features of paracoccidioidomycosis. Budding cells of *Paracoccidioides brasiliensis* (methenamine silver stain). Courtesy of Centers for Disease Control and Prevention.

CHAPTER 97

Paragonimiasis

CLINICAL MANIFESTATIONS

There are 2 major forms of paragonimiasis. Primary pulmonary disease with or without extrapulmonary manifestations is principally attributable to *Paragonimus westermani, Paragonimus heterotremus, Paragonimus africanus, Paragonimus uterobilateralis,* and *Paragonimus kellicotti.* Extrapulmonary disease caused by aberrant migrating immature flukes, sometimes resulting in a visceral larva migrans syndrome similar to that caused by *Toxocara canis,* is attributable to other species of *Paragonimus,* most notably *Paragonimus skrjabini,* for which humans are unintentional hosts.

Pulmonary infections are mostly asymptomatic or result in mild symptoms but may be associated with chronic cough and dyspnea, often of insidious onset. During worm migration in the lungs, migratory infiltrates may be noted on serial imaging. Heavy infestations cause paroxysms of coughing, which often produce blood-tinged sputum that is brown because of the presence of the pigmented *Paragonimus* eggs and hemosiderin. Hemoptysis can be severe. Eosinophilic pleural effusion, pneumothorax, bronchiectasis, and pulmonary fibrosis with clubbing can develop.

Extrapulmonary manifestations may involve the liver, spleen, abdominal cavity, intestinal wall, intra-abdominal lymph nodes, skin, or central nervous system (CNS), with meningoencephalitis, seizures, and space-occupying tumors attributable to invasion of the brain by adult flukes. Cerebral paragonimiasis is the most common extrapulmonary manifestation and is more common in children. Extrapulmonary paragonimiasis is also associated with migratory subcutaneous nodules, which contain juvenile worms. Symptoms tend to subside after approximately 5 years but can persist for as many as 20 years.

ETIOLOGY

Paragonimiasis is caused by the lung fluke (trematode, flat worm) *Paragonimus.* In Asia, classic paragonimiasis is caused by adult flukes and eggs of *P westermani* and *P heterotremus.* In Africa, the adult flukes and eggs of *P africanus* and *P uterobilateralis* produce the disease. *P kellicotti* is the endemic species in North America, where it parasitizes mink, opossums, and other animals, and it can cause infection in humans.

The adult flukes of *P westermani* are up to 12 mm long and 7 mm wide and occur throughout Asia. A triploid parthenogenetic form of *P westermani,* which is larger, produces more eggs, and elicits greater disease, has been described in Japan, Korea, Taiwan, and parts of eastern China. *P heterotremus* occurs in Southeast Asia and adjacent parts of China.

Extrapulmonary paragonimiasis (ie, visceral larva migrans syndrome) can be caused by larval stages of *P skrjabini* and *Paragonimus miyazakii.* The worms rarely mature in infected human tissues. *P skrjabini* occurs in China, whereas *P miyazakii* occurs in Japan. *Paragonimus mexicanus* and *Paragonimus ecuadoriensis* occur in Mexico, Costa Rica, Ecuador, and Peru.

EPIDEMIOLOGY

Transmission occurs when raw or undercooked freshwater crabs or crayfish, including pickled and soy sauce–marinated products, containing larvae (metacercariae) are ingested. Numerous cases of *P kellicotti* infection have occurred when people have ingested uncooked or undercooked crayfish while canoeing or camping in the Midwestern United States. In North America, disease has also been caused by *P westermani* in imported crab. A less common mode of transmission that may also occur is human infection through ingestion of meat from a paratenic host, most commonly ingestion of raw pork, usually from wild pigs, containing the juvenile stages of *Paragonimus* species (described as occurring in Japan). Humans are unintentional (dead-end) hosts for *P skrjabini* and *P miyazakii* in visceral larva migrans. These flukes cannot mature in humans and do not produce eggs. *Paragonimus* species also infect a variety of other mammals, such as canids, mustelids, felids, and rodents, which serve as animal reservoir hosts.

The **incubation period** is variable. Egg production begins by approximately 8 weeks after ingestion of *P westermani* metacercariae.

DIAGNOSIS

Paragonimiasis should be considered in patients with unexplained fever, cough, eosinophilia, and pleural effusion or other chest radiographic abnormalities who have eaten raw or undercooked crayfish. Microscopic examination of stool, sputum, pleural fluid, cerebrospinal fluid, and other tissue specimens may reveal operculate eggs. A Western blot serological antibody test based on *P westermani* antigen, available at the Centers for Disease Control and Prevention, is sensitive and specific; antibody concentrations detected by immunoblot decrease slowly after the infection is cured by treatment. Charcot-Leyden crystals and eosinophils in sputum are useful diagnostic elements. Peripheral blood eosinophilia is also characteristic. Chest radiographs may appear normal or may resemble radiographs from patients with tuberculosis or malignancy.

TREATMENT

Praziquantel in a 2-day course is the treatment of choice and is associated with high cure rates, as demonstrated by disappearance of egg production and resolution of radiographic lesions in the lungs. The drug is also effective for some extrapulmonary manifestations. An alternative drug for patients unable to take praziquantel (eg, because of previous allergic reaction) is triclabendazole, given in 1 or 2 doses. Triclabendazole is a narrow-spectrum anthelmintic with activity against *Fasciola* and *Paragonimus*. A short course of steroids may be beneficial in addition to the praziquantel, for patients with CNS paragonimiasis, to reduce the inflammatory response associated with dying flukes. Other supportive care, including antiepileptics and shunt placement, may be needed.

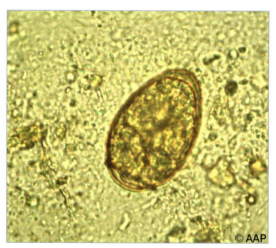

Image 97.1
Paragonimus westermani ova in stool preparation (original magnification ×400).

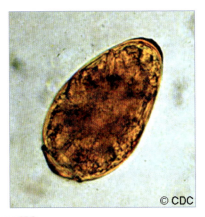

Image 97.2
Ovum of *Paragonimus westermani*. The average ovum size is 85 × 53 μm (range, 68–118 μm × 39–67 μm). They are yellow-brown and ovoid or elongate, with a thick shell, and often asymmetrical, with one end slightly flattened. At the large end, the operculum is clearly visible. The opposite (abopercular) end is thickened. The ova of *P westermani* are excreted unembryonated and may be found in the stool or sputum. Courtesy of Centers for Disease Control and Prevention.

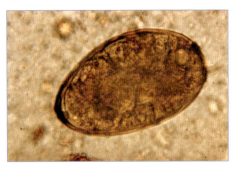

Image 97.3
This micrograph depicts an egg from the trematode parasite *Paragonimus westermani*. This parasite's eggs range in size from 68–118 μm × 39–67 μm. They are yellow-brown and ovoidal or elongated, with a thick shell, and often asymmetrical, with one end slightly flattened. At the large end, the operculum (lid or covering) is visible. Courtesy of Centers for Disease Control and Prevention.

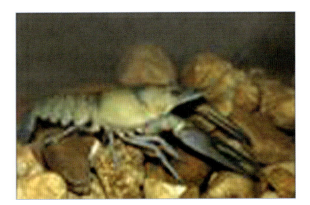

Image 97.4
Eating raw or undercooked crabs or crayfish can result in human paragonimiasis, a parasitic disease caused by *Paragonimus westermani* and *Paragonimus heterotrema*. Courtesy of Centers for Disease Control and Prevention.

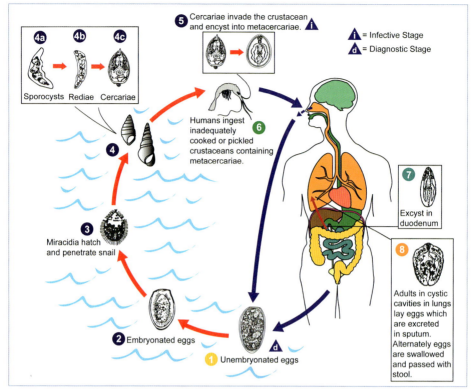

Image 97.5

Life cycle of *Paragonimus westermani*. The eggs are excreted unembryonated in the sputum, or, alternatively, they are swallowed and passed with stool (1). In the external environment, the eggs become embryonated (2), and miracidia hatch and seek the first intermediate host, a snail, and penetrate its soft tissues (3). Miracidia go through several developmental stages inside the snail (4): sporocysts (4a) and rediae (4b), with the latter giving rise to many cercariae (4c), which emerge from the snail. The cercariae invade the second intermediate host, a crustacean such as a crab or crayfish, where they encyst and become metacercariae. This is the infective stage for the mammalian host (5). Human infection with *P westermani* occurs by eating inadequately cooked or pickled crab or crayfish that harbor metacercariae of the parasite (6). The metacercariae excyst in the duodenum (7), penetrate through the intestinal wall into the peritoneal cavity, and then penetrate through the abdominal wall and diaphragm into the lungs, where they become encapsulated and develop into adults (8) (7.5–12 mm × 4–6 mm). The worms can also reach other organs, such as the brain, and other tissues, such as striated muscles. However, when this takes place, completion of the life cycles is not achieved because the eggs laid cannot exit these sites. Time from infection to oviposition is 65–90 days. Infections may persist for 20 years in humans. Animals such as pigs, dogs, and a variety of feline species can also harbor *P westermani*. Courtesy of Centers for Disease Control and Prevention.

CHAPTER 98

Parainfluenza Viral Infections

CLINICAL MANIFESTATIONS

Parainfluenza viruses (PIVs) are the major cause of laryngotracheobronchitis (croup) and may be the cause of bronchiolitis and pneumonia as well as upper respiratory tract infection. PIV type 1 (PIV-1) and, to a lesser extent, PIV type 2 (PIV-2) are the most common pathogens associated with croup. PIV type 3 (PIV-3) is most commonly associated with bronchiolitis and pneumonia in infants and young children. Infections with PIV type 4 (PIV-4) are less well characterized but have been associated with both upper and lower respiratory tract infections. Longitudinal studies have demonstrated that upper respiratory tract infections caused by viruses, including PIVs, can be associated with acute otitis media, which is frequently a mixed viral-bacterial infection. Rarely, PIVs have been isolated from patients with parotitis, myopericarditis, aseptic meningitis, encephalitis, febrile seizures, and Guillain-Barré syndrome. PIV infections can exacerbate symptoms of chronic lung disease and asthma in children and adults. In children with immunodeficiency and recipients of hematopoietic stem cell transplants, PIVs, most commonly PIV-3, can cause refractory infections with persistent shedding, severe pneumonia with viral dissemination, and even fatal disease. PIV infections do not confer complete protective immunity; therefore, reinfections can occur with all serotypes and at any age, but reinfections are usually mild and limited to the upper respiratory tract.

ETIOLOGY

PIVs are enveloped, single-stranded negative-sense RNA viruses classified in the family *Paramyxoviridae*. Four antigenically distinct types—1, 2, 3, and 4 (with 2 subtypes, 4A and 4B)—that infect humans have been identified. PIV-1 and PIV-3 are in the genus *Respirovirus* and PIV-2 and PIV-4 are classified in the genus *Rubulavirus*.

EPIDEMIOLOGY

PIVs are transmitted from person to person by direct contact with contaminated nasopharyngeal secretions through large respiratory tract droplets and fomites. PIV infections can be sporadic or associated with outbreaks of acute respiratory tract disease. Seasonal patterns of infection are distinct, predictable, and cyclic in temperate regions. Different serotypes have distinct epidemiological patterns. PIV-1 tends to produce outbreaks of respiratory tract illness, usually croup, in the autumn of every other year. A major increase in the number of cases of croup in the autumn usually indicates a PIV-1 outbreak. PIV-2 can also cause outbreaks of respiratory tract illness in the autumn, but PIV-2 outbreaks tend to be less severe, irregular, and less common. PIV-3 is endemic and is usually prominent during spring and summer in temperate climates but often continues into autumn, especially in years when autumn outbreaks of PIV-1 or PIV-2 are absent. PIV-4 seasonal patterns are not as well characterized, but studies have shown that infections with PIV-4 had year-round prevalence with peaks during the fall and winter.

The age of primary infection varies with serotype. Primary infection with all types usually occurs by 5 years of age. Infection with PIV-3 more often occurs in infants and frequently causes bronchiolitis and pneumonia in this age-group. By 12 months of age, 50% of infants have acquired PIV-3 infection. Infections with PIV-1 and, to a lesser extent, PIV-2 are more likely to occur between 1 and 5 years of age. Acquisition of PIV-4 also occurs more often during preschool years.

Immunocompetent children with primary PIV infection may shed virus for up to 1 week before onset of clinical symptoms and for 1 to 3 weeks after symptoms have disappeared, depending on serotype. Severe lower respiratory tract disease with prolonged shedding of the virus can occur in immunocompromised individuals. In these patients, infection may disseminate.

The **incubation period** ranges from 2 to 6 days.

DIAGNOSTIC TESTS

Reverse transcriptase–polymerase chain reaction assays are the preferred diagnostic method for detection and differentiation of PIVs and have become the standard method in clinical practice. PIVs are included in many multiplex polymerase chain reaction–based respiratory pathogen panels, although PIV-4 is less commonly included. PIVs may be isolated from nasopharyngeal secretions in cell culture, usually within 4 to 7 days of culture inoculation. Serological diagnosis, made by a significant increase in antibody titer between acute and convalescent serum specimens, is less useful.

TREATMENT

Specific antiviral therapy is unavailable. Racemic epinephrine aerosol is commonly given to severely affected hospitalized patients with laryngotracheobronchitis (croup) to decrease airway obstruction. Parenteral, oral, and nebulized corticosteroids have been demonstrated to lessen the severity and duration of symptoms and hospitalization in patients with moderate to severe laryngotracheobronchitis. Oral steroids are also effective for outpatients with less severe croup. Management is otherwise supportive.

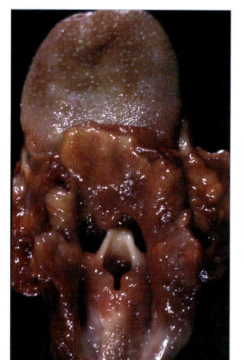

Image 98.1
Fatal croup. Edema, congestion, and inflammation of larynx and pharynx. Courtesy of Dimitris P. Agamanolis, MD.

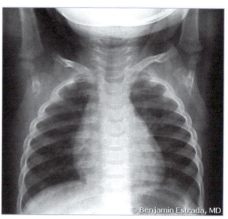

Image 98.2
Parainfluenza laryngotracheitis in a 2-year-old boy. Courtesy of Benjamin Estrada, MD.

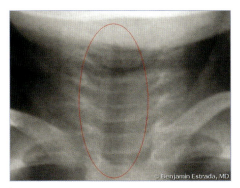

Image 98.3
Parainfluenza laryngotracheitis with the steeple sign (circled) in a 2-year-old. Courtesy of Benjamin Estrada, MD.

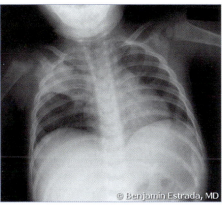

Image 98.4
Parainfluenza pneumonia in a 2-year-old boy. Courtesy of Benjamin Estrada, MD.

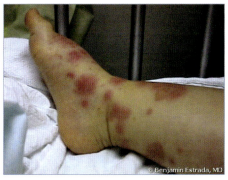

Image 98.5
Erythema multiforme minor in a 2-year-old boy with parainfluenza. Courtesy of Benjamin Estrada, MD.

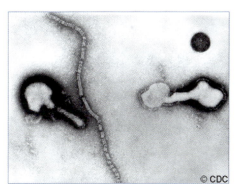

Image 98.6
Transmission electron micrograph of parainfluenza virus showing 2 intact particles and a free filamentous nucleocapsid. Courtesy of Centers for Disease Control and Prevention.

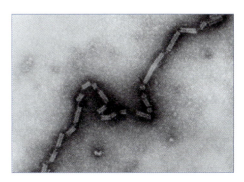

Image 98.7
This electron micrograph depicts the paramyxovirus 4A nucleocapsid with its herringbone-shaped RNA core. Courtesy of Centers for Disease Control and Prevention.

CHAPTER 99

Parasitic Diseases

Parasites are among the most common causes of morbidity and mortality in various and diverse geographic locations worldwide. Outside the tropics and subtropics, parasitic diseases are common in travelers, immigrants, and immunocompromised people. Toxocariasis occurs in the United States, most commonly in the South. Malaria infections in the United States occur in people who have traveled to regions with ongoing malaria transmission, and the diagnosis should be considered when evaluating fever in a returned traveler. Certain parasitic infections have long latency periods, and the diseases they cause, such as Chagas disease, neurocysticercosis, schistosomiasis, and strongyloidiasis, are encountered in immigrants from regions with endemic infection. Clinicians need to be aware of where these infections may be acquired, their clinical manifestations, methods of diagnosis, and how to prevent infection. Table 99.1 details some infrequently encountered parasitic diseases not discussed elsewhere.

Consultation and assistance in diagnosis and management of parasitic diseases are available from the Centers for Disease Control and Prevention (CDC), state health departments, and university departments or hospitals that have divisions of travel medicine, tropical medicine, infectious diseases, international or global health, and public health.

Specific expertise or multiple sources should be consulted, especially when there is a lack of familiarity with the parasite or the drugs recommended for treatment. The CDC distributes several drugs that are not available commercially in the United States for treatment of parasitic diseases. To request these drugs, a physician must contact the CDC Parasitic Diseases Inquiries office (404/718-4745; email: **parasites@cdc.gov**). Consultation with a medical officer from the CDC is required before a drug is released for a patient. For drugs and consultation regarding malaria, a separate CDC hotline is available (770/488-7788).

Table 99.1
Selected Parasitic Diseases Not Covered Elsewhere

Disease and/or Agent	Where Infection May Be Acquired	Definitive Host	Intermediate Host	Modes of Human Infection	Diagnostic Laboratory Tests in Humans	Parasitic Form Causing Human Disease	Common Manifestations in Humans
Angiostrongylus cantonensis (neurotropic disease)	Widespread in the tropics, particularly Pacific Islands and Southeast Asia, Central and South America, the Caribbean, and the United States	Rats	Snails and slugs	Eating improperly cooked infected mollusks or food contaminated by mollusk secretions containing larvae; possibly other modes	Eosinophils in CSF: rarely, identification of larvae in CSF; serological testing or CSF PCR not available commercially	Larval worms	Eosinophilic meningitis, peripheral eosinophilia
Angiostrongylus costaricensis (gastrointestinal tract disease)	Central and South America	Rodents	Snails and slugs	Eating improperly cooked infected mollusks or food contaminated by mollusk secretions containing larvae	Identification of larvae and eggs in tissue; serological testing not commercially available	Larval worms	Abdominal pain, nausea, vomiting, diarrhea (may mimic appendicitis) eosinophilia
Anisakiasis	Cosmopolitan, most commonly where eating raw fish is practiced	Marine mammal	Certain saltwater fish, squid, and octopus	Eating raw or undercooked infected marine fish or squid or octopus	Identification of recovered larvae on endoscopy or within tissue biopsies; serological testing available	Larval worms	Abdominal pain, nausea, vomiting, diarrhea
Capillariasis of intestine (*Capillaria philippinensis*)	Philippines, Thailand	Humans, fish-eating birds	Fish	Ingestion of uncooked infected fish	Eggs and parasite in feces or biopsies of small intestine	Larvae and mature worms	Abdominal pain, diarrhea, vomiting, weight loss
Clonorchis sinensis, *Opisthorchis viverrini*, *Opisthorchis felineus* (liver flukes)	East Asia, eastern Europe, Russian Federation	Humans, cats, dogs, other mammals	Certain freshwater snails	Eating raw or undercooked infected freshwater fish, crabs, or crayfish	Eggs in stool or duodenal fluid; serological testing not commercially available	Larvae and mature flukes	Abdominal pain; hepatobiliary disease; cholangiocarcinoma

(continues)

Table 99.1 (continued)

Disease and/or Agent	Where Infection May Be Acquired	Definitive Host	Intermediate Host	Modes of Human Infection	Diagnostic Laboratory Tests in Humans	Parasitic Form Causing Human Disease	Common Manifestations in Humans
Dracunculiasis (*Dracunculus medinensis*) (guinea worm)	Foci in Africa; global eradication nearly achieved, with only 54 human cases worldwide in 2019	Humans	Crustacea (copepods)	Drinking water infested with infected copepods	Identification of emerging or adult worm in subcutaneous tissues; serology available but not necessary	Adult female worms	Emerging roundworm; inflammatory response; systemic and local blister or ulcer in skin
Fascioliasis (liver flukes; *Fasciola hepatica*)	Worldwide; predominantly in the tropics	Sheep and cattle most important; other ruminants	Snails	Eating raw freshwater plants (eg, watercress) or drinking water contaminated with larvae	Identifying eggs in stool, duodenal fluid, or bile; serological testing; examination of surgical specimens	Larvae and mature flukes	Abdominal pain, nausea, vomiting; hepatobiliary disease
Fasciolopsiasis (intestinal flukes; *Fasciolopsis buski*)	East Asia	Humans, pigs, dogs	Certain freshwater snails, plants	Eating uncooked infected plants	Eggs or worm in feces or duodenal fluid; serological testing not commercially available	Larvae and mature flukes	Diarrhea, constipation, vomiting, anorexia, edema of face and legs, ascites

CSF indicates cerebrospinal fluid; PCR, polymerase chain reaction.

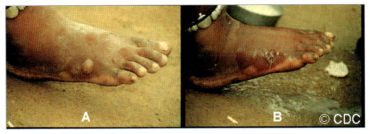

Image 99.1
Dracunculiasis. The female *Dracunculus medinensis* (guinea worm) induces a painful blister (A); after rupture of the blister, the worm emerges as a whitish filament (B) in the center of a painful ulcer, which is often secondarily infected. Courtesy of Centers for Disease Control and Prevention.

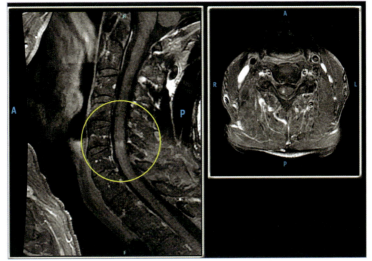

Image 99.2
Sagittal and axial T2-weighted magnetic resonance images of a focal lesion of the cervical spine in an 18-year-old patient with spinal cord involvement of infection with *Gnathostoma spinigerum*, a nematode found throughout Asia that can be acquired by humans through consumption of undercooked shellfish or meat. Courtesy of James Sejvar, MD.

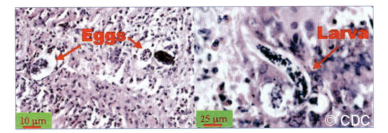

Image 99.3
Eggs and larva of *Angiostrongylus costaricensis*. In humans, eggs and larvae are not normally excreted but remain sequestered in tissues. Eggs and larvae (and, occasionally, adult worms) of *A costaricensis* can be identified in biopsy or surgical specimens of intestinal tissue. The larvae need to be distinguished from the larvae of *Strongyloides stercoralis*; however, the presence of granulomas containing thin-shelled eggs and/or larvae serves to distinguish *A costaricensis* infections. The larval infection can cause mesenteric arteritis and abdominal pain, occurring primarily in people in Central and South America. Courtesy of Centers for Disease Control and Prevention.

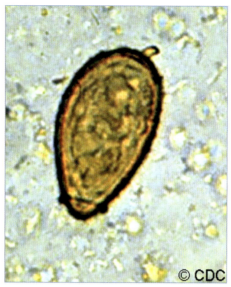

Image 99.4
Opisthorchis (formerly *Clonorchis*) *sinensis* (Chinese liver fluke) egg. These are small, operculated eggs, 27–35 μm × 11 to 20 μm. The operculum, at the smaller end of the egg, is convex and rests on a visible "shoulder." At the opposite (larger, abopercular) end, a small knob or hooklike protrusion is often visible (as is shown). The miracidium is visible inside the egg. (Also referred to as *opisthorchiasis*.) Courtesy of Centers for Disease Control and Prevention.

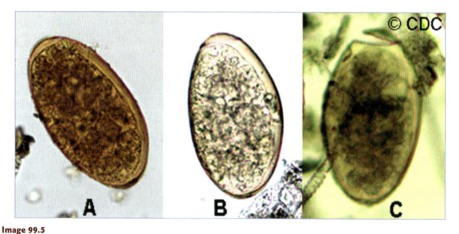

Image 99.5
Fasciola hepatica eggs (wet mounts with iodine). The eggs are ellipsoidal. They have a small, barely distinct operculum (A and B, upper end of the eggs). The operculum can be opened (egg C), for example, when a slight pressure is applied to the coverslip. The eggs have a thin shell that is slightly thicker at the abopercular end. They are passed unembryonated. The size ranges from 120–150 μm × 63–90 μm. Fascioliasis is caused by the sheep liver fluke infecting the liver and biliary system. Courtesy of Centers for Disease Control and Prevention.

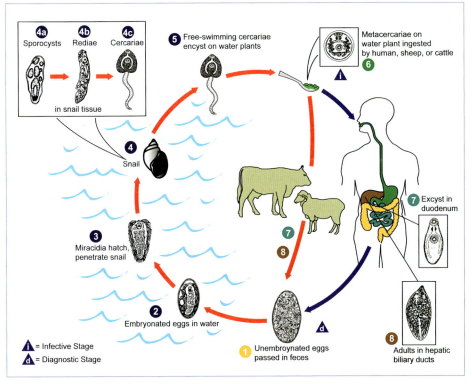

Image 99.6

Fasciola hepatica (life cycle). Immature eggs are discharged in the biliary ducts and in the stool (1). Eggs become embryonated in water (2) and release miracidia (3), which invade a suitable snail intermediate host (4), including many species of the genus *Lymnaea*. In the snail, the parasites undergo several developmental stages (sporocysts [4a], rediae [4b], and cercariae [4c]). The cercariae are released from the snail (5) and encyst as metacercariae on aquatic vegetation or other surfaces. Mammals acquire the infection by eating vegetation containing metacercariae. Humans can become infected by ingesting metacercariae-containing freshwater plants, especially watercress (6). After ingestion, the metacercariae excyst in the duodenum (7) and migrate through the intestinal wall, the peritoneal cavity, and the liver parenchyma into the biliary ducts, where they develop into adults (8). In humans, maturation from metacercariae into adult flukes takes approximately 3–4 months. The adult flukes (*F hepatica*, up to 30 × 13 mm; *Fasciola gigantica*, up to 75 mm) reside in the large biliary ducts of the mammalian host. *F hepatica* infect various animal species, mostly herbivores. Courtesy of Centers for Disease Control and Prevention.

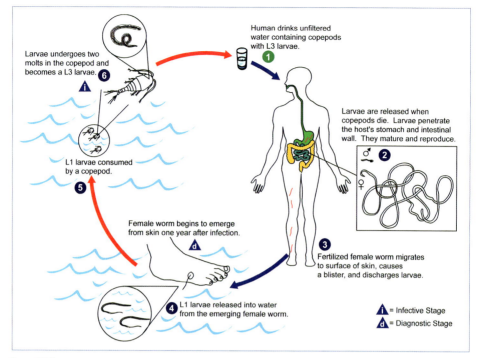

Image 99.7

Dracunculus medinensis. Humans become infected by drinking unfiltered water containing copepods (small crustaceans) that are infected with larvae of *D medinensis* (1). Following ingestion, the copepods die and release the larvae, which penetrate the host stomach and intestinal wall and enter the abdominal cavity and retroperitoneal space (2). After maturation into adults and copulation, the male worms die and the females (length, 70–120 cm) migrate in the subcutaneous tissues toward the skin surface (3). Approximately 1 year after infection, the female worm induces a blister on the skin, generally on the distal lower extremity, which ruptures. When this lesion comes into contact with water, a contact that the patient seeks to relieve the local discomfort, the female worm emerges and releases larvae (4). The larvae are ingested by a copepod (5) and after 2 weeks (and 2 molts) have developed into infective larvae (6). Ingestion of the copepods closes the cycle. Courtesy of Centers for Disease Control and Prevention.

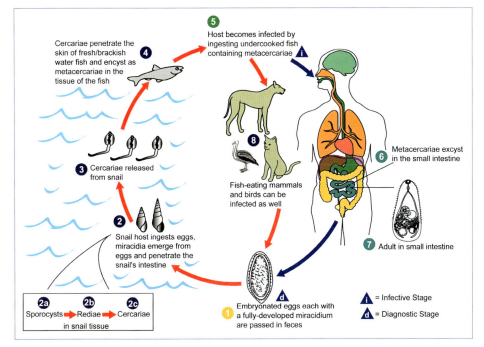

Image 99.8

Heterophyes heterophyes. Adults release embryonated eggs, each with a fully developed miracidium, and eggs are passed in the host's feces (1). After ingestion by a suitable snail (first intermediate host), the eggs hatch and release miracidia, which penetrate the snail's intestine (2). Genus *Cerithidia* is an important snail host is Asia; *Pironella*, in the Middle East. The miracidia undergo several developmental stages in the snail (sporocysts [2a], rediae [2b], and cercariae [2c]). Many cercariae are produced from each redia. The cercariae are released from the snail (3) and encyst as metacercariae in the tissues of a suitable freshwater or brackish water fish (second intermediate host) (4). The definitive host becomes infected by ingesting undercooked or salted fish containing metacercariae (5). After ingestion, the metacercariae excyst, attach to the mucosa of the small intestine (6), and mature into adults (measuring 1.0–1.7 mm × 0.3–0.4 mm) (7). In addition to humans, various fish-eating mammals (eg, cats, dogs) and birds can be infected by *H heterophyes* (8). Geographic distribution: Egypt, the Middle East, and the Far East. Courtesy of Centers for Disease Control and Prevention.

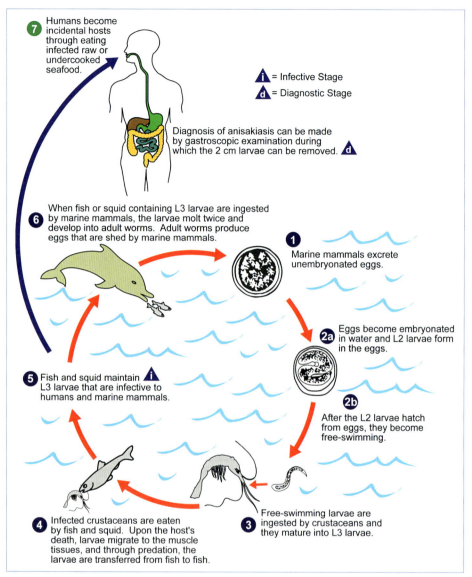

Image 99.9

Anisakiasis is caused by the unintentional ingestion of larvae of the nematodes (roundworms) *Anisakis simplex* or *Pseudoterranova decipiens*. Adult stages of *Anisakis simplex* or *P decipiens* reside in the stomach of marine mammals, where they are embedded in the mucosa, in clusters. Unembryonated eggs produced by adult females are passed in the feces of marine mammals (1). The eggs become embryonated in water, and first-stage larvae are formed in the eggs. The larvae molt, becoming second-stage larvae (2a), and after the larvae hatch from the eggs, they become free-swimming (2b). Larvae released from the eggs are ingested by crustaceans (3). The ingested larvae develop into third-stage larvae that are infective to fish and squid (4). The larvae migrate from the intestine to the tissues in the peritoneal cavity and grow up to 3 cm in length. On the host's death, larvae migrate to the muscle tissues and, through predation, are transferred from fish to fish. Fish and squid maintain third-stage larvae that are infective to humans and marine mammals (5). When fish or squid containing third-stage larvae are ingested by marine mammals, the larvae molt twice and develop into adult worms. The adult females produce eggs that are shed by marine mammals (6). Humans become infected by eating raw or undercooked infected marine fish (7). After ingestion, the *Anisakis* larvae penetrate the gastric and intestinal mucosa, causing the symptoms of anisakiasis. Courtesy of Centers for Disease Control and Prevention.

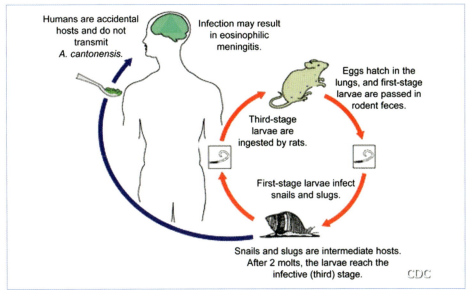

Image 99.10
Life cycle of *Angiostrongylus cantonensis*. Courtesy of Centers for Disease Control and Prevention/*Emerging Infectious Diseases*.

CHAPTER 100
Parechovirus Infections

CLINICAL MANIFESTATIONS

Parechoviruses (PeVs) primarily cause disease in young infants and manifest in a similar manner to that of enterovirus, disseminated herpes simplex virus, or bacterial infections, with a febrile illness, exanthem (maculopapular and/or generalized erythema or erythroderma, often with palmar and plantar erythema and at times in a distribution limited to the hands and feet), sepsis-like syndrome (frequently with leukopenia), and/or central nervous system (CNS) manifestations. CNS manifestations include meningitis (typically with little or no pleocytosis), encephalitis, seizures, and apnea, often with brain imaging abnormalities primarily affecting white matter; long-term neurodevelopmental sequelae may occur. Infections (particularly with PeV-A3) may be severe, with manifestations that include sepsis, hepatitis and coagulopathy, myocarditis, pneumonia, and/or meningoencephalitis, with long-term sequelae or death. PeV infections in older infants and toddlers have been associated with generally mild upper and lower respiratory tract disease and gastroenteritis (although causation has not been established consistently) and a variety of other less common manifestations, including acute flaccid paralysis, acute disseminated encephalomyelitis, myalgia and myositis, herpangina, hand-foot-and-mouth disease, sudden infant death syndrome, and hemophagocytic lymphohistiocytosis.

ETIOLOGY

PeVs are a group of small nonenveloped, single-stranded positive-sense RNA viruses in the family *Picornaviridae*. The *Parechovirus* genus consists of 4 species, *Parechovirus* A through D. *Parechovirus* A (formerly named human *Parechovirus*) includes at least 19 PeV types (designated 1–19) and is the only species known to cause human disease. PeV-A1 was previously classified as echovirus 22; PeV-A2, as echovirus 23. PeV-A1 and PeV-A3 have most frequently been implicated in disease.

EPIDEMIOLOGY

Humans are the primary reservoir for PeVs, although zoonotic infection in a number of animals hosts has been demonstrated for different PeV species. PeV-A infections have been reported worldwide. Seroepidemiologic studies suggest that PeV-A infections occur commonly during early childhood. In some studies, most school-aged children have serological evidence of prior infection, but seroprevalence appears to vary by geographic region and specific PeV-A type. Overall, PeV-A1 and PeV-A3 infections are most commonly reported in childhood and tend to infect children up to several years of age. PeV infections are frequently asymptomatic. Symptomatic infection is most frequent in children younger than 2 years, with the most severe disease occurring in infants (especially <6 months of age with PeV-A3) and young children. Disease infrequently occurs in older children and adults.

Transmission appears to occur via the fecal-oral and respiratory routes, from symptomatic or asymptomatic individuals. On the basis of reports of very early-onset neonatal disease, in utero transmission may also occur. Certain PeV-A types may circulate throughout the year, whereas infections by other types (eg, PeV-A3) occur more commonly during summer and fall months, with cyclic peaks described. Multiple PeV-A types may circulate in a community during the same period, and community outbreaks have been described. Epidemiological observations suggest household transmission, and health care–associated transmission in neonatal and pediatric hospital units has also been observed. Virus is shed from the upper respiratory tract for 1 to 3 weeks and in stool for less than 2 weeks to as long as 6 months. Shedding may occur in the absence of illness.

The **incubation period** for PeV infections has not been defined.

DIAGNOSTIC TESTS

Reverse transcriptase–polymerase chain reaction (RT-PCR) assays that detect PeVs, available at the Centers for Disease Control and Prevention and select reference and hospital-based laboratories, represent the best diagnostic modality currently available. Some of the assays may not detect all

PeV-A types. Enterovirus RT-PCR assays do not detect PeVs (and vice versa). PeVs can be detected by RT-PCR in stool, throat swab specimens, nasopharyngeal aspirates, tracheal secretions, blood, and cerebrospinal fluid (CSF). Multiplex PCR assays designed to detect a number of bacterial and viral agents of meningitis and encephalitis, including PeVs, in CSF are available. As with the enteroviruses, the PeVs can be shed from the respiratory and gastrointestinal tract for prolonged periods, so detection at these sites does not necessarily represent a current disease attributable to PeVs. Viral culture can be used, but recovery in culture is less sensitive than RT-PCR assay.

TREATMENT

No specific therapy is available for PeV infections. Immune globulin intravenous has been used in some published case reports of neonates with severe PeV infections.

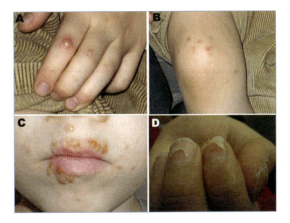

Image 100.1
Vesicular eruptions in hand (A), foot (B), and mouth (C) of a 6-year-old with coxsackievirus A6 infection. Several of the fingernails shed (D) 2 months after the pictures were taken. Courtesy of Centers for Disease Control and Prevention/ *Emerging Infectious Diseases.*

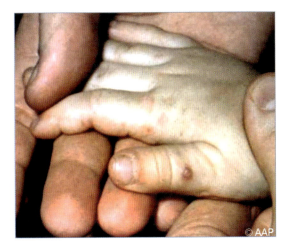

Image 100.2
Enterovirus infection in a preschool-aged child. Hand-foot-and-mouth disease lesions are caused by coxsackievirus A16 and enterovirus 71.

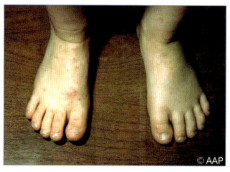

Image 100.3
Enterovirus infection (hand-foot-and-mouth disease) affecting the feet.

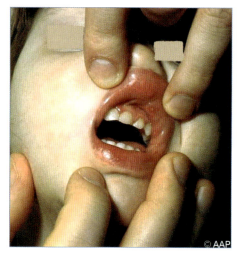

Image 100.4
Enterovirus infection (hand-foot-and-mouth disease) affecting the anterior buccal mucosa. These lesions are generally less painful than herpes simplex lesions.

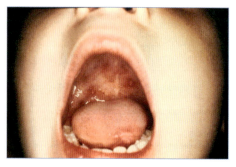

Image 100.5
Characteristic papulovesicular lesions of hand-foot-and-mouth disease in a 2-year-old. Courtesy of George Nankervis, MD.

CHAPTER 101

Parvovirus B19
(Erythema Infectiosum, Fifth Disease)

CLINICAL MANIFESTATIONS

Infection with parvovirus B19 is clinically recognized most often as erythema infectiosum (EI), or fifth disease, which is characterized by a distinctive rash that may be preceded by mild systemic symptoms, including fever in 15% to 30% of patients. The facial rash can be intensely red with a "slapped cheek" appearance that is often accompanied by circumoral pallor. A symmetrical, macular, lacelike, and often pruritic rash occurs on the trunk, moving peripherally to involve the arms, buttocks, and thighs. The rash can fluctuate in intensity and can recur with environmental changes, such as temperature and exposure to sunlight, for weeks to months. A brief, mild, nonspecific illness consisting of fever, malaise, myalgia, and headache often precedes the characteristic exanthem by approximately 7 to 10 days. Arthralgia and arthritis occur in less than 10% of infected children but commonly occur in adults, especially women. Knees are involved most commonly in children, but a symmetrical polyarthropathy of knees, fingers, and other joints is common in adults.

Parvovirus B19 can cause asymptomatic or subclinical infections. Other manifestations (Table 101.1) include a mild respiratory tract illness with no rash, a rash atypical for EI that may be rubelliform or petechial, papular-purpuric gloves-and-socks syndrome (PPGSS; painful and pruritic papules, petechiae, and purpura of hands and feet, often with fever and an enanthem), polyarthropathy syndrome (arthralgia and arthritis in adults in the absence of other manifestations of EI), chronic erythroid hypoplasia with severe anemia in patients with immunodeficiency (eg, patients with HIV infection, patients receiving immunosuppressive therapy), and transient aplastic crisis lasting 7 to 10 days in patients with hemolytic anemias (eg, sickle cell disease and autoimmune hemolytic anemia). For children with other conditions associated with low hemoglobin concentrations, including hemorrhage and severe anemia, parvovirus B19 infection does not usually result in aplastic crisis but might result in prolongation of recovery from the anemia. Patients with transient aplastic crisis may have a prodromal illness with fever, malaise, and myalgia, but rash is usually absent. In addition, parvovirus B19 infection has sometimes been associated with fewer platelets, lymphocytes, and neutrophils. In rare cases, parvovirus B19 infection has been associated with acute hepatitis, myocarditis, encephalopathies, and hemophagocytic lymphohistiocytosis in children and young adults. Parvovirus B19 infection occurring during pregnancy can cause fetal hydrops, intrauterine growth restriction, isolated pleural and pericardial effusions, and death, but the virus is not a proven cause of congenital anomalies. The risk of fetal death is between 2% and 6% when infection occurs during pregnancy. The greatest risk appears to occur during the first half of pregnancy.

ETIOLOGY

Parvovirus B19 is a small, nonenveloped, single-stranded DNA virus in the family *Parvoviridae*, genus *Erythroparvovirus*. Three distinct genotypes of the virus have been described, but there is no evidence of differences of virological or disease characteristics among the genotypes. Parvovirus B19 replicates in human erythrocyte

Table 101.1
Clinical Manifestations of Parvovirus B19 Infection

Conditions	Usual Hosts
Erythema infectiosum (fifth disease)	Immunocompetent children
Polyarthropathy syndrome	Immunocompetent adults (more common in women)
Chronic anemia/pure red cell aplasia	Immunocompromised hosts
Transient aplastic crisis	People with hemolytic anemia (ie, sickle cell disease)
Fetal hydrops/congenital anemia	Fetus (first 20 weeks of pregnancy)
Petechial, papular-purpuric gloves-and-socks syndrome	Immunocompetent children and young adults

precursors, which accounts for some of the clinical manifestations following infection. Parvovirus B19–associated red blood cell aplasia is related to caspase-mediated apoptosis of erythrocyte precursors.

EPIDEMIOLOGY

Parvovirus B19 is distributed worldwide and is a common cause of infection in humans, who are the only known hosts. Modes of transmission include contact with respiratory tract secretions, percutaneous exposure to blood or blood products, and vertical transmission from mother to fetus. Parvovirus B19 infections are ubiquitous, and cases of EI can occur sporadically or in outbreaks in schools during late winter and early spring. Secondary spread among susceptible household members is common, with infection occurring in approximately 50% of susceptible contacts in some studies. The transmission rate in schools is lower, but infection can be an occupational risk for school and child care personnel, with approximately 20% of susceptible contacts becoming infected. In young children, antibody seroprevalence is generally 5% to 10%. In most communities, approximately 50% of young adults and often more than 90% of elderly people are seropositive.

The **incubation period** from acquisition of parvovirus B19 to onset of initial symptoms (rash or symptoms of aplastic crisis) is between 4 and 14 days but can be as long as 21 days. Timing of the presence of high-titer parvovirus B19 DNA in serum and respiratory tract secretions indicates that people with EI are infectious before rash onset and are unlikely to be infectious after onset of the rash and/or joint symptoms. In contrast, patients with aplastic crises are contagious from before the onset of symptoms through at least the week after onset. Symptoms of PPGSS can occur in association with viremia and before development of antibody response, and affected patients should be considered infectious.

DIAGNOSTIC TESTS

In the immunocompetent host, detection of serum parvovirus B19–specific immunoglobulin M (IgM) antibodies is the preferred diagnostic test for an acute or recent parvovirus B19–associated rash illness. A positive IgM test result indicates that infection probably occurred within the previous 2 to 3 months. On the basis of immunoassay results, IgM antibodies may be detected in 90% or more of patients at the time of the EI rash and by the third day of illness in patients with transient aplastic crisis. Serum immunoglobulin G (IgG) antibodies appear by approximately day 2 of EI and persist for life; therefore, presence of parvovirus B19 IgG is not necessarily indicative of acute infection. IgM assays have variable sensitivity and specificity.

Serum IgM and IgG assays are unreliable in immunocompromised patients. The optimal method for detecting transient aplastic crisis or chronic infection in the immunocompromised patient is demonstration of high titer of viral DNA by polymerase chain reaction (PCR) assays. Such patients generally have greater than 10^6 copies/mL of parvovirus B19 DNA in plasma. With the availability of a World Health Organization nucleic acid standard for parvovirus B19 DNA, assay results can be reported in international units per milliliter (IU/mL) to allow for comparison across assays. False-negative results can occur with PCR assays that do not detect all 3 genotypes. Because parvovirus B19 DNA can be detected at low levels by PCR assay in serum for months and even years after the acute viremic phase, detection does not necessarily indicate acute infection. Low levels of parvovirus B19 DNA can also be detected by PCR in tissues (skin, heart, liver, and bone marrow), independent of active disease. Qualitative PCR may be used on amniotic fluid as an aid to diagnosis of fetal hydrops. Parvovirus B19 cannot be propagated in standard cell culture.

TREATMENT

For most patients, only supportive care is indicated. Patients with aplastic crisis may require transfusions of blood products. Immune globulin intravenous therapy is often effective and should be used for the treatment of parvovirus B19 infection in immunodeficient patients. Reduction of immunosuppression should also be attempted, if possible. Some cases of parvovirus B19 infection in pregnancy concurrent with fetal hydrops have been treated successfully with intrauterine blood transfusions of the fetus.

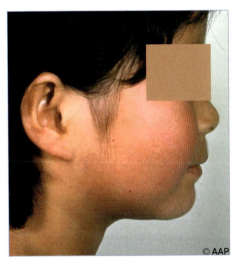

Image 101.1
Parvovirus B19 infection (erythema infectiosum, fifth disease) with typical facial erythema, commonly referred to as the "slapped cheek" sign.

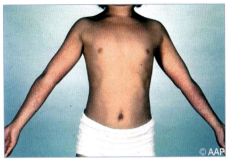

Image 101.2
Parvovirus B19 infection. Note lacelike pattern of the rash on the volar aspect of the child's arms. This is the same patient as in Image 101.1.

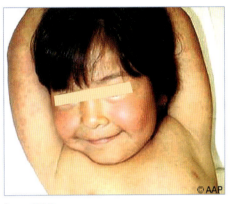

Image 101.4
Characteristic "slapped cheek" appearance of the face in a child who has fifth disease. The characteristic rash is also present on the arms.

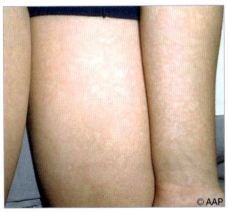

Image 101.3
Parvovirus B19 infection (erythema infectiosum, fifth disease). Three preschool-aged female siblings manifested the rash on the same day.

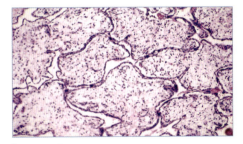

Image 101.5
Parvovirus infection in pregnancy. Hydropic placental villi. Courtesy of Dimitris P. Agamanolis, MD.

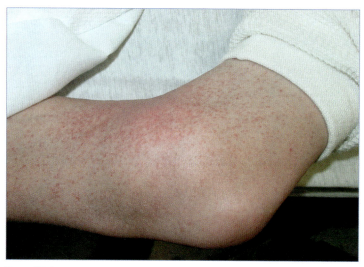

Image 101.6
Parvovirus B19 infection with a rash in a 10-year-old boy. Courtesy of Benjamin Estrada, MD.

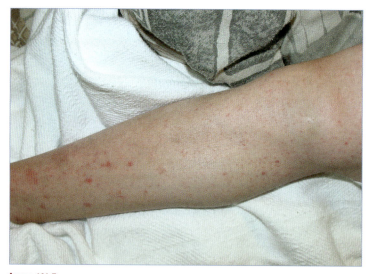

Image 101.7
Parvovirus B19 infection with a rash in a 10-year-old boy. Courtesy of Benjamin Estrada, MD.

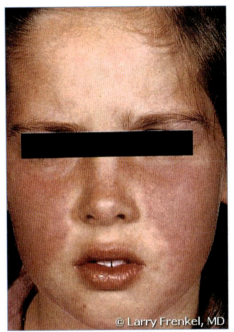

Image 101.8
An 8-year-old girl with the facial erythema of erythema infectiosum. Courtesy of Larry Frenkel, MD.

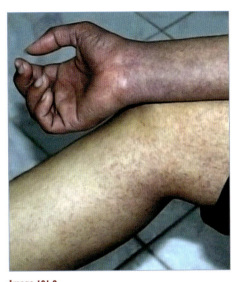

Image 101.9
Stocking glove purpura. This 18-year-old young woman awoke one morning with asymptomatic symmetrical purpura of the hands and feet, which spread to involve the proximal extremities. The exanthem faded over 7–10 days. Although an enanthem is not usually reported with parvovirus infection, she also developed some erythema of the buccal mucosa and white plaques on a red base on the dorsum of the tongue. Courtesy of H. Cody Meissner, MD, FAAP.

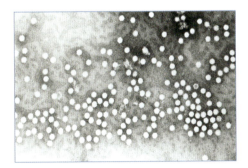

Image 101.10
This electron micrograph depicts a number of parvovirus H1 virions of the *Parvoviridae* family. These are nonenveloped, single-stranded DNA viruses. The *Parvoviridae* family of viruses also contains the parvovirus B19 virion, which is responsible for causing erythema infectiosum, or fifth disease. Courtesy of Centers for Disease Control and Prevention.

CHAPTER 102

Pasteurella Infections

CLINICAL MANIFESTATIONS

The most common manifestation is cellulitis at the site of a bite or scratch of a cat, a dog, or another domestic or wild animal. Cellulitis typically develops within 24 hours of the injury and includes swelling, erythema, tenderness, and serosanguinous to purulent drainage at the wound site. Regional lymphadenopathy, chills, and fever can occur. The most frequent local complications are abscesses and tenosynovitis, but septic arthritis and osteomyelitis also occur. Other less common manifestations that are not always associated with an animal bite include septicemia, central nervous system infections (meningitis is the most common; however, brain abscess and subdural empyema have been observed), ocular infections (eg, conjunctivitis, corneal ulcer, endophthalmitis), endocarditis, respiratory tract infections (eg, pneumonia, pulmonary abscesses, pleural empyema, epiglottitis), appendicitis, hepatic abscess, peritonitis, and urinary tract infection. People with liver disease, solid organ transplant, or underlying host defense abnormalities are predisposed to bacteremia with *Pasteurella multocida*.

ETIOLOGY

The genus *Pasteurella* is one of 4 genera of human pathogens classified in the family *Pasteurellaceae*; the other genera are *Actinobacillus*, *Aggregatibacter*, and *Haemophilus*. Members of the genus *Pasteurella* are nonmotile, facultatively anaerobic, mostly catalase and oxidase positive, gram-negative coccobacilli that are primarily respiratory tract colonizers and pathogens in animals. The most common human pathogen is *P multocida*. Most human infections are caused by the following species or subspecies (subsp): *P multocida* subsp *multocida* (causing >50% of infections), *P multocida* subsp *septica*, *Pasteurella canis*, *Pasteurella stomatis*, and *Pasteurella dagmatis*.

EPIDEMIOLOGY

Pasteurella species have a worldwide distribution. They colonize the upper respiratory tract of 70% to 90% of cats, 25% to 50% of dogs, and many other wild and domestic animals. Transmission most frequently occurs from the bite or scratch or licking of a previous wound by a cat or dog. Infected cat bite wounds contain *Pasteurella* species more often than do dog bite wounds. Rarely, respiratory tract spread occurs from animals to humans, and in a significant proportion of cases, no animal exposure can be identified. Human-to-human transmission has been documented vertically from mother to neonate, horizontally from colonized humans, and by contaminated blood products.

The **incubation period** is usually less than 24 hours.

DIAGNOSTIC TESTS

The isolation of *Pasteurella* species from a normally sterile body site (eg, blood, joint fluid, cerebrospinal fluid, pleural fluid, suppurative lymph nodes) establishes the diagnosis of systemic infection. Recovery of the organism from a superficial site, such as drainage from a skin lesion subsequent to an animal bite, must be interpreted in the context of other potential pathogens isolated, and mixed infection may occur. *Pasteurella* species are somewhat fastidious but may be cultured on several media generally used in clinical laboratories, including tryptic soybean digest agar with 5% sheep blood and chocolate agars, at 35 to 37 °C (95–99 °F) without increased carbon dioxide concentration. Although they resemble several other organisms morphologically, laboratory identification to the genus level is generally not difficult. Newer laboratory methods, including polymerase chain reaction amplification of the 16S ribosomal RNA gene followed by sequencing and identification of cellular components by MALDI-TOF (matrix-assisted laser desorption/ionization–time-of-flight) mass spectroscopy, have significantly improved specific identification.

TREATMENT

The drug of choice is penicillin. Penicillin resistance is rare, but β-lactamase–producing strains have been recovered. Other oral agents that are usually effective include ampicillin, amoxicillin, amoxicillin-clavulanate, cefuroxime, cefixime, cefpodoxime, doxycycline, and fluoroquinolones. Parenteral third-generation cephalosporins, including ceftriaxone and cefotaxime, demonstrate excellent in vitro activity. Oral and parenteral antistaphylococcal penicillins and first-generation cephalosporins including cephalexin are not as active and are not recommended for treatment. *Pasteurella* species are usually resistant to vancomycin, clindamycin, and erythromycin. For patients who are allergic to β-lactam agents, azithromycin, trimethoprim-sulfamethoxazole, and the fluoroquinolones are alternative choices, but clinical experience with these agents is limited. For suspected polymicrobial infected bite wounds, oral amoxicillin-clavulanate or, for severe infection, intravenous ampicillin-sulbactam or piperacillin-tazobactam can be given. The duration of therapy is usually 7 to 10 days for local infections and 10 to 14 days for more severe infections. Antimicrobial therapy should be continued for 4 to 6 weeks for bone and joint infections. Wound drainage or debridement may be necessary.

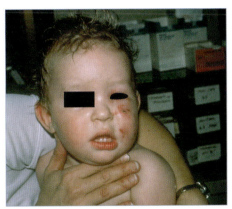

Image 102.1
Pasteurella multocida cellulitis secondary to multiple cat bites around the face of a 1-year-old. Courtesy of George Nankervis, MD.

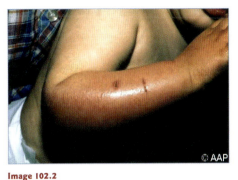

Image 102.2
Right forearm of a 1-year-old boy bitten by a stray cat. The child developed fever, redness, and swelling 10 hours after the bite. He was taking amoxicillin for otitis media at the time of the bite. The child responded to treatment with intravenous cefuroxime, although the fever persisted for 36 hours. *Pasteurella multocida* was cultured from purulent material obtained from the wound the day after admission. Courtesy of Larry I. Corman, MD.

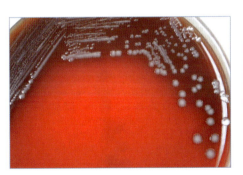

Image 102.3
This photograph depicts the colonial morphological features displayed by gram-negative *Yersinia pestis* bacteria, which was grown on a medium of sheep blood agar for a 72-hour period at a temperature of 37 °C (98.6 °F). Courtesy of Centers for Disease Control and Prevention/Todd Parker, MD, and Audra Marsh.

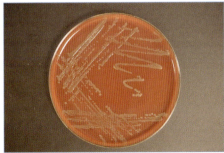

Image 102.4
Pasteurella multocida on chocolate agar. Colonies are small, gray, smooth, and nonhemolytic. Courtesy of Julia Rosebush, DO; Robert Jerris, PhD; and Theresa Stanley, M(ASCP).

CHAPTER 103

Pediculosis Capitis
(Head Lice)

CLINICAL MANIFESTATIONS

Itching is the most common symptom of head lice infestation, but many children are asymptomatic. Adult lice (2–3 mm long, tan to grayish-white, with claws on all 6 legs) or eggs (match hair color) and nits (empty egg casings, white) are found on the hair and are most readily apparent behind the ears and near the nape of the neck. Excoriations and crusting caused by secondary bacterial infection may occur and are often associated with regional lymphadenopathy. Head lice usually deposit their eggs on a hair shaft 1 to 2 mm from the scalp. Because hair grows at a rate of approximately 1 cm per month, duration of infestation can be estimated by the distance of the nit from the scalp.

ETIOLOGY

Pediculus humanus capitis is the head louse. Both nymphs and adult lice feed on human blood.

EPIDEMIOLOGY

Head lice infestation in the United States is most common in children attending child care, preschool, and elementary school and is not a sign of poor hygiene. All income groups are affected. Head lice infestation is not influenced by hair length, hair texture, or frequency of shampooing or brushing. Head lice are not a health hazard and are not responsible for spread of any disease. Transmission occurs mainly by direct head-to-head contact with hair of infested people. Transmission by contact with personal belongings, such as combs, hairbrushes, sporting gear, and hats, is uncommon. Head lice survive less than 1 day at room temperature away from the scalp, and their eggs generally become nonviable within a week and cannot hatch at a lower ambient temperature than that near the scalp.

The **incubation period** from the laying of eggs to the hatching of the first nymph is usually about 1 week (range, 6–9 days). Lice mature to the adult stage approximately 7 days later. Adult females may then lay eggs, but these will develop only if the female has mated.

DIAGNOSTIC TESTS

Identification of eggs, nymphs, and adult lice with the naked eye is possible; diagnosis can be confirmed by using a hand lens, dermatoscope (epiluminescence microscope), or traditional microscope. Nymphal and adult lice shun light and move rapidly to conceal themselves. Wetting the hair with water, oil, or a conditioner to "slow down" the movement of the lice and using a fine-tooth comb may improve ability to diagnose infestation and shorten inspection time. It is important to differentiate nits from dandruff, hair casts (a layer of follicular cells that slide easily off the hair shaft), plugs of desquamated cells, external hair debris, and fungal infections of the scalp. Finding nits attached firmly within 0.64 cm (0.25 inches) of the base of the hair shaft suggests that a person has had infestation, but because nits remain affixed firmly to hair even after hatching or dying, their mere presence (particularly >1 cm from the scalp) is not a conclusive sign of an active infestation.

TREATMENT

Treatment is recommended for people who have an active infestation. A number of effective pediculicidal agents are available to treat head lice infestation (Table 103.1). Costs and recommended age ranges vary by product (Table 103.1). Safety is a major concern with pediculicides, because lice infestation itself presents minimal risk to the host. Pediculicides should be used only as directed and with care and only when there is concern for active infestation. Instructions on proper use of any product should be explained carefully. Extra amounts should not be used, and multiple products should not be used concurrently. If medication gets into a child's eyes, it should be flushed out immediately with water. Skin exposure to pediculicide should be limited. Hair should be rinsed over a sink rather than during a shower or bath after topical pediculicide application, and warm rather than hot water should be used to minimize skin absorption attributable to vasodilatation. Therapy can be initiated with over-the-counter permethrin, 1%, lotion or with pyrethrin combined with piperonyl butoxide, both of which have good safety profiles. Resistance to these compounds has been documented in the United States, and clinical resistance may vary by region.

Table 103.1
Pediculicides for the Treatment of Head Lice

Product	Brand Name	Recommended Age Range	Re-treatment Interval (If Needed)	Availability	Cost Estimate[a]
Permethrin, 1%, lotion	Multiple products	≥2 mo	9–10 days	Over the counter	$
Pyrethrins + piperonyl butoxide shampoo	Example: Rid	≥24 mo	9–10 days	Over the counter	$
Malathion, 0.5%	Ovide	≥2 y (safety not established for 2–6 y)	7–9 days if live lice are observed after initial dose	Prescription	$$$$
Spinosad, 0.9%, suspension	Natroba	≥6 mo	7 days if live lice are observed after initial dose	Prescription	$$$$
Abametapir, 0.74%, lotion	Xeglyze	≥6 mo	Single use	Prescription	$$$$
Ivermectin, 0.5%, lotion	Sklice	≥6 mo	Single use	Over the counter	$$$$
Ivermectin (oral)	Stromectol	Any age, if weight ≥15 kg	9–10 days	Prescription	$$$$

[a] $ = ≤$25; $$ = $26–$99; $$$ = $100–$199; $$$$ = $200–$299.

Drugs vary in their residual activity, and no treatment is 100% ovicidal. Re-treatment may be needed after eggs present at the time of initial treatment have hatched but before new eggs are produced; re-treatment intervals vary by product.

- **Permethrin, 1%, lotion.** Permethrin is available without a prescription in a 1% lotion. Infested hair and scalp are washed first with a nonconditioning shampoo and towel dried. Permethrin is then applied to the scalp and entire length of wet hair, left on for 10 minutes, and then rinsed off with water. Permethrin has a low potential for toxic effects and can be highly effective. Although residual permethrin is designed to kill emerging nymphs, many experts advise a second treatment 9 to 10 days after the first treatment, especially if hair is washed within a week after the first treatment or if live lice are observed.

- **Pyrethrin-based shampoo products.** Pyrethrins are natural extracts from the chrysanthemum flower, formulated with piperonyl butoxide, and are available without a prescription as shampoos or mousse preparations. The product is applied to dry hair in sufficient amounts to saturate the scalp and entire length of the hair, left on for 10 minutes, and then rinsed off with water. Pyrethrins have no residual activity; repeated application 9 to 10 days after the first application is necessary to kill newly hatched lice. Pyrethrins are contraindicated in people who are allergic to chrysanthemums or ragweed.

- **Malathion, 0.5%, lotion.** This organophosphate pesticide, which is both pediculicidal and partially ovicidal, is available only by prescription as a lotion. Malathion lotion is applied to dry hair in sufficient amounts to saturate the scalp and entire length of the hair, left on to dry naturally, and then removed 8 to 12 hours later by washing and rinsing the hair. The product can be reapplied 7 to 9 days later only if live lice are still observed. The high alcohol content of the lotion makes it highly flammable; therefore, the lotion or lotion-coated hair during treatment should not be exposed to lighted cigarettes (no smoking around the individual during hair treatment), open flames, or electric heat sources such as hair dryers or curling irons. Malathion lotion should not be used in children younger than 2 years.

- **Spinosad, 0.9%, suspension.**
  Spinosad is a novel neurotoxin derived from *Saccharopolyspora spinosa*. Spinosad suspension contains benzyl alcohol and is pediculicidal. The suspension is applied to dry hair in sufficient amounts to saturate the scalp and entire length of the hair, left on for 10 minutes, and then rinsed off with water. A second treatment is applied at 7 days if live lice are still observed. This product should not be used in infants younger than 6 months because systemic absorption may lead to benzyl alcohol toxicity.

- **Abametapir, 0.74%, lotion.** Abametapir inhibits metalloproteinases, which have a role in physiological processes critical to egg development and survival of lice. Abametapir lotion contains benzyl alcohol and is ovicidal. Abametapir lotion is applied to dry hair in sufficient amounts to thoroughly coat the hair and scalp, left on for 10 minutes, and then rinsed off with warm water. Treatment involves a single application. This product should not be used in infants younger than 6 months because systemic absorption may lead to benzyl alcohol toxicity.

- **Ivermectin, 0.5%, lotion.** Ivermectin interferes with the function of invertebrate nerve and muscle cells and is used widely as an anthelmintic agent. Ivermectin lotion is not ovicidal, but it appears to prevent newly hatched lice (nymphs) from surviving. The lotion is applied to dry hair in sufficient amounts to saturate the scalp and entire length of the hair, left on for 10 minutes, and then rinsed off with water. It is effective in most patients when given as a single application on dry hair without nit combing and may be used in children 6 months and older.

- **Oral ivermectin.** Ivermectin may be effective against head lice if sufficient concentration is present in the blood at the time a louse feeds. It has been given as a single oral dose of 200 μg/kg or 400 μg/kg, with a second dose given after 9 to 10 days. Fewer failures occur at the 400-μg/kg dose than at the lower dose. Ivermectin should not be used in children weighing less than 15 kg because it blocks essential neural transmission if it crosses the blood-brain barrier and young children have higher risk for this adverse drug reaction.

Detection of living lice on scalp inspection 24 hours or more after treatment suggests incorrect use of pediculicide, hatching of lice after treatment, reinfestation, or resistance to therapy, because pediculicides kill lice shortly after application. After exclusion of incorrect use, re-treatment with a different pediculicide followed by a second application (except for single-use topical ivermectin) at the intervals specified above is recommended in these situations.

Itching or mild burning of the scalp caused by inflammation of the skin in response to topical therapeutic agents can persist for many days after lice are killed; this is not a reason for re-treatment. Topical corticosteroid and oral antihistamine agents may be beneficial for relieving these signs and symptoms.

Manual removal of nits after successful treatment with a pediculicide is helpful to decrease diagnostic confusion and to decrease the small risk of self-reinfestation and social stigmatization. Fine-tooth nit combs designed for this purpose are available, although the type of comb is less important than the actual action of combing. Other products, such as vinegar, should not be used to help remove nits, because these may interfere with effectiveness of the pediculicide.

PEDICULOSIS CAPITIS

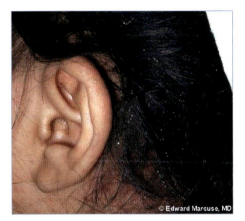

Image 103.1
Nits on the hair shafts. Copyright Edgar K. Marcuse, MD.

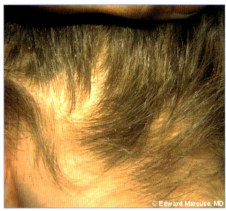

Image 103.2
Nits on the hair shaft. Copyright Edgar K. Marcuse, MD.

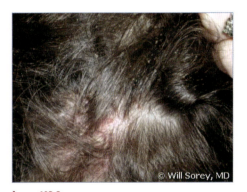

Image 103.3
An 8-year-old girl with an earache. This child reported otalgia. During the course of otoscopic evaluation, she was noted to have a very large number of nits in her hair as well as active lice. On questioning, she stated she had had itching of the scalp. She was treated with topical permethrin with temporary resolution. Reinfestation occurred after sharing a riding helmet with a cousin. Courtesy of Will Sorey, MD.

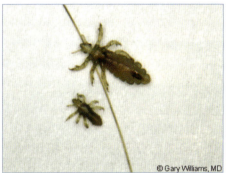

Image 103.4
Head louse, baby louse, and hair. Copyright Gary Williams, MD.

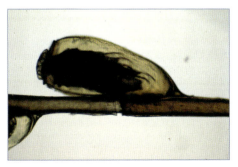

Image 103.5
Lice nit. Copyright James Brien, DO.

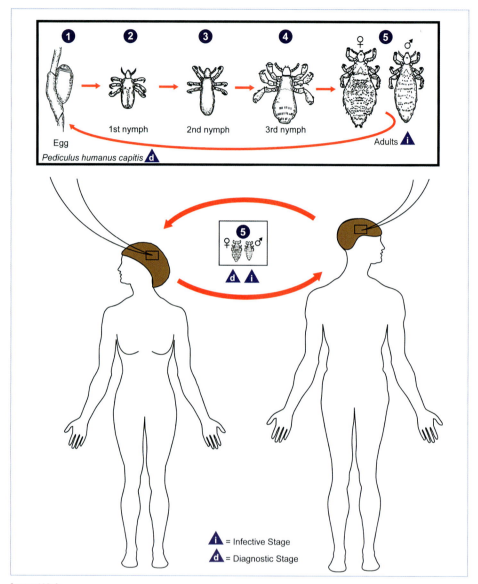

Image 103.6

The life cycle of the head louse has 3 stages: egg, nymph, and adult. Eggs: Nits are head lice eggs. They are hard to see and are often confused for dandruff or hair spray droplets. Nits are laid by the adult female and are cemented at the base of the hair shaft nearest the scalp (1). They are 0.8×0.3 mm, oval, and usually yellow to white. Nits take about 1 week to hatch (range, 6–9 days). Viable eggs are usually located within 6 mm of the scalp. Nymphs: The egg hatches to release a nymph (2). The nit shell then becomes a more visible dull yellow and remains attached to the hair shaft. The nymph looks like an adult head louse but is about the size of a pinhead. Nymphs mature after 3 molts (3, 4) and become adults about 7 days after hatching. Adults: The adult louse is about the size of a sesame seed, has 6 legs (each with claws), and is tan to grayish-white (5). In people with dark hair, the adult louse appears darker. Females are usually larger than males and can lay up to 8 nits per day. Adult lice can live up to 30 days on a person's head. To live, adult lice need to feed on blood several times daily. Without blood meals, the louse will die within 1–2 days off the host. Courtesy of Centers for Disease Control and Prevention.

CHAPTER 104
Pediculosis Corporis
(Body Lice)

CLINICAL MANIFESTATIONS

Patients affected with pediculosis corporis characteristically come to medical attention because of intense itching, particularly at night. Bites manifest as small erythematous macules, papules, and excoriations, primarily on the trunk. In heavily bitten areas, typically around the midsection of the body (waist, groin, and upper thighs), the skin can become thickened and discolored. Secondary bacterial infection of the skin (pyoderma) caused by scratching is common.

ETIOLOGY

Pediculus humanus corporis (or *humanus*) is the body louse. Both nymphs and adult lice feed on human blood.

EPIDEMIOLOGY

Body lice are generally restricted to people living in crowded conditions without access to regular bathing (at least weekly) or changes of clean clothing (refugees, survivors of war or natural disasters, people facing homelessness). Under these conditions, body lice can spread rapidly through direct contact or contact with contaminated clothing or bedding. Body lice live in clothes or bedding used by infested people, lay their eggs on or near the seams of clothing, and move to the skin only to feed. Body lice cannot survive away from a blood source for longer than approximately 5 to 7 days at room temperature. In contrast with head and pubic lice, body lice are well-recognized vectors of disease (eg, epidemic typhus, trench fever, epidemic relapsing fever, and bacillary angiomatosis).

The **incubation period** from the laying of eggs to the hatching of the first nymph is approximately 1 to 2 weeks, depending on ambient temperature. Lice mature and are capable of reproducing 9 to 19 days after hatching, depending on whether infested clothing is removed for sleeping.

DIAGNOSTIC TESTS

Seams of clothing should be examined for eggs (nits), nymphs, and adult lice (2–4 mm) if body louse infestation is suspected. Nits and lice may be observed with the naked eye; diagnosis can be confirmed by using a hand lens, a dermatoscope (epiluminescence microscope), or a traditional microscope. Adult and nymphal body lice are seldom observed on the body, because they are generally sequestered in clothing.

TREATMENT

Treatment consists of improving hygiene, including bathing and regular (at least weekly) changes to clean clothes and bedding. Infested materials can be either discarded or decontaminated by machine washing with the hot water cycle and machine drying with the hot air cycle, by dry cleaning, by sealing in a plastic bag and placing into storage for 2 weeks, or by pressing with a hot iron. Temperatures exceeding 54 °C (130 °F) for 5 minutes are lethal to lice and eggs. Pediculicides for patients are usually not necessary if materials are laundered sufficiently hot at least weekly. People with abundant body hair may require full-body treatment with a pediculicide, because lice and eggs may occasionally adhere to body hair. Guidance for the choice of pediculicide (if desired for treatment) is the same as for head lice.

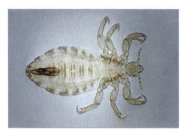

Image 104.1
This body louse, *Pediculus humanus humanus*, family *Pediculidae*, is a parasitic insect that lives on the body and in the clothing or bedding of infested humans. Infestation is common and is found worldwide. Itching and rash are common with lice infestation. Courtesy of Centers for Disease Control and Prevention.

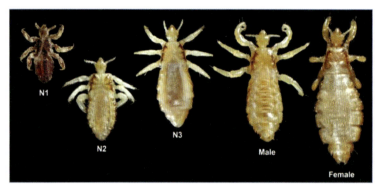

Image 104.2
This image depicts 5 body lice, *Pediculus humanus humanus*, which, from left to right, include 3 nymphal-staged lice, beginning with an N1-staged nymph, moving to an N2, and ending with an N3, followed by an adult male louse and, finally, an adult female louse. Courtesy of Centers for Disease Control and Prevention/Joseph Strycharz, PhD; Kyong Sup Yoon, PhD; and Frank Collins, PhD.

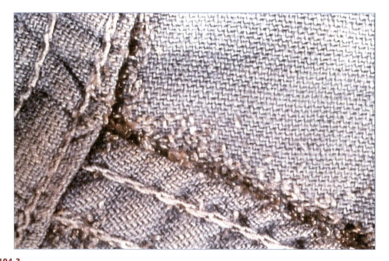

Image 104.3
This is a piece of clothing, the seams of which contained lice eggs from the body louse *Pediculus humanus humanus*. The most important factor in the control of body lice infestation is the ability to change and wash clothing. Courtesy of Centers for Disease Control and Prevention/Reed & Carnrick Pharmaceuticals.

CHAPTER 105
Pediculosis Pubis
(Pubic Lice, Crab Lice)

CLINICAL MANIFESTATIONS

Pruritus of the anogenital area is a common symptom in pubic lice infestations ("crabs" or "phthiriasis"). Adult lice (1–2 mm long and flattened, tan to grayish-white, with 4 of its 6 legs terminating in crab-like claws) or eggs (match hair color) and nits (empty egg casings, white) are found on hair, particularly near the hair-skin junction. The parasite is most frequently found in the pubic region, but infestation can involve other coarse body hair, including the eyelashes, eyebrows, beard, axilla, legs, perianal area, and, rarely, scalp. A characteristic sign of heavy pubic lice infestation is the presence of bluish or slate-colored macules (maculae ceruleae) on the chest, abdomen, or thighs.

ETIOLOGY

Phthirus pubis is the pubic or crab louse. Both nymphs and adult lice feed on human blood. Pubic lice are not a health hazard and are not responsible for the spread of any disease.

EPIDEMIOLOGY

Pubic lice infestations are more prevalent among teenagers and young adults and are usually spread through sexual contact. Transmission by contact with contaminated items, such as bed linens, towels, or shared clothing, can occur. Pubic lice on the eyelashes or eyebrows of children (likely the only areas of coarse hair) may be evidence of sexual abuse. People with pubic lice infestation should be examined for the presence of other sexually transmitted infections (STIs). Animals do not get or spread pubic lice.

The **incubation period** from the laying of eggs to the hatching of the first nymph is 6 to 10 days. Adult lice become capable of reproducing 2 to 3 weeks after hatching. Adult pubic lice can survive away from a host for up to 48 hours, and their eggs can remain viable for up to 10 days under suitable environmental conditions.

DIAGNOSTIC TESTS

Identification of eggs (nits), nymphs, and lice with the naked eye is possible, although it can be difficult to detect lice unless they have had a recent blood meal. The diagnosis can be confirmed by using a hand lens, traditional microscope, or dermatoscope (epiluminescence microscope) to examine hair shafts. Pubic lice may be difficult to find because of low numbers, and they do not crawl as quickly as head and body lice. If crawling lice are not observed, finding nits in the pubic area strongly suggests infestation and should lead to treatment.

TREATMENT

All areas of the body with coarse hair should be examined for evidence of pubic lice infestation. Lice and their eggs can be removed manually, or the hairs can be shaved to eliminate infestation immediately (although topical pediculicides should still be used even when the affected area is shaved). Caution should be used when inspecting, removing, or treating lice on or near the eyelashes. Recommended therapies include either permethrin, 1%, cream rinse (applied to affected areas and washed off after 10 minutes) or pyrethrins with piperonyl butoxide (applied to the affected area and washed off after 10 minutes). Reported resistance to permethrin and pyrethrins has been increasing and is widespread. Evaluation should be performed after 1 week if symptoms persist. Re-treatment might be necessary if lice are found or if eggs are observed at the hair-skin junction. If no clinical response is achieved to one of the recommended regimens, treatment with malathion (0.5% lotion applied to affected areas and washed off after 8–12 hours) or oral ivermectin (250 μg/kg orally, repeated in 7–14 days) is recommended.

Infested people should be examined for other STIs. Pubic lice on the eyelashes or eyebrows of children should prompt evaluation for sexual abuse.

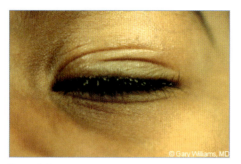

Image 105.1
Pubic lice (*Phthirus pubis*) in the eyelashes of a 3-year-old boy. The diagnosis can be confirmed by the use of a hand lens or microscope. Copyright Gary Williams, MD.

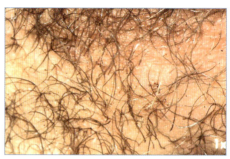

Image 105.2
This photograph reveals the presence of pubic or crab lice, *Phthirus pubis,* with reddish-brown feces. Pubic lice are generally found in the genital area on pubic hair but may occasionally be found on other coarse body hair, such as leg hair, armpit hair, mustache, beard, eyebrows, and eyelashes. Courtesy of Centers for Disease Control and Prevention/Reed & Carnrick Pharmaceuticals.

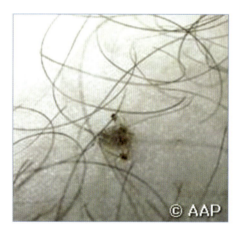

Image 105.3
Pediculosis, the infestation of humans by lice, has been documented for millennia. Three species of lice infest humans: *Pediculus humanus humanus*, the body louse; *Pediculus humanus capitis*, the head louse; and *Phthirus pubis,* the pubic or crab louse. The hallmark of louse infestation is pruritus at the site of bites. Lice are more active at night, frequently disrupting the sleep of the host, which is the derivation of the term "feeling lousy." Adult pubic lice can survive without a blood meal for 36 hours. Unlike head lice, which may travel up to 23 cm per minute, pubic lice are sluggish, traveling a maximum of 10 cm per day. Viable eggs on pubic hairs may hatch up to 10 days later. Pubic louse infestation is localized most frequently to the pubic and perianal regions but may spread to the mustache, beard, axillae, eyelashes, or scalp hair. Infestation is usually acquired through sexual contact, and the finding of pubic lice in children (often limited to the eyelashes) should raise concern for possible sexual abuse. Courtesy of H. Cody Meissner, MD, FAAP.

CHAPTER 106

Pelvic Inflammatory Disease

CLINICAL MANIFESTATIONS

Pelvic inflammatory disease (PID) comprises a spectrum of inflammatory disorders of the female upper genital tract, including any combination of endometritis, parametritis, salpingitis, oophoritis, tubo-ovarian abscess, and pelvic peritonitis. Acute PID is difficult to diagnose because of the wide variation in symptoms and signs. Symptoms of acute PID include unilateral or bilateral lower abdominal or pelvic pain, fever, vomiting, abnormal vaginal discharge, irregular vaginal bleeding, and pain with intercourse. The severity of symptoms varies widely and may range from indolent to severe. Patients occasionally present with right upper quadrant abdominal pain resulting from peritoneal adhesions related to perihepatitis (Fitz-Hugh–Curtis syndrome). Many episodes of PID go undiagnosed and untreated because the patient and/or health care professional fails to recognize the implications of mild or nonspecific symptoms and signs. Subclinical PID is defined as inflammation of the upper reproductive tract in the absence of signs and symptoms of acute PID, and there is a growing body of evidence that this represents a large proportion of all PID cases. In both clinically apparent and subclinical PID, inflammation occurs within the reproductive tract that scars or damages the fallopian tubes or surrounding structures. Clinicians need to maintain a high degree of suspicion for PID when a woman of reproductive age presents with mild or nonspecific findings, particularly in a young female who might provide an incomplete or inaccurate sexual history.

Examination findings vary but may include oral temperature higher than 38.3 °C (>101 °F), lower abdominal tenderness with or without peritoneal signs, abnormal cervical or vaginal discharge, tenderness with lateral motion of the cervix, uterine tenderness, unilateral or bilateral adnexal tenderness, and adnexal fullness. Pyuria (presence of white blood cells [WBCs] on urine microscopy), abundant WBCs on saline microscopy of vaginal fluid, an elevated erythrocyte sedimentation rate, an elevated C-reactive protein level, and an adnexal mass demonstrated by abdominal or transvaginal ultrasonography are all findings that support a diagnosis of PID.

Complications of PID include perihepatitis (Fitz-Hugh–Curtis syndrome) and tubo-ovarian abscess/complex formation. Long-term sequelae include tubal scarring that can cause infertility in an estimated 10% to 20% of affected females, ectopic pregnancy in an estimated 9%, and chronic pelvic pain in an estimated 18%. Factors that may increase the likelihood of infertility are delay in diagnosis or delay in initiation of antimicrobial therapy, younger age at time of infection, chlamydial infection, recurrent PID, and PID determined to be severe by laparoscopic examination.

Any prepubertal girl with PID needs to be assessed for sexual abuse.

ETIOLOGY

Neisseria gonorrhoeae and *Chlamydia trachomatis* are the pathogens most commonly associated with PID, although in recent studies, less than half of PID cases have evidence of these bacterial pathogens. A number of organisms other than *N gonorrhoeae* and *C trachomatis* have been isolated from upper genital tract cultures of females with PID, including anaerobes (such as *Prevotella* species), *Gardnerella vaginalis, Haemophilus influenzae, Streptococcus agalactiae,* enteric gram-negative rods, cytomegalovirus, *Mycoplasma hominis,* and *Ureaplasma urealyticum.* Therefore, PID is managed as a polymicrobial infection. In more than half of cases, however, no organism is identified from routine lower genital tract swab specimens (ie, endocervical or vaginal swab specimens). *Mycoplasma genitalium* has also been implicated in the etiology of PID in some studies, although the natural history of *M genitalium* in females remains unclear. PID may also be secondary to other causes of peritonitis, such as ruptured appendicitis.

EPIDEMIOLOGY

Although many of the issues pertaining to high-risk sexual behavior and acquisition of sexually transmitted infections (STIs) are common to both adolescents and adults, they are often intensified in adolescents because of both behavioral and biological predispositions. Adolescents and young women can have higher risk for STIs and PID because of behavioral factors such as inconsistent barrier contraceptive use, douching, greater number of current and lifetime sexual partners, and use of alcohol and other substances that may impair judgment while engaging in sexual activity. Use of condoms may reduce the risk of PID. Adolescent and young adult females also have an increased biological susceptibility to STIs. Cervical ectopy increases risk of chlamydia and gonorrhea infection by exposing columnar epithelium to a potential infectious inoculum.

An **incubation period** for PID is undefined.

DIAGNOSTIC TESTS

Centers for Disease Control and Prevention (CDC) criteria for clinical diagnosis and presumptive treatment of PID are presented in Box 106.1. Acute PID is difficult to diagnose because of its wide variation in symptoms and signs. Many women with PID have subtle or nonspecific symptoms or no symptoms, and a diagnosis of PID is usually based on imprecise clinical findings. A clinical diagnosis of symptomatic PID has a positive predictive value for salpingitis of 65% to 90% compared to that of laparoscopy. No single historical, physical, or laboratory finding is both sensitive and specific for the diagnosis of acute PID. Because of the difficulty of diagnosis and the potential for damage to the reproductive health of women, health care professionals should maintain a low threshold for the clinical diagnosis of PID.

A cervical or vaginal swab specimen should be obtained from all patients with suspected PID to perform a nucleic acid amplification test (NAAT) for *C trachomatis* and *N gonorrhoeae*. A swab specimen for culture of *N gonorrhoeae* may be collected from the cervix or vagina to allow susceptibility testing to be performed. The most specific criteria for diagnosing PID include endometrial biopsy with histopathologic evidence of endometritis; transvaginal ultrasonography or magnetic

---

Box 106.1
Criteria for Clinical Diagnosis and Presumptive Treatment of Pelvic Inflammatory Disease[a]

Minimum criteria

Presumptive treatment of PID should be initiated in sexually active young women and other women with risk for STIs if they are experiencing pelvic or lower abdominal pain, if no cause for the illness other than PID can be identified, and if one or more of the following **minimum clinical criteria** are present on pelvic examination:

- Cervical motion tenderness
- Uterine tenderness
- Adnexal tenderness

One or more of the following **additional criteria** can be used to enhance the specificity of the minimum clinical criteria and support a diagnosis of PID:

- Oral temperature >38.3 °C (>101 °F);
- Abnormal cervical mucopurulent discharge or cervical friability
- Presence of abundant numbers of WBCs on saline microscopy of vaginal fluid
- Elevated erythrocyte sedimentation rate
- Elevated C-reactive protein level
- Laboratory documentation of cervical infection with *Neisseria gonorrhoeae* or *Chlamydia trachomatis*

Most women with PID have either mucopurulent cervical discharge or evidence of WBCs on a microscopic evaluation of a saline preparation of vaginal fluid (ie, wet mount). If the cervical discharge appears normal and no WBCs are observed on the wet mount of vaginal fluid, the diagnosis of PID is unlikely, and alternative causes of pain should be considered. A wet mount of vaginal fluid can also detect the presence of concomitant infections (eg, bacterial vaginosis and trichomoniasis).

PID indicates pelvic inflammatory disease; STI, sexually transmitted infection; and WBC, white blood cell.

[a] Adapted from Workowski KA, Bachmann LH, Chan PA, et al. Sexually transmitted infections treatment guidelines, 2021. *MMWR Recomm Rep.* 2021;70(4):1–187.

resonance imaging techniques showing thickened, fluid-filled tubes with or without free pelvic fluid or tubo-ovarian complex, or Doppler ultrasonography suggesting pelvic infection (eg, tubal hyperemia); or laparoscopic findings consistent with PID. A diagnostic evaluation that includes some of these more extensive procedures might be warranted in some cases. Endometrial biopsy is warranted in women who are undergoing laparoscopy and do not have visual evidence of salpingitis, because endometritis is the only sign of PID for some women.

In addition to determining whether WBCs are present in cervicovaginal secretions, a wet mount assists in the diagnosis or exclusion of the commonly associated trichomonas or bacterial vaginosis. Serological testing for HIV and syphilis should also be performed.

TREATMENT

A sexually active adolescent or young adult female who has lower abdominal pain and exhibits uterine, adnexal, or cervical motion tenderness on bimanual examination should be treated for PID if no other cause is identified. To minimize risks of progressive infection and subsequent infertility, treatment should be initiated at the time of clinical diagnosis, and therapy should be completed, regardless of the STI test results.

Among females with mild to moderate PID, there is no difference in clinical course, recurrent PID, chronic pelvic pain, or infertility rates between females hospitalized and those treated on an outpatient basis for PID. The decision to hospitalize adolescent or young adult females with acute PID should be based on the professional's judgment and whether the patient meets any of the following suggested criteria:

- Surgical emergencies (eg, appendicitis) cannot be excluded.
- Tubo-ovarian abscess.
- Pregnancy.
- Severe illness, nausea and vomiting, or high fever.
- Inability to follow or tolerate an outpatient oral regimen.
- No clinical response to oral antimicrobial therapy.

Whether the patient is treated on an inpatient or outpatient basis, the antimicrobial regimen chosen should provide empirical, broad-spectrum coverage directed against the most common causative agents, including *N gonorrhoeae* and *C trachomatis*, even if these pathogens are not identified in lower genital tract specimens. If the *N gonorrhoeae* culture is positive, antimicrobial susceptibility testing should guide subsequent therapy. If the isolate is determined to be quinolone-resistant *N gonorrhoeae* or if antimicrobial susceptibility cannot be assessed (eg, if only NAAT testing is available), consultation with an infectious disease specialist is recommended.

Parenteral regimens are recommended by the CDC for the treatment of patients in the hospital, and intramuscular/oral regimens are recommended for the treatment of patients in the outpatient setting. For women hospitalized and treated initially with parenteral therapy, transition to oral therapy can usually be initiated within 24 to 48 hours of clinical improvement. For women with tubo-ovarian abscesses, at least 24 hours of inpatient observation is recommended.

Intramuscular/oral therapy can be considered for women with mild to moderately severe acute PID who can be treated in the outpatient setting from the outset, because the clinical outcomes of women treated with these regimens are similar to those treated with intravenous therapy. Women who do not respond to intramuscular/oral therapy within 72 hours should be reevaluated to confirm the diagnosis and be administered intravenous therapy. Women should demonstrate clinical improvement (eg, defervescence; reduction in direct or rebound abdominal tenderness; and reduction in uterine, adnexal, cervical motion tenderness) within 3 days after initiation of therapy. If no clinical improvement has occurred within 72 hours after outpatient intramuscular/oral therapy, then hospitalization, assessment of the antimicrobial regimen, and additional diagnostics (including consideration of diagnostic laparoscopy for alternative diagnoses) are recommended.

If an adolescent or young woman with an intrauterine device (IUD) receives a diagnosis of PID, the IUD does not need to be removed. However, the patient should undergo close clinical follow-up, and if there is no clinical improvement 48 to 72 hours after treatment initiation, removal of the IUD may be considered.

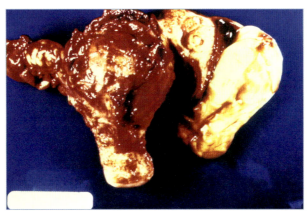

Image 106.1
A uterus and ovary that had been excised, because of the presence of an ovarian abscess in a case of pelvic inflammatory disease, which had been caused by an undisclosed anaerobic bacterium. Courtesy of Centers for Disease Control and Prevention.

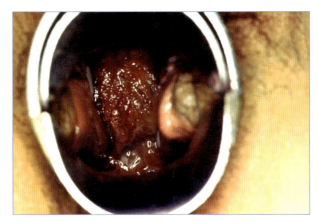

Image 106.2
A colposcopic view of a female patient's cervix, which had manifested signs of erosion and erythema, because of a *Chlamydia trachomatis* infection. If left untreated, chlamydial infection can cause severe, costly reproductive and other health problems. Both short- and long-term consequences can ensue, including pelvic inflammatory disease, infertility, and potentially fatal tubal ectopic pregnancies. Courtesy of Centers for Disease Control and Prevention.

CHAPTER 107

Pertussis
(Whooping Cough)

CLINICAL MANIFESTATIONS

Pertussis begins with mild upper respiratory tract symptoms similar to those of the common cold (catarrhal stage) and progresses to cough, usually paroxysms of cough (paroxysmal stage), characterized by inspiratory whoop (gasping) after repeated cough on the same breath, which is commonly followed by vomiting. Fever is absent or minimal. Symptoms wane gradually over weeks to months (convalescent stage). Cough illness in immunized children and adults can range from typical to very mild. The duration of classic pertussis is 6 to 10 weeks. Complications in adolescents and adults include syncope, weight loss, sleep disturbance, incontinence, rib fractures, and pneumonia; in adults, complications may increase with age. Pertussis is most severe when it occurs during the first 6 months after birth, particularly in preterm and unimmunized infants. Disease in infants younger than 6 months can be atypical with a short catarrhal stage, followed by gagging, gasping, bradycardia, or apnea as prominent early manifestations; absence of whoop; and prolonged convalescence. Sudden unexpected death can be caused by pertussis. Complications in infants include pneumonia, pulmonary hypertension, and severe coughing spells with associated conjunctival bleeding, hernia, and hypoxia. Seizures (0.9%), encephalopathy (<0.5%), apnea, and death can occur in infants with pertussis. Approximately half of infants with pertussis in the United States are hospitalized. Case-fatality rates are approximately 1.6% in infants younger than 2 months and less than 1.2% in infants 2 through 11 months of age. Maternal immunization during pregnancy and infant receipt of at least some doses of pertussis vaccine reduce morbidity and mortality in young infants.

ETIOLOGY

Pertussis is caused by a fastidious, gram-negative, pleomorphic bacillus, *Bordetella pertussis*. Other *Bordetella* species can cause sporadic prolonged cough illness in people, including *Bordetella parapertussis*, *Bordetella bronchiseptica* (the cause of canine kennel cough), and *Bordetella holmesii*.

EPIDEMIOLOGY

Humans are the only known hosts of *B pertussis*. Transmission occurs by close contact with infected individuals via large respiratory droplets generated by coughing or sneezing. Cases occur year round, typically with a late summer–autumn peak. Neither infection nor immunization provides lifelong immunity. Waning immunity, particularly when acellular pertussis vaccine is used for the entire immunization series, is predominantly responsible for increased cases reported in school-aged children, adolescents, and adults. Additionally, waning maternal immunity of mothers who have not received Tdap vaccine during that pregnancy results in low concentrations of transplacentally transmitted antibody and an increased risk of pertussis in very young infants. Pertussis incidence is cyclic and in the United States has increased between 2000 and 2016. Pertussis is highly contagious. As many as 80% of susceptible household contacts of symptomatic infant cases are infected with *B pertussis*, with symptoms in these contacts varying from mild to classic pertussis. Siblings and adults with cough illness are important sources of pertussis infection in young infants. Infected people are most contagious during the catarrhal stage through the third week after onset of paroxysms or until 5 days after the start of effective antimicrobial treatment. Factors affecting the length of communicability include age, immunization status or previous infection, and receipt of appropriate antimicrobial therapy.

The **incubation period** is 7 to 10 days, with a range of 5 to 21 days.

DIAGNOSTIC TESTS

Culture was previously considered the gold standard for laboratory diagnosis of pertussis but is not optimally sensitive and has largely been replaced by nucleic acid amplification tests (NAATs). Culture requires collection of an appropriate nasopharyngeal swab specimen, obtained either by aspiration or with polyester or flocked rayon swabs or calcium alginate swabs. Specimens must not be allowed to dry during prompt transport to the laboratory. Culture results can be negative if taken from a previously immunized person, if antimicrobial therapy has been started, if more than 2 weeks has elapsed since cough onset, or if the specimen is not collected or handled appropriately.

NAATs cleared by the US Food and Drug Administration, including polymerase chain reaction (PCR) assays, are commercially available as stand-alone tests or as multiplex assays and are the most commonly used laboratory method for detection of *B pertussis* because of greater sensitivity and more rapid turnaround time. The PCR test requires collection of an adequate nasopharyngeal specimen by using a Dacron swab or nasopharyngeal wash or aspirate. Calcium alginate swabs can be inhibitory to PCR and should not be used. The PCR test has optimal sensitivity during the first 3 weeks of cough and is unlikely to be useful if antimicrobial therapy has been given for more than 5 days. Most PCR assays target only a multicopy insertion gene sequence (IS 481) found in *B pertussis* as well as the less commonly encountered *B holmesii* and some strains of *B bronchiseptica*. Multiple DNA target sequences are required to distinguish among clinically relevant *Bordetella* species.

Serological tests for pertussis infection may be helpful for diagnosis, especially late in illness. In the absence of recent immunization, an elevated serum immunoglobulin G (IgG) antibody to pertussis toxin (PT) present 2 to 8 weeks after onset of cough suggests recent *B pertussis* infection. For single serum specimens, an IgG anti-PT value of approximately 100 IU/mL or greater (by using standard reference sera as a comparator) has been recommended. Positive paired serological results based on the World Health Organization pertussis case definition may also be considered diagnostic. immunoglobulin A and immunoglobulin M assays lack adequate sensitivity and specificity and should not be used for the diagnosis of pertussis. Direct fluorescent antibody testing is not recommended.

An increased white blood cell (WBC) count attributable to absolute lymphocytosis is suggestive of pertussis in infants and young children but is often absent in older people with pertussis and may be only mildly abnormal in some infants. A markedly elevated WBC count is associated with a poor prognosis in young infants.

TREATMENT

Antimicrobial therapy administered during the catarrhal stage may ameliorate the disease. Antimicrobial therapy is indicated before test results are received if the clinical history strongly suggests pertussis or the patient has high risk for severe or complicated disease (eg, is an infant). A 5-day course of azithromycin is the appropriate first-line choice for treatment and for postexposure prophylaxis (Table 107.1). After the paroxysmal cough is established, antimicrobial agents have no discernible effect on the course of illness but are recommended to limit spread of organisms to others. Resistance of *B pertussis* to macrolide antimicrobial agents has been reported but rarely in the United States. Penicillins and first- and second-generation cephalosporins are ineffective against *B pertussis*.

Orally administered erythromycin and, to a lesser degree, azithromycin, when given in the first 6 weeks after birth, are associated with increased risk of infantile hypertrophic pyloric stenosis, but azithromycin remains the drug of choice for treatment or prophylaxis of pertussis in very young infants.

Trimethoprim-sulfamethoxazole (TMP-SMX) is an alternative for patients older than 2 months who cannot tolerate macrolides or who are infected with a macrolide-resistant strain, but studies evaluating TMP-SMX as treatment of pertussis are limited.

Young infants have increased risk for respiratory failure attributable to apnea or secondary bacterial pneumonia and have risk for cardiopulmonary failure and death from severe pulmonary hypertension. Illness characteristics that suggest the need for hospitalization of infants with pertussis include respiratory distress, inability to feed, cyanosis or apnea, and seizures. Some experts believe that age younger than 4 months is itself an indication for hospitalization of infants with pertussis or suspected pertussis infection. Hospitalized young infants with pertussis should be treated in a setting/facility where these complications can be recognized and managed urgently. Exchange transfusions or leukopheresis has been reported to be lifesaving in infants with progressive pulmonary hypertension and markedly elevated lymphocyte counts.

Because data on the clinical effectiveness of antibiotic treatment on *B parapertussis* are limited, treatment decisions should be based on clinical judgment, with particular attention toward special populations that may have increased risk for severe *B parapertussis* disease, including infants, elderly people, and immunocompromised people. Limited available data suggest that *B parapertussis* is less susceptible to antimicrobial agents than *B pertussis*, although some studies indicate that macrolides, TMP-SMX, and ciprofloxacin generally have activity against *B parapertussis*. *B bronchiseptica* has intrinsic resistance to macrolide antibiotics.

Table 107.1
Recommended Antimicrobial Therapy and Postexposure Prophylaxis for Pertussis in Infants, Children, Adolescents, and Adults[a]

Age	Recommended Drugs			Alternative
	Azithromycin	Erythromycin	Clarithromycin	TMP-SMX
<1 month	10 mg/kg/day as a single dose daily for 5 days[b,c]	40 mg/kg/day in 4 divided doses for 14 days	Not recommended	Contraindicated at <2 months
1–5 months	10 mg/kg/day as a single dose daily for 5 days[b]	40 mg/kg/day in 4 divided doses for 14 days	15 mg/kg/day in 2 divided doses for 7 days	≥2 months: TMP, 8 mg/kg/day; SMX, 40 mg/kg/day in 2 doses for 14 days
≥6 months and children	10 mg/kg as a single dose on day 1 (maximum 500 mg), then 5 mg/kg/day as a single dose on days 2–5 (maximum 250 mg/day)[b,d]	40 mg/kg/day in 4 divided doses for 7–14 days (maximum 2 g/day)	15 mg/kg/day in 2 divided doses for 7 days (maximum 1 g/day)	≥2 months: TMP, 8 mg/kg/day; SMX, 40 mg/kg/day in 2 doses for 14 days
Adolescents and adults	500 mg as a single dose on day 1, then 250 mg as a single dose on days 2–5[b,d]	2 g/day in 4 divided doses for 7–14 days	1 g/day in 2 divided doses for 7 days	TMP, 320 mg/day; SMX, 1,600 mg/day in 2 divided doses for 14 days

SMX indicates sulfamethoxazole; TMP, trimethoprim.
[a] Centers for Disease Control and Prevention. Recommended antimicrobial agents for the treatment and postexposure prophylaxis of pertussis: 2005 CDC guidelines. *MMWR Recomm Rep.* 2005;54(RR-14):1–16.
[b] Azithromycin should be used with caution in people with prolonged QT interval and certain proarrhythmic conditions.
[c] Preferred macrolide for this age because of risk of idiopathic hypertrophic pyloric stenosis associated with erythromycin.
[d] A 3-day course of azithromycin for postexposure prophylaxis or treatment has not been validated and is not recommended.

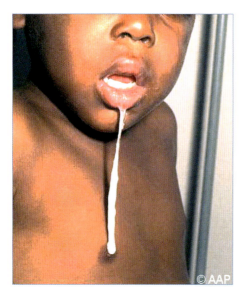

Image 107.1
A preschool-aged boy with pertussis. Thick respiratory secretions were produced by a paroxysmal coughing spell. Courtesy of Edgar O. Ledbetter, MD, FAAP.

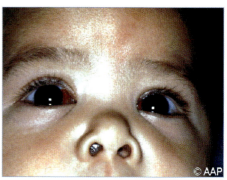

Image 107.2
Bilateral subconjunctival hemorrhages and thick nasal mucus in an infant with pertussis.

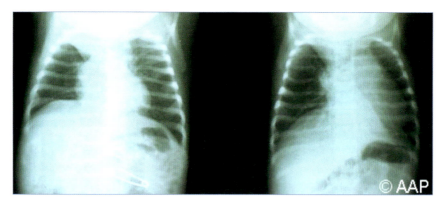

Image 107.3
A 4-week-old with pertussis pneumonia with pulmonary air trapping and progressive atelectasis confirmed at autopsy. The neonate acquired the infection from the mother shortly after birth. Segmented and lobar atelectasis are not uncommon complications of pertussis.

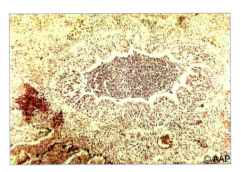

Image 107.4
Bronchiolar plugging in the neonate in Image 107.3, who died of pertussis pneumonia. Neonates, infants, and children often acquire pertussis from an infected adult or sibling contact.

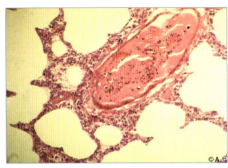

Image 107.5
Plugging and alveolar dilatation of pertussis pneumonia in an infant who died. Courtesy of Edgar O. Ledbetter, MD, FAAP.

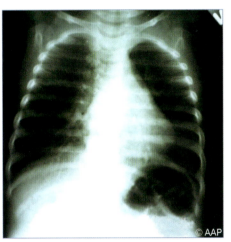

Image 107.6
Pertussis pneumonia with hyperaeration (air trapping) caused by inability to cough out thick pulmonary secretions.

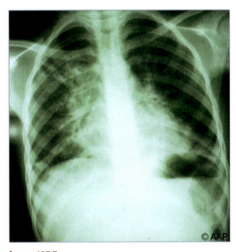

Image 107.7
Pertussis pneumonia in a 7-year-old who was exhausted from persistent coughing. Obliteration of cardiac borders on the chest radiograph is a common radiographic change of pertussis pneumonia.

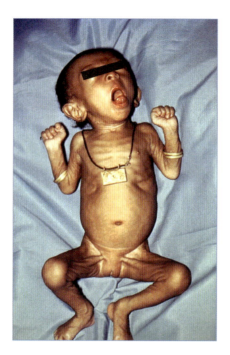

Image 107.8
This image depicts an infant girl who presented to a clinic with malnutrition as well as what was diagnosed as pertussis. Pertussis is a highly communicable, vaccine-preventable disease caused by *Bordetella pertussis*, a gram-negative coccobacillus, that lasts for many weeks and typically affects children with severe coughing, whooping, and posttussive vomiting. Courtesy of Centers for Disease Control and Prevention.

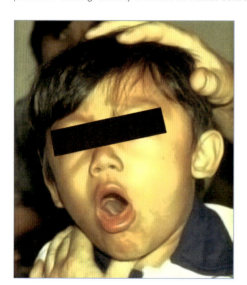

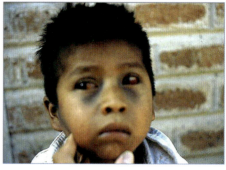

Image 107.10
This child has broken blood vessels in his eyes and bruising on his face because of coughing from pertussis. Courtesy of Thomas Schlenker, MD, MPH, chief medical officer, Children's Hospital of Wisconsin.

Image 107.9
This child has pertussis (whooping cough). He has severe coughing spasms, which are often followed by a whooping sound. It is difficult for him to stop coughing and catch his breath. Courtesy of Centers for Disease Control and Prevention.

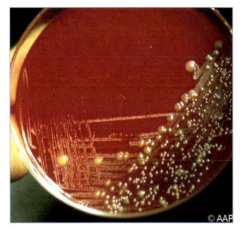

Image 107.11
Colonies of *Bordetella pertussis* growing on Bordet-Gengou media. Courtesy of Edgar O. Ledbetter, MD, FAAP.

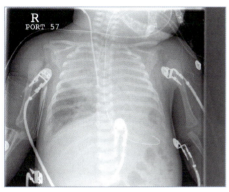

Image 107.12
Pertussis pneumonia in a 2-month-old 2 days after hospital admission. His mother had been coughing since shortly after delivery. Courtesy of Carol J. Baker, MD, FAAP.

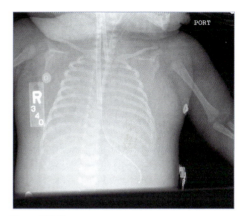

Image 107.13
The infant in Image 107.12 required mechanical ventilation because of respiratory failure. Courtesy of Carol J. Baker, MD, FAAP.

CHAPTER 108
Pinworm Infection
(Enterobius vermicularis)

CLINICAL MANIFESTATIONS

Pinworm infection (enterobiasis) is commonly asymptomatic but may cause pruritus ani and, rarely, pruritus vulvae. Pruritus ani can be severe enough to cause sleep disturbance. Bacterial superinfections can result from scratching and excoriation of the irritated area. Pinworms have been found in the lumen of the appendix, and in some cases, these intraluminal parasites have been associated with signs of acute appendicitis, but they have also been observed in histologically normal appendices removed for incidental reasons. Urethritis, vaginitis, salpingitis, or pelvic peritonitis may occur from aberrant migration of an adult worm from the perineum. Eosinophilic enterocolitis has been reported, although peripheral eosinophilia is generally not found.

ETIOLOGY

Enterobius vermicularis is a nematode or roundworm.

EPIDEMIOLOGY

Enterobiasis occurs worldwide and commonly clusters within families. Prevalence rates are higher among preschool and school-aged children, among primary caregivers of infected children, and in institutions. An estimated 40 million people in the United States have been infected with pinworms, with a prevalence of 20% to 30% among some age-groups and communities.

Initial infection occurs by ingestion of contaminated food or by contact with hands, clothing, bedding, or other items contaminated with eggs. Alternative modes of transmission include person-to-person or sexual transmission. Eggs hatch and release larvae in the small intestine, and adult worms then usually locate themselves in the cecum, appendix, and ascending colon. Adult males die soon after copulating. Gravid females migrate, usually at night while the host is resting, to the perianal area to deposit eggs containing larvae, which mature in 6 to 8 hours. Females have an overall life span of up to 100 days. Adult females and eggs may induce intense perianal pruritus, leading to an autoinfection cycle during which the area is scratched and the eggs are lodged on the hands and under the fingernails and are ingested when the hands are put into the mouth. A person remains infectious as long as female nematodes are discharging eggs on perianal skin. Eggs may remain infective in an indoor environment for up to 2 weeks. Humans are the only known natural hosts. Pets are not reservoirs of infection.

The **incubation period** from ingestion of an egg until an adult gravid female migrates to the perianal region is 2 to 6 weeks or longer.

DIAGNOSTIC TESTS

Diagnosis is established via the classic cellulose tape test ("Scotch tape test") or with a commercially available pinworm paddle test, which is a clear plastic paddle coated with an adhesive surface on one side that is pressed on both sides of the perianal region during the night or at the time of waking and before bathing. The tape or paddle is then pressed on a slide, and eggs can be visualized by microscopy. Eggs are 50 to 60 × 20 to 30 μm and flattened on one side, giving them a bean-shaped appearance. Testing on 3 different days will increase the sensitivity from approximately 50% for a single test to approximately 90%. Adult females, which are white and measure 8 to 13 mm, can also be found in the perineal region. Stool examination is unhelpful, because worms or eggs are found infrequently in the stool. Neither peripheral eosinophilia nor elevated immunoglobulin E concentrations are typical.

TREATMENT

Several drugs will treat pinworms including over-the-counter pyrantel pamoate and prescription mebendazole and albendazole. Mebendazole and albendazole are significantly more costly than pyrantel pamoate in the United States. Each medication is recommended to be given in a single dose and repeated in 2 weeks, because these drugs are not completely effective against the egg or developing larvae stages. Ivermectin has been evaluated and is partially effective; the safety of ivermectin in children weighing less than 15 kg and in pregnant women has not been established. Because reinfection is common even when effective therapy is given, treatment of the entire household as a group should be considered. Repeated infections should be treated by the same method as the first infection. Vaginitis is self-limited and does not require separate treatment. "Pulse" treatment with a single dose of mebendazole every 14 days for 16 weeks has been used in refractory cases with multiple recurrences. Alternative diagnoses in cases being attributed to recurrent pinworm infections can include *Dipylidium caninum*, which is diagnosed by stool ova and parasite analysis and treated with praziquantel as well as delusional parasitosis.

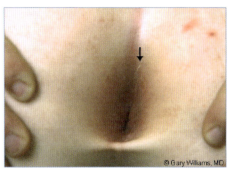

Image 108.1
Adult pinworm (*Enterobius vermicularis*; arrow) in the perianal area of a 14-year-old boy. Perianal inspection 2–3 hours after the child goes to sleep may reveal pinworms that have migrated outside the intestinal tract. Copyright Gary Williams, MD.

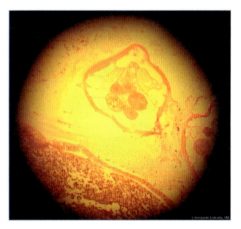

Image 108.2
Enterobius vermicularis in the lumen of the appendix of a 10-year-old. Pinworms can be found in the lumen of the appendix, but most evidence indicates that they do not cause acute appendicitis. Courtesy of Benjamin Estrada, MD.

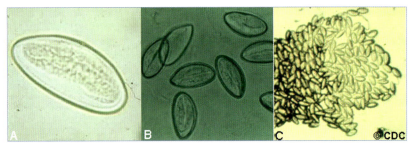

Image 108.3
A and B, Enterobius egg(s). C, Enterobius eggs on cellulose tape preparation. Courtesy of Centers for Disease Control and Prevention.

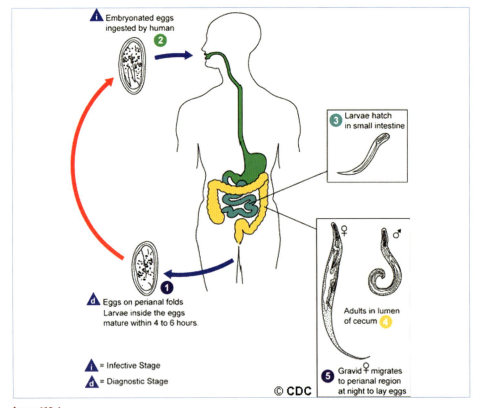

Image 108.4
Eggs are deposited on perianal folds (1). Self-infection occurs by transferring infective eggs to the mouth with hands that have scratched the perianal area (2). Person-to-person transmission can also occur through handling of contaminated clothes or bed linens. Enterobiasis may also be acquired through surfaces in the environment that are contaminated with pinworm eggs (eg, curtains, carpeting). Some small number of eggs may become airborne and inhaled. These could be swallowed and follow the same development as ingested eggs. Following ingestion of infective eggs, the larvae hatch in the small intestine (3) and the adults establish themselves in the colon (4). The time interval from ingestion of infective eggs to oviposition by the adult females is about 1 month. The life span of the adults is about 2 months. Gravid females migrate nocturnally outside the anus and oviposit while crawling on the skin of the perianal area (5). The larvae contained inside the eggs develop (the eggs become infective) in 4–6 hours under optimal conditions (1). Retroinfection, or the migration of newly hatched larvae from the anal skin back into the rectum, may occur, but the frequency with which this happens is unknown. Courtesy of Centers for Disease Control and Prevention.

CHAPTER 109
Pityriasis Versicolor
(Formerly Tinea Versicolor)

CLINICAL MANIFESTATIONS

Pityriasis versicolor (formerly tinea versicolor) is a common and benign superficial infection of the skin, classically manifesting on the upper trunk and neck. Most patients are asymptomatic, although some may experience pruritus. In infants and children, the infection is likely to involve the face, particularly the temples. Infection can include other areas, including the scalp, genital area, and thighs. Symmetrical involvement with ovoid discrete or coalescent lesions of varying size is typical; these macules or patches vary in color, even in the same person. White, pink, tan, or brown coloration is often surmounted by faint, dusty scales. Lesions fail to tan during the summer and are relatively darker than the surrounding skin during the winter, hence the term *versicolor*. The differential diagnosis includes pityriasis alba, vitiligo, seborrheic dermatitis, pityriasis rosea, pityriasis lichenoides, progressive macular hypopigmentation, and dyschromatosis universalis hereditaria. Folliculitis can also occur, particularly in immunocompromised patients. Invasive infections can occur in neonates, particularly those receiving total parenteral nutrition with lipids.

ETIOLOGY

The cause of pityriasis versicolor is a number of species of the *Malassezia furfur* complex, a group of lipid-dependent yeasts that exist on healthy skin in yeast phase and cause clinical lesions only when substantial growth of hyphae occurs. Moisture, heat, and the presence of lipid-containing sebaceous secretions encourage rapid overgrowth of hyphae.

EPIDEMIOLOGY

Pityriasis versicolor can occur in any climate or age-group but tends to favor adolescents and young adults. Living in hot and humid climates, sweating excessively, or having a weakened immune system allows the fungus to flourish. Pityriasis versicolor is not contagious.

The **incubation period** is unknown.

DIAGNOSTIC TESTS

The presence of symmetrically distributed faintly scaling macules and patches of varying color concentrated on the upper back and chest is close to diagnostic. The "evoked scale" sign is when the clinician uses their thumb and forefinger to stretch the skin, eliciting a visible white patch of scale overlying the affected area, which is still visible when the affected area is released. Another technique to evoke scales is scraping the involved skin with a scalpel blade or glass microscope slide, again yielding a pale and fuzzy scale that is confined to the lesion. Involved areas fluoresce yellow-green under Wood lamp evaluation. Potassium hydroxide wet mount of scraped scales reveals the classic "spaghetti and meatballs" short hyphae and clusters of yeast forms. Because this yeast is a common inhabitant of the skin, fungal culture from the skin surface is nondiagnostic. To grow the fungus in the laboratory, samples from pustules (if folliculitis is present) or sterile sites should be placed into media enriched with olive oil or another long-chain fatty acid.

TREATMENT

Multiple topical and systemic agents are efficacious, and recommendations vary substantially. For uncomplicated cases, most experts recommend initiating therapy with topical agents. The most cost-effective treatments are selenium sulfide shampoo/lotion and clotrimazole cream. Selenium sulfide shampoo is used for 3 to 7 days; application is once daily for 5 to 10 minutes, followed by rinsing. Topical azole therapy (eg, clotrimazole cream) is applied twice daily for 2 to 3 weeks. Adherence with these agents may be low because of unpleasant adverse effects (the shampoo has a sulfur-like odor) or duration and anatomical extent of required therapy. Other effective topical agents include ketoconazole, ciclopirox, econazole, oxiconazole, and off-label bifonazole, miconazole, econazole, oxiconazole, clotrimazole, terbinafine, and ciclopirox, as well as zinc pyrithione shampoo. Shampoos are easier to disperse, particularly on wet skin, than topical creams and may increase adherence. Treatment response is measured by resolution of scale and/or disappearance of spaghetti and meatball microscopic findings. Restoration of normal pigmentation may take months after successful treatment.

Recurrence following discontinuation of therapy may approach 60% to 80%, and preventive treatments are sometimes used to decrease recurrences. Off-label regimens to decrease recurrence include use of the aforementioned shampoos/lotions weekly or monthly.

Systemic therapy is reserved for resistant infection or extensive involvement. Medications, including fluconazole, itraconazole, and pramiconazole, are not approved by the US Food and Drug Administration for pityriasis versicolor. Fluconazole (preferred) can be administered at 300 mg weekly for 2 to 4 weeks, or itraconazole can be administered at 200 mg daily for 1 week. Although oral agents may be easier to use than topical agents, they are not necessarily more effective and have possible serious adverse effects. Drug interactions can occur when using oral drugs, and monitoring for liver toxicity must be considered for patients receiving systemic therapy, particularly if they receive multiple courses. In several studies, topical therapy has appeared to be equivalent or superior to systemic therapy.

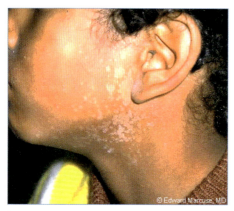

Image 109.1
Pityriasis versicolor.

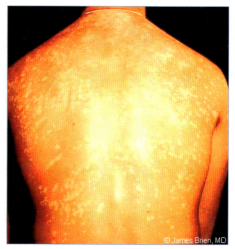

Image 109.2
Pityriasis versicolor of the posterior surface of the neck and trunk. Courtesy of James Brien.

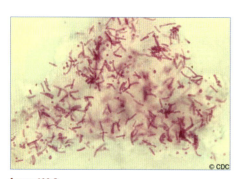

Image 109.3
This photomicrograph of a skin scale reveals the presence of the fungus *Malassezia furfur*. Usually *M furfur* grows sparsely without causing a rash. In some individuals, it grows more actively for reasons unknown, resulting in pale brown, flaky patches on the trunk, neck, or arms, a condition called *pityriasis versicolor* (formerly called *tinea versicolor*).

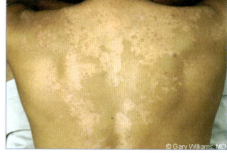

Image 109.4
Pityriasis versicolor in a 16-year-old boy. Copyright Gary Williams, MD.

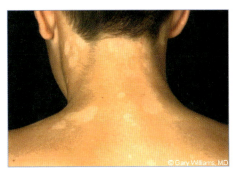

Image 109.5
Pityriasis versicolor in a 14-year-old boy. Copyright Gary Williams, MD.

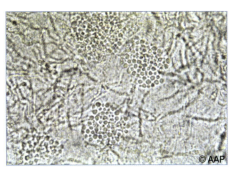

Image 109.6
The spores and pseudohyphae of *Malassezia furfur* (a yeast that can cause pityriasis versicolor) resemble spaghetti and meatballs on a potassium hydroxide slide.

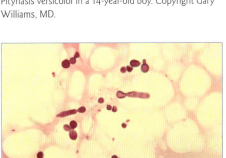

Image 109.7
Note the yeast-like fungal cells and short hyphae of *Malassezia furfur* in skin scale from a patient with pityriasis versicolor. Usually, *M furfur* grows sparsely without causing a rash. In some individuals, it grows more actively for reasons unknown, resulting in pale brown, flaky patches on the trunk, neck, or arms, a condition called *pityriasis versicolor* (formerly called *tinea versicolor*). Courtesy of Centers for Disease Control and Prevention.

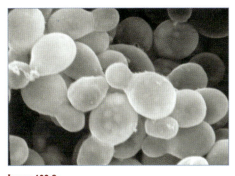

Image 109.8
Scanning electron micrograph of *Malassezia furfur*. Courtesy of Centers for Disease Control and Prevention.

CHAPTER 110

Plague

CLINICAL MANIFESTATIONS

Naturally acquired plague most commonly manifests in the primary **bubonic form,** with fever and a painful swollen regional lymph node (bubo). Buboes develop most commonly in the inguinal region but also occur in axillary or cervical areas. Plague manifests less commonly in the primary **septicemic form** without localizing signs (fever, hypotension, purpuric skin lesions, intravascular coagulopathy, and organ failure) or as primary **pneumonic plague** (cough, fever, dyspnea, and hemoptysis) and rarely as **meningitic, pharyngeal, cutaneous, ocular,** or **gastrointestinal plague.** Occasionally, patients have symptoms of mild lymphadenitis or prominent gastrointestinal tract symptoms, which may obscure the correct diagnosis. Secondary septicemic, pneumonic, or other forms of plague can occur via hematogenous dissemination of bacteria. Untreated, plague often progresses to overwhelming sepsis and death. Plague has been referred to as the *black death* because of the tissue necrosis that it induces.

ETIOLOGY

Plague is caused by *Yersinia pestis,* a pleomorphic, bipolar-staining (with Giemsa, Wright, and Wayson stains), facultative intracellular gram-negative coccobacillus. *Y pestis* is a member of the *Enterobacteriaceae* family, along with more common *Yersinia* species and other enteric bacteria.

EPIDEMIOLOGY

Plague is a zoonotic infection primarily maintained in rodents and their fleas. Humans are incidental hosts who develop bubonic or primary septicemic manifestations, typically through the bite of infected rodent fleas or through direct contact with tissues of infected animals. Primary pneumonic plague is acquired by inhalation of respiratory tract droplets from a human or animal with pneumonic plague. Only the pneumonic form has been shown to be transmitted from person to person. Plague occurs worldwide with enzootic foci in parts of Asia, Africa, and the Americas. Most human plague cases are reported from rural, underdeveloped areas and mainly occur as isolated cases or in small focal clusters. In the United States, plague is endemic in western states, with most cases reported from New Mexico, Colorado, Arizona, and California. Cases of plague in states without endemic plague have been identified in travelers returning from these states.

Y pestis has also been identified as a potential bioterrorism agent, through widespread dispersal of an aerosolized form. Such an event would have potential for a large number of pneumonic plague cases.

The **incubation period** is 2 to 8 days for bubonic plague and 1 to 6 days for primary pneumonic plague.

DIAGNOSTIC TESTS

Diagnosis of plague is usually confirmed by culture of *Y pestis* from blood, bubo aspirate, sputum, or another clinical specimen. The organism is slow growing but not fastidious and can be isolated on sheep blood and chocolate agars with typical "fried egg" colonies appearing after 48 to 72 hours of incubation. *Y pestis* has a bipolar (safety-pin) appearance when stained with Wright-Giemsa or Wayson stain. A positive direct fluorescent antibody test result for the presence of *Y pestis* in direct smears or cultures of blood, bubo aspirate, sputum, or another clinical specimen provides presumptive evidence of *Y pestis* infection. Automated, commercially available biochemical identification systems are not recommended, because they can misidentify *Y pestis.* Polymerase chain reaction assay and immunohistochemical staining for rapid diagnosis of *Y pestis* are available in some reference or public health laboratories.

A single positive serological test result from a passive hemagglutination assay or enzyme immunoassay provides presumptive evidence of infection. Seroconversion, defined as a 4-fold increase in antibody titer between serum specimens obtained 4 to 6 weeks apart, also confirms the diagnosis of plague.

TREATMENT

After diagnostic specimens are obtained, appropriate antibiotic therapy should be started immediately for any patient suspected of having plague. Pediatric treatment recommendations are as follows:

- For naturally acquired primary bubonic or pharyngeal plague without signs of secondary pneumonic or septicemic plague and for early/mild primary pneumonic or septicemic plague, monotherapy with gentamicin, streptomycin, ciprofloxacin, or levofloxacin is recommended.
- Doxycycline is also a first-line option for treatment of naturally acquired bubonic or pharyngeal plague but is second-line therapy for naturally acquired pneumonic plague.
- Dual therapy with 2 distinct antimicrobial classes is recommended for initial treatment of patients with naturally acquired primary bubonic disease with large buboes or with naturally acquired moderate-severe septicemic or pneumonic plague. The recommended drugs are those listed in the first bulleted item.
- For naturally acquired plague meningitis, chloramphenicol should be added to the patient's existing treatment regimen. If chloramphenicol is unavailable, moxifloxacin or levofloxacin should be added to the treatment regimen.
- For bioterrorism-related plague, dual therapy with 2 distinct classes of antimicrobials should be used for all patients until sensitivity patterns are known.

Neonates of pregnant women with plague at or around the time of delivery should be treated if they are symptomatic, by using the antibiotic selections in the first 3 bulleted items. If the neonate is asymptomatic but the mother is untreated or has only recently begun treatment, the neonate should receive antimicrobial prophylaxis, with the same antibiotic choices. If the neonate is asymptomatic and the mother has been sufficiently treated and is improving, observation of the neonate is acceptable.

The duration of antimicrobial treatment is 10 to 14 days; treatment duration can be extended for patients with ongoing fever or other concerning signs or symptoms. Drainage of abscessed buboes may be necessary; drainage material is considered infectious.

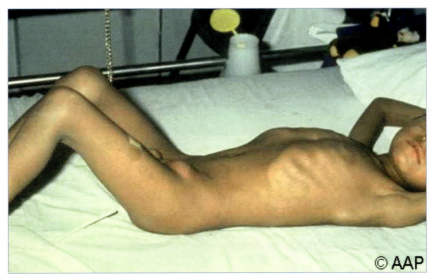

Image 110.1
Inguinal plague buboes in an 8-year-old boy. If left untreated, bubonic plague often becomes septicemic, with meningitis occurring in 6% of cases.

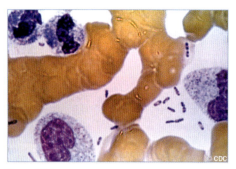

Image 110.2
Dark-stained bipolar ends of *Yersinia pestis* can clearly be observed in this Wright stain of blood from an individual with plague. The actual cause of the disease is the plague bacillus, *Y pestis*. It is a nonmotile, nonspore-forming, gram-negative, nonlactose-fermenting, bipolar, ovoid, safety-pin–shaped bacterium. Courtesy of Centers for Disease Control and Prevention.

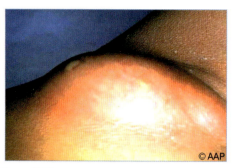

Image 110.3
Close-up view of inguinal buboes of the patient in Image 110.1. Surgical excision of infected lymph nodes without appropriate antimicrobial treatment may result in septicemic plague. When left untreated, plague often progresses to overwhelming sepsis and death.

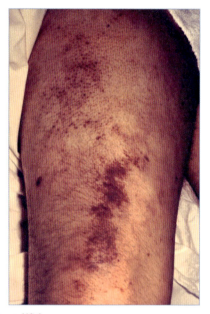

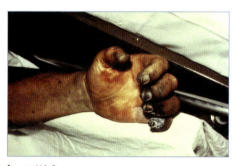

Image 110.5
This patient presented with symptoms of plague that included gangrene of the right hand, causing necrosis of the fingers. Courtesy of Centers for Disease Control and Prevention.

Image 110.4
This patient acquired a plague infection through abrasions on his upper right leg. Bubonic plague is transmitted through the bite of an infected flea or, as in this case, exposure to inoculated material through a break in the skin. Symptoms include swollen, tender lymph glands known as buboes. Courtesy of Centers for Disease Control and Prevention.

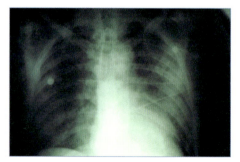

Image 110.6
This anteroposterior radiograph demonstrates bilaterally progressive plague infection involving both lung fields. The first signs of plague are fever, headache, weakness, and rapidly developing pneumonia with shortness of breath, chest pain, cough, and, sometimes, bloody or watery sputum, eventually progressing for 2–4 days into respiratory failure and shock. Courtesy of Centers for Disease Control and Prevention.

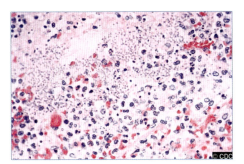

Image 110.7
Photomicrograph of lung tissue (Giemsa stain) from a patient with fatal human plague, revealing pneumonia and an abundance of *Yersinia pestis* organisms. Courtesy of Centers for Disease Control and Prevention.

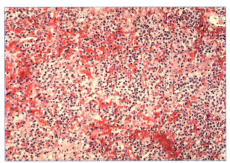

Image 110.8
Histopathologic features of lung in fatal human plague. Area of marked fibrinopurulent pneumonia. Courtesy of Centers for Disease Control and Prevention.

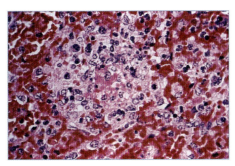

Image 110.9
This photomicrograph depicts the histopathologic changes in splenic tissue in a case of fatal human plague (hematoxylin-eosin stain, magnification ×400). Note the presence of general arteriolar inflammation, or arteriolitis, and an accompanying surrounding hemorrhage indicative of an acute infection associated with fatal human plague. Courtesy of Centers for Disease Control and Prevention.

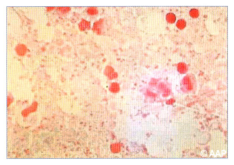

Image 110.10
Bubo aspirate (Gram stain) showing many gram-negative bacilli, *Yersinia pestis*.

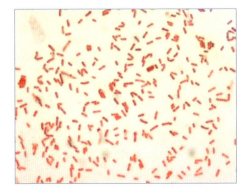

Image 110.11
Yersinia pestis is a small (0.5 × 1.0 μm) gram-negative bacillus (magnification ×1,000). Bipolar staining occurs when using Wayson, Wright, Giemsa, or methylene-blue stain and may occasionally be observed in Gram-stained preparations. Courtesy of Centers for Disease Control and Prevention.

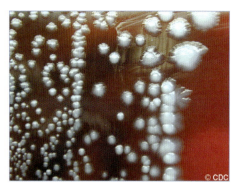

Image 110.12
Yersinia pestis on sheep blood agar, 72 hours. *Y pestis* grows well on most standard laboratory media, after 48–72 hours, with gray-white to slightly yellow opaque raised, irregular "fried egg" morphological features; alternatively, colonies may have a "hammered copper" shiny surface. Courtesy of Centers for Disease Control and Prevention.

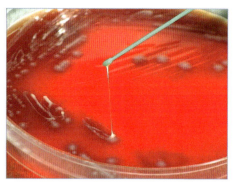

Image 110.13
This photograph depicts the colonial morphological features displayed by gram-negative *Yersinia pestis* bacteria, which were grown on a medium of sheep blood agar for a 48-hour period at a temperature of 37 °C (98.6 °F). There is a tenacious nature of these colonies when touched by an inoculation loop, and they tend to form stringy, sticky strands. Morphological characteristics after 48 hours of *Y pestis* colonial growth include an average colonial diameter of 1.0–2.0 mm and an opaque coloration that ranges from gray-white to yellowish. If permitted to continue growing, *Y pestis* colonies take on what is referred to as a "fried egg" appearance, which becomes more prominent as the colonies age. Older colonies also display what is termed a "hammered copper" texture to their surfaces. Courtesy of Centers for Disease Control and Prevention.

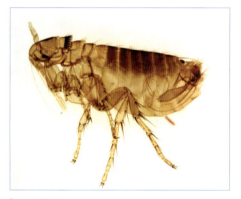

Image 110.14
This photograph depicts an adult male *Diamanus montana* flea, formerly known as *Oropsylla montana*. This flea is a common ectoparasite of the rock squirrel, *Citellus variegatus*, and in the western United States, it is an important vector for the bacterium *Yersinia pestis*, the pathogen responsible for causing plague. Courtesy of Centers for Disease Control and Prevention.

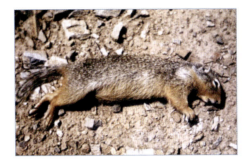

Image 110.15
This photograph shows a ground squirrel that died because of plague, *Yersinia pestis*. Field rodents, such as western ground squirrels and prairie dogs, may be a threat when their burrows are beside labor camps and residential areas because they and their fleas are carriers of the plague bacteria. Courtesy of Centers for Disease Control and Prevention.

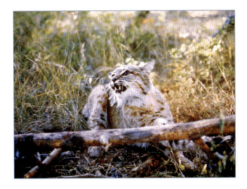

Image 110.16
The bobcat, *Felis rufus*, can be a source of plague infection for humans. People involved in trapping and skinning wild carnivores, especially bobcats, should be extremely cautious about exposure to *Yersinia pestis* vectors. Courtesy of Centers for Disease Control and Prevention.

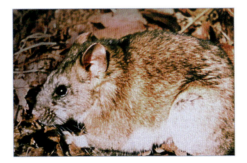

Image 110.17
The bushy-tailed wood rat, *Neotoma cinerea*, is known to carry fleas inoculated with the plague bacteria *Yersinia pestis*. All wood rat species are quick to occupy and construct nests in human habitations or outbuildings within their range, thereby bringing vector fleas into close contact with humans and their pets. Courtesy of Centers for Disease Control and Prevention.

CHAPTER 111
Pneumocystis jirovecii Infections

CLINICAL MANIFESTATIONS

Symptomatic infection with *Pneumocystis jirovecii* is extremely rare in healthy people. However, in immunocompromised infants and children, *P jirovecii* causes a respiratory illness characterized by dyspnea, tachypnea, significant hypoxemia, nonproductive cough, chills, fatigue, and fever. The intensity of these signs and symptoms may vary, and in some immunocompromised children and adults, the onset may be acute and fulminant. Most children with *Pneumocystis* pneumonia are significantly hypoxic. Chest radiographs often show bilateral diffuse interstitial or alveolar disease but may appear normal in early disease. Atypical radiographic findings may include lobar, miliary, cavitary, and nodular lesions. The mortality rate among immunocompromised patients ranges from 5% to 40% in treated patients and approaches 100% without therapy.

ETIOLOGY

Nomenclature for *Pneumocystis* species has evolved. Human *Pneumocystis* is called *P jirovecii*, although the familiar initialism PCP (originally *Pneumocystis carinii* pneumonia) is still used commonly among clinicians. *P jirovecii* is an atypical fungus (on the basis of DNA sequence analysis) with several morphological and biological similarities to protozoa, including susceptibility to a number of antiprotozoal agents but resistance to most antifungal agents. In addition, the organism exists as 2 distinct morphological forms: the 5- to 7-μm–diameter cysts, which contain up to 8 intracystic bodies or sporozoites, and the smaller, 1- to 5-μm–diameter trophozoite or trophic form.

EPIDEMIOLOGY

Pneumocystis species are ubiquitous in mammals worldwide and have a tropism for respiratory tract epithelium. Asymptomatic or mild human infection occurs early in life, with more than 85% of healthy children showing seropositivity by 20 months of age. Animal models and studies of patients with AIDS do not support the existence of latency, and they suggest that disease after the second year after birth is likely reinfection.

The single most important factor in susceptibility to PCP is the status of cell-mediated immunity of the host, reflected by a marked decrease in percentage and numbers of $CD4^+$ T lymphocytes or a decrease in $CD4^+$ T-lymphocyte function. In resource-limited countries and in times of famine, *Pneumocystis* pneumonia (also referred to as PCP, maintaining the same initialism as was previously used for the organism) can occur in epidemics, primarily affecting malnourished infants and children. In industrialized countries, PCP occurs almost entirely in immunocompromised people with deficient cell-mediated immunity, particularly people with HIV infection, recipients of immunosuppressive therapy after solid organ transplant and hematopoietic stem cell transplant (HSCT), people undergoing treatment for hematologic malignancy, and children with primary immunodeficiency syndromes. Although onset of disease can occur at any age, PCP most commonly occurs in HIV-infected children in the first year after birth, with peak incidence at 3 through 6 months of age. In patients with cancer, the disease can occur during remission or relapse of the malignancy.

The incidence of PCP has dramatically decreased in the United States because of combination antiretroviral therapy (ART) for people with HIV and the general adoption of recommendations for prophylaxis (Table 111.1). Despite this decrease, it is still one of the leading opportunistic infections in people with HIV infection, particularly those not aware of their infection and not receiving ART.

Animal studies have demonstrated animal-to-animal transmission by the airborne route; human-to-human transmission has been suggested by molecular epidemiology and global clustering of PCP cases in several studies. Outbreaks in hospitals have been reported. Vertical transmission has been postulated but never proven. The period of communicability is unknown.

The **incubation period** is unknown, but outbreaks of PCP in transplant recipients have demonstrated a median of 53 days from exposure to clinically apparent infection.

Table III.1
Recommendations for *Pneumocystis jirovecii* Pneumonia Prophylaxis for HIV-Exposed Infants and Children, by Age and HIV Infection Status[a]

Age and HIV Infection Status	Initiation of PCP Prophylaxis[b]	Discontinuation of PCP Prophylaxis[b]
Birth through 4–6 weeks of age, HIV exposed or infected	No prophylaxis	Not applicable
4–6 weeks through 12 months of age HIV infected or indeterminate HIV infection presumptively or definitively excluded	Prophylaxis No prophylaxis	Throughout first year after birth Not applicable
1 through 5 years of age, HIV infected	Prophylaxis if CD4$^+$ T-lymphocyte count is <500/μL or percentage is <15%.[c]	Discontinue if combination ART administered for >6 months, and the following values have been sustained for >3 consecutive months: CD4$^+$ T-lymphocyte count is ≥500/μL or percentage is ≥15%.
≥6 years, HIV infected	Prophylaxis if CD4$^+$ T-lymphocyte count is <200/μL or percentage is <15%.	Discontinue if combination ART administered for >6 months, and the following values have been sustained for >3 consecutive months: CD4$^+$ T-lymphocyte count is ≥200/μL or percentage is ≥15%.

ART indicates antiretroviral therapy; PCP, *Pneumocystis jirovecii* pneumonia.

[a] Panel on Opportunistic Infections in HIV-Exposed and HIV-Infected Children. *Guidelines for the Prevention and Treatment of Opportunistic Infections in HIV-Exposed and HIV-Infected Children.* US Dept of Health and Human Services. Accessed June 28, 2022. https://clinicalinfo.hiv.gov/en/guidelines/pediatric-opportunistic-infection/whats-new.

[b] Children who have had PCP should receive lifelong ("secondary") PCP prophylaxis unless/until their CD4$^+$ T-lymphocyte cell counts and percentages are achieved and maintained at designated age-specific values greater than those indicative of severe immunosuppression (Immune Category 3) for at least 6 months.

[c] Prophylaxis should be considered on a case-by-case basis for children who might otherwise have risk for PCP, such as children with rapidly declining CD4$^+$ T-lymphocyte counts or percentages or children with Clinical Category C status of HIV infection.

DIAGNOSTIC TESTS

A definitive diagnosis of PCP is made by visualization of organisms (*Pneumocystis* cysts) in lung tissue or respiratory tract secretion specimens. Bronchoscopy with bronchoalveolar lavage is the diagnostic procedure of choice for most infants and children. Methenamine silver stain, toluidine blue stain, and fluorescently conjugated monoclonal antibody are useful tools for identifying the thick-walled cysts of *P jirovecii*. Sporozoites (within cysts) and trophozoites are identified with Giemsa or modified Wright-Giemsa stain. The sensitivity of all microscopy-based methods depends on the skill of the laboratory technician.

Polymerase chain reaction (PCR) assays to diagnose PCP are becoming more widely available. They are highly sensitive with a variety of specimen types from the respiratory tract, including nasopharyngeal aspirates. Because highly sensitive PCR assays may detect colonization with these organisms, results from such assays must be interpreted in the context of clinical manifestation.

Limited data suggest that serum 1,3-β-D-glucan assay, which is available as a US Food and Drug Administration–cleared test in the United States for invasive fungal infections, may be a potential marker for *Pneumocystis* infection. This compound is a component of the cell wall of the cyst stage of the organism and may be found in high concentrations in serum of patients infected with *P jirovecii*; however, most other fungi also secrete the compound during infection, so correlation with clinical manifestation is imperative.

TREATMENT

The drug of choice is trimethoprim-sulfamethoxazole (TMP-SMX), usually administered intravenously. Oral therapy should be reserved for patients with mild disease who do not have malabsorption or diarrhea and for patients with a favorable clinical response to initial intravenous therapy. Duration of therapy is 21 days. The rate of adverse reactions to TMP-SMX (eg, rash, neutropenia, anemia, thrombocytopenia, renal toxicity, hepatitis, nausea, vomiting, and diarrhea) is higher in HIV-infected children than in non–HIV-infected patients. It is unnecessary to discontinue therapy for mild adverse reactions (eg, vomiting). At least half of patients with more severe reactions that include rash require interruption of therapy. Desensitization to TMP-SMX may be considered after the acute reaction has abated.

Pentamidine, administered intravenously, is an alternative drug for treatment of *Pneumocystis* infection in children and adults who cannot tolerate TMP-SMX or who have severe disease and have not responded to TMP-SMX after 5 to 7 days of therapy. The therapeutic efficacy of intravenous pentamidine in adults with PCP is similar to that of TMP-SMX. Pentamidine is associated with a high incidence of adverse reactions, including renal toxicity, pancreatitis, diabetes mellitus, electrolyte abnormalities, hypoglycemia, hyperglycemia, hypotension, cardiac arrhythmias, fever, and neutropenia. Aerosolized pentamidine should not be used for treatment, because its efficacy is limited.

Atovaquone is approved for oral treatment of mild to moderate PCP in adults who are intolerant of TMP-SMX. Experience with use of atovaquone in children is limited, although a study comparing the efficacy of bacterial prophylaxis of atovaquone-azithromycin to that of TMP-SMX noted that prevention of PCP was equivalent between the 2 drug regimens. Adverse reactions to atovaquone are limited to rash, nausea, and diarrhea.

Other potentially useful drugs for mild to moderate PCP in adults include clindamycin with primaquine (adverse reactions are rash, nausea, and diarrhea), dapsone with trimethoprim (associated with neutropenia, anemia, thrombocytopenia, methemoglobinemia, rash, and elevation of aminotransferase level), and trimetrexate with leucovorin. Experience with the use of these combinations in children is limited.

On the basis of studies in both adults and children, a course of corticosteroids is recommended in patients with moderate to severe PCP (as defined by an arterial oxygen pressure <70 mm Hg when in ambient air or an arterial-alveolar gradient ≥35 mm Hg), starting within 72 hours of diagnosis.

Coinfection with other organisms, such as cytomegalovirus (CMV) or *Streptococcus pneumoniae*, has been reported in HIV-infected children. Children with dual infections may have more severe disease.

Chemoprophylaxis

Chemoprophylaxis is highly effective in preventing PCP in groups with high risk. Prophylaxis against a first episode of PCP is indicated for many patients with significant immunosuppression, including people with HIV infection and people with primary or acquired cell-mediated immunodeficiency.

The recommended drug regimen for PCP prophylaxis for all immunocompromised patients is TMP-SMX (Box 111.1). For patients who cannot tolerate TMP-SMX, alternative oral choices include atovaquone or dapsone. Atovaquone is effective and safe but expensive. Dapsone is effective and inexpensive but associated with more serious adverse effects than atovaquone. Aerosolized pentamidine is recommended for children who cannot tolerate TMP-SMX, atovaquone, or dapsone and are old enough to use a Respirgard II nebulizer. Intravenous pentamidine has been used but is not generally recommended for prophylaxis. Other drug combinations with potential for prophylaxis include pyrimethamine plus dapsone plus leucovorin or pyrimethamine-sulfadoxine. Experience with these drugs in adults and children for this indication is limited. These agents should be considered only when recommended regimens are not tolerated or cannot be used for other reasons.

Prophylaxis for PCP is recommended for children who have received HSCTs or solid organ transplants; children with hematologic malignancies (eg, leukemia or lymphoma) and some

Box III.1
Drug Regimens for *Pneumocystis jirovecii* Pneumonia Prophylaxis for Children 4 Weeks and Older[a]

Recommended daily dose

TMP-SMX (TMP, 5–10 mg/kg per day; and SMX, 25–50 mg/kg per day, orally). The total daily dose should not exceed 320 mg TMP and 1,600 mg SMX.

Acceptable dosing intervals and schedules
- In divided doses twice daily, given 3 days per week on consecutive days or on alternate days
- In divided doses twice daily, given 2 days per week on consecutive days or on alternate days
- Total dose once daily, given 7 days per week

Alternative regimens if TMP-SMX is not tolerated
- **Atovaquone**
  - **Children 1–3 months of age and >24 months–12 years of age:** 30 mg/kg (maximum 1,500 mg), orally, once a day
  - **Children 4–24 months of age:** 45 mg/kg (maximum 1,500 mg), orally, once a day
  - **Children >12 years:** 1,500 mg, orally, once a day
- **Dapsone (children ≥1 month)**
  2 mg/kg (maximum 100 mg), orally, once a day, or 4 mg/kg (maximum 200 mg), orally, every week
- **Aerosolized pentamidine (children ≥5 years)**
  300 mg, inhaled monthly via Respirgard II nebulizer

SMX indicates sulfamethoxazole; TMP, trimethoprim.

[a] Panel on Opportunistic Infections in HIV-Exposed and HIV-Infected Children. *Guidelines for the Prevention and Treatment of Opportunistic Infections in HIV-Exposed and HIV-Infected Children.* US Dept of Health and Human Services. Accessed June 28, 2022. https://clinicalinfo.hiv.gov/en/guidelines/pediatric-opportunistic-infection/whats-new.

nonhematologic malignancies; children with severe cell-mediated immunodeficiency, including children who received adrenocorticotropic hormone for treatment of infantile spasms; and children who are otherwise immunocompromised and who have had a previous episode of PCP. For this diverse group of immunocompromised hosts, the risk of PCP varies with duration and intensity of chemotherapy, with other immunosuppressive therapies, with coinfection with immunosuppressive viruses (eg, CMV), and with local epidemiological rates of PCP. Guidelines for allogeneic HSCT recipients recommend that PCP prophylaxis be initiated at engraftment (or before engraftment, if engraftment is delayed) and administered for at least 6 months in autologous HSCT patients and for at least 1 year in allogeneic transplant recipients, especially matched unrelated or haploidentical transplants who may receive in vivo T-lymphocyte depletion with antithymocyte globulin or Campath. It should be continued in all children receiving ongoing or intensified immunosuppressive therapy (eg, prednisone, cyclosporine) or in children with chronic graft-versus-host disease. In general, PCP prophylaxis is recommended for all solid organ transplant recipients for at least 6 to 12 months posttransplant, although longer durations should be considered. For lung and small-bowel transplant recipients, as well as any transplant patient with a history of prior PCP infection or chronic CMV disease, lifelong prophylaxis may be indicated.

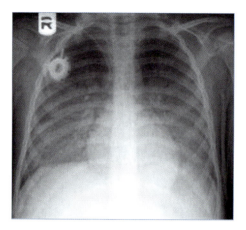

Image III.1

Pneumocystis jirovecii pneumonia. This pathogen is an important cause of pulmonary infections in patients who are immunocompromised. Characteristic signs and symptoms include dyspnea at rest, tachypnea, nonproductive cough, fever, and hypoxia with an increased oxygen requirement. The intensity of the signs and symptoms can vary, and onset may be acute and fulminant. Chest radiographs frequently demonstrate diffuse bilateral interstitial or alveolar disease. This is a chest radiograph from a 5-year-old boy demonstrating bilateral perihilar infiltrates caused by *P jirovecii*. Courtesy of Beverly P. Wood, MD, FAAP, MSEd, PhD.

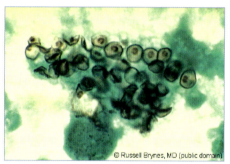

Image III.2

Cysts of *Pneumocystis jirovecii* in a smear from bronchoalveolar lavage (Grocott-Gomori methenamine–silver nitrate stain). Courtesy of Russell Byrnes, MD.

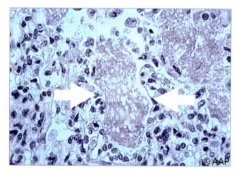

Image III.3

Foamy intra-alveolar exudate in lung biopsy specimen from a patient with *Pneumocystis jirovecii* pneumonia (hematoxylin-eosin stain).

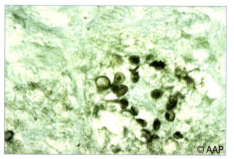

Image III.4

Pneumocystis jirovecii organisms in lung biopsy specimen (Grocott-Gomori methenamine–silver nitrate stain).

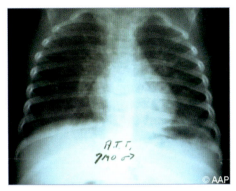

Image III.5
Pneumocystis jirovecii pneumonia with hyperaeration in an infant with congenital agammaglobulinemia.

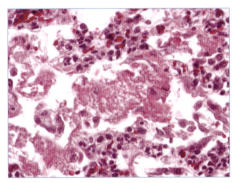

Image III.6
Pneumocystis jirovecii in the lung. Frothy exudate in alveolar spaces. Courtesy of Dimitris P. Agamanolis, MD.

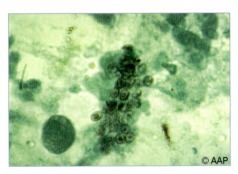

Image III.7
Pneumocystis jirovecii organisms in tracheal aspirate (Grocott-Gomori methenamine–silver nitrate stain).

CHAPTER 112
Poliovirus Infections

CLINICAL MANIFESTATIONS

Approximately 70% of poliovirus infections in susceptible children are asymptomatic. Nonspecific illness with low-grade fever and sore throat (minor illness) occurs in approximately 25% of infected people, and viral meningitis (nonparalytic polio), sometimes accompanied by paresthesias, occurs in 1% to 5% of patients a few days after the minor illness has resolved. Rapid onset of asymmetrical acute flaccid paralysis with areflexia of the involved limb (paralytic poliomyelitis) occurs in less than 1% of infections, with residual paresis in approximately two-thirds of patients. Classical paralytic polio begins with a minor illness characterized by fever, sore throat, headache, nausea, constipation, and/or malaise for several days, followed by a symptom-free period of 1 to 3 days. Rapid onset of paralysis then follows. Typically, paralysis is asymmetrical and affects the proximal muscles more than the distal muscles. Cranial nerve involvement (bulbar poliomyelitis) and paralysis of the diaphragm and intercostal muscles may lead to impaired respiration requiring assisted ventilation. Sensation is usually intact. The cerebrospinal fluid (CSF) profile is characteristic of viral meningitis, with mild pleocytosis and lymphocytic predominance.

Adults who contracted paralytic poliomyelitis during childhood may develop the noninfectious postpolio syndrome 15 to 40 years later, characterized by slow and irreversible exacerbation of weakness in the muscle groups affected during the original infection. Muscle and joint pain are also common manifestations. The estimated incidence of postpolio syndrome in poliomyelitis survivors is 25% to 40%.

ETIOLOGY

Polioviruses are classified as members of the family *Picornaviridae*, genus *Enterovirus*, in the species enterovirus C, and include 3 serotypes. They are nonenveloped, single-stranded positive-sense RNA viruses that are highly stable in a liquid environment. Acute paralytic disease may be caused by naturally occurring (wild) polioviruses and, rarely, by oral poliovirus (OPV) vaccine viruses.

OPV-associated cases of vaccine-associated paralytic poliomyelitis (VAPP) may occur in vaccine recipients or their close contacts or may be associated with circulating vaccine-derived polioviruses (cVDPVs) that have acquired virulence properties that are indistinguishable from naturally occurring polioviruses because of sustained person-to-person transmission in the absence of adequate population immunity. People with primary (but not acquired) B-lymphocyte immunodeficiencies have increased risk for VAPP and for persistent infection (immunodeficiency-associated vaccine-derived polioviruses, or iVDPVs) from vaccine virus. With continuing progress toward polio eradication, more global cases of paralytic disease are now caused by vaccine-related viruses (VAPP and cVDPV) than by wild polioviruses.

EPIDEMIOLOGY

Humans are the only natural reservoir for poliovirus. Spread is by contact with feces and/or respiratory secretions. Infection is more common in infants and young children and occurs at an earlier age in children living in poor hygienic conditions. In temperate climates, poliovirus infections are most common during summer and autumn; in the tropics, the seasonal pattern is less pronounced.

The last cases of poliomyelitis attributable to indigenously acquired, naturally occurring wild poliovirus in the United States were reported in 1979. Except for very rare imported cases, all poliomyelitis cases acquired in the United States have been attributable to VAPP, which, until 1998, occurred in an average of 6 to 8 people annually. Fewer VAPP cases were reported in 1998 and 1999, after a shift in US immunization policy in 1997 from use of OPV to a sequential inactivated poliovirus (IPV) vaccine/OPV schedule. Implementation of an all-IPV vaccine schedule in 2000 halted the occurrence of VAPP cases in the United States.

The risk of contact in the United States with imported wild polioviruses and cVDPV viruses has decreased in parallel with the success of the global eradication program. Of the 3 poliovirus serotypes, type 2 wild poliovirus was declared eradicated in 2015, with the last naturally occurring case detected in 1999 in India, and type 3 wild poliovirus was declared eradicated in October

2019, with the last naturally occurring case having occurred in Nigeria in 2012. Type 1 poliovirus now accounts for all polio cases attributable to wild poliovirus. Because the only source of disease from type 2 poliovirus is now related only to vaccine use, there was a global switch from trivalent OPV to bivalent OPV in April 2016, thus ending all routine immunization with live type 2 poliovirus–containing oral vaccines. Concurrent recommendations were made for all countries to provide at least one dose of IPV to all vaccinees. Similarly, following this vaccine change, the only remaining risk of type 2 infection would come from continued transmission of type 2 OPV viruses administered before the switch, long-term iVDPV type 2 excretors, and breach of containment at facilities maintaining type 2 polioviruses (both wild-type and OPV strains). For this reason, containment of all type 2 poliovirus infectious and potentially infectious materials into accredited essential facilities has been initiated globally.

On August 25, 2020, the World Health Organization (WHO) African Region was certified as wild poliovirus–free after 4 years without a case. With this historic milestone, 5 of the 6 WHO regions, representing more than 90% of the world's population, are now free of the wild poliovirus, moving the world closer to achieving global polio eradication.

Communicability of poliovirus is greatest shortly before and after onset of clinical illness, when the virus is present in the throat and excreted in high concentrations in feces. Virus persists in the throat for approximately 1 to 2 weeks after onset of illness and is excreted in feces for an average of 3 to 6 weeks. In recipients of OPV, virus also persists in the throat for 1 to 2 weeks and is excreted in feces for several weeks, although in rare cases, excretion for longer than 2 months can occur. Immunocompromised patients with significant primary B-lymphocyte immunodeficiencies have excreted iVDPV for periods of longer than 30 years.

The **incubation period of nonparalytic poliomyelitis** is 3 to 6 days. For the onset of poliomyelitis, the **incubation period to paralysis** is usually 7 to 21 days (range, 3–35 days).

DIAGNOSTIC TESTS

Poliovirus can be detected in specimens from the pharynx and feces; less commonly, from urine; and rarely, from CSF by isolation in cell culture or polymerase chain reaction (PCR). The relatively low sensitivity of isolation in cell culture from CSF is likely attributable to low viral load. Fecal material and pharyngeal swab specimens are most likely to yield virus in cell culture.

The diagnostic test of choice for confirming poliovirus disease is viral culture of stool specimens and throat swab specimens obtained as early in the course of illness as possible. There are currently nucleic acid amplification tests for enteroviruses from CSF and at least several multiplexed assays that detect enteroviruses, in addition to a number of other bacterial and viral agents. Such commonly used molecular tests for enteroviruses detect poliovirus but do not differentiate poliovirus from other enteroviruses and, therefore, are insufficient to demonstrate that poliovirus is the etiology of disease. In these situations, additional virus testing is necessary to confirm the diagnosis of poliovirus-related disease. Interpretation of acute and convalescent serological test results can be difficult because of high levels of population immunity.

Real-time reverse transcriptase–PCR (RT-PCR) assays generally have sensitivity that is nearly comparable to or better than that of cell culture and may be more likely to help identify polioviruses in CSF. Two or more stool and throat swab specimens for enterovirus isolation should be obtained or detection by RT-PCR should be demonstrated at least 24 hours apart from patients with suspected paralytic poliomyelitis as early in the course of illness as possible, ideally within 14 days of onset of symptoms. Poliovirus may be excreted intermittently, and a single negative test result does not rule out infection.

Molecular methods have replaced neutralization for identification and typing to differentiate wild-type from vaccine-derived virus strains.

TREATMENT

Management is supportive.

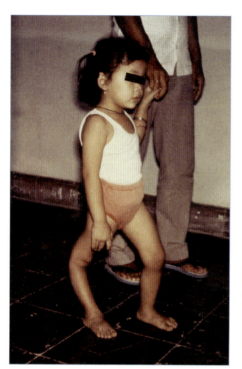

Image 112.1
This child is displaying a deformity of her right lower extremity caused by the poliovirus. Courtesy of Centers for Disease Control and Prevention.

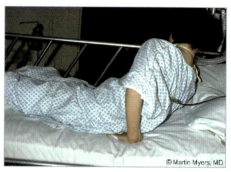

Image 112.2
A young girl with bulbar poliomyelitis with tripod sign attempts to sit upright. Copyright Martin G. Myers, MD.

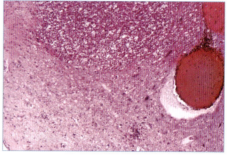

Image 112.3
Pontine histopathologic features caused by the effects of poliomyelitis. Photomicrograph of the pons at the level of the sixth cranial nerve nucleus (abducens nerve) from a patient with type 3 poliomyelitis. Courtesy of Centers for Disease Control and Prevention.

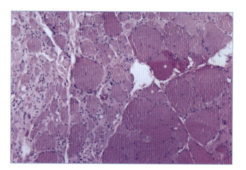

Image 112.4
A photomicrograph of skeletal muscle tissue revealing myotonic dystrophic changes resulting from poliovirus type 3. When spinal neurons die, wallerian degeneration takes place, resulting in muscle weakness of those muscles once innervated by the now-dead neurons (denervated). The degree of paralysis is directly correlated to the number of deceased neurons. Courtesy of Centers for Disease Control and Prevention.

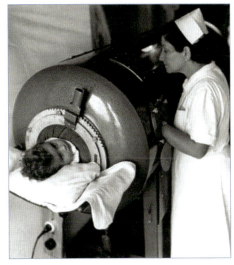

Image 112.5
Patients whose respiratory muscles were affected by poliomyelitis were placed into an iron lung to enable them to breathe. Courtesy of World Health Organization.

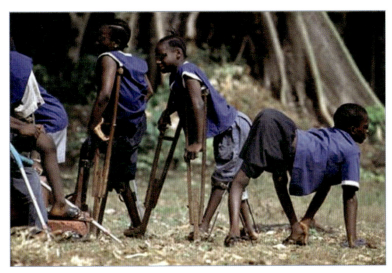

Image 112.6
Cheshire Home for Handicapped Children, Freetown, Sierra Leone. Courtesy of World Health Organization/Immunization Action Coalition.

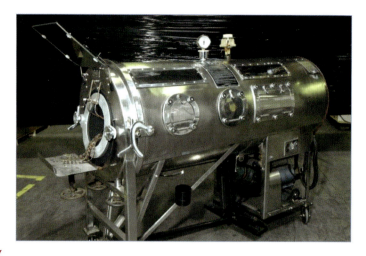

Image 112.7
Made of stainless steel and still in good working order, this Emerson Respirator, also known as an iron lung, was used by patients who had poliomyelitis and whose ability to breathe was paralyzed because of this crippling viral disease. This iron lung was donated to the David J. Sencer Centers for Disease Control and Prevention Museum by the family of patient Barton Hebert of Covington, LA, who had poliomyelitis and used the device from the late 1950s until his death in 2003. Iron lungs encase the thoracic cavity externally in an airtight chamber. The chamber is used to create a negative pressure around the thoracic cavity, thereby causing air to rush into the lungs to equalize intrapulmonary pressure. Courtesy of Centers for Disease Control and Prevention.

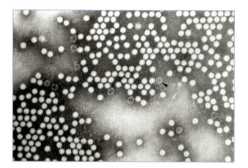

Image 112.8
Transmission electron micrograph of poliovirus type 1. Virions are 20–30 nm in diameter and have icosahedral symmetry. Courtesy of Centers for Disease Control and Prevention.

CHAPTER 113

Polyomaviruses
(BK, JC, and Other Polyomaviruses)

CLINICAL MANIFESTATIONS

BK virus (BKV) infection and JC virus (JCV) infection in humans usually occur in childhood and seemingly result in lifelong persistence. More than 80% of adults are seropositive for BKV. Primary infection with BKV in immunocompetent children is generally asymptomatic, although it may result in mild upper respiratory tract symptoms. BKV is more likely to cause disease in immunocompromised people, including hemorrhagic cystitis in hematopoietic stem cell transplant recipients and interstitial nephritis and ureteral stenosis in renal transplant recipients. The primary symptom of BKV-associated hemorrhagic cystitis in immunocompromised children is painful hematuria; blood clots in the urine and secondary obstructive nephropathy can also occur. BKV-associated nephropathy occurs in 3% to 8% of renal transplant recipients and, less frequently, in other solid organ transplant recipients. BKV-associated nephropathy should be suspected in any renal transplant recipient with allograft dysfunction. More than half of renal allograft patients with BKV-associated nephropathy may experience allograft loss.

JCV causes progressive multifocal leukoencephalopathy (PML), a demyelinating disease of the central nervous system that occurs in severely immunocompromised patients, including patients with AIDS, patients receiving intensive chemotherapy, recipients of hematopoietic stem cell or solid organ transplants, and patients receiving various monoclonal antibody therapies for treatment of autoimmune, oncological, and neurological diseases. PML, the only known disease caused by JCV, occurs in approximately 3% to 5% of untreated adults with AIDS but rarely occurs in children with AIDS. Symptoms include cognitive disturbance, hemiparesis, ataxia, cranial nerve dysfunction, and aphasia. Lytic infection of oligodendrocytes by JCV is the primary mechanism of pathogenesis for PML. In the absence of restored T-lymphocyte function, PML is almost always fatal. PML is an AIDS-defining illness in HIV-infected people. Approximately 50% to 60% of adults are infected by JCV, with infections being acquired during adolescence and early adulthood.

To date, 14 polyomaviruses have been detected in humans, but only a few have been associated with disease, including BK and JC viruses. The Merkel cell polyomavirus (MCPyV) has been detected in more than 80% of cases of Merkel cell carcinomas, which are rare neuroendocrine tumors of the skin. The trichodysplasia spinulosa–associated polyomavirus (TSPyV) has been identified in tissue from patients with trichodysplasia spinulosa, a rare follicular disease of immunocompromised patients that primarily affects the face. The KI polyomavirus (KIPyV) and WU polyomavirus (WUPyV) have been identified in respiratory tract secretions, primarily in association with known pathogenic viruses of the respiratory tract. Human polyomaviruses 6 and 7 (HPyV6 and HPyV7) have been detected as asymptomatic inhabitants of human skin. Human polyomavirus 9 (HPyV9) has been detected in the serum of some renal transplant recipients. The natural history, prevalence, and pathogenic potential of these recently discovered human polyomaviruses have not yet been established.

ETIOLOGY

Polyomaviruses are members of the family *Polyomaviridae*. BKV, JCV, WUPyV, and KIPyV are members of the genus *Betapolyomavirus;* MCPyV, TSPyV, HPyV9, human polyomavirus 12, and New Jersey polyomavirus are members of the genus *Alphapolyomavirus;* HPyV6, HPyV7, Malawi polyomavirus, and St Louis polyomavirus are members of the genus *Deltapolyomavirus*. They are nonenveloped viruses with a circular double-stranded DNA genome with icosahedral symmetry of the capsid ranging 40 to 50 nm in diameter. One of the biological characteristics of the polyomaviruses is the maintenance of a chronic viral infection in their host with few or no symptoms. Symptomatic disease caused by human polyomavirus infections occurs almost exclusively in immunosuppressed people.

EPIDEMIOLOGY

Humans are the only known natural hosts for BKV and JCV. The mode of transmission of BKV and JCV is uncertain, but the respiratory route and the oral route by water or food have been postulated. BKV and JCV are ubiquitous in the human population, with BKV infection occurring in early childhood and JCV infection occurring primarily in adolescence and adulthood. BKV persists in the kidney and gastrointestinal tract of healthy subjects, with urinary excretion occurring in 3% to 5% of healthy adults. JCV persists in the kidney, gastrointestinal tract, and brain of healthy people. The prevalence of urinary excretion of JCV increases with age.

DIAGNOSTIC TESTS

Detection of BKV T antigen by immunohistochemical analysis of renal biopsy material is the gold standard for diagnosis of BKV-associated nephropathy, but nucleic acid–based polymerase chain reaction (PCR) assays are the most sensitive tools for rapid viral screening for polyomaviruses and quantification of viral load. Prospective monitoring of BK viral load in plasma by using PCR assay is common after renal transplant to monitor for BKV-associated nephropathy. Detection of BKV nucleic acid in plasma by PCR assay is associated with an increased risk of BKV-associated nephropathy, especially when BKV viral loads exceed 10,000 genomes/mL, but detection of BKV in urine of renal transplant recipients is common and does not predict BKV disease after renal transplant. Both BKV and JCV can be propagated in cell culture, but culture plays no role in the laboratory diagnosis of infection attributable to these agents. Antibody assays are commonly used to detect the presence of specific antibodies against individual viruses.

The diagnosis of BKV-associated hemorrhagic cystitis is made clinically when other causes of urinary tract bleeding are excluded. In hematopoietic stem cell transplant recipients, detection of BKV by PCR assay in urine is common (>50%), but BKV-associated hemorrhagic cystitis is much less common (10%–15%). Prolonged urinary shedding of BKV and detection of BKV in plasma after hematopoietic stem cell transplant has been associated with increased risk of developing BKV-associated hemorrhagic cystitis. Urine cytological testing may suggest urinary shedding of BKV on the basis of presence of decoy cells, which resemble renal carcinoma cells, but decoy cells do not have high sensitivity or specificity for BKV disease.

A confirmed diagnosis of PML attributable to JCV requires a compatible clinical syndrome and magnetic resonance imaging or computed tomographic findings showing lesions in the brain white matter coupled with brain biopsy findings. JCV can be demonstrated by in situ hybridization, electron microscopy, or immunohistochemistry of brain biopsy or autopsy material. There are no US Food and Drug Administration–cleared nucleic acid amplification tests (NAATs) for detection of JCV. Diagnosis of PML can be facilitated when JCV DNA is detected in cerebrospinal fluid (CSF) by a NAAT, which may obviate the need for a brain biopsy. Early in the course of PML, false-negative PCR assay results have been reported, so repeated testing is warranted when clinical suspicion of PML is high. Measurement of JCV DNA concentrations in CSF samples may be a useful marker for managing PML in patients with AIDS who are receiving combination antiretroviral therapy (ART).

TREATMENT

Fluoroquinolones or immune globulin intravenous provide little to no benefit in the treatment of BKV-associated nephropathy. Judicious reduction of immunosuppression has been shown to prevent development of BKV-associated nephropathy without increasing the risk of rejection in renal transplant patients with BKV plasma viral loads greater than 10,000 genomes/mL.

Most patients with BKV-hemorrhagic cystitis after hematopoietic stem cell transplant require only supportive care, because restoration of immune function by stem cell engraftment ultimately controls BKV replication. In severe cases, surgical intervention may be required to stop bladder hemorrhage. Parenteral and/or intravesicular cidofovir have been used for treatment. Use of systemic cidofovir must be balanced against its high risk of nephrotoxicity. Adoptive transfer of BKV-specific T lymphocytes has been used with varying success at some transplant centers.

Restoration of immune function (eg, combination ART for patients with AIDS) is necessary for survival of patients with PML. Cidofovir has not been shown to be effective for treatment of PML. For patients with monoclonal antibody–associated PML, plasmapheresis and/or immune stimulatory agents (eg, granulocyte colony-stimulating factor) may be useful to improve outcomes.

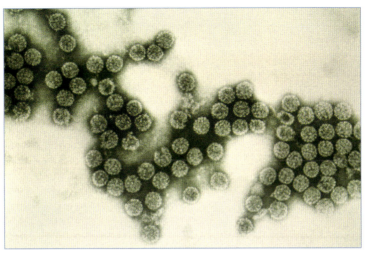

Image 113.1
This digitally colorized transmission electron micrograph reveals some of the ultrastructural morphological features exhibited by a number of unspecified DNA-based, icosahedral-shaped polyomavirus virions, a member of the family *Polyomaviridae*. Courtesy of Centers for Disease Control and Prevention.

CHAPTER 114

Prion Diseases: Transmissible Spongiform Encephalopathies

CLINICAL MANIFESTATIONS

Prion diseases, or transmissible spongiform encephalopathies (TSEs), constitute a group of rare, rapidly progressive, universally fatal, transmissible neurodegenerative diseases of humans and animals characterized by neuronal degeneration, reactive gliosis, and, most often, spongiform degeneration in the cerebral cortical, subcortical, and cerebellar gray matter. Those findings are accompanied by accumulation of an abnormal misfolded, partially protease-resistant prion (proteinaceous infectious) protein. The normal protease-sensitive isomer of the protein is called *cellular* prion protein, or PrP^C. The protease-resistant prion protein is variably called PrP^{res}, *scrapie* prion protein (PrP^{sc}, named for the first known prion disease affecting sheep), or, as suggested by the World Health Organization, *TSE-associated* prion protein (PrP^{TSE}). PrP^{TSE} distributes widely, albeit unevenly, throughout the central nervous system, sometimes forming plaques of varying morphologies.

Human prion diseases include several sporadic, familial, and acquired diseases: Creutzfeldt-Jakob disease (CJD), Gerstmann-Sträussler-Scheinker disease, fatal familial insomnia and fatal sporadic insomnia, kuru, and variant CJD (vCJD), caused by the agent of bovine spongiform encephalopathy [BSE], commonly called "mad cow disease"). Classic CJD can be sporadic (approximately 85% of cases), familial (approximately 15% of cases), or iatrogenic (<1% of cases). Sporadic CJD is most commonly a disease of older adults (median age of death in the United States, 68 years) but has also been described in adolescents and young adults. Iatrogenic CJD has been acquired through intramuscular injection of contaminated cadaveric pituitary hormones (growth hormone and human gonadotropin), dura mater allografts, corneal transplant, contaminated instruments used in neurosurgery, and electroencephalographic probe electrodes. In 1996, an outbreak of a new variant of CJD (vCJD) was linked to consumption of beef from BSE-infected cattle in the United Kingdom and France, with index cases occurring in teenagers. Since the end of 2003, 4 presumptive cases of transfusion-transmitted vCJD have been reported: 3 clinical cases as well as 1 asymptomatic case in which PrP^{TSE} was detected in the spleen and lymph nodes but not brain tissues. A fifth possible iatrogenic vCJD infection was reported in the United Kingdom, affecting a hemophiliac patient, also asymptomatic, who had PrP^{TSE} in the spleen; pre-clinical vCJD was attributed to treatment with plasma-derived coagulation factor fractionated in the United Kingdom; the plasma product implicated in transmitting vCJD was never marketed in the United States.

The best known prion diseases affecting animals include scrapie of sheep and goats, BSE, and a chronic wasting disease (CWD) of North American deer, elk, and moose. CWD was recently detected in reindeer and moose (European elk) in Norway, Sweden, and Finland. Except for vCJD, no human prion disease has yet been attributed convincingly to infection with an agent of animal origin.

CJD most typically manifests as a rapidly progressive neurological disease with escalating defects in memory, personality, and other higher cortical functions. At presentation, approximately one-third of patients have cerebellar dysfunction, including ataxia, incoordination, and dysarthria. Iatrogenic CJD may also manifest as dementia with cerebellar signs. Myoclonus develops in at least 80% of affected patients at some point in the course of disease. Death usually occurs in weeks to months (median, 4–5 months); only 10% to 15% of patients with sporadic CJD survive for more than 1 year.

vCJD is distinguished from classic CJD by younger age of onset (median age at death, around 28 years), early "psychiatric" manifestations, and other features such as painful sensations in the limbs, delayed onset of overt neurological signs, relative absence of diagnostic electroencephalographic changes, and a more prolonged duration of illness (median, 13–14 months). In vCJD, but not in classic CJD, a high proportion of people exhibit high signal abnormalities on T2-weighted brain magnetic resonance imaging (MRI) in the pulvinar region of the posterior thalamus (known as the pulvinar sign). In vCJD, the neuropathologic examination reveals highly reproducible pathology with spongiform vacuolation and numerous florid plaques (compact flowerlike amyloid plaques surrounded by vacuoles) and exceptionally striking punctate deposition of PrP^{TSE} in the basal ganglia. In addition, PrP^{TSE} is detectable by immunohistochemistry in the tonsils, appendix, spleen, and lymph nodes of patients with vCJD.

ETIOLOGY

The proteinaceous infectious particle (or prion), widely believed to cause human and animal prion diseases, consists of PrP^{TSE}, the misfolded form of PrP^C, a ubiquitous normal sialoglycoprotein of unknown function found on the surfaces of neurons and many other cells of humans and animals. It has been postulated by some authorities that sporadic CJD and atypical forms of BSE may result from a spontaneous structural change of host-encoded PrP^C into the self-replicating pathogenic PrP^{TSE} form. Prion propagation is proposed to occur by a recruitment reaction in which abnormal PrP^{TSE} serves as a template to convert PrP^C molecules into misfolded PrP^{TSE} molecules that precipitate in saline-detergent solutions, resist digestion with some proteolytic enzymes, and have a high potential to aggregate.

EPIDEMIOLOGY

Classic sporadic CJD is rare, occurring in the United States at a rate of approximately 1 to 1.5 cases per million people annually. Lifetime risk of CJD probably exceeds 1 in 10,000 people. Onset of disease peaks in the 60- through 74-year age-group. Case-control studies of sporadic CJD have helped identify no consistent environmental risk factor. No increase in cases of sporadic CJD has been observed in people previously transfused with blood or blood components or injected with human plasma derivatives. Rate of sporadic CJD is not increased in patients with several diseases treated by repeated blood transfusions (eg, thalassemia and sickle cell disease) or in patients with hemophilia treated with human plasma derivatives. The American Red Cross traced a number of recipients of blood transfusions from donors later diagnosed with sporadic CJD; no cases of CJD were identified in recipients, some of whom survived for many years. This information suggests that any risk of transfusion-transmitted classic sporadic CJD must be very low and appropriately regarded as theoretical. Except in families with familial forms of the disease, CJD has not been reported in progeny of mothers who died with CJD. Familial forms of prion diseases are expressed as autosomal dominant disorders with variable penetrance associated with a variety of mutations of the prion protein–encoding gene (*PRNP*) located on chromosome 20. On average, familial CJD begins approximately 10 years earlier than does sporadic CJD, but age at onset varies widely, even for members of the same family harboring identical mutations.

As of May 2019 (**www.cjd.ed.ac.uk/surveillance**), the total number of vCJD cases reported was 178 patients in the United Kingdom, 28 in France, 5 in Spain, 4 in Ireland, 4 in the United States, 3 in the Netherlands, 3 in Italy, 2 in Portugal, 2 in Canada, and 1 each in Taiwan, Japan, and Saudi Arabia. Two of the 4 patients in the United States, 2 of the 4 in Ireland, and 1 each of the patients in France, Canada, and Taiwan are believed to have acquired vCJD during residence in the United Kingdom. Researchers using statistical analysis of probability density of exposure to BSE concluded that 2 vCJD patients in the United States and another in Canada were probably infected during childhood residence in the Kingdom of Saudi Arabia. On the basis of animal inoculation studies, comparative prion protein immunoblotting, and epidemiological investigations, almost all cases of vCJD are believed to have resulted from exposure to tissues from cattle infected with BSE. Authorities suspect that the Japanese patient was infected during a short visit of 24 days to the United Kingdom in 1990, 12 years before onset of vCJD. Most patients with vCJD were younger than 30 years at onset, and several were adolescents. Median age at death of the 175 primary vCJD cases was 27 years. The ages at death of the 3 iatrogenic vCJD transfusion-transmitted cases were 32, 69, and 75 years; they developed typical vCJD 6.3 to 8.5 years after transfusions with nonleukoreduced red blood cells from apparently healthy individuals who donated the blood 1.4 to 3.5 years before onset of vCJD, demonstrating that blood contained the infectious agent during a substantial part of the asymptomatic incubation period. One patient with hemophilia, also showing no clinical signs of prion disease, was probably infected through injections of human plasma–derived clotting factors.

The **incubation periods** for iatrogenic classic CJD vary by route of exposure and range, from about 14 months to at least 42 years. No transfusion-transmitted cases of classic CJD have been recognized.

DIAGNOSTIC TESTS

The diagnosis of human prion diseases can be made with certainty only by neuropathologic examination of affected brain tissue, usually obtained at autopsy. Immunodetection methods for prion protein, such as immunohistochemistry with sections and Western blot with saline-detergent extracts, can be used to test brain tissues. Electroencephalography (EEG), MRI, and cerebrospinal fluid (CSF) testing can be used to diagnose prion disease in living patients. In most patients with classic CJD, characteristic 1- to 2-cycle-per-second triphasic sharp-wave discharges on EEG tracing indicate CJD. The likelihood of finding this abnormality is enhanced by serial EEG recordings. Validated assays that detect 2 protein markers, 14-3-3 and tau, in CSF showed 83% to 90% sensitivity and 78% specificity. These proteins, sometimes detected in other neurological diseases, are surrogate nonspecific markers found in CSF, probably because of the death of neurons. No validated blood test is available. Recent promising developments exploit the in vivo prion replication process to amplify and detect even minute amounts of prions in biological samples. One such technique, real-time quaking-induced conversion (RT-QuIC), has been applied successfully in the clinical diagnosis of CJD in CSF samples with high specificity and sensitivity. RT-QuIC has also been applied to diagnose CJD in olfactory epithelium brushings and, with additional validation, may be used in clinical settings. RT-QuIC has not yet been applied successfully to blood samples. Some success has been reported with blood samples tested by using another PrP^{TSE} amplification technique, called *protein misfolding cyclic amplification*. These are currently research-use–only tests not marketed for human diagnosis. Any person bearing a pathogenic mutation of the *PRNP* gene (not a normal polymorphism) with progressive neurological signs suggestive of a TSE can be presumed to have a prion disease. Brain biopsies for patients with possible CJD should be considered only when other potentially treatable diseases remain in the differential diagnosis. Complete postmortem examination of the brain is encouraged to confirm the clinical diagnosis of prion disease; to detect emerging forms of CJD, such as vCJD; and to survey for potential zoonotic transmission of CWD.

TREATMENT

No treatment has stopped or slowed the progressive neurodegeneration in prion diseases. Experimental treatments are being studied. Supportive therapy aids in managing dementia, spasticity, rigidity, and seizures occurring during the course of illness.

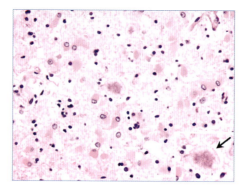

Image 114.1
Histopathologic changes in frontal cerebral cortex of the patient who died of variant Creutzfeldt-Jakob disease in the United States. Marked astroglial reaction is shown, occasionally with relatively large florid plaques surrounded by vacuoles (arrow in inset) (hematoxylin-eosin stain, original magnification ×40). Courtesy of *Emerging Infectious Diseases*.

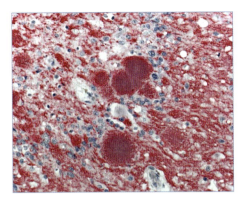

Image 114.2
Immunohistochemical staining of cerebellar tissue of the patient who died of variant Creutzfeldt-Jakob disease in the United States. Stained amyloid plaques are shown with surrounding deposits of abnormal prion protein (immunoalkaline phosphatase stain, naphthol fast red substrate with light hematoxylin counterstain; original magnification ×158). Courtesy of *Emerging Infectious Diseases*.

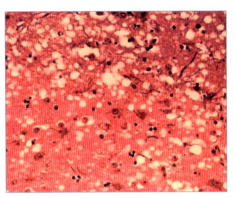

Image 114.3
This micrograph of brain tissue reveals the cytoarchitectural histopathologic changes found in bovine spongiform encephalopathy (BSE). The presence of vacuoles (ie, microscopic "holes" in the gray matter) gives the brain of BSE-affected cows a spongelike appearance when tissue sections are examined in the laboratory. Courtesy of Centers for Disease Control and Prevention.

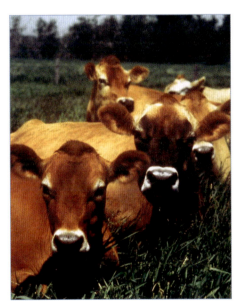

Image 114.4
These cattle will be inspected by the US Department of Agriculture (USDA) Food Safety and Inspection Service before slaughter. USDA Animal and Plant Health Inspection Service leads an ongoing, comprehensive interagency surveillance program for bovine spongiform encephalopathy in the United States to ensure the health of America's cattle herd. Courtesy of Centers for Disease Control and Prevention.

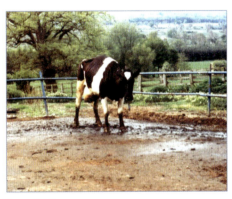

Image 114.5
Cattle affected by bovine spongiform encephalopathy (BSE) experience progressive degeneration of the nervous system. Behavioral changes in temperament (eg, nervousness, aggression), abnormal posture, incoordination and difficulty in rising, decreased milk production, and/or weight loss despite continued appetite are followed by death in cattle affected by BSE. Courtesy of Centers for Disease Control and Prevention.

CHAPTER 115
Pseudomonas aeruginosa Infections

CLINICAL MANIFESTATIONS

Pseudomonas aeruginosa causes a variety of localized and systemic infections including otitis externa, mastoiditis, folliculitis, cellulitis, ecthyma gangrenosum, wound infection, ocular infection, pneumonia, osteomyelitis, bacteremia, endocarditis, meningitis, and urinary tract infection. It is a common cause of health care–associated infections (particularly in the presence of invasive devices), infections in immunocompromised children, pulmonary infections in children with cystic fibrosis (CF), and infections in children with burns. *Pseudomonas* ophthalmia occurs predominantly in preterm infants and manifests with eyelid edema and erythema, purulent discharge, and pannus formation. It can progress to corneal perforation, endophthalmitis, sepsis, and meningitis.

ETIOLOGY

P aeruginosa is an aerobic, gram-negative, nonfermenting bacillus that is commonly found in the environment. The organism has a number of virulence factors, including the ability to form biofilms. *P aeruginosa* can convert to a mucoid phenotype, particularly in the setting of prolonged colonization, such as in individuals with CF.

EPIDEMIOLOGY

P aeruginosa is an opportunistic pathogen, causing infections in people with immunocompromise (particularly those with neutropenia or poor granulocyte function) and those with indwelling devices, burns, or CF. Children with CF commonly develop chronic endobronchial infection with *P aeruginosa*, which is often associated with a more rapid decline in pulmonary function. Children with CF can share epidemic strains of *P aeruginosa*. Hospital-acquired *P aeruginosa* infections include ventilator-associated pneumonia, catheter-associated urinary tract infections, and surgical site infections. Community-associated infections include hot tub folliculitis, otitis externa after swimming in fresh water, osteomyelitis after a puncture wound (particularly through a sneaker), and endocarditis in people who inject drugs. It is a common cause of "contact lens" keratitis. Auricular chondritis has occurred after upper ear piercing. Outbreaks of infection have occurred because of contaminated bronchoscopes.

P aeruginosa has intrinsic resistance to a variety of antibiotics, and circulating strains are often multidrug resistant. Resistance may emerge during therapy. Production of β-lactamases, loss of outer membrane proteins, and multidrug efflux pumps are common. Carbapenemase-producing strains (most commonly IMP and VIM) have occurred in the United States in recent years.

The **incubation period** is variable, depending on the host and site of colonization/infection. Incubation period for folliculitis following immersion in a whirlpool is a few hours to several days after exposure.

DIAGNOSTIC TESTS

Diagnosis is established by growth of *P aeruginosa*. Isolates may be identified by traditional biochemical tests, by a variety of commercially available biochemical test systems, by mass spectrometry of bacterial cell components, or by molecular methods.

TREATMENT

- Empirical combination therapy from different antimicrobial classes (eg, adding a fluoroquinolone or an aminoglycoside to an antipseudomonal β-lactam) may be indicated in patients with severe sepsis, in patients with neutropenia, in patients who recently received broad-spectrum β-lactams, or in settings where antibiotic resistance is high to increase the probability of covering the infecting organism before knowing its identification and susceptibility.

- Cultures and susceptibilities should be sent before initiation of empirical therapy and therapy adjusted as per susceptibility data. In most patients, therapy can be simplified to a single active agent; there are no data to support continuation of combination therapy for an isolate susceptible to an appropriate antipseudomonal drug. When the clinical course is complicated or when there is multidrug resistance, it is recommended that an infectious disease expert assist in the management, particularly in the setting of carbapenem resistance.

- An important component of treatment is source control (ie, removal of catheters and devices, drainage of abscesses).

- Antimicrobial agents that have activity against *P aeruginosa* include piperacillin-tazobactam, ceftazidime, cefepime, aztreonam, ciprofloxacin, levofloxacin, meropenem, and imipenem-cilastatin; however, susceptibility patterns vary regionally. Aminoglycosides are often used as adjunctive therapy (but not as monotherapy beyond urinary tract infections). Polymyxins (ie, colistin, polymyxin B) can be considered in the setting of highly resistant organisms but should not be used as first-line treatments if newer agents (eg, imipenem-cilastatin-relebactam, ceftazidime-avibactam, or ceftolozane-tazobactam) are available because of their generally lower efficacy and higher adverse event rates compared with those of these newer agents.

- Treatment of children with CF should occur in conjunction with an expert in CF. Treatment of pulmonary exacerbation often includes 2 antipseudomonal agents in patients known to be chronically infected with *P aeruginosa*. The Cystic Fibrosis Foundation recommends early eradication of *P aeruginosa* with inhaled tobramycin (300 mg twice daily for 28 days). Once *P aeruginosa* becomes established, it can persist for years. Chronic suppressive treatment with inhaled antibiotics can decrease the bacterial burden. Inhaled antibiotics are not generally indicated for pulmonary exacerbations.

- Management of *Pseudomonas* neonatal ophthalmia urgently requires a combination of systemic and topical therapy, because systemic antibiotics alone have poor penetration in the anterior chamber of the eye. The diagnosis should be suspected when gram-stained specimens of exudate contain gram-negative bacilli and should be confirmed by culture.

- Duration of therapy is based on clinical and bacteriologic response of the patient and the site(s) of infection. Most bloodstream infections, ventilator-associated pneumonias, and urinary tract infections can be treated with 7 to 14 days of antibiotic therapy.

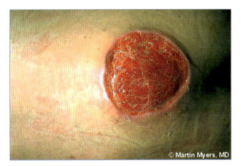

Image 115.1
Rapidly progressive necrotizing *Pseudomonas* lesion (ecthyma gangrenosum). Copyright Martin G. Myers, MD.

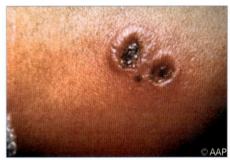

Image 115.2
Bullous, necrotic, umbilicated lesions in an infant with septicemia caused by *Pseudomonas aeruginosa*.

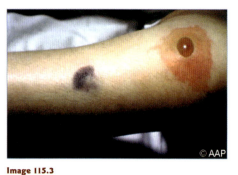

Image 115.3
Skin lesions caused by *Pseudomonas aeruginosa* in a child with neutropenia and septicemia.

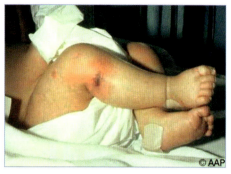

Image 115.4
Sepsis caused by *Pseudomonas aeruginosa* with early ecthyma gangrenosum.

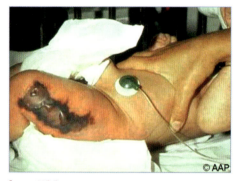

Image 115.5
Sepsis caused by *Pseudomonas aeruginosa* with rapidly progressing ecthyma gangrenosum.

CHAPTER 116
Q Fever
(*Coxiella burnetii* Infection)

CLINICAL MANIFESTATIONS

Approximately half of acute Q fever infections result in symptoms. Acute and persistent (chronic) forms of the disease exist, and both can manifest as fever of unknown origin. Acute Q fever in children is typically characterized by abrupt onset of fever and is often accompanied by chills, headache, weakness, cough, and other nonspecific systemic symptoms. Illness is typically self-limited, although a relapsing febrile illness lasting for several months has been documented in children. Gastrointestinal tract symptoms, such as diarrhea, vomiting, abdominal pain, and anorexia, are reported in 50% to 80% of children. Rash has been observed in some patients with Q fever. Q fever pneumonia usually manifests with a mild cough and shortness of breath but can progress to respiratory distress. Chest radiographic patterns are variable. In immunocompromised patients, a nodular pattern accompanied by a halo of ground-glass opacification and vessel connection, or findings suggestive of a necrotizing process, may be visualized. More severe manifestations of acute Q fever are rare but include hepatitis, hemolytic-uremic syndrome, myocarditis, pericarditis, cerebellitis, encephalitis, meningitis, hemophagocytosis, lymphadenitis, cholecystitis, and rhabdomyolysis. The presence of anticardiolipin antibodies during acute Q fever has been associated with severe complications in adults. There appears to be a small link between Q fever and subsequent development of lymphoma in adulthood because of the risk factor of lymphadenitis. Persistent, localized (chronic) Q fever in children is rare but can manifest as blood culture–negative endocarditis, vascular infection, chronic relapsing or multifocal osteomyelitis, or chronic hepatitis. Osteomyelitis is a common manifestation of persistent, localized Q fever in children. Children who are immunocompromised or have underlying valvular heart disease may have higher risk for persistent, localized Q fever.

ETIOLOGY

Coxiella burnetii, the cause of Q fever, was previously considered to be a rickettsial organism but is a gram-negative intracellular bacterium that belongs to the order *Legionellales*, family *Coxiellaceae*. It shares many features, including relatedness of several virulence genes, with *Legionella pneumophila*. The infectious form of *C burnetii* is highly resistant to heat, desiccation, and disinfectant chemicals and can persist for long periods in the environment. *C burnetii* is classified as a category B bioterrorism agent.

EPIDEMIOLOGY

Q fever is a zoonotic infection that has been reported worldwide, including in every state in the United States. The Q comes from *query* fever, the name of the disease until its etiologic agent was identified in the 1930s. *C burnetii* infection is usually asymptomatic in animals. Many different species can be infected, although cattle, sheep, and goats are the primary reservoirs for human infection. Tick vectors may be important for maintaining animal and bird reservoirs but are not believed to be important in transmission to humans. Humans most often acquire infection by inhalation of fine-particle aerosols of *C burnetii* generated from birthing fluids or other excreta of infected animals or through inhalation of dust contaminated by these materials. Infection can occur by exposure to contaminated materials, such as wool, straw, bedding, or laundry. Windborne particles containing infectious organisms can travel prolonged distances, contributing to sporadic cases for which no apparent animal contact can be demonstrated. Unpasteurized dairy products can also contain the organism. Seasonal trends occur in farming areas with predictable frequency, and the disease often coincides with the livestock birthing season in spring.

The **incubation period** is 14 to 22 days, with a range from 9 to 39 days, depending on the inoculum size. Persistent, localized (chronic) Q fever can develop months to years after initial infection.

DIAGNOSTIC TESTS

Serological evidence of a 4-fold increase in phase II immunoglobulin G (IgG) via immunofluorescent assay (IFA) tests between paired sera taken 3 to 6 weeks apart is the most commonly used method to diagnose acute Q fever. A single high serum phase II IgG titer (≥1:128) by IFA in the convalescent stage may be considered evidence of probable infection. Confirmation of persistent (chronic)

Q fever is based on an increasing phase I IgG titer (typically ≥1:1,024) that is often higher than the phase II IgG titer *and* an identifiable nidus of infection (eg, endocarditis, vascular infection, osteomyelitis, chronic hepatitis). Polymerase chain reaction (PCR) testing on whole blood or serum may be useful in the first 2 weeks of symptom onset and before antimicrobial administration. Although a positive PCR assay result can confirm the diagnosis, a negative PCR test result will not rule out Q fever. PCR and serological testing for *C burnetii* are available through state public health laboratories and from some commercial diagnostic laboratories. Detection of *C burnetii* in tissues (eg, heart valve) by immunohistochemistry or PCR assay can also confirm a diagnosis of chronic Q fever. However, PCR test results may be negative in up to 66% of patients with endocarditis attributable to Q fever.

TREATMENT

Acute Q fever is generally a self-limited illness, and many patients recover without antimicrobial therapy. However, early treatment is effective in shortening illness duration and symptom severity and should be initiated in all symptomatic patients. For symptomatic patients with suspected Q fever, immediate empirical therapy should be given, because laboratory results are often negative early in illness onset pending production of quantifiable antibody. Doxycycline, administered for 14 days, is the drug of choice for severe infections in patients and can be used for acute Q fever regardless of patient age. Pregnant women and patients allergic to doxycycline can be treated with trimethoprim-sulfamethoxazole.

Persistent (chronic) Q fever is much more difficult to treat, and relapses can occur despite appropriate therapy, necessitating repeated courses of therapy. For Q fever endocarditis in adults, the recommended therapy is a combination of doxycycline and hydroxychloroquine for a minimum of 18 months. There are limited data available on effective treatment of chronic Q fever in children, but in some cases, surgical replacement of infected tissue and/or surgical debridement may be required.

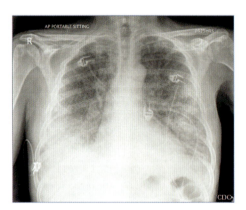

Image 116.1
Chest radiograph of a patient at admission to the hospital, before intubation, demonstrating extensive bilateral airspace disease. The first cases of Q fever in Nova Scotia were recognized in 1979 during a study of atypical pneumonia. This observation led to a series of studies that showed Q fever was common in Nova Scotia (50–60 cases per year in a population of approximately 950,000) and the epidemiological finding was unique; exposure to infected parturient cats or newborn kittens was the major risk factor for infection. At about the same time, cat-related outbreaks were noted in neighboring Prince Edward Island and New Brunswick. In the early 1990s, cases began to decline, but to our knowledge, since 1999, Q fever in this area has not been systematically studied. Courtesy of *Emerging Infectious Diseases*.

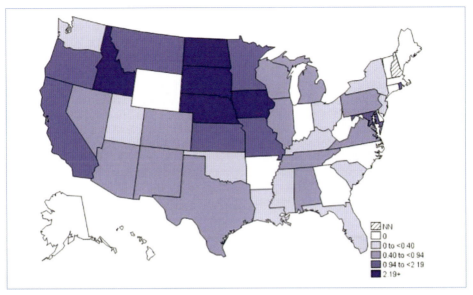

Image 116.2
Annual incidence (per million population) of reported Q fever—United States, 2019. NN indicates not notifiable. Courtesy of Centers for Disease Control and Prevention.

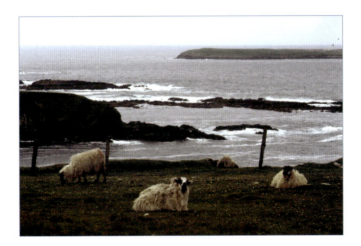

Image 116.3
These domestic sheep were lying on a hillside in Glencolumbkille, County Donegal, Ireland, with the Atlantic Ocean in the background. In 2004, Ireland had almost 7 million domestic sheep. That year, the Irish state exported approximately 51,500 tons of sheep meat valued at 165 million euros. While important to national economies, livestock industries can present health hazards for producers and consumers. Diseases that can be transmitted from animals to humans are called *zoonoses*. Q fever, *Coxiella burnetii*, is a disease passed to humans from sheep. People working around domestic sheep should consider getting immunized against this disease. The disease can be acquired from the inhalation of aerosolized barnyard dust should it contain infected dried urine, manure particles, or dried fluids from the birth of calves or lambs. Domestic animals present problems not only for their handlers (ie, farmers) but for consumers when animals are used for food. Food products made from animals include not only meat but meat derivatives that are added to sweets and other foods and, therefore, are less obvious to consumers. Courtesy of Centers for Disease Control and Prevention/Edwin P. Ewing Jr, MD.

Rabies

CLINICAL MANIFESTATIONS

Infection with rabies virus and other lyssaviruses characteristically produces an acute illness with rapidly progressive central nervous system manifestations, including anxiety, radicular pain, dysesthesia or pruritus, hydrophobia, and dysautonomia. Some patients may have paralysis. Illness almost invariably progresses to death. The differential diagnosis of acute encephalitic illnesses of unknown cause or with features of Guillain-Barré syndrome should include rabies.

ETIOLOGY

Rabies virus is a single-stranded RNA virus classified in the *Rhabdoviridae* family, *Lyssavirus* genus. The genus *Lyssavirus* currently contains 14 species divided into 3 phylogroups.

EPIDEMIOLOGY

Understanding the epidemiology of rabies has been aided by viral variant identification with monoclonal antibodies and nucleotide sequencing. In the United States, human cases have decreased steadily since the 1950s, reflecting widespread immunization of dogs and the availability of effective prophylaxis after exposure to a rabid animal. From 2000 through 2017, 34 of 49 cases of human rabies reported in the United States were acquired indigenously. Of the 34 indigenously acquired cases, all but 5 were associated with bats. Despite the large focus of rabies in raccoons in the eastern United States, only 3 human deaths have been attributed to the raccoon rabies virus variant. Historically, 2 cases of human rabies were attributable to probable aerosol exposure in laboratories, and 2 unusual cases have been attributed to possible airborne exposures in caves inhabited by millions of bats, although alternative infection routes cannot be discounted. Transmission has also occurred by transplant of organs, corneas, and other tissues from patients dying of undiagnosed rabies. Person-to-person transmission by bite has not been documented in the United States, although the virus has been isolated from saliva of infected patients.

Wildlife rabies perpetuates throughout all of the 50 United States except Hawaii, which remains "rabies-free." Wildlife, including bats, raccoons, skunks, foxes, coyotes, bobcats, and mongoose, are the most important potential sources of infection for humans and domestic animals in the United States and its territories. Rabies in small rodents (squirrels, hamsters, guinea pigs, gerbils, chipmunks, rats, and mice) and lagomorphs (rabbits, pikas, and hares) is rare. Rabies may occur in woodchucks or other large rodents in areas where raccoon rabies is common. The virus is present in saliva and is transmitted by bites or, rarely, by contamination of mucosa or skin lesions by saliva or other potentially infectious material (eg, neural tissue). Worldwide, most rabies cases in humans result from dog bites in areas where canine rabies is enzootic. Most rabid dogs, cats, and ferrets shed virus for a few days before there are obvious signs of illness. No case of human rabies in the United States has been attributed to a dog, cat, or ferret that has remained healthy throughout the standard 10-day period of confinement after an exposure.

The **incubation period** in humans averages 1 to 3 months but ranges from days to years.

DIAGNOSTIC TESTS

Infection in animals can be diagnosed by demonstration of the presence of rabies virus antigen in brain tissue with a direct fluorescent antibody (DFA) test. Suspected rabid animals should be euthanized in a manner that preserves brain tissue for appropriate laboratory diagnosis. Virus can be isolated in suckling mice or in tissue culture from saliva, brain, and other specimens and can be detected by identification of viral antigens by immunofluorescence or immunoperoxidase staining or nucleotide sequences by reverse transcriptase–polymerase chain reaction (RT-PCR) in affected tissues. Diagnosis in suspected human cases can be made post-mortem by either immunofluorescent or immunohistochemical examination of brain tissue or by detection of viral nucleotide sequences; RT-PCR is performed together with DFA. Antemortem diagnosis can be made by DFA testing on skin biopsy specimens from the nape of the neck, by isolation of the virus from saliva, by detection of antibody in serum (neutralization or indirect fluorescent antibody methods are generally used) in unvaccinated people and in cerebrospinal fluid in all infected people, and by detection of viral nucleotide sequences in saliva, skin, or other tissues. RT-PCR assay plays a greater role in the diagnosis of rabies in such antemortem specimens in the absence of a brain biopsy specimen. No single test is sufficiently sensitive because of the unique nature of rabies pathobiology. State or local health departments should be consulted before submission of specimens to the Centers for Disease Control and Prevention. Consultation with public health authorities facilitates cases inconsistent with rabies to be identified before specimens are collected and enables appropriate collection and transport of materials to be arranged when rabies testing is indicated.

TREATMENT

There is no specific treatment. Once symptoms have developed, neither rabies vaccine nor rabies immune globulin improves the prognosis. A combination of sedation and intensive medical intervention may be valuable adjunctive therapy. Details of one management protocol used can be found at **www.mcw.edu/rabies.** Eleven people have survived rabies in association with incomplete rabies vaccine schedules. Eight people who had not received rabies postexposure prophylaxis survived rabies. Approximately half of survivors have normal cognition.

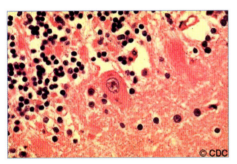

Image 117.1
Characteristic Negri bodies are present within a Purkinje cell of the cerebellum in this patient who died of rabies. Courtesy of Centers for Disease Control and Prevention.

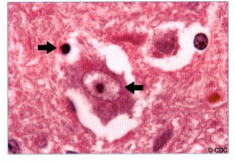

Image 117.2
Photomicrograph of brain tissue from a patient with rabies encephalitis (hematoxylin-eosin stain). Histopathologic brain tissue from a patient with rabies displaying the pathognomonic finding of Negri bodies (arrows) within the neuronal cytoplasm (hematoxylin-eosin stain). Courtesy of Centers for Disease Control and Prevention.

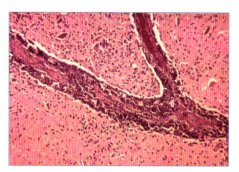

Image 117.3
This micrograph depicts the histopathologic changes associated with rabies encephalitis (hematoxylin-eosin stain). Note the perivascular cuffing caused by the accumulation of inflammatory cell infiltrates, including lymphocytes and polymorphonuclear leukocytes. Courtesy of Centers for Disease Control and Prevention.

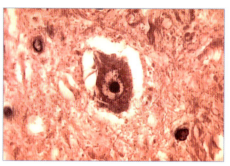

Image 117.4
This micrograph depicts the histopathologic changes associated with rabies encephalitis (hematoxylin-eosin stain). Note the Negri bodies, which are cellular inclusions found most frequently in the pyramidal cells of hippocampus proper and in the Purkinje cells of the cerebellum. They are also found in the cells of the medulla and various other ganglia. Courtesy of Centers for Disease Control and Prevention.

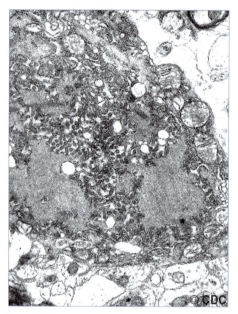

Image 117.5
Electron micrograph of the rabies virus. This electron micrograph shows the rabies virus as well as Negri bodies, or cellular inclusions. Courtesy of Centers for Disease Control and Prevention.

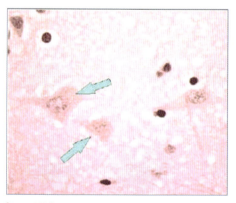

Image 117.6
Neurons without Negri bodies in hematoxylin-eosin–stained tissue. Courtesy of Centers for Disease Control and Prevention.

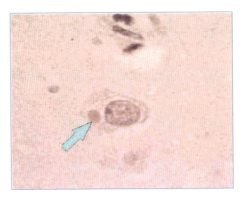

Image 117.7
Negri body in infected tissue in hematoxylin-eosin–stained tissue. Courtesy of Centers for Disease Control and Prevention.

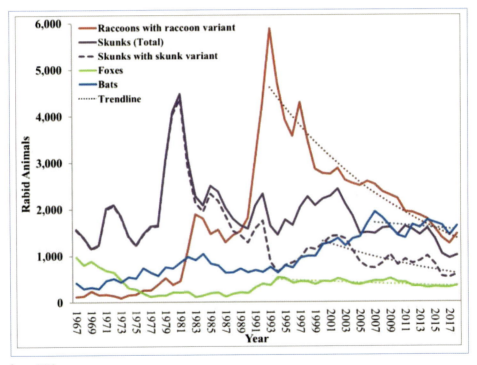

Image 117.8
Wild animals accounted for 92.7% of reported cases of rabies in 2018. Bats were the most frequently reported rabid wildlife species (33% of all animal cases during 2018), followed by raccoons (30.3%), skunks (20.3%), and foxes (7.2%). Courtesy of Centers for Disease Control and Prevention.

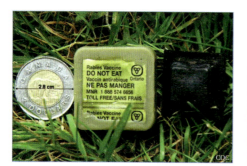

Image 117.9
Aerial distribution of rabies vaccine bait has been a feasible tactic for controlling rabies in foxes in some urban areas, including Toronto, Canada. Courtesy of Centers for Disease Control and Prevention/*Emerging Infectious Diseases* and R. C. Rosatte.

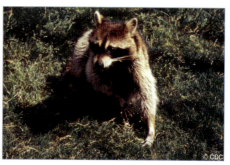

Image 117.10
Raccoons can be vectors of the rabies virus, transmitting the virus to humans and other animals. Rabies virus belongs to the order *Mononegavirales*. Raccoons continue to be the most frequently reported rabid wildlife species and involved 37.7% of all animal-transmitted cases during 2000. Courtesy of Centers for Disease Control and Prevention.

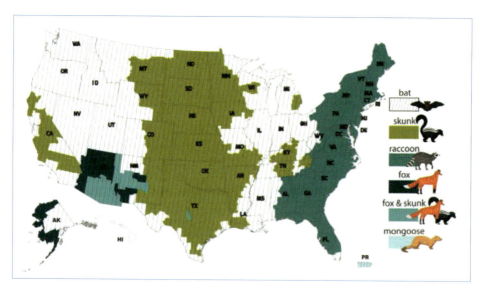

Image 117.11
Between 2013 and 2017, bats with rabies were found in every state except for Hawaii. Skunks with rabies have been found in parts of California, the Midwest, Texas, Kentucky, Virginia, North Carolina, and Tennessee. Raccoons with rabies have been found in the southern and eastern states. Foxes with rabies have been found in Alaska, Arizona, and New Mexico. Foxes and skunks with rabies have been found in Arizona, New Mexico, and Texas. Mongoose with rabies have been found in Puerto Rico. Courtesy of Centers for Disease Control and Prevention.

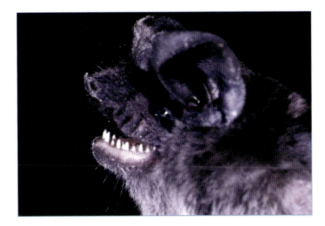

Image 117.12
This bat, *Artibeus jamaicensis*, is also known as the Jamaican fruit bat. Most of the recent human rabies cases in the United States have been caused by rabies virus that was transmitted through a bat vector. Courtesy of Centers for Disease Control and Prevention.

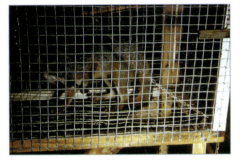

Image 117.13
This wild fox exhibited symptoms including agitation and excessive salivation and was diagnosed as having rabies. Courtesy of Centers for Disease Control and Prevention.

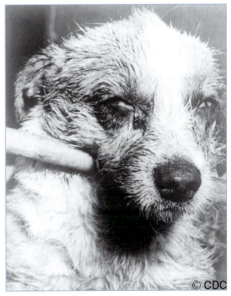

Image 117.14
Close-up of a dog's face during late-stage "dumb" (paralytic) rabies. Animals with dumb rabies appear depressed, lethargic, and uncoordinated. Gradually, they become completely paralyzed. When their throat and jaw muscles are paralyzed, the animals drool and have difficulty swallowing. Courtesy of Centers for Disease Control and Prevention.

CHAPTER 118
Rat-Bite Fever

CLINICAL MANIFESTATIONS

Rat-bite fever is caused by *Streptobacillus moniliformis* or *Spirillum minus*. *S moniliformis* infection (streptobacillary fever or Haverhill fever) is characterized by relapsing fever, rash, and migratory polyarthritis. There is an abrupt onset of fever, chills, muscle pain, vomiting, headache, and, rarely (unlike *S minus*), lymphadenopathy. A maculopapular, purpuric, or petechial rash develops, predominantly on the peripheral extremities including the palms and soles, typically within a few days of fever onset. The skin lesions may become purpuric or confluent and may desquamate. The bite site usually heals promptly and exhibits no or minimal inflammation. Nonsuppurative migratory polyarthritis or arthralgia follows in approximately 50% of patients. Symptoms of untreated infection may resolve within 2 weeks, but fever can occasionally relapse for weeks or months, and infection can lead to serious complications including soft tissue and solid organ abscesses (ie, brain, myocardium), septic arthritis, pneumonia, endocarditis, myocarditis, pericarditis, sepsis, and meningitis. The case-fatality rate is 7% to 13% in untreated patients, and fatal cases have been reported in children.

With *S minus* infection (sodoku), a period of initial apparent healing at the site of the bite is usually followed by fever and ulceration, discoloration, swelling, and pain at the site (approximately 1–4 weeks later), regional lymphangitis and lymphadenopathy, and a distinctive rash of red or purple plaques. Arthritis is rare.

ETIOLOGY

The causes of rat-bite fever are *S moniliformis*, a microaerophilic, facultatively anaerobic, gram-negative, pleomorphic bacillus, and *S minus*, a small gram-negative, spiral-shaped bacterium with bipolar flagellar tufts.

EPIDEMIOLOGY

Rat-bite fever is a zoonotic illness. The natural habitat of *S moniliformis* and *S minus* is the oropharynx and nasopharynx of rodents. *S moniliformis* is transmitted by bites or scratches from or exposure to oral secretions of infected rats (eg, kissing pet rodents), other rodents (eg, mice, gerbils, squirrels, weasels), and rodent-eating animals, including cats and dogs. Haverhill fever refers to infection after ingestion of unpasteurized milk, water, or food contaminated with urine containing *S moniliformis* and may be associated with an outbreak of disease. *S minus* is transmitted by bites of rats and mice. *S moniliformis* infection accounts for almost all cases of rat-bite fever in the United States; *S minus* infections occur primarily in Asia.

The **incubation period** for *S moniliformis* is usually less than 7 days but can range from 3 days to 3 weeks; for *S minus*, the **incubation period** is 7 to 21 days.

DIAGNOSTIC TESTS

S moniliformis is a fastidious, slow-growing organism isolated from blood, synovial fluid, abscesses, or aspirates from the bite lesion. Growth is best in bacteriologic media enriched with blood (15% rabbit blood seems optimal), serum, and ascitic fluid; cultures should be kept in 5% to 10% carbon dioxide atmosphere at 37 °C (99 °F). The laboratory should be alerted that *S moniliformis* is suspected and to hold the culture for at least 1 week. A nucleic acid amplification–based assay may be available in research laboratories. The use of 16S ribosomal RNA gene sequencing and MALDI-TOF (matrix-assisted laser desorption/ionization–time-of-flight) mass spectrometry improves the diagnostic sensitivity and specificity of culture-based practices.

S minus has not been recovered on artificial media but can be visualized by darkfield microscopy in wet mounts of blood, exudate of a lesion, and lymph nodes. Blood specimens should also be viewed with Giemsa or Wright stain.

TREATMENT

Penicillin G procaine administered intramuscularly or penicillin G administered intravenously for 7 to 10 days is the treatment of rat-bite fever caused by either agent; currently in the United States and other countries, intravenous administration is the more acceptable route. Initial intravenous penicillin G therapy for 5 to 7 days followed by oral penicillin V for 7 days has also been successful. Limited experience exists for ampicillin, cefuroxime, ceftriaxone, and cefotaxime. Doxycycline or streptomycin can be substituted when a patient has a serious allergy to penicillin. Patients with endocarditis should receive intravenous high-dose penicillin G for at least 4 weeks. The addition of streptomycin or gentamicin for initial therapy may be useful in severe infections including endocarditis.

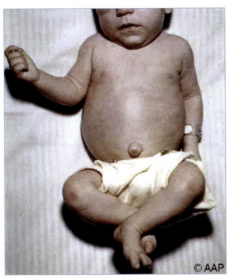

Image 118.1
The rash of rat-bite fever (*Streptobacillus moniliformis*) in an infant bitten by a rat on the right side of the face while sleeping.

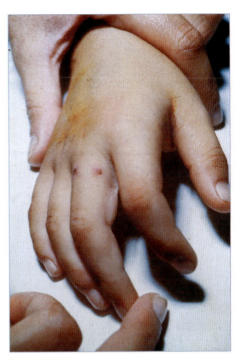

Image 118.2
Rat-bite wounds on the finger of a 5-year-old boy 12 hours after the bite appears noninflammatory. Because of fever, chills, headache, and rash 5 days later, blood cultures were obtained that grew *Streptobacillus moniliformis*. Courtesy of George Nankervis, MD.

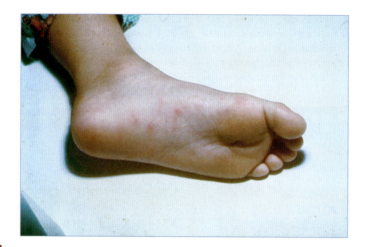

Image 118.3
Five days after being bitten by a rat, the child in Image 118.2 developed fever, chills, and headache, followed 5 days later by a papulovesicular rash on the hands and feet. *Streptobacillus moniliformis* was isolated from blood cultures, and the patient responded to intravenous penicillin therapy without complication. Courtesy of George Nankervis, MD.

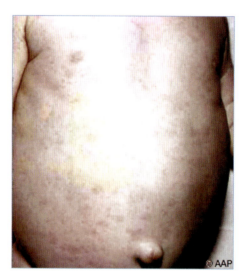

Image 118.4
Close-up view of the rash of the same infant as in Image 118.1, who was bitten on the right cheek by a rat. Sodoku, or rat-bite fever caused by *Spirillum minus*, rarely occurs in the United States.

CHAPTER 119

Respiratory Syncytial Virus

CLINICAL MANIFESTATIONS

Respiratory syncytial virus (RSV) causes acute respiratory tract infections in people of all ages and is one of the most common diseases of early childhood. Most infants infected with RSV experience upper respiratory tract symptoms, and 20% to 30% develop lower respiratory tract disease (eg, bronchiolitis and/or pneumonia) with the first infection. Signs and symptoms of bronchiolitis typically begin with rhinitis and cough, which may progress to increased respiratory effort with tachypnea, wheezing, rales, crackles, intercostal and/or subcostal retractions, grunting, and nasal flaring. Fever may occur. Infection with RSV during the first few weeks after birth, particularly in preterm neonates, may manifest with more general symptoms such as lethargy, irritability, and poor feeding, accompanied with minimal respiratory tract symptoms. However, these infants have risk for developing apnea, even in the absence of other respiratory symptoms.

Most previously healthy infants who develop RSV bronchiolitis do not require hospitalization, and most who are hospitalized improve with supportive care and are discharged after 2 or 3 days. However, approximately 1% to 3% of all children in the first 12 months after birth are hospitalized because of severe RSV lower respiratory tract disease, with the highest rate of RSV hospitalizations occurring in the first 6 months after birth. Factors that increase the risk of severe RSV lower respiratory tract illness include preterm birth, especially of infants born before 29 weeks of gestation; chronic lung disease of prematurity (formerly called *bronchopulmonary dysplasia*); certain types of hemodynamically significant congenital heart disease, especially conditions associated with pulmonary hypertension; certain immunodeficiency states; and neurological and neuromuscular conditions. Identified risk factors with a more limited correlation with disease severity include low birth weight, maternal smoking during pregnancy, exposure to secondhand smoke in the household, family history of atopy, lack of breastfeeding, and household crowding. Mortality is rare when supportive care is available.

The association between RSV infection early in life and subsequent asthma remains incompletely understood. Infants who experience severe lower respiratory tract disease (eg, bronchiolitis, pneumonia) from RSV have an increased risk for developing asthma later in life. This association is also found with other respiratory viral infections, particularly those caused by rhinoviruses. The unresolved question is whether the association between severe infection and reactive airway disease is causal and attributable to direct damage caused by viral replication and the host response. Alternatively, the association may reflect a common genotype, indicating that the same anatomical or immunologic abnormalities that predispose to asthma also predispose to severe viral lower respiratory tract disease. Results from 2 randomized, placebo-controlled trials demonstrate that providing RSV immunoprophylaxis to full-term and preterm infants had no measurable effect on medically attended wheezing, physician-diagnosed asthma, or lung function at 3 to 6 years of age.

Almost all children are infected by RSV at least once by 24 months of age, and reinfection throughout life is common. Subsequent infections are usually less severe than a primary infection. Particularly in otherwise healthy older children and adults, recurrent RSV infection manifests as mild upper respiratory tract illness and seldom involves the lower respiratory tract. However, serious disease involving the lower respiratory tract may develop in older children and adults, especially in immunocompromised people and frail, elderly people, particularly those with cardiopulmonary comorbidities.

ETIOLOGY

RSV is an enveloped, nonsegmented, negative-strand RNA virus of the genus *Orthopneumovirus* of the family *Pneumoviridae*. Human RSV exists as 2 antigenic subgroups, A and B, and often these co-circulate during the same RSV season. A consistent correlation between RSV subgroup and disease severity is unclear. The RSV envelope contains 3 surface glycoproteins: glycoprotein G, fusion protein F, and a small hydrophobic protein. Antibodies directed against F and G are protective and neutralizing. G glycoprotein is involved in viral attachment to the cell and assists in the ability of the virus to evade host immunity. F protein enables viral penetration of the epithelial cell once viral attachment occurs.

EPIDEMIOLOGY

Humans are the only source of infection. RSV is usually transmitted by direct or close contact with contaminated secretions, which may occur from exposure to large-particle droplets at short distances (typically <2 m [6 ft]) or by self-inoculation after touching contaminated surfaces or fomites. Viable RSV can persist on environmental surfaces for several hours and for 30 minutes or more on hands.

RSV occurs in annual epidemics, generally beginning in fall and continuing through early spring in temperate climates. Spread among households and people in child care facilities, including adults, is common. Spread can also occur in the health care setting. The usual period of viral shedding is 3 to 8 days, but it may be longer, especially in young infants and immunosuppressed children, whose shedding may continue for 3 to 4 weeks or longer.

The **incubation period** ranges from 2 to 8 days; 4 to 6 days is most common.

DIAGNOSTIC TESTS

For many years, laboratory diagnosis of RSV respiratory tract disease required viral isolation in cell culture. Although cell culture is still used, this approach requires a specialized laboratory and several days of incubation before characteristic cytopathic changes (syncytia formation) are observed. Centrifugation-enhanced, shell vial techniques shorten the time to results to 24 to 48 hours. Rapid diagnostic assays, including direct fluorescent antibody assays and enzyme or chromatographic immunoassays, are available for detection of viral antigen in nasopharyngeal specimens and are reliable in infants and young children. Sensitivity in older children and adults is lower, because less virus is shed in the upper airways. As with all antigen detection assays, the predictive value is high during the peak season, but false-positive test results are more likely to occur when the incidence of disease is low, such as in the summer in temperate areas.

Molecular diagnostic tests via reverse transcriptase–polymerase chain reaction (RT-PCR) assays have largely replaced both culture and antigen detection assays. Some commercially available assays are designed as multiplex assays to facilitate testing for multiple respiratory viruses from a single nasopharyngeal specimen. Some complex multiplex tests can distinguish between RSV A and B subgroups. With RT-PCR assays, as many as 30% of symptomatic children demonstrate the presence of a viral coinfection with 2 or more viruses. Whether symptomatic children who are coinfected with more than one virus experience more severe or even less severe disease is unclear.

In most outpatient settings for children with bronchiolitis, routine specific respiratory viral testing has little effect on management and is not recommended. For hospitalized children with bronchiolitis, testing for viral etiology is not routinely recommended. However, if patient cohorts are necessary, identification of the specific viral etiology of a respiratory infection will aid hospital infection prevention efforts.

TREATMENT

No available treatment shortens the course of bronchiolitis or hastens the resolution of symptoms. Treatment of young children hospitalized with bronchiolitis is supportive and should include hydration, careful assessment of respiratory status, and suction of the upper airway, as necessary. Supplemental oxygen is recommended only when oxyhemoglobin saturation persistently decreases below 90% in a previously healthy infant. Nasal continuous positive airway pressure and heliox have been used for respiratory support in hospitalized infants with bronchiolitis.

Early studies with aerosolized ribavirin therapy demonstrated a small increase in oxygen saturation in small clinical trials; however, a decrease in the need for mechanical ventilation or a decrease in the length of stay was not shown. Because of limited evidence for a clinically relevant benefit, potential toxic effects, and high cost, routine use of aerosolized ribavirin is not recommended.

α- and β-Adrenergic Agents

β-Adrenergic agents are not recommended for care of wheezing associated with RSV bronchiolitis, and a trial of albuterol is no longer recommended as an option in the management of RSV bronchiolitis. Evidence does not support the use of nebulized epinephrine in children hospitalized with bronchiolitis. Insufficient data are available to recommend routine use of epinephrine for outpatient treatment of children with bronchiolitis.

Glucocorticoid Therapy

Controlled clinical trials in children with bronchiolitis have demonstrated that corticosteroids do not reduce hospital admissions and do not reduce length of stay for inpatients. Corticosteroid treatment should not be used for infants and children with RSV bronchiolitis.

Antimicrobial Therapy

Antimicrobial therapy is not indicated for infants with RSV bronchiolitis or pneumonia unless there is evidence of concurrent bacterial infection. A young child with a distinct viral lower respiratory tract infection (bronchiolitis) has a low risk (<1%) of bacterial infection of the cerebrospinal fluid or blood. Bacterial lung infections and bacteremia are uncommon in this setting. Acute otitis media caused by RSV or bacterial superinfection may occur in infants with RSV bronchiolitis. Oral antimicrobial therapy for treatment of otitis media may be considered if bulging of the tympanic membrane is present.

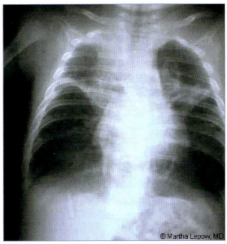

Image 119.1
Respiratory syncytial virus bronchiolitis and pneumonia. Note the bilateral infiltrates and striking hyperaeration. Copyright Martha Lepow, MD.

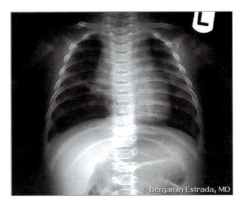

Image 119.2
An anteroposterior radiograph of a 2-month-old girl with respiratory syncytial virus bronchiolitis. Note the wide intercostal spaces, hyperaeration of the lung fields, and flattening of the diaphragm. Courtesy of Benjamin Estrada, MD.

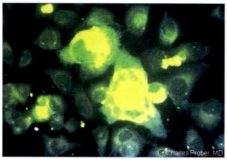

Image 119.3
Direct fluorescent antibody staining of respiratory syncytial virus in cell culture. Copyright Charles Prober, MD.

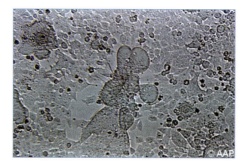

Image 119.4
The characteristic cytopathic effect of respiratory syncytial virus in tissue culture includes the formation of large multinucleated syncytial cells.

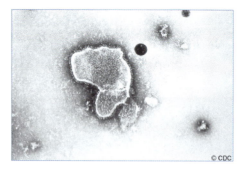

Image 119.5
Electron micrograph of a respiratory syncytial virus. The virion is variable in shape and size (average diameter between 120 and 300 nm). Respiratory syncytial virus is the most common cause of bronchiolitis and pneumonia in infants <1 year of age. Courtesy of Centers for Disease Control and Prevention.

CHAPTER 120

Rhinovirus Infections

CLINICAL MANIFESTATIONS

Rhinoviruses (RVs) are the most frequent cause of the common cold, or rhinosinusitis. Typical clinical manifestations include sore throat, nasal congestion, and nasal discharge that is initially watery and clear but often becomes mucopurulent and viscous after a few days. Malaise, headache, myalgia, low-grade fever, cough, and sneezing may occur. Symptoms typically peak in severity after 2 to 3 days and have a median duration of 7 days but may persist for more than 10 days in approximately 25% of illnesses. Rhinoviruses also cause otitis media and lower respiratory tract infections (eg, bronchiolitis, pneumonia), particularly in infants, and are associated with approximately 60% to 70% of acute exacerbations of asthma in school-aged children.

ETIOLOGY

Rhinoviruses are small, nonenveloped, single, positive-stranded RNA viruses classified into 3 species (RV-A, RV-B, and RV-C) in the family *Picornaviridae*, genus *Enterovirus*. More than 160 RV types have been identified by immunologic and molecular methods. Infection confers type-specific immunity, but protection is temporary.

EPIDEMIOLOGY

Rhinovirus infection is ubiquitous in human populations. Children have an average of 2 RV infections each year, and 93% of adults experience at least 1 RV infection annually. Rhinoviruses cause approximately two-thirds of cases of the common cold and, thus, are responsible for more episodes of human illness than any other infectious agent. They can cause sinusitis and otitis media, either as the sole pathogen or with secondary bacterial infections. Rhinovirus infections are a major viral cause of exacerbations of asthma, cystic fibrosis, and chronic obstructive pulmonary disease and have been detected in lower respiratory tract infections in patients of all ages hospitalized with wheezing or pneumonia.

Person-to-person transmission occurs predominantly by self-inoculation by contaminated secretions on hands or by large-particle aerosol spread. Infections occur throughout the year, but peak activity occurs during autumn and spring. Multiple types circulate simultaneously, and the prevalent types circulating in a given population change from season to season. Viral shedding in nasopharyngeal secretions is most abundant during the first 2 to 3 days of infection and usually ceases by 7 to 10 days. Viral RNA may be detectable in nasal secretions by molecular testing for as long as 30 days, although low amounts of virus detected by polymerase chain reaction (PCR) assay in an asymptomatic person are unlikely to result in transmission.

The **incubation period** is usually 2 to 3 days.

DIAGNOSTIC TESTS

Rhinovirus infection is diagnosed by detection of virus in respiratory secretions. Reverse transcriptase–PCR assays are the preferred method to identify RV infections. Most of these assays are designed as multiplexed tests that detect a wide variety of viral and, in some cases, bacterial respiratory pathogens. In general, these assays cannot clearly distinguish RVs from enteroviruses because of the genetic similarity of the 2 groups. Given the prevalence of RV infection and the occurrence of shedding following infection, RV detection, even in symptomatic patients, may not be causal.

TREATMENT

Treatment is supportive. Antimicrobial agents should not be used for prevention of secondary bacterial infection, because their use may promote the emergence of resistant bacteria and subsequently complicate treatment of a bacterial infection and because there is risk of antibiotic-associated adverse effects.

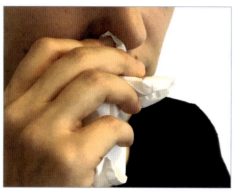

Image 120.1
Rhinoviruses are the most frequent cause of the common cold. Typical clinical manifestations include sore throat, nasal congestion, and nasal discharge. Courtesy of National Institute of Allergy and Infectious Diseases.

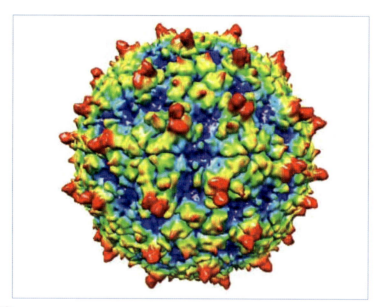

Image 120.2
The structure of a rhinovirus C, showing the spikelike fingers in red. Rhinovirus C, along with rhinoviruses A and B, is a leading cause of common colds. These viruses can also cause severe respiratory infections in infants and young children and cause serious illness for those with asthma and other chronic respiratory conditions. Courtesy of the National Institutes of Health.

CHAPTER 121

Rickettsial Diseases

Rickettsial diseases comprise infections caused by bacterial species of the genera *Rickettsia* (endemic and epidemic typhus and spotted fever group rickettsioses), *Orientia* (scrub typhus), *Ehrlichia* (ehrlichiosis), *Anaplasma* (anaplasmosis), *Neoehrlichia*, and *Neorickettsia*. The genus *Rickettsia* is further divided into 4 groups on the basis of serological and genomic analysis: typhus group, spotted fever group, ancestral group, and transitional group.

CLINICAL MANIFESTATIONS

Early signs and symptoms can be nonspecific and often mimic viral illness. Rickettsial infections have many features in common. Fever, rash (especially in spotted fever and typhus group rickettsiae), headache, myalgia, and respiratory symptoms are prominent features. The classic rash of Rocky Mountain spotted fever (RMSF) may not appear until 3 to 5 days after onset of symptoms, and approximately 10% of patients do not develop an identifiable rash. One or more inoculation eschars occur with many rickettsial diseases, especially most spotted fever group rickettsioses, rickettsialpox, and scrub typhus. Systemic endothelial damage of small blood vessels resulting in increased vascular permeability is the hallmark pathological feature of most severe spotted fever and typhus group rickettsial infections. Some rickettsial diseases, particularly RMSF and Mediterranean spotted fever, can rapidly become life threatening. Risk factors for severe disease include glucose-6-phosphate dehydrogenase deficiency, male sex, and antecedent exposure to sulfonamides.

Immunity against reinfection by the same agent after natural infection is not well studied, but some anecdotal information suggests that prior infection confers immunity for at least 1 year. Documented reinfections with *Rickettsia* and *Ehrlichia* species have been described only rarely.

ETIOLOGY

Rickettsiae are small coccobacillary gram-negative bacteria that are obligate intracellular pathogens and cannot be grown in cell-free media. *Orientia* and *Rickettsia* organisms reside free within the cytoplasm, and *Anaplasmataceae* organisms reside in phagosomes. Currently recognized rickettsial pathogens of humans include more than 20 species of *Rickettsia*, 5 species of *Ehrlichia*, 2 species each of *Orientia* and *Anaplasma*, and *Neorickettsia sennetsu*. Tickborne neoehrlichiosis caused by *Candidatus Neoehrlichia mikurensis*, which features rodents as the primary host, is an emerging disease in Asia and Europe.

EPIDEMIOLOGY

Rickettsial diseases have various hematophagous arthropod vectors that include ticks, fleas, mites, and lice. Except for *Rickettsia prowazekii*, the cause of epidemic typhus, humans are incidental hosts for rickettsial pathogens. Rickettsial life cycles typically involve one or more arthropod species as well as various mammalian reservoirs or amplifying hosts, and transmission to humans occurs during environmental or occupational exposures to infected arthropods. Geographic and seasonal occurrences of each rickettsial disease are related directly to distributions and life cycles of the specific vector.

Incubation periods vary according to organism.

Other Global Rickettsial Spotted Fever Infections

A number of other epidemiologically distinct fleaborne and tickborne spotted fever infections caused by rickettsiae have been recognized. These diseases may affect people living in, traveling to, or returning from areas where these agents are endemic. These infections have clinical and pathological features that vary widely in severity. Many manifest with an eschar at the site of the tick bite and without rash. Causative agents of spotted fevers in the United States and of other rickettsial diseases most important for travelers include

- *Rickettsia africae*, the causative agent of African tick–bite fever that is endemic in sub-Saharan Africa, Oceania, and some Caribbean islands

- *Rickettsia akari*, the causative agent of rickettsialpox, which occurs sporadically throughout the United States but is often reported from the Northeast, particularly New York City

- *Rickettsia conorii* and subspecies, the causative agents of Mediterranean spotted fever, India tick typhus, Israeli tick typhus, and Astrakhan spotted fever, that are endemic in southern Europe, Africa, the Middle East, and the Indian subcontinent
- *Rickettsia parkeri*, a causative agent of eschar-associated infections in the Americas
- *Rickettsia* species 364D, the causative agent of eschar, headache, and fever in California (Pacific coast tick fever)

DIAGNOSTIC TESTS

Group-specific antibodies are detectable in the serum of most patients by 7 to 10 days after onset of illness, but slower antibody responses may occur, particularly in some diseases of lesser severity, such as African tick–bite fever. The utility of serological testing during the acute illness is generally of limited value, and a negative serological test result during the initial stage of the illness should never be used to exclude a diagnosis of rickettsial disease. Serological assays provide an excellent method of retrospective confirmation when paired serum samples collected during the illness and 2 to 6 weeks later are tested in tandem. The indirect immunofluorescent antibody assay is recommended in most circumstances but cannot determine the causative agent to the species level. Treatment early in the course of illness can blunt or delay serological responses. Polymerase chain reaction (PCR) assays can detect rickettsiae in whole blood or tissues collected during the acute stage of illness and before administration of antimicrobial agents; availability of these tests is often limited to reference and research laboratories. Immunohistochemical staining and PCR testing of skin biopsy specimens from patients with rash or eschar lesions can help diagnose rickettsial infections early in the course of disease. PCR assays and sequencing of DNA collected during acute infection provide more accurate identification of the etiologic agent than serological testing.

TREATMENT

Prompt initiation of treatment is indicated for all patients in all age-groups with presumptive evidence of any rickettsial disease and is of paramount importance when there is clinical suspicion of a potentially life-threatening infection such as RMSF, ehrlichiosis, epidemic typhus, murine typhus, or scrub typhus. Treatment decisions should be made on the basis of clinical findings and epidemiological data and should never be delayed until test results are known. Therapy is less effective in preventing complications when disease remains untreated into the second week of illness. For all ages, the drug of choice for all rickettsioses, including RMSF and ehrlichiosis, is doxycycline, and the treatment course is generally 7 to 14 days.

CHAPTER 122

Rickettsialpox

CLINICAL MANIFESTATIONS

Rickettsialpox is a febrile, eschar-associated illness characterized by generalized, relatively sparse, erythematous, papulovesicular eruptions on the trunk, face, extremities (less often on the palms and soles), and oral mucous membranes. The rash develops 1 to 4 days after onset of fever and 3 to 10 days after appearance of an eschar at the site of the bite of an infected house mouse mite. Regional lymph nodes in the area of the inoculation eschar typically become enlarged. Without specific antimicrobial therapy, systemic disease lasts approximately 7 to 14 days; manifestations include fever, headache, malaise, and myalgia. Less frequent manifestations include anorexia, vomiting, conjunctivitis, hepatitis, nuchal rigidity, and photophobia. The disease is milder than Rocky Mountain spotted fever (RMSF), and although no rickettsialpox-associated deaths have been described, disease is occasionally severe enough to warrant hospitalization.

ETIOLOGY

Rickettsialpox is caused by *Rickettsia akari*, a gram-negative intracellular bacillus now classified along with *Rickettsia felis* and *Rickettsia australis* within the transitional group, which has features of both the spotted fever and typhus groups.

EPIDEMIOLOGY

The natural host for *R akari* in the United States is *Mus musculus*, the common house mouse. The organism is transmitted by the house mouse mite, *Liponyssoides sanguineus*. Disease risk is heightened in areas infested with house mice. The disease can occur wherever the hosts, pathogens, and humans coexist but is most frequently reported in large urban settings. In the United States, rickettsialpox has been described predominantly in northeastern metropolitan centers, especially in New York City. It has been confirmed in many other countries, including the Netherlands, Croatia, Ukraine, Turkey, Russia, South Korea, South Africa, and Mexico. All age-groups can be affected. No seasonal pattern of disease occurs.

The disease is not communicable but occurs occasionally in families or people cohabiting in a house mouse mite–infested dwelling.

The **incubation period** is 6 to 15 days.

DIAGNOSTIC TESTS

R akari can be isolated in cell culture from blood and eschar biopsy specimens during the acute stage of disease, but culture is not attempted routinely. Because antigens of *R akari* have extensive cross-reactivity with antigens of *Rickettsia rickettsii* (the cause of RMSP) and other spotted fever–group rickettsiae, an indirect immunofluorescent antibody assay for *R rickettsii* can be used to demonstrate a 4-fold or greater change in antibody titers between acute and convalescent serum specimens taken 2 to 6 weeks apart. Use of *R akari* antigen is recommended for a more accurate serological diagnosis but may be available only in specialized research laboratories. Immunoglobulin M and immunoglobulin G are detected 7 to 15 days after illness onset. Immunohistochemical testing of formalin-fixed, paraffin-embedded eschars or papulovesicle biopsy specimens can detect rickettsiae in the samples and are useful diagnostic techniques, but because of antigenic cross-reactivity, these assays are not able to confirm the etiologic agent. A polymerase chain reaction assay for detection of rickettsial DNA with subsequent sequence identification can confirm *R akari* infection but is currently not cleared by the US Food and Drug Administration for use in the United States.

TREATMENT

Doxycycline is the drug of choice in all age-groups. The minimum course of therapy is 5 days. Doxycycline shortens the course of disease, and symptoms typically resolve within 12 to 48 hours after initiation of therapy. Chloramphenicol is an alternative drug but carries a risk of serious adverse events and is not available as an oral formulation in the United States. Use of chloramphenicol should be considered only in rare cases, such as for patients with an absolute contraindication to receiving doxycycline, because rickettsialpox is usually mild and self-limited. Untreated rickettsialpox usually resolves within 2 weeks.

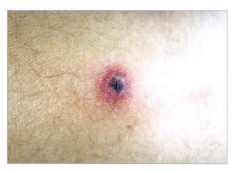

Image 122.1
Eschar on the posterior right calf of patient with rickettsialpox. This type of lesion is not encountered with Rocky Mountain spotted fever. Courtesy of *Emerging Infectious Diseases*.

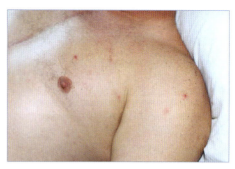

Image 122.2
Multiple papulovesicular lesions involving the upper trunk of a patient with rickettsialpox. Courtesy of *Emerging Infectious Diseases*.

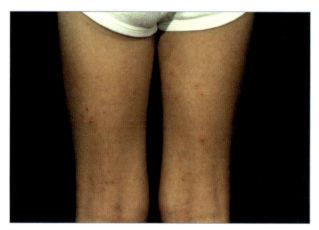

Image 122.3
Rickettsialpox on the legs. Copyright James Brien, DO.

CHAPTER 123

Rocky Mountain Spotted Fever

CLINICAL MANIFESTATIONS

Rocky Mountain spotted fever (RMSF) is a systemic, small-vessel vasculitis that often involves a characteristic rash. High fever, myalgia, headache (less commonly reported in young children), nausea, vomiting, and malaise are typical manifesting symptoms. Abdominal pain and diarrhea can be present and obscure the diagnosis. The rash usually begins within the first 2 to 4 days of symptoms; a faint maculopapular rash appears on the wrists and ankles and then spreads centripetally to include the trunk. The rash associated with RMSF can also involve the palms and soles. Although development of a rash is a useful diagnostic sign, the early rash may be faint, and rash can be absent altogether in up to 10% of patients. As the rash progresses, it becomes petechial, a sign reflective of the small-vessel vasculitis and indicative of progression to severe disease. Delayed onset or atypical appearance of the rash is a risk factor for misdiagnosis and poor outcome. Meningismus, altered mental status, and coma may occur. Children may experience peripheral or periorbital edema. Thrombocytopenia, elevated liver aminotransferase levels, and hyponatremia (serum sodium concentrations <130 mg/dL are observed in 20%–50% of cases) are the laboratory abnormalities measured most frequently and worsen as disease progresses. White blood cell count is often normal until later stages of disease, but leukopenia and anemia can occur. Patients treated early in the course of symptoms may have a mild illness, with fever resolving in the first 48 hours of treatment. If appropriate antimicrobial treatment is not initiated or is delayed past the fifth day of symptoms, the illness can be severe, with prominent central nervous system, cardiac, pulmonary, gastrointestinal tract, and renal involvement; disseminated intravascular coagulation; necrosis of digits and gangrene; and shock leading to death. RMSF can progress rapidly, even in previously healthy people. Case-fatality rates of untreated RMSF range from 20% to 80%, with a median time to death of 8 days. Significant long-term sequelae can occur in patients with severe RMSF, even if treated with appropriate antibiotics; these include neurological (paraparesis, hearing loss, peripheral neuropathy, bladder and bowel incontinence, developmental and language delays, and cerebellar, vestibular, and motor dysfunction) and non-neurological (disability from limb or digit amputation) sequelae.

ETIOLOGY

Rickettsia rickettsii, an obligate intracellular gram-negative bacillus and a member of the spotted fever group of rickettsiae, is the causative agent. The primary targets of infection in mammalian hosts are endothelial cells lining the small blood vessels of all major tissues and organs. Diffuse small-vessel vasculitis leads to poor perfusion, infarction, and increased permeability.

EPIDEMIOLOGY

The pathogen is transmitted to humans by the bite of a tick of the *Ixodidae* family (hard ticks). The principal recognized vectors of *R rickettsii* are *Dermacentor variabilis* (the American dog tick) in the eastern and central United States and *Dermacentor andersoni* (the Rocky Mountain wood tick) in the northern and western United States. Another emergent vector is *Rhipicephalus sanguineus* (the brown dog tick), which feeds on dogs and has been confirmed as a vector of *R rickettsii* in Arizona and Mexico and may play a role in other regions. Ticks and their small mammal hosts serve as reservoirs of the pathogen in nature. Other wild animals and dogs have been found with antibodies to *R rickettsii*, but their role as natural reservoirs is unclear. People with occupational or recreational exposure to the tick vector (eg, pet owners, animal handlers, and people who spend more time outdoors) have increased risk for exposure to the organism. People of all ages can be infected. The period of highest incidence in the United States is from April to September, although RMSF can occur year round in certain areas with endemic disease. Laboratory-acquired infection is rare. Transmission has occurred on rare occasions by blood transfusion. RMSF is the most severe and frequently fatal rickettsial illness in the United States.

Spotted fever rickettsiosis (SFR) is widespread in the United States, with most cases reported in the south Atlantic, southeastern, and south-central states. The southwestern United States is reporting increasing amounts of SFR, which is largely believed to be RMSF. During 2016 to 2017, reported cases of SFR increased 46% from 4,269 to 6,248 cases. It is unknown how many of those cases are RMSF.

The **incubation period** is approximately 1 week (typical range, 3–12 days).

DIAGNOSTIC TESTS

The diagnosis of RMSF must be made on the basis of clinical signs and symptoms and can be confirmed later by using diagnostic tests. Treatment should never be delayed while awaiting laboratory confirmation or because of lack of history of tick bite: approximately half of RMSF patients do not report tick bite. The gold standard confirmatory test is indirect immunofluorescent antibody to *R rickettsii* antigen. Both immunoglobulin G (IgG) and immunoglobulin M (IgM) antibodies begin to increase around 7 to 10 days after onset of symptoms; IgM is a less specific test, and IgG is the preferred test. Confirmation requires a 4-fold or greater increase in antigen-specific IgG between acute (first 1–2 weeks of illness while symptomatic) and convalescent (2–4 weeks later) sera. An elevated acute titer may represent prior exposure rather than acute infection, and a negative serological test result in the acute phase does not rule out diagnosis of RMSF. Cross-reactivity may be observed between antibodies to other spotted fever group rickettsiae, including *Rickettsia parkeri* and *Rickettsia africae*. Enzyme-linked immunosorbent assays can also be used for assessing antibody presence in acute and convalescent sera but are less useful for quantifying changes in titer values.

RMSF may be diagnosed by detection of *R rickettsii* DNA in acute whole blood, tissue, and serum specimens by polymerase chain reaction (PCR) assay. *R rickettsii* does not typically circulate in large numbers in whole blood until advanced stages of disease; assays relying on detection of DNA may lack sensitivity, and a negative result does not rule out RMSF. Specimens used for PCR assay should be obtained before doxycycline administration when possible. Diagnosis may be confirmed by detection of rickettsial DNA in biopsy or autopsy specimens by PCR assay or immunohistochemical visualization of rickettsiae in tissues.

R rickettsii may also be isolated from acute blood specimens or through tissue culture, but culture requires specialized procedures (not routine blood culture). Cell culture cultivation of the organism must be confirmed by molecular methods.

TREATMENT

Doxycycline is the drug of choice for treatment of RMSF in patients of any age and should be started as soon as RMSF is suspected. Physicians should treat empirically if RMSF is being considered and should not postpone treatment while awaiting laboratory confirmation. The doxycycline dose for RMSF is 2.2 mg/kg of body weight per dose, twice daily, orally or intravenously (maximum 100 mg per dose); the adult dose is 100 mg, twice daily. Treatment is most effective if initiated in the first 5 days of symptoms, and treatment started after that time is less likely to prevent death or other adverse outcomes. Antimicrobial treatment should be continued until the patient has been afebrile for at least 3 days and has demonstrated clinical improvement; the usual duration of therapy is 5 to 7 days but may be longer in severe cases. Chloramphenicol can be found in some references as an alternative treatment; however, its use is associated with a higher risk of fatal outcome. In the case of severe doxycycline allergy, a specialist should be consulted to discuss risks, benefits, and alternatives.

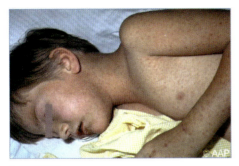

Image 123.1
Rocky Mountain spotted fever in an 8-year-old boy. Sixth day of rash without treatment.

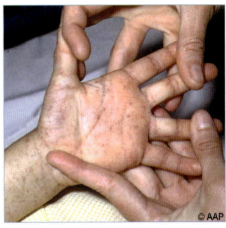

Image 123.2
Rocky Mountain spotted fever. Sixth day of rash without treatment. This is the same patient as in Image 123.1.

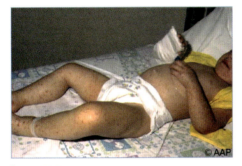

Image 123.3
A 2-year-old boy with obtundation, disorientation, and petechial rash of Rocky Mountain spotted fever, with facial and generalized edema secondary to generalized vasculitis. Rocky Mountain spotted fever is the most severe and frequently reported rickettsial illness in the United States.

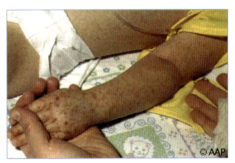

Image 123.4
This is the same patient as in Image 123.3, showing petechial rash and edema of the upper extremity. The rickettsiae multiply in the endothelial cells of small blood vessels, resulting in vasculitis.

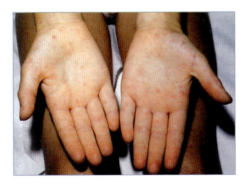

Image 123.5
This 8-year-old girl presented with a history of "chickenpox" for 11 days. She had numerous lesions on her chest, face, arms, and proximal legs. There were subcutaneous erythematous lesions on the hands, and she had 5 or 6 lesions on her feet. The diagnosis of Rocky Mountain spotted fever was confirmed serologically, and she was treated without any complications. Courtesy of Neal Halsey, MD.

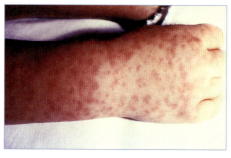

Image 123.6
A child's right hand and wrist displaying the spotted rash and edema of Rocky Mountain spotted fever. Courtesy of Centers for Disease Control and Prevention.

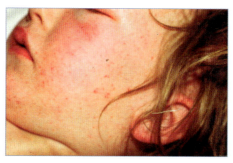

Image 123.7
A 7-year-old girl with severe Rocky Mountain spotted fever. Note the rash and edema secondary to diffuse vasculitis. Courtesy of Larry Frenkel, MD.

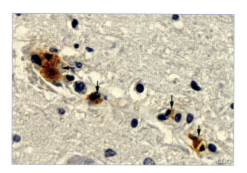

Image 123.8
Immunohistochemical analysis shows the presence of spotted fever group rickettsiae (brown; arrows) in vessels of the brain of a patient with fatal Rocky Mountain spotted fever (magnification ×400). Courtesy of Centers for Disease Control and Prevention/*Emerging Infectious Diseases* and Marylin Hidalgo.

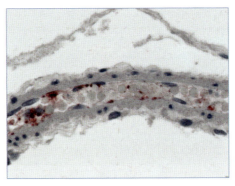

Image 123.9
Immunohistochemical staining of *Rickettsia rickettsii* in vascular endothelial cells in the cerebellum of a child with fatal Rocky Mountain spotted fever. Immunoalkaline phosphatase with naphthol fast red and hematoxylin counterstain (original magnification ×158). Courtesy of Christopher Paddock, MD.

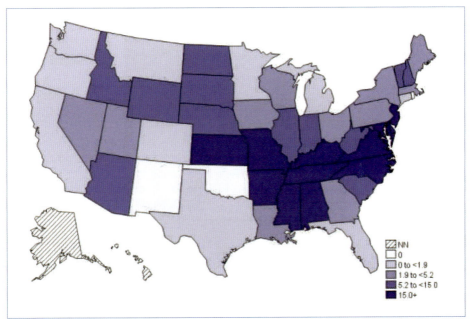

Image 123.10
Annual incidence (per million population) of reported spotted fever rickettsiosis—United States, 2019. NN indicates not notifiable. Courtesy of Centers for Disease Control and Prevention.

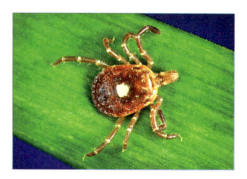

Image 123.11
This is a female lone star tick, *Amblyomma americanum*, and is found in the southeastern and mid-Atlantic United States. This tick is a vector of several zoonotic diseases, including human monocytic ehrlichiosis and Rocky Mountain spotted fever. Courtesy of Centers for Disease Control and Prevention.

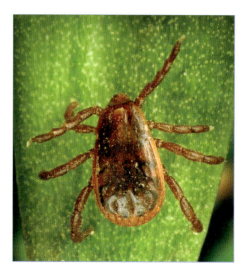

Image 123.12
This image depicts a male brown dog tick, *Rhipicephalus sanguineus*, from a superior, or dorsal, view looking down on this hard tick's scutum, which entirely covers its back, identifying it as a male. In the female, the dorsal abdomen is only partially covered, thereby offering room for abdominal expansion when she becomes engorged with blood while ingesting her blood meal obtained from her host. Courtesy of Centers for Disease Control and Prevention/James Gathany; William Nicholson.

CHAPTER 124
Rotavirus Infections

CLINICAL MANIFESTATIONS

The clinical manifestations vary and depend on whether it is the first infection or reinfection. After 3 months of age, the first infection is generally the most severe. Infection begins with acute onset of vomiting followed 24 to 48 hours later by watery diarrhea; up to one-third of patients have high fevers. Symptoms usually last for 3 to 7 days but improve over time. In moderate to severe cases or with prolonged diarrhea, dehydration, electrolyte abnormalities, and acidosis may occur. In certain immunocompromised children, including children with congenital cellular immunodeficiencies or severe combined immunodeficiency and children with hematopoietic stem cell or solid organ transplants, severe, prolonged, and sometimes fatal rotavirus diarrhea may occur. The presence of rotavirus RNA in cerebrospinal fluid has been detected in children with rotavirus-associated seizures.

ETIOLOGY

Rotaviruses are segmented, nonenveloped, double-stranded RNA viruses belonging to the family *Reoviridae*, with at least 10 distinct groups (A–J). Group A viruses are the major causes of human disease, although rotaviruses of groups B and C have also been associated with acute gastroenteritis. A binomial genotyping system, Gx-P[x], based on the 2 outer capsid viral proteins, VP7 glycoprotein (G) and VP4 protease-cleaved protein (P), is being replaced with an 11-gene typing system where the notation Gx-P[x]-Ix-Rx-Cx-Mx-Ax-Nx-Tx-Ex-Hx indicates the genotypes of the 6 structural viral proteins (ie, VP7, VP4, VP6, VP1, VP2, VP3) and the 6 nonstructural proteins (ie, NSP1, NSP2, NSP3, NSP4, NSP5/6), respectively. Before introduction of the rotavirus vaccine, genotypes G1P[8], G2P[4], G3P[8], G4P[8], and G9P[8] were the most common genotypes circulating in the United States. However, since 2012, G12P[8] has been the most common genotype identified.

EPIDEMIOLOGY

Rotavirus is present in high titer in stools of infected patients several days before and may continue for at least 10 days after onset of clinical disease. A small inoculum (100 colony-forming units/g) is needed for transmission, which occurs via the fecal-oral route. Rotavirus can remain viable for weeks to months on contaminated environmental surfaces and fomites (such as toys), which can also lead to transmission. Airborne droplet transmission has not been proven but may play a minor role in disease transmission. Spread within families and institutions is common. Rarely, common-source outbreaks from contaminated water or food have been reported.

In temperate climates, rotavirus disease is most prevalent during the cooler months. Before licensure of rotavirus vaccines in North America, the annual rotavirus epidemic usually started during the fall in Mexico and the southwest United States and moved eastward, reaching the northeast United States and Maritime Provinces by spring. Such a seasonal pattern of disease is less pronounced in tropical climates.

The epidemiology and burden of rotavirus disease in the United States has changed dramatically following the introduction of rotavirus vaccines in 2006 and 2008. Before widespread use of these vaccines, rotavirus was the most common cause of community-acquired gastroenteritis and health care–associated diarrhea in young children. Since the introduction of rotavirus vaccines in the United States, a biennial pattern has emerged, with small, short seasons (median, 9 weeks) beginning in late winter/early spring (eg, 2009, 2011, 2013, 2015, 2017), alternating with years with extremely low circulation (eg, 2008, 2010, 2012, 2014, 2016). Beginning in 2008, annual hospitalizations for rotavirus disease in US children younger than 5 years declined by approximately 75%, with an estimated 40,000 to 50,000 fewer rotavirus hospitalizations nationally each year. In case-control evaluations in the United States, the rotavirus vaccines (full series) have been found to be approximately 80% to 90% effective against rotavirus disease resulting in hospitalization. The vaccines are also highly effective in reducing emergency department visits for rotavirus disease. During a 4-year period after vaccine introduction, an estimated 177,000 hospitalizations, 242,000 emergency department visits, and 1.1 million outpatient visits for diarrhea were averted among US children younger than 5 years.

The **incubation period** for rotavirus is short, usually less than 48 hours.

DIAGNOSTIC TESTS

It is not possible to diagnose rotavirus infection by clinical manifestation or nonspecific laboratory tests. Diagnostic enzyme immunoassays and rapid chromatographic immunoassays for group A rotavirus antigen detection in stool are available commercially. Polymerase chain reaction (PCR)–based multipathogen detection systems that test stool for a panel of viral, bacterial, and parasitic gastrointestinal tract pathogens, including rotavirus, are being increasingly used. Although the advantages of such PCR-based systems are increased sensitivity and the ability to test for multiple pathogens in a single sample, the probability of coincidental detection of rotaviruses or other potential pathogens that may not be causing current symptoms complicates test interpretation. The virus from approved rotavirus vaccines can be detected in stool for at least 10 days after immunization.

The following tests are available in some research and reference laboratories: electron microscopy, polyacrylamide gel electrophoresis of viral RNA with silver staining, and viral culture. However, these tests are not generally used for clinical diagnosis of rotavirus disease.

TREATMENT

No specific antiviral therapy is available. Oral or parenteral fluids and electrolytes are given to prevent or correct dehydration. Orally administered human immune globulin, administered as an investigational therapy in immunocompromised patients with prolonged infection, has decreased viral shedding and shortened the duration of diarrhea.

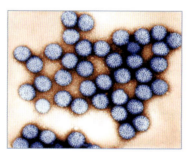

Image 124.1
Electron micrograph of intact rotavirus particles, double-shelled. Note the characteristic wheel-like appearance. Courtesy of Centers for Disease Control and Prevention.

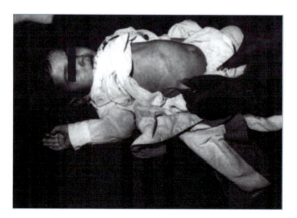

Image 124.2
Doctor examining a child dehydrated from rotavirus infection. In developing countries, rotavirus causes approximately 600,000 deaths each year in children <5 years of age. Courtesy of World Health Organization.

CHAPTER 125
Rubella

CLINICAL MANIFESTATIONS

Postnatal Rubella

Many cases of postnatal rubella are subclinical, with 25% to 50% of adults being asymptomatic. Clinical disease is usually mild and characterized by a generalized erythematous maculopapular rash, lymphadenopathy, and slight fever. The rash starts on the face, becomes generalized in 24 hours, and lasts a median of 3 days. Lymphadenopathy, which may precede rash, often involves posterior auricular or suboccipital lymph nodes, can be generalized, and lasts between 5 and 8 days. In addition, conjunctivitis, cough, headache, coryza, and palatal enanthema may occur 1 to 5 days before the rash. Transient polyarthralgia and polyarthritis rarely occur in children but commonly occur in adolescents and adults, especially in females. Encephalitis (1 in 6,000 cases) and thrombocytopenia (1 in 3,000 cases) are complications.

Congenital Rubella Syndrome

Maternal rubella during pregnancy can result in miscarriage, fetal death, or a constellation of congenital anomalies (congenital rubella syndrome [CRS]). The most commonly described anomalies/manifestations associated with CRS are ophthalmologic (ie, cataracts, pigmentary retinopathy, microphthalmos, congenital glaucoma), cardiac (ie, patent ductus arteriosus, peripheral pulmonary artery stenosis), auditory (sensorineural hearing impairment), or neurological (ie, behavioral disorders, meningoencephalitis, microcephaly, developmental disabilities). Neonatal manifestations of CRS include growth restriction, interstitial pneumonitis, radiolucent bone disease, hepatosplenomegaly, thrombocytopenia, and dermal erythropoiesis (so-called blueberry muffin lesions). Mild forms of the disease can be associated with few or no obvious clinical manifestations at birth. Congenital defects primarily occur in women infected during the first trimester. CRS is one of the few known causes of autism.

ETIOLOGY

Rubella virus is an enveloped, positive-stranded RNA virus classified as a *Rubivirus* in the *Togaviridae* family.

EPIDEMIOLOGY

Humans are the only natural host. Postnatal rubella is transmitted primarily through direct or droplet contact from nasopharyngeal secretions. The peak incidence of infection is during late winter and early spring. Immunity from wild-type or vaccine virus is usually lifelong, but reinfection has rarely been demonstrated and has rarely resulted in CRS. The period of maximal communicability extends from a few days before to 7 days after onset of rash.

Rubella virus has been recovered in high titer from lens aspirates in children with congenital cataracts for several years, and a small proportion of infants with congenital rubella continue to shed virus in nasopharyngeal secretions and urine for 1 year or longer, with transmission to susceptible contacts. Rubella has also been associated with Fuchs heterochromic uveitis, sometimes decades after the initial infection.

Before widespread use of rubella vaccine, rubella was an epidemic disease, occurring in 6- to 9-year cycles, with most cases occurring in children. In the postvaccine era, most cases in the mid-1970s and 1980s occurred in young unimmunized adults in outbreaks on college campuses and in occupational settings. More recent outbreaks have occurred among people who are born outside the United States or among populations who are underimmunized. The incidence of rubella in the United States has decreased by more than 99% from the prevaccine era.

The United States was determined to no longer have endemic rubella in 2004, and from 2004 through 2017, 107 cases of rubella and 17 cases of CRS were reported in the United States; all the cases were import associated or from unknown sources. A national serological survey from 2009–2010 indicated that among children, adolescents, and young adults 6 through 19 years of age, seroprevalence was greater than 97%. Epidemiological studies of rubella and CRS in the United States have helped identify that seronegativity is higher among people born outside the United States or from areas with poor vaccine coverage, and the risk of CRS is highest among infants of women born outside the United States.

In 2003, the Pan American Health Organization (PAHO) adopted a resolution calling for elimination of rubella and CRS in the Americas by the year 2010. The strategy consisted of achieving high levels of measles-rubella vaccination coverage in the routine immunization program and in the supplemental vaccination campaigns to rapidly reduce the number of people in the country susceptible to acute infection. The last confirmed endemic rubella case in the Americas was diagnosed in Argentina in February 2009, and the last confirmed endemic CRS case was diagnosed in Brazil in August 2009. In April 2015, the PAHO International Expert Committee for Verification of Measles and Rubella Elimination verified that the region of the Americas had achieved the rubella and CRS elimination goals.

The average **incubation period** of rubella virus is 17 days, with a range of 12 to 23 days. People infected with rubella are most contagious when the rash is erupting.

DIAGNOSTIC TESTS

Rubella

Detection of rubella-specific immunoglobulin M (IgM) antibody usually indicates recent postnatal infection, but both false-negative and false-positive results occur, requiring additional specialized testing in a reference laboratory. Most postnatal cases are IgM positive by 5 days after symptom onset. For diagnosis of postnatally acquired rubella, a 4-fold or greater increase in antibody titer between acute and convalescent periods or seroconversion between acute and convalescent immunoglobulin G (IgG) serum titers also indicate infection. Acute serum must be collected as close to rash onset as possible, preferably in the first 3 days after symptom onset.

Congenital Rubella Syndrome

CRS can be confirmed by detection of rubella-specific IgM antibody usually within the first 6 months after birth. Congenital infection can also be confirmed by stable or increasing serum concentrations of rubella-specific IgG over the first 7 to 11 months after birth. Diagnosis of congenital rubella infection in children older than 1 year is difficult because of routine vaccination with measles-mumps-rubella vaccine; serological testing is usually nondiagnostic, and viral isolation, although confirmatory, is possible in only the small proportion of congenitally infected children who are still shedding virus at this age.

The most commonly used methods of serological screening for previous rubella infection are enzyme immunoassays (EIAs) and latex agglutination tests. As a general rule, both IgM and IgG antibody testing should be performed for suspected cases of both congenital and postnatal rubella, because both their results may aid diagnosis.

A false-positive IgM test result may be caused by a number of factors including rheumatoid factor, parvovirus IgM, and heterophile antibodies. The use of IgM-capture EIA may reduce the occurrence of false-positive IgM results. The presence of high-avidity IgG or a lack of increase in IgG titers can be useful in identifying false-positive rubella IgM results. Low-avidity IgG is associated with recent primary rubella infection, whereas high-avidity IgG is associated with past infection or reinfection or with previous vaccination. The avidity assay is not a routine test and should be performed at reference laboratories such as the Centers for Disease Control and Prevention.

Rubella virus can be isolated most consistently from throat or nasal swab specimens (and less consistently from urine) by inoculation of appropriate cell culture. Detection of rubella virus RNA by real-time reverse transcriptase–polymerase chain reaction (RT-PCR) assay of a throat/nasal swab or urine specimen with subsequent genotyping of strains may be valuable for diagnosis and molecular epidemiology. RT-PCR assays are generally available in commercial and public health laboratories. In most postnatal cases, viral detection is possible by culture or RT-PCR assay on the day of symptom onset. In most congenital cases, viral detection is possible at birth; in some, for up to 12 months. Laboratory personnel should be notified immediately that rubella is suspected, because specialized cell culture methods are required to isolate and identify the virus. Blood, urine, and cataract specimens may also yield virus, particularly in infants with congenital infection. With the successful elimination of indigenous rubella and CRS in the Western hemisphere, molecular typing of viral isolates is critical in defining a source in outbreak scenarios as well as for sporadic cases.

TREATMENT

Management is supportive.

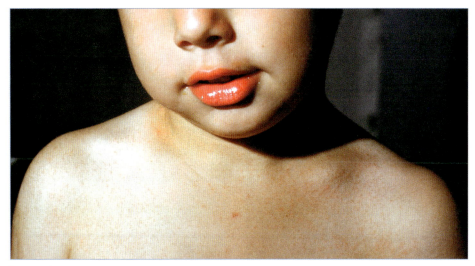

Image 125.1
This 5-year-old Hawaiian boy developed the fine macular rash noted on his face and chest. He had serologically confirmed rubella. Courtesy of Neal Halsey, MD.

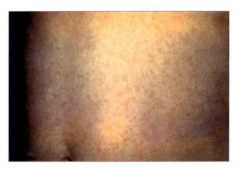

Image 125.2
This patient presented with a generalized rash on the abdomen caused by rubella. The rash usually lasts about 3 days and may be accompanied by a low-grade fever. Rubella is caused by a different virus than the one that causes regular measles. Immunity to rubella does not protect a person from measles or vice versa. Courtesy of Centers for Disease Control and Prevention

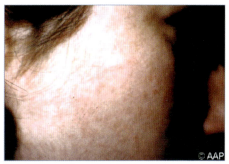

Image 125.3
Rubella rash (face) in a previously unimmunized female. Adenovirus and enterovirus infections can cause exanthema that mimics rubella. Serological testing is important if the patient is pregnant.

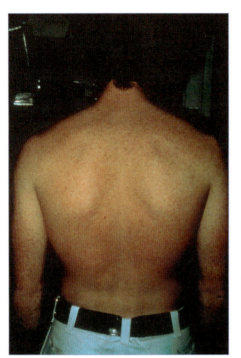

Image 125.4
A generalized, nonpruritic rash of rubella over the posterior trunk and arms of a 17-year-old boy with rubella. Courtesy of George Nankervis, MD.

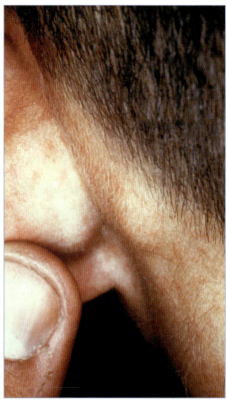

Image 125.5
Postauricular lymphadenopathy in the same 17-year-old with rubella as in Image 125.4. Courtesy of George Nankervis, MD.

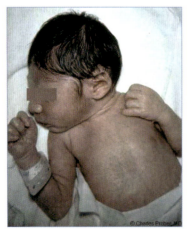

Image 125.6
Infant boy with congenital rubella with microcephaly. Copyright Charles Prober, MD.

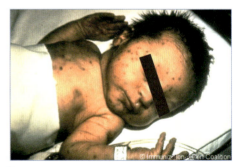

Image 125.7
Newborn with congenital rubella rash. Courtesy of Immunization Action Coalition.

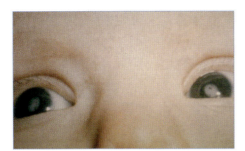

Image 125.8
This photograph shows the cataracts in an infant's eyes caused by congenital rubella syndrome. Rubella is a viral disease that can affect susceptible people of any age. Although rubella generally produces a mild rash, if it is contracted in early pregnancy, there can be a high rate of fetal wastage or birth defects, known as congenital rubella syndrome. Courtesy of Centers for Disease Control and Prevention.

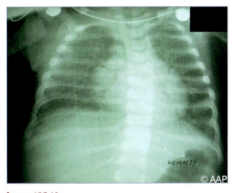

Image 125.10
Radiograph of the chest and upper abdomen of an infant with congenital rubella pneumonia with hepatosplenomegaly.

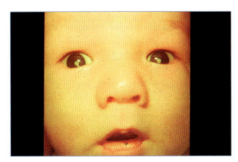

Image 125.12
A 1-month-old with congenital rubella syndrome with bilateral cataracts. Courtesy of Larry Frenkel, MD.

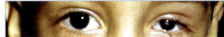

Image 125.9
A 4-year-old boy with congenital rubella syndrome with unilateral microphthalmos and cataract formation in the left eye.

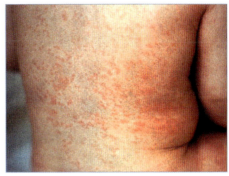

Image 125.11
Rubella rash on a child's back. The distribution is similar to that of measles, although the lesions are less intensely red. Courtesy of Centers for Disease Control and Prevention.

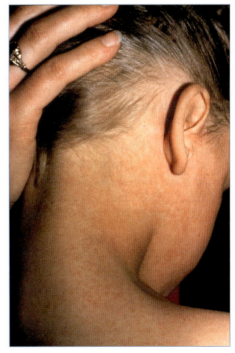

Image 125.13
Rubella on the neck. Courtesy of James Brien, DO.

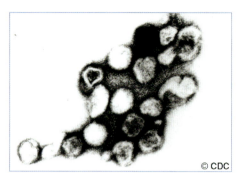

Image 125.14
Transmission electron micrograph of rubella virus. Rubella virus is an enveloped, positive-stranded RNA virus classified as a *Rubivirus* in the *Togaviridae* family. Courtesy of Centers for Disease Control and Prevention.

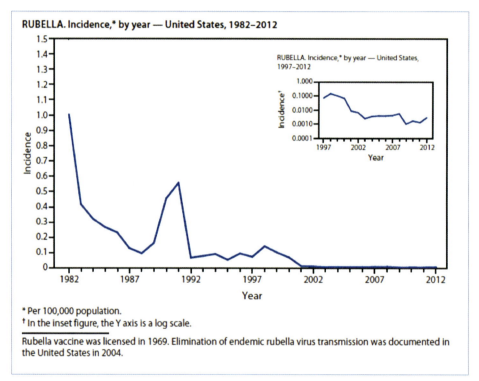

* Per 100,000 population.
† In the inset figure, the Y axis is a log scale.

Rubella vaccine was licensed in 1969. Elimination of endemic rubella virus transmission was documented in the United States in 2004.

Image 125.15
Rubella. Incidence, by year—United States, 1982–2012. Since 2012, <10 people in the United States are reported to have rubella each year. Courtesy of *Morbidity and Mortality Weekly Report*.

CHAPTER 126

Salmonella Infections

CLINICAL MANIFESTATIONS

Nontyphoidal *Salmonella* Infection

Nontyphoidal *Salmonella* (NTS) infection is associated with a spectrum of illness, ranging from asymptomatic gastrointestinal tract carriage to gastroenteritis, urinary tract infection, bacteremia, and focal infections, including meningitis, brain abscess, and osteomyelitis (to which people with sickle cell anemia are predisposed). The most common illness associated with NTS infection is gastroenteritis, with manifestations of diarrhea, abdominal cramps, and fever. The site of infection is usually the distal small intestine as well as the colon. Sustained or intermittent bacteremia can occur, and focal infections are recognized in up to 10% of patients with NTS bacteremia. In the United States, the incidence of invasive NTS is highest among infants. Certain NTS serovars (eg, Dublin, Choleraesuis), although rare, are more likely to result in invasive infection than in gastroenteritis. Invasive NTS disease in infants and toddlers, manifesting as severe clinical illness and accompanied by high case-fatality rates, is prevalent in many parts of sub-Saharan Africa. *Salmonella* Typhimurium, *Salmonella* Enteritidis, and *Salmonella* I:4,[5],12:i:- (and, to a lesser extent, *Salmonella* Dublin) are the most frequent NTS serovars isolated from blood and cerebrospinal fluid. Severe anemia, malaria, HIV, and malnutrition are known risk factors that contribute to the high case-fatality rate (10%–30%).

Enteric Fever

Salmonella enterica serovars Typhi, Paratyphi A, Paratyphi B, and Paratyphi C (which occurs rarely) can cause a protracted bacteremic illness referred to, respectively, as typhoid and paratyphoid fever and collectively as enteric fever. In older children, the onset of enteric fever is typically gradual, with manifestations such as fever, constitutional symptoms (eg, headache, malaise, anorexia, and lethargy), abdominal pain, hepatomegaly, splenomegaly, dactylitis, and rose spots (present in approximately 30% of patients). Change in mental status and shock may ensue. Myocarditis or endocarditis occurs rarely. In infants and toddlers, invasive infection with enteric fever serovars can manifest as a mild, nondescript febrile illness accompanied by self-limited bacteremia or as an invasive infection associated with more severe clinical symptoms and signs, sustained bacteremia, and meningitis. Diarrhea (resembling pea soup) or constipation can be an early feature. Gastrointestinal tract bleeding occurs in approximately 10% of hospitalized adults and children with enteric fever. Relative bradycardia (pulse rate slower than would be expected for a given body temperature) has been considered a common feature of typhoid fever in adults but in children is not a discriminating feature. The propensity to become a chronic *S* Typhi carrier (excretion >1 year) following acute typhoid infection correlates with the prevalence of cholelithiasis, increases with age, and is greater in females than males. Chronic carriage in children is uncommon.

ETIOLOGY

Salmonella organisms are gram-negative bacilli that belong to the family *Enterobacteriaceae*. Current taxonomy recognizes 2 *Salmonella* species: *S enterica* with 6 subspecies and *Salmonella bongori*. *S enterica* subspecies enterica (also called subspecies I) is responsible for most infections in humans and other warm-blooded animals; the other *S enterica* subspecies and *S bongori* are usually isolated from cold-blooded animals. More than 2,600 *Salmonella* serovars have been described. In 2016, the most commonly reported human isolates in the United States were *Salmonella* serovars Enteritidis, Newport, Typhimurium, Javiana, and I 4,[5],12:i:-; these 5 serovars accounted for approximately 45% of all *Salmonella* infections in the United States. *S* Typhi belongs to O serogroup 9, along with many other common serovars including Enteritidis and Dublin. The relative prevalence of other serovars varies by country.

EPIDEMIOLOGY

Nontyphoidal *Salmonella* Infection

Every year, NTS organisms are among the most common causes of laboratory-confirmed cases of enteric disease. The incidence of NTS infection is highest among children younger than 4 years. In the United States, rates of invasive infections and mortality are higher among infants, elderly people, and people with hemoglobinopathies (including sickle cell disease) and immunocompromising conditions (eg, malignant neoplasms, HIV infection).

Most reported cases are sporadic, but widespread outbreaks, including health care–associated and institutional outbreaks, have been reported.

The principal reservoirs for NTS organisms include birds, mammals, reptiles, and amphibians. The major food vehicles of transmission to humans in industrialized countries include seeded vegetables and other produce, as well as food of animal origin (eg, poultry, beef, eggs, and dairy products). Multiple other food vehicles (eg, peanut butter, frozen potpies, powdered infant formula, cereal, and bakery products) have been implicated in outbreaks in the United States and Europe. Other modes of transmission include ingestion of contaminated water or close contact with infected animals, mainly poultry (eg, chicks, chickens, ducks), reptiles or amphibians (eg, pet turtles, iguanas, geckos, bearded dragons, lizards, snakes, frogs, toads, newts, salamanders), and rodents (eg, hamsters, mice, guinea pigs) or other mammals (eg, hedgehogs). Reptiles and amphibians that live in tanks or aquariums can contaminate the water with bacteria, which can spread to people. Small turtles with a shell length of less than 10 cm (4 inches) are a well-known source of *Salmonella* organisms. Because of this risk, the US Food and Drug Administration has banned the interstate sale and distribution of these turtles since 1975. Animal-derived pet foods and treats have been linked to *Salmonella* infections as well, especially in young children.

A risk of transmission of infection to others persists for as long as an infected person sheds NTS organisms. Twelve weeks after infection with the most common NTS serovars, approximately 45% of children younger than 5 years shed organisms, compared with 5% of older children and adults; antimicrobial therapy can prolong shedding. Approximately 1% of adults continue to shed NTS organisms for more than 1 year.

Enteric Fever

Although typhoid fever (approximately 300–400 cases annually) and paratyphoid fever (approximately 100 cases annually) are uncommon in the United States, these infections are highly endemic in many resource-limited countries, particularly in Asia. Consequently, most typhoid fever infections in US residents are acquired during international travel. Unlike NTS serovars, the enteric fever serovars (ie, *S* Typhi, *S* Paratyphi A, *S* Paratyphi B) are restricted to human hosts, in whom they cause both clinical and subclinical infections. Chronic human *S* Typhi carriers (mostly involving chronic infection of the gall bladder but occasionally involving infection of the urinary tract) constitute the long-term reservoir in areas with endemic infection. Infection with enteric fever serovars implies ingestion of a food or water vehicle contaminated by a chronic carrier or person with acute infection.

The **incubation period** for NTS gastroenteritis is usually 6 to 48 hours, but incubation periods of a week or more have been reported. For enteric fever, the **incubation period** is usually 7 to 14 days (range, 3–60 days).

DIAGNOSTIC TESTS

Isolation of *Salmonella* organisms from cultures of stool, blood, urine, bile (including duodenal fluid containing bile), and material from foci of infection is diagnostic. Gastroenteritis is diagnosed by stool culture or molecular testing; stool cultures should be obtained in all children with bloody diarrhea or unexplained persistent or severe diarrhea. Blood and stool cultures (positive in up to 30%) should be obtained for all children who present with unexplained fever after travel to resource-poor countries. In addition, blood cultures should be considered for patients with risk for severe illness (eg, age <3 months, those who are immunocompromised or have hemolytic anemia) and in patients with evidence of disseminated infection, septicemia, or enteric fever. Optimum recovery of *Salmonella* from stool is achieved with the use of enrichment broth and multiple selective agar plate media. Definitive identification requires confirmation by phenotypic methods (biochemical profiling), molecular methods such as whole genome sequencing or polymerase chain reaction (PCR) assays, or mass spectrometry of cellular components and O serogroup determination. Serovar determination is helpful from an epidemiological perspective and is usually performed at public health laboratories.

Diagnostic tests to detect *Salmonella* antigens by enzyme immunoassay, latex agglutination, and monoclonal antibodies have been developed, as have commercial immunoassays that detect antibodies to antigens of enteric fever serovars. The latter tests are more important in areas of the world where typhoid fever is endemic.

Several multiplex PCR platforms for detection of multiple viral, parasitic, and bacterial pathogens, including *Salmonella*, directly in stool are available. Laboratories should maintain culture capabilities for *Salmonella* species, because antimicrobial susceptibility testing requires an isolate. In addition, isolates are useful for state public health laboratories to conduct genomic characterization of strains for outbreak detection and investigation.

If enteric fever is suspected, multiple cultures may be needed to isolate the pathogen. Blood, bone marrow, or bile cultures are often diagnostic, because organisms are often absent from stool. The sensitivity of blood culture in children with enteric fever is approximately 60%; of bone marrow culture, approximately 90%. The combination of a single blood culture plus culture of bile (collected from a bile-stained duodenal string) is 90% sensitive in detecting *S* Typhi infection in children with clinical enteric fever. Isolate recovery remains important for guiding antimicrobial therapy for enteric fever. Serological testing may be helpful in identification of chronic carriers in outbreak situations.

TREATMENT

Nontyphoidal *Salmonella* Infection

- Antimicrobial therapy is not usually indicated for patients with either asymptomatic infection or uncomplicated gastroenteritis caused by NTS serovars, because therapy does not shorten the duration of diarrheal disease, can prolong duration of fecal shedding, and increases symptomatic relapse rate. Antimicrobial therapy is recommended for gastroenteritis caused by NTS serovars in people with increased risk for invasive disease, including infants younger than 3 months and people with chronic gastrointestinal tract disease, malignant neoplasms, hemoglobinopathies, HIV infection, or other immunosuppressive illnesses or therapies. It should also be considered for those experiencing severe symptoms such as severe diarrhea or prolonged or high fever.

- If antimicrobial therapy is initiated in patients in the United States with presumed or proven NTS gastroenteritis, blood and stool cultures should be obtained before antibiotic administration and an initial dose of ceftriaxone should be given. The patient who does not appear ill or have evidence of disseminated infection can be discharged with oral azithromycin pending blood culture results. Once susceptibilities are available, ampicillin or trimethoprim-sulfamethoxazole (TMP-SMX) may be considered for susceptible strains. A fluoroquinolone is an alternative option. For those who appear ill or have evidence of disseminated infection, hospitalization is required.

- For bacteremia caused by NTS, disseminated disease (ie, meningitis, osteoarticular infection, endocarditis) should be excluded. Blood cultures should be repeated until negative. Initial therapy with ceftriaxone should be given. Transition from intravenous ceftriaxone to oral azithromycin or a fluoroquinolone may be considered after the blood culture has cleared and focal disease has been excluded, for a total 7- to 10-day course. Aminoglycosides are not recommended for the treatment of any invasive *Salmonella* infections (including those attributable to *S* Typhi) despite in vitro sensitivity of strains, because the clinical effectiveness is poor.

- For meningitis, the duration of treatment should be 4 weeks, and for osteomyelitis or other focal metastatic infections, a duration of 4 to 6 weeks is recommended. Evaluation for underlying immunodeficiency (eg, asplenia, HIV) should be considered.

- Antibiotic-resistant NTS strains are increasing. Ciprofloxacin-nonsusceptible strains increased from 2% in 2009 to 8% in 2017.

Enteric Fever

- Travel history and regional antibiotic resistance patterns should be carefully considered when choosing empirical antibiotic therapy for enteric fever. Most typhoid fever infections diagnosed in the United States are fluoroquinolone nonsusceptible; therefore, clinicians should not use fluoroquinolones as empirical therapy, especially in returning travelers from South Asia.

- Since 2016, in Pakistan there has been an ongoing large epidemic of extensively drug-resistant (XDR) S Typhi with resistance to ceftriaxone, ampicillin, ciprofloxacin, and TMP-SMX; isolates are susceptible only to azithromycin and carbapenems. More than 5,000 cases of XDR S Typhi have been reported in Pakistan since the start of the outbreak, and multiple confirmed cases of XDR typhoid have been documented in travelers returning to the United States and the United Kingdom from Pakistan.

- For enteric fever caused by S Typhi that is known or likely to be multidrug resistant (but not XDR), empirical therapy with a parenteral third-generation cephalosporin or azithromycin should be initiated. The optimal duration of therapy is unclear and depends on the antibiotic used. Most experts would treat for at least 7 to 10 days for people with uncomplicated disease; if amoxicillin or TMP-SMX is considered on the basis of susceptibility testing, a 14-day course of therapy should be considered. Consultation with an expert in infectious diseases may be useful for management of severe and complicated cases.

- Relapse of typhoidal Salmonella infection can occur in up to 17% of patients within 4 weeks and is a particular risk for immunocompromised patients, who may require longer duration of treatment as well as re-treatment. Relapse rates appear to be lower in those treated with azithromycin than with fluoroquinolones or ceftriaxone.

- The chronic carrier state may be eradicated by 4 weeks of oral therapy with ciprofloxacin or norfloxacin, both of which are antimicrobial agents that are highly concentrated in bile. High-dose parenteral ampicillin can also be used if 4 weeks of oral fluoroquinolone therapy is not well tolerated and if the strain is susceptible. Cholecystectomy followed by another course of antimicrobial agents may be indicated in some adults if antimicrobial therapy alone fails.

- Corticosteroids may be beneficial in children with severe enteric fever, which is characterized by delirium, obtundation, stupor, coma, or shock. These drugs should be reserved for critically ill patients in whom relief of manifestations of toxemia may be lifesaving. The usual regimen is high-dose dexamethasone, administered intravenously at an initial dose of 3 mg/kg, followed by 1 mg/kg, every 6 hours, for a total course of 48 hours.

- For enteric fever caused by S Typhi acquired from overseas travel, a stool culture should be performed on all people who traveled with the index person(s). If results are positive, treatment should be initiated with azithromycin or a fluoroquinolone and the patient should be monitored for development of any symptoms. Asymptomatic people in the United States who had contact with the index person(s) but did not travel overseas with them should be evaluated on a case-by-case basis to determine necessity for culture of stool samples.

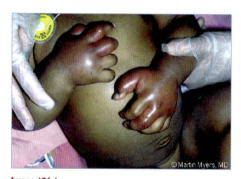

Image 126.1
A young child with sickle cell disease and Salmonella sepsis with swelling of the hands. Probable diagnosis: acute sickle cell dactylitis with septicemia. Copyright Martin G. Myers, MD.

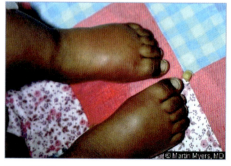

Image 126.2
A young child with sickle cell dactylitis of the foot and Salmonella sepsis. This is the same patient as in Image 126.1. Copyright Martin G. Myers, MD.

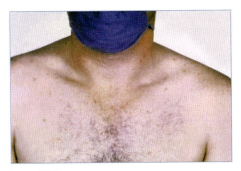

Image 126.3
Rose spots on the chest of a patient with typhoid fever caused by the bacterium *Salmonella* serovar Typhi. Symptoms of typhoid fever may include a sustained fever as high as 39.4–40.0 °C (103–104 °F), weakness, stomach pains, headache, and loss of appetite. In some cases, patients have a rash of flat, rose-colored spots. Courtesy of Centers for Disease Control and Prevention.

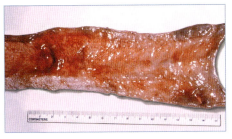

Image 126.4
Typhoid fever cholecystitis with an ulceration and perforation of the gallbladder into the jejunum. *Salmonella* serovar Typhi, the bacterium responsible for causing typhoid fever, has a preference for the gallbladder and, if present, will colonize the surface of gallstones, which is how people become long-term carriers of the disease. Courtesy of Centers for Disease Control and Prevention.

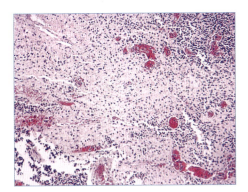

Image 126.5
Histopathologic features of the gallbladder in a case of typhoid fever. *Salmonella* serovar Typhi, the bacterium responsible for causing typhoid fever, has a preference for the gallbladder and, if present, will colonize the surface of gallstones, which is how people become long-term carriers of the disease. Courtesy of Centers for Disease Control and Prevention.

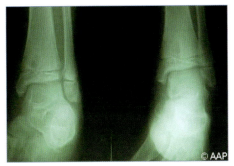

Image 126.6
Osteomyelitis caused by *Salmonella* infection of the distal tibia.

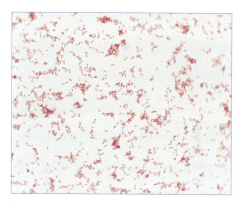

Image 126.7
Gram stain of *Salmonella* species. Courtesy of Rita Yee, MT(ASCP)SM.

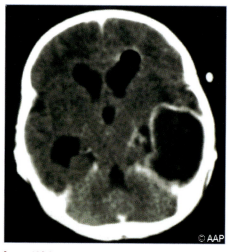

Image 126.8
A computed tomographic scan showing a large brain abscess in the posterior parietal region as a complication of *Salmonella* meningitis in a neonate.

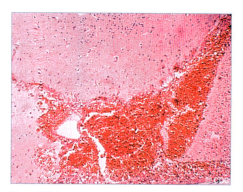

Image 126.9
Histopathologic changes in brain tissue caused by *Salmonella* serovar Typhi meningitis. *Salmonella* septicemia has been associated with subsequent infection of virtually every organ system, and the nervous system is no exception. Courtesy of Centers for Disease Control and Prevention.

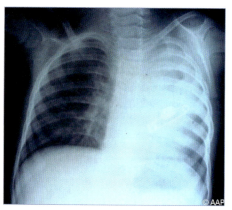

Image 126.10
Salmonella pneumonia with empyema in a 3-year-old girl who had congenital neutropenia and required chest tube drainage and prolonged antibiotic treatment to control extensive pneumonia caused by a nontyphoidal *Salmonella* species. Courtesy of Edgar O. Ledbetter, MD, FAAP.

SALMONELLA INFECTIONS

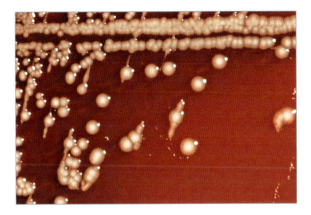

Image 126.11
This image depicts the colonial growth pattern displayed by *Salmonella enterica* subspecies *arizonae* grown on blood agar, also known as *S arizonae* or *Arizona hinshawii*. *Salmonella* species are gram-negative, aerobic, rod-shaped, zoonotic bacteria that can infect people, birds, reptiles, and other animals. Courtesy of Centers for Disease Control and Prevention.

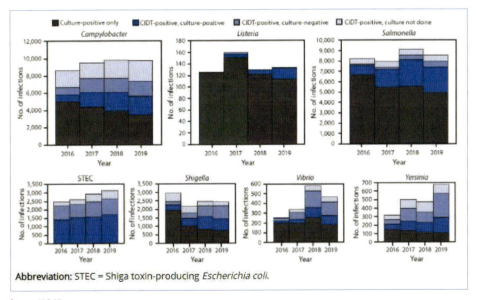

Image 126.12
Number of infections diagnosed via culture or culture-independent diagnostic tests (CIDTs), by pathogen, year, and culture status—10 US sites, Foodborne Diseases Active Surveillance Network,* 2016–2019.[†] *Data collected from laboratories in Connecticut, Georgia, Maryland, Minnesota, New Mexico, Oregon, Tennessee, and selected counties in California, Colorado, and New York. [†]Data for 2019 are preliminary. Courtesy of Centers for Disease Control and Prevention.

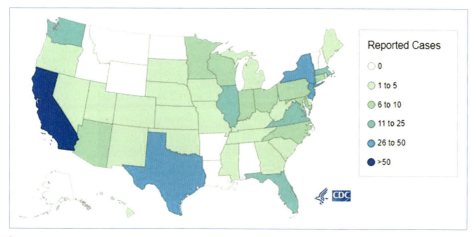

Image 126.13
Typhoid fever cases reported to National Typhoid and Paratyphoid Fever Surveillance, by jurisdiction, 2016 (n = 349). Courtesy of Centers for Disease Control and Prevention.

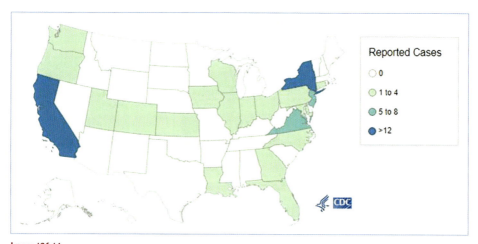

Image 126.14
Paratyphoid fever cases reported to National Typhoid and Paratyphoid Fever Surveillance, by jurisdiction, 2016 (n = 80). Courtesy of Centers for Disease Control and Prevention.

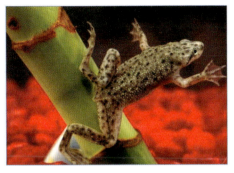

Image 126.15
African dwarf frog. *Salmonella* infection can be acquired through contact with reptiles and amphibians in homes, petting zoos, parks, child care facilities, and other locations. Courtesy of Centers for Disease Control and Prevention.

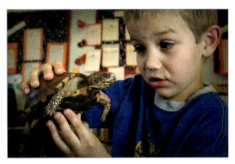

Image 126.16
Turtles carry *Salmonella*. The sale of turtles <10 cm (4 inches) in length has been banned in the United States since 1975. The ban by the US Food and Drug Administration has prevented an estimated 100,000 cases of salmonellosis annually in children. Courtesy of Centers for Disease Control and Prevention/James Gathany.

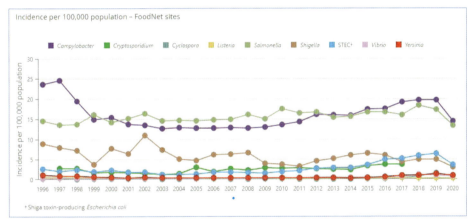

Image 126.17
Foodborne diseases, infections by year. Courtesy of Centers for Disease Control and Prevention.

CHAPTER 127
Scabies

CLINICAL MANIFESTATIONS

Scabies is characterized by an intensely pruritic, erythematous eruption that may include papules, nodules, vesicles, or bullae that is caused by burrowing of adult female mites in upper layers of the epidermis, creating serpiginous burrows. Itching is most intense at night. In older children and adults, the sites of predilection are interdigital folds, flexor aspects of wrists, extensor surfaces of elbows, anterior axillary folds, waistline, thighs, navel, genitalia, areolae, abdomen, intergluteal cleft, and buttocks. In children younger than 2 years, the eruption is more often vesicular and often occurs in areas usually spared in older children and adults, such as the scalp, face, neck, palms, and soles. The eruption is caused by a hypersensitivity reaction to proteins of the parasite.

Characteristic scabietic burrows appear as thin, gray or white, serpiginous, threadlike lines. Excoriations are common, and most burrows are obliterated by scratching before a patient seeks medical attention. Occasionally, 2- to 5-mm red-brown nodules are present, particularly on covered parts of the body, such as the genitalia, groin, and axilla. These scabies nodules are a granulomatous response to dead mite antigens and feces; the nodules can persist for weeks and even months after effective treatment. Cutaneous secondary bacterial infection is a frequent complication and is usually caused by *Streptococcus pyogenes* or *Staphylococcus aureus*. Studies have demonstrated a rare correlation between scabies and development of poststreptococcal glomerulonephritis.

Crusted (formerly called *Norwegian*) scabies is an uncommon clinical syndrome characterized by a large number of mites and widespread, crusted, hyperkeratotic lesions. Crusted scabies usually occurs in people with debilitating conditions, people with developmental disabilities, or people with immunocompromise, including patients receiving biologic response modifiers. Crusted scabies can also occur in otherwise healthy children after long-term use of topical corticosteroid therapy.

Postscabietic pustulosis is a reactive phenomenon that may follow successful treatment of primary infestation with scabies. Affected infants and young children manifest episodic crops of sterile, pruritic papules, and pustules predominantly in an acral distribution, but lesions may extend to a lesser degree onto the torso.

ETIOLOGY

The mite *Sarcoptes scabiei* subspecies (subsp) *hominis* causes scabies. The adult female burrows in the stratum corneum of the skin and lays eggs. Larvae emerge from the eggs in 2 to 4 days and molt to nymphs and then to adults, which mate and produce new eggs. The entire cycle takes approximately 10 to 17 days. *S scabiei* subsp *canis*, acquired from dogs with clinical mange, can cause a self-limited and mild infestation in humans, usually involving the area in direct contact with the infested animal.

EPIDEMIOLOGY

Humans are the source of infestation. Transmission usually occurs through prolonged close, personal contact. Even minimal contact with patients with crusted scabies or their immediate environment can result in transmission because of the large number of mites in exfoliating scales. Infestation acquired from dogs and other animals is uncommon, and these mites do not replicate in humans. Scabies of human origin can be transmitted as long as the patient remains infested and untreated, including during the interval before symptoms develop. Scabies is endemic in many countries and occurs worldwide sporadically and in epidemics, which may be cyclical in some settings. Scabies affects people from all socioeconomic levels without regard to age, gender, or standards of personal hygiene. Scabies in adults may be acquired sexually.

The **incubation period** in people without previous exposure is usually 4 to 6 weeks. People who were previously infested are sensitized and develop symptoms 1 to 4 days after repeated infestation with the mite; these reinfestations are usually milder than the original episode.

DIAGNOSTIC TESTS

Diagnosis of scabies is typically made by clinical examination. Diagnosis can be confirmed by identification of the mite, mite eggs, or scybala (feces) from scrapings of papules or intact burrows, preferably from the terminal portion where the mite is generally found. Mineral oil, microscope immersion oil, or water applied to skin facilitates collection of scrapings. A broad-blade scalpel is used to scrape the burrow. Scrapings and oil can be placed on a slide under a glass coverslip and examined microscopically under low power. Adult female mites average 330 to 450 μm in length. Skin scrapings provide definitive evidence of infestation but have low sensitivity. Handheld dermoscopy (epiluminescence microscopy) has been used to identify in vivo the pigmented mite parts or air bubbles corresponding to infesting mites within the stratum corneum. Reflectance in vivo microscopy and polymerase chain reaction assays on swabbed skin material are promising techniques with improved sensitivity and specificity.

TREATMENT

Topical 5% permethrin cream and off-label use of oral ivermectin are both effective agents for treatment of scabies. Most experts recommend starting with topical 5% permethrin cream as the drug of choice, particularly for infants (not approved for infants <2 months of age), young children, and pregnant or nursing women. Permethrin cream should be removed by bathing after 8 to 14 hours. Children and adults with infestation should apply lotion or cream containing this scabicide over their entire body below the head. Permethrin kills the scabies mite and eggs. Two (or more) applications, each about a week apart, may be necessary to eliminate all mites. Because scabies can affect the face, scalp, and neck in infants and young children, treatment of the entire head, neck, and body in this age-group is required. Special attention should be given to trimming fingernails and ensuring application of medication to these areas.

A Cochrane review showed that oral ivermectin is as effective as topical permethrin for treating scabies. Because ivermectin is not ovicidal, it is given as 2 doses, 7 to 14 days apart. Oral ivermectin should be considered for patients whose treatment has failed or who cannot tolerate topical medications for the treatment of scabies. The safety of ivermectin in children weighing less than 15 kg and in pregnant women has not been established.

Alternative drugs include 10% crotamiton cream or lotion or 5% to 10% precipitated sulfur compounded into petrolatum. Lindane lotion should not generally be used for treatment of scabies.

Because scabietic lesions result from a hypersensitivity reaction to the mite, itching may not subside for several weeks despite successful treatment. The use of oral antihistamines and topical corticosteroids can help relieve this itching. Topical or systemic antimicrobial therapy is indicated for secondary bacterial infections of excoriated lesions.

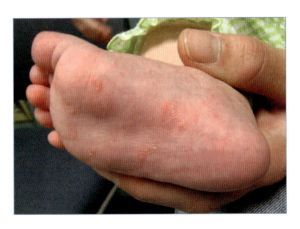

Image 127.1
A 2-year-old girl who had scabies and was adopted from an orphanage in eastern Europe. Courtesy of Daniel P. Krowchuk, MD, FAAP.

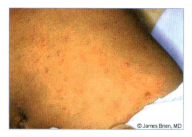

Image 127.2
Scabies rash in an infant. Copyright James Brien.

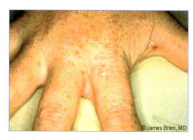

Image 127.3
Scabies in the hands of the mother of the infant in Image 127.2. Copyright James Brien.

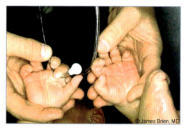

Image 127.4
Scabies in an infant with striking hand involvement. Copyright James Brien.

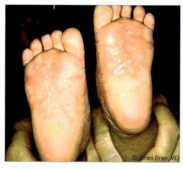

Image 127.5
Scabies in an infant with striking involvement of the feet. Copyright James Brien.

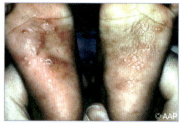

Image 127.6
Papulopustules and excoriation of the soles of the feet of an infant with severe scabies.

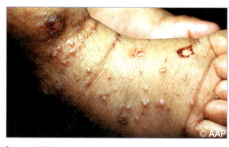

Image 127.7
Papulopustules and a widespread eczematous eruption, which represents a hypersensitivity reaction to a scabies infestation.

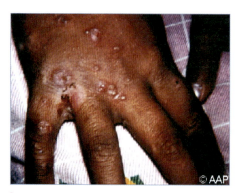

Image 127.8
Older children, adolescents, and adults with scabies exhibit erythematous papules, nodules, or burrows in the interdigital webs, as in this patient.

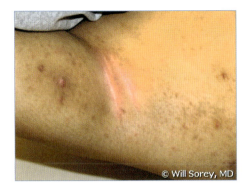

Image 127.9
A 12-year-old with itching in the axillae and groin for 2 weeks. She recently returned from a family camping trip, where she shared a tent with "dozens of cousins." Since returning home, she has had itching in the armpits and in her pubic area. She now has papules and pustules on her fingers, toes, and gluteal furrow. The family is reluctant to inquire about relatives with similar lesions. Examination of scrapings of the lesions indicated a few oval structures suggestive of scabies eggs. She responded to treatment with topical sulfur and oil in lieu of pesticide-based therapy. Courtesy of Will Sorey, MD.

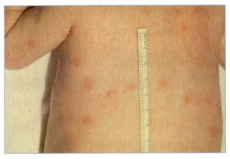

Image 127.10
A 9-month-old boy with atypical, eczema-like papulovesicular lesions of scabies on the trunk and extremities. Courtesy of George Nankervis, MD.

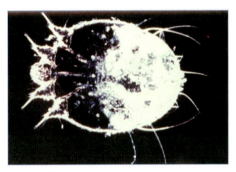

Image 127.11
This is a *Sarcoptes scabiei* subspecies *hominis*, or itch mite, which is the cause of scabies. Females are 0.3- to 0.4-mm long and 0.25- to 0.35-mm wide. Male mites are slightly more than half that size. Scabies is a highly contagious infestation of the skin caused by a mite affecting humans and animals. Scabies is usually transmitted by intimate interpersonal contact, often sexual in nature, but transmission through casual contact can occur. Courtesy of Centers for Disease Control and Prevention.

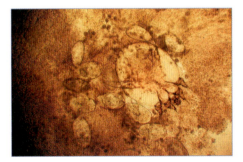

Image 127.12
The mite *Sarcoptes scabiei* subspecies *hominis* is responsible for scabies in humans. Courtesy of Larry Frenkel, MD.

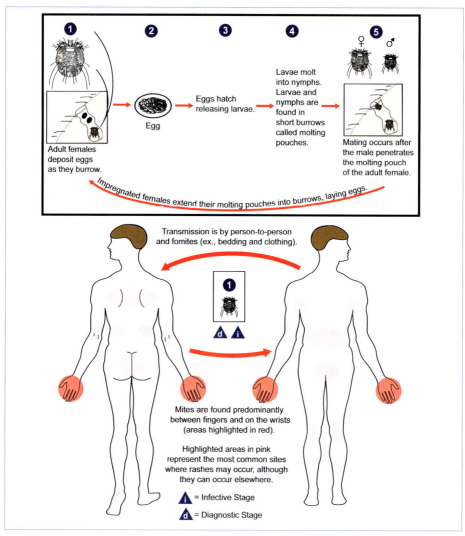

Image 127.13

Life cycle. *Sarcoptes scabiei* undergoes 4 stages in its life cycle: egg, larva, nymph, and adult. Females deposit eggs at 2- to 3-day intervals as they burrow through the skin (1). Eggs are oval and 0.1–0.15 mm in length (2) and incubation time is 3–8 days. After the eggs hatch, the larvae migrate to the skin surface and burrow into the intact stratum corneum to construct almost invisible, short burrows called *molting pouches*. The larval stage, which emerges from the eggs, has only 3 pairs of legs (3), and this form lasts 2–3 days. After larvae molt, the resulting nymphs have 4 pairs of legs (4). This form molts into slightly larger nymphs before molting into adults. Larvae and nymphs may often be found in molting pouches or in hair follicles and look similar to adults, only smaller. Adults are round, saclike eyeless mites. Females are 0.3- to 0.4-mm long and 0.25- to 0.35-mm wide, and males are slightly more than half that size. Mating occurs after the nomadic male penetrates the molting pouch of the adult female (5). Impregnated females extend their molting pouches into the characteristic serpentine burrows, laying eggs in the process. The impregnated females burrow into the skin and spend the remaining 2 months of their lives in tunnels under the surface of the skin. Males are rarely seen. They make a temporary gallery in the skin before mating. Transmission occurs by the transfer of ovigerous females during personal contact. Mode of transmission is primarily person-to-person contact, but transmission may also occur via fomites (eg, bedding, clothing). Mites are found predominantly between the fingers and on the wrists. The mites hold on to the skin by using suckers attached to the 2 most anterior pairs of legs. Courtesy of Centers for Disease Control and Prevention.

CHAPTER 128

Schistosomiasis

CLINICAL MANIFESTATIONS

Schistosomiasis (bilharzia) is established by skin penetration of infecting larvae (cercariae, shed by freshwater snails). Initial infections are often asymptomatic. Skin manifestations include pruritus at the penetration site a few hours after water exposure, followed in 5 to 14 days by an intermittent pruritic, sometimes papular, eruption. More intense papular eruptions may occur more quickly and last for 7 to 10 days after exposure in people sensitized previously. Cercarial dermatitis (swimmer's itch) can also be caused by larvae of schistosome parasites of birds or other wildlife. These larvae can penetrate human skin but eventually die in the dermis and do not cause systemic disease.

Parasites capable of causing intestinal and urogenital schistosomiasis enter the bloodstream after penetration of the skin, migrate through the lungs, and eventually mature into adult worms that reside in the venous plexus that drains the intestines or, in the case of *Schistosoma haematobium*, the urogenital tract. Four to 8 weeks after exposure, worms develop into adults and females begin egg deposition, which can lead to an acute serum sickness–like illness (Katayama syndrome) that manifests as fever, malaise, cough, rash, abdominal pain, hepatosplenomegaly, diarrhea, nausea, lymphadenopathy, and eosinophilia. This syndrome is most common in nonimmune hosts, such as travelers. Severity of symptoms associated with chronic infection is related to worm burden. People with low to moderate worm burdens may have only subclinical disease or relatively mild manifestations, such as growth stunting or anemia. Higher worm burdens are associated with a range of symptoms primarily caused by inflammation and local fibrosis triggered by the immune response to eggs produced by adult worms. Severe forms of chronic intestinal schistosomiasis (*Schistosoma mansoni* and *Schistosoma japonicum* infections) can result in hepatosplenomegaly, abdominal pain, bloody diarrhea, portal hypertension, ascites, esophageal varices, and hematemesis. Urogenital schistosomiasis (*S haematobium* infections) can result in the bladder becoming inflamed and fibrotic. Urinary tract symptoms and signs include dysuria, urgency, terminal microscopic and gross hematuria, secondary urinary tract infections, hydronephrosis, and nonspecific pelvic pain. *S haematobium* is associated with lesions of the lower genital tract (vulva, vagina, and cervix) in women, prostatitis and hematospermia in men, and certain forms of bladder cancer. Other organ systems can be involved (eg, eggs can embolize to the lungs, causing pulmonary hypertension). Less commonly, eggs can lodge in the central nervous system, causing severe neurological complications.

ETIOLOGY

The trematodes (flukes) *S mansoni, S japonicum, Schistosoma mekongi, Schistosoma guineensis,* and *Schistosoma intercalatum* cause intestinal schistosomiasis, and *S haematobium* causes urogenital disease. All species have similar life cycles.

EPIDEMIOLOGY

Persistence of schistosomiasis depends on presence of an appropriate snail as an intermediate host. Eggs excreted in stool (*S mansoni, S japonicum, S mekongi, S intercalatum,* and *S guineensis*) or urine (*S haematobium*) into fresh water hatch into motile miracidia, which infect snails. After development and asexual replication in snails, cercariae emerge and penetrate the skin of humans in contact with water. In areas with endemic schistosomiasis, children are infected first when they accompany their mothers to lakes, ponds, and other open freshwater sources. School-aged children are typically the most heavily infected people in the community because of prolonged wading and swimming in infected waters. Children have greater susceptibility to infection than older people because of a lack of high preexisting immunity to these parasites and are important in maintaining transmission through behaviors such as uncontrolled defecation and urination. Animals play an important zoonotic role (as a source of eggs) in maintaining the life cycle of *S japonicum*. Infection is not transmissible by person-to-person contact or blood transfusion.

The distribution of schistosomiasis is focal and limited by the presence of appropriate snail vectors, infected human reservoirs, and freshwater sources. *S mansoni* occurs throughout tropical Africa, in parts of several Caribbean islands, and in areas of Venezuela, Brazil, Suriname, and the Arabian Peninsula. *S japonicum* is found in China, the Philippines, and Indonesia. *S haematobium* occurs in Africa and the Middle East; in 2014, local transmission was reported in Corsica. *S mekongi* is found in Cambodia and Laos. *S intercalatum* is found in Central Africa; *S guineensis*, in West Africa. Adult worms of *S mansoni* usually survive for 5 to 7 years but can live as long as 30 years in the human host. Schistosomiasis can be diagnosed in patients many years after they have left an area with endemic transmission. Immunity is incomplete, and reinfection occurs commonly. Swimmer's itch can occur in all regions of the world after exposure to fresh water, brackish water, or salt water.

The **incubation period** is variable but is approximately 4 to 6 weeks for *S japonicum*, 6 to 8 weeks for *S mansoni*, and 10 to 12 weeks for *S haematobium*.

DIAGNOSTIC TESTS

Eosinophilia is common and may be intense in Katayama syndrome (acute schistosomiasis). Infection with *S mansoni* and other intestinal species is diagnosed by microscopic examination of stool specimens to detect characteristic eggs containing fully differentiated larvae, but results may be negative if performed too early in the course of infection. In light infections, several stool specimens examined by a concentration technique may be needed before eggs are found, or eggs may be found in a biopsy of the rectal mucosa. *S haematobium* is diagnosed by examining urine for eggs; filtration or centrifugation and examination of the urinary sediment are required for optimum sensitivity. Egg excretion in urine often peaks between noon and 3:00 pm. Biopsy of the bladder mucosa may be used to diagnose *S haematobium* infection. Urine reagent dipsticks are commonly positive for blood. Serological tests, available through the Centers for Disease Control and Prevention and some commercial laboratories, may be helpful for detecting light infections; results of these antibody-based tests remain positive for many years and are not useful in differentiating ongoing infection from past infection or reinfection. Serological test results are negative during acute infection, turn positive 6 to 12 weeks or more after infection, and may be positive before eggs are detectable. Polymerase chain reaction and antigen tests for detection of schistosomes have been developed but are considered to be research tools.

Swimmer's itch, which is caused by the cercariae of certain schistosome species whose normal hosts are birds and nonhuman mammals, can be difficult to differentiate from other causes of dermatitis. A skin biopsy may demonstrate larvae, but their absence does not exclude the diagnosis. A history of exposure to water used by waterfowl may be helpful in making the diagnosis.

TREATMENT

The drug of choice for schistosomiasis caused by any species is praziquantel. The alternative drug for *S mansoni* is oxamniquine, which is no longer available in the United States. Optimal timing of treatment after known exposures is uncertain, but it is reasonable to give treatment with praziquantel within 6 to 8 weeks of exposure. Praziquantel does not kill developing worms, so treatment administered early (eg, 4–8 weeks after exposure) should be repeated 2 to 4 weeks later to improve parasitological cure. Initial management of acute schistosomiasis and neuroschistosomiasis includes reduction of inflammation with steroids, although optimal dose and duration are uncertain. Initial treatment with praziquantel may exacerbate symptoms. The optimal timing of adding praziquantel is unknown; treating with this drug when inflammation has subsided is generally favored. Swimmer's itch is a self-limited disease that may require symptomatic treatment of the rash. More intense reactions may require a course of oral corticosteroids.

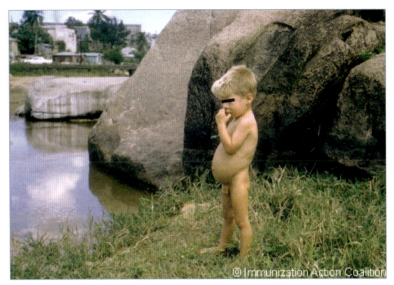

Image 128.1
A boy with a swollen abdomen caused by schistosomiasis with hepatosplenomegaly. Courtesy of Immunization Action Coalition.

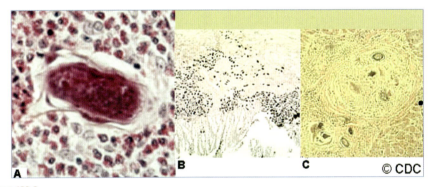

Image 128.2
A–C, Cross section of different human tissues showing *Schistosoma* species eggs. A, *Schistosoma mansoni* eggs in intestinal wall. B, *Schistosoma japonicum* eggs in colon. C, *S japonicum* eggs in liver. Courtesy of Centers for Disease Control and Prevention.

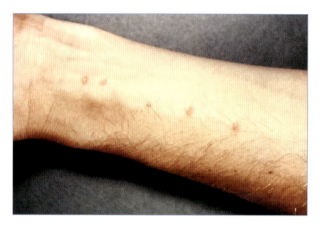

Image 128.3

Schistosome dermatitis, or swimmer's itch, occurs when skin is penetrated by a free-swimming, fork-tailed infective cercaria. On release from the snail host, the infective cercariae swim, penetrate the skin of the human host, and shed their forked tail, becoming schistosomula. The schistosomula migrate through several tissues and stages to their residence in the veins. Courtesy of Centers for Disease Control and Prevention.

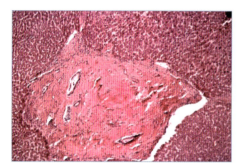

Image 128.4

This micrograph reveals signs of schistosomiasis of the liver, also known as pipestem cirrhosis (magnification ×500). Pipestem cirrhosis occurs when schistosomes infect the liver (ie, hepatic schistosomiasis), which causes scarring to occur, thereby entrapping parasites and their ova in and around the hepatic portal circulatory vessels. Courtesy of Centers for Disease Control and Prevention.

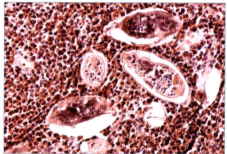

Image 128.5

Histopathologic features of *Schistosoma haematobium*, bladder. Histopathologic features of the bladder show eggs of *S haematobium* surrounded by intense infiltrates of eosinophils. Courtesy of Centers for Disease Control and Prevention/Edwin P. Ewing Jr, MD.

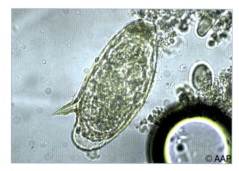

Image 128.6

Schistosoma haematobium ova (original magnification ×400).

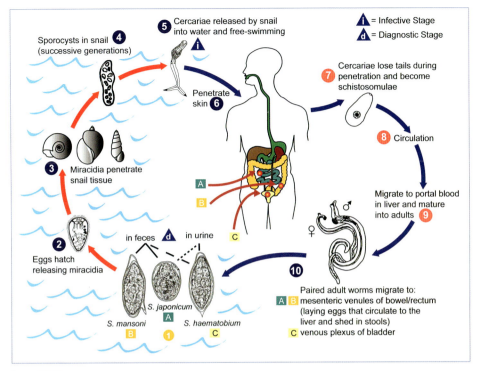

Image 128.7

Life cycle. Eggs are eliminated with feces or urine (1). Under optimal conditions, the eggs hatch and release miracidia (2), which swim and penetrate specific snail intermediate hosts (3). The stages in the snail include 2 generations of sporocysts (4) and the production of cercariae (5). On release from the snail, the infective cercariae swim, penetrate the skin of the human host (6), and shed their forked tail, becoming schistosomula (7). The schistosomula migrate through several tissues and stages to their residence in the veins (10). Adult worms in humans reside in the mesenteric venules in various locations, which, at times, seem to be specific for each species (10). For instance, *Schistosoma japonicum* is more frequently found in the superior mesenteric veins draining the small intestine (A), and *Schistosoma mansoni* occurs more often in the superior mesenteric veins draining the large intestine (B). However, both species can occupy either location, and they are capable of moving between sites, so it is not possible to state unequivocally that one species occurs in only one location. *Schistosoma haematobium* most often occurs in the venous plexus of the bladder (C), but it can also be found in the rectal venules. The females (size 7–20 mm; males slightly smaller) deposit eggs in the small venules of the portal and perivesical systems. The eggs are moved progressively toward the lumen of the intestine (*S mansoni* and *S japonicum*) and are eliminated with feces or toward the lumen of the bladder and ureters (*S haematobium*) and are eliminated with urine (1). Pathological manifestations of *S mansoni* and *S japonicum* schistosomiasis include Katayama fever, presinusoidal egg granulomas, Symmers pipestem periportal fibrosis, portal hypertension, and occasional embolic egg granulomas in the brain or spinal cord. Pathological manifestations of *S haematobium* schistosomiasis include hematuria, scarring, calcification, squamous cell carcinoma, and occasional embolic egg granulomas in the brain or spinal cord. Human contact with water is thus necessary for infection by schistosomes. Various animals, such as dogs, cats, rodents, pigs, horses, and goats, serve as reservoirs for *S japonicum*; dogs, for *S mekongi*. Courtesy of Centers for Disease Control and Prevention.

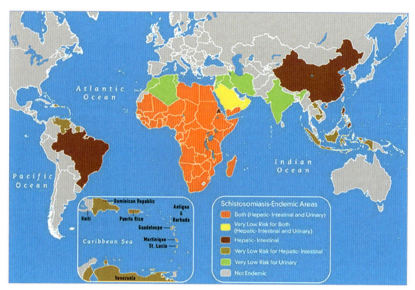

Image 128.8
Geographic distribution of schistosomiasis. Courtesy of Centers for Disease Control and Prevention.

CHAPTER 129

Shigella Infections

CLINICAL MANIFESTATIONS

Shigella species primarily infect the large intestine, causing clinical manifestations that range from watery or loose stools with minimal or no constitutional symptoms to more severe symptoms including high fever, abdominal cramps or tenderness, tenesmus, and mucoid stools with or without blood. *Shigella dysenteriae* serotype 1 often causes a more severe illness than other *Shigella* species, with a higher risk of complications, including septicemia, pseudomembranous colitis, toxic megacolon, intestinal perforation, hemolysis, and hemolytic-uremic syndrome (HUS). Infection attributable to *S dysenteriae* serotype 1 has become rare in industrialized countries. Generalized seizures have been reported in young children with shigellosis attributable to any serotype; although the pathophysiology and incidence are poorly understood, such seizures are usually self-limited and are usually associated with high fever or electrolyte abnormalities. Septicemia is rare during the course of illness and is caused by *Shigella* organisms or by other gut flora that gain access to the bloodstream through intestinal mucosa damaged during shigellosis. Septicemia occurs most often in neonates, children with malnourishment, and people with *S dysenteriae* serotype 1 infection but may occur in healthy children with non–*S dysenteriae* shigellosis. Reactive arthritis with possible extraarticular manifestations is a rare complication that can develop weeks or months after shigellosis, especially in patients expressing HLA-B27. Postinfectious irritable bowel syndrome can occur and last weeks to months.

ETIOLOGY

Shigella species are facultative aerobic, gram-negative bacilli in the family *Enterobacteriaceae*. Four species (with >40 serotypes) have been identified, with *Shigella sonnei* being most common in the United States. The other species are *Shigella flexneri*, *S dysenteriae*, and *Shigella boydii*. In resource-limited countries, especially in Africa and Asia, *S flexneri* predominates, and *S dysenteriae* serotype 1 often causes outbreaks. Shiga toxin, a potent cytotoxin produced by *S dysenteriae* serotype 1, enhances the virulence of this serotype at the colonic mucosa and can cause small blood vessel and renal damage, leading to HUS in some individuals. The Shiga toxin genes are phage encoded and have been found in a small number of strains belonging to other *Shigella* species and serotypes, including *S flexneri* serotype 2a, *S dysenteriae* serotype 4, and *S sonnei*. HUS has been associated with an infection attributable to *S sonnei* in an adult, although the non–*S dysenteriae* species are not commonly associated with HUS.

EPIDEMIOLOGY

Humans are the natural host for *Shigella* organisms. Whereas the primary mode of transmission is the fecal-oral route, transmission can also occur via contact with a contaminated inanimate object, ingestion of contaminated food or water, or sexual contact. Houseflies and cockroaches may also be vectors through physical transport of infected feces. Ingestion of as few as 10 organisms, depending on the species, is sufficient for infection to occur. Prolonged organism survival in water (up to 6 months) and food (up to 30 days) can occur with *Shigella* species. Children 5 years or younger in child care settings and their caregivers and people living in crowded conditions have increased risk for infection. Men who have sex with men also have increased risk for shigellosis, including infections with multidrug-resistant strains. Infections attributable to *S flexneri*, *S boydii*, and *S dysenteriae* are slightly more common in adults than in children. Travel to resource-limited countries with inadequate sanitation can place travelers at risk of infection. Even without antimicrobial therapy, the carrier state usually ceases within 1 to 4 weeks after onset of illness; long-term carriage is uncommon.

Antibiotic resistance is increasing among *Shigella* isolates. From 1999–2015, 59% of 7,391 *Shigella* isolates in the United States were resistant to ampicillin, 43% were resistant to trimethoprim-sulfamethoxazole (TMP-SMX), 3% were resistant to amoxicillin-clavulanate, less than 1% were resistant to ciprofloxacin, and less than 0.3% were resistant to ceftriaxone. From 2011–2015, 6% of 2,085 isolates demonstrated decreased susceptibility to azithromycin. By 2017, 10% of *Shigella* isolates were resistant to ciprofloxacin and 24% had decreased susceptibility to azithromycin. The Centers for Disease Control and Prevention has been monitoring *Shigella* isolates that harbor one or more quinolone resistance mechanisms (ie, those with a minimum inhibitory concentration [MIC] of ≥0.12 μg/mL for ciprofloxacin) but that have in vitro susceptibility to fluoroquinolones. Data from the National Antimicrobial Resistance Monitoring System indicate that many *Shigella* isolates with a quinolone resistance mechanism are nonsusceptible or resistant to many other commonly used treatment agents, such as azithromycin, TMP-SMX, amoxicillin-clavulanic acid, and ampicillin.

The **incubation period** varies from 1 to 7 days but is typically 1 to 3 days.

DIAGNOSTIC TESTS

Isolation of *Shigella* organisms from feces or rectal swab specimens containing feces is diagnostic; sensitivity is improved by testing stool as soon as possible after it is passed, along with the use of enrichment broth media and selective agar plate media. If specimens cannot be transported to the testing laboratory within 2 hours, they should be transferred to appropriate transport media (eg, Cary-Blair or similar media) and kept and transported at 4 °C (39 °F). Definitive identification of the organism requires both biochemical profiling and serogrouping to differentiate *Shigella* from *Escherichia* species. The presence of fecal lactoferrin (or fecal leukocytes) demonstrated on a methylene-blue stained stool smear is fairly sensitive for the diagnosis of colitis but is nonspecific for shigellosis. Although bacteremia is rare, blood should be cultured in severely ill, immunocompromised, or malnourished children. Multiplex polymerase chain reaction (PCR) platforms for detection of multiple bacterial (including *Shigella*), viral, and parasitic pathogens have high sensitivity but do not distinguish between viable and nonviable organisms. To guide treatment, stool cultures are recommended if shigellosis is diagnosed by using multiplex PCR platforms or other nonculture-based diagnostic tests. Other tests for bacterial detection, including qualitative and quantitative PCR assays, are available in research laboratories and some clinical laboratories.

TREATMENT

- Although severe dehydration is rare with shigellosis, correction of fluid and electrolyte losses, preferably by oral rehydration solutions, is the mainstay of treatment.

- Most clinical infections with *S sonnei* are self-limited (48–72 hours), and mild episodes do not require antimicrobial therapy.

- Antimicrobial treatment is recommended for patients with severe disease or with underlying immunosuppressive conditions; in these patients, empirical therapy should be given while awaiting culture and susceptibility results. Available evidence suggests that antimicrobial therapy is somewhat effective in shortening duration of diarrhea and in hastening eradication of organisms from feces.

- Antimicrobial susceptibility testing of clinical isolates is indicated to guide therapy, because resistance to antimicrobial agents is common and increasing. *Shigella* strains with decreased susceptibility to azithromycin and resistance to ciprofloxacin have been reported in the United States. Ceftriaxone resistance has been reported recently, although it is still relatively uncommon in the United States. When antibiotic treatment is required, oral administration is recommended, except for seriously ill patients. First-line therapy should consist of one of the following antibiotics:

  ○ A fluoroquinolone (eg, ciprofloxacin) for 3 days. Fluoroquinolones should be avoided if the *Shigella* strain has an MIC of 0.12 μg/mL or greater for ciprofloxacin, even if the laboratory indicates that the isolate is "susceptible," until more is known about the clinical outcomes of ciprofloxacin treatment when MICs are 0.12 μg/mL or greater.

  ○ Azithromycin for 3 days. Clinical laboratories are often unable to perform azithromycin susceptibilities for *Shigella* species, because the clinical break points have not been established.

  ○ Parenteral ceftriaxone for 2 to 5 days. Oral cephalosporins (eg, cefixime) are of unclear efficacy.

- For susceptible strains, oral ampicillin or TMP-SMX for 5 days is an alternative; amoxicillin is ineffective because of its rapid absorption from the gastrointestinal tract.
- Antidiarrheal compounds that inhibit intestinal peristalsis are contraindicated, because they can prolong the clinical and bacteriologic course of disease and can increase the rate of complications.
- Nutritional supplementation, including vitamin A (200,000 IU) and zinc (elemental zinc, orally daily for 10–14 days, 10 mg/day for newborns to 6 months of age, and 20 mg/day for those >6 months), can be given to hasten clinical resolution in geographic areas where children have risk for malnutrition.

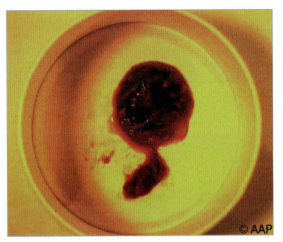

Image 129.1
Characteristic bloody mucoid stool of a child with shigellosis.

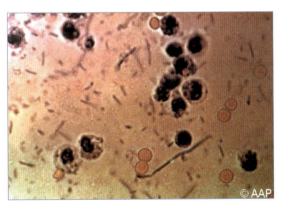

Image 129.2
Fecal leukocytes (shigellosis) (methylene-blue stain). The presence of fecal leukocytes suggests a bacterial diarrhea, although nonspecific for *Shigella* infection. Courtesy of Edgar O. Ledbetter, MD, FAAP.

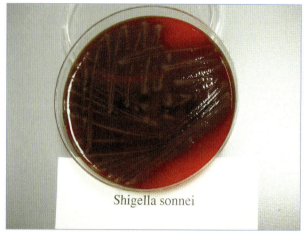

Image 129.3
Culture of *Shigella sonnei* grown on a blood agar plate. Courtesy of Rita Yee, MT(ASCP) SM.

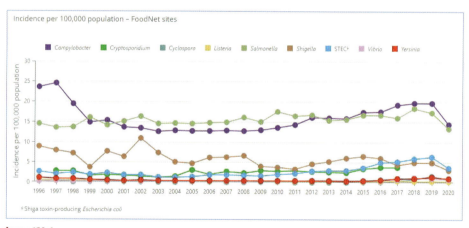

Image 129.4
Foodborne diseases, infections by year. Courtesy of Centers for Disease Control and Prevention.

CHAPTER 130

Smallpox (Variola)

The last naturally occurring case of smallpox occurred in Somalia in 1977, followed by 2 cases with 1 death in 1978 after a photographer was infected during a laboratory exposure and later transmitted smallpox to her mother in the United Kingdom. In 1980, the World Health Assembly declared that smallpox (variola virus) had been eradicated successfully worldwide, and no subsequent human cases have been confirmed. The United States discontinued routine childhood immunization against smallpox in 1972 and routine immunization of health care professionals in 1976. Immunization of US military personnel continued until 1990. Following eradication, 2 World Health Organization reference laboratories were authorized to maintain stocks of variola virus. Because of terrorism events on September 11, 2001, and concern that the virus might be used as a weapon of bioterrorism, the smallpox immunization policy was revisited. In 2002, the United States resumed immunization of military personnel deployed to certain areas of the world and in 2003 initiated a civilian smallpox immunization program for first responders to facilitate preparedness and response to a possible smallpox bioterrorism event. Such a bioterrorism event has not occurred.

CLINICAL MANIFESTATIONS

People infected with variola major strains develop a severe prodromal illness characterized by high fever (38.9–40 °C [102–104 °F]) and constitutional symptoms, including malaise, severe headache, backache, abdominal pain, and prostration, lasting for 2 to 5 days. Infected children may experience vomiting and seizures during this prodromal period. Most patients with smallpox are severely ill and bedridden during the febrile prodrome. The prodromal period is followed by development of lesions on mucosa of the mouth or pharynx, which may not be noticed by the patient. This stage occurs less than 24 hours before onset of rash, which is usually the first recognized manifestation of smallpox. With onset of oral lesions, the patient becomes infectious and remains so until all skin crust lesions have separated. The rash typically begins on the face and rapidly progresses to involve the forearms, trunk, and legs, with the greatest concentration of lesions on the face and distal extremities. Most patients have lesions on the palms and soles. With rash onset, fever decreases but does not resolve. Lesions begin as macules that progress to papules, followed by firm vesicles and then deep-seated, hard pustules described as "pearls of pus." Each stage lasts 1 to 2 days. By the sixth or seventh day of rash, lesions may begin to umbilicate or become confluent. Lesions increase in size for approximately 8 to 10 days, after which they begin to crust. Once all the crusts have separated, 3 to 4 weeks after the onset of rash, the patient is no longer infectious. Variola major in unimmunized people is associated with case-fatality rates of approximately 30% during epidemics of smallpox. The mortality rate is highest among pregnant women, children younger than 1 year, and adults older than 40 years. The potential for improved outcomes because of modern supportive therapy is unknown.

Variola minor strains cause a disease that is indistinguishable clinically from variola major, except that they cause less severe systemic symptoms and more rapid rash evolution, reduced scarring, and fewer fatalities.

In addition to the typical manifestation of smallpox (≥90% of cases), there are 2 uncommon severe forms of variola major: hemorrhagic (characterized by a hemorrhagic diathesis before onset of the typical smallpox rash [early hemorrhagic smallpox] or by hemorrhage into skin lesions and disseminated intravascular coagulation [late hemorrhagic smallpox]) and malignant or flat type (in which the skin lesions do not progress to the pustular stage but remain flat and soft). Each variant occurs in approximately 5% of cases and is associated with a 95% to 100% mortality rate. Pregnancy is a risk factor for hemorrhagic variola. Defects in cellular immunity may be responsible for flat-type variola major, which is observed more commonly in children than adults.

Varicella (chickenpox) is the condition most likely to be mistaken for smallpox. Generally, children with varicella do not have a febrile prodrome, but adults may have a brief, mild prodrome. Although the 2 diseases are confused easily in the first few days of the rash, smallpox lesions develop into pustules that are firm and deeply embedded in the dermis, whereas varicella lesions develop into superficial vesicles. Because varicella erupts in crops of lesions that evolve quickly, lesions on any one part of the body will be in different stages of evolution (papules, vesicles, and crusts), whereas all smallpox lesions on any one part of the body are in the same stage of development. The rash distribution of the 2 diseases differs. Varicella most commonly starts on the trunk and moves peripherally with less involvement of the extremities as compared with the trunk (centripetal). Variola lesions can be found distributed on all parts of the body but are generally found in higher numbers on the face and extremities as compared with the trunk (centrifugal). Monkeypox could also be mistaken for smallpox because it produces a clinically similar but milder illness. Prominent lymphadenopathy can be a distinguishing feature of monkeypox virus infection, and its diagnosis should be considered only in the United States in the appropriate epidemiological setting.

ETIOLOGY

Variola, the virus that causes smallpox, is a member of the *Poxviridae* family (genus *Orthopoxvirus*). Other members of this genus that can infect humans include monkeypox virus, cowpox virus, vaccinia virus, and several putative novel species. Cowpox virus is believed to have been used by Benjamin Jesty in 1774 and by Edward Jenner in 1796 as material for the first smallpox vaccine. Later, cowpox virus was replaced with vaccinia virus.

EPIDEMIOLOGY

Humans are the only natural reservoir for variola virus (smallpox). Smallpox is spread most commonly by large respiratory droplets from the oropharynx of infected people, although rare transmission from aerosol spread has been reported. Infection from direct contact with lesion material or indirectly via fomites, such as clothing and bedding, has also been reported. Because most patients with smallpox are extremely ill and bedridden, spread is generally limited to household contacts, hospital workers, and other health care professionals. Secondary household attack rates for smallpox were considerably lower than for measles and similar to or lower than rates for varicella.

In 2003, an outbreak caused by monkeypox virus that was linked to prairie dogs exposed to rodents imported from Ghana occurred in the United States. In 2017–2018, Nigeria reported the largest ever outbreak of monkeypox in West Africa, with cases epidemiologically linked to Nigeria subsequently reported in the United Kingdom, Israel, and Singapore. Ongoing sporadic monkeypox cases within and linked to Nigeria continued to be reported through 2019. Novel putative orthopox species with clinical manifestations like those of cowpox virus and vaccinia virus have been reported in Alaska and in the country of Georgia.

The **incubation period** for smallpox is 7 to 17 days (mean, 10–12 days).

DIAGNOSTIC TESTS

Variola virus can be detected in vesicular or pustular fluid by a number of different methods, including electron microscopy, immunohistochemistry, culture, or polymerase chain reaction (PCR) assay. Only PCR assay can diagnose infection with variola virus definitively; all other methods simply screen for orthopoxviruses. Screening is available through the US Laboratory Response Network and through state or local public health departments. Final, confirmatory variola-specific laboratory testing is available only at the Centers for Disease Control and Prevention. Diagnostic workup includes exclusion of varicella-zoster virus or other common conditions that cause a vesicular/pustular rash illness.

TREATMENT

Tecovirimat (TPOXX or ST-246) was licensed by the US Food and Drug Administration in July 2018 for the treatment of smallpox in people who weigh at least 13 kg. It has been shown to be active against monkeypox and rabbitpox in animal models, although effectiveness against variola in humans is unknown. It inhibits the function of an envelope protein required for extracellular transmission of virus. Cidofovir, a nucleotide analogue of cytosine, has demonstrated antiviral activity against certain orthopoxviruses in vitro and in animal models. Its effectiveness in treatment of variola in humans is unknown. Tecovirimat and cidofovir are included in the US Strategic National Stockpile that is managed by the US Department of Health and Human Services, Office of the Assistant Secretary for Preparedness and Response. Brincidofovir (a lipophilic derivative of cidofovir) is an investigational agent with broad-spectrum antiviral activity including against poxviruses in vitro and in animal studies.

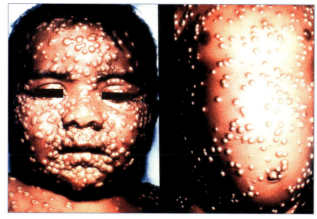

Image 130.1
Smallpox in a 2-year-old boy demonstrating greater density of commonplace lesions on the face than that on the child's body. Courtesy of Paul Wehrle, MD.

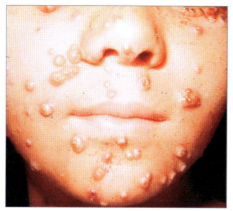

Image 130.2
Variola minor lesions on the face of a 2-year-old boy. Courtesy of Paul Wehrle, MD.

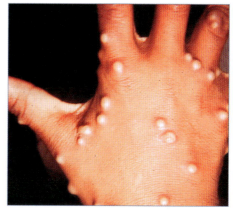

Image 130.3
Variola minor lesions on the hand of the boy in Image 130.2. Courtesy of Paul Wehrle, MD.

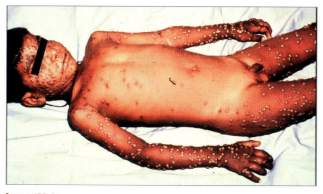

Image 130.4
A 7-year-old boy residing in India with smallpox lesions in a typical centripetal distribution. Courtesy of Paul Wehrle, MD.

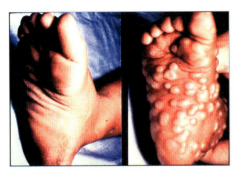

Image 130.5
The right foot of two 6-year-old boys: one (right) with smallpox, the other (left) with varicella. The palms and soles are characteristically involved in patients with smallpox and infrequently involved in varicella. Courtesy of Paul Wehrle, MD.

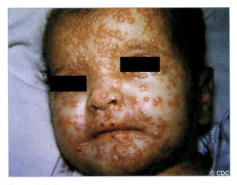

Image 130.6
Early smallpox pustules on the face of an infant. If this infant survives, smallpox lesions, or pustules, will eventually form scabs that fall off, leaving marks on the skin. The patient is contagious to others until all the scabs have fallen off. Courtesy of Centers for Disease Control and Prevention.

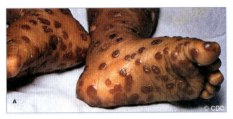

Image 130.7
Numerous healing smallpox lesions on the feet of a young child. Courtesy of Centers for Disease Control and Prevention.

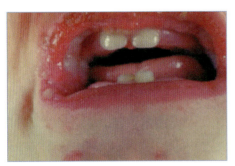

Image 130.9
Subsequent to receiving a vaccine, this 1-year-old developed erythema multiforme. Erythema multiforme major, also known as Stevens-Johnson syndrome, is a toxic or allergic rash in response to the smallpox vaccine that can take various forms and range from moderate to severe. Courtesy of Centers for Disease Control and Prevention.

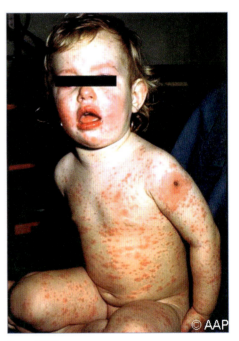

Image 130.8
Generalized vaccinia reaction secondary to smallpox vaccination. No vaccinia immunoglobulin treatment was required for resolution. Note the primary vaccination reaction on the left deltoid area. Courtesy of Edgar O. Ledbetter, MD, FAAP.

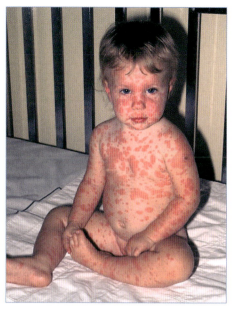

Image 130.10
After receiving a smallpox vaccine, this 1-year-old developed erythema multiforme. Erythema multiforme major, also known as Stevens-Johnson syndrome, is a toxic or allergic rash in response to the smallpox vaccine that can take various forms and range from moderate to severe. Courtesy of Centers for Disease Control and Prevention.

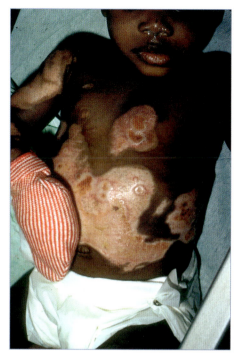

Image 130.11
Generalized vaccinia in a 6-month-old boy; he had experienced burns and was then unintentionally inoculated by contact with a vaccinated sibling. Courtesy of George Nankervis, MD.

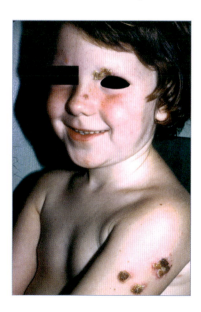

Image 130.12
Multiple secondary vaccinia lesions from autoinoculation in a 5-year-old girl, one of the more common complications of smallpox vaccination. Courtesy of George Nankervis, MD.

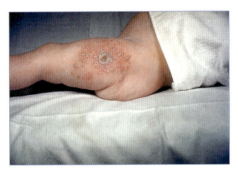

Image 130.13
After receiving a smallpox vaccine, this child developed a cluster of satellite lesions surrounding the vaccination site. Courtesy of Centers for Disease Control and Prevention.

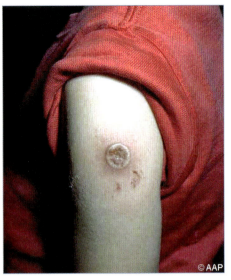

Image 130.14
Primary smallpox vaccination site with satellite vaccinia lesions in an 18-month-old girl. No treatment was required for resolution in conjunction with the primary vaccination lesion.

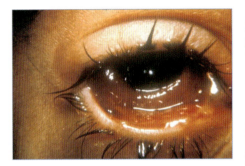

Image 130.15
This conjunctivitis was caused by the unintentional implantation of vaccinia virus on the eyelid of this 6-year-old primary vaccinee. Vaccinia vaccine is a highly effective immunizing agent that brought about the global eradication of smallpox. However, because the smallpox vaccine is live, it can be spread to other people, as well as to other parts of one's own body. Courtesy of Centers for Disease Control and Prevention.

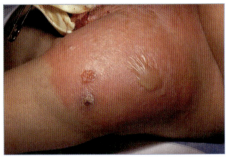

Image 130.16
This child developed a secondary staphylococcal infection at the smallpox vaccination site. Note the signs of cellulitis, including spreading erythema that envelopes the smallpox vaccination site; swelling; and accompanying areas of cutaneous purulence. Courtesy of Centers for Disease Control and Prevention.

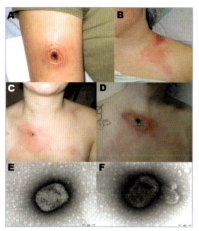

Image 130.17
A–F, Cowpox virus infection in a person in northern France caused by transmission from infected pet rats. Courtesy of Centers for Disease Control and Prevention.

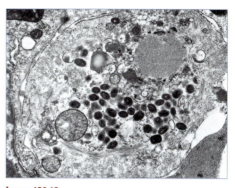

Image 130.18
A transmission electron micrograph of a tissue section containing variola virus. Smallpox is a serious, highly contagious, and sometimes fatal infectious disease. There is no specific treatment of smallpox, and the only prevention is immunization. Courtesy of Centers for Disease Control and Prevention.

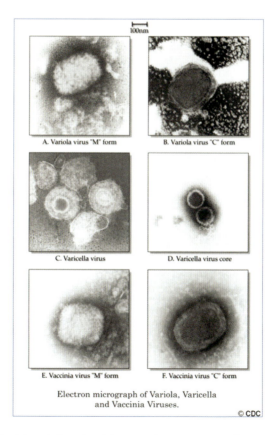

Image 130.19
Electron micrographs of variola, varicella, and vaccinia virions. Electron micrographs from top to bottom: variola virion (forms M and C), varicella virion and virion core, vaccinia virion (forms M and C). Courtesy of Centers for Disease Control and Prevention.

CHAPTER 131
Sporotrichosis

CLINICAL MANIFESTATIONS

There are 3 **cutaneous** patterns described for sporotrichosis. The classic lymphocutaneous process with multiple nodules is found more commonly in adults. Inoculation occurs at a site of minor trauma, causing a painless papule that enlarges slowly to become a firm, slightly tender subcutaneous nodule that can develop a violaceous hue or ulcerate. Secondary lesions follow the same evolution and develop along the lymphatic distribution proximal to the initial lesion. A localized cutaneous form of sporotrichosis, also called *fixed cutaneous form*, is found more commonly in children and manifests as a solitary crusted papule or papuloulcerative or nodular lesion in which lymphatic spread is not observed. The extremities and face are the most common sites of infection. A disseminated cutaneous form with multiple lesions is rare, usually occurring in immunocompromised patients.

Extracutaneous sporotrichosis accounts for 20% of all cases and usually occurs in the setting of unusual areas of trauma or in immunocompromised patients. Osteoarticular infection results from hematogenous spread or local inoculation. The most commonly affected joints are the knees, elbows, wrists, and ankles. Pulmonary sporotrichosis clinically resembles tuberculosis and occurs after inhalation or aspiration of aerosolized conidia. Disseminated disease generally occurs after hematogenous spread from primary skin or lung infection. Disseminated sporotrichosis can involve multiple foci (eg, eyes, pericardium, genitourinary tract, central nervous system) and occurs predominantly in immunocompromised patients. Pulmonary and disseminated forms of sporotrichosis are uncommon in children.

ETIOLOGY

Sporothrix schenckii is a thermally dimorphic fungus that grows as a mold or mycelial form at room temperature and as a budding yeast at 35 to 37 °C (95–99 °F) and in host tissues. *S schenckii* is a complex of at least 6 species. Within this complex, *S schenckii sensu stricto* is responsible for most infections, followed by *Sporothrix globosa*; in South America, *Sporothrix brasiliensis* is a major cause of infection.

EPIDEMIOLOGY

S schenckii is a ubiquitous organism that has worldwide distribution but is most common in tropical and subtropical regions of Central and South America and parts of North America and Asia. The fungus has been isolated from soil and plant material, including hay, straw, sphagnum moss, and decaying vegetation. Thorny plants such as rose bushes and pine trees are commonly implicated, because pricks from their thorns or needles inoculate the organism from the soil or moss around the bush or tree. Zoonotic spread from cats infected with *S brasiliensis* is responsible for hyperendemic cutaneous sporotrichosis involving mostly women and children in Rio de Janeiro.

The **incubation period** is 7 to 30 days after cutaneous inoculation but can be as long as 6 months.

DIAGNOSTIC TESTS

Culture of *Sporothrix* species from a tissue, wound drainage, or sputum specimen is diagnostic. The mold phase of the organism can be isolated on a variety of fungal media, including Sabouraud dextrose agar at 25 to 30 °C (77–86 °F). Filamentous colonies generally appear within 1 week. Definitive identification requires conversion to the yeast phase by subculture to enriched media, such as brain-heart infusion agar with 5% blood and incubation at 35 to 37 °C (95–99 °F). In some cases, repeated subcultures are required for conversion. Culture of *Sporothrix* species from a blood specimen is definite evidence for the disseminated form of infection associated with immunodeficiency. Histopathologic examination of tissue may be helpful but is often not, because the organism is seldom abundant, but may exclude clinically similar infections such as cutaneous leishmaniasis. Fungal stains including periodic acid–Schiff reagent or Grocott-Gomori methenamine–silver nitrate stain to visualize the oval or cigar-shaped organism are required. Antibody tests that are offered by some reference laboratories have been useful in a few cases of extracuteneous sporotrichosis. Molecular testing on tissue samples is available only in a few reference laboratories and is not standardized.

TREATMENT

Sporotrichosis does not usually resolve without treatment. Itraconazole is the drug of choice for children with lymphocutaneous and localized cutaneous disease; many experts prefer using the oral solution, which is taken on an empty stomach and appears to achieve better concentrations. The duration of therapy is 2 to 4 weeks after all lesions have resolved, usually for a total duration of 3 to 6 months. Serum trough concentrations of itraconazole should be 1 to 2 μg/mL. Concentrations should be checked after several days of therapy to ensure adequate drug exposure. When measured by high-pressure liquid chromatography, both itraconazole and its bioactive hydroxy-itraconazole metabolite are reported, the sum of which should be considered in assessing drug levels. Saturated solution of potassium iodide (1 drop, 3 times daily, increasing as tolerated to a maximum of 1 drop/kg of body weight or 40–50 drops, 3 times daily, whichever is lowest) is an alternative therapy for nonsevere forms.

Amphotericin B is recommended as the initial therapy for visceral or disseminated sporotrichosis in children. After clinical response to amphotericin B therapy is documented, itraconazole can be substituted and should be continued for at least 12 months. Itraconazole may be required for lifelong therapy in children with HIV infection. Pulmonary and disseminated infections respond less well than cutaneous infection, despite prolonged therapy.

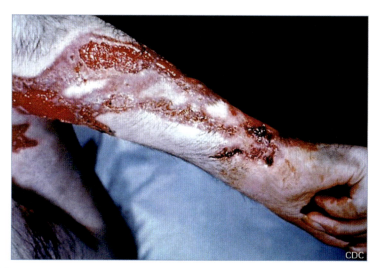

Image 131.1
This patient's arm shows the effects of the fungal disease sporotrichosis, caused by the fungus *Sporothrix schenckii*. Courtesy of Centers for Disease Control and Prevention.

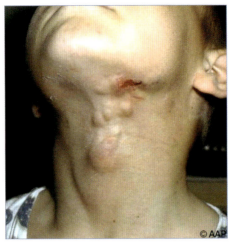

Image 131.2
Sporothrix schenckii was cultured from the biopsy specimen from an abscessed cervical lymph node of this 10-year-old boy. Test results were negative on stained smears of purulent material aspirated from a cervical lymph node.

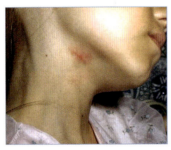

Image 131.3
The cervical lesions of a younger sister of the patient in Image 131.2 also responded to an oral-saturated solution of potassium iodide. There was no evidence of systemic sporotrichosis in these 3 siblings. The origin of their infections was not determined.

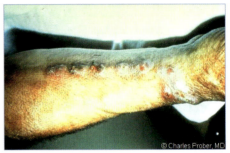

Image 131.4
Linear lymphadenitis secondary to sporotrichosis infection of the foot and foreleg. Copyright Charles Prober, MD.

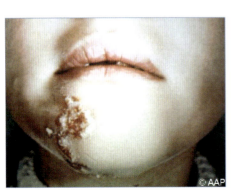

Image 131.5
Cutaneous sporotrichosis of the face in a preschool-aged child. Courtesy of Edgar O. Ledbetter, MD, FAAP.

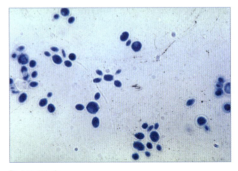

Image 131.6
This micrograph is taken from a slant culture of *Sporothrix schenckii* during its yeast phase. Courtesy of Centers for Disease Control and Prevention.

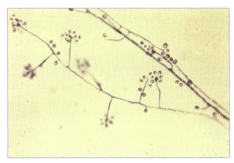

Image 131.7
Sporothrix schenckii, mold phase (48-hour potato dextrose agar, lactophenol cotton blue preparation); small tear-shaped conidia forming rosette-like clusters. Courtesy of Centers for Disease Control and Prevention.

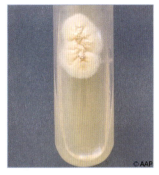

Image 131.8
Sporothrix schenckii on Sabouraud agar slant (specimen from the patient in Image 131.2).

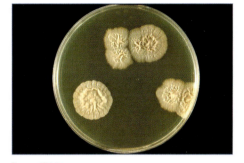

Image 131.9
This is an image of a Sabhi agar plate culture of *Sporothrix schenckii* grown at 20 °C (68 °F). *S schenckii* is the causative agent for the fungal infection sporotrichosis, also known as rose handler's disease, which affects individuals who handle thorny plants, sphagnum moss, or baled hay. Courtesy of Centers for Disease Control and Prevention.

CHAPTER 132

Staphylococcal Food Poisoning

CLINICAL MANIFESTATIONS

Staphylococcal foodborne illness is characterized by abrupt and sometimes violent onset of severe nausea, abdominal cramps, vomiting, and prostration, often accompanied by diarrhea. Low-grade fever or mild hypothermia can occur. The illness typically lasts no longer than 1 day, but symptoms are intense and can require hospitalization. The short incubation period, brevity of illness, and usual lack of fever help distinguish staphylococcal from other infectious causes of food poisoning, except for the vomiting syndrome caused by *Bacillus cereus*. *Clostridium perfringens* food poisoning usually has a longer incubation period, and chemical food poisoning usually has a shorter incubation period. Patients with foodborne *Salmonella*, *Campylobacter*, or *Shigella* infection are more likely to have fever and a longer incubation period.

ETIOLOGY

Enterotoxins produced by strains of *Staphylococcus aureus* and, rarely, *Staphylococcus epidermidis* and *Staphylococcus intermedius* cause the symptoms of staphylococcal food poisoning.

EPIDEMIOLOGY

Illness is caused by ingestion of food containing heat-stable staphylococcal enterotoxins. The most commonly implicated foods are pork, beef, and chicken. Meats can be contaminated by staphylococci carried by animals. Foods may also be contaminated by enterotoxigenic strains of *S aureus* via contact with food handlers; approximately 25% of people are asymptomatically colonized with *S aureus*. When contaminated foods remain at room temperature for several hours, the toxin-producing staphylococcal organisms multiply and produce toxins that are heat stable (ie, not inactivated by reheating). Much less commonly, the toxigenic staphylococci are of bovine origin (eg, from cows with mastitis) from contaminated milk or milk products, especially cheeses.

The **incubation period** ranges from 30 minutes to 8 hours after ingestion, typically 2 to 4 hours.

DIAGNOSTIC TESTS

In most cases, given the short duration of illness and rapid recovery with supportive care, diagnostic testing to confirm the diagnosis is unnecessary. However, tests for enterotoxin are commercially available. In an outbreak, recovery of large numbers of staphylococci ($\geq 10^5$ *S aureus* per gram) from stool or vomitus or detection of enterotoxin in an implicated food can confirm the diagnosis, as can identification of the same subtype of *S aureus* from the stool or vomitus of 2 or more ill people.

TREATMENT

Treatment is supportive. Antimicrobial agents are not indicated.

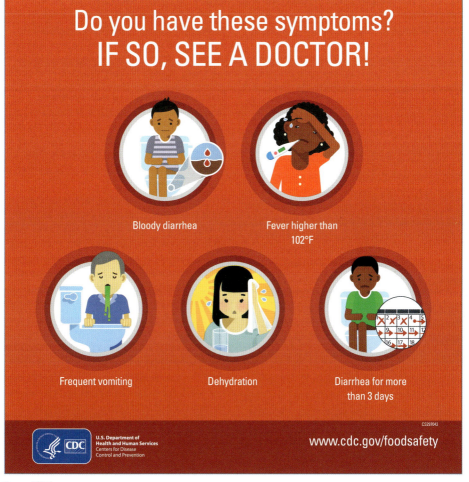

Image 132.1
Staph food poisoning is a gastrointestinal illness caused by eating foods contaminated with toxins produced by the bacterium *Staphylococcus aureus* (Staph) bacteria. Courtesy of Centers for Disease Control and Prevention.

CHAPTER 133
Staphylococcus aureus

CLINICAL MANIFESTATIONS

Staphylococcus aureus causes a variety of localized and invasive suppurative infections and 3 toxin-mediated syndromes: toxic shock syndrome, scalded skin syndrome, and food poisoning. Localized infections include cellulitis, skin and soft tissue abscesses, furuncles, carbuncles, pustulosis, impetigo (bullous and nonbullous), paronychia, mastitis, hordeola, omphalitis, sinusitis, orbital cellulitis/abscess, peritonsillar abscesses (quinsy), parotitis, lymphadenitis, and wound infections. Bacteremia can be associated with focal complications including osteomyelitis; septic arthritis; endocarditis; pneumonia; pleural empyema; septic pulmonary emboli; pericarditis; soft tissue, muscle, or visceral abscesses; and septic thrombophlebitis of small and large vessels. In patients with neutropenia, ecthyma gangrenosum may occur. Primary *S aureus* pneumonia can also occur after aspiration of organisms from the upper respiratory tract and can occur in the context of concurrent or antecedent viral infections from the community (eg, influenza) or in ventilated patients. Meningitis may occur in preterm infants but is otherwise rare unless accompanied by an intradermal foreign body (eg, ventriculoperitoneal shunt) or a congenital or acquired defect in the dura. *S aureus* also causes infections with and without bacteremia associated with foreign bodies, including intravascular catheters or grafts, peritoneal catheters, cerebrospinal fluid shunts, spinal instrumentation or intramedullary rods, pressure equalization tubes, pacemakers and other intracardiac devices, vagal nerve stimulators, and prosthetic joints. *S aureus* infections can be fulminant. Certain chronic diseases, conditions, and events, such as diabetes mellitus, malignancy, preterm birth, immunodeficiency, kidney disease, nutritional disorders, dialysis, surgery, and transplant, increase the risk for severe *S aureus* infections. Metastatic foci and abscess formation need to be drained and foreign bodies should be removed when possible. Prolonged antimicrobial therapy is often necessary to achieve cure.

Staphylococcal toxic shock syndrome (TSS), a toxin-mediated disease, is usually caused by strains producing TSS toxin-1 or possibly other related staphylococcal enterotoxins. Characterized by acute onset of fever, generalized erythroderma, rapid-onset hypotension, and signs of multisystem organ involvement, including profuse watery diarrhea, vomiting, conjunctival injection, and severe myalgia (see Box 133.1 for clinical case definition). TSS can occur in menstruating females using tampons or following childbirth or abortion. TSS can also occur in males and females after surgical procedures, in association with cutaneous lesions, or without a readily identifiable focus of infection. Prevailing clones (eg, USA300) of methicillin-resistant *S aureus* (MRSA) rarely produce TSS toxin. People with TSS, especially menses-associated illness, have risk for a recurrent episode.

Staphylococcal scalded skin syndrome (SSSS) is a toxin-mediated disease caused by circulation of exfoliative toxins A and B. The manifestations of SSSS are age related and include Ritter disease (generalized exfoliation) in the neonate, a tender scarlatiniform eruption and localized bullous impetigo in older children, or a combination of these with thick white/brown flaky desquamation of the entire skin, especially on the face and neck, in older infants and toddlers. The hallmark of SSSS is the toxin-mediated cleavage of the stratum granulosum layer of the epidermis (ie, Nikolsky sign). Proper pain management is a mainstay of therapy for SSSS. Healing occurs without scarring. Bacteremia is rare, but dehydration and superinfection can occur with extensive exfoliation.

ETIOLOGY

Staphylococci are catalase-positive, gram-positive cocci that appear microscopically as grapelike clusters. Staphylococci are ubiquitous and can survive extreme conditions of drying, heat, and low-oxygen and high-salt environments. *S aureus* has many surface proteins, including the microbial surface components recognizing adhesive matrix molecule receptors, which allow the organism to bind to tissues and foreign bodies coated with fibronectin, fibrinogen, and collagen. This permits a low inoculum of organisms to adhere to sutures, catheters, prosthetic valves, and other devices.

EPIDEMIOLOGY

S aureus is the most common cause of skin and soft tissue infections and musculoskeletal infections in otherwise healthy children. *S aureus*

Box 133.1
Staphylococcus aureus Toxic Shock Syndrome: Clinical Case Definition[a]

Clinical findings
- Fever: temperature ≥38.9 °C (≥102 °F)
- Rash: diffuse macular erythroderma
- Desquamation: 1–2 weeks after onset of rash, particularly on palms, soles, fingers, and toes
- Hypotension: systolic pressure ≤90 mm Hg for adults; <5th percentile for age for children <16 years
- Multisystem organ involvement: 3 or more of the following signs:
  1. Gastrointestinal tract: vomiting or diarrhea at onset of illness
  2. Muscular: severe myalgia or creatinine phosphokinase concentration greater than twice the upper limit of reference
  3. Mucous membrane: vaginal, oropharyngeal, or conjunctival hyperemia
  4. Renal: serum urea nitrogen or serum creatinine concentration greater than twice the upper limit of reference or urinary sediment with ≥5 white blood cells/high-power field in the absence of urinary tract infection
  5. Hepatic: total bilirubin, aspartate aminotransferase, or alanine aminotransferase concentration greater than twice the upper limit of reference
  6. Hematologic: platelet count ≤100,000/μL
  7. Central nervous system: disorientation or alterations in consciousness without focal neurological signs when fever and hypotension are absent

Laboratory criteria
- *Negative* results on the following tests, if obtained:
  1. Blood, throat, or cerebrospinal fluid cultures; blood culture may rarely be positive for *S aureus*.
  2. Serological tests for Rocky Mountain spotted fever, leptospirosis, or measles.

Case classification
- **Probable:** a case that meets the laboratory criteria and in which 4 of 5 clinical findings are present
- **Confirmed:** a case that meets laboratory criteria and in which all 5 of the clinical findings, including desquamation, are present unless the patient dies before desquamation occurs

[a] Adapted from wwwn.cdc.gov/nndss/conditions/toxic-shock-syndrome-other-than-streptococcal/case-definition/2011.

colonizes the skin and mucous membranes of 30% to 50% of healthy adults and children. The anterior nares, throat, axilla, perineum, vagina, and rectum are usual sites of colonization. *S aureus* is second only to coagulase-negative staphylococci as a cause of health care–associated bacteremia, is one of the most common causes of health care–associated pneumonia in children, and is the most common pathogen responsible for surgical site infections. Patients with neutrophil dysfunction, such as those with chronic granulomatous disease, also have risk for *S aureus* infections.

S aureus–mediated TSS was recognized in 1978, and many early cases were associated with tampon use. Although changes in tampon composition and use have resulted in a decreased proportion of cases associated with menses, menstrual and nonmenstrual cases of TSS continue to occur and are reported with similar frequency. Risk factors for TSS include absence of antibody to TSS toxin-1 and focal *S aureus* infection with a TSS toxin-1–producing strain. TSS toxin-1–producing strains can be part of normal flora of the anterior nares or vagina, and colonization at these sites is believed to result in protective antibody in greater than 90% of adults.

Transmission of *S aureus*

Rates of skin carriage of greater than 50% occur among children with desquamating skin disorders or burns and among people with frequent needle use (eg, diabetes mellitus, hemodialysis, people who inject drugs, people who take allergy shots). Although domestic animals can be colonized, data suggest that colonization is acquired from other humans. Hospitalized children who are colonized with MRSA on admission or acquire MRSA colonization in the hospital have increased risk for subsequent MRSA infection as compared to noncolonized children.

S aureus is transmitted most often by direct contact in community settings and indirectly from patient to patient via transiently colonized hands of health care professionals in health care settings. Health care professionals and family members who are colonized with *S aureus* in the nares or on skin can also serve as a reservoir for transmission. Contaminated environmental surfaces and objects can also play a role in transmission of *S aureus*. Although not transmitted routinely by the droplet route, *S aureus* can be dispersed into the air over short distances. Dissemination of *S aureus* from people with nasal carriage, including infants, is related to density of colonization, and increased dissemination occurs during viral upper respiratory tract infections. Maternal *S aureus* colonization at a variety of body sites has been associated with neonatal colonization.

Health Care–Associated MRSA

MRSA has been endemic in most US hospitals since the 1980s and in 2016 accounted for approximately 40% of health care–associated *S aureus* bloodstream infections in pediatric inpatients. Risk factors for health care–associated MRSA infections include hospitalization, surgery, dialysis, long-term care stay within the previous year, presence of an indwelling device, presence of wounds, and history of prior MRSA infection or colonization. The incidence of invasive health care–associated MRSA infections has decreased in many communities since the mid-2000s.

Health care–associated MRSA strains (ie, those that were historically responsible for most health care–associated MRSA infections) are usually multidrug resistant and are predictably susceptible only to vancomycin, ceftaroline, linezolid, daptomycin, and agents not approved for use in children.

Community-Associated MRSA

Community-associated MRSA infections attributable to strains different from traditional health care–associated MRSA emerged in the 1990s. These strains most commonly cause skin and soft tissue abscesses, although they can also cause more severe infections. Clinical infections are more common in settings where there is crowding; frequent skin-to-skin contact; sharing of personal items, such as towels and clothing; and poor personal hygiene and among those with nonintact skin including body piercings. Outbreaks have been reported among athletic teams, in correctional facilities, and in military training facilities. Community-associated MRSA strains can also circulate in hospitals and cause health care–associated MRSA infections. Unlike health care–associated strains, community-associated MRSA strains are usually susceptible to a variety of non–β-lactam antibiotics (eg, trimethoprim-sulfamethoxazole [TMP-SMX], clindamycin, tetracycline), and the antibiotics used to treat health care–associated MRSA strains.

Vancomycin–Intermediately Susceptible *S aureus*

Vancomycin–intermediately susceptible *S aureus* (VISA) strains (minimum inhibitory concentration [MIC], 4–8 μg/mL) have been isolated from people (historically, dialysis patients) who have received multiple courses of vancomycin. Strains of MRSA can be heterogeneous for vancomycin resistance. Extensive vancomycin use allows VISA strains to develop during therapy. Control measures have included using proper methods to detect VISA, using appropriate infection-control measures, and adopting measures to ensure appropriate vancomycin use.

Vancomycin-Resistant *S aureus*

Vancomycin-resistant *S aureus* infections (MIC >8 μg/mL) are very rare, and in all confirmed cases, reported patients had underlying medical conditions, a history of MRSA infections, and prolonged exposure to vancomycin.

The **incubation period** is variable for staphylococcal disease. A long delay can occur between acquisition of the organism and onset of disease. For SSSS, the **incubation period** is usually 1 to 10 days; for postoperative TSS, the **incubation period** can be as short as 12 hours. Menses-related cases can develop at any time during menstruation.

DIAGNOSTIC TESTS

Gram stains of specimens from skin lesions or pyogenic foci showing gram-positive cocci in clusters can provide presumptive evidence of staphylococcal infection. Isolation of organisms from culture of otherwise sterile body fluid is the method for definitive diagnosis. Molecular assays have been approved by the US Food and Drug Administration for detection of *S aureus* from blood cultures growing gram-positive organisms. These assays include nonamplified molecular assays, such as peptide nucleic acid fluorescent in situ hybridization and Verigene (Luminex), as well as nucleic acid amplification tests, such as BD GenOhm Staph SR (BD Molecular Diagnostics), Xpert MRSA/SA BC (Cepheid), and the FilmArray Blood Culture Identification Panel (BCID) (Biofire). MALDI-TOF (matrix-assisted laser desorption/ionization–time-of-flight) mass spectrometry can rapidly identify *S aureus* colonies on culture plates or from growth in blood cultures. *S aureus* is almost never a contaminant when isolated from a blood culture.

S aureus–mediated TSS is a clinical diagnosis; *S aureus* is isolated from blood cultures in less than 5% of patients with TSS. Specimens for culture should be obtained from an identified focus of infection, because these sites usually yield the organism. Because approximately one-third of isolates of *S aureus* from nonmenstrual cases produce toxins other than TSS toxin-1, and TSS toxin-1–producing organisms can be present as normal flora, TSS toxin-1 production by an isolate is not a useful diagnostic test.

Antimicrobial susceptibility testing should be performed for all *S aureus* specimens isolated from normally sterile sites. Laboratory practice includes routine screening (D-testing) to exclude inducible clindamycin resistance. Another phenomenon that has been described is heteroresistance to antibiotics, in which the heterogeneous or heterotypic strains appear susceptible by disk diffusion but contain resistant subpopulations that are apparent only when cultured with antibiotic-containing media. When these resistant subpopulations are cultured on antibiotic-free media, they can continue as stable resistant mutants or revert to susceptible strains (heterogeneous resistance). Bacteria expressing heteroresistance grow more slowly than the susceptible bacteria and can be missed at growth conditions greater than 35 °C (>95 °F).

S aureus strain genotyping, in conjunction with epidemiological information, can facilitate identification of the source, extent, and mechanism of transmission in an outbreak. A number of molecular typing methods are available for *S aureus*, including pulsed-field gel electrophoresis, spa typing, and whole genome sequencing.

TREATMENT

Skin and Soft Tissue Infection

Skin and soft tissue infection, such as diffuse impetigo or cellulitis attributable to methicillin-susceptible *S aureus* (MSSA), is optimally treated with oral penicillinase-resistant β-lactam drugs, such as a first- or second-generation cephalosporin. For the penicillin-allergic patient and in cases in which MRSA is considered, TMP-SMX, doxycycline, or clindamycin can be used if the isolate is susceptible. Topical mupirocin is recommended for localized impetigo.

The most frequent manifestation of community-associated MRSA infection is skin and soft tissue infection, which can range from mild to severe. Drainage is an important part of managing these types of infections. A randomized, placebo-controlled study evaluating treatment strategies for uncomplicated skin infections included children with simple abscesses 3 cm or smaller (6–11 months of age), 4 cm or smaller (1–8 years of age), or 5 cm or smaller (>8 years of age) in diameter and showed that drainage plus systemic oral therapy with either clindamycin or TMP-SMX is associated with better outcomes than those of drainage alone. Applying mupirocin to the nares and bathing with chlorhexidine for 5 consecutive days for all family members have been associated with decreased recurrences. Studies in adults have reported success with a 7-day course of the combination of oral rifampin and doxycycline plus nasal mupirocin.

Invasive Staphylococcal Infections

Empirical therapy for suspected invasive staphylococcal infection, including pneumonia, osteoarticular infection, visceral abscesses, and foreign body–associated infection with bacteremia, is vancomycin plus a semisynthetic β-lactam (eg, nafcillin, oxacillin). Subsequent therapy should be based on antimicrobial susceptibility results. Serious MSSA infections require intravenous therapy with an antistaphylococcal β-lactam antimicrobial agent, such as nafcillin, oxacillin, or cefazolin, because most *S aureus* strains produce β-lactamase enzymes and resist penicillin and ampicillin. The addition of rifampin may be considered for those with invasive disease associated with an indwelling foreign body, especially if removal of the infected implant or device is not feasible. Vancomycin is not recommended for treatment of serious MSSA infections (including endocarditis), because it is weakly bactericidal and outcomes are inferior with vancomycin compared with antistaphylococcal β-lactams. First- or second-generation cephalosporins (eg, cefazolin) or vancomycin is less effective than nafcillin or oxacillin for treatment of MSSA meningitis. Clindamycin is bacteriostatic and should not be used for treatment of primary bacteremia or endovascular infection.

For MRSA pneumonia complicating influenza in children, vancomycin monotherapy in the first 24 hours of treatment was associated with higher mortality than that of vancomycin combined with a second antibiotic (clindamycin, linezolid, or ceftaroline) in a retrospective, multicenter study. Thus, a combination of vancomycin plus one of these agents is recommended for empirical treatment of children with life-threatening pneumonia complicating influenza. Antibiotic therapy can be de-escalated to a single agent if there is clinical improvement and antibiotic susceptibility information to guide treatment.

VISA infection is rare in children. For seriously ill patients who have a history of recurrent MRSA infections or for patients whose vancomycin therapy is failing and in whom VISA strains are a consideration, initial therapy could include linezolid or TMP-SMX, with or without gentamicin. If antimicrobial susceptibility results document multidrug resistance, alternative agents, such as ceftaroline, daptomycin (except for pneumonia, for which daptomycin should not be used because of inhibition by pulmonary surfactant), tigecycline, or quinupristin-dalfopristin, could be considered. In addition, in children younger than 8 years, there may be reversible inhibition of bone growth and adverse effects on tooth development with tigecycline use.

Duration of therapy for serious MSSA or MRSA infections depends on the site and severity of infection but is usually 4 weeks or longer for endocarditis, osteomyelitis, necrotizing pneumonia, or disseminated infection, assuming a documented clinical and microbiological response. In assessing whether modification of therapy is necessary, clinicians should consider whether the patient is improving clinically, should identify and drain sequestered foci of infection and remove foreign material (eg, a central catheter) when possible, and for MRSA strains should consider the vancomycin MIC and the achievable vancomycin exposure. The area under the curve to MIC (AUC:MIC) has been identified as the most appropriate pharmacokinetic/pharmacodynamic target for vancomycin in patients with MRSA. Dosing in children should be designed to achieve an AUC of 400 to 600 μg-hour/L (assuming MIC of 1) and/or trough levels less than 15 μg/mL to minimize acute kidney injury risks. Bayesian estimation can be completed with 2 levels, with one level being recommended 1 to 2 hours after end of vancomycin infusion and the second level being drawn 4 to 6 hours after end of infusion. Levels can be obtained as early as after the second dose. It is recommended to avoid AUC greater than 800 and troughs greater than 15. Most children younger than 12 years require higher doses to achieve optimal AUC:MIC as compared to older children.

Completion of the treatment course with an oral drug can be considered in children if an endovascular infection (ie, endocarditis, infected thrombus) or central nervous system (CNS) infection is not a concern. For endovascular and CNS infections, parenteral therapy is recommended for the entire treatment course (Table 133.1). Drainage of large abscesses, often more than once, and removal of foreign bodies are almost always required in addition to medical therapy. In some cases, multiple debridement procedures are necessary for children with complicated S aureus osteoarticular infection.

Duration of therapy for S aureus central catheter–associated bloodstream infections is controversial and is dependent on a number of factors (ie, the type and location of the catheter, the site of infection [exit site vs tunnel vs line], the feasibility of using an alternative vascular access site at a later date, the presence or absence of a catheter-related thrombus, and host immunity). Infections are more difficult to treat when associated with a thrombus, thrombophlebitis, or an intra-atrial thrombus, and a longer course is suggested if the patient is immunocompromised. Expert opinion differs on recommended treatment duration, but

Table 133.1
Parenteral Antimicrobial Agent(s) for Treatment of Bacteremia and Other Serious *Staphylococcus aureus* Infections

Antimicrobial Agents	Comments
I. Initial empirical therapy (organism of unknown susceptibility)	
Drugs of choice: Vancomycin (15 mg/kg, every 6 h) + nafcillin or oxacillin[a,b]	For life-threatening infections (ie, septicemia, endocarditis, CNS infection); ceftaroline or linezolid are alternatives, but there are limited efficacy data in children.
Vancomycin (15 mg/kg, every 6–8 h)[b]	For non-life-threatening infection without signs of sepsis (eg, skin infection, cellulitis, osteomyelitis, pyarthrosis) when rates of MRSA colonization and infection in the community are substantial; ceftaroline or linezolid are alternatives.
Clindamycin	For non-life-threatening infection without signs of sepsis when rates of MRSA colonization and infection in the community are substantial and prevalence of clindamycin resistance is <15%
II. Methicillin-susceptible S aureus	
Drugs of choice: Nafcillin or oxacillin[c]	
Cefazolin	
Alternatives: Clindamycin	Only for patients with a serious penicillin allergy and clindamycin-susceptible strain
Vancomycin[b]	Only for patients with a serious penicillin and cephalosporin allergy
Ampicillin + sulbactam	For patients with polymicrobial infections caused by susceptible isolates
III. Methicillin-resistant S aureus (oxacillin MIC, ≥4 μg/mL)	
A. Health care–associated (multidrug resistant)	
Drugs of choice: Vancomycin ± gentamicin[b,c]	
Alternatives: susceptibility testing results available before alternative drugs are used — TMP-SMX	
Ceftaroline[d]	
Linezolid[d]	
Daptomycin[d,e]	
B. Community-associated (not multidrug resistant)	
Drugs of choice: Vancomycin ± gentamicin[b,c]	For life-threatening infections or endovascular infections including those complicated by venous thrombosis
Clindamycin (if strain susceptible)	For pneumonia,[a] septic arthritis, osteomyelitis, or skin or soft tissue infections
TMP-SMX	For skin or soft tissue infections
Doxycycline (if strain susceptible)	

(continues)

Table 133.1 (continued)

Antimicrobial Agents		Comments
B. Community-associated (not multidrug resistant) (continued)		
Alternative:	Vancomycin[b]	For serious infections
	Linezolid	For serious infections caused by clindamycin-resistant isolates in patients with renal dysfunction or those with intolerance of vancomycin
IV. Vancomycin–intermediately susceptible S aureus (MIC, 4–16 μg/mL)[d]		
Drugs of choice:	Optimal therapy unknown	Dependent on in vitro susceptibility test results
	Linezolid[d]	
	Ceftaroline[d]	
	Daptomycin[e]	
	Quinupristin-dalfopristin[d]	
	Tigecycline[d]	
Alternatives:	Vancomycin[b] + linezolid ± gentamicin	
	Vancomycin[b] + TMP-SMX[c]	

AUC indicates area under the curve; CNS, central nervous system; MIC, minimum inhibitory concentration; MRSA, methicillin-resistant *S aureus*; SMX, sulfamethoxazole; and TMP, trimethoprim.

[a] For suspected MRSA pneumonia complicating influenza in critically ill children, add clindamycin, ceftaroline, or linezolid to vancomycin empirical treatment. Empirical selection of antibiotics highly depends on the local/regional susceptibility data.

[b] The AUC:MIC has been identified as the most appropriate pharmacokinetic/pharmacodynamic target for vancomycin in adult patients with MRSA. Although there are limitations in prospective outcomes data in pediatric patients with serious MRSA infections, the most recent consensus guideline from the American Society of Health-System Pharmacists, the Infectious Diseases Society of America, the Pediatric Infectious Diseases Society, and the Society of Infectious Diseases Pharmacists recommend AUC-guided therapeutic monitoring, preferably with bayesian estimation, for all pediatric age-groups receiving vancomycin.[f–h] This estimation accounts for developmental changes of vancomycin clearance from newborn to adolescent. Dosing in children should be designed to achieve an AUC of 400 to 600 μg·hour/L (assuming MIC of 1) and/or trough levels <15 μg/mL to minimize acute kidney injury risks. Bayesian estimation can be completed with 2 levels, with one level being recommended 1–2 hours after end of vancomycin infusion and the second level being drawn 4–6 hours after end of infusion. Levels can be obtained as early as after the second dose. Software to assist with these calculations is available online and for purchase. It is recommended to avoid AUC >800 and troughs >15. Most children <12 years require higher doses to achieve optimal AUC:MIC as compared to older children. Consultation with an infectious diseases specialist should be considered to determine which agent to use and duration of use.

[c] Gentamicin and rifampin for the first 2 weeks should be added for endocarditis of a prosthetic device. Addition of rifampin is recommended for other device-related infections (ie, spinal instrumentation, prosthetic joint).

[d] Linezolid, ceftaroline, quinupristin-dalfopristin, and tigecycline are agents with activity in vitro and efficacy in adults with multidrug-resistant, gram-positive organisms, including *S aureus*. Because experience with these agents in children is limited, consultation with a specialist in infectious diseases should be considered before use. Further, tigecycline should not be used in children <8 years if there are effective alternatives, because there may be reversible inhibition of bone growth and adverse effects on tooth development.

[e] Daptomycin is active in vitro against multidrug-resistant, gram-positive organisms, including *S aureus*. Daptomycin is approved by the US Food and Drug Administration only for treatment of complicated skin and skin structure infections and for *S aureus* bloodstream infections. Daptomycin is ineffective for treatment of pneumonia. Because experience with these agents in children is limited, consultation with a specialist in infectious diseases should be considered before use.

[f] Rybak MJ, Le J, Lodise TP, et al. Therapeutic monitoring of vancomycin for serious methicillin-resistant *Staphylococcus aureus* infections: a revised consensus guideline and review by the American Society of Health-System Pharmacists, the Infectious Diseases Society of America, the Pediatric Infectious Diseases Society, and the Society of Infectious Diseases Pharmacists. *Am J Health Syst Pharm.* 2020;77(11):835–864.

[g] Rybak MJ, Le J, Lodise TP, et al. Executive summary: therapeutic monitoring of vancomycin for serious methicillin-resistant *Staphylococcus aureus* infections: a revised consensus guideline and review by the American Society of Health-System Pharmacists, the Infectious Diseases Society of America, the Pediatric Infectious Diseases Society, and the Society of Infectious Diseases Pharmacists. *J Pediatr Infect Dis Soc.* 2020;9(3):281–284.

[h] Heil EL, Claeys KC, Mynatt RP, et al. Making the change to area under the curve-based vancomycin dosing. *Am J Health Syst Pharm.* 2018;75(24):1986–1995.

many suggest a minimum of 14 days provided there is no evidence of a metastatic focus and the patient responds to antimicrobial therapy with rapid sterilization of the blood cultures. If the patient needs a new central catheter, waiting 48 to 72 hours after bacteremia has apparently resolved before insertion is optimal. If a tunneled catheter is needed for ongoing care, treatment of the infection without removal of the catheter can be attempted but may not always be successful. Vegetations or a thrombus in the heart or great vessels should always be considered when a central catheter becomes infected and should be suspected more strongly if blood cultures remain positive for longer than 2 days on appropriate antimicrobial therapy following removal of the central catheter or if there are other clinical manifestations associated with endocarditis. Transesophageal echocardiography is the most sensitive technique for identifying vegetations, but transthoracic echocardiography is generally adequate for children younger than 10 years and/or weighing less than 60 kg.

Management of *S aureus* Toxin-Mediated Diseases

The principles of therapy for TSS include aggressive fluid management (and vasoactive agents, as needed) to maintain adequate venous return and cardiac filling to prevent end-organ damage, source control that includes prompt identification and removal of any indwelling foreign body (eg, tampon) or drainable focus, and anticipation and management of the commonly observed multiorgan complications of TSS (eg, acute respiratory distress syndrome, renal dysfunction). Initial antimicrobial therapy should include a parentally administered antistaphylococcal β-lactam antimicrobial agent and a protein synthesis-inhibiting drug, such as clindamycin, at maximum dosages. Vancomycin should be added to the β-lactam agent in regions where MRSA infections are common, although MRSA-associated TSS is rare in the United States. Empirical antibiotic therapy should be modified to targeted therapy once antibiotic susceptibilities are known. An active antimicrobial agent should be continued for 10 to 14 days. Administration of antimicrobial agents can be changed to the oral route once the patient is tolerating oral alimentation. The total duration of therapy is based on the usual duration of established foci of infection (eg, pneumonia, osteomyelitis). Immune globulin intravenous (IGIV) can be considered in patients with severe staphylococcal TSS unresponsive to other therapeutic measures, because IGIV may neutralize circulating toxin. Although data on the use of IGIV are not robust, it may be considered for critically ill children with shock that is unresponsive to fluid resuscitation, an undrainable focus of infection, or persistent oliguria with pulmonary edema. The optimal IGIV regimen is unknown, but 150 to 400 mg/kg per day for 5 days or a single dose of 1 to 2 g/kg has been used. SSSS in infants should be treated with a parenteral antistaphylococcal β-lactam antimicrobial agent or clindamycin, depending on local susceptibility patterns and the severity of the disease. If MRSA is a consideration, vancomycin or clindamycin (depending on local susceptibility patterns) can be used. Transition to an oral agent is appropriate in nonneonates who have demonstrated excellent clinical response to parenteral therapy.

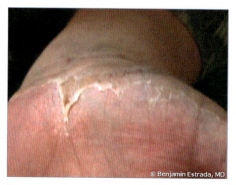

Image 133.1
Skin desquamation of the hand in a 7-year-old boy with staphylococcal scalded skin syndrome. Courtesy of Benjamin Estrada, MD.

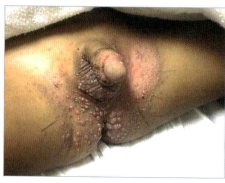

Image 133.2
Newborn with pustulosis of the perineum and genitalia caused by *Staphylococcus aureus*. Copyright Michael Rajnik, MD, FAAP.

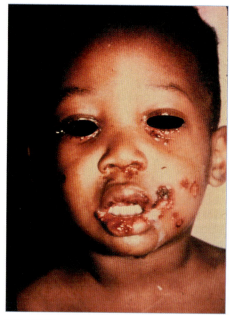

Image 133.3
Staphylococcal bullous impetigo lesions around the eyes, nose, and mouth in a 6-year-old boy. Also, note the secondary anterior cervical lymphadenopathy. Courtesy of George Nankervis, MD.

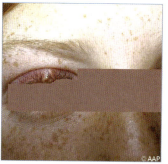

Image 133.4
Staphylococcus aureus hordeolum (sebaceous gland abscess) in an adolescent girl.

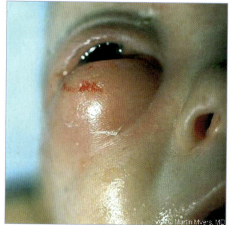

Image 133.5
An infant with orbital cellulitis and ethmoid sinusitis caused by *Staphylococcus aureus*. Copyright Martin G. Myers, MD.

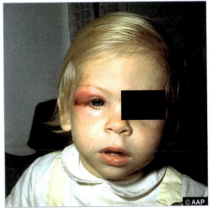

Image 133.6
Periorbital cellulitis caused by *Staphylococcus aureus*–infected lesion adjacent to the orbit (most likely secondary to a recent insect bite). Courtesy of Edgar O. Ledbetter, MD, FAAP.

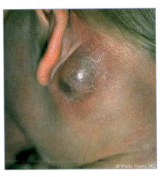

Image 133.7
A 1½-year-old boy, atopic, with subauricular lymphadenitis caused by *Staphylococcus aureus*. Copyright Martin G. Myers, MD.

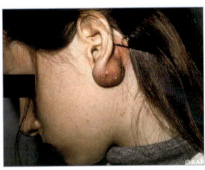

Image 133.8
Staphylococcus aureus abscess of the lobe of the left ear secondary to ear piercing in an adolescent girl. Courtesy of Edgar O. Ledbetter, MD, FAAP.

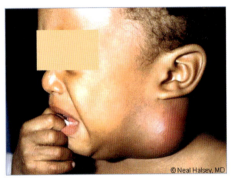

Image 133.9
Subauricular cervical adenitis *Staphylococcus aureus* in a 2-year-old boy. Copyright Neal Halsey, MD.

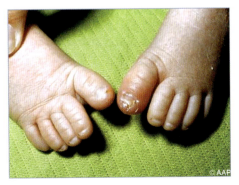

Image 133.10
Posttraumatic paronychia caused by *Staphylococcus aureus* of the left great toe of an infant. Courtesy of Edgar O. Ledbetter, MD, FAAP.

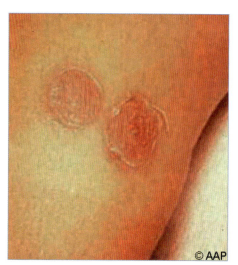

Image 133.11
Impetigo (bullous) caused by *Staphylococcus aureus*.

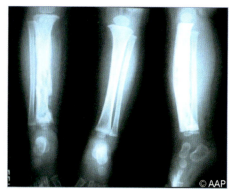

Image 133.13
Chronic osteomyelitis of the right tibia caused by *Staphylococcus aureus*.

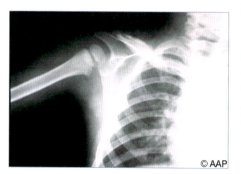

Image 133.15
In a 12-year-old boy, chronic osteomyelitis of the clavicle caused by *Staphylococcus aureus*.

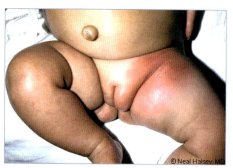

Image 133.12
Cellulitis, inguinal, caused by *Staphylococcus aureus*. Copyright Neal Halsey, MD.

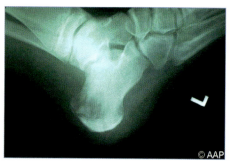

Image 133.14
Osteomyelitis of the calcaneus caused by *Staphylococcus aureus* with no history of injury.

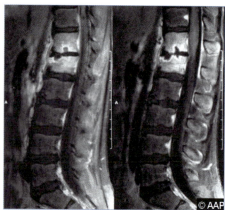

Image 133.16
Vertebral osteomyelitis in a 13-year-old with a 6-week history of back pain. Magnetic resonance imaging revealed osteolytic changes of the anterior segments of the first and second lumbar vertebrae. A culture of the biopsy specimen grew methicillin-resistant *Staphylococcus aureus*.

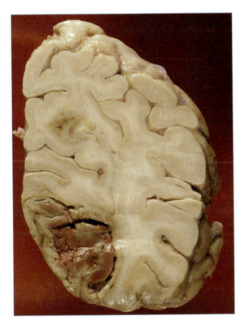

Image 133.17
Cerebral infarct in a patient with bacterial endocarditis.
Courtesy of Dimitris P. Agamanolis, MD.

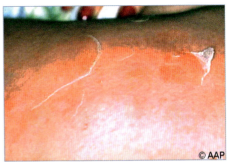

Image 133.18
Staphylococcal scalded skin syndrome with a positive Nikolsky sign.

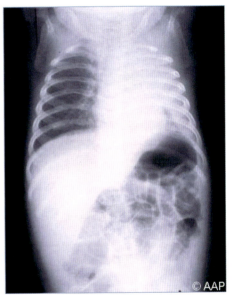

Image 133.20
Staphylococcal pneumonia, primary, with rapid progression with empyema. This is the same patient as in Image 133.19.

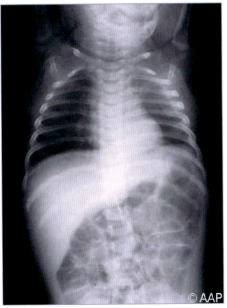

Image 133.19
Staphylococcal pneumonia, primary, with rapid progression and empyema. The infant had only mild respiratory distress and paralytic ileus without fever when first examined.

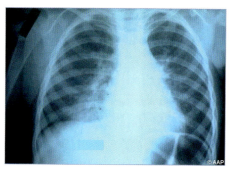

Image 133.21
Pneumonia caused by *Staphylococcus aureus* with right lower lobe infiltrate in a preschool-aged child (day 1). Courtesy of Edgar O. Ledbetter, MD, FAAP.

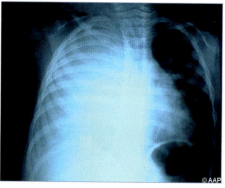

Image 133.22
Staphylococcal pneumonia with massive empyema demonstrating the rather rapid progression typical of staphylococcal infection. This is the same patient as in Image 133.21 (day 4). Courtesy of Edgar O. Ledbetter, MD, FAAP.

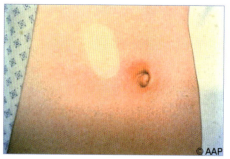

Image 133.23
Erythroderma that blanches on pressure in a patient with toxic shock syndrome. The mortality rate for staphylococcal toxic shock syndrome is lower than that for streptococcal toxic shock syndrome.

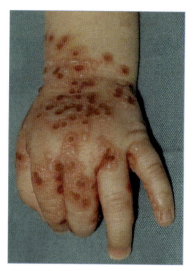

Image 133.24
Children who have atopic dermatitis are prone to recurrent skin infections, particularly with *Staphylococcus aureus* and herpes simplex virus, for several reasons. Exacerbations of eczema disrupt the skin's protective barrier. The failure to produce endogenous antimicrobial peptides has been offered as a reason.

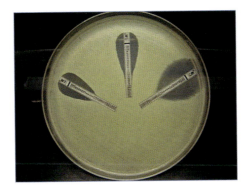

Image 133.25
A *Staphylococcus aureus* isolate tested by the gradient diffusion method with vancomycin, daptomycin, and linezolid on Mueller-Hinton-IH agar. The minimum inhibitory concentration of each agent is determined by the intersection of the organism growth with the strip as measured by use of the scale inscribed on the strip. Used with permission from *Clinical Infectious Diseases*.

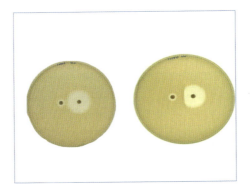

Image 133.26
D zone test for clindamycin-induced resistance by *Staphylococcus aureus*. The left shows a negative result, and the right shows a positive one. Courtesy of Sarah Long, MD, FAAP.

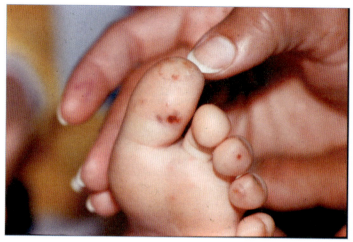

Image 133.27
Janeway lesions on the toes of a 4-year-old with subacute bacterial endocarditis caused by *Staphylococcus aureus*. Courtesy of Carol J. Baker, MD, FAAP.

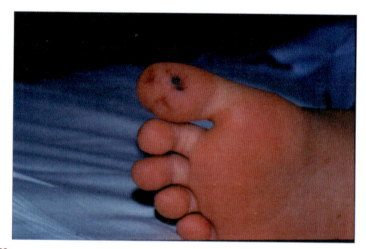

Image 133.28
Nontender, small erythematous or hemorrhagic macular or nodular lesions (Janeway lesions) of the toe in a 10-year-old boy who had acute *Staphylococcus aureus* bacterial endocarditis of the aortic valve. Courtesy of Carol J. Baker, MD, FAAP.

CHAPTER 134
Coagulase-Negative Staphylococcal Infections

CLINICAL MANIFESTATIONS

Most coagulase-negative staphylococci (CoNS) isolates from patient specimens represent contamination of culture material. Of the isolates that do not represent contamination, most come from infections associated with health care, such as obvious disruptions of host defenses caused by surgery, medical device insertion, immunosuppression, or preterm birth (eg, very low birth weight). CoNS are the most common cause of late-onset bacteremia and septicemia in preterm infants, typically infants weighing less than 1,500 g at birth, and of episodes of health care–associated bacteremia in all age-groups. CoNS are responsible for bacteremia in children with intravascular catheters, vascular grafts, intracardiac patches, prosthetic cardiac valves, or pacemaker wires. Infection may also be associated with other indwelling foreign bodies, including cerebrospinal fluid (CSF) shunts, peritoneal catheters, spinal instrumentation, baclofen pumps, pacemakers, or prosthetic joints. Mediastinitis after open-heart surgery, endophthalmitis after intraocular trauma, and omphalitis and scalp abscesses in preterm neonates have been described. CoNS can also enter the bloodstream from the respiratory tract of mechanically ventilated preterm infants or from the gastrointestinal tract of infants with necrotizing enterocolitis. Some species of CoNS are associated with urinary tract infection, including *Staphylococcus saprophyticus* in adolescent girls and young adult women, often after sexual intercourse, and *Staphylococcus epidermidis* and *Staphylococcus haemolyticus* in hospitalized patients with urinary tract catheters. *Staphylococcus lugdunensis* is particularly virulent and may cause infections resembling *Staphylococcus aureus*, including skin and soft tissue infection and bacteremia with or without endocarditis.

ETIOLOGY

There are more than 40 named coagulase-negative *Staphylococcus* species in the family; *S epidermidis*, *S haemolyticus*, *S saprophyticus*, *Staphylococcus schleiferi*, and *S lugdunensis* are most often associated with human infections. Many CoNS produce an exopolysaccharide slime biofilm that enables these organisms to bind to medical devices (eg, catheters) and makes them relatively inaccessible to host defenses and antimicrobial agents.

EPIDEMIOLOGY

CoNS are common inhabitants of the skin and mucous membranes. Virtually all neonates are colonized with CoNS at multiple sites by 2 to 4 days of age. The most frequently isolated CoNS organism is *S epidermidis*, which is found widely in most areas of skin. Different species colonize specific areas of the body. *S haemolyticus* is found on areas of skin with numerous apocrine glands, and *S lugdunensis* has a predilection for colonization of the inguinal and groin areas. Infants and children in intensive care units, including neonatal intensive care units, have the highest incidence of CoNS bloodstream infections. CoNS can be introduced at the time of medical device placement, through mucous membrane or skin breaks, through loss of bowel wall integrity (eg, necrotizing enterocolitis in very low birth weight neonates), or during catheter manipulation. Less often, health care professionals with environmental CoNS colonization on their hands transmit the organism.

The **incubation period** is variable for CoNS disease. A long delay can occur between acquisition of the organism and onset of disease.

DIAGNOSTICS TESTS

CoNS are readily isolated in culture by using the same media and incubation conditions used for *S aureus*. Tests for coagulase by traditional methods or by latex agglutination are the same as are used for *S aureus*. CoNS isolated from a single blood culture are commonly classified as skin contaminants introduced into the blood culture bottle during venipuncture, and full identification and antimicrobial susceptibility testing are not performed by most clinical laboratories. Fluorescent in situ hybridization probes or multiplex polymerase chain reaction panel assays can rapidly differentiate CoNS and *S aureus* in positive blood cultures. In a very preterm neonate, a person with immunocompromise, or a patient with an indwelling catheter or prosthetic device, repeated isolation of the same species of CoNS from blood cultures or another normally sterile body fluid suggests true infection. For central catheter–associated bloodstream infection, blood cultures drawn from the catheter generally become positive 2 or more hours before cultures from a peripheral blood vessel. This type of analysis requires that both peripheral and catheter blood cultures be performed at the same time by using equal volumes of blood.

Criteria that suggest CoNS as bloodstream pathogens, rather than contaminants, include

- Two or more positive blood cultures with the same *Staphylococcus* species from different collection sites
- A positive culture from blood and from another sterile site (eg, CSF, joint) with the same *Staphylococcus* species and identical antimicrobial susceptibility patterns for each isolate
- Growth in a continuously monitored blood culture system within 15 hours of incubation
- Clinical findings of infection
- An intravascular catheter that has been in place for 3 days or more
- Similar or identical genotypes among all isolates

TREATMENT

Greater than 90% of health care–associated CoNS strains are methicillin resistant. Methicillin-resistant strains are resistant to all β-lactam drugs, including cephalosporins (except ceftaroline), and usually several other drug classes. Intravenous vancomycin is recommended for treatment of serious infections caused by CoNS strains resistant to β-lactam antimicrobial agents. Ceftaroline, daptomycin, and linezolid are alternative agents when vancomycin cannot be used. An exception to this is *S lugdunensis*, which is generally methicillin susceptible. Treatment of infected foreign bodies often involves removal of the device, in addition to antibiotic therapy. Prolonged therapy is likely necessary when there is endocarditis or when the infected device (eg, spinal hardware) cannot be removed entirely. Antimicrobial lock therapy of tunneled central catheters may result in a higher rate of catheter salvage among adults with CoNS infections, but experience with this approach is limited in children. If blood cultures remain positive for more than 3 to 5 days after initiation of appropriate antimicrobial therapy for CoNS or if the patient's condition fails to improve, the central catheter should be removed, parenteral therapy should be continued, and the patient should be evaluated for metastatic foci of infection. If a central catheter is removed, there is no demonstrable thrombus, and bacteremia resolves promptly, a 5-day course of therapy is generally appropriate for CoNS infections in immunocompetent hosts. The exception is *S lugdunensis*, which should be managed similarly to *S aureus* catheter-related infections.

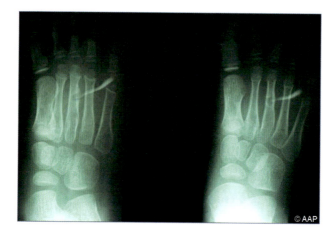

Image 134.1
Osteomyelitis caused by *Staphylococcus epidermidis* secondary to foreign body penetration of the third metatarsal of the right foot in a 5-year-old boy. Coagulase-negative staphylococcal infections are often associated with disruption of normal defense mechanisms. Courtesy of Edgar O. Ledbetter, MD, FAAP.

CHAPTER 135

Group A Streptococcal Infections

CLINICAL MANIFESTATIONS

The most common group A streptococcal (GAS) infection is acute pharyngotonsillitis (pharyngitis), which manifests as sore throat with tonsillar inflammation and, often, tender anterior cervical lymphadenopathy, palatal petechiae, or a strawberry tongue. Purulent complications of pharyngitis include peritonsillar or retropharyngeal abscesses, suppurative cervical adenitis, and, rarely, sinusitis and otitis media. Nonsuppurative complications include acute rheumatic fever (ARF) and acute glomerulonephritis (AGN). The goal of antimicrobial therapy for GAS pharyngitis is to reduce acute morbidity, suppurative and nonsuppurative (ARF) complications, and transmission to close contacts. Antimicrobial therapy to prevent AGN after pyoderma or pharyngitis is ineffective.

Scarlet fever occurs most often with pharyngitis and rarely with pyoderma or an infected wound. Scarlet fever, which has reemerged in the United Kingdom, China, and Hong Kong, involves a characteristic confluent erythematous sandpaper-like rash caused by one or more GAS erythrogenic exotoxins. Other than rash, the epidemiological features, symptoms, signs, sequelae, and treatment of scarlet fever are the same as those of streptococcal pharyngitis.

Acute streptococcal pharyngitis is uncommon in children younger than 3 years. Instead, they may present with rhinitis and a protracted illness with moderate fever, irritability, and anorexia (streptococcal fever or streptococcosis). The second most common site of GAS infection is the skin. Streptococcal skin infections (eg, pyoderma or impetigo) can be followed by AGN, occasionally in epidemics. GAS skin infection has not been proven to lead to ARF.

Other GAS infections include erysipelas, cellulitis (including perianal), vaginitis, bacteremia, sepsis, pneumonia, endocarditis, pericarditis, septic arthritis, necrotizing fasciitis (NF), purpura fulminans, osteomyelitis, myositis, puerperal sepsis, surgical wound infection, mastoiditis, and neonatal omphalitis. Invasive GAS infections often encompass bacteremia with or without a focus of infection and can manifest as streptococcal toxic shock syndrome (TSS), overwhelming sepsis, or NF. Necrotizing fasciitis can follow minor or unrecognized trauma but uncommonly follows pharyngitis, often involves an extremity, and manifests as pain out of proportion to examination findings.

Streptococcal TSS is caused by infection of normally sterile body site(s) (eg, blood, pleura, cerebrospinal fluid) with a toxin-producing GAS strain, typically manifesting as a severe acute illness with fever, generalized erythroderma, rapid-onset hypotension, and signs of multiorgan involvement, including renal failure. Local soft tissue infection (eg, cellulitis, myositis, NF) associated with severe, rapidly increasing pain is common, although streptococcal TSS can occur without an identifiable focus of infection.

Rheumatic fever is a nonsuppurative sequela of GAS pharyngitis and is endemic in parts of Africa, Asia, and the Pacific, including the Australian and New Zealand Indigenous populations. The United States, Canada, and most countries of Europe are considered ARF low-risk areas, although sporadic cases continue to occur.

An association between GAS infection and sudden onset of obsessive-compulsive behavior, tic disorders, or other unexplained acute neurological changes (ie, pediatric autoimmune neuropsychiatric disorders associated with streptococcal infections [PANDAS], as a subset of pediatric acute-onset neuropsychiatric syndrome [PANS]) has been proposed. Data for an association with GAS infection and either PANDAS or PANS rely on a number of small and as yet unduplicated studies. In the absence of acute clinical symptoms and signs of pharyngitis, GAS testing (by culture, antigen detection, or serology) is not recommended for such patients. There is also insufficient evidence to support antibiotic treatment or prophylaxis, immune globulin, or plasmapheresis for children suspected to have PANDAS or PANS. Management is best directed by specialists with experience with the manifesting symptoms and signs, such as child psychiatrists, behavioral and developmental pediatricians, or child neurologists.

ETIOLOGY

More than 240 distinct serotypes or genotypes of group A streptococci (*Streptococcus pyogenes*) have been identified on the basis of M-protein serotype or M-protein gene sequence (*emm* types). In general, *emm* typing is more discriminating than M-protein serotyping. Epidemiological studies indicate an association between certain *emm* types (eg, types 1, 3, 5, 6, 14, 18, 19, and 24) and rheumatic fever, but a specific rheumatogenic factor remains unidentified. Several *emm* types (eg, types 2, 49, 55, 57, 59, 60, and 61) are more commonly associated with pyoderma and AGN. Other serotypes (eg, types 1, 6, and 12) are associated with pharyngitis and AGN. Although many M types can cause streptococcal TSS, most cases are caused by *emm* 1 and *emm* 3 strains producing at least 1 pyrogenic exotoxin, most commonly streptococcal pyrogenic exotoxin A (*speA*). These toxins are superantigens, stimulating production of tumor necrosis factor and other inflammatory mediators causing capillary leak and other physiological changes including hypotension and multiorgan damage. In the United Kingdom, an increase in scarlet fever cases since 2016 has been associated with a new strain of *emm*1 (M1UK lineage).

EPIDEMIOLOGY

Pharyngitis usually results from contact with respiratory secretions of someone with GAS pharyngitis. Fomites and household pets, such as dogs, are not vectors. Pharyngitis and impetigo (and their nonsuppurative complications) can be associated with crowding, often present in socioeconomically disadvantaged populations. Close contact in schools, child care centers, contact sports (eg, wrestling), boarding schools, and military installations facilitates transmission. Rare foodborne outbreaks of pharyngitis are a consequence of human contamination of food with improper food preparation or refrigeration.

GAS pharyngitis occurs at all ages but is most common in school-aged children and adolescents, peaking at 7 to 8 years of age. GAS pharyngitis and pyoderma are substantially less common in adults than children.

Geographically, GAS pharyngitis and pyoderma are ubiquitous. Pyoderma is more common in tropical climates and warm seasons, in part because of antecedent insect bites and other minor skin trauma. Streptococcal pharyngitis is more common during late autumn, winter, and spring in temperate climates, in part because of close contact in schools. Communicability of streptococcal pharyngitis peaks during acute infection and when untreated gradually diminishes over weeks.

Throat culture surveys of healthy asymptomatic children during the streptococcal season and during school outbreaks of pharyngitis yield GAS infection prevalence rates as high as 25%. GAS carriage can persist for many months, but the risk of transmission is low.

In streptococcal impetigo, the organism is usually acquired by direct contact from another person. GAS colonization of healthy skin usually precedes impetigo. Impetiginous lesions occur at the site of breaks in skin (eg, insect bites, burns, traumatic wounds, varicella lesions). After development of impetiginous lesions, the upper respiratory tract can become colonized with GAS organisms. Infection of surgical wounds and postpartum (puerperal) sepsis usually result from transmission through direct contact. Health care workers who are pharyngeal, anal, or vaginal GAS carriers and those with skin infection or skin colonization can transmit GAS infection to patients, particularly surgical and obstetric patients, resulting in health care–associated outbreaks. Infections in neonates, uncommon in the United States but common in many developing countries, result from intrapartum or contact transmission; the latter infection can begin as omphalitis, cellulitis, or NF. In the United States, the incidence of invasive GAS infections is highest among infants and elderly people. Fatal cases in children are uncommon, but they can progress very rapidly (eg, overwhelming sepsis). Before varicella vaccine, varicella infection (chickenpox) was the most common predisposing factor for invasive GAS infection in children. Other risk factors include exposure to other children and household crowding. The portal of entry is unknown in most invasive GAS infections but is presumably skin or mucous membranes. Such infections very rarely follow symptomatic GAS pharyngitis. An association between nonsteroidal anti-inflammatory drugs and invasive GAS infections in children with varicella has been suggested, but a causal relationship has not been established.

Streptococcal TSS can occur at any age. Less than 5% of invasive streptococcal infections in children are associated with streptococcal TSS. Childhood streptococcal TSS has been reported with focal lesions (eg, varicella, cellulitis, trauma, osteomyelitis, pneumonia), and with bacteremia without a defined focus. Mortality rates are substantially lower for children than for adults with streptococcal TSS.

During GAS epidemics on military bases in the 1950s, ARF developed in up to 3% of cases of untreated acute GAS pharyngitis; rare cases have occurred in treated patients. The current incidence in the United States is not precisely known but is believed to be less than 0.5%, with higher rates reported among people of Samoan ancestry living in Hawaii or residents of American Samoa. Focal outbreaks of ARF in school-aged children occurred in several areas in the 1990s, and small clusters continue to be reported periodically, most likely related to circulation of particularly rheumatogenic strains.

The **incubation period** for streptococcal pharyngitis is 2 to 5 days. For impetigo, a 7- to 10-day period between GAS acquisition on healthy skin and development of lesions has been demonstrated. The **incubation period** for streptococcal TSS is unknown but is as short as 14 hours when associated with subcutaneous inoculation of organisms (eg, puerperal sepsis, penetrating trauma).

DIAGNOSTIC TESTS

Testing for Group A Streptococci in Pharyngitis

Children with acute onset of sore throat and clinical signs and symptoms such as pharyngeal exudate, pain on swallowing, fever, and enlarged tender anterior cervical nodes are more likely to have GAS infection and should be tested. Children with pharyngitis and obvious viral symptoms (eg, rhinorrhea, cough, hoarseness, oral ulcers) should not be tested or treated for GAS infection; testing is also not generally recommended for children younger than 3 years. Laboratory confirmation before initiation of antimicrobial treatment is required for children with pharyngitis without viral symptoms, because many do not have GAS pharyngitis. A specimen should be obtained by vigorously swabbing both tonsils and the posterior pharynx for rapid antigen testing or other diagnostic tests, as discussed below. A second swab specimen from a child with a negative rapid antigen test result should be submitted for culture. Culture on sheep blood agar can confirm GAS infection, with latex agglutination differentiating group A streptococci from other β-hemolytic streptococci (eg, group C or G). False-negative culture results occur in less than 10% of symptomatic patients when an adequate throat swab specimen is obtained and cultured by trained personnel. Recovery of GAS organisms from the pharynx, including the number of colonies on a culture plate, does not distinguish patients with true acute streptococcal infection from chronic streptococcal carriers with intercurrent viral pharyngitis. Cultures negative for GAS organisms after 18 to 24 hours' incubation should be reincubated for a second day to optimize recovery from GAS infection.

Several rapid tests for GAS pharyngitis are available. The specificity of these tests is generally high (very few false-positive results), but reported sensitivities vary considerably and are generally 80% to 85% (ie, false-negatives occur). As with throat cultures, the sensitivity of these tests highly depends on the quality of the throat swab specimen, the experience of the test performer, and the rigor of the culture method used for comparison.

Because of very high specificity of rapid antigen tests, a positive result does not require culture confirmation, but negative results require a confirmatory test in children. Other diagnostic tests by using techniques such as polymerase chain reaction assay, chemiluminescent DNA probes, and isothermal nucleic acid amplification tests (NAATs) have been developed. The US Food and Drug Administration has cleared some NAATs for detection of group A streptococci from throat swab specimens as stand-alone tests that, because of high sensitivity, do not require routine culture confirmation of negative test results. Some studies suggest that in addition to providing more timely results, these tests may be more sensitive than standard throat swab cultures on sheep blood agar, although the device labeling states that culture is still required if the test result is negative and the patient's symptoms persist or if there is an outbreak of rheumatic fever.

Testing Contacts for GAS Infection

Indications for testing contacts for GAS infection are few. Testing asymptomatic household contacts is not recommended, except when the contacts have increased risk for sequelae of GAS infection, such as ARF or AGN; if test results are positive, the contacts should be treated.

In schools, child care centers, or other environments where many people are in close contact, the prevalence of GAS pharyngeal carriage in healthy children can reach 25% in the absence of an outbreak of streptococcal disease. Therefore, classroom or more widespread culturing is not generally indicated.

Follow-up Throat Cultures

Posttreatment throat cultures are indicated only for those with particularly high risk for ARF (eg, with previous history of ARF).

Patients with repeated episodes of pharyngitis at short intervals in whom GAS infection is documented by culture or rapid antigen test or NAAT present a special problem. Most often, they are chronic GAS carriers experiencing frequent viral illnesses for whom repeated testing and antimicrobials are unnecessary. In assessment of these patients, inadequate adherence to oral treatment should also be considered. Testing asymptomatic household contacts is not usually helpful. However, if multiple household members have pharyngitis or other GAS infections, simultaneous cultures of all household members and treatment following all positive test results may be of value.

Testing for Group A Streptococci in Nonpharyngitis Infections

Cultures of impetigo lesions often yield both streptococci and staphylococci, and determination of the primary pathogen is generally difficult. Culture is useful to determine *Staphylococcus aureus* susceptibility. In suspected invasive GAS infections, cultures of blood and focal sites of possible infection are indicated. In NF, imaging studies may delay, rather than facilitate, establishment of the diagnosis. Clinical suspicion of NF should prompt urgent surgical evaluation with possible urgent debridement of affected tissues, with Gram stain and culture of surgical specimens. Streptococcal TSS is diagnosed on the basis of clinical and laboratory findings and isolation of GAS organisms (Box 135.1); greater than 50% of patients with streptococcal TSS have blood cultures positive for group A streptococci. Cultures of focal sites of infection are also usually positive and can remain positive for several days after initiation of an appropriate antimicrobial agent.

TREATMENT

S pyogenes is uniformly susceptible to all β-lactam antibiotics (penicillins and cephalosporins); thus, susceptibility testing is needed only for non–β-lactam agents, such as a macrolide or clindamycin, to which *S pyogenes* can be resistant.

Pharyngitis

- Penicillin V is the drug of choice for GAS pharyngitis. Prompt administration of penicillin shortens the clinical course, decreases risk of transmission and suppurative sequelae, and prevents ARF, even when administered up to 9 days after illness onset. All patients with ARF should receive a complete course of penicillin or another appropriate antimicrobial agent for GAS pharyngitis, even if group A streptococci are not recovered from the throat.

- Amoxicillin, orally as a single daily dose (50 mg/kg; maximum, 1,000–1,200 mg) for 10 days, is as effective as penicillin V or amoxicillin administered orally multiple times per day for 10 days and is a more palatable suspension than penicillin V. This regimen is endorsed by the American Heart Association and the Infectious Disease Society of America in its guidelines for the treatment of GAS pharyngitis and the prevention of ARF. Adherence is particularly important for once-daily dosing regimens.

- The dose of oral penicillin V is 400,000 U (250 mg), 2 to 3 times per day, for 10 days for children weighing less than 27 kg and 800,000 U (500 mg), 2 to 3 times per day, for those weighing 27 kg or greater, including adolescents and adults. To prevent ARF, oral penicillin or amoxicillin should be taken for 10 full days, regardless

Box 135.1
Streptococcal Toxic Shock Syndrome: Clinical Case Definition[a]

I. Isolation of group A streptococci (*Streptococcus pyogenes*)
  A. From a normally sterile site (eg, blood; cerebrospinal, peritoneal, joint, pleural, or pericardial fluid)
  B. From a nonsterile site (eg, throat, sputum, vagina, open surgical wound, superficial skin lesion)
II. Clinical signs of severity
  A. Hypotension: systolic pressure ≤90 mm Hg in adults or <5th percentile for age in children <16 years

AND

  B. Two or more of the following signs of multiorgan involvement:
  - Renal impairment: creatinine concentration ≥177 μmol/L (≥2 mg/dL) for adults or at least 2 times the upper limit of reference for age[b]
  - Coagulopathy: platelet count ≤100,000/μL and/or disseminated intravascular coagulation defined by prolonged clotting times, low fibrinogen level, and presence of fibrin degradation products
  - Hepatic involvement: elevated alanine aminotransferase, aspartate aminotransferase, or total bilirubin concentrations at least 2 times the upper limit of reference for age[b]
  - Acute respiratory distress syndrome defined by acute onset of diffuse pulmonary infiltrates and hypoxemia in absence of cardiac failure or by evidence of diffuse capillary leak
  - A generalized erythematous macular rash that may desquamate
  - Soft tissue necrosis, including necrotizing fasciitis or myositis, or gangrene

[a] An illness fulfilling criteria IA and IIA and IIB can be defined as a *confirmed* case. An illness fulfilling criteria IB and IIA and IIB can be defined as a *probable* case if no other cause for the illness is identified. Manifestations need not be detected within the first 48 hours of illness or hospitalization.
[b] In patients with preexisting renal or hepatic disease, concentrations ≥2-fold patient's baseline.

Adapted from The Working Group on Severe Streptococcal Infections. Defining the group A streptococcal toxic shock syndrome: rationale and consensus definition. *JAMA*. 1993;269(3):390–391.

---

of promptness of clinical recovery. Treatment failures occur more often with oral penicillin than with intramuscular penicillin G benzathine because of inadequate adherence. Notably, short-course treatment (<10 days) of GAS pharyngitis, particularly with penicillin V, is associated with inferior bacteriologic eradication rates.

- Intramuscular penicillin G benzathine is appropriate therapy, helping ensure adequate blood concentrations and prevent adherence issues, but administration may be painful. Discomfort is decreased if the preparation of penicillin G benzathine is brought to room temperature before intramuscular injection. Mixtures containing shorter-acting penicillins (eg, penicillin G procaine) in addition to penicillin G benzathine are not more effective than penicillin G benzathine alone but are less painful. Although supporting data are limited, the combination of 900,000 U (562.5 mg) of penicillin G benzathine and 300,000 U (187.5 mg) of penicillin G procaine is satisfactory for most children; however, the efficacy of this combination for heavier patients has not been documented.

- For patients who have a history of nonanaphylactic allergy to penicillin, a 10-day course of a narrow-spectrum (first-generation) oral cephalosporin (eg, cephalexin) is indicated. Patients with immediate (anaphylactic) or type I hypersensitivity to penicillin should receive oral clindamycin (20 mg/kg/day in 3 divided doses; maximum, 900 mg/day for 10 days) rather than a cephalosporin.

- An oral macrolide (eg, erythromycin, azithromycin, clarithromycin) is also acceptable for penicillin-allergic patients. This should not be used in patients who can take a β-lactam agent. Therapy for 10 days is indicated, except for azithromycin, which is given for 5 days. GAS strains resistant to macrolides have been highly prevalent in some countries and have resulted in treatment failures. In some areas in the United States, macrolide resistance rates of greater than 20% have been reported. Testing for macrolide resistance may help decide the best antimicrobial agent for specific penicillin-allergic patients.

- Tetracyclines, sulfonamides, and fluoroquinolones should not be used for treating GAS pharyngitis.

Shortly after a full course of a recommended oral agent, children with recurrent GAS pharyngitis can be re-treated with the same antimicrobial agent (if it is a β-lactam), an alternative β-lactam oral drug (eg, cephalexin, amoxicillin-clavulanate), or an intramuscular dose of penicillin G benzathine. Susceptibility testing should be performed when considering a macrolide or clindamycin.

Frequent Acute Pharyngitis With Positive GAS Testing

Treatment of a patient with frequently repeated episodes of acute pharyngitis and repeatedly positive test results for group A streptococci is complex. To determine whether the patient is a long-term streptococcal pharyngeal carrier who is experiencing repeated episodes of intercurrent viral pharyngitis (the most common situation), it should be determined (1) whether clinical findings are more suggestive of GAS or viral infection; (2) whether household or community epidemiological factors support group A streptococci or a virus as the cause; (3) what the nature of the clinical response to antimicrobial therapy is (in bona fide GAS pharyngitis, response to therapy is usually <24 hours); and (4) whether test results are positive for group A streptococci between episodes of acute pharyngitis (suggesting the patient is a carrier). Measurement of serological response to GAS extracellular antigens (eg, antistreptolysin O) is discouraged, because interpretation can be very difficult. Typing (M or *emm* typing) of GAS isolates is generally available only in research laboratories, but if this typing is performed, repeated isolation of the same type suggests carriage; isolation of differing types indicates repeated infections.

Pharyngeal Carriers

Antimicrobial therapy is not indicated for most GAS pharyngeal carriers. The few specific situations in which eradication of carriage may be indicated include (1) a local outbreak of ARF or poststreptococcal glomerulonephritis; (2) an outbreak of GAS pharyngitis in a closed or semiclosed community; (3) a family history of ARF; (4) multiple (ping-pong) episodes of documented symptomatic GAS pharyngitis occurring within a family for many weeks despite appropriate therapy; or (5) a patient being seriously considered for tonsillectomy solely because of frequent GAS isolations.

GAS carriage is difficult to eradicate with conventional antimicrobial therapy. Several agents, including clindamycin, cephalosporins, amoxicillin-clavulanate, azithromycin, or a combination that includes either 10 days of penicillin V or intramuscular penicillin G benzathine with rifampin for the last 4 days of treatment, are more effective than penicillin alone in terminating chronic streptococcal carriage. Of these drugs, oral clindamycin, 20 to 30 mg/kg/day in 3 doses (maximum, 900 mg/day) for 10 days, has been reported to be most effective. Documented eradication of carriage is helpful in evaluation of subsequent episodes of acute pharyngitis; however, carriage can recur after reacquisition of GAS infection, as some individuals are "carrier prone."

Nonbullous Impetigo

Topical mupirocin or retapamulin ointment may be useful for limiting person-to-person spread of nonbullous impetigo and for eradicating localized disease. With multiple lesions or nonbullous impetigo in multiple family members, child care groups, or athletic teams, treatment should include oral agents active against both group A streptococci and *S aureus*.

Toxic Shock Syndrome

As outlined in boxes 135.2 and 135.3, most aspects of management are the same for TSS caused by group A streptococci or by *S aureus*. Paramount are immediate aggressive fluid resuscitation; management of respiratory and cardiac failure, if present; and prompt surgical debridement of any deep-seated infection. Because *S pyogenes* and *S aureus* TSS are difficult to distinguish clinically, initial therapy should include an antistaphylococcal agent and a protein synthesis–inhibiting agent, such as clindamycin. Addition of clindamycin to penicillin is recommended for serious GAS infections, because its antimicrobial activity is unaffected by inoculum size (does not have the Eagle effect that occurs with β-lactam antibiotics), has a long postantimicrobial effect, and inhibits bacterial protein synthesis, which results in suppression of synthesis of *S pyogenes* antiphagocytic M-protein and bacterial toxins. Clindamycin **should not be used alone** as initial antimicrobial therapy in life-threatening

Box 135.2
Management of Streptococcal Toxic Shock Syndrome Without Necrotizing Fasciitis

- Fluid management to maintain adequate venous return and cardiac filling pressures to prevent end-organ damage.
- Anticipatory management of multisystem organ failure.
- Parenteral antimicrobial therapy at maximum doses with the capacity to
  - Kill organism with bactericidal cell wall inhibitor (eg, β-lactamase–resistant antimicrobial agent)
  - Decrease enzyme, toxin, or cytokine production with protein synthesis inhibitor (eg, clindamycin)
- IGIV is often used as an adjunct, typically at 1 g/kg on day 1, followed by 0.5 g/kg on 1–2 subsequent days.

IGIV indicates immune globulin intravenous.

Box 135.3
Management of Streptococcal Toxic Shock Syndrome With Necrotizing Fasciitis

- Principles outlined in Box 135.2.
- Immediate surgical evaluation.
  - Exploration or incisional biopsy for diagnosis and culture
  - Resection of all necrotic tissue
- Repeated resection of tissue may be needed if infection persists or progresses.

situations because of the potential for resistance. In 2017, 22% of invasive GAS case isolates from the Active Bacterial Core surveillance system in the United States were resistant to clindamycin.

Once GAS infection is confirmed, antimicrobial therapy should be tailored to penicillin and clindamycin. Intravenous therapy should be continued at least until the patient's condition is afebrile and stable hemodynamically and their blood is documented to be sterile. Clindamycin may be discontinued after a few days if there is adequate source control and clinical improvement. The total duration of therapy is based on duration established for the primary site of infection.

Aggressive drainage and irrigation of accessible sites of infection should be performed as soon as possible. If NF is suspected, immediate surgical exploration or biopsy is crucial to identify and debride deep soft tissue infection.

Immune globulin intravenous (IGIV) should be strongly considered as adjunctive therapy for streptococcal TSS or NF if the patient is moderately to severely ill, although its use is supported by limited data.

Other Infections

Parenteral antimicrobial therapy is required for severe GAS infections, such as endocarditis, pneumonia, empyema, deep abscess, septicemia, meningitis, arthritis, osteomyelitis, erysipelas, NF, and neonatal omphalitis. Treatment is often prolonged (2–6 weeks).

Acute Rheumatic Fever

Jones criteria for diagnosis of ARF were established in 1944 and revised and modified several times, most recently in 2015. The 2015 Jones criteria revision (Box 135.4) differentiates major and minor criteria on the basis of whether the child is from an area with low or high risk for ARF. Laboratory evidence of antecedent GAS infection should be confirmed in suspected cases of ARF and includes an increased or increasing antistreptolysin O or anti-DNAase B titer or a positive rapid antigen or streptococcal throat culture. Because of the long latency between GAS infection and chorea, laboratory evidence may be lacking when chorea is the major criterion (see Box 135.4 for the major and minor criteria).

Box 135.4
Revised Jones Criteria (2015)

1. All patients require evidence of antecedent GAS infection for diagnosis of ARF (except in case of chorea, where evidence of antecedent GAS infection is not required).
2. To confirm an initial diagnosis of ARF, need 2 major OR 1 major and 2 minor criteria.
3. To confirm recurrent ARF diagnosis, need 2 major OR 1 major and 2 minor OR 3 minor criteria.
4. Criteria for diagnosis depend on whether patient is from a low- or moderate-/high-risk area. Moderate- and high-risk areas include countries where ARF remains endemic (Africa, Asia-Pacific, Indigenous Australia). The United States, Canada, and Europe are examples of low-risk areas.
5. Major and minor criteria are listed below, by risk categorization; differences for moderate-/high-risk populations are **bolded.**

Low-risk area

Major criteria
- Carditis (clinical or subclinical)
- Arthritis (only polyarthritis)
- Chorea
- Subcutaneous nodules
- Erythema marginatum

Minor criteria
- Polyarthralgia
- Fever ≥38.5 °C (101.3 °F)
- ESR ≥60 mm/h and/or CRP level ≥3 mg/dL
- Prolonged PR interval (in absence of carditis)

Moderate- and high-risk areas

Major criteria
- Carditis (clinical or subclinical)
- Arthritis (polyarthritis or **monoarthritis,** or **polyarthralgia**)
- Chorea
- Subcutaneous nodules
- Erythema marginatum

Minor criteria
- **Monoarthralgia**
- **Fever ≥38 °C (100 °F)**
- **ESR ≥30 mm/h** and/or CRP level ≥3 mg/dL
- Prolonged PR interval (in absence of carditis)

ARF indicates acute rheumatic fever; CRP, C-reactive protein; ESR, erythrocyte sedimentation rate; and GAS, group A streptococcal.
Modified from Table 7. In: Gewitz MH, Baltimore RS, Tani LY, et al. Revision of the Jones criteria for the diagnosis of acute rheumatic fever in the era of Doppler echocardiography: a scientific statement from the American Heart Association. *Circulation.* 2015;131(20):1806–1818.

Treatment of ARF includes eradication of group A streptococci with a standard pharyngitis regimen, treatment of acute manifestations (eg, arthritis or valvulitis-associated heart failure), education for parents and patient, and initiation of secondary prophylaxis to prevent future GAS infection. Following initial treatment of ARF, patients with well-documented history of ARF (including cases manifested solely as Sydenham chorea) and patients with documented rheumatic heart disease (RHD) should be given continuous antimicrobial prophylaxis to prevent recurrent ARF attacks (secondary prophylaxis), because asymptomatic and symptomatic GAS infections can trigger recurrence of ARF. Continuous secondary prophylaxis should be initiated as soon as the diagnosis of ARF or RHD is made and should be long-term, perhaps for life, for patients with RHD (even after prosthetic valve replacement), because they continue to have risk for ARF recurrence. Risk of recurrence decreases as the interval from the most recent acute episode increases, and patients without RHD have lower risk for recurrence than patients with residual cardiac involvement. These considerations and the estimate of future exposure to GAS infection influence the duration of secondary prophylaxis in adults but should not alter the duration of secondary prophylaxis for children and adolescents. Secondary prophylaxis for all who have had ARF should be continued for at least 5 years or until the person is 21 years of age, whichever is longer (Table 135.1). Prophylaxis should also be continued if the risk of contact with people with GAS infection is high (eg, for parents with school-aged children, teachers, and others in frequent contact with children).

The antibiotic regimens in Table 135.2 are effective for secondary prophylaxis. The intramuscular regimen is the most reliable, because success of

Table 135.1
Duration of Prophylaxis for People Who Have Had Acute Rheumatic Fever: Recommendations of the American Heart Association[a]

Category	Duration
Rheumatic fever without carditis	5 years since last episode of ARF or until 21 years of age, whichever is longer
Rheumatic fever with carditis but without residual heart disease (no valvular disease[b])	10 years since last episode of ARF or until 21 years of age, whichever is longer
Rheumatic fever with carditis and residual heart disease (persistent valvular disease[b])	10 years since last episode of ARF or until 40 years of age, whichever is longer; consider lifelong prophylaxis for people with severe valvular disease or likelihood of ongoing exposure to group A streptococcal infection.

ARF indicates acute rheumatic fever.

[a] Modified from Gerber M, Baltimore R, Eaton C, et al. Prevention of rheumatic fever and diagnosis and treatment of acute streptococcal pharyngitis. A scientific statement from the American Heart Association Rheumatic Fever, Endocarditis, and Kawasaki Disease Committee of the Council on Cardiovascular Disease in the Young; Interdisciplinary Council on Functional Genomics and Translational Biology; and Interdisciplinary Council on Quality of Care and Outcomes Research. Circulation. 2009;119(11):1541–1551.
[b] Clinical or echocardiographic evidence.

Table 135.2
Chemoprophylaxis for Recurrences of Acute Rheumatic Fever[a]

Drug	Dose	Route
Penicillin G benzathine	1.2 million U, every 4 weeks[b]; 600,000 U, every 4 weeks for patients weighing <27 kg (60 lb)	Intramuscular
OR		
Penicillin V	250 mg, twice a day	Oral
OR		
Sulfadiazine or sulfisoxazole	0.5 g, once a day for patients weighing ≤27 kg (60 lb)	Oral
	1.0 g, once a day for patients weighing >27 kg (60 lb)	
For people who are allergic to penicillin and sulfonamide drugs		
Macrolide or azalide	Variable (See text.)	Oral

[a] Gerber M, Baltimore R, Eaton C, et al. Prevention of rheumatic fever and diagnosis and treatment of acute streptococcal pharyngitis. A scientific statement from the American Heart Association Rheumatic Fever, Endocarditis, and Kawasaki Disease Committee of the Council on Cardiovascular Disease in the Young; Interdisciplinary Council on Functional Genomics and Translational Biology; and Interdisciplinary Council on Quality of Care and Outcomes Research. Circulation. 2009;119(11):1541–1551.
[b] In particularly high-risk situations (usually non-US sites), administration every 3 weeks is recommended.

oral prophylaxis depends primarily on patient adherence; however, inconvenience and pain of injection may cause some patients to discontinue intramuscular prophylaxis. In non-US populations whose risk for ARF is particularly high, administration of penicillin G benzathine every 3 weeks is justified and recommended, because serum penicillin concentrations can decrease below a protective level in the fourth week after a dose. In the United States, administration every 4 weeks is likely adequate, except for those who have developed recurrent ARF despite adherence to an every-4-week regimen. Oral sulfadiazine is as effective as oral penicillin for secondary prophylaxis but may not be as readily available in the United States. By extrapolation from sulfadiazine, sulfisoxazole has been deemed an appropriate alternative; it is available in combination with erythromycin as a generic version.

Allergic reactions to oral penicillin are less common and usually less severe than reactions to parenteral penicillin and occur much more often in adults than in children. Severe allergic reactions rarely occur with intramuscular penicillin G benzathine prophylaxis, but the incidence may be higher among patients older than 12 years with severe RHD. Most severe reactions seem to be vasovagal responses rather than anaphylaxis. A serum sickness–like reaction characterized by fever and joint pains can occur in those receiving prophylaxis and can be mistaken for recurrence of ARF.

Reactions to continuous sulfadiazine or sulfisoxazole prophylaxis are rare and usually minor; evaluation of blood cell counts may be advisable after 2 weeks of prophylaxis, because leukopenia has been reported. Prophylaxis with a sulfonamide during late pregnancy is contraindicated because of interference with fetal bilirubin metabolism. Febrile mucocutaneous syndromes (erythema multiforme, Stevens-Johnson syndrome, or toxic epidermal necrolysis) have rarely been associated with penicillin and sulfonamides.

When an adverse event occurs with any prophylactic regimen, the drug should be stopped immediately and an alternative drug selected. For the rare patient allergic to both penicillins and sulfonamides, erythromycin is recommended. Other macrolides, such as azithromycin or clarithromycin, are also acceptable; they present less risk of gastrointestinal tract intolerance but increased cost.

Poststreptococcal Reactive Arthritis

After an episode of acute GAS pharyngitis, reactive arthritis may develop without sufficient clinical and laboratory findings to fulfill the Jones criteria for diagnosis of ARF. This syndrome has been termed *poststreptococcal reactive arthritis* (PSRA). The precise relationship of PSRA to ARF is unclear. In contrast to arthritis of ARF, PSRA does not respond dramatically to nonsteroidal anti-inflammatory agents. Because a very small proportion of patients with PSRA have been reported to develop late valvular heart disease, they should be observed carefully for 1 to 2 years for evidence of carditis, and some experts recommend secondary prophylaxis during the observation period. If carditis develops, the patient should be considered to have had ARF, and secondary prophylaxis should be initiated (see Acute Rheumatic Fever).

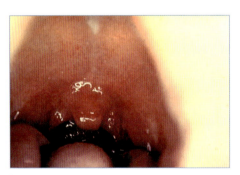

Image 135.1
Group A streptococcal pharyngitis with inflammation of the tonsils and uvula. Courtesy of Centers for Disease Control and Prevention.

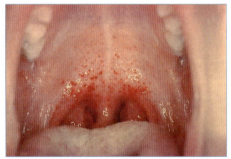

Image 135.2
Note inflammation of the oropharynx with petechiae on the soft palate, small red spots caused by group A streptococcal pharyngitis. Courtesy of Centers for Disease Control and Prevention.

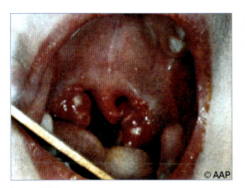

Image 135.3
Erythematous tonsils in a child with group A streptococcal pharyngitis.

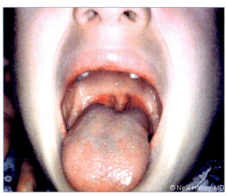

Image 135.4
Group A streptococcal pharyngitis with localized erythema and edema of the tonsils and soft palate. Copyright Neal Halsey, MD.

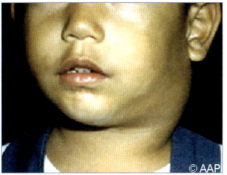

Image 135.5
Group A streptococcal nasopharyngitis in a toddler, which is often associated with tender anterior cervical lymphadenopathy. A throat culture result is not always positive when the infection has localized to the cervical lymph nodes.

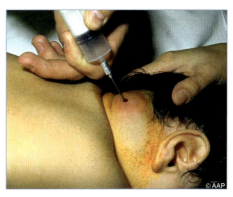

Image 135.6
Posterior cervical lymph node aspiration. Culture result was positive for group A streptococci. Courtesy of Edgar O. Ledbetter, MD, FAAP.

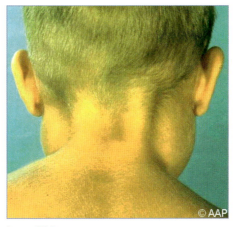

Image 135.7
Bilateral cervical lymphadenitis (posterior view).

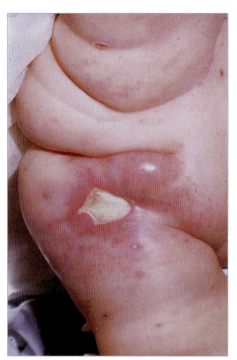

Image 135.8
Group A streptococcal cellulitis and necrotizing fasciitis in the perineal area of a 7-month-old girl, complicating varicella. Courtesy of George Nankervis, MD.

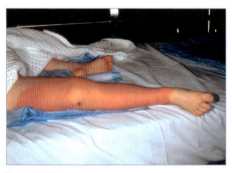

Image 135.10
Group A streptococcal cellulitis (erysipelas) of the right leg in a school-aged child, secondary to impetigo. Courtesy of George Nankervis, MD.

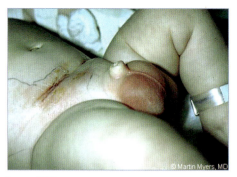

Image 135.9
A 5-month-old boy with group A streptococcal cellulitis 12 hours after herniorrhaphy. Copyright Martin G. Myers, MD.

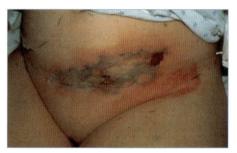

Image 135.11
Group A streptococcal necrotizing fasciitis complicating varicella in a 3-year-old girl. Courtesy of George Nankervis, MD.

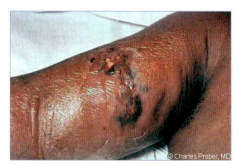

Image 135.12
Necrotizing fasciitis of the left upper arm and shoulder secondary to group A streptococci. Copyright Charles Prober, MD.

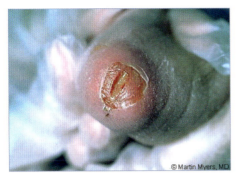

Image 135.13
An infant boy with group A streptococcal infection at a heel-stick site. Copyright Martin G. Myers, MD.

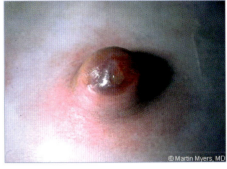

Image 135.14
A newborn with group A streptococcal omphalitis and peritonitis. Copyright Martin G. Myers, MD

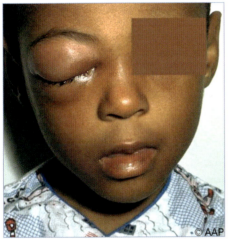

Image 135.15
Group A streptococcal ethmoid sinusitis with periorbital cellulitis.

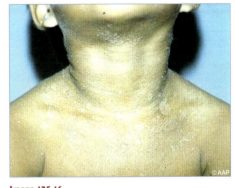

Image 135.16
Group A streptococcal scarlet fever with characteristic sandpaper-like rash with desquamation in a 6-year-old boy. Courtesy of Edgar O. Ledbetter, MD, FAAP.

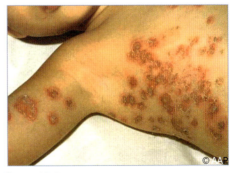

Image 135.18
Group A streptococcal impetigo.

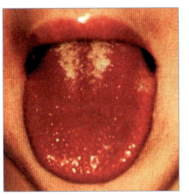

Image 135.17
The characteristic inflammatory changes in the tongue (ie, the strawberry tongue) of scarlet fever. Courtesy of Paul Wehrle, MD.

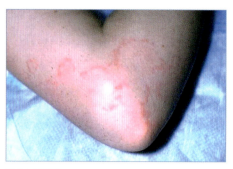

Image 135.19
Erythema marginatum in a 12-year-old girl. Although a characteristic rash of rheumatic fever, it is noted in <3% of cases. Its serpiginous border and evanescent nature serve to distinguish it from erythema migrans lesions of Lyme disease. Copyright Martin G. Myers, MD.

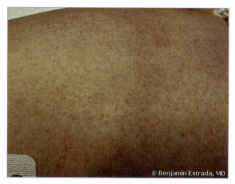

Image 135.20
Petechial rash in a 6-year-old girl with *Streptococcus pyogenes* septicemia. Courtesy of Benjamin Estrada, MD.

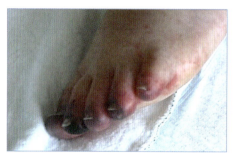

Image 135.21
Purpura fulminans in a 6-year-old girl with *Streptococcus pyogenes* septicemia. Courtesy of Benjamin Estrada, MD.

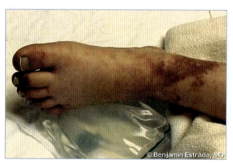

Image 135.22
Purpura fulminans in a 6-year-old girl with *Streptococcus pyogenes* septicemia. Courtesy of Benjamin Estrada, MD.

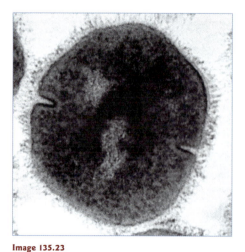

Image 135.23
Electron micrograph (magnification ×70,000) of an ultrathin section of *Streptococcus pyogenes*. Courtesy of Centers for Disease Control and Prevention/Dr Vincent A. Fischetti, Rockefeller University.

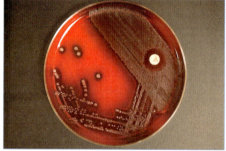

Image 135.24
Streptococcus pyogenes on blood agar. The bacitracin disk has been placed to help distinguish group A streptococci from other β-hemolytic streptococci. The formation of any zone of inhibition is considered a positive test result. Courtesy of Julia Rosebush, DO; Robert Jerris, PhD; and Theresa Stanley, M(ASCP).

CHAPTER 136
Group B Streptococcal Infections

CLINICAL MANIFESTATIONS

Group B streptococci are a major cause of perinatal infections, including bacteremia, intra-amniotic infection (formerly called *chorioamnionitis*), and endometritis in pregnant and postpartum women, as well as systemic and focal infections in neonates and young infants (Figure 136.1). In newborns, early-onset disease (EOD) usually occurs within the first 24 hours after birth (range, 0–6 days), manifesting with respiratory distress, apnea, shock, pneumonia, and, less often, meningitis (5%–10% of cases). Late-onset disease (LOD), which typically occurs at 3 to 4 weeks of age (range, 7–89 days), commonly manifests as bacteremia or meningitis (approximately 30% of cases); other focal infections, such as osteomyelitis, septic arthritis, necrotizing fasciitis, pneumonia, adenitis, and cellulitis, occur less commonly. Approximately 20% of survivors of neonatal group B streptococcal (GBS) meningitis have moderate to severe neurodevelopmental impairment. Cases in infants older than 90 days are reported rarely, usually in very preterm infants requiring prolonged hospitalization.

ETIOLOGY

Group B streptococci (*Streptococcus agalactiae*) are gram-positive diplococci that typically produce a narrow zone of beta hemolysis on 5% sheep blood agar. These organisms are divided into 10 types on the basis of capsular polysaccharides structures. Types Ia, Ib, II, III, IV, and V account for approximately 99% of cases in infants in the United States. Type III causes approximately 30% of EOD and 60% of LOD.

EPIDEMIOLOGY

Group B streptococci colonize the human gastrointestinal and genitourinary tracts and, less commonly, the pharynx. The vaginal/rectal colonization rate among pregnant women ranges from 15% to 35% and can be persistent or intermittent. In the 1990s, recommendations were made for prevention of early-onset GBS disease through maternal intrapartum antibiotic prophylaxis (IAP). Because of widespread implementation of IAP, the incidence of EOD has decreased by approximately 80% to an estimated 0.25 cases per 1,000 live births in 2018. The use of IAP has had no measurable effect on late-onset GBS disease incidence. In 2018, LOD incidence exceeded that of EOD at 0.28 cases per 1,000 live births. The case-fatality rate for GBS disease in full-term infants ranges from 1% to 3% but is higher in preterm neonates (estimated to be 20% for EOD and 8% for LOD). Approximately 70% of EOD and 50% of LOD affect full-term neonates.

Transmission from mother to infant generally occurs shortly before or during delivery in mothers who are colonized with GBS organisms. Less commonly, GBS infection may be transmitted in the nursery from health care professionals or visitors or in the community via colonized family members or caregivers. The risk of EOD is increased for preterm infants, infants born 18 hours or more after membrane rupture, and infants born to women with intrapartum fever (temperature ≥38 °C [≥100.4 °F]), intra-amniotic infection, GBS bacteriuria during the current pregnancy, or a history of a previous infant with invasive GBS disease. A higher incidence of EOD has also been associated with mothers younger than 20 years and mothers of Black race. However, the independent contribution of these factors is unclear, because both maternal age and race have also been associated with higher rates of both GBS colonization and preterm birth. Infants can remain colonized for several months despite treatment of systemic infection. Recurrent GBS disease affects an estimated 1% to 3% of appropriately treated infants.

The **incubation period** of EOD is less than 7 days. In LOD, the **incubation period** is unknown.

DIAGNOSTIC TESTS

Visualization of gram-positive cocci in pairs or short chains from a normally sterile body fluid provides presumptive evidence of infection, but growth of the organism in culture establishes the diagnosis. Meningitis/encephalitis multiplex panel polymerase chain reaction assays are available in many clinical laboratories for direct testing of cerebrospinal fluid (CSF) for GBS organisms.

For prenatal GBS screening, maternal swab specimens from vaginal and rectal sites are collected (vaginal swab specimens alone underestimate GBS colonization by up to 10%–15%). Culture yield can be increased with the use of commercially available selective broth enrichment media for 18 to 24 hours of incubation before being plated on tryptic soy blood agar or other selective agars for an additional 24 to 48 hours. Alternatively, DNA probe assays, latex agglutination assays, and nucleic acid amplification tests (NAATs) are available to detect GBS organisms from enriched broth specimens. Several NAATs are approved for antepartum or intrapartum detection of GBS organisms from vaginal/rectal swab specimens collected from pregnant women.

TREATMENT

- Ampicillin plus an aminoglycoside is the initial empirical treatment of choice for a **newborn 7 days or younger** with presumptive early-onset GBS infection; this reflects the need for coverage of other pathogens, such as *Escherichia coli*, which is the second most common cause of EOD. In a critically ill neonate, particularly one with low birth weight, broader-spectrum empirical therapy should be considered when there is concern about non-GBS ampicillin-resistant infection.

- For empirical therapy for late-onset GBS disease in **newborns 8 through 28 days of age** who are not critically ill and do not have evidence of meningitis, ampicillin plus either gentamicin or cefotaxime (or ceftazidime or cefepime if cefotaxime is unavailable) is recommended. If meningitis is suspected, ampicillin plus cefotaxime (or ceftazidime or cefepime if cefotaxime is unavailable) should be used; gentamicin should not be used if meningitis is suspected.

- For **newborns and infants 29 to 90 days of age,** ceftriaxone is recommended. If there is evidence of meningitis or critical illness, vancomycin should be added to expand empirical coverage.

- For a **preterm infant hospitalized beyond 72 hours,** empirical treatment of sepsis should take into account the potential for health care–associated pathogens as well as coverage for pathogens associated with neonatal sepsis, including group B streptococci.

- When GBS infection is identified definitively, penicillin G or ampicillin is recommended.

- For meningitis, especially in the neonate, some experts recommend that a second lumbar puncture (LP) be performed approximately 24 to 48 hours after initiation of therapy to assist in management and prognosis. If CSF sterility is not achieved or if increasing protein concentration is noted, a complication (eg, cerebral infarcts, cerebritis, ventriculitis, subdural empyema, ventricular obstruction) is more likely. Additional LPs and intracranial imaging may be indicated if neurological abnormalities persist or focal neurological deficits occur. A failed hearing screening or abnormal neurological examination findings at discharge mandate careful clinical follow-up.

- For infants with **bacteremia without a defined focus** or with an **isolated urinary tract infection** without bacteremia, treatment should be continued parenterally for 10 days. Shorter intravenous courses have been reported, sometimes with an oral component; however, prospective clinical studies are lacking. For infants with uncomplicated **meningitis,** 14 days of parenteral treatment is recommended, with longer courses of treatment provided for infants with prolonged or complicated courses. **Septic arthritis or osteomyelitis** requires treatment for 3 to 4 weeks. Patients who have **endocarditis or ventriculitis** require treatment for at least 4 weeks.

- Because of the reported increased risk of infection, the birth mates of a multiple-birth index patient with EOD or LOD should be observed carefully and evaluated and treated empirically for suspected systemic infection if signs of illness occur; treatment should be continued for a full course for those with confirmed infection.

Figure 136.1
Risk Assessment for Early-Onset Group B Streptococcal Disease Among Infants Born at ≤34 Weeks' Gestation

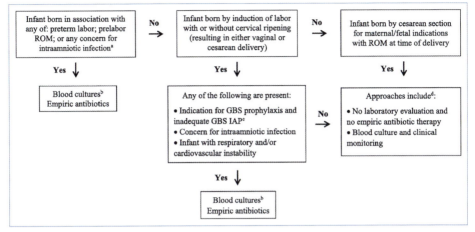

CSF indicates cerebrospinal fluid; GBS, group B streptococcal; IAP, intrapartum antibiotic prophylaxis; and ROM, rupture of membranes.

Reproduced from Puopolo KM, Lynfield R, Cummings JJ; American Academy of Pediatrics Committee on Fetus and Newborn and Committee on Infectious Diseases. Management of infants at risk for group B streptococcal disease. *Pediatrics.* 2019;144(2): e20191881.

[a] Intraamniotic infection should be considered when a pregnant woman presents with unexplained decreased fetal movement and/or there is sudden and unexplained poor fetal testing.

[b] Lumbar puncture and CSF culture should be performed before initiation of empiric antibiotics for infants who are at the highest risk of infection unless the procedure would compromise the infant's clinical condition. Antibiotics should be administered promptly and not deferred because of procedural delays.

[c] Adequate GBS IAP is defined as the administration of penicillin G, ampicillin, or cefazolin ≥4 hours before delivery.

[d] For infants who do not improve after initial stabilization and/or those who have severe systemic instability, the administration of empiric antibiotics may be reasonable but is not mandatory.

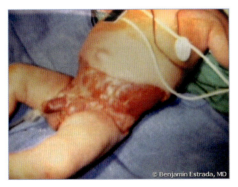

Image 136.1
Streptococcus agalactiae necrotizing fasciitis in a 3-month-old. Courtesy of Benjamin Estrada, MD.

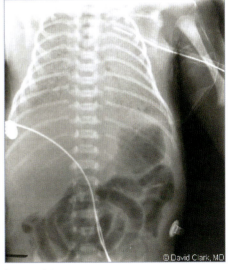

Image 136.2
Bilateral, severe group B streptococcal pneumonia in a neonate. Copyright David Clark, MD.

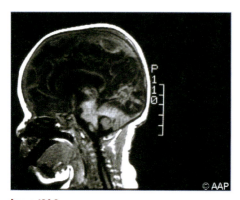

Image 136.3
Magnetic resonance imaging after group B streptococcal meningitis.

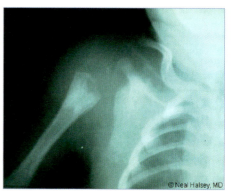

Image 136.4
Neonatal group B streptococcal septic arthritis of the right shoulder joint and osteomyelitis of the right proximal humerus. Copyright Neal Halsey, MD.

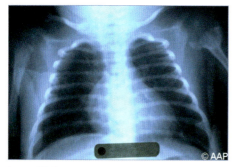

Image 136.5
Neonatal group B streptococcal septic arthritis of the left shoulder joint and osteomyelitis of the left proximal humerus. Courtesy of Edgar O. Ledbetter, MD, FAAP.

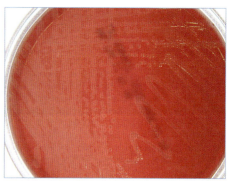

Image 136.6
Streptococcus agalactiae, 24-hour sheep blood agar plate, beta hemolysis, close-up view. Courtesy of Robert Jerris, PhD.

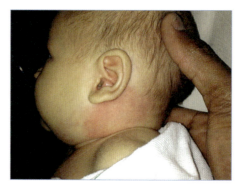

Image 136.7
A full-term 3-week-old who had poor feeding and irritability followed 2 hours later by fever to 38.1 °C (100.6 °F). On admission to the hospital 3 hours later, he required fluid resuscitation and intravenous antibiotic therapy. His spinal fluid was within reference range, but the blood culture grew group B streptococci. At admission, the physical examination revealed the classic facial and submandibular erythema, tenderness, and swelling characteristic of group B streptococcal cellulitis. Courtesy of Nate Serazin, MD, and C. Mary Healy, MD.

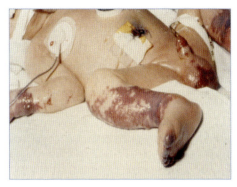

Image 136.8
A full-term 3-day-old with fatal group B streptococcal sepsis and peripheral gangrene. Courtesy of Carol J. Baker, MD, FAAP.

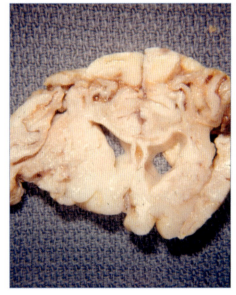

Image 136.9
The brain of a 3-week-old full-term boy with late-onset group B streptococcal meningitis and fatal status epilepticus. Courtesy of Carol J. Baker, MD, FAAP

CHAPTER 137

Non–group A or B Streptococcal and Enterococcal Infections

CLINICAL MANIFESTATIONS

Streptococci other than Lancefield groups A or B can be associated with invasive disease in infants, children, adolescents, and adults. The principal clinical syndromes of groups C and G streptococci (most belong to the *Streptococcus dysgalactiae* group) are bacteremia, septicemia, upper and lower respiratory tract infections (eg, pharyngitis, sinusitis, and pneumonia), skin and soft tissue infections, septic arthritis, osteomyelitis, meningitis with a parameningeal focus, brain abscess, toxic shock syndrome, pericarditis, and endocarditis with various clinical manifestations. Viridans streptococci are the most common cause of bacterial endocarditis in children, especially children with congenital or valvular heart disease. Viridans streptococci are a common cause of bacteremia in neutropenic patients with cancer, especially following intensive induction chemotherapy for acute myeloid leukemia, after hematopoietic stem cell transplant, and as a cause of central catheter–associated bacteremia. Among the viridans streptococci, group F streptococci (most belong to the *Streptococcus anginosus* group) are an implication in complicated sinus infections but are an infrequent cause of invasive infection. More serious *S anginosus* group infections include brain or dental abscesses or abscesses in other sites, including lymph nodes, liver, pelvis, and lung. These organisms may also cause sinusitis and other head and neck infections, meningitis, spondylodiskitis, spinal epidural abscesses, subdural empyema, peritonitis, complicated intra-abdominal infections, and cholangitis. Enterococci are associated with bacteremia in neonates and immunocompromised hosts, device-associated infections, intra-abdominal abscesses, and urinary tract infections in patients with anatomical anomalies.

ETIOLOGY

Changes in taxonomy and nomenclature of the *Streptococcus* genus have evolved with advances in molecular technology (Table 137.1). Among gram-positive organisms that are catalase negative and display chains by Gram stain, the genera associated most often with human disease are *Streptococcus* and *Enterococcus*.

The genus *Streptococcus* has been subdivided into 6 species groups on the basis of 16S ribosomal RNA gene sequencing. Members of the genus that are β-hemolytic on blood agar plates include *Streptococcus pyogenes*, *Streptococcus agalactiae*, and groups C and G streptococci; *S dysgalactiae* subspecies (subsp) *equisimilis* is the group C subsp most often associated with human infections. Streptococci that are non–β-hemolytic (β-hemolytic or nonhemolytic) on blood agar plates include (1) *Streptococcus pneumoniae;* (2) the *Streptococcus gallolyticus* (formerly *Streptococcus bovis*) group; and (3) viridans streptococci clinically relevant in humans, which include 5 *Streptococcus* species groups (*S anginosus* group, *Streptococcus mitis* group, *Streptococcus sanguinis* group, *Streptococcus salivarius* group, and *Streptococcus mutans* group). The *S anginosus* group (formerly *Streptococcus milleri* group) includes *S anginosus*, *Streptococcus constellatus*, and *Streptococcus intermedius*. This group can vary in hemolysis, and approximately one-third possess group A, C, F, or G antigens. Nutritionally variant streptococci, once believed to be viridans streptococci, are now classified in the genera *Abiotrophia* and *Granulicatella*. Group D streptococci include *S gallolyticus*, *Streptococcus infantarius*, and *Streptococcus pasteurianus*, now classified under the *S gallolyticus* group.

The genus *Enterococcus* contains at least 25 species, with *Enterococcus faecalis* and *Enterococcus faecium* accounting for most human enterococcal infections. Outbreaks and health care–associated spread of vancomycin-resistant enterococcal species including *Enterococcus gallinarum*, *Enterococcus casseliflavus*, or *Enterococcus flavescens* have occurred.

EPIDEMIOLOGY

The habitats that non–group A and B streptococci and enterococci occupy in humans include the skin (groups C and G streptococci), oropharynx (groups C and G streptococci and the *S mutans* group), gastrointestinal tract (groups C and G streptococci, the *S gallolyticus* group, and *Enterococcus* species), and vagina (groups C, D, and G streptococci and *Enterococcus* species).

Table 137.1
Classification of Streptococci Most Commonly Associated With Disease, by Lancefield Group and by Hemolysis

Species	Lancefield Group	Hemolysis
Streptococcus pyogenes	A	β
Streptococcus agalactiae	B	β
Streptococcus dysgalactiae subsp equisimillis, Streptococcus equi subsp zooepidemicus	C	β
Enterococcus faecalis, Enterococcus faecium, Streptococcus gallolyticus	D	β
Streptococcus canis	G	β
Streptococcus pneumoniae, viridans streptococci	Not groupable[a]	β

subsp indicates subspecies.
[a] Occasional viridans streptococci have variable hemolysis and can possess Lancefield group A, C, F, or G antigens.

Typical human habitats of species of viridans streptococci are the oropharynx, epithelial surfaces of the oral cavity, teeth, skin, and gastrointestinal and genitourinary tracts. Intrapartum transmission is responsible for most cases of early-onset neonatal infection caused by non–group A and B streptococci and enterococci. Environmental contamination or transmission via hands of health care professionals can lead to colonization of patients. Groups C and G streptococci can cause foodborne outbreaks of pharyngitis.

The **incubation period** and the period of communicability are unknown.

DIAGNOSTIC TESTS

Diagnosis is established by culture of usually sterile body sites or abscesses with appropriate biochemical testing and serological analysis for definitive identification. Mass spectrometry is unreliable in differentiation of S pneumoniae from viridans streptococci. Genomic methods are being used increasingly, particularly for rapid identification of positive blood cultures. Antimicrobial susceptibility testing of isolates from usually sterile sites should be performed to guide treatment of infections caused by viridans streptococci or enterococci. The proportion of vancomycin-resistant enterococci (VRE; most of which are E faecium) among hospitalized patients can be as high as 30%. Selective agars are available for screening of vancomycin-resistant enterococcus from stool specimens. Molecular assays are available for direct detection of vanA and vanB genes (which confer vancomycin resistance) from rectal and blood specimens to identify VRE.

TREATMENT

Penicillin G is the drug of choice for groups C and G streptococci. Other agents with good activity include ampicillin, third- and fourth-generation cephalosporins, vancomycin, and linezolid. The combination of gentamicin (when high level resistance is not present) with a β-lactam antimicrobial agent (eg, penicillin, ampicillin) or vancomycin may enhance bactericidal activity needed for treatment of life-threatening infections (eg, endocarditis and meningitis).

Many viridans streptococci remain susceptible to penicillin (minimum inhibitory concentration [MIC] ≤0.12 μg/mL). Infections caused by strains susceptible to penicillin, including endocarditis, can be treated with penicillin or ceftriaxone. Strains with an MIC greater than 0.12 μg/mL and less than 0.5 μg/mL are considered relatively resistant to penicillin by criteria in the American Heart Association guidelines for treatment of infective endocarditis in childhood. In this situation, penicillin, ampicillin, or ceftriaxone for 4 weeks, combined for the first 2 weeks with gentamicin, is recommended for endocarditis treatment. Strains with a penicillin MIC 0.5 μg/mL or greater are considered resistant. Nonpenicillin antimicrobial agents with good activity against viridans streptococci include cephalosporins (especially ceftriaxone), vancomycin, linezolid, and tigecycline.

Abiotrophia and *Granulicatella* organisms can exhibit relative or high-level resistance to penicillin. The combination of high-dose penicillin or vancomycin and an aminoglycoside can enhance bactericidal activity.

Enterococci exhibit uniform resistance to cephalosporins (except ceftaroline and, where available, ceftobiprole), aztreonam, and antistaphylococcal penicillins. Most are intrinsically resistant to clindamycin and trimethoprim-sulfamethoxazole even if in vitro susceptibility indicates otherwise. The vast majority of *E faecalis* strains are susceptible to ampicillin (which can be extrapolated to amoxicillin, piperacillin-tazobactam, and imipenem but not to penicillin). *E faecium* strains may be multidrug resistant. Two types of vancomycin resistance are identified: intrinsic low-level resistance that occurs with *E gallinarum* and *E casseliflavus/E flavescens* (these strains are ampicillin susceptible) and acquired resistance, which has been found in *E faecium* and some *E faecalis* strains but also has been recognized in *Enterococcus raffinosus*, *Enterococcus avium*, and *Enterococcus durans*.

Systemic enterococcal infections, such as endocarditis or meningitis, should be treated with penicillin or ampicillin (if the isolate is susceptible) combined with ceftriaxone or gentamicin (see endocarditis guidelines); vancomycin plus an aminoglycoside (with appropriate monitoring of renal function) is suggested for patients who are unable to tolerate penicillins and who cannot be desensitized. Gentamicin should not be used if in vitro susceptibility testing demonstrates high-level resistance. In general, children with a central catheter–associated bloodstream infection caused by enterococci should have the device removed promptly. Linezolid or daptomycin is an option for treatment of other systemic infections caused by vancomycin-resistant *E faecium*. Linezolid is approved for use in children, including neonates. Isolates of VRE that are resistant to linezolid have been described, and resistance can develop during prolonged linezolid treatment. Most vancomycin-resistant isolates of *E faecalis* and *E faecium* are daptomycin susceptible. Daptomycin should not be used to treat pneumonia, because tissue concentrations are poor and daptomycin is inactivated by surfactants. Tigecycline is approved for use in adults with complicated skin and skin structure infections caused by vancomycin-susceptible *E faecalis*. Tigecycline is bacteriostatic against both vancomycin-resistant *E faecalis* and vancomycin-resistant *E faecium*.

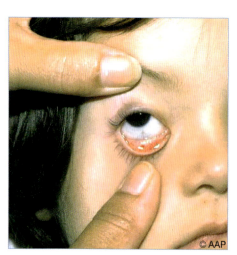

Image 137.1
Conjunctival (palpebral) petechiae in an adolescent girl with *Streptococcus viridans* subacute bacterial endocarditis.

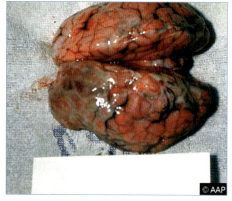

Image 137.2
Brain from a neonate with *Enterococcus faecalis* meningitis showing copious purulent exudate covering the meninges. Courtesy of Edgar O. Ledbetter MD, FAAP.

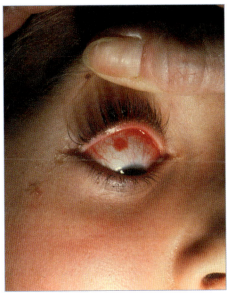

Image 137.3
A conjunctival hemorrhage in an adolescent girl with enterococcal endocarditis. Courtesy of George Nankervis, MD.

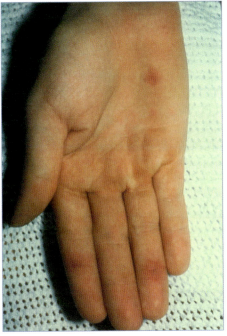

Image 137.4
Osler nodes on the fingers and a Janeway lesion in the palm of the same patient as in Image 137.3, with enterococcal endocarditis. Courtesy of George Nankervis, MD.

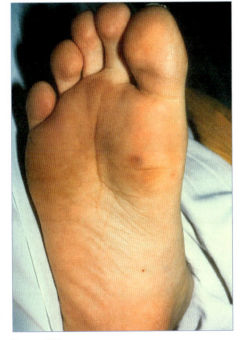

Image 137.5
A Janeway lesion on the sole of the same patient as in images 137.3 and 137.4, with enterococcal endocarditis. Courtesy of George Nankervis, MD.

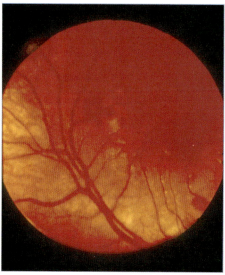

Image 137.6
Hemorrhagic retinitis with Roth spots in the adolescent girl in images 137.3–137.5, with enterococcal endocarditis. Courtesy of George Nankervis, MD.

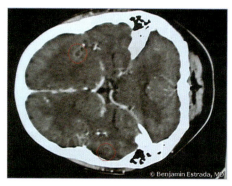

Image 137.7
Brain abscesses in a 13-year-old with *Streptococcus viridans* endocarditis. Courtesy of Benjamin Estrada, MD.

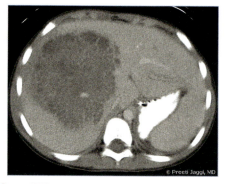

Image 137.8
Computed tomographic scan showing a large liver abscess in a previously healthy 5-year-old girl with abdominal pain and nausea. Culture results were positive for *Streptococcus anginosus* (formerly *Streptococcus milleri*). Courtesy of Preeti Jaggi, MD.

CHAPTER 138

Streptococcus pneumoniae (Pneumococcal) Infections

CLINICAL MANIFESTATIONS

Streptococcus pneumoniae is a common bacterial cause of acute otitis media, sinusitis, community-acquired pneumonia (CAP), and pediatric conjunctivitis; pleural empyema, mastoiditis, and periorbital cellulitis occur. It is the most common cause of bacterial meningitis in infants and children aged 2 months to 11 years in the United States. *S pneumoniae* may also cause endocarditis, pericarditis, peritonitis, pyogenic arthritis, osteomyelitis, soft tissue infection, and neonatal septicemia. Overwhelming septicemia in patients with splenic dysfunction is noted, and hemolytic-uremic syndrome can accompany pneumococcal infection.

ETIOLOGY

S pneumoniae organisms (pneumococci) are lancet-shaped gram-positive, catalase-negative diplococci. More than 90 pneumococcal serotypes have been identified on the basis of unique polysaccharide capsules.

EPIDEMIOLOGY

Nasopharyngeal carriage rates in children range from 21% in industrialized settings to more than 90% in resource-limited settings. Transmission is from person to person by respiratory droplet contact. Viral upper respiratory tract infections, including influenza, can predispose to pneumococcal infection and transmission. Pneumococcal infections are most prevalent during winter months. The period of communicability is unknown and may be as long as the organism is present in respiratory tract secretions but is probably less than 24 hours after effective antimicrobial therapy is begun.

The incidence and severity of infections are increased in people with congenital or acquired humoral immunodeficiency, HIV infection, absent or deficient splenic function (eg, sickle cell disease, congenital or surgical asplenia), certain complement deficiencies, diabetes mellitus, chronic liver disease, chronic renal failure or nephrotic syndrome, or abnormal innate immune responses.

HIV-exposed uninfected infants also have increased risk for severe pneumococcal infections. Children with cochlear implants, particularly those who had placement of an older model that involved a cochlear electrode, have high rates of pneumococcal meningitis, as do children with congenital or acquired cerebrospinal fluid (CSF) leaks. Other categories of children with presumed high risk or with moderate risk for developing invasive pneumococcal disease (IPD) are outlined in Table 138.1. Infection rates are highest among infants, young children, elderly people, and Black, Alaska Native, and some American Indian populations. Since introduction of the heptavalent pneumococcal conjugate vaccine (PCV7) in 2000 and the 13-valent pneumococcal conjugate vaccine (PCV13) in 2010, racial disparities have diminished; however, rates of IPD among some American Indian (Alaska Native, Navajo, and White Mountain Apache) populations remain more than 4-fold higher than the rate among children in the general US population. Recent data from Alaska and the southwestern United States indicate that most IPD cases in American Indian/Alaska Native children are now caused by serotypes not contained in the PCV13 vaccine.

By 2016, 6 years after the introduction of PCV13, the incidence of vaccine-type invasive pneumococcal infections decreased by 98% as compared to the incidence before introduction of PCV7, and the incidence of all IPD decreased by 95% among children younger than 5 years. In adults 65 years and older, IPD caused by PCV13 serotypes decreased 87% as compared with baseline, and all IPD decreased by 61%. The reduction in cases in this latter group indicates the significant indirect (ie, herd) benefits of PCV13 immunization achieved by interruption of transmission of pneumococci from vaccinated children to adults. Although *S pneumoniae* strains that are nonsusceptible to penicillin G, ceftriaxone, and other antimicrobial agents have been identified throughout the United States and worldwide, a reduction in the proportion of isolates that are penicillin resistant and ceftriaxone resistant has been observed since introduction of PCV7 and PCV13.

The **incubation period** varies by type of infection but can be as short as 1 day.

Table 138.1
Underlying Medical Conditions That Indicate Immunization With 23-Valent Pneumococcal Polysaccharide Vaccine (PPSV23)[a] in Children, by Risk Group[b]

Risk Group	Condition
Children with immunocompetence	Chronic heart disease[c]
	Chronic lung disease[d]
	Diabetes mellitus
	Cerebrospinal fluid leaks
	Cochlear implant
Children with functional or anatomical asplenia	Sickle cell disease and other hemoglobinopathies
	Chronic or acquired asplenia, or splenic dysfunction
Children with immunocompromising conditions	HIV infection
	Chronic renal failure and nephrotic syndrome
	Diseases associated with treatment with immunosuppressive drugs or radiation therapy, including malignant neoplasms, leukemias, lymphomas, and Hodgkin disease; or solid organ transplant
	Congenital immunodeficiency[e]

[a] PPSV23 is indicated starting at 24 months of age.
[b] Centers for Disease Control and Prevention. Licensure of a 13-valent pneumococcal conjugate vaccine (PCV13) and recommendations for use among children. Advisory Committee on Immunization Practices (ACIP). MMWR Morb Mortal Wkly Rep. 2010;59(9):258–261; and Centers for Disease Control and Prevention. Use of 13-valent pneumococcal conjugate vaccine and 23-valent pneumococcal polysaccharide vaccine among children aged 6-18 years with immunocompromising conditions: recommendation of the ACIP. MMWR Morb Mortal Wkly Rep. 2013;62(25):521–524.
[c] Particularly cyanotic congenital heart disease and cardiac failure.
[d] Including asthma if treated with prolonged high-dose oral corticosteroids.
[e] Includes B- (humoral) or T-lymphocyte deficiency; complement deficiencies, particularly C1, C2, C3, and C4 deficiencies; and phagocytic disorders (excluding chronic granulomatous disease).

DIAGNOSTIC TESTS

Recovery of *S pneumoniae* from a normally sterile site confirms the diagnosis. The finding of lancet-shaped gram-positive organisms and white blood cells in expectorated sputum (older children and adults) or pleural exudate suggests pneumococcal pneumonia. Recovery of pneumococci by culture of an upper respiratory tract swab specimen is not sufficient to assign an etiologic diagnosis of pneumococcal disease involving the middle ear, upper or lower respiratory tract, or sinus.

There are at least 2 multiplexed nucleic acid amplification tests designed to identify *S pneumoniae* and other bacterial and fungal pathogens from positive blood culture bottles. At least 1 real-time polymerase chain reaction (PCR) assay is available for detection of *S pneumoniae* in CSF. The assay is a multiplexed PCR designed to detect a number of agents of bacterial, fungal, and viral meningitis or encephalitis. PCR testing should be accompanied by culture of CSF to obtain an isolate, which is needed for antimicrobial susceptibility testing.

Detection of C polysaccharide (common to all pneumococci) in urine for diagnosis of pneumococcal pneumonia may have some utility in adults but is not useful in children, because asymptomatically colonized children may have positive test results. Similarly, commercially available antigen detection tests performed on CSF or blood are not recommended for routine use because of low sensitivity.

Susceptibility Testing

All *S pneumoniae* isolates from normally sterile body fluids should be tested for antimicrobial susceptibility to determine the minimum inhibitory concentration (MIC) of penicillin, cefotaxime or ceftriaxone, and clindamycin. CSF isolates should also be tested for susceptibility to vancomycin, meropenem, and rifampin. If the patient has a non-meningeal infection caused by an isolate that is nonsusceptible to penicillin, cefotaxime, and ceftriaxone, susceptibility testing to other agents such as clindamycin, erythromycin, trimethoprim-sulfamethoxazole, levofloxacin, linezolid, meropenem, and vancomycin should be performed.

TREATMENT

Bacterial Meningitis Possibly or Proven to Be Caused by *S pneumoniae*

For children with bacterial meningitis possibly or known to be caused by *S pneumoniae*, vancomycin should be administered in addition to cefotaxime (or ceftriaxone for patients >1 month of age) because of the possibility of *S pneumoniae* resistant to penicillin and third-generation cephalosporins. In neonates, when cefotaxime is unavailable, ceftazidime or cefepime can be used in addition to vancomycin. Vancomycin should be stopped if susceptibility to third-generation cephalosporins is documented (by using central nervous system break points for thresholds of resistance), if another organism not requiring vancomycin is identified, or if the CSF culture is negative. If the *S pneumoniae* isolate is nonsusceptible (intermediate or resistant) to penicillin or third-generation cephalosporins, treatment options are provided in Table 138.2. Consultation with an infectious diseases specialist should be considered for all children with bacterial meningitis.

For children with serious proven hypersensitivity reactions to third- or fourth-generation cephalosporins, a pediatric infectious diseases specialist should be consulted for consideration of use of vancomycin plus either meropenem or rifampin.

A repeated lumbar puncture should be considered after 48 hours of therapy in any of the following circumstances:

- The organism is penicillin nonsusceptible by oxacillin disk or quantitative (MIC) testing, and results from cefotaxime and ceftriaxone quantitative susceptibility testing are not yet available or the isolate is cefotaxime and ceftriaxone nonsusceptible.

- The patient's condition has not improved or has worsened.

- The child has received dexamethasone, which can interfere with the ability to interpret the clinical response, such as resolution of fever.

Dexamethasone

For infants and children 6 weeks and older, adjunctive therapy with dexamethasone may be considered after weighing the potential benefits and risks. Some experts recommend use of corticosteroids in pneumococcal meningitis, but this issue is controversial and data are not sufficient to make a routine recommendation for children. If used, dexamethasone should be administered before or concurrently with the first dose of parenteral antimicrobial agents.

Table 138.2
Antimicrobial Therapy for Infants and Children With Meningitis Caused by *Streptococcus pneumoniae* on the Basis of Susceptibility Test Results

Susceptibility Test Results	Antimicrobial Management[a]
Susceptible to penicillin	Discontinue vancomycin **AND EITHER** Continue cefotaxime or ceftriaxone alone[b] **OR** Begin penicillin (and discontinue cephalosporin)
Nonsusceptible to penicillin (*intermediate* or *resistant*) **AND** *Susceptible* to cefotaxime and ceftriaxone	Discontinue vancomycin **AND** Continue cefotaxime or ceftriaxone
Nonsusceptible to penicillin (*intermediate* or *resistant*) **AND** *Nonsusceptible* to cefotaxime and ceftriaxone (*intermediate* or *resistant*) **AND** *Susceptible* to rifampin	Continue vancomycin and high-dose cefotaxime or ceftriaxone **AND** Rifampin may be added in selected circumstances (See text.)

[a] Initial empirical therapy of nonallergic children >1 month of age with presumed bacterial meningitis should be vancomycin and cefotaxime or ceftriaxone. Some experts recommend the maximum dosages.
[b] Some physicians may choose this alternative for convenience and cost savings but only in treatment of meningitis.

Nonmeningeal Invasive Pneumococcal Infections Requiring Hospitalization

For nonmeningeal invasive infections in previously healthy children who are not critically ill, antimicrobial agents currently used to treat infections with S pneumoniae and other potential pathogens should be initiated at the usually recommended dosages.

For critically ill infants and children with invasive infections potentially attributable to S pneumoniae, vancomycin, in addition to empirical antimicrobial therapy (eg, cefotaxime or ceftriaxone or others), can be considered. These patients include those with presumed septic shock, severe pneumonia with empyema, or significant hypoxia or myopericardial involvement. If vancomycin is administered, it should be discontinued as soon as antimicrobial susceptibility test results demonstrate effective alternative agents.

If the organism has in vitro resistance to penicillin, cefotaxime, and ceftriaxone, therapy should be modified on the basis of clinical response, susceptibility to other antimicrobial agents, and results of follow-up cultures of blood and other infected body fluids. Consultation with an infectious diseases specialist should be considered.

For children with severe hypersensitivity to β-lactam antimicrobial agents (penicillins and cephalosporins), initial management should include vancomycin or clindamycin, in addition to antimicrobial agents for other potential pathogens, as indicated. Consultation with an infectious diseases specialist should be considered.

Acute Otitis Media

According to clinical practice guidelines of the American Academy of Pediatrics and the American Academy of Family Physicians on suppurative acute otitis media (AOM), amoxicillin (80–90 mg/kg/day) is recommended for infants younger than 6 months, for those 6 through 23 months of age with bilateral disease, and for those older than 6 months with severe signs and symptoms. A watch-and-wait option can be considered for older children and those with nonsevere disease. Optimal duration of therapy is uncertain. For younger children and children with severe disease at any age, a 10-day course is recommended; for children 6 years and older with mild or moderate disease, a duration of 5 to 7 days is appropriate. Otalgia should be treated symptomatically.

Patients whose initial management fails should be reassessed at 48 to 72 hours to confirm the diagnosis of suppurative AOM and exclude other causes of illness. If suppurative AOM is confirmed in the patient treated initially with observation, amoxicillin should be administered. If the patient's initial antibacterial therapy has failed, a change in antibacterial agent is indicated. Suitable alternative agents should be active against penicillin-nonsusceptible pneumococci as well as β-lactamase–producing Haemophilus influenzae and Moraxella catarrhalis. Such agents include high-dose oral amoxicillin-clavulanate; oral cefdinir, cefpodoxime, or cefuroxime; or once-daily doses of intramuscular ceftriaxone for 3 consecutive days. Macrolide resistance among S pneumoniae is high, so clarithromycin and azithromycin are not considered appropriate alternatives for initial therapy even in patients with a type I (immediate, anaphylactic) reaction to a β-lactam agent. In these cases, treatment with clindamycin (if susceptibility is known) or levofloxacin is preferred. For patients with a history of non–type I allergic reaction to penicillin, agents such as cefdinir, cefuroxime, or cefpodoxime can be used orally.

Myringotomy or tympanocentesis should be considered for children whose second-line therapy fails, for severe cases to obtain cultures to guide therapy, and for patients with invasive pneumococcal infection. For multidrug-resistant strains of S pneumoniae, use of levofloxacin or other agents should be considered in consultation with an infectious diseases specialist and on the basis of the specific susceptibility profile.

Sinusitis

Antimicrobial agents effective for treatment of suppurative AOM are also likely to be effective for acute sinusitis and are recommended when a child's condition meets clinical criteria for diagnosis.

Pneumonia

Oral amoxicillin at a dose of 45 mg/kg/day in 3 equally divided doses or 90 mg/kg/day in 2 divided portions is likely to be effective in ambulatory children with pneumonia caused by susceptible and relatively resistant pneumococci, respectively. Ampicillin is recommended for intravenous therapy for CAP. Cefotaxime or ceftriaxone is recommended for treatment of inpatients infected with pneumococci suspected or proven to be penicillin-resistant strains, for serious infections including empyema, or in those not fully immunized with PCV13. Vancomycin should be included in those with life-threatening infection. For patients with isolates resistant to penicillin (MICs of ≥4.0 μg/mL) or significant allergy to β-lactam antimicrobials, treatment with clindamycin (if susceptible) or levofloxacin should be considered, assuming that concurrent meningitis has been excluded.

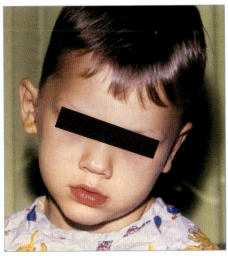

Image 138.1
A 3½-year-old boy with acute suppurative otitis media and mastoiditis caused by *Streptococcus pneumoniae*. Note the protuberance of the right external ear secondary to mastoid swelling. Courtesy of George Nankervis, MD.

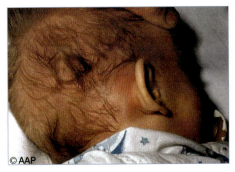

Image 138.2
Child with acute mastoiditis caused by *Streptococcus pneumoniae*.

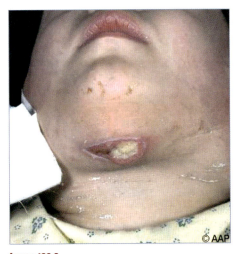

Image 138.3
Streptococcus pneumoniae submental abscess in a 5-year-old girl with dysgammaglobulinemia. There is an increased incidence of pneumococcal disease among children with immunocompromise. Courtesy of Edgar O. Ledbetter, MD, FAAP.

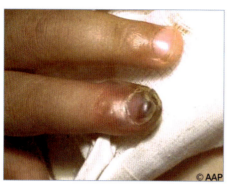

Image 138.4
Perionychial abscess caused by *Streptococcus pneumoniae* in a child with acute lymphoblastic leukemia.

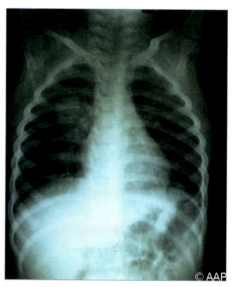

Image 138.5
Segmental (nodular) pneumonia caused by *Streptococcus pneumoniae*.

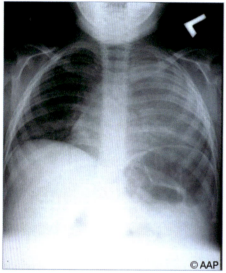

Image 138.6
Acute pneumococcal pneumonia of the left upper lobe proven by a positive result from blood culture. Courtesy of Edgar O. Ledbetter, MD, FAAP.

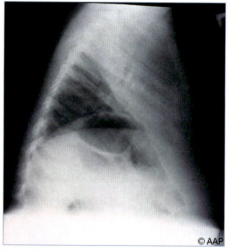

Image 138.7
Acute pneumococcal pneumonia of the left upper lobe proven by a positive result from blood culture. This is the same patient as in Image 138.6. Courtesy of Edgar O. Ledbetter, MD, FAAP.

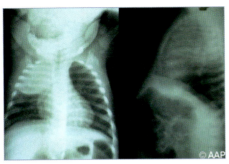

Image 138.8
Streptococcus pneumoniae pneumonia of the upper lobe of the right lung. The blood culture result was positive, and the infant promptly responded to penicillin therapy.

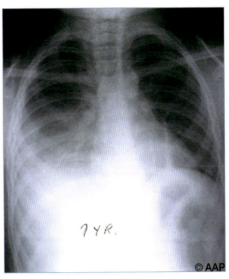

Image 138.9
Pneumococcal pneumonia with pleural effusion on the right. Courtesy of Edgar O. Ledbetter, MD, FAAP.

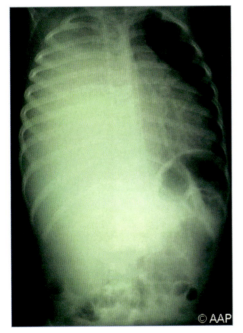

Image 138.10
Pneumococcal pneumonia with massive effusion pushing the mediastinal structures into the left area of the chest. A delayed clinical response to treatment was not surprising. Courtesy of Edgar O. Ledbetter, MD, FAAP.

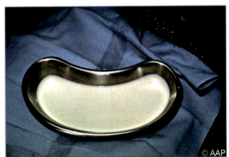

Image 138.11
Purulent pleural fluid of pneumococcal empyema removed from the patient in Image 138.10. Courtesy of Edgar O. Ledbetter, MD, FAAP.

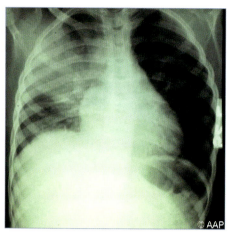

Image 138.12
Pneumonia with right subpleural empyema caused by *Streptococcus pneumoniae* in a child with sickle cell disease.

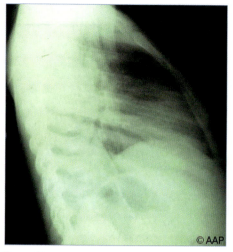

Image 138.13
Pneumonia with subpleural empyema caused by *Streptococcus pneumoniae* evident on lateral chest radiograph. This is the same patient as in Image 138.12. Note the difference in the level of the right and left hemidiaphragms.

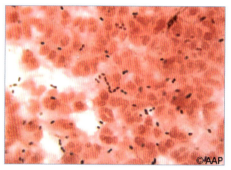

Image 138.14
Streptococcus pneumoniae in pleural exudate (Gram stain).

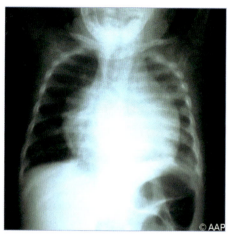

Image 138.15
Pneumonia and purulent pericarditis caused by *Streptococcus pneumoniae* in a previously healthy infant. Despite clinical improvement with penicillin therapy and repeated needle aspiration of the pericardial space, the infant died of constrictive pericarditis.

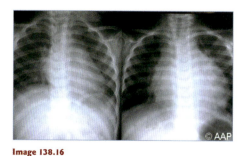

Image 138.16
Pneumonia and pericarditis caused by *Streptococcus pneumoniae*. Despite pericardial drainage by needle aspiration followed by pericardiostomy drainage, the child died. Surgical drainage is imperative in the management of purulent pericarditis.

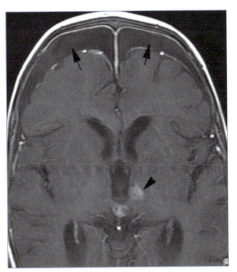

Image 138.17
An axial T1-weighted magnetic resonance image following contrast shows frontal subdural hygromas (arrows). Also note the enhancing left thalamic infarction secondary to penetrating artery spasm (arrowhead) in a patient with pneumococcal meningitis.

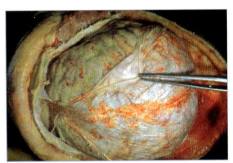

Image 138.18
Skull opened at autopsy revealing purulent inflammation of leptomeninges beneath reflected dura in a patient who died of pneumococcal meningitis. Courtesy of Centers for Disease Control and Prevention.

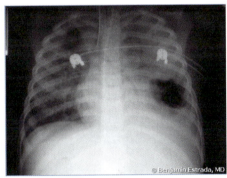

Image 138.20
Streptococcus pneumoniae pneumonia with pneumatocele formation in the left lung. Courtesy of Benjamin Estrada, MD.

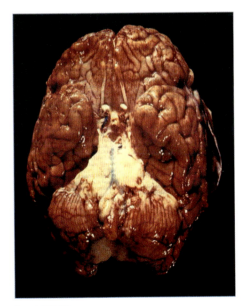

Image 138.19
A ventral view of the brain depicting purulent exudate from fatal *Streptococcus pneumoniae* meningitis. Courtesy of Centers for Disease Control and Prevention.

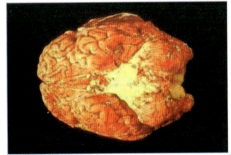

Image 138.21
This is a photo of the brain of a person who died of pneumococcal meningitis. Note the purulence (pus) that covers the brain surface. Courtesy of Centers for Disease Control and Prevention.

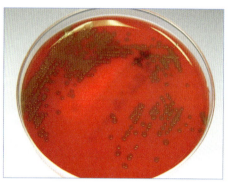

Image 138.22
Streptococcus pneumoniae, 24-hour sheep blood agar plate, with alpha hemolysis. Courtesy of Robert Jerris, PhD.

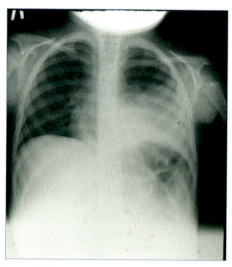

Image 138.23
A 3-year-old boy who presented with high fever, tachypnea, left-sided chest pain, and his chest radiograph. Note the left lower consolidation, pleural fluid, and rounded air-filled cavities. Courtesy of Carol J. Baker MD, FAAP.

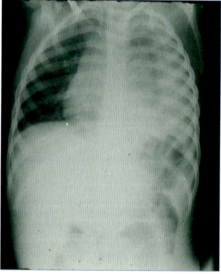

Image 138.24
Same patient as in Image 138.23 after 48 hours of antibiotic therapy. He had continued to have high fever, tachypnea, and no audible breath sounds in the left side of his chest. Courtesy of Carol J. Baker, MD, FAAP.

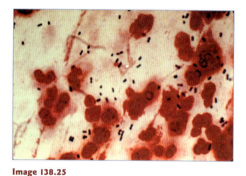

Image 138.25
Gram stain from pleural fluid on day 5 of antibiotic therapy for the patient in images 138.23 and 138.24. The gram-positive, lancet-shaped diplococci are abundant in this empyema fluid, which grew *Streptococcus pneumoniae*, as did his admission blood culture. Two days after chest tube drainage, he became afebrile. Courtesy of Carol J. Baker, MD, FAAP.

CHAPTER 139

Strongyloidiasis
(Strongyloides stercoralis)

CLINICAL MANIFESTATIONS

Most infections with *Strongyloides stercoralis* are asymptomatic. When symptoms occur, they are related most often to larval tissue migration and/or the presence of adult worms in the intestine. Infective (filariform) larvae are acquired from skin contact with contaminated soil, which may produce transient pruritic papules at the site of penetration. Larvae then migrate to the lungs, where they may cause a transient pneumonitis or Löffler-like syndrome. After ascending the tracheobronchial tree, larvae are swallowed and mature into adult forms within the gastrointestinal tract. Symptoms of intestinal infection may include nonspecific abdominal pain, malabsorption, vomiting, and diarrhea. Larval migration may produce migratory serpiginous pruritic erythematous skin lesions. These tracks are referred to as *larva currens* and are pathognomonic for *Strongyloides*. The most feared complication is *Strongyloides* hyperinfection syndrome and disseminated disease, in which larvae migrate via the systemic circulation to distant organs, including the brain, liver, kidney, heart, and skin. Hyperinfection syndrome typically occurs in immunocompromised people, most often those receiving immunosuppressive agents, particularly glucocorticoids, for underlying disease (eg, malignancy, autoimmunity) but also recipients of solid organ or hematopoietic stem cell transplants (through either reactivation of prior asymptomatic infection in the recipient or donor-derived infection) and patients with human T-lymphotropic virus I coinfection. *Strongyloides* hyperinfection syndrome is characterized by fever, abdominal pain, diffuse pulmonary infiltrates, and septicemia or meningitis caused by enteric gram-negative bacilli and may be fatal.

ETIOLOGY

S stercoralis is a nematode (roundworm).

EPIDEMIOLOGY

Strongyloidiasis is endemic in the tropics and subtropics, including the southeastern United States, wherever suitable moist soil and improper disposal of human waste coexist. Humans are the principal hosts, but dogs, cats, and other animals can serve as reservoirs. Transmission involves penetration of skin by filariform larvae from contact with contaminated soil. Infections can also be acquired via fecal-oral route with ingestion of food contaminated with human feces containing larvae or from inadvertent coprophagy. Adult females release eggs in the small intestine, where they hatch as first-stage (rhabditiform) larvae that are excreted in feces. A small percentage of larvae molt to the infective (filariform) stage during intestinal transit, at which point they can penetrate the bowel mucosa or perianal skin, thus maintaining the life cycle within a single person (autoinfection). Because of the capacity for autoinfection, people can remain infected for decades even after leaving an endemic area.

The **incubation period** in humans is unknown.

DIAGNOSTIC TESTS

Strongyloidiasis can be difficult to diagnose. Testing may be performed on stool or serologically. Visualization through direct microscopy for larvae (rhabditiform, or, less often, filariform) in the stool (or from duodenal biopsy or fluid, obtained by using the string test [Entero-Test] or a direct aspirate through a flexible endoscope) confirms the diagnosis. At least 3 consecutive stool specimens should be examined microscopically by using a concentration method (eg, sedimentation techniques) for characteristic larvae (not eggs), but a negative test result does not exclude infection because larvae excretion can be intermittent and of low intensity. Filariform larvae may be identified in disseminated strongyloidiasis from other specimens such as sputum or bronchoalveolar lavage fluid, spinal fluid, pleural fluid, peritoneal fluid or in skin biopsies. Serological tests, including enzyme-linked immunosorbent assays that detect immunoglobulin G to filariform larvae, are highly sensitive but cross-reactivity may occur in patients with filariasis and other nematode infections. Serological tests with recombinant antigens have similar high sensitivity but greater specificity for strongyloidiasis. Serological testing has several limitations. Detection does not confirm active infection, because antibodies may remain positive for a period following infection resolution. False-negative results may also occur, so a negative test result does not eliminate the possibility of ongoing infection. Serological monitoring may be useful in following treatment in immunocompetent patients.

Eosinophilia (blood eosinophil count >500/µL) is generally present during acute and chronic infection, but its absence does not eliminate infection from consideration. When eosinophilia is absent in hyperinfection syndrome, it may predict poor outcome. Gram-negative bacillary meningitis and bacteremia may occur with disseminated disease and carry a high mortality rate.

TREATMENT

Ivermectin is the treatment of choice for all forms of strongyloidiasis. Ivermectin is contraindicated in people with confirmed or suspected coinfection with *Loa loa*. An alternative agent is albendazole, although it is associated with lower cure rates. Mebendazole is not recommended. Prolonged or repeated treatment may be necessary in people with hyperinfection and disseminated strongyloidiasis, and relapse can occur.

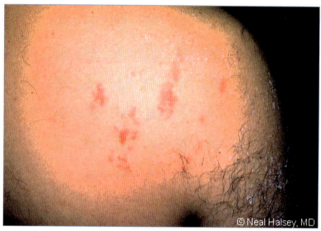

Image 139.1
Cutaneous migration sites of *Strongyloides stercoralis* over the left shoulder area. Copyright Neal Halsey, MD.

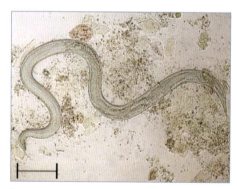

Image 139.2
Adult female of *Strongyloides stercoralis* collected in bronchial fluid of a patient with disseminated disease (scale bar = 400 µm). Courtesy of Centers for Disease Control and Prevention/*Emerging Infectious Diseases*.

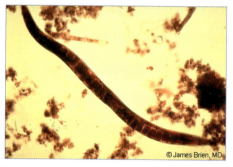

Image 139.3
Strongyloides stercoralis larvae (oil immersion magnification). Copyright James Brien.

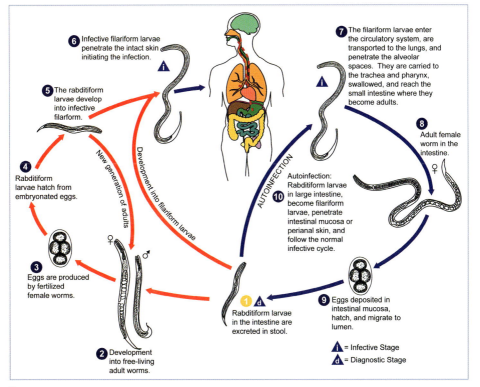

Image 139.4

The *Strongyloides* life cycle is complex among helminths with its alternation between free-living and parasitic cycles and its potential for autoinfection and multiplication within the host. Two types of cycles exist. Free-living cycle: The rhabditiform larvae passed in the stool (1) (see Parasitic cycle) can either molt twice and become infective filariform larvae (direct development) (6) or molt 4 times and become free-living adult males and females (2) that mate and produce eggs (3), from which rhabditiform larvae hatch (4). The latter, in turn, can develop (5) into either a new generation of free-living adults (as represented in 2) or infective filariform larvae (6). The filariform larvae penetrate the human host skin to initiate the parasitic cycle. Parasitic cycle: Filariform larvae in contaminated soil penetrate human skin (6) and are transported to the lungs, where they penetrate the alveolar spaces; they are carried through the bronchial tree to the pharynx, are swallowed, and then reach the small intestine (7). In the small intestine, they molt twice and become adult female worms (8). The females live threaded in the epithelium of the small intestine and by parthenogenesis produce eggs (9), which yield rhabditiform larvae. The rhabditiform larvae can be passed in the stool (1) (see Free-living cycle) or can cause autoinfection (10). In autoinfection, the rhabditiform larvae become infective filariform larvae, which can penetrate the intestinal mucosa (internal autoinfection) or the skin of the perianal area (external autoinfection); in either case, the filariform larvae may follow the previously described route, being carried successively to the lungs, bronchial tree, pharynx, and small intestine, where they mature into adults, or they may disseminate widely in the body. To date, occurrence of autoinfection in humans with helminthic infections is recognized only in *Strongyloides stercoralis* and *Capillaria philippinensis* infections. In the case of *Strongyloides*, autoinfection may explain the possibility of persistent infections for many years in people who have not been in an endemic area and of hyperinfections in individuals with immunodepression.

CHAPTER 140
Syphilis

CLINICAL MANIFESTATIONS

Congenital Syphilis

Intrauterine infection with *Treponema pallidum* can result in stillbirth, fetal hydrops, or preterm birth or may be asymptomatic at birth. Infected infants can have hepatosplenomegaly; snuffles (copious nasal secretions); lymphadenopathy; mucocutaneous lesions; pneumonia; osteochondritis, periostitis, and pseudoparalysis; edema; rash (maculopapular consisting of small dark red–copper spots that is most severe on the hands and feet); hemolytic anemia; or thrombocytopenia at birth or within the first 4 to 8 weeks of age. Untreated infants, including those asymptomatic at birth, may develop late manifestations, which usually appear after 2 years of age and involve the central nervous system (CNS), bones and joints, teeth, eyes, and skin. Some findings may not become apparent until many years after birth, such as interstitial keratitis, eighth cranial nerve deafness, Hutchinson teeth (peg-shaped, notched central incisors), anterior bowing of the shins, frontal bossing, mulberry molars, saddle nose, rhagades (perioral fissures), and Clutton joints (symmetrical, painless swelling of the knees). Late manifestations can be prevented by treatment of early infection.

Acquired Syphilis

Acquired disease can be divided into 3 stages. The **primary stage** (or **primary syphilis**) appears as painless indurated ulcers (chancres) of the skin or mucous membranes at the site of inoculation. These lesions appear, on average, 3 weeks after exposure (10–90 days) and heal spontaneously in a few weeks. Adjacent lymph nodes are frequently enlarged but are nontender. The **secondary stage** (or **secondary syphilis**), beginning 1 to 2 months later, is characterized by fever, sore throat, muscle aches, rash, mucocutaneous lesions, hepatitis, and generalized lymphadenopathy. The polymorphic maculopapular rash is generalized and typically includes the palms and soles. In moist areas of the perineum, hypertrophic papular lesions (condyloma lata) can be confused with condyloma acuminata secondary to human papillomavirus (HPV) infection. Malaise, splenomegaly, headache, alopecia, and arthralgia can be present. This stage resolves spontaneously without treatment in approximately 3 to 12 weeks. A variable asymptomatic latent period follows but may be interrupted during the first few years by recurrences of symptoms of secondary syphilis. **Latent syphilis** is the period after infection when patients are seroreactive but demonstrate no clinical manifestations of disease. Development of latent syphilis within the preceding year is referred to as **early latent syphilis;** if beyond 1 year's duration, it is known as **late latent syphilis.** If the duration of infection is unknown, the patient should be considered to have late latent syphilis for the purposes of management. The **tertiary stage** of syphilis occurs 15 to 30 years after the initial infection and can include gumma formation (soft, noncancerous, granulomatous growths that can destroy tissue) or cardiovascular involvement (including aortitis). Neurosyphilis infection of the CNS can occur at any stage of infection, especially in people with HIV and in neonates with congenital syphilis; manifestations include meningitis, uveitis, seizures, optic atrophy, hearing loss, and, typically years after infection, dementia and posterior spinal cord degeneration (tabes dorsalis, including a characteristic high-stepping gait with the feet slapping the ground with each step because of loss of proprioception).

ETIOLOGY

T pallidum subspecies (subsp) *pallidum* (*T pallidum*) is a thin, motile spirochete that is extremely fastidious, surviving only briefly outside the host. It is very closely related to 3 other organisms causing nonvenereal human disease in distinct geographic regions of the world: *T pallidum* subsp *pertenue*, which causes yaws; *T pallidum* subsp *endemicum*, which causes endemic syphilis; and *Treponema carateum*, which causes pinta. The genus *Treponema* is classified in the family *Spirochaetaceae*.

EPIDEMIOLOGY

During 2013–2017, the primary and secondary syphilis rate increased 72.7% nationally, and 155.6% among women, from 5.5 to 9.5 cases per 100,000 population. Syphilis rates increased by 17.6% overall from 2015 to 2016, with most primary and secondary cases occurring among men, particularly gay, bisexual, and other men who have sex with men (MSM). Also, half of MSM in whom syphilis was diagnosed had a diagnosis of HIV infection. In 2017, among women 15 through 24 years of age, the rate of reported primary and secondary syphilis was 5.5 cases per 100,000, which was a 7.8% increase from 2016 (5.1 cases per 100,000) and an 83.3% increase from 2013 (3.0 cases per 100,000). Among men 15 through 24 years of age, the rate was 26.1 cases per 100,000, which was an 8.3% increase from 2016 (24.1 cases per 100,000) and a 50.9% increase from 2013 (17.3 cases per 100,000). During 2016–2017, the rate of reported syphilis cases increased 9.8% among people 15 through 19 years of age and 7.8% among people 20 through 24 years of age.

In 2018, the number of infants born with syphilis was the highest since 1997, increasing from 9.2 cases per 100,000 live births to 33.1 per 100,000 live births from 2013 to 2018, with an absolute increase in cases over that period from 362 to 1,306 in 2018. This trend mirrors the rise in primary and secondary syphilis cases encountered in women of reproductive age. From 2013 to 2018, rates of early syphilis among girls and women of reproductive age (15–44 years) increased from 2.5 to 15.1 per 100,000 population, reflecting an increase from 3,386 to 9,651 per year.

Congenital syphilis may be contracted at any stage of maternal infection via transplacental transmission at any time during pregnancy or via contact with maternal lesions at the time of delivery. In pregnant women with untreated early syphilis, up to 40% of pregnancies result in spontaneous abortion, stillbirth, or perinatal death. The rate of maternal-fetal transmission is 60% to 100% in the setting of primary and secondary syphilis during pregnancy and decreases with later stages of maternal infection (approximately 40% with early latent infection and <8% with late latent infection). Among women who acquire syphilis during pregnancy, the risk of transmission to the infant increases directly with the gestational age at the time of maternal infection. HIV-infected women, in particular, have a higher prevalence of untreated or inadequately treated syphilis during pregnancy; therefore, their newborns may have higher risk for congenital syphilis. In addition, syphilis coinfection during pregnancy may also increase the rate of mother-to-child transmission of HIV.

T pallidum is not transmitted through human milk, but transmission may occur if the breastfeeding mother has an infectious lesion (chancre) on her breast.

Acquired syphilis is almost always contracted through direct sexual contact with ulcerative lesions of the skin or mucous membranes of infected people. Open, moist lesions of the primary or secondary stages are highly infectious. Syphilis acquired beyond the neonatal period should be considered diagnostic of sexual abuse in infants and young children once rare vertical transmission is excluded.

The **incubation period** for acquired primary syphilis is typically 3 weeks but ranges from 10 to 90 days.

DIAGNOSTIC TESTS

Definitive diagnosis is made when spirochetes are identified by microscopic darkfield examination of lesion exudate, nasal discharge, or tissue, such as placenta, lymph node, umbilical cord, or autopsy specimens. *T pallidum* can be detected by polymerase chain reaction (PCR) assay. Specimens from mouth lesions can contain nonpathogenic treponemes that are difficult to distinguish from *T pallidum* by darkfield microscopy.

Presumptive diagnosis requires the use of both nontreponemal and treponemal serological tests. Nontreponemal tests for syphilis include the Venereal Disease Research Laboratory (VDRL) slide test and the rapid plasma reagin (RPR) test. These tests are inexpensive, can be performed across a range of laboratory levels of complexity with fairly rapid turnaround times for analysis, and provide semiquantitative results that can both help define disease activity and monitor response to therapy. Nontreponemal test results may be falsely negative (ie, nonreactive) in early primary syphilis, latent acquired syphilis of long duration, and late congenital syphilis. Occasionally, the result of a nontreponemal test performed on serum containing high concentrations of antibody is weakly reactive or falsely negative, a reaction termed the *prozone phenomenon;* if the serum being tested is diluted, the result will be positive. The prozone phenomenon may be observed more often in HIV-coinfected individuals. When nontreponemal tests are used serially to monitor treatment response, the same test (RPR or VDRL), ideally from the same laboratory, must be used throughout the follow-up period to ensure comparability of results.

Except for congenital infection, a reactive nontreponemal test result should be confirmed by one of the specific treponemal tests to exclude a false-positive test result. False-positive nontreponemal results can be caused by certain viral infections (eg, Epstein-Barr virus infection, hepatitis, HIV infection, varicella, measles), lymphoma, tuberculosis, malaria, endocarditis, connective tissue disease, pregnancy, older age, use of injection drugs, or laboratory or technical error. When a cord blood sample is being used to test a newborn's RPR status, Wharton jelly has been shown to be a potential confounder for results, and an actual neonatal blood sample, when feasible, is a preferred specimen for testing. Treponemal tests in use include the *T pallidum* particle agglutination (TP-PA) test (which is the preferred treponemal test), *T pallidum* enzyme immunoassay (TP-EIA), *T pallidum* chemiluminescence assay (TP-CIA), and fluorescent treponemal antibody absorption (FTA-ABS) test. Most people who have reactive treponemal test results remain reactive for life, even after successful therapy. However, 15% to 25% of patients treated during primary syphilis revert to being serologically nonreactive on treponemal testing after 2 to 3 years. Treponemal test results may also be variably positive in patients with other spirochetal diseases, such as yaws, pinta, leptospirosis, rat-bite fever, relapsing fever, and Lyme disease.

In most cases, if a patient has a positive RPR or VDRL result in low titer and has a negative treponemal test result, the nontreponemal test result will be a false positive. However, because false-negative test results can occur in early syphilis, retesting in 2 to 4 weeks and again later if clinically indicated should be considered in people with increased risk for syphilis, especially in pregnant women.

The Centers for Disease Control and Prevention and the US Preventive Services Task Force recommend syphilis serological screening with a nontreponemal test; this screening is followed by confirmation with one of the several available treponemal tests (*conventional diagnostic approach*). Some clinical laboratories and blood banks, however, have begun to screen samples with treponemal tests first rather than begin with a nontreponemal test. This *reverse-sequence screening* approach may result in false-positive results, especially in low-prevalence populations. When the reverse-sequence algorithm is used, people with a positive treponemal test result and a negative nontreponemal test result (eg, EIA positive, RPR negative) should undergo a second treponemal test targeting a different *T pallidum* antigen to confirm the results of the original test. If the second treponemal-specific test result is negative (eg, EIA positive, RPR negative, then TP-PA negative) and the person has low risk for syphilis, the original treponemal test result was likely a false positive.

Cerebrospinal Fluid Tests

Cerebrospinal fluid (CSF) abnormalities in patients with neurosyphilis can include increased protein concentration, increased white blood cell (WBC) count, and/or a reactive CSF-VDRL test result. Outside the neonatal period, the CSF-VDRL is highly specific but insensitive; therefore, a negative result does not exclude a diagnosis of neurosyphilis. Conversely, a reactive CSF-VDRL test result in a neonate can be caused by nontreponemal immunoglobulin G antibodies that cross the blood-brain barrier. The CSF leukocyte count is usually elevated in neurosyphilis (>5 WBCs/μL). Interpretation of CSF test results requires a nontraumatic lumbar puncture (LP) (ie, a CSF sample that is not contaminated with blood). CSF test results obtained during the neonatal period can be difficult to interpret; normal values differ by gestational age and are higher in preterm infants. Studies suggest that 95% of healthy neonates have values of 16 to 19 WBCs/μL or less and/or protein 115 to 118 mg/dL or less on CSF examination. During the second month after birth, 95% of normal infants have values of 9 to 11 WBCs/μL or less and/or protein 89 to 91 mg/dL or less. Lower values (ie, 5 WBCs/μL and protein 40 mg/dL) might be considered the upper limits of reference in older infants. Other causes of elevated values should be considered when an infant is being evaluated for congenital syphilis. A positive CSF FTA-ABS or TP-PA result can support the diagnosis of neurosyphilis but does not establish the diagnosis definitively. Fewer data exist for the EIA or RPR test for CSF, and these tests should not be used for CSF evaluation.

Testing During Pregnancy

Prevention of congenital syphilis requires that pregnant women be screened serologically early in pregnancy. False-negative test results are possible in recent infection, and syphilis may be acquired later in pregnancy. Therefore, in communities and populations in which the prevalence of syphilis is high and for women with high risk for infection, serological testing should also be performed at 28 weeks' gestation and again at delivery. A nontreponemal test (RPR or VDRL) is recommended for screening, followed by a treponemal test if the screening result is positive. In most cases, if the treponemal antibody test result is negative, the nontreponemal test result is falsely positive and no further evaluation is necessary. However, retesting in 2 to 4 weeks, and again later if clinically indicated, should be considered for pregnant women who have high risk for syphilis.

If the reverse-sequence screening algorithm is used, pregnant women with reactive treponemal screening test results should undergo confirmatory testing with a quantitative nontreponemal test. If the nontreponemal test result is negative (eg, EIA positive, RPR negative), a second treponemal-specific test by using a different *T pallidum* antigen should be obtained to determine whether the initial treponemal test result was a false positive (TP-PA preferred). If the second treponemal test result is negative (eg, EIA positive, RPR negative, then TP-PA negative) and the person has low risk for syphilis, the original treponemal test result was likely a false positive. However, retesting in 2 to 4 weeks and again later if clinically indicated should be considered for pregnant women who are at high risk for syphilis.

Ultrasonographic evaluation of the fetus from the second trimester onward should be performed when syphilis is diagnosed at any time during pregnancy, even if appropriate maternal treatment has been administered. Pathological examination of the placenta and/or umbilical cord at delivery should also be performed.

Evaluation of Infants for Congenital Infection During the Newborn Period to 1 Month of Age

No newborn should be discharged from the hospital without determination of the mother's serological status for syphilis. All infants born to seropositive mothers require a careful examination and nontreponemal testing. A negative maternal RPR or VDRL test result at delivery does not rule out the possibility of the infant having congenital syphilis, although such a situation is rare. The diagnostic approach to infants being evaluated for congenital syphilis is presented in Figure 140.1.

Evaluation of Infants Older Than 1 Month and Children

When infants and children are identified as having reactive serological tests for syphilis, maternal serological test results and records should be reviewed to assess whether the mother has congenital or acquired syphilis. Evaluation for congenital syphilis after 1 month of age includes (1) CSF analysis for VDRL, cell count, and protein; (2) complete blood cell count, differential count, and platelet count; (3) other tests as clinically indicated (eg, long-bone radiographs, chest radiograph, liver function tests, abdominal ultrasonography, ophthalmologic examination, neuroimaging, and auditory brainstem response); and (4) testing for HIV infection.

TREATMENT

Parenteral penicillin G is the preferred drug for treatment of syphilis at any stage. The type and duration of penicillin G therapy vary depending on the stage of disease and clinical manifestations. Parenteral penicillin G is the only documented effective therapy for patients who have neurosyphilis, congenital syphilis, or syphilis during pregnancy and is also recommended for people with HIV infection.

Penicillin Allergy

Infants and children who have a history of penicillin allergy or who develop presumed penicillin allergy during treatment should be desensitized and then treated with penicillin whenever possible. Data to support the use of alternatives to penicillin are limited, but options for nonpregnant patients who are allergic to penicillin may include doxycycline, tetracycline, and, for neurosyphilis, ceftriaxone. These therapies should be used with close clinical and laboratory follow-up to ensure expected serological response and cure. In pregnancy, desensitization and treatment with doses of intramuscular benzathine

Figure 140.1
Algorithm for Diagnostic Approach of Infants Born to Mothers With Reactive Serological Tests for Syphilis

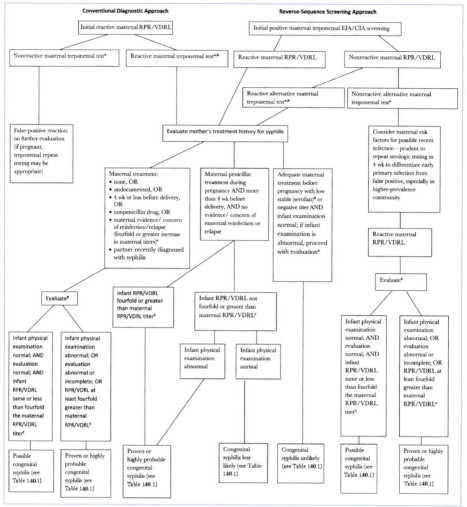

CIA indicates chemiluminescence assay; EIA, enzyme immunoassay; RPR, rapid plasma reagin; and VDRL, Venereal Disease Research Laboratory.

[a] *Treponema pallidum* particle agglutination (which is the preferred treponemal test) or fluorescent treponemal antibody absorption.
[b] Test for HIV antibody. Infants of HIV-infected mothers do not require different evaluation or treatment of syphilis.
[c] A 4-fold change in titer is the same as a change of 2 dilutions. For example, a titer of 1:64 is 4-fold greater than a titer of 1:16, and a titer of 1:4 is 4-fold lower than a titer of 1:16. When comparing titers, the same type of nontreponemal test should be used (eg, if the initial test was an RPR, the follow-up test should also be an RPR).
[d] Stable VDRL titers ≤1:2 or RPR ≤1:4 beyond 1 year after successful treatment is considered low serofast.
[e] Complete blood cell count and platelet count; cerebrospinal fluid examination for cell count, protein, and quantitative VDRL; other tests as clinically indicated (eg, chest radiographs, long-bone radiographs, eye examination, liver function tests, neuroimaging, and auditory brainstem response). For neonates, pathological examination of the placenta or umbilical cord with specific fluorescent antitreponemal antibody staining, if possible.

penicillin, guided by the stage of syphilis diagnosed, are the only appropriate therapy in the setting of a maternal penicillin allergy. Erythromycin and azithromycin, which have been suggested as extended-course alternatives in nonpregnant adults with penicillin allergy, are not appropriate for treatment in pregnancy because they may suboptimally treat the mother and do not cross the placenta adequately to treat the fetus. Similarly, doxycycline is not appropriate for extended use in pregnancy, especially in the second and third trimesters.

Congenital Syphilis

Newborn Period to 1 Month of Age

The management of congenital syphilis is based on whether the infant has proven or probable congenital syphilis, has possible congenital syphilis, or is considered less likely or unlikely to have syphilis, as detailed in Table 140.1. If more than 1 day of therapy is missed, the entire course should be restarted. Data supporting use of other antimicrobial agents (eg, ampicillin) for treatment of congenital syphilis are unavailable. When possible, a full 10-day course of penicillin is preferred, even if ampicillin was initially provided for possible sepsis. Use of agents other than penicillin requires close serological follow-up to assess adequacy of therapy.

Infants 1 Month and Older and Children

Infants 1 month and older who possibly have congenital syphilis and children older than 2 years who have late and previously untreated congenital syphilis should be treated with intravenous aqueous crystalline penicillin (200,000–300,000 U/kg/day, intravenously, administered as 50,000 U/kg, every 4–6 hours for 10 days). Some experts suggest giving such patients a single dose of penicillin G benzathine (50,000 U/kg, intramuscularly, not to exceed 2.4 million U) after the 10-day course of intravenous aqueous crystalline penicillin. If the patient has no clinical manifestations of disease, the CSF examination findings are normal, and the CSF-VDRL test result is negative, some experts would treat with 3 weekly doses of penicillin G benzathine (50,000 U/kg, intramuscularly, not to exceed 2.4 million U).

Penicillin Shortage

When the availability of penicillin G aqueous crystalline is compromised, check local sources for penicillin G aqueous crystalline (potassium or sodium).

For infants with proven or highly probably congenital syphilis, if intravenous penicillin G is limited, substitute some or all daily doses with penicillin G procaine (50,000 U/kg/dose intramuscularly in a single daily dose for 10 days). If penicillin G aqueous or procaine is unavailable, ceftriaxone (50–75 mg/kg/day intravenously every 24 hours) can be considered with careful clinical and serological follow-up and in consultation with a pediatric infectious diseases specialist, because evidence is insufficient to support the use of ceftriaxone for the treatment of congenital syphilis. In neonates 28 days and younger, ceftriaxone is contraindicated if they have hyperbilirubinemia or if they require treatment with calcium-containing intravenous solutions, because of the risk of precipitation of ceftriaxone-calcium.

For infants who have possible congenital syphilis or in whom congenital syphilis is less likely, with penicillin G procaine (50,000 U/kg/dose intramuscularly a day in a single dose for 10 days) or penicillin G benzathine (50,000 U/kg intramuscularly as a single dose) should be used. If any part of the evaluation for congenital syphilis is abnormal or was not performed, CSF examination is uninterpretable, or follow-up is uncertain, penicillin G procaine is recommended. A single dose of ceftriaxone is inadequate therapy. However, for preterm infants who might not tolerate intramuscular injections because of decreased muscle mass, intravenous ceftriaxone can be considered with careful clinical and serological follow-up and in consultation with a pediatric infectious diseases specialist.

Syphilis in Pregnancy

Regardless of stage of pregnancy, women should be treated with penicillin according to the dosage schedules appropriate for the stage of syphilis as recommended for nonpregnant patients (Table 140.2). Nonpenicillin treatment of syphilis during pregnancy cannot be considered reliable to cure infection in the mother and does not cross the placenta adequately to ensure fetal treatment.

Table 140.1
Evaluation and Treatment of Infants Up To 1 Month of Age With Possible, Probable, or Confirmed Congenital Syphilis

Category	Findings	Recommended Evaluation	Treatment
Proven or highly probable congenital syphilis	Abnormal physical examination findings consistent with congenital syphilis OR A serum quantitative nontreponemal serological titer 4-fold higher than the maternal titer OR A positive result of darkfield test or PCR assay of lesions or body fluid(s)	CSF analysis (for VDRL, cell count, and protein) CBC count with differential count and platelet count Other tests (as clinically indicated): • Long-bone radiography • Chest radiography • Aminotransferase levels • Neuroimaging • Ophthalmologic examination • Auditory brainstem response	Penicillin G aqueous crystalline, 50,000 U/kg, IV, every 12 hours (age ≤1 week), then every 8 hours for infants >1 week, for a total of 10 days of therapy[a] (**preferred**) OR Penicillin G procaine, 50,000 U/kg, IM, as single daily dose for 10 days
Possible congenital syphilis	Normal infant examination findings AND A serum quantitative nontreponemal serological titer equal to or less than 4-fold the maternal titer AND ONE OF THE FOLLOWING FINDINGS: Mother was not treated, was inadequately treated, or had no documentation of receiving treatment OR Mother was treated with a regimen other than recommended in the guideline (ie, a nonpenicillin regimen) OR Mother received recommended treatment <4 weeks before delivery	CSF analysis (for VDRL, cell count, and protein) CBC count with differential count and platelet count Long-bone radiography	Penicillin G aqueous crystalline, 50,000 U/kg, IV, every 12 hours (age ≤1 week), then every 8 hours for infants >1 week, for a total of 10 days of therapy[b] (**preferred**) OR Penicillin G procaine, 50,000 U/kg, IM, as single daily dose for 10 days OR Penicillin G benzathine, 50,000 U/kg, IM, single dose (recommended by some experts, but **only** if all components of the evaluation are obtained and are normal[c] and follow-up is certain)

Scenario	Criteria	Evaluation	Treatment
Congenital syphilis less likely	Normal infant examination findings AND A serum quantitative nontreponemal serological titer equal to or less than 4-fold the maternal titer AND Mother was treated during pregnancy, treatment was appropriate for stage of infection, and treatment was administered >4 weeks before delivery AND Mother has no evidence of reinfection or relapse	Not recommended	Penicillin G benzathine, 50,000 U/kg, IM, single dose (**preferred**) Alternatively, infants whose mothers' nontreponemal titers decreased at least 4-fold after appropriate therapy for early syphilis or remained stable at low titer (eg, VDRL ≤1:2; RPR ≤1:4) may be followed up every 2–3 months without treatment until the nontreponemal test result becomes nonreactive. Nontreponemal antibody titers should decrease by 3 months of age and should be nonreactive by 6 months of age; patients with increasing titers or with persistent stable titers 6–12 months after initial treatment should undergo reevaluation, including a CSF examination, and treatment with a 10-day course of parenteral penicillin G, even if they were treated previously.
Congenital syphilis unlikely	Normal infant examination findings AND A serum quantitative nontreponemal serological titer ≤4-fold the maternal titer AND Mother was treated adequately before pregnancy AND Mother's nontreponemal serological titer remained low and stable (ie, serofast) before and during pregnancy and at delivery (eg, VDRL ≤1:2; RPR ≤1:4)	Not recommended	None, but infants with reactive nontreponemal test results should be followed up serologically to ensure test result returns to negative. Penicillin G benzathine, 50,000 U/kg, IM, single dose, can be considered if follow-up is uncertain and infant has a reactive test result (some experts). Neonates who have a negative nontreponemal test result at birth and whose mothers were seroreactive at delivery should be retested at 3 months to rule out incubating congenital syphilis.

CBC indicates complete blood cell count; CSF, cerebrospinal fluid; PCR, polymerase chain reaction; IM, intramuscularly; IV, intravenously; RPR, rapid plasma reagin; and VDRL, Venereal Disease Research Laboratory.
Adapted and modified from Centers for Disease Control and Prevention. Sexually transmitted diseases treatment guidelines, 2015. *MMWR Recomm Rep.* 2015;64(RR-3):45–47.
[a] If ≥24 hours of therapy is missed, the entire course must be restarted.
[b] If CSF is not obtained or uninterpretable (eg, bloody tap), a 10-day course is recommended.

Acquired Primary, Secondary, and Early Latent Syphilis; Late Latent Syphilis; Tertiary Syphilis; and Neurosyphilis

Treatment recommendations for children and adults are detailed in Table 140.2.

Other Considerations

- All nonneonatal patients with syphilis should be tested for other sexually transmitted infections (STIs), including *Neisseria gonorrhoeae*, *Chlamydia trachomatis*, HIV, hepatitis B, and hepatitis C. Patients who have syphilis should be retested for HIV infection after 3 months if the first HIV test result is negative. Immunization status for hepatitis B and HPV should be reviewed and vaccines should be administered if not up to date.

- All recent sexual contacts of people with acquired syphilis should be evaluated for other STIs as well as syphilis.

- Children with acquired primary, secondary, or latent syphilis should be evaluated for possible sexual assault or abuse.

Follow-up and Management

Congenital Syphilis

All infants who have reactive serological tests for syphilis or were born to mothers who were seroreactive at delivery should receive careful follow-up evaluations during well-child visits at 2, 4, 6, and 12 months of age. Serological nontreponemal tests should be performed every 2 to 3 months until the test result becomes nonreactive. Nontreponemal antibody titers typically decrease by 3 months of age and should be nonreactive by 6 months of age, whether the infant was infected and adequately treated or was not infected and initially seropositive because of transplacentally acquired maternal antibody. The serological response after therapy may be slower for infants treated after the neonatal period. Patients with increasing titers or with persistent stable titers 6 to 12 months after initial treatment should undergo reevaluation, including a CSF examination. Re-treatment with a 10-day course of parenteral penicillin G may be indicated, even if they were treated previously. Neonates with a negative nontreponemal test result at birth whose mothers were seroreactive at delivery should be retested at 3 months to rule out incubating congenital syphilis.

Treponemal tests should not be used to evaluate treatment response, because results can remain positive despite effective therapy. Passively transferred maternal treponemal antibodies can persist in an infant until 15 months of age. A reactive treponemal test result after 18 months of age is diagnostic of congenital syphilis and should be followed by evaluation and, if necessary, treatment of congenital syphilis. If the treponemal test result is nonreactive at this time, no further evaluation or treatment is necessary.

Neonates whose initial CSF evaluation findings are abnormal do not need repeated LP unless they exhibit persistent nontreponemal serological test titers at age 6 to 12 months. After 2 years of follow-up, a reactive CSF VDRL test result or abnormal CSF indices that cannot be attributed to another ongoing illness at the 6-month interval are indications for re-treatment.

Acquired Syphilis

People with acquired primary or secondary syphilis should undergo clinical and serological evaluations at 6 and 12 months after treatment. More frequent evaluation might be necessary if adherence to follow-up or reinfection is a concern. If signs or symptoms persist or recur, or a 4-fold or greater increase in nontreponemal titers occurs, treatment failure or reinfection may be responsible. CSF analysis, HIV testing, and re-treatment based on CSF findings are indicated. Failure of nontreponemal titers to decline 4-fold within 6 to 12 months may also indicate treatment failure.

Following treatment, people with acquired latent syphilis should undergo serological evaluation at 6, 12, and 24 months after treatment; HIV-infected people should also undergo serological testing at 3 and 9 months in addition to 6, 12, and 24 months. Patients should experience a 4-fold or greater decline in nontreponemal titers within 12 to 24 months. If titers increase at least 4-fold or initial high titers fail to fall 4-fold, or symptoms of syphilis develop, reevaluation, including a CSF examination, is warranted.

Table 140.2
Recommended Treatment of Acquired Primary, Secondary, and Early Latent Syphilis; Late Latent Syphilis; Tertiary Syphilis; and Neurosyphilis[a]

Status	Children	Adults
Primary, secondary, and early latent[b]	Penicillin G benzathine,[c] 50,000 U/kg, IM, up to the adult dose of 2.4 million U in a single dose *If allergic to penicillin and not pregnant*, doxycycline, 4.4 mg/kg divided in 2 doses, max 200 mg/day, orally, twice a day for 14 days **OR** Tetracycline, 25–50 mg/kg divided in 4 doses, max 2 g/day, orally, for 14 days (**for age ≥8 y**)	Penicillin G benzathine, 2.4 million U, IM, in a single dose **OR** *If allergic to penicillin and not pregnant*, doxycycline, 100 mg, orally, twice a day for 14 days **OR** Tetracycline, 500 mg, orally, 4 times/day for 14 days
Late latent[d]	Penicillin G benzathine, 50,000 U/kg, IM, up to the adult dose of 2.4 million U, administered as 3 single doses at 1-wk intervals (total 150,000 U/kg, up to the adult dose of 7.2 million U) *If allergic to penicillin and not pregnant*, doxycycline, 4.4 mg/kg divided in 2 doses, max 200 mg/day, orally, twice a day for 4 wk (**for age ≥8 y**) **OR** Tetracycline, 25–50 mg/kg divided in 4 doses, max 2 g/day, orally, for 4 wk (**for age ≥8 y**)	Penicillin G benzathine, 7.2 million U total, administered as 3 doses of 2.4 million U, IM, each at 1-wk intervals; pregnant women who have delays in any dose of therapy beyond 9 days between doses should repeat the full course of therapy **OR** *If allergic to penicillin and not pregnant*, doxycycline, 100 mg, orally, twice a day for 4 wk **OR** Tetracycline, 500 mg, orally, 4 times/day for 4 wk
Tertiary	…	Penicillin G benzathine, 7.2 million U total, administered as 3 doses of 2.4 million U, IM, at 1-wk intervals *If allergic to penicillin and not pregnant, consult an infectious diseases expert.*
Neurosyphilis[e]	Penicillin G aqueous crystalline, 200,000–300,000 U/kg/day, IV, administered as 50,000 U/kg every 4–6 h for 10–14 days, in doses not to exceed the adult dose	Penicillin G aqueous crystalline, 18–24 million U/day, administered as 3–4 million U, IV, every 4 h for 10–14 days[f] **OR** Penicillin G procaine,[c] 2.4 million U, IM, once daily **PLUS** probenecid, 500 mg, orally, 4 times/day, both for 10–14 days[f]

IM indicates intramuscularly; IV, intravenously; and max, maximum.
[a] Excludes patients with either early or late recognition of congenital syphilis.
[b] Early latent syphilis is defined as being acquired within the preceding year.
[c] Penicillin G benzathine and penicillin G procaine are approved only for intramuscular administration.
[d] Late latent syphilis is defined as syphilis beyond 1 year's duration.
[e] Patients who are allergic to penicillin should be desensitized.
[f] Some experts administer penicillin G benzathine, 2.4 million U, IM, once per week for up to 3 weeks after completion of these neurosyphilis treatment regimens.

Patients with neurosyphilis associated with acquired syphilis must undergo periodic serological testing, clinical evaluation at 6-month intervals, and repeated CSF examinations. If the CSF WBC count has not decreased after 6 months or if the CSF WBC count or protein concentration is not normal after 2 years, re-treatment should be considered. CSF abnormalities may persist for extended periods in people with HIV infection with neurosyphilis.

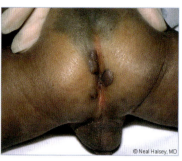

Image 140.1
Cutaneous syphilis in a 6-month-old. Courtesy of Neal Halsey, MD.

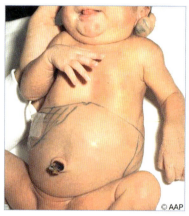

Image 140.2
Congenital syphilis in a 2-week-old boy with marked hepatosplenomegaly. The neonate kept his upper extremities in a flail-like position because of painful periostitis. Courtesy of Edgar O. Ledbetter, MD, FAAP.

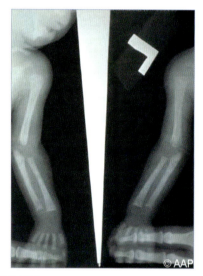

Image 140.3
Upper extremities of the patient in Image 140.2, with early periostitis. Note radiolucency of the distal radius and ulna occurring bilaterally. Courtesy of Edgar O. Ledbetter, MD, FAAP.

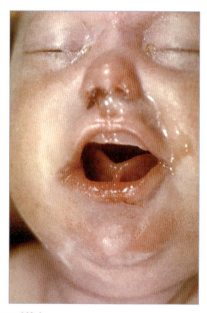

Image 140.4
The face of a newborn displaying pathological morphology indicative of congenital syphilis with striking mucous membrane involvement. Courtesy of Centers for Disease Control and Prevention.

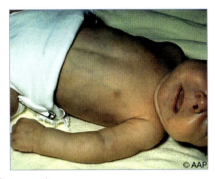

Image 140.5
A newborn with congenital syphilis with bleeding from the nares and tender swelling of the wrists and elbows secondary to luetic periostitis.

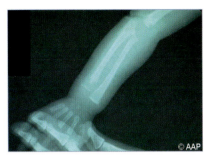

Image 140.6
Congenital syphilis with metaphyseal destruction of the distal humerus, radius, and ulna.

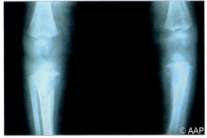

Image 140.7
Congenital syphilis with proximal tibial metaphysitis (Wimberger sign).

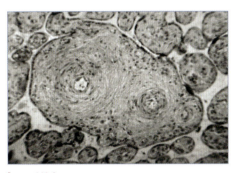

Image 140.8
A photomicrograph revealing cytoarchitectural changes of the placenta found in congenital syphilis. The chorionic villi are enlarged and contain dense laminated connective tissue, and the capillaries distributed throughout the villi are compressed by this connective tissue proliferation (hematoxylin-eosin stain, magnification ×450). Courtesy of Centers for Disease Control and Prevention.

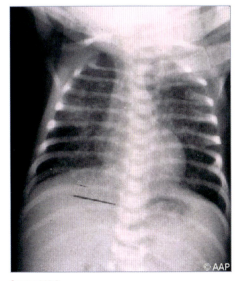

Image 140.9
Congenital syphilis with pneumonia alba. The infant survived with penicillin treatment.

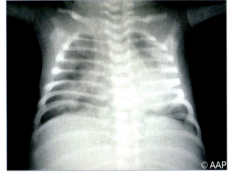

Image 140.10
A 3-day-old with severe pneumonia alba.

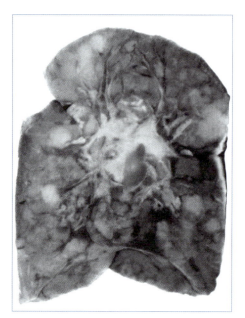

Image 140.11
This pathological condition of the lungs, known as pneumonia alba, is caused by congenital syphilis. The lungs are enlarged, heavy, uniformly firm, and yellow-white. Seventy percent of all pregnant women with untreated primary syphilis may transmit the infection to their fetuses. Courtesy of Centers for Disease Control and Prevention.

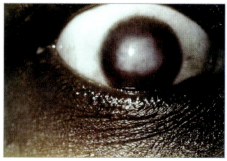

Image 140.12
This photograph depicts the presence of a diffuse stromal haze in the cornea of a female patient, known as interstitial keratitis, which was caused by her late-stage congenital syphilitic condition. Interstitial keratitis, which is an inflammation of the cornea's connective tissue elements and usually affects both eyes, can occur as a complication brought on by congenital or acquired syphilis. Interstitial keratitis usually occurs in children >2 years of age. Courtesy of Centers for Disease Control and Prevention.

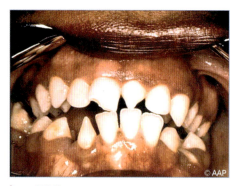

Image 140.13
Hutchinson teeth, a late manifestation of congenital syphilis. Changes occur in secondary dentition. The central incisors are smaller than normal and have sloping sides. Courtesy of Edgar O. Ledbetter, MD, FAAP.

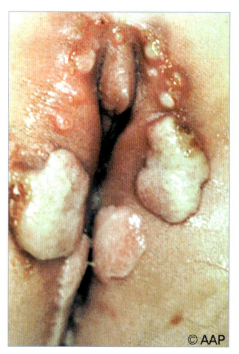

Image 140.14
Condyloma latum in a 7-year-old girl who had been sexually abused. These whitish-gray, moist lesions are caused by *Treponema pallidum* and are highly contagious.

SYPHILIS

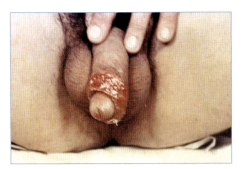

Image 140.15
This image shows an extensive chancre, located on the penile shaft, that resulted from a primary syphilitic infection caused by *Treponema pallidum*. The primary stage of syphilis is usually marked by the appearance of a single lesion, called a *chancre*. The chancre is usually firm, round, small, and painless. It appears at the spot where *T pallidum* entered the body and lasts 3–6 weeks, healing on its own. Courtesy of Centers for Disease Control and Prevention.

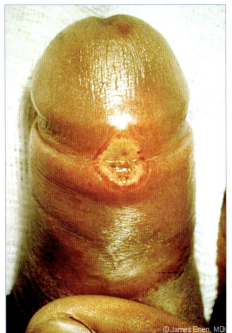

Image 140.16
Syphilis with penile chancre. Copyright James Brien.

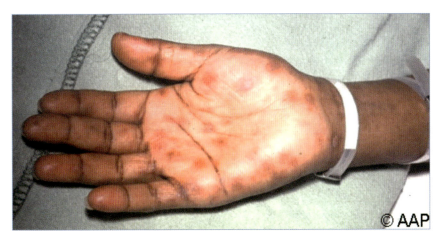

Image 140.17
A 16-year-old girl with rash of secondary syphilis noticed at 3 months' gestation of her pregnancy. The sign and symptoms of secondary syphilis generally occur 6–8 weeks after the primary infection when primary lesions have usually healed.

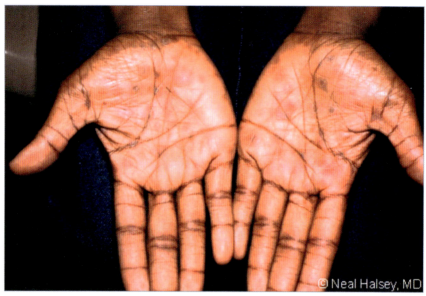

Image 140.18
Secondary syphilis in a different patient than in Image 140.17 with discrete palmar lesions. The diagnosis was suspected because of the palmar lesions. Copyright Neal Halsey, MD.

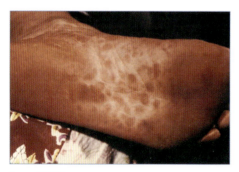

Image 140.19
This patient presented with a papular rash on the sole of the foot caused by secondary syphilis. The second stage of syphilis starts when ≥1 areas of the skin break into a rash that appears as rough red or reddish-brown spots on the palms of the hands and the bottoms of the feet. Even without treatment, the rash clears up spontaneously. Courtesy of Centers for Disease Control and Prevention.

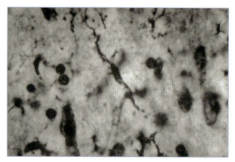

Image 140.20
Elongated microglia (rod cells) caused by untreated syphilis, leading to general paresis called *paretic neurosyphilis*. Neurosyphilis is a slowly progressive and destructive infection of the brain and spinal cord that occurs in untreated syphilis. This image shows bipolar, elongated microglia (rod cells) characteristic of paretic neurosyphilis (Hortega method, magnification ×950). Courtesy of Centers for Disease Control and Prevention.

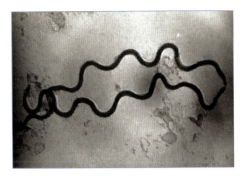

Image 140.21
An electron photomicrograph of 2 spiral-shaped *Treponema pallidum* bacteria (magnification ×36,000). Courtesy of Centers for Disease Control and Prevention.

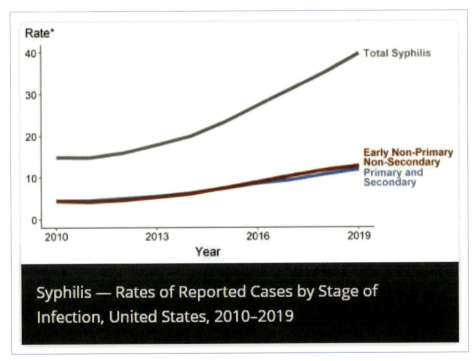

Image 140.22
Rates of reported syphilis cases by stage of infection, United States, 2010–2019. *Per 100,000. Courtesy of Centers for Disease Control and Prevention.

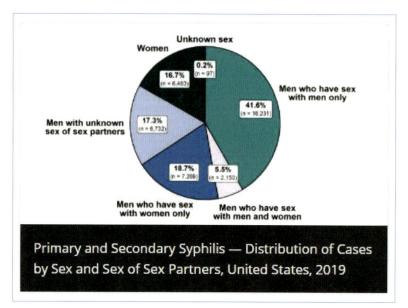

Image 140.23
Distribution of primary and secondary syphilis cases by sex and sex of sex partners, United States, 2019. Courtesy of Centers for Disease Control and Prevention.

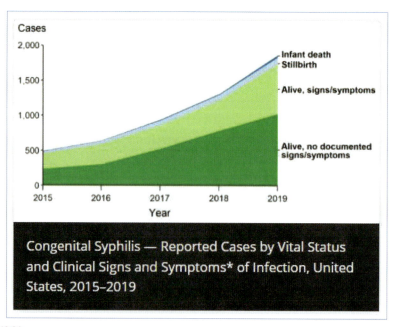

Image 140.24
Reported cases of congenital syphilis by vital status and clinical signs and symptoms of infection, United States, 2015-2019. *Infants with signs/symptoms of congenital syphilis have documentation of at least one of the following: long bone changes consistent with congenital syphilis, snuffles, condyloma lata, syphilitic skin rash, pseudoparalysis, hepatosplenomegaly, edema, jaundice due to syphilitic hepatitis, reactive cerebrospinal fluid (CSF)–VDRL, elevated CSF WBC or protein, or evidence of direct detection of *T Pallidum*. VDRL indicates Venereal Disease Research Laboratory; WBC, white blood cell. Courtesy of Centers for Disease Control and Prevention.

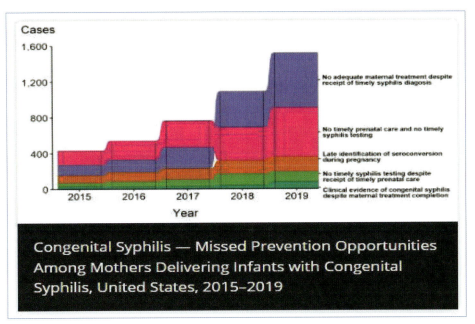

Image 140.25
Congenital syphilis: missed prevention opportunities among mothers delivering infants with congenital syphilis, United States, 2015–2019. Courtesy of Centers for Disease Control and Prevention.

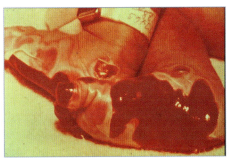

Image 140.26
Cutaneous lesions of congenital syphilis in a full-term newborn. Courtesy of Carol J. Baker, MD, FAAP.

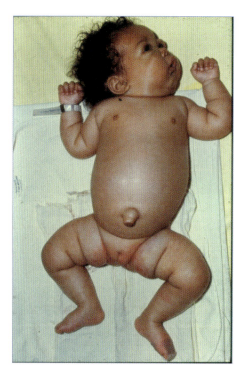

Image 140.27
A full-term newborn with ascites, hepatosplenomegaly, adenopathy, and periostitis caused by congenital syphilis. Although rare, nephrotic syndrome can result from congenital syphilis. Courtesy of Carol J. Baker, MD, FAAP.

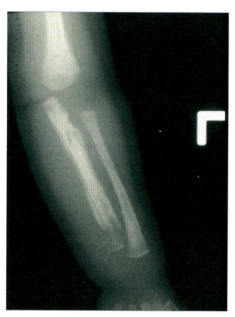

Image 140.28
Radiograph of the forearm of the newborn in Image 140.27 illustrating the periostitis of the radius and ulna. Courtesy of Carol J. Baker, MD, FAAP.

CHAPTER 141

Tapeworm Diseases
(Taeniasis and Cysticercosis)

CLINICAL MANIFESTATIONS

Taeniasis

Infection with adult tapeworms is often asymptomatic. The most common symptom is noting passing tapeworm segments from the anus or in feces. Other mild gastrointestinal tract symptoms, such as nausea or diarrhea, can occur.

Cysticercosis

Cysticercosis, caused by larval pork tapeworm (*Taenia solium*) infection, can have serious consequences. Manifestations depend on the location and number of pork tapeworm larval cysts (cysticerci) and on the host response. Cysticerci may be found anywhere in the body. The most common and serious clinical manifestations are caused by cysticerci in the central nervous system (CNS). Larval cysts of *T solium* in the brain (neurocysticercosis) can result in seizures, headache, obstructive hydrocephalus, and other neurological signs and symptoms. Neurocysticercosis is the leading infectious cause of epilepsy in the developing world. Most symptoms result from the host reaction to degenerating cysticerci. Cysts in the spinal column can cause gait disturbance, pain, or transverse myelitis. Subcutaneous cysticerci produce palpable nodules, and ocular involvement can cause visual impairment.

ETIOLOGY

Taeniasis is caused by intestinal infection by the adult tapeworm, *Taenia saginata* (beef tapeworm) or *T solium* (pork tapeworm). *Taenia asiatica* causes taeniasis in Asia. Human cysticercosis is caused only by the larvae of *T solium*.

EPIDEMIOLOGY

Tapeworm diseases have worldwide distribution. Prevalence is high in areas with poor sanitation and human fecal contamination in areas where cattle graze or where swine are fed. Most cases of *T solium* infection in the United States are imported from Latin America, although the disease is prevalent in parts of Asia and sub-Saharan Africa as well. *T saginata* infection occurs at high rates in East Africa and the Middle East and is also prevalent in Latin America, much of Asia, and eastern Europe. *T asiatica* is common in China, Taiwan, and Southeast Asia. Taeniasis is acquired by eating undercooked beef (*T saginata*), pork (*T solium*), or pig viscera (*T asiatica*) that contain encysted larvae.

Cysticercosis in humans is acquired by ingesting eggs of the pork tapeworm (*T solium*). Transmission is fecal-oral, usually by ingestion of food contaminated by feces from a person harboring the adult tapeworm. Autoinfection, in which tapeworm carriers infect themselves, also occurs. Humans are the obligate definitive host and the only host to shed the eggs. Eggs liberate oncospheres in the intestine that migrate through the blood and lymphatics to tissues throughout the body, including the CNS, where the oncospheres develop into cysticerci. Although nearly all cases of cysticercosis in the United States are imported, cysticercosis can be acquired in the United States from tapeworm carriers who emigrated from an area with endemic infection and still have *T solium* intestinal-stage infection. *T saginata* and *T asiatica* do not cause cysticercosis.

The **incubation period** for taeniasis (the time from ingestion of the larvae until the time segments are passed in the feces) is 2 to 3 months. For cysticercosis, the time between infection and onset of symptoms is typically several years.

DIAGNOSIS

Diagnosis of taeniasis (adult tapeworm infection) is based on demonstration of the proglottids or ova in feces or the perianal region, although these techniques are insensitive. Species identification of the parasite is based on the different structures of gravid proglottids and scolex or on polymerase chain reaction assay.

Diagnosis of neurocysticercosis typically depends on clinical manifestation and imaging of the CNS. Serological testing can also be helpful in certain cases. Computed tomography (CT) scanning or magnetic resonance imaging (MRI) of the brain or spinal cord is used to demonstrate lesions compatible with cysticerci. CT scans are helpful in identifying calcifications. MRI is better at helping identify extraparenchymal cysts (eg, in ventricles or the subarachnoid space) and the invaginated scolex within the parasite cysticercus. Antibody assays that detect specific antibodies to larval *T solium* in serum can be useful to confirm the diagnosis. In the United States, immunoblot assays (including the enzyme-linked immunotransfer blot) are available through the Centers for Disease Control and Prevention (CDC) and a few commercial laboratories and are the antibody tests of choice. In general, immunoblot assays are more sensitive with serum specimens than with cerebrospinal fluid specimens. Even immunoblot tests can have limited sensitivity if only one cysticercus or only calcified cysticerci are present, and results are often negative in children with solitary parenchymal lesions. A negative serological test result does not exclude the diagnosis of neurocysticercosis when clinical suspicion is high. Antigen-detection assays are available from the CDC and National Institutes of Health for selected cases.

TREATMENT

Taeniasis

Praziquantel is highly effective for eradicating infection with the adult tapeworm. Praziquantel is not approved for this indication, but dosing recommendations are available for children 4 years and older. Niclosamide is an alternative agent for treatment of taeniasis but is not available commercially in the United States.

Cysticercosis

Neurocysticercosis treatment should be individualized on the basis of the number, location, and viability of cysticerci as assessed by neuroimaging studies (MRI or CT) and clinical manifestations. Symptomatic therapy is critical and should include antiseizure medications for patients with seizures and surgery for patients with hydrocephalus. Two antiparasitic drugs, albendazole and praziquantel, are available. Both drugs are cysticercidal and hasten radiological resolution of cysts, but symptoms result from host inflammatory response and may be exacerbated by treatment. In symptomatic patients with a single cyst within brain parenchyma, controlled studies demonstrate that clinical resolution and seizure recurrence rates are slightly improved when children are treated with albendazole along with corticosteroids. Two studies demonstrated that in those with more than 2 lesions, the response rate was better when albendazole was coadministered with praziquantel and corticosteroids. When a single agent is used, albendazole is preferred over praziquantel, because it has fewer drug-drug interactions with anticonvulsants and steroids. Patients with calcified cysts do not benefit from antiparasitic treatment. An ophthalmic examination should be performed before antiparasitic treatment to rule out intraocular cysticerci. Coadministration of corticosteroids during antiparasitic therapy decreases adverse effects during treatment and is required for some forms of the disease (eg, basilar or subarachnoid, extensive parenchymal, or spinal involvement). Duration of corticosteroid therapy is longer in patients with subarachnoid disease, vasculitis, or encephalitis. Arachnoiditis, vasculitis, or diffuse cerebral edema (cysticercal encephalitis) is treated with corticosteroid therapy until the cerebral edema is controlled. Corticosteroids can affect the tissue concentrations of albendazole. Patients requiring steroids may need screening for strongyloidiasis, latent tuberculosis, and vitamin D deficiency.

Medical and surgical management of cysticercosis can be highly complex and often needs to be conducted in consultation with a neurologist or neurosurgeon and an infectious diseases or other specialist with experience treating neurocysticercosis. Seizures may recur for months or years. Anticonvulsant therapy is recommended until there is neuroradiological evidence of resolution and seizures have not occurred for 6 months (for a single lesion) or 1 to 2 years (for multiple lesions). Calcification of cysts may require prolonged or indefinite use of anticonvulsants. Subarachnoid cysticercosis does not respond well to the regimens used for parenchymal disease and should generally be treated with prolonged courses of antiparasitic and anti-inflammatory medications. Methotrexate and/or tumor necrosis factor inhibitors have been used as steroid-sparing agents. Intraventricular cysticerci and hydrocephalus should usually be treated surgically. Surgical removal of intraventricular cysticerci is the treatment of choice when possible and can often be accomplished by endoscopic surgery (lateral, third, and, sometimes, fourth ventricles) or open surgery (fourth ventricle). If cysticerci cannot be removed easily, hydrocephalus should be corrected with placement of intraventricular shunts. Adjunctive chemotherapy with antiparasitic agents and corticosteroids may decrease the rate of subsequent shunt failure. Ocular cysticercosis is treated by surgical excision of the cysticerci. Ocular cysticercosis is not generally treated with anthelminthic drugs, which can exacerbate inflammation. Spinal cysticercosis may be treated with medical and/or surgical therapy. There is not adequate evidence to guide the choice of medical versus surgical therapy.

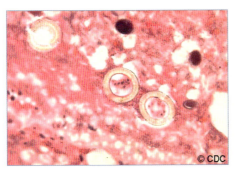

Image 141.1
Histopathologic features of *Taenia saginata* in the appendix.

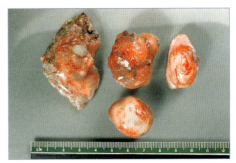

Image 141.2
Gross pathological features of the membrane and hydatid daughter cysts excised from a human lung. Hydatid disease is a parasitic infestation caused by a tapeworm of the genus *Echinococcus*. Endemic areas usually involve low-income countries. The liver is the most common organ involved, followed by the lungs. Courtesy of Centers for Disease Control and Prevention.

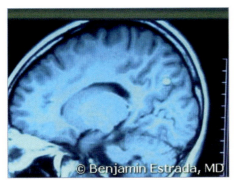

Image 141.3
Neurocysticercosis in an 11-year-old girl apparent on a computed tomographic scan. Courtesy of Benjamin Estrada, MD.

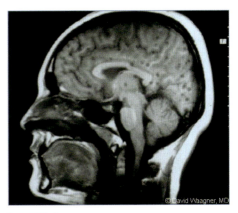

Image 141.4
Cerebral neurocysticercosis with diffuse, scattered, ring-enhancing lesions throughout the brain parenchyma with focal edema evident on a computed tomographic scan. Copyright David Waagner, MD.

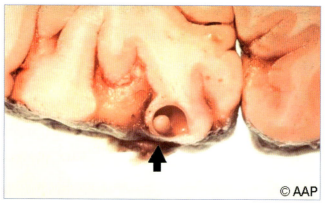

Image 141.5
Cross section showing cysticercosis of the brain at autopsy.

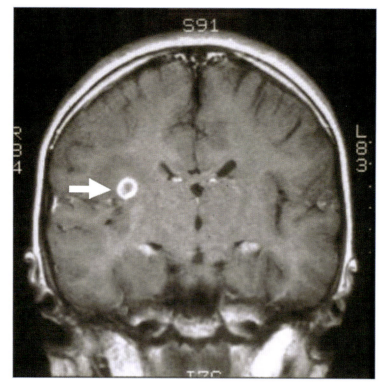

Image 141.6
A young boy with a seizure. Magnetic resonance imaging of the brain revealed a ringlike lesion (arrow) characteristic of neurocysticercosis. Copyright Barbara Ann Jantausch, MD, FAAP.

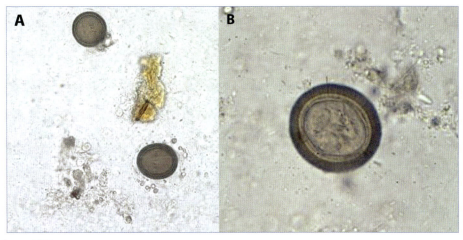

Image 141.7
A and B, The eggs of *Taenia solium* and *Taenia saginata* are indistinguishable from each other, as well as from other members of the *Taeniidae* family. The eggs measure 30–35 μm in diameter and are radially striated. The internal oncosphere contains 6 refractile hooks. *Taenia* species eggs in unstained wet mounts. Courtesy of Centers for Disease Control and Prevention.

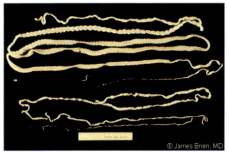

Image 141.8
Taenia saginata adult tapeworm. Copyright James Brien.

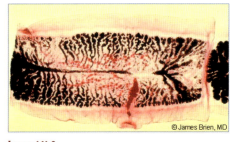

Image 141.9
Taenia saginata gravid proglottid. Courtesy of James Brien.

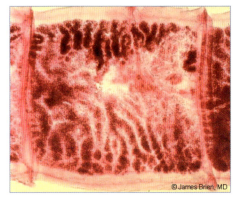

Image 141.10
Taenia solium gravid proglottid. Courtesy of James Brien.

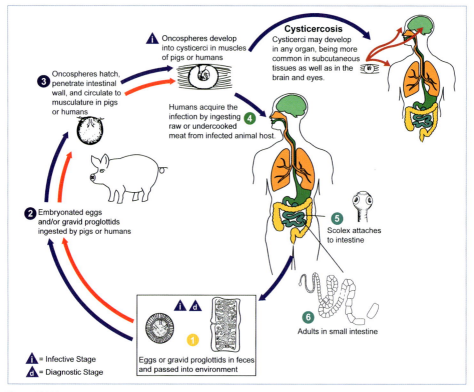

Image 141.11

Cysticercosis is an infection of humans and pigs with the larval stages of the parasitic cestode, *Taenia solium*. This infection is caused by ingestion of eggs shed in the feces of a human tapeworm carrier (1). Pigs and humans become infected by ingesting eggs or gravid proglottids (2). Humans are infected by ingestion of food contaminated with feces or by autoinfection. In the latter case, a human infected with adult *T solium* can ingest eggs produced by that tapeworm through fecal contamination or, possibly, from proglottids carried into the stomach by reverse peristalsis. Once eggs are ingested, oncospheres hatch in the intestine (3), invade the intestinal wall, and migrate to striated muscles, as well as the brain, liver, and other tissues, where they develop into cysticerci. In humans, cysts can cause serious sequelae if they localize in the brain, resulting in neurocysticercosis. The parasite life cycle is completed, resulting in human tapeworm infection when humans ingest undercooked pork containing cysticerci (4). Cysts evaginate and attach to the small intestine by their scolex (5). Adult tapeworms develop (up to 2–7 m in length and produce <1,000 proglottids, each with approximately 50,000 eggs) and reside in the small intestine for years (6). Courtesy of Centers for Disease Control and Prevention/Alexander J. da Silva, PhD/Melanie Moser.

CHAPTER 142

Other Tapeworm Infections
(Including Hydatid Disease)

Most tapeworm (cestode) infections are asymptomatic, but nausea, abdominal pain, and diarrhea have been observed in people who are heavily infected.

ETIOLOGIES, DIAGNOSIS, AND TREATMENT

Hymenolepis nana

This tapeworm, also known as the dwarf tapeworm because it is the smallest of the adult human tapeworms (about 3–4 cm long), can complete its entire life cycle within humans. Transmission occurs by ingestion of eggs present in feces of infected people resulting in human-to-human spread via the fecal-oral route or, rarely, by ingestion of infected arthropods (certain species of beetles and fleas) present in food. Autoinfection, in which eggs can hatch within the intestine and reinitiate the life cycle, leads to development of new worms and increases the worm burden. Most infections are asymptomatic. Young children may develop abdominal cramps, diarrhea, and irritability with heavy infection. Anal pruritus and difficulty sleeping mimic pinworm infections. Diagnosis is by identification of the characteristic eggs in stool. Praziquantel is the treatment of choice, with nitazoxanide as an alternative drug; niclosamide is another therapeutic option but is not available commercially in the United States. If infection persists, re-treatment with praziquantel is indicated.

Dipylidium caninum

This is the most common tapeworm of dogs and cats and has a wide geographic distribution. Children develop infection with *Dipylidium caninum* after inadvertently swallowing a dog or cat flea (the intermediate host). Most cases are asymptomatic and come to attention when motile proglottids are passed in stool. Some children have abdominal pain, diarrhea, and anal pruritus. Diagnosis is made by finding the characteristic eggs or motile proglottids in stool. Proglottids resemble rice kernels and may be mistaken for maggots or fly larvae. Their appearance can be mistaken for recurrent pinworm infections.

Infection is self-limiting in the human host and typically clears spontaneously by 6 weeks. Therapy with praziquantel is effective. Niclosamide is an alternative therapeutic option but is not available commercially in the United States.

Diphyllobothrium Species (and Related Species)

These are the largest tapeworms that can infect humans. Fish are intermediate hosts of the *Diphyllobothrium* tapeworm, also known as the fish tapeworm or broad tapeworm (because of the shape of the proglottids). Consumption of infected, raw, or undercooked fresh water (including trout and pike), salt water (at least 17 species including one shark), or anadromous (salmon) fish leads to infection. Within 3 to 6 weeks after ingestion, the adult tapeworm matures and begins to lay eggs. The most common symptom is noting passage of proglottids. Abdominal pain and diarrhea may occur. The worm may rarely cause mechanical obstruction of the bowel or gallbladder, diarrhea, or abdominal pain. Megaloblastic anemia secondary to vitamin B_{12} deficiency has been noted only with the species *Diphyllobothrium latum* (found in northern Europe and North America and also known as *Dibothriocephalus latus*). Diagnosis is made by recognition of the characteristic proglottids or eggs passed in stool. Therapy with praziquantel is effective; niclosamide is an alternative but is not available commercially in the United States.

Echinococcus granulosus and *Echinococcus multilocularis*

The larval forms of these tapeworms cause human echinococcosis. *Echinococcus granulosus* causes the disease cystic echinococcosis, also known as hydatid disease. The distribution of *E granulosus* is related to areas where sheep or cattle are raised and where dogs, the definitive host, are used for herding. Areas of high prevalence include parts of South America, East Africa, eastern Europe, the Middle East, the Mediterranean region, China, and central Asia. The parasite is also endemic in Australia and New Zealand. In the United States, small foci of endemic transmission have been reported historically in Arizona, California, New Mexico, and Utah, and a strain of the parasite has adapted to wolves, moose, and caribou in Alaska and Canada. Dogs, coyotes, wolves, dingoes, and jackals can become infected by swallowing protoscolices of the parasite within hydatid cysts in the organs of slaughtered sheep or other intermediate hosts. Dogs pass embryonated eggs in their feces, and humans become intermediate hosts by ingesting the viable parasite eggs. Humans then develop cysts in various organs, such as the liver, lungs, kidneys, and spleen. Cysts caused by larvae of *E granulosus* usually grow slowly (1 cm in diameter per year in the liver) and can eventually contain several liters of fluid. If a cyst ruptures, anaphylaxis and multiple secondary cysts from seeding of protoscolices can result. Clinical diagnosis is often difficult. A history of contact with dogs in an area with endemic infection is helpful. Cystic lesions can be demonstrated by radiography, ultrasonography, or computed tomography of various organs. Serological testing is helpful, but false-negative results occur. Treatment depends on ultrasonographic staging and may include antiparasitic therapy, PAIR (**p**uncture, **a**spiration, **i**njection of protoscolicidal agents, and **r**easpiration), surgical excision, or no treatment but with watchful waiting. Optimal therapy varies with the location, size, and stage of the parasite. Small cysts in the liver may respond to antiparasitic drugs alone. For larger, uncomplicated liver cysts, treatment of choice is PAIR. Contraindications to PAIR include communication of the cyst with the biliary tract (eg, bile staining after initial aspiration), superficial cysts, and heavily septated cysts. Surgical therapy is indicated for complicated cases and requires meticulous care to prevent spillage, including preparations such as soaking of surgical drapes in hypertonic saline. In general, the cyst should be removed intact, because leakage of contents is associated with a higher rate of complications, including anaphylactic reactions to cyst contents. Treatment with albendazole should generally be initiated days to weeks before surgery or PAIR and continued for several weeks to months thereafter. Degenerating cysts can be managed by watchful waiting with follow-up imaging studies. For lung lesions, small cysts often resolve with antiparasitic drugs alone. Larger cysts are best removed surgically.

Echinococcus multilocularis, the causative agent for alveolar echinococcosis, has definitive hosts (foxes, coyotes, and other wild canines) and intermediate hosts (rodents). Alveolar echinococcosis is characterized by invasive growth of the larvae in the liver (which may mimic neoplasm) with occasional metastatic spread, most worrisomely to the brain. Alveolar echinococcosis is limited to the Northern hemisphere and is usually diagnosed in people 50 years or older. The disease has been reported frequently from western China and is also endemic in central Europe. Diagnosis can be confirmed by imaging and serological testing. The preferred treatment is surgical removal of the entire larval mass followed by treatment with albendazole. In nonresectable cases, continuous treatment with albendazole has been associated with clinical improvement. Two other species, *Echinococcus vogeli* and *Echinococcus oligarthrus*, infect humans; they cause polycystic echinococcosis.

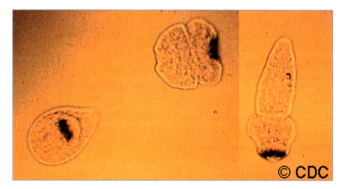

Image 142.1
Hydatid sand. Fluid aspirated from a hydatid cyst will show multiple protoscolices (size, approximately 100 μm), each of which has typical hooklets. The protoscolices, which are normally invaginated (left), evaginate (middle, then right) when put into saline.

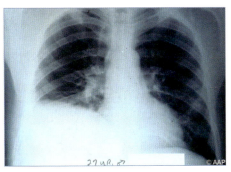

Image 142.2
Echinococcus cyst in the right lobe of the liver in a 27-year-old man. Note the striking elevation of the right hemidiaphragm. Courtesy of Edgar O. Ledbetter, MD, FAAP.

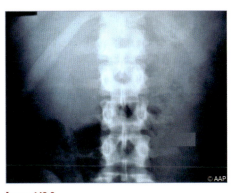

Image 142.3
Abdominal radiograph showing hepatic mass (echinococcus cyst). This is the same patient as in Image 142.2. Courtesy of Edgar O. Ledbetter, MD, FAAP.

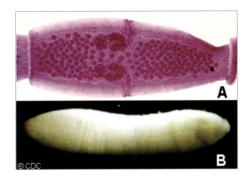

Image 142.4
A and B, Proglottids of *Dipylidium caninum*. Such proglottids (average mature size, 12 × 3 mm) have 2 genital pores, one in the middle of each lateral margin. Proglottids may be passed singly or in chains and, occasionally, may be found dangling from the anus. They are pumpkin seed–shaped when passed and often resemble rice grains when dried. Courtesy of Centers for Disease Control and Prevention.

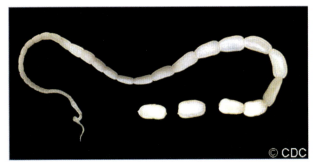

Image 142.5
Adult tapeworm, *Dipylidium caninum*. The scolex of the worm is very narrow, and the proglottids, as they mature, get larger.

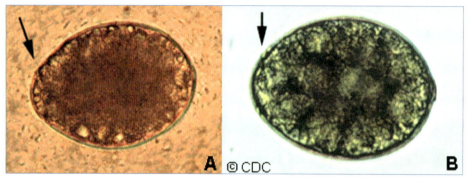

Image 142.6
Eggs of *Diphyllobothrium latum*. These eggs are oval or ellipsoidal, with an operculum (arrows) at one end that can be inconspicuous (A). At the opposite (abopercular) end is a small knob that can be barely discernible (B). The eggs are passed in the stool unembryonated. Size range, 58–76 μm × 40–51 μm. Courtesy of Centers for Disease Control and Prevention.

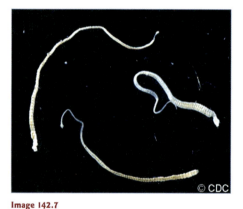

Image 142.7
Three adult *Hymenolepis nana* tapeworms. Each tapeworm (length, 15–40 mm) has a small, rounded scolex at the anterior end, and proglottids can be distinguished at the posterior, wider end. Courtesy of Centers for Disease Control and Prevention.

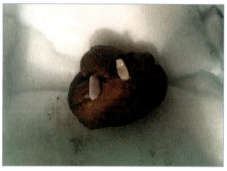

Image 142.8
Dog tapeworm, *Dipylidium caninum*, in the stool of a 7-month-old boy. Courtesy of Carol J. Baker, MD, FAAP.

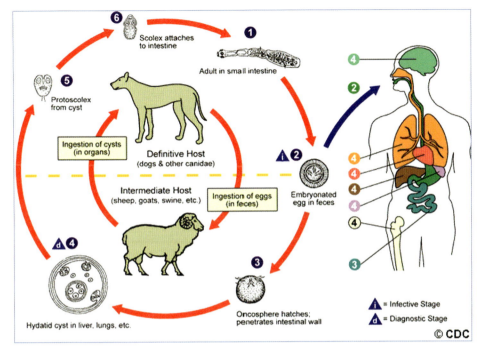

Image 142.9

The adult *Echinococcus granulosus* (3–6 mm long) (1) resides in the small bowel of the definitive hosts (dogs or other canids). Gravid proglottids release eggs (2) that are passed in the feces. After ingestion by a suitable intermediate host (under natural conditions, sheep, goat, swine, cattle, horses, or camel), the egg hatches in the small bowel and releases an oncosphere (3) that penetrates the intestinal wall and migrates through the circulatory system into various organs, especially the liver and lungs. In these organs, the oncosphere develops into a cyst (4) that enlarges gradually, producing protoscolices and daughter cysts that fill the cyst interior. The definitive host becomes infected by ingesting the cyst-containing organs of the infected intermediate host. After ingestion, the protoscolices (1) evaginate, attach to the intestinal mucosa (6), and develop into adult stages (1) in 32–80 days. The same life cycle occurs with *Echinococcus multilocularis* (1.2–3.7 mm long), with the following differences: the definitive hosts are foxes and, to a lesser extent, dogs, cats, coyotes, and wolves; the intermediate host are small rodents; and larval growth (in the liver) remains indefinitely in the proliferative stage, resulting in invasion of the surrounding tissues. With *Echinococcus vogeli* (up to 5.6 mm long), the definitive hosts are bush dogs and dogs, the intermediate hosts are rodents, and the larval stage (in the liver, lungs, and other organs) develops externally and internally, resulting in multiple vesicles. *Echinococcus oligarthrus* (up to 2.9 mm long) has a life cycle that involves wild felids as definitive hosts and rodents as intermediate hosts. Humans become infected by ingesting eggs (2), with resulting release of oncospheres (3) in the intestine and the development of cysts (4) in various organs.

CHAPTER 143
Tetanus
(Lockjaw)

CLINICAL MANIFESTATIONS

Tetanus is caused by neurotoxin produced by the anaerobic bacterium *Clostridium tetani* in a contaminated wound and can manifest in 3 overlapping clinical forms: generalized, local, and cephalic.

Generalized tetanus (lockjaw) is a neurological disease manifesting as trismus and severe muscular spasms, including risus sardonicus, which is a facial expression characterized by raised eyebrows and grinning distortion of the face resulting from spasm of facial muscles. Onset is gradual, occurring over 1 to 7 days, and symptoms progress to severe painful generalized muscle spasms, which are often aggravated by any external stimulus. Autonomic dysfunction, manifesting as diaphoresis, tachycardia, labile blood pressure, and arrhythmias, is often present. Other potential complications include fractures associated with muscle spasms, laryngospasm, pulmonary embolism, and aspiration pneumonia. Severe spasms persist for 1 week or longer and subside over several weeks in people who recover. Neonatal tetanus is a form of generalized tetanus occurring in newborns lacking protective passive immunity because their mothers are not immune. Early symptoms include inability to suck or breastfeed and excessive crying that progress to findings typical of generalized tetanus.

Local tetanus manifests as local muscle spasms in areas contiguous to a wound. **Cephalic tetanus** is the rarest form of tetanus and usually causes flaccid cranial nerve palsies, although trismus can occur. It is associated with infected wounds on the head and neck including, rarely, suppurative otitis media. Local and cephalic tetanus can precede generalized tetanus.

ETIOLOGY

C tetani is a spore-forming, obligate anaerobic, gram-positive bacillus. This organism is a wound contaminant that causes neither tissue destruction nor an inflammatory response. The vegetative form of *C tetani* produces a potent plasmid-encoded exotoxin (tetanospasmin). The heavy chain of tetanospasmin binds to the presynaptic motor neuron and facilitates entry of the light chain, a zinc-dependent protease, into the cytosol. As a result, gamma-aminobutyric acid- and glycine-containing vesicles are not released, and inhibitory action on motor and autonomic neurons is lost.

EPIDEMIOLOGY

Tetanus occurs worldwide and is more common in warmer climates and during warmer months, in part because of higher frequency of contaminated wounds associated with those locations and seasons. The organism, a normal inhabitant of soil and animal and human intestines, is ubiquitous in the environment, especially where contamination by excreta is common. Organisms multiply in wounds, recognized or unrecognized, and elaborate toxins in the presence of anaerobic conditions. Contaminated wounds, especially wounds with devitalized tissue and deep-puncture trauma, pose the greatest risk. Neonatal tetanus is common in many resource-limited countries where pregnant women are not immunized appropriately against tetanus and nonsterile umbilical cord–care practices are followed. Globally, activities are ongoing to eliminate maternal and neonatal tetanus by improving vaccination coverage among pregnant women and promoting safe delivery practices. During 2000–2018, 45 countries achieved maternal and neonatal tetanus elimination, reported cases of neonatal tetanus decreased 90%, and estimated deaths declined 85%.

Widespread active immunization against tetanus has modified the epidemiology of disease in the United States, where it is now rare. Tetanus is not transmissible from person to person.

In the United States, nearly all cases of tetanus occur in individuals who have never received a tetanus vaccine or who have not received their 10-year booster vaccine. At particular risk are people with immunocompromising conditions, people with diabetes mellitus, or people who use intravenous drugs.

The **incubation period** ranges from 3 to 21 days, with most cases occurring within 8 days. In general, the farther the injury site from the central nervous system, the longer the incubation period. Shorter incubation periods have been associated with more heavily contaminated wounds, more severe disease, and a worse prognosis. In neonatal tetanus, symptoms usually appear from 4 to 14 days after birth, averaging 7 days. Cephalic tetanus may have an **incubation period** as short as 1 to 2 days.

DIAGNOSTIC TESTS

The diagnosis of tetanus is made clinically by excluding other causes of tetanic spasms, such as hypocalcemic tetany, phenothiazine reaction, strychnine poisoning, and conversion disorder. Attempts to culture *C tetani* are associated with poor yield, and a negative culture does not rule out disease. A protective serum antitoxin concentration should not be used to exclude the diagnosis of tetanus.

TREATMENT

Human tetanus immune globulin (TIG) binds circulating unbound toxin and prevents further progression of disease, but it does not reverse the effects of already bound toxin. A single dose of human TIG is recommended for treatment. However, the optimal therapeutic dose has not been established. Most experts recommend 500 IU, which appears to be as effective as higher doses ranging from 3,000 to 6,000 IU and causes less discomfort. Available preparations must be administered intramuscularly. Infiltration of part of the dose locally around the wound is recommended, although the efficacy of this approach has not been proven. If TIG is unavailable (as in some countries), immune globulin intravenous can be used at a dose of 200 to 400 mg/kg. In some countries, equine tetanus antitoxin may be considered if TIG is unavailable and the patient is tested for sensitivity and desensitized as necessary.

- All wounds should be cleaned and debrided properly, especially if extensive necrosis is present. In neonatal tetanus, wide excision of the umbilical stump is not indicated.

- Supportive care and pharmacotherapy to control tetanic spasms and autonomic instability are of major importance.

- Oral (or intravenous) metronidazole is effective in decreasing the number of vegetative forms of *C tetani* and is the antimicrobial agent of choice. Parenteral penicillin G is an alternative treatment. Therapy for 7 to 10 days is recommended.

- Active immunization against tetanus should always be undertaken during convalescence from tetanus. Because of the extreme potency of tiny amounts of toxin, tetanus disease may not result in immunity.

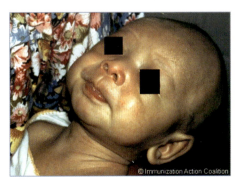

Image 143.1
This infant with tetanus has spasm of the facial muscles with trismus. Copyright Immunization Action Coalition.

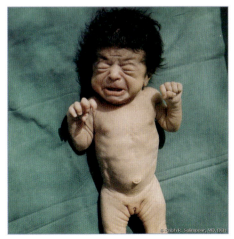

Image 143.2
Severe muscular spasms with trismus in a newborn who acquired neonatal tetanus from contamination of the umbilical stump. Courtesy of Ralph R. Salimpour, MD, DCH, FAAP.

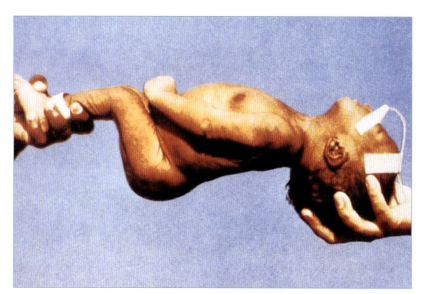

Image 143.3
This neonate is displaying a body rigidity produced by *Clostridium tetani* exotoxin. Neonatal tetanus may occur in neonates born without protective passive immunity, when the mother is not immune. It usually occurs through infection of the unhealed umbilical stump, particularly when the stump is cut with an unsterile instrument. Courtesy of Centers for Disease Control and Prevention.

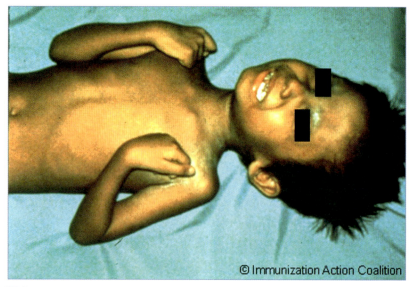

Image 143.4
A preschool-aged boy with tetanus with severe muscle contractions, generalized, caused by tetanospasmin action in the central nervous system. Courtesy of Immunization Action Coalition.

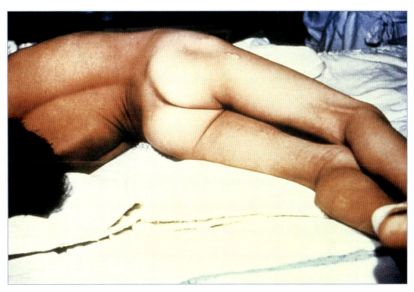

Image 143.5
This patient is displaying a bodily posture, known as opisthotonos, caused by *Clostridium tetani* exotoxin. Generalized tetanus, the most common type (about 80%), usually manifests with a descending pattern, starting with trismus or lockjaw, followed by stiffness of the neck, difficulty in swallowing, and rigidity of abdominal muscles. Courtesy of Centers for Disease Control and Prevention.

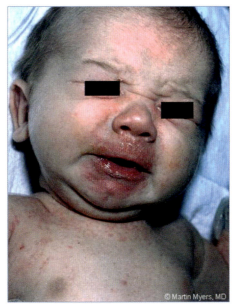

Image 143.6
The face of an infant with neonatal tetanus with risus sardonicus. Copyright Martin G. Myers, MD.

CHAPTER 144
Tinea Capitis
(Ringworm of the Scalp)

CLINICAL MANIFESTATIONS

Dermatophytic fungal infections of the scalp usually manifest with an area of localized alopecia and scaling but may include subtle findings of mild hair loss with faint scaling or a large hairless, boggy erythematous area (kerion). Other manifestations include a common "black dot" pattern reflecting stubs of broken-off hairs at the scalp surface; a less common "gray patch" pattern with prominent, well-demarcated alopecic areas of scaling and erythema; or a vesiculopustular pattern resembling bacterial folliculitis. Regional lymphadenopathy may be present.

The differential diagnosis for tinea capitis depends on the clinical manifestation. In the classic scaling manifestation, clinicians should consider atopic dermatitis, seborrheic dermatitis, and psoriasis. Alopecia should raise the possibility of trichotillomania and alopecia areata, although these disorders are not usually associated with scaling. When vesiculopustular in nature, lice infestation and bacterial infection should be considered. A boggy fluctuant mass likely represents a kerion, but primary (or secondary) bacterial infection can be considered. Although scalp scarring can result from tinea, particularly when a kerion suppurates, presence of scalp scarring should raise the possibility of an autoimmune disorder, such as discoid lupus.

An associated skin eruption, known as a dermatophytic or id reaction, can occur as a hypersensitivity reaction to the infecting fungus and can manifest as diffuse, pruritic, papular, vesicular, and/or eczematous lesions occurring at sites distant from the fungal infection. Id reactions may begin after starting therapy but do not represent a drug allergy.

Tinea capitis can occur in association with tinea corporis. Examination of the body (face, trunk, and limbs) should be performed, particularly in wrestlers and others engaged in contact sports.

ETIOLOGY

Tinea capitis develops when dermatophyte fungal elements invade the scalp hair follicle and shaft. The specific pathogen varies by geographic region and mode of transmission. The primary causes are fungi of the genus *Trichophyton*, including *Trichophyton tonsurans* and *Trichophyton violaceum*, as well as *Microsporum*, including *Microsporum canis* and *Microsporum audouinii*.

EPIDEMIOLOGY

Tinea capitis primarily occurs in prepubertal children but may occur in children of all ages and in adults. In the United States, *T tonsurans* is responsible for up to 95% of tinea capitis and is most common in Black school-aged children but occurs in all racial and ethnic groups. Infection with *T tonsurans* is contracted from direct contact with an infected individual, animal, or contaminated object such as a hat or brush. *T violaceum* is the dominant organism in eastern Europe and South Asia and is found more frequently in immigrant populations in the United States.

M canis is associated with less than 5% of infections in the United States but is distributed more evenly among racial and ethnic groups. *M canis* infection almost always results from contact with infected pets, particularly kittens or puppies. *M canis* outbreaks in schools and child care facilities have followed visits from infected animals.

The dermatophyte organism remains viable for prolonged periods on fomites (eg, brushes, combs, hats, towels), and rate of asymptomatic carriage and infected individuals among family members of index individuals is high. Asymptomatic carriers almost certainly serve as a reservoir of infection within families, schools, and communities.

Immunocompromised people and those with trisomy 21 syndrome have an increased susceptibility to dermatophyte infections.

The **incubation period** is unknown but is believed to be 1 to 3 weeks.

DIAGNOSTIC TESTS

The presence of alopecia, pruritus, scale, and posterior cervical lymphadenopathy makes the diagnosis of tinea capitis almost certain. Most clinicians choose to treat empirically. Diagnosis can be confirmed by dermatoscopic examination of the affected area, by microscopic evaluation of a potassium hydroxide wet mount of cutaneous scrapings, or by isolation in culture. Dermatoscopic evaluation of areas of alopecia with a lighted magnifier may show comma, corkscrew, or elbow-shaped hairs. Potassium hydroxide wet mount microscopy may be used to examine hairs and scale obtained by gentle scraping of a moistened area of the scalp with a blunt scalpel, hairbrush, toothbrush, or cotton swab or by plucking with tweezers. Visualization of spores filling the interior of the hair shaft indicates an endothrix infection caused by *T tonsurans*, whereas coating of the outside of the hair shaft with spores indicates an ectothrix infection, such as from *M canis*. In both forms, septate hyphae may be visualized in scrapings from the scalp surface. Fungal culture can establish a diagnosis, in conjunction with or instead of microscopy. If fungal culture is desired, a cotton-tipped applicator can be used to swab an affected area. The sample is transported to a mycology laboratory for processing; 2 to 4 weeks of incubation on Sabouraud dextrose agar are required for results. Polymerase chain reaction assay is very useful but expensive and not yet widely available. Under Wood lamp, tinea lesions are not fluorescent unless the etiologic agent is of the *Microsporum* genus, in which blue-green fluorescence is noted because it is an ectothrix infection.

TREATMENT

Tinea capitis always requires systemic medication, because the fungal infection is found within the hair follicles, where topical agents do not reach (Table 144.1). Optimal treatment of tinea capitis includes consideration of drug tolerability, availability, and cost.

Griseofulvin is approved for children 2 years and older, is available in either liquid or tablet form, can be administered daily, and should be taken with fatty foods. Experts generally use higher doses of griseofulvin than have been approved by the US Food and Drug Administration (FDA) or that were used in clinical trials. Laboratory testing of serum hepatic enzymes is not required if duration of griseofulvin therapy is less than 8 weeks (but treatment of >8 weeks is often required for resolution of infection). High-dose griseofulvin is considered standard of care for *M canis* infection.

Table 144.1
Recommended Systemic Therapy for Tinea Capitis

Drug	Dosage	Duration	FDA Approved for Tinea Capitis
Griseofulvin microsize (liquid, 125 mg/5 mL)	20–25 mg/kg/day (max 1 g/day)	≥6 wk; continue until clinically clear.	Yes (children ≥2 y)
Griseofulvin ultramicrosize (tablets of varying size)	10–15 mg/kg/day (max 750 mg/day)		
Terbinafine tablets (250 mg)[a]	4–6 mg/kg/day (max 250 mg) or 10–20 kg: 62.5 mg 20–40 kg: 125 mg >40 kg: 250 mg	*Trichophyton tonsurans*: 4–6 wk *Microsporum canis*: 8–12 wk	No
Terbinafine granules (125 mg and 187.5 mg)[b]	<25 kg: 125 mg 25–35 kg: 187.5 mg >35 kg: 250 mg	*T tonsurans*: 4–6 wk *M canis*: 8–12 wk	Yes (children ≥4 y)
Fluconazole (liquid, 10 mg/mL; tablet, 50 and 100 mg)	6 mg/kg/day (max 400 mg/day)	3–6 wk	No (but approved for pediatric patients ≥6 mo for other indications)
Itraconazole solution (10 mg/mL)	3 mg/kg/day (max 600 mg/day)	2–4 wk	No
Itraconazole capsule (100 mg)	5 mg/k/day (max 600 mg/day)		

FDA indicates US Food and Drug Administration; max, maximum.
[a] Some experts use "higher" dosing listed for terbinafine granules instead.
[b] Terbinafine granules have been discontinued in the United States.

Terbinafine granules are approved for use in children 4 years and older and can be split and mixed with foods such as pudding and peanut butter to increase palatability (although bioavailability does not depend on food). Advantages of terbinafine for *T tonsurans* infection include possibility of shorter duration of therapy and equal or superior effectiveness as compared with griseofulvin.

Fluconazole is the only oral antifungal agent approved by the FDA for children younger than 2 years, albeit not for tinea capitis. It had lower cure rates than other oral agents in a large randomized controlled trial. Accumulating evidence supports that itraconazole (currently not FDA approved for use in children or for tinea capitis) can be effective and safe for this disease. Liver function testing need not be assessed at baseline unless the child has preexisting liver disease or is receiving concomitant hepatotoxic medications. Monitoring while on therapy need not occur unless treatment duration is longer than 4 weeks or the child develops symptoms while receiving treatment.

Topical treatment, such as shampoos containing selenium sulfide, ketoconazole, or ciclopirox, may be useful as an adjunct to systemic therapy to decrease carriage of viable conidia for all forms of tinea capitis. Shampoo can be applied 2 to 3 times per week and left in place for 5 to 10 minutes. Treatments should continue for at least 2 weeks, and some experts recommend continuing topical treatments until clinical and mycological cure occurs.

Affected patients receiving therapy should be reassessed in 1 month for clinical response. Fungal cultures may be obtained to evaluate for a mycological response. Poor response may prompt re-treatment with a different agent, if adherence with the initial drug is confirmed.

Kerion is managed by systemic antifungal treatment as outlined previously. Removal of crusts with wet compresses is thought to decrease the risk of secondary bacterial infection. Combined antifungal and corticosteroid therapy (either oral or intralesional) has not been shown to be superior to antifungal therapy alone. Nonetheless, if the condition is unresponsive to traditional therapy, most experts will add systemic prednisone, 1 mg/kg/day for 2 weeks, to decrease likelihood of scarring. Treatment with antimicrobial agents is unnecessary unless secondary bacterial infection occurs.

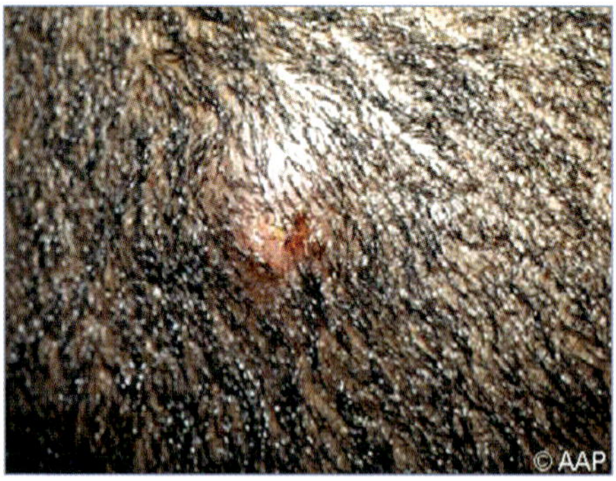

Image 144.1
Tinea capitis may cause hair loss. Remnants of infected hairs ("black dots") that have broken at the scalp line may be noted within areas of alopecia.

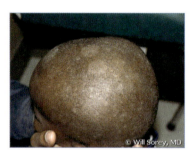

Image 144.2
A 4-year-old with multiple areas of alopecia and hair loss. This boy had a 3-week history of "dandruff." The scaling became more apparent following a shaved haircut. The barber saw areas of hair loss and was concerned about ringworm. He recommended medical evaluation. Physical examination indicated multiple patches of alopecia with a light appearance to the broken hair stubs in the areas of alopecia. Wood lamp examination indicated numerous patches of fluorescence. Culture result was positive for *Microsporum canis*. He was treated with griseofulvin for a total of 7 weeks. His hair has grown back without scarring. Follow-up examination result with Wood lamp was negative, although a sibling was noted to have a kerion and required treatment. Courtesy of Will Sorey, MD.

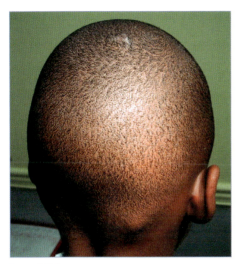

Image 144.3
An 8-year-old boy with a bald spot, hair loss, and enlarging posterior cervical lymph node for 2 weeks. The node was described as tender, not fluctuant, and without erythema of the overlying scalp. The area of hair loss was boggy and fluctuant. The patient responded well to treatment with griseofulvin. Copyright Stan Block, MD, FAAP.

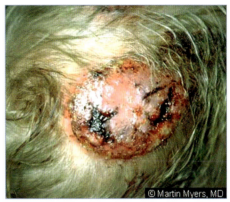

Image 144.4
A 2½-year-old boy with a kerion secondary to chronic, progressive tinea capitis. Copyright Martin G. Myers, MD.

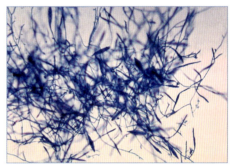

Image 144.6
Microsporum audouinii. Microsporum canis, a zoophilic dermatophyte often found in cats and dogs, is a common cause of tinea corporis and tinea capitis in humans. Other dermatophytes are included in the genera *Epidermophyton* and *Trichophyton*. Courtesy of Centers for Disease Control and Prevention.

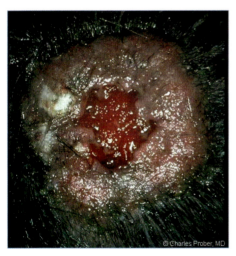

Image 144.5
Close-up of tinea capitis (*Microsporum audouinii*). Copyright Charles Prober, MD.

CHAPTER 145
Tinea Corporis
(Ringworm of the Body)

CLINICAL MANIFESTATIONS

Superficial tinea infections of the nonhairy (glabrous) skin, termed *tinea corporis*, involve the face, trunk, or limbs. Lesions are often ring shaped or circular (hence, the lay term "ringworm") and are sharply marginated. Involved skin is slightly erythematous and scaly, with color variations from red to brown. The classic eruption displays a scaly, vesicular, or pustular border (often serpiginous) with central clearing. Small confluent plaques or papules as well as multiple lesions can occur, particularly in wrestlers (tinea gladiatorum).

The differential diagnosis for tinea corporis includes pityriasis rosea (particularly the herald patch), candidiasis, psoriasis, other dermatitides (seborrheic, atopic, irritant, or allergic, generally caused by therapeutic agents applied to the area), pityriasis versicolor (tinea versicolor), nummular eczema, erythema annulare centrifugum, and erythrasma (an eruption of reddish-brown patches resulting from superficial bacterial skin infection caused by *Corynebacterium minutissimum*).

The typical appearance of the lesions is altered in patients who have been treated erroneously with topical corticosteroids. Known as tinea incognito, this altered appearance includes diminished erythema and absence of typical scaling borders. These patients can also develop Majocchi granuloma, a fungal invasion of the hair shaft and surrounding dermis, which causes a granulomatous dermal reaction that can extend into the surrounding subcutaneous fat. Majocchi granuloma can also occur without prior use of corticosteroids.

An associated dermatophytic or id reaction can be present as a hypersensitivity reaction to the infecting fungus, manifesting as diffuse, pruritic, papular, vesicular, or eczematous lesions, which can occur at sites distant from the fungal infection. Sometimes id reactions first appear following institution of therapy, but they do not represent a drug allergy.

Skin lesions can occur as grouped papules or pustules without erythema or scaling in patients with diminished T-lymphocyte function (eg, HIV infection).

Tinea corporis can occur in association with tinea capitis. The scalp should be examined, particularly in wrestlers and others engaged in contact sports.

ETIOLOGY

Tinea corporis develops when dermatophytic fungi invade the outer skin layers at the affected body region. Primary etiologic agents are *Trichophyton* species, especially *Trichophyton tonsurans, Trichophyton rubrum,* and *Trichophyton mentagrophytes; Microsporum* species, especially *Microsporum canis;* and *Epidermophyton floccosum.*

EPIDEMIOLOGY

Causative fungi occur worldwide and are transmissible by direct contact with infected humans, animals, soil, or fomites (eg, brushes, combs, hats, towels), where organisms can remain viable for prolonged periods.

Immunocompromised people have an increased susceptibility to dermatophyte infections.

The **incubation period** is believed to be 1 to 3 weeks but can be shorter.

DIAGNOSTIC TESTS

Tinea corporis is diagnosed by clinical manifestations and can be confirmed by microscopic examination of a potassium hydroxide wet mount of skin scrapings or fungal culture. Skin scrapings, ideally at the scaly edges of lesions for best recovery of organisms, are obtained by gentle scraping of a moistened area with a glass coverslip, blunt scalpel, toothbrush, or brush or by plucking with tweezers. If fungal culture is desired, a cotton-tipped applicator can be used to swab an affected area gently. The sample is transported to a mycology laboratory for processing; 2 to 4 weeks of incubation on Sabouraud dextrose agar are required for results. Polymerase chain reaction of specimens is available but expensive and is not generally necessary. Under Wood lamp, tinea is not fluorescent unless the etiologic agent is of the genus *Microsporum,* in which case a blue-green fluorescence can be seen because it is an ectothrix infection.

TREATMENT

A myriad of topical antifungal options are available for treatment and should be applied on the lesions and 1 to 2 cm beyond the borders. Some topical agents are approved by the US Food and Drug Administration only for certain lesion locations and age-groups and with applications specified as once or twice daily. Any of the following products (applied twice daily) are reasonable first-line therapies if appropriate for age: miconazole, clotrimazole, tolnaftate, or ciclopirox. Any of the following products can also be used (applied once daily) if appropriate for age: ketoconazole, terbinafine, econazole, naftifine, luliconazole, or butenafine. Oxiconazole and sulconazole can be used (once or twice daily) if appropriate for age.

Although clinical resolution may be evident within 2 weeks of therapy, continuing therapy for another 2 to 4 weeks is generally recommended. If significant clinical improvement is not observed after 2 weeks of treatment, an alternative diagnosis and/or systemic therapy should be considered. Topical preparations of antifungal medication combined with a corticosteroid should not be used because of inferior effectiveness, the possibility of leading to Majocchi granuloma, and increase in the rate of relapse, higher cost, and potential for adverse corticosteroid effects.

If lesions are extensive or unresponsive to topical therapy, griseofulvin (for children ≥2 years) or terbinafine (for children ≥4 years; oral formulation not approved for this indication but approved for tinea capitis [granules] and onychomycosis in adults [tablets]) may be administered orally for 4 to 6 weeks. Oral fluconazole is approved for other indications in infants and children 6 months and older. If a Majocchi granuloma is present, oral antifungal therapy is recommended, because topical therapy is unlikely to penetrate adequately to eradicate infection.

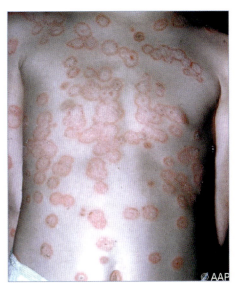

Image 145.1
Generalized tinea corporis in a 5-year-old girl.

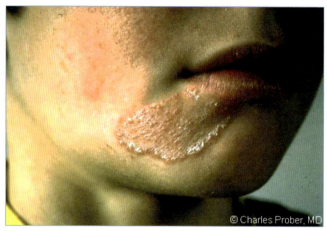

Image 145.2
Tinea corporis of the face. These annular erythematous lesions have a scaly center. Copyright Charles Prober, MD.

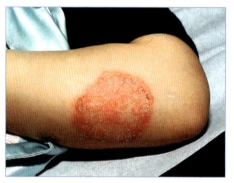

Image 145.3
Tinea corporis of the arm. This 6-year-old girl had an enlarging skin lesion that had been present for 1 week. Copyright Larry I. Corman.

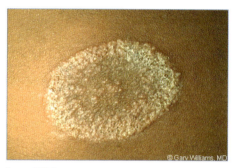

Image 145.4
Tinea corporis lesion in a 10-year-old girl. Copyright Gary Williams, MD.

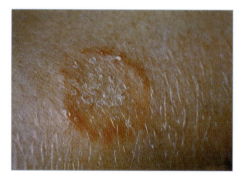

Image 145.5
This patient presented with ringworm on the arm, or tinea corporis, caused by *Trichophyton* mentagrophytes. The genus *Trichophyton* inhabits the soil, humans, or animals and is one of the leading causes of hair, skin, and nail infections, or dermatophytosis, in humans. Courtesy of Centers for Disease Control and Prevention.

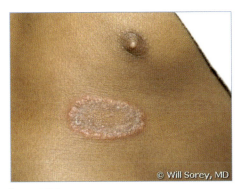

Image 145.6
A 16-month-old with a pruritic patch on his trunk. It had gotten larger over 3 days. He had a cat with dandruff and hair loss. The cat slept on his bed during the sunny part of the day. The child was treated with antifungal cream. The cat was evaluated by a veterinarian and cultured positive for *Microsporum canis*. This represents tinea corporis, commonly known as ringworm. Courtesy of Will Sorey, MD.

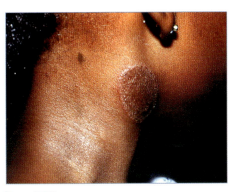

Image 145.8
Tinea corporis involving the neck of a 10-year-old girl with an enlarging lesion that had been present for 9 days. Courtesy of Larry I. Corman.

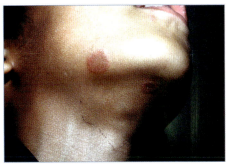

Image 145.7
Tinea corporis of the chin on a 6-year-old girl with enlarging lesions. The patient was successfully treated with clotrimazole. Copyright Larry I. Corman.

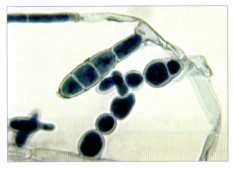

Image 145.9
This photomicrograph reveals a number of macroconidia of the dermatophytic fungus *Epidermophyton floccosum*, which is known to be a cause of dermatophytosis leading to tinea corporis (ringworm), tinea cruris (jock itch), tinea pedis (athlete's foot), and onychomycosis or tinea unguium, a fungal infection of the nail bed. Courtesy of Centers for Disease Control and Prevention.

CHAPTER 146
Tinea Cruris
(Jock Itch)

CLINICAL MANIFESTATIONS

Tinea cruris is a common superficial fungal disorder of the groin, pubic/perianal area, and upper thighs. It is more common in male adults and adolescents and uncommon in prepubertal children. The lesions are often ring shaped or circular (hence, the lay term "ringworm"), are sharply marginated, and can be intensely pruritic (jock itch). The involved skin is slightly erythematous and scaly, with color variations from red to brown. Lesions can display a scaly, vesicular, or pustular border (often serpiginous) with central clearing. Maceration may also develop. The disorder usually spares the scrotum unless candidiasis is also present. The margins can be subtle in chronic infections, and lichenification may be present.

The differential diagnosis for tinea cruris includes intertrigo, candidiasis, psoriasis, other dermatitides (seborrheic, atopic, irritant, or allergic, generally caused by therapeutic agents applied to the area), pityriasis versicolor (tinea versicolor), nummular eczema, erythema annulare centrifugum, and erythrasma (an eruption of reddish-brown patches resulting from superficial bacterial skin infection caused by *Corynebacterium minutissimum*).

An altered appearance known as tinea incognito can occur in patients who have been treated erroneously with topical corticosteroids, which includes diminished erythema and absence of typical scaling borders. Such patients can also develop Majocchi granuloma when fungi invade the hair shaft and surrounding dermis, causing a granulomatous dermal reaction that can extend into the surrounding subcutaneous fat. Majocchi granuloma can also occur without prior use of topical corticosteroid.

An associated skin eruption, known as a dermatophytic or id reaction, can occur as a hypersensitivity reaction to the infecting fungus and manifests as diffuse, pruritic, papular, vesicular, or eczematous lesions at sites distant from the fungal infection. An id reaction can first occur following institution of therapy but does not represent a drug allergy.

Concomitant tinea pedis, tinea unguium, and tinea corporis have been reported in patients with tinea cruris.

ETIOLOGY

Tinea cruris develops when dermatophyte fungi invade the outer skin layers of the affected body region. The fungi *Epidermophyton floccosum*, *Trichophyton rubrum*, and *Trichophyton mentagrophytes* are the most common causes. *Trichophyton tonsurans*, *Trichophyton verrucosum*, and *Trichophyton interdigitale* have also been identified as causes.

EPIDEMIOLOGY

Tinea cruris occurs predominantly in adolescent and adult males and is acquired principally through indirect contact with desquamated epithelium or hair. Direct person-to-person transmission also occurs. Moisture, close-fitting garments, noncotton underwear, friction, and obesity are predisposing factors. Recurrence is common.

Immunocompromised patients have increased susceptibility to dermatophyte infections. In patients with diminished T-lymphocyte function (eg, HIV infection), skin lesions can appear as grouped papules or pustules unaccompanied by scaling or erythema.

The **incubation period** is unknown but is thought to be approximately 1 to 3 weeks.

DIAGNOSTIC TESTS

Confirmatory diagnostic modalities for tinea cruris are similar to those for tinea corporis.

TREATMENT

Treatment is similar to that of tinea corporis. Treatment of concurrent onychomycosis (tinea unguium) and tinea pedis may reduce recurrence. Recurrence is common, particularly if predisposing factors such as moisture and friction are not minimized. Loose-fitting clothing and use of antifungal powders, such as tolnaftate and miconazole, should aid in recovery and prevent recurrence.

Oral terbinafine, itraconazole, and fluconazole are options. Griseofulvin, administered orally for 4 to 6 weeks, may be effective if lesions are unresponsive to topical therapy. Oral antifungal therapy is recommended if a Majocchi granuloma (deep folliculitis) is present. Dermatophyte infections in other locations, if present, should be treated concurrently.

Topical steroids are not recommended, even in formulations coupled with antifungal agents, as these may exacerbate the infection.

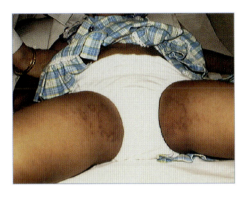

Image 146.1
Symmetrical, confluent, annular, scaly red, and hyperpigmented plaques. This 10-year-old girl developed a chronic itchy eruption on the groin that spread to the anterior thighs. A potassium hydroxide preparation showed hyphae, and she was treated successfully with topical antifungal cream.

CHAPTER 147

Tinea Pedis and Tinea Unguium (Onychomycosis)
(Athlete's Foot, Ringworm of the Feet)

CLINICAL MANIFESTATIONS

Tinea pedis can have a variety of clinical manifestations in children. Lesions can involve all areas of the foot but are usually patchy in distribution, with a predisposition to cause fissures, macerated areas, and scaling between toes, particularly in the third and fourth interdigital spaces. A pruritic, fine scaly, or vesiculopustular eruption is most common. "Moccasin foot" exhibits confluent, hyperkeratotic, dry scaling of the soles. Recurrence of tinea pedis is common, and it can be a chronic infection. Toenails can be infected (onychomycosis or tinea unguium) and become distorted, discolored, and thickened with accumulation of subungual debris. A superficial white form of foot and toenail fungal infection can occur in children. Toenails may be the source for recurrent tinea pedis.

Tinea pedis must be differentiated from dyshidrotic eczema, atopic dermatitis, contact dermatitis, juvenile plantar dermatosis, palmoplantar keratoderma, and erythrasma (reddish-brown patches that can affect the feet and axillae and that result from superficial bacterial skin infection caused by *Corynebacterium minutissimum*).

An associated skin eruption, known as a dermatophytic or id reaction, can occur as a hypersensitivity reaction to the infecting fungus and manifests as diffuse, pruritic, papular, vesicular, or eczematous lesions at sites distant from the fungal infection. An id reaction can occur first following institution of therapy but does not represent a drug allergy.

Skin lesions may appear as grouped papules or pustules unaccompanied by erythema or scaling in patients with diminished T-lymphocyte function (eg, HIV infection).

The differential diagnosis of tinea unguium includes trauma (particularly if only 1 nail is involved), psoriasis, twenty-nail dystrophy (trachyonychia), and, occasionally, subungual exostosis if only 1 nail is involved.

ETIOLOGY

Tinea pedis and unguium develop when dermatophytic fungi invade the skin layers and nails of the affected body region. The fungi *Trichophyton rubrum*, *Trichophyton mentagrophytes*, and *Epidermophyton floccosum* are the most common causes of tinea pedis.

EPIDEMIOLOGY

Tinea pedis is a common infection worldwide in adolescents and adults but is less common in young children. Fungi are acquired by contact with infected skin scales or organisms present in damp areas, such as swimming pools, locker rooms, and showers. Tinea pedis may spread among family members in the household; this may represent enhanced genetic susceptibility as well as increased exposure to the organism. The incidence of onychomycosis, which is more common in toenails, increases with age, with worldwide prevalence estimated to be from 0.1% to 0.87%. The increased use of occlusive footwear earlier in childhood and exposure to high-risk areas (eg, swimming pools, gyms) earlier in life may be associated with an increase of tinea pedis in children. Childhood onychomycosis is associated with a history of tinea pedis, a history of family member infection, increased number of siblings, and male sex.

Immunocompromised people and those with trisomy 21 syndrome have increased susceptibility to dermatophyte infections.

The **incubation period** is unknown, although it is believed to be approximately 1 to 3 weeks.

DIAGNOSTIC TESTS

Confirmatory diagnostic tests for tinea pedis are similar to those for tinea corporis. Fungal infection of the nail (tinea unguium or onychomycosis) can be verified by direct microscopic examination with potassium hydroxide, fungal culture of desquamated subungual material, or fungal stain of nail clippings fixed in formalin.

TREATMENT

A myriad of topical options are available for treatment of tinea pedis. Therapy duration of 2 weeks is usually sufficient for milder cases of tinea pedis in children. Acute vesicular lesions can be treated with intermittent use of open wet compresses (eg, with Burow solution, diluted 1:80). Tinea pedis that is severe, chronic, or refractory to topical treatment can be treated with oral therapy similar to that for tinea capitis.

Recurrence of tinea pedis is prevented by proper foot hygiene of the patient, which includes keeping the feet dry and cool, cleaning them gently, drying between the toes, using absorbent antifungal foot powder, exposing affected areas to air frequently, and avoiding occlusive footwear, nylon socks, and other fabrics that interfere with dissipation of moisture. Protective footwear should be worn in common areas such as pools, gyms, and other public facilities.

Topical antifungal lacquers and solutions that are effective for distal toenail infections that do not involve the nail matrix are now available. Despite lower cure rates, topical agents are preferred because of substantially lower adverse effects, lack of drug-drug interactions, and avoidance of need for laboratory test monitoring for toxicity. Topical ciclopirox, 8%, lacquer, can be used in patients 12 years and older and can be applied to affected toenail(s) twice daily for up to 48 weeks. Efinaconazole, 10%, solution and tavaborole, 5%, solution can be used for tinea unguium in adults; both have higher cure rates for adults than ciclopirox. Topical therapies appear to show a higher cure rate for children than for adults, possibly because of thinner nail plates and faster nail growth rate of children.

Studies in adults have demonstrated that the best cure rates for onychomycosis (tinea unguium) are with oral terbinafine or itraconazole. Although oral therapies are more likely to lead to cure, they also require laboratory monitoring and can induce drug-drug interactions. The duration of therapy is the same as for adults (6 weeks for fingernail infection, 12 weeks for toenail infection). Pediatric dosing of oral itraconazole is not established for superficial mycoses.

Factors that influence choice of therapy include severity of infection, results of fungal culture or potassium hydroxide preparation (if performed), prior treatments, concomitant drug therapy for other illnesses, patient preference, and cost. Topical and systemic therapy may be used concurrently to increase therapeutic response. Cure rates following oral or combined therapy approach 80% for children. Mechanical and chemical debridement of the nail, by using urea, 40%, ointment daily under occlusion for 10 days to soften the nail, should be performed when cases are refractory or when severe thickening of the nail is likely to decrease absorption and response to therapy.

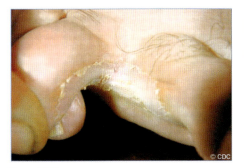

Image 147.1
This patient presented with ringworm of the feet (specifically the toes), or tinea pedis, which is also known as athlete's foot. Tinea pedis is a fungal infection of the feet, principally involving the toe webs and soles. Athlete's foot can be caused by the fungi *Epidermophyton floccosum* or by numerous members of the *Trichophyton* genus. Courtesy of Centers for Disease Control and Prevention.

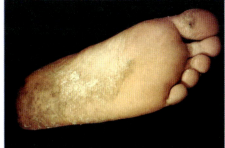

Image 147.2
This patient presented with ringworm of the foot (tinea pedis) caused by the dermatophytic fungus *Trichophyton rubrum*. Individuals who practice generally poor hygiene, wear enclosed footwear such as tennis shoes, experience prolonged wetting of the skin (ie, sweating during exercise), and experience minor skin or nail injuries are more prone to experience tinea infections. Courtesy of Centers for Disease Control and Prevention.

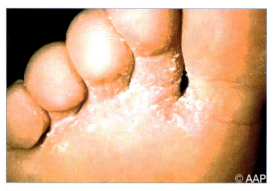

Image 147.3
Tinea pedis and tinea unguium.

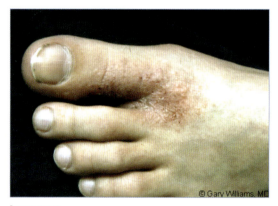

Image 147.4
Tinea pedis and tinea unguium. Copyright Gary Williams, MD.

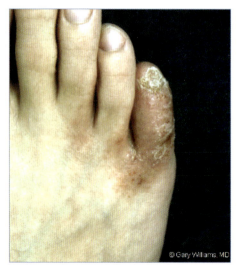

Image 147.5
Tinea pedis and tinea unguium infection. This is the same patient as in Image 147.4. Copyright Gary Williams, MD.

CHAPTER 148

Toxocariasis

CLINICAL MANIFESTATIONS

Clinical disease is caused by parasitic nematode larval migration through tissues. Signs and symptoms differ depending on the affected organ and host inflammatory response. Toxocariasis can be of the following types: covert toxocariasis, visceral larval migrans, neurotoxocariasis, or ocular larval migrans. Most infected children are asymptomatic. Covert disease most often manifests with simple, persistent eosinophilia and may be attributed to the continuation of the migratory phase, which may last for many years. Symptoms of visceral toxocariasis include fever, cough, wheezing, abdominal pain, and malaise and may uncommonly include myocarditis and rash. Neurotoxocariasis may manifest with an eosinophilic meningoencephalitis, space-occupying lesions, myelitis, or cerebral vasculitis and may manifest with seizures. Laboratory abnormalities include leukocytosis, eosinophilia, and hypergammaglobulinemia. Ocular invasion (resulting in uveitis, endophthalmitis, or retinal granulomas) most often manifests as unilateral vision loss, often without other systemic signs of infection.

ETIOLOGY

Toxocariasis is caused by *Toxocara* species, which are nematode parasites (roundworms) of dogs and cats (especially puppies or kittens), specifically *Toxocara canis* and *Toxocara cati,* respectively; most cases are caused by *T canis.*

EPIDEMIOLOGY

A nationally representative survey revealed that 5% of the US population 6 years and older to have serological evidence of *Toxocara* infection. Visceral toxocariasis typically occurs in children 2 to 7 years of age but can occur in older children and adults. Ocular toxocariasis usually occurs in older children and adolescents, and most reported cases of ocular toxocariasis occur in patients living in southern states. Infection is more likely in people who own dogs and people who live in poverty and is more prevalent in hot and humid regions where eggs remain viable in soil. Humans are infected by ingestion of soil containing infective eggs of the parasite. Eggs may be found wherever dogs and cats defecate, often in sandboxes and on playgrounds. Eggs become infective after 2 to 4 weeks in the environment and may persist in the long term in the soil.

The **incubation period** cannot be determined accurately.

DIAGNOSTIC TESTS

Laboratory findings include marked leukocytosis with eosinophilia and, occasionally, anemia and hypergammaglobulinemia. Patients with visceral disease frequently have increased titers of isohemagglutinin to the A and B blood group antigens. An enzyme-linked immunosorbent assay for *Toxocara* antibodies in serum or vitreous fluid is available through the Centers for Disease Control and Prevention and is preferred over testing by commercial laboratories. A positive antibody test result does not distinguish between past and current infection, and the test is less sensitive for diagnosis of ocular toxocariasis. For visceral disease, imaging of the liver by using ultrasonography, computed tomography, or magnetic resonance imaging may reveal diffuse nodular lesions measuring less than 2 cm in diameter. Microscopic identification of larvae in a liver biopsy specimen is diagnostic, but this test is not sensitive or specific and therefore rarely indicated.

TREATMENT

Albendazole is recommended for treatment of visceral and ocular toxocariasis. Mebendazole is an alternative. In severe cases with myocarditis or involvement of the central nervous system, corticosteroid therapy administered concurrently with albendazole is warranted. Control of inflammation of the eye with oral or topical corticosteroids may be warranted; surgical therapy may be helpful in complicated cases.

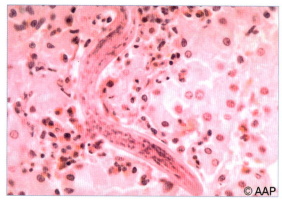

Image 148.1
Visceral toxocariasis (previously visceral larval migrans) with *Toxocara canis* larvae on liver biopsy.

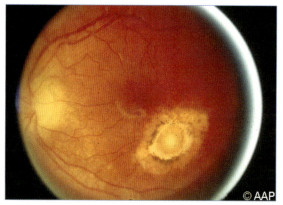

Image 148.2
Toxocara canis. Fundus damage from larval invasion. Courtesy of Hugh Moffet, MD.

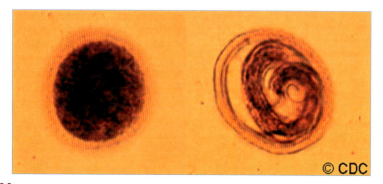

Image 148.3
Eggs of *Toxocara canis*. These eggs are passed in dog feces, especially puppy feces. Humans do not produce or excrete eggs; therefore, eggs are not a diagnostic finding in human toxocariasis. The egg to the left is fertilized but not yet embryonated, whereas the egg to the right contains a well-developed larva. The latter egg would be infective if ingested by a human (frequently, a child).

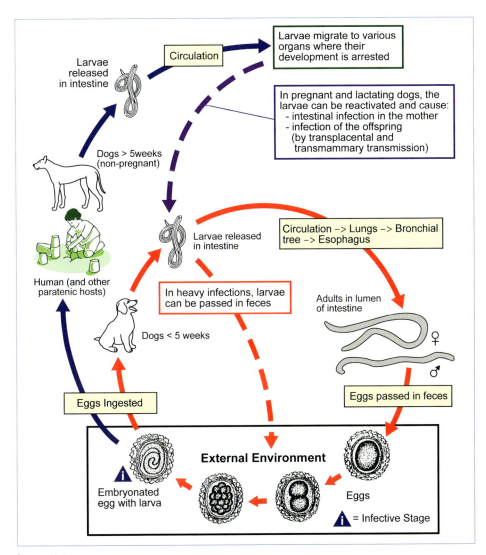

Image 148.4

Toxocara canis accomplishes its life cycle in dogs, with humans acquiring the infection as unintentional hosts. Following ingestion by dogs, the infective eggs yield larvae that penetrate the gut wall and migrate into various tissues, where they encyst if the dog is >5 weeks of age. In younger dogs, the larvae migrate through the lungs, bronchial tree, and esophagus; adult worms develop and oviposit in the small intestine. In the older dogs, the encysted stages are reactivated during pregnancy and infect by the transplacental and transmammary routes of the puppies, whose small intestine adult worms become established. Thus, infective eggs are excreted by lactating adult female dogs and puppies. Humans are paratenic hosts who become infected by ingesting infective eggs in contaminated soil. After ingestion, the eggs yield larvae that penetrate the intestinal wall and are carried by the circulation to a wide variety of tissues (ie, liver, heart, lungs, brain, muscle, eyes). Although the larvae do not undergo any further development in these sites, they can cause severe local reactions that are the basis of toxocariasis. Courtesy of Centers for Disease Control and Prevention/Alexander J. da Silva, PhD/Melanie Moser.

CHAPTER 149
Toxoplasma gondii Infections
(Toxoplasmosis)

CLINICAL MANIFESTATIONS

Up to 50% of patients with acute *Toxoplasma* infection are asymptomatic. When present, common signs and symptoms of acute *Toxoplasma* infection can include flulike symptoms, lymphadenopathy with atypical lymphocytosis, fever, myalgia, arthralgia, sweats, chills, fatigue, headache, chorioretinitis, hepatic dysfunction, pneumonitis, meningoencephalitis, myocarditis, myositis, acute disseminated encephalomyelitis, and myelitis. Reactivation of chronic *Toxoplasma* infection in immunocompromised patients may result in fever, pneumonia, septic shock, brain abscesses, diffuse encephalitis without brain-space occupying lesions, seizures, chorioretinitis, myocarditis, myelitis, and polymyositis.

Congenital Infection

Mothers are not screened routinely for toxoplasmosis during pregnancy in the United States. Clinically apparent signs and symptoms of congenital toxoplasmosis are found on routine physical examination in a minority of infected infants at birth, but more specific testing (of cerebrospinal fluid [CSF], dilated eye examination, or central nervous system imaging) can reveal evidence of infection. Visual or hearing impairment, learning disabilities, or severe developmental delay become apparent later in life in a large proportion of congenitally infected infants. Chorioretinitis occurs in approximately 70% of congenitally infected infants whose mothers were not treated during pregnancy and in up to 25% of those whose mothers were treated.

Clinical illness is more likely to be severe when infection occurs in the first trimester and is not treated during gestation. The classic triad of chorioretinitis, cerebral calcifications, and hydrocephalus is highly suggestive of congenital toxoplasmosis. Additional signs at birth include microcephaly, seizures, hearing loss, strabismus, petechial rash, jaundice, generalized lymphadenopathy, hepatomegaly, splenomegaly, pneumonia, thrombocytopenia, and anemia. Meningoencephalitis may be associated with CSF abnormalities including high protein concentrations, hypoglycorrhachia, and eosinophilia. Some severely affected fetuses/neonates with disseminated congenital toxoplasmosis die in utero or within a few days of birth. Cerebral calcifications can be demonstrated by plain radiography, ultrasonography, computed tomography (CT), or magnetic resonance imaging (MRI) of the head. CT is the radiological technique of choice because it is the most sensitive for calcifications and can reveal brain abnormalities when ultrasonographic study findings are normal.

Postnatally Acquired Primary Infection

Postnatally acquired *Toxoplasma gondii* infections in immunocompetent patients are usually asymptomatic. When symptoms develop, they may be nonspecific and can include malaise, fever, headache, sore throat, arthralgia, and myalgia. Lymphadenopathy, frequently cervical, is the most common sign. Patients occasionally have a mononucleosis-like illness associated with a maculopapular rash, hepatosplenomegaly, hepatic dysfunction, and atypical lymphocytosis. The clinical course is usually benign and self-limited.

In a subset of patients, primary infection may be severe and/or persistent disease including fever, myocarditis, pericarditis, myositis, hepatitis, pneumonia, encephalitis with and without brain abscesses, and skin lesions (maculopapular rash). These severe syndromes are especially common in patients who acquired primary *T gondii* infections with high parasite loads and/or in areas where atypical, more virulent strains are present (eg, Mexico, French Guiana, Brazil, and Colombia).

Chorioretinitis

Toxoplasmic chorioretinitis can occur (a) with congenital infection; (b) from a postnatally acquired acute infection; and (c) from reactivation of a congenital or postnatally acquired infection. Acute onset of blurred vision, eye pain, decreased visual acuity, floaters, scotoma, photophobia, epiphora, nystagmus, or strabismus is noted. Ocular findings in toxoplasmic eye disease include white focal retinitis with overlying vitreous inflammation ("headlight in the fog"), nearby prior pigmented retinochoroidal scar, retinal vasculitis, vitreous inflammation, cataracts, iridocyclitis and stellate keratic precipitates (accompanying chorioretinitis), and elevated intraocular pressure. Complications can include retinal detachment, cystoid macular edema, optic atrophy, chronic iridocyclitis, cataract formation, secondary glaucoma, or band keratopathy.

Reactivation of Chronic Infection in Immunocompromised Patients

Reactivation of latent infection may occur in immunosuppressed patients. Reactivation can result in encephalitis, brain abscesses, seizures, pneumonia, myocarditis, hepatitis, skin lesions, posterior uveitis or panuveitis with chorioretinitis, fever of unknown origin, and disseminated disease and death. Toxoplasmic encephalitis (TE) can manifest as a single brain lesion or multiple brain lesions on MRI or as a diffuse form with a rapidly progressive clinical course leading to death despite apparently normal brain imaging findings. MRI is superior to CT for the diagnosis of TE. In patients with AIDS, TE is the most common cause of space-occupying brain lesions and typically manifests with acute to subacute neurological or psychiatric symptoms and multiple ring-enhancing brain lesions. In these patients, a clear improvement in the neurological examination within 7 to 10 days of beginning empirical anti-*Toxoplasma* therapy is considered diagnostic of TE. Lack of radiographic response 2 weeks after initiation of anti-*Toxoplasma* therapy is an indication to consider alternative diagnoses. Non-AIDS patients with multiple brain lesions should not be treated empirically for only toxoplasmosis, and other etiologies should be entertained for diagnostic and empirical treatment purposes.

Seropositive hematopoietic stem cell transplant and solid organ transplant recipients have risk for reactivation of latent infection in the absence of appropriate prophylaxis. Toxoplasmosis in this setting manifests as pneumonia, unexplained fever or seizures, myocarditis, hepatitis, hepatosplenomegaly, lymphadenopathy, skin lesions, or brain abscesses and diffuse encephalitis. Transplant donors and recipients should be screened pretransplant for *Toxoplasma* infection, including heart, other solid organ, and hematopoietic stem cell/bone marrow donors.

ETIOLOGY

T gondii is a protozoan and obligate intracellular parasite. The infectious forms include tachyzoites, tissue cysts containing bradyzoites, and oocysts containing sporozoites. The tachyzoite and the corresponding host immune reaction are responsible for observed symptoms. The tissue cyst is responsible for latent infection and is usually present in brain, eye, cardiac tissue, and skeletal muscle.

EPIDEMIOLOGY

Seroprevalence of *T gondii* infection varies by geographic locale and socioeconomic strata of the population. The overall *T gondii* seropositivity rate in the United States among people older than 6 years is 11.1% and among women 15 to 44 years of age is 7.5%.

Congenital transmission occurs in most cases because of acute primary maternal infection acquired during pregnancy or within 3 months before conception. In utero infection can rarely result from reactivated parasitemia in a latently infected immunocompromised woman in the absence of prophylaxis. Rarely, congenital toxoplasmosis is acquired from an immunocompetent pregnant women reinfected with a different *T gondii* strain. Incidence of acute primary *T gondii* infection during pregnancy in the United States is estimated to be 0.2 to 1.1 per 1,000 pregnant women.

The **incubation period** of postnatally acquired infection is approximately 7 days, with a range of 4 to 21 days. Parasites can be detected in the blood for up to 2 weeks after acute infection; prolonged parasitemia has also been reported.

DIAGNOSTIC TESTS

Serological tests are the primary means of diagnosis. *Toxoplasma* immunoglobulin G (IgG) and immunoglobulin M (IgM) tests can be performed by commercial laboratories in most situations; exceptions are testing of pregnant women with suspected acute *Toxoplasma* infections during gestation and neonates with suspected congenital toxoplasmosis, for whom testing should be performed at a reference laboratory. *Toxoplasma* IgM results from commercial laboratories can be falsely positive; confirmation should be obtained from reference laboratories with special expertise such as the Palo Alto Medical Foundation Toxoplasma Serology Laboratory (PAMF-TSL; Palo Alto, CA; **www.sutterhealth.org/RemingtonLab;** telephone: 650/853-4828; email: **RemingtonLab@sutterhealth.org**). Confirmatory testing at the reference laboratory may include IgM antibody testing; immunoglobulin A (IgA), immunoglobulin E (IgE), and IgG avidity testing; and the differential agglutination (of acetone [AC]-fixed versus that of formalin [HS]-fixed tachyzoites) test (AC/HS test).

IgG-specific antibodies achieve a peak concentration 3 to 5 months after infection and remain positive indefinitely. IgM-specific antibodies can be detected 1 to 2 weeks after infection (Tests for IgG-specific antibodies usually produce negative results during this period), achieve peak concentrations in 1 month, and usually become undetectable within 6 to 9 months, but they may also persist for years without apparent clinical significance. The lack of *T gondii*–specific IgM antibodies in a person with low-positive titers of IgG antibodies (eg, a dye test at PAMF-TSL ≤1:512) indicates infection of at least 6 months' duration. In contrast, detectable *T gondii*–specific IgM antibodies can indicate recent infection, chronic (latent) infection, or a false-positive reaction. If timing of infection is clinically important (eg, in a pregnant woman), sera with positive *T gondii* IgM test results can be sent to PAMF-TSL to establish acute versus chronic infection by using an additional panel of tests such as IgG avidity, AC/HS, and IgA- and IgE-specific antibody tests.

Polymerase chain reaction (PCR) detection has been applied to body fluid or tissue, and *T gondii*–specific immunoperoxidase staining can be performed with any tissue, depending on the clinical scenario. A positive PCR test result in tissue must be interpreted with caution, because it may amplify tachyzoite or bradyzoite DNA and cannot distinguish between tachyzoites with acute infection or reactivation or bradyzoites with chronic latent infection. CSF PCR assay for *T gondii* has high specificity (96%–100%) but sensitivity is only 50%.

Congenital Toxoplasmosis

During pregnancy, PCR assay of amniotic fluid is the method of choice to confirm fetal infection. Fetal ultrasonography can assess for anatomical abnormalities. Examination of the placenta by histological testing and PCR assay may provide additional information but is not sufficiently sensitive or specific for diagnostic purposes. At birth or postnatally, serological tests for IgG, IgM, and IgA should be performed on the neonate, and CSF, urine, and whole blood should be sent for *T gondii* PCR assay. Positive neonatal serum *Toxoplasma* IgM (after 5 days after birth) and/or IgA (after 10 days after birth), along with a positive IgG, is considered diagnostic of congenital toxoplasmosis. IgM immunosorbent agglutination assay results can be falsely positive after transfusion of blood products but usually become negative 14 days after transfusion. Occasionally, false-positive results for IgG, IgM, and IgA can be observed because of platelet transfusions or immune globulin intravenous infusions. The diagnosis of congenital toxoplasmosis can also be made definitively in an infant who remains *Toxoplasma* IgG positive at 12 months after birth.

Newborns being evaluated for toxoplasmosis should also undergo complete blood cell count (CBC) with differential count, liver function tests, and CSF cell count, differential count, protein level measurement, and glucose measurement (in addition to *T gondii* PCR assay, as above). Ophthalmologic and audiological assessments should be conducted, and head ultrasonography or brain MRI should be performed. Abdominal ultrasonography can be considered to evaluate for hepatosplenomegaly or intrahepatic calcifications.

Asymptomatic newborns with low suggestion of congenital toxoplasmosis but who were initially IgG positive but IgM and IgA negative should undergo follow-up serological testing with IgG only at 4- to 6-week intervals until complete disappearance of IgG antibodies, usually within 6 to 12 months. In the absence of postnatal treatment, disappearance of IgG antibodies in the infant safely excludes the diagnosis of congenital toxoplasmosis.

Expert advice for evaluation and treatment of neonates/infants with suspected or confirmed congenital toxoplasmosis is available at the PAMF-TSL (**www.sutterhealth.org/RemingtonLab;** telephone: 650/853-4828; email: **RemingtonLab@sutterhealth.org**) and the Toxoplasmosis Center,

University of Chicago, Chicago, IL (**www.uchicagomedicine.org/conditions-services/ophthalmology/toxoplasmosis-center;** telephone: 773/834-4131; email: **rmcleod@bsd.uchicago.edu**).

TREATMENT

Most cases of acquired acute *T gondii* infections in immunocompetent hosts do not require specific therapy unless (a) infection occurs during pregnancy; (b) there is ocular involvement; or (c) symptoms are severe or persistent. Treatment of acute *T gondii* infections in immunocompromised patients is always recommended.

Newborns and infants with confirmed/strongly suspected congenital toxoplasmosis should receive oral therapy with pyrimethamine, sulfadiazine, and folinic acid (P/S/FA), usually for 12 months, as outlined in Table 149.1. While receiving pyrimethamine, neonates/infants should be monitored for development of neutropenia weekly for 4 weeks; if the absolute neutrophil count (ANC) is stable, CBCs should be obtained every 2 weeks for 2 to 3 months and then every 3 to 4 weeks for the remainder of treatment. If the ANC decreases to less than 750, the frequency of folinic acid administration should be increased to daily dosing and pyrimethamine therapy should be held temporarily.

Ophthalmologic evaluations should be continued at least every 3 to 6 months during the first 3 years after birth for children with confirmed/probable congenital toxoplasmosis, even if the initial evaluation findings at or near birth were normal. Long-term neurodevelopmental evaluation is also required.

Infected neonates/infants with asymptomatic congenital toxoplasmosis with normal findings in fetal ultrasonography and normal findings in all postnatal evaluations, including head ultrasonography or head MRI, abdominal ultrasonography, eye examination, hearing test, CBC, and liver function tests, should be treated with the regimen used for symptomatic infants (P/S/FA). Treatment duration may be shorter than 12 months (but should be at least 3 months) and should be discussed with a congenital toxoplasmosis expert. Ophthalmologic and neurodevelopmental follow-up should be performed.

Older children with active toxoplasmic chorioretinitis represent a medical emergency, and treatment should be initiated as soon as possible, as outlined in Box 149.1. Close monitoring by a retinal specialist with expertise in management of toxoplasmic eye disease and a toxoplasmosis infectious diseases expert is recommended. Treatment of eye disease is usually given for 1 to 2 weeks beyond complete resolution of all clinical signs and symptoms and is usually approximately 4 to 6 weeks total. Treatment courses up to 3 months total are required occasionally.

Immunocompetent and immunocompromised children with severe primary (acute) toxoplasmosis and immunocompromised children with reactivation of latent (chronic) *Toxoplasma* infection should receive oral therapy with P/S/FA, as outlined in Table 149.2. In patients for whom P/S/FA is not immediately available, who are allergic or unable to take pyrimethamine or sulfadiazine, or who have significant issues with absorption of oral medications, alternative regimens are listed in Table 149.2.

While children are receiving pyrimethamine, weekly monitoring with CBC and differential count is recommended. If neutropenia is detected, the dose of leucovorin should be increased.

Table 149.1

Treatment of Neonates/Infants With Confirmed or Strongly Suspected Congenital Toxoplasmosis

Regimen	Dosing and Duration
Pyrimethamine PLUS Sulfadiazine PLUS Folinic acid[a]	Doses: Pyrimethamine[b]: 1 mg/kg every 12 hours orally for 2 days, followed by 1 mg/kg once daily for 2–6 months (6 months should be considered for symptomatic cases), followed by 1 mg/kg once per day every Monday, Wednesday, and Friday to complete a total course of 12 months PLUS Sulfadiazine: 50 mg/kg every 12 hours orally for 12 months PLUS Folinic acid (leucovorin): 10 mg/dose 3 times per week orally (during and up to 1 week after completing pyrimethamine) Duration: Treatment is usually recommended for 1 year.[c] Prednisone (if CSF protein level ≥1 g/dL or severe chorioretinitis in vision-threatening area): 0.5 mg/kg (maximum 20 mg/dose) every 12 hours orally until CSF protein level <1 g/dL or resolution of severe chorioretinitis (If prednisone is used, it should be started 48–72 hours after the initiation of anti-*Toxoplasma* therapy.)

CSF indicates cerebrospinal fluid.

[a] Folic acid should not be used as a substitute for folinic acid (leucovorin).

[b] In some centers in Europe, the regimen of pyrimethamine-sulfadoxine (Fansidar) every 10 days, plus folinic acid, is used for subclinical/mild forms of congenital toxoplasmosis and/or for poor adherence and/or frequent hematologic adverse effects. This regimen is used after the first 2 months of daily therapy with pyrimethamine-sulfadiazine (plus folinic acid 2–3 times per week). No other alternative medications have been studied adequately for treatment of congenital toxoplasmosis.

[c] For infants with delayed diagnosis of congenital toxoplasmosis (several months after birth), optimal duration of treatment should be discussed with a toxoplasmosis expert.

Box 149.1
Treatment of Older Children With Active Toxoplasmic Chorioretinitis

- Active toxoplasmic chorioretinitis, particularly in patients with severe eye disease in vision-threatening areas, is a medical emergency and treatment should begin as soon as possible.
- Duration: Treatment is usually given for 1–2 weeks beyond resolution of clinical manifestations and is usually approximately 4–6 weeks total; prolonged treatment courses up to 3 months may sometimes be needed.
- Consultation with a retinal specialist (with experience in treatment of patients with toxoplasmic chorioretinitis) AND with a toxoplasmosis infectious diseases expert should be requested to assist with optimal medication dosing, duration of therapy, and necessary monitoring.

Doses:
Pyrimethamine[a–c]:
Loading dose: 1 mg/kg once every 12 hours orally (max 50 mg/day) for 2 days,
followed by maintenance dose: 1 mg/kg once per day orally (max 25 mg/day)

PLUS

Sulfadiazine:
Loading dose: 75 mg/kg (first dose),
followed (12 hours later) by maintenance dose: 50 mg/kg every 12 hours orally (max 4 g/day)

PLUS

Folinic acid (leucovorin)[d]:
10–20 mg/dose daily orally (during and 1 week after therapy with pyrimethamine)

Prednisone (for severe eye disease in vision-threatening areas [eg, fovea/macula]): 0.5 mg/kg every 12 hours orally (max 40 mg/day). If steroids are used, they should be started after 48–72 hours of anti-*Toxoplasma* therapy, with rapid taper. Use steroids at the lowest possible dose and for the shortest possible duration.

<u>Suppressive therapy for recurrent toxoplasmic chorioretinitis:</u>
Although there are no pediatric clinical trials for primary or secondary prophylaxis (suppressive therapy), 2 adult randomized trials in Brazil for secondary prophylaxis showed that after recurrent active toxoplasmic chorioretinitis, initiation of chronic suppressive anti-*Toxoplasma* therapy (1 double-strength TMP-SMX every 2–3 days, for 12–20 months) significantly decreased the incidence of recurrences.[e]

G6PD indicates glucose-6-phosphate dehydrogenase; max, maximum; SMX, sulfamethoxazole; and TMP, trimethoprim.

[a] If pyrimethamine tablets cannot be obtained immediately, compounded pyrimethamine can be obtained by calling Imprimis Rx at 844/446-6979. Treatment should change back to pyrimethamine tablets as soon as they are acquired.

[b] TMP-SMX can also be used when the first-line therapy (pyrimethamine-sulfadiazine) is not readily available but ONLY until the first-line therapy with pyrimethamine, sulfadiazine, and folinic acid becomes available. In those cases, the highest doses should be used (15–20 mg/kg TMP; 75–100 mg/kg SMX per day divided every 6–8 hours).

[c] While children are receiving pyrimethamine therapy, a complete blood cell count should be performed weekly. Screening for G6PD deficiency before starting sulfadiazine or TMP-SMX should be performed for patients from regions with high prevalence of severe G6PD deficiency.

[d] Folic acid should not be used as a substitute for folinic acid (leucovorin).

[e] Silveira C, Belfort R Jr, Muccioli C, et al. The effect of long-term intermittent trimethoprim/sulfamethoxazole treatment on recurrences of toxoplasmic retinochoroiditis. *Am J Ophthalmol.* 2002;134(1):41–46; and Fernandez Felix JP, Cavalcanti Lira RP, Santos Zacchia R, et al. Trimethoprim-sulfamethoxazole versus placebo to reduce the risk of recurrences of *Toxoplasma gondii* retinochoroiditis: randomized controlled clinical trial. *Am J Ophthalmol.* 2014;157(4):762–766.e1.

Table 149.2
Treatment Regimens for Children and Adolescents With Severe Primary (Acute) Toxoplasmosis[a] and Immunocompromised Children and Adolescents With Severe Toxoplasmosis Attributable to Reactivation[b]

Regimen	Dose
PREFERRED REGIMEN Pyrimethamine[c,d] (oral) PLUS Folinic acid[e] (oral) PLUS Sulfadiazine (oral)	Loading dose: 1 mg/kg every 12 h (max 100 mg/day) for 2 days, followed by 1 mg/kg once per day (up to 50 mg/day) [if <60 kg] or up to 75 mg/day [if ≥60 kg] in older patients with severe disease) 10–20 mg/dose once per day (up to 50 mg/day) (during and 1 week after therapy with pyrimethamine) 100–200 mg/kg/day divided every 6 h (max 4–6 g/day for severe disease)
PREFERRED ALTERNATIVE REGIMEN TMP-SMX[d] (IV or oral)	
ALTERNATIVE REGIMENS (WITH LIMITED DATA) Pyrimethamine + folinic acid + clindamycin Pyrimethamine + folinic acid + atovaquone Pyrimethamine + folinic acid + clarithromycin Pyrimethamine + folinic acid + azithromycin Atovaquone + sulfadiazine	

IV indicates intravenous; max, maximum; SMX, sulfamethoxazole; and TMP, trimethoprim.

[a] Includes immunocompetent or immunocompromised children with severe acute *Toxoplasma gondii* infection, particularly in the setting of myocarditis, myositis, hepatitis, pneumonia, brain lesions, and lymphadenopathy accompanied by severe or persisting symptoms (**for drug dosing for ocular toxoplasmosis, see Box 149.1**). For toxoplasmic encephalitis in HIV patients, treatment should be continued for 3–6 weeks followed by suppressive therapy.

[b] Expert advice is available at the Palo Alto Medical Foundation Toxoplasma Serology Laboratory, Palo Alto, CA (**www.sutterhealth.org/RemingtonLab**; telephone: 650/853-4828; email: **RemingtonLab@sutterhealth.org**) and the Toxoplasmosis Center, University of Chicago, Chicago, IL (**www.uchicagomedicine.org/conditions-services/ophthalmology/toxoplasmosis-center**; telephone: 773/834-4131; email: **rmcleod@bsd.uchicago.edu**).

[c] If pyrimethamine tablets cannot be obtained immediately, compounded pyrimethamine can be obtained by calling Imprimis Rx at 844/446-6979. Treatment should change back to pyrimethamine tablets as soon as they are acquired.

[d] TMP-SMX can also be used when the first-line therapy (pyrimethamine-sulfadiazine) is not readily available and ONLY until the first-line therapy with pyrimethamine, sulfadiazine, and folinic acid becomes available. In those cases, the highest doses of TMP-SMX should be used (10–15 mg/kg/day of the TMP component, divided every 8–12 hours).

[e] Folinic acid = leucovorin; folic acid must not be used as a substitute for folinic acid.

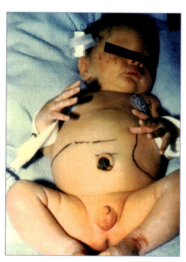

Image 149.1
A 12-day-old boy with congenital toxoplasmosis with marked hepatosplenomegaly. Courtesy of George Nankervis, MD.

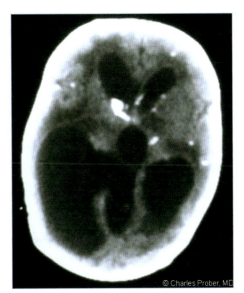

Image 149.2
Congenital infection evident on a computed tomographic scan of the head that shows diffuse calcifications and hydrocephaly. Copyright Charles Prober, MD.

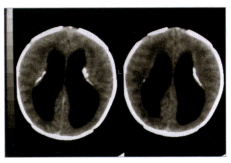

Image 149.3
A 3-day-old boy presented with a seizure. His computed tomographic scan demonstrated hydrocephalus and periventricular calcification, suggestive of congenital infection, such as toxoplasmosis, rubella, cytomegalovirus infection, or herpes simplex. *Toxoplasma* serological test result was positive, and the neonate was treated for congenital toxoplasmosis with pyrimethamine, sulfadiazine, and folinic acid. Copyright Barbara Jantausch, MD, FAAP.

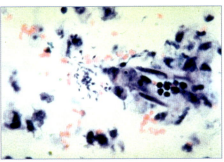

Image 149.4
Brain biopsy shows multiple *Toxoplasma gondii* organisms (Giemsa stain, original magnification ×400). Copyright Jerri Ann Jenista, MD.

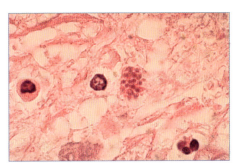

Image 149.5
Histopathologic features of toxoplasmosis of the brain in fatal AIDS. Pseudocyst contains numerous tachyzoites of *Toxoplasma gondii*. Courtesy of Centers for Disease Control and Prevention.

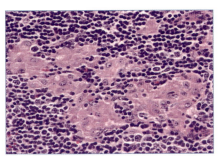

Image 149.6
Toxoplasma lymphadenitis. Noncaseating epithelioid cell granulomas in lymph node. Courtesy of Dimitris P. Agamanolis, MD.

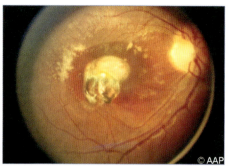

Image 149.7
Toxoplasma gondii retinitis. Note well-defined areas of chorioretinitis with pigmentation and irregular scarring.

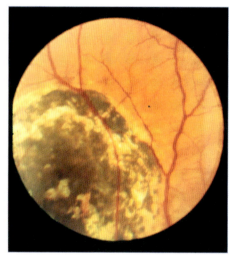

Image 149.8
Extensive chorioretinitis in an infant with congenital toxoplasmosis. Courtesy of George Nankervis, MD.

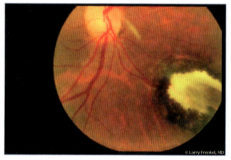

Image 149.9
A neonate with congenital toxoplasmosis with chorioretinitis. Courtesy of Larry Frenkel, MD.

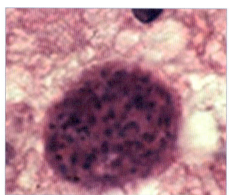

Image 149.10
Cysts of *Toxoplasma gondii* usually range from 5–50 μm in diameter. Cysts are usually spherical in the brain but more elongated in cardiac and skeletal muscles. They may be found in various sites throughout the body of the host but are most common in the brain and skeletal and cardiac muscles. *T gondii* cyst in brain tissue (hematoxylin-eosin stain). Courtesy of Centers for Disease Control and Prevention.

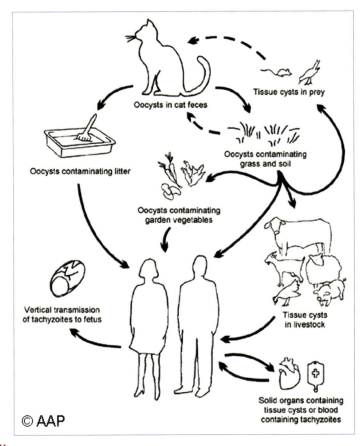

Image 149.11

Pathways for infection with *Toxoplasma gondii*. The only source for the production of *T gondii* oocysts is the feline intestinal tract. Humans usually acquire the disease by direct ingestion of oocysts from contaminated sources (eg, soil, cat litter, garden vegetables) or the ingestion of tissue cysts present in undercooked tissues from infected animals. Fetal infection occurs most commonly following acute maternal infection in pregnancy, but it can also occur following reactivation of latent infection in women with immunocompromise. Pathways leading to human disease (solid arrow); pathways leading to feline infection (dashed arrow).

CHAPTER 150

Trichinellosis
(*Trichinella spiralis* and Other Species)

CLINICAL MANIFESTATIONS

The clinical spectrum of *Trichinella* infection ranges from inapparent infection to fulminant and fatal illness; most infections are asymptomatic. Severity of disease is proportional to the infective dose and varies with the causative species of *Trichinella*. During the first week after ingesting infected meat, a person may experience abdominal discomfort, nausea, vomiting, and/or diarrhea as excysted larvae penetrate the intestinal mucosa. Two to 8 weeks later, as progeny larvae migrate into tissues, fever, myalgia, periorbital edema, urticarial rash, and conjunctival and subungual hemorrhages may develop. In severe infections, myocarditis, neurological involvement, and pneumonitis can occur in 1 or 2 months. Larvae may remain viable in tissues for years; calcification of some larvae in skeletal muscle usually occurs within 6 to 24 months and may be detected by using various imaging modalities.

ETIOLOGY

Infection is caused by nematodes (roundworms) of the genus *Trichinella*. Seven species have been implicated in human disease; worldwide, *Trichinella spiralis* is the most common cause of human infection.

EPIDEMIOLOGY

Animal infections occur worldwide in carnivores and omnivores, especially scavengers. Humans acquire the infection following ingestion of raw or insufficiently cooked meat containing larvae of *Trichinella* species. Commercial and home-raised pork remain a source of human infections, but meats other than pork, such as venison, horse meat, and particularly meats from wild carnivorous or omnivorous game (especially bear, boar, seal, and walrus), are now the most common sources of infection. The disease is not transmitted from person to person.

The **incubation period** is usually less than 1 month.

DIAGNOSTIC TESTS

Eosinophilia of up to 70% in the setting of compatible symptoms and dietary history suggests the diagnosis. Increases in concentrations of muscle enzymes, such as creatinine phosphokinase and lactic dehydrogenase, may occur. Larvae can be detected in suspect meat. Encapsulated larvae in a skeletal muscle biopsy specimen (particularly deltoid and gastrocnemius) are visible under light microscopy beginning 2 weeks after infection by examining hematoxylin-eosin–stained slides or sediment from digested muscle tissue. Serological testing is available through the Centers for Disease Control and Prevention, some state reference laboratories, and commercial laboratories. Serum antibodies are detectable at 3 or more weeks postinfection and may remain for years. Testing of paired acute and convalescent serum specimens showing an increase in titer is diagnostic, but a single positive test result in the appropriate clinical setting makes the diagnosis likely.

TREATMENT

Albendazole and mebendazole are each recommended for treatment of acute trichinellosis, although anthelmintics do not typically kill larvae that have already encysted within muscles. Coadministration of corticosteroids with anthelmintics is recommended when systemic symptoms are severe. Corticosteroids can be lifesaving when the central nervous system or heart is involved.

TRICHINELLOSIS

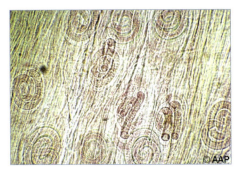

Image 150.1
Larvae of *Trichinella spiralis* in skeletal muscle biopsy. This disease is acquired by eating undercooked meat, usually pork, containing encysted *Trichinella* larvae.

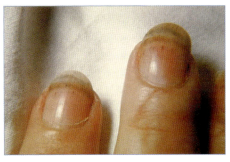

Image 150.3
The parasitic disease trichinosis is manifested by splinter hemorrhages under the fingernails as shown. Trichinosis, or trichinellosis, is caused by eating raw or undercooked pork infected with the larvae of a species of worm called *Trichinella*. Initial symptoms include nausea, diarrhea, vomiting, fatigue, fever, and abdominal discomfort. Courtesy of Centers for Disease Control and Prevention/ Dr Thomas F. Sellers, Emory University.

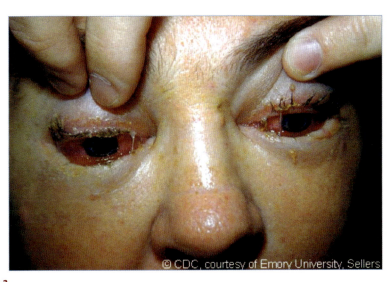

Image 150.2
This patient with trichinosis had periorbital swelling, muscle pain, diarrhea, and 28% (0.28) eosinophils. Courtesy of Centers for Disease Control and Prevention/Dr Thomas F. Sellers, Emory University.

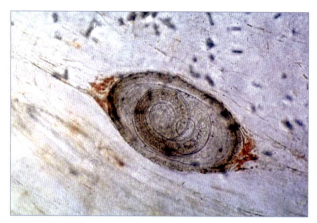

Image 150.4
Trichinella larvae in a sample of infected meat (light microscopy, magnification ×100). Courtesy of *Emerging Infectious Diseases*.

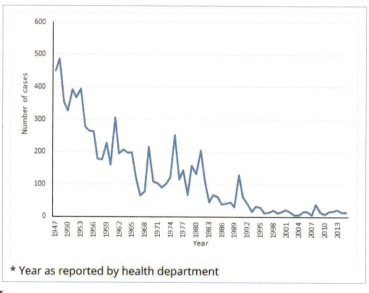

Image 150.5
Number of reported cases of trichinellosis, by year,* 1947–2015, in the United States. Courtesy of Centers for Disease Control and Prevention.

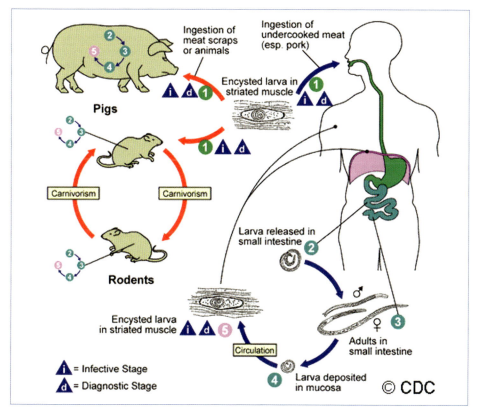

Image 150.6

Life cycle. Trichinosis is acquired by ingesting meat containing cysts (encysted larvae) (1) of *Trichinella*. After exposure to gastric acid and pepsin, the larvae are released (2) from the cysts and invade the small bowel mucosa, where they develop into adult worms (3) (female, 2.2 mm in length; males, 1.2 mm in length; life span in the small bowel, 4 weeks). After 1 week, the females release larvae (4) that migrate to the striated muscles, where they encyst (5). *Trichinella pseudospiralis*, however, do not encyst. Encystment is completed in 4–5 weeks, and the encysted larvae may remain viable for several years. Ingestion of the encysted larvae perpetuates the cycle. Rats and rodents are primarily responsible for maintaining the endemicity of this infection. Carnivorous or omnivorous animals, such as pigs or bears, feed on infected rodents or meat from other animals. Different animal hosts are implicated in the life cycle of the different species of *Trichinella*. Humans are unintentionally infected when eating improperly processed meat of these carnivorous animals (or eating food contaminated with such meat). Courtesy of Centers for Disease Control and Prevention.

CHAPTER 151

Trichomonas vaginalis Infections

(Trichomoniasis)

CLINICAL MANIFESTATIONS

Infection with *Trichomonas vaginalis* (TV), which has been described as the most common nonviral sexually transmitted infection affecting approximately 3.7 million people in the United States, is asymptomatic in 70% to 85% of infected individuals. Untreated infections may persist for months to years. Clinical manifestations in symptomatic pubertal or postpubertal females may include a diffuse vaginal discharge, odor, and vulvovaginal pruritus and irritation. Dysuria and, less often, lower abdominal pain can occur. Vaginal discharge may be any color but is classically yellow-green, frothy, and malodorous. The vulva and vaginal mucosa can be erythematous and edematous. The cervix can be inflamed and is sometimes covered with numerous punctate cervical hemorrhages and swollen papillae, referred to as *strawberry cervix*. This finding occurs in less than 5% of infected females but is highly suggestive of trichomoniasis. Clinical manifestations in symptomatic men include urethritis and, rarely, epididymitis or prostatitis. Reinfection is common, and resistance to treatment is uncommon but increasing. Rectal infections are uncommon, and oral infections have not been described.

TV infections in pregnant females have been associated with increased risks of premature rupture of the membranes and preterm delivery, although direct causation has not been clearly established. Perinatal infection may occur in up to 5% of neonates of infected mothers. TV in female newborns may cause vaginal discharge during the first weeks after birth but is usually self-limited. Respiratory infections in newborns may occur as well.

ETIOLOGY

T vaginalis is a flagellated protozoan about the size of a leukocyte. It requires adherence to host cells for survival.

EPIDEMIOLOGY

The United States population-based TV prevalence is 2.1% among females and 0.5% among males, with the highest rate among Black women (9.6%) and Black men (3.6%), compared with non-Hispanic white females (0.8%) and Hispanic females (1.4%). Unlike chlamydia and gonorrhea, TV prevalence rates are as high among women 24 years and older as they are among women younger than 24 years. Other risk factors for *T vaginalis* include having 2 or more sex partners in the past year, having less than a high school education, and living below the poverty level. Women with bacterial vaginosis have higher risk for TV. Male partners of women with TV are likely to have infection, although the prevalence of trichomoniasis in men who have sex with men is low. TV commonly coexists with other infections, particularly with *Neisseria gonorrhoeae* and herpes simplex virus infections. Transmission results almost exclusively from sexual contact. The presence of TV in a child or preadolescent beyond the perinatal period is considered indicative of sexual abuse. TV infection can increase both the acquisition and the transmission of HIV.

The **incubation period** averages 1 week but ranges from 5 to 28 days.

DIAGNOSTIC TESTS

Wet mount microscopy of vaginal discharge has traditionally been used as the preferred diagnostic test for TV in women, but its sensitivity is lower (44%–68%) than that of culture. TV culture in Diamond media or other trichomonas-specific culture systems is a specific method of diagnosis in females with a sensitivity of 75% to 96% but has lower sensitivity in males. In women, vaginal secretions are the preferred specimen type for culture, because urine culture is less sensitive. In men, culture specimens require a urethral swab, urine sediment, and/or semen specimen.

In contrast, nucleic acid amplification tests are highly sensitive, detecting more TV infections in women than wet mount microscopy. Sensitivities and specificities are generally in the 95% to 100% range. Some, but not all, are cleared for use in both women (vaginal, endocervical, and urine) and men (urine). There are also several US Food and Drug Administration–cleared rapid tests available to detect TV with improved sensitivities and specificities than those of wet mount. These rapid tests detect TV antigen or nucleic acid (via DNA hybridization) and produce results within 15 to 45 minutes. Sensitivity of antigen tests is generally in the 85% to 95% range; specificity, in the 97% to 100% range. For the nucleic acid rapid tests, they are generally 90% to 98%. These rapid tests are not currently cleared for use in men.

Some commercially available molecular-based diagnostic tests can simultaneously detect several different pathogens that cause vaginitis, typically *Candida*, TV, and bacterial vaginosis.

TREATMENT

The recommended treatment of TV infection in women is metronidazole, 500 mg, orally, twice daily for 7 days. In men, the recommended treatment is metronidazole, 2 g, orally in a single dose. An alternative regimen in both women and men is tinidazole, 2 g, orally, in a single dose. Tinidazole is generally more expensive than metronidazole, reaches higher concentrations in serum and the genitourinary tract, has a longer half-life (12.5 hours vs 7.3 hours), and has fewer gastrointestinal adverse effects.

If treatment failure occurs in a woman after completion of a treatment course of metronidazole, 500 mg, twice daily for 7 days, and she has been reexposed to an untreated partner, a repeated course of the same regimen is recommended. If there has been no reexposure, she should be treated with 2 g of metronidazole or tinidazole, once daily for 7 days. If a man is still infected with TV after a single dose of 2 g of metronidazole and has been reexposed to an untreated partner, he should be given another single dose of 2 g of metronidazole. If he has not been reexposed, he should be given a course of metronidazole, 500 mg, twice daily for 7 days.

Pregnancy

TV infection in pregnant females has been associated with adverse pregnancy outcomes, particularly premature rupture of membranes, preterm delivery, and delivery of an infant with low birth weight. Although metronidazole treatment produces parasitological cure, trials have shown no significant difference in perinatal morbidity following metronidazole treatment. In symptomatic infected pregnant females, regardless of pregnancy stage, consideration should be given to treatment with metronidazole. Metronidazole is secreted in human milk. Although several reported case series showed no evidence of adverse effects in infants exposed to metronidazole in human milk, some clinicians advise deferring breastfeeding for 12 to 24 hours following maternal treatment with metronidazole. Tinidazole should be avoided in pregnant women, and breastfeeding should be deferred for 72 hours after a single 2-g dose of tinidazole.

Neonatal

For newborns, infection with TV acquired maternally is self-limited, and treatment is not generally recommended.

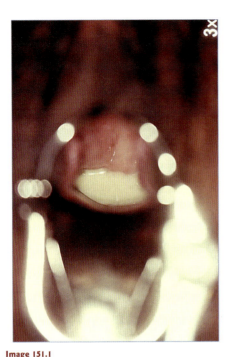

Image 151.1
This was a case of *Trichomonas* vaginitis revealing a copious purulent discharge emanating from the cervical os. *Trichomonas vaginalis*, a flagellate, is the most common pathogenic protozoan of humans in industrialized countries. This protozoan resides in the female lower genital tract and the male urethra and prostate, where it replicates by binary fission. Courtesy of Centers for Disease Control and Prevention.

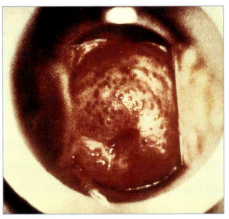

Image 151.2
This patient presented with a strawberry cervix (colpitis macularis) caused by a *Trichomonas vaginalis* infection, or trichomoniasis. The term *strawberry cervix* is used to describe the appearance of the cervix caused by the presence of *T vaginalis* protozoa. The cervical mucosa reveals punctate hemorrhages along with accompanying vesicles or papules. Courtesy of Centers for Disease Control and Prevention.

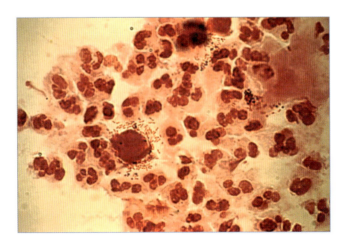

Image 151.3
This Gram-stained micrograph of a urethral discharge revealed the presence of trichomonads and gram-negative rods. *Trichomonas vaginalis*, a flagellate, is the most common pathogenic protozoan of humans in industrialized countries. This protozoan resides in the female lower genital tract and the male urethra and prostate, where it replicates by binary fission. Courtesy of Centers for Disease Control and Prevention.

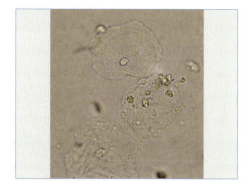

Image 151.4
An asymptomatic vaginal discharge in a premenarcheal girl who has other signs of the effects of estrogen is most likely caused by physiological leukorrhea. The discharge is caused by the desquamation of vaginal epithelial cells in response to the effect of estrogen on the vaginal mucosa. Before puberty, the vaginal mucosa is atrophic, the pH of vaginal secretions is 6.5–7.5, and the bacterial flora are mixed. Following the onset of puberty, *Lactobacillus* becomes the predominant organism in the vagina. These gram-positive bacilli metabolize sloughed epithelial cells, producing lactic acid and decreasing the pH of the vagina to <4.5. Courtesy of H. Cody Meissner, MD, FAAP.

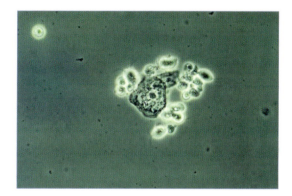

Image 151.5
This phase-contrast wet mount micrograph of a vaginal discharge revealed the presence of *Trichomonas vaginalis* protozoa. *T vaginalis*, a flagellate, is the most common pathogenic protozoan of humans in industrialized countries. This protozoan resides in the female lower genital tract and the male urethra and prostate, where it replicates by binary fission. Courtesy of Centers for Disease Control and Prevention.

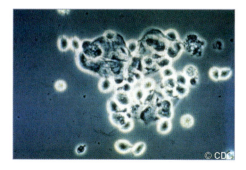

Image 151.6
Wet mount showing the presence of motile trichomonads in vaginal secretions. This indicates an infection caused by *Trichomonas vaginalis*. Courtesy of Centers for Disease Control and Prevention.

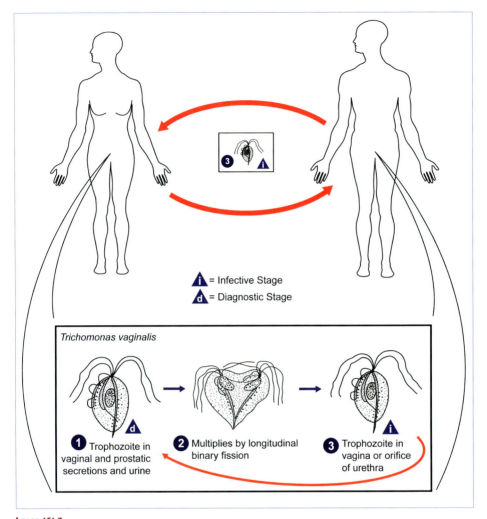

Image 151.7
Trichomonas vaginalis resides in the female lower genital tract and the male urethra and prostate (1), where it replicates by binary fission (2). The parasite does not appear to have a cyst form and does not survive well in the external environment. *T vaginalis* is transmitted among humans, its only known host, primarily by sexual intercourse (3). Courtesy of Centers for Disease Control and Prevention/Alexander J. da Silva, PhD/Melanie Moser.

CHAPTER 152

Trichuriasis
(Whipworm Infection)

CLINICAL MANIFESTATIONS

Disease caused by the whipworm *Trichuris trichiura* is generally proportional to the intensity of the infection. Most infected children are asymptomatic, but those with heavy infestations can develop a colitis that mimics inflammatory bowel disease and can lead to anemia, chronic abdominal pain and diarrhea, physical growth restriction, and clubbing. A more serious condition is *Trichuris* dysentery syndrome, which is characterized by severe abdominal pain, tenesmus, bloody diarrhea, and, occasionally, rectal prolapse.

ETIOLOGY

T trichiura, the human whipworm, is the causative agent of trichuriasis. Adult worms are 30 to 50 mm long with a large, threadlike anterior end that embeds in the mucosa of the large intestine. Adult worms typically reside in the cecum and ascending colon; with heavy infection, worms may extend further into the colon and rectum.

EPIDEMIOLOGY

T trichiura is the second most prevalent soil-transmitted helminth in the world, with approximately 600 to 800 million people infected worldwide, most of whom reside in tropical regions that lack proper sanitation infrastructure. It is frequently coendemic with *Ascaris* and hookworm species. Humans are the natural reservoir. Eggs excreted in moist soil require a range of 10 days to 4 weeks of incubation, depending on temperature, before they are infectious. Children become infected by unintentional ingestion of infective eggs in food or on hands contaminated with soil. The disease is not communicable directly from person to person.

The time between infection and appearance of eggs in the stool (**incubation period**) is approximately 12 weeks; worms may live 1 to 3 years or more.

DIAGNOSTIC TESTS

Quantitative techniques such as the Kato-Katz, McMaster, and FLOTAC methods are typically used in research settings to quantify fecal egg excretion as a measure of infection intensity. Direct microscopic visualization of eggs by using stool concentrating techniques is recommended in routine clinical settings and in screening populations with risk such as immigrants, refugees, and international adoptees. Adult worms may be visualized on proctoscopy or colonoscopy.

TREATMENT

Mebendazole and albendazole administered for 3 days are first-line therapies in the treatment of trichuriasis; some recommend mebendazole over albendazole given its higher early cure rate (11% vs 2%). Ivermectin is an alternative treatment. Longer duration of therapy (5–7 days) is recommended for heavy infections.

The cure rate for any single drug is low; stool specimens should be reexamined approximately 2 weeks after therapy to document cure. Those whose therapy fails should be re-treated. In clinical studies, combination therapy with 2 anthelmintics (eg, albendazole plus ivermectin or albendazole plus oxantel pamoate) has been associated with higher cure rates than single-drug therapy with mebendazole and should be considered in patients who persistently test positive following single-agent treatment. Iron supplements should be prescribed in patients with severe or symptomatic anemia.

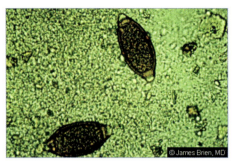

Image 152.1
Trichuris trichiura ova. Copyright James Brien.

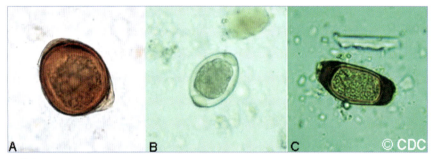

Image 152.2
Trichuris trichiura ova. A–C, Atypical *Trichuris* species eggs. Courtesy of Centers for Disease Control and Prevention.

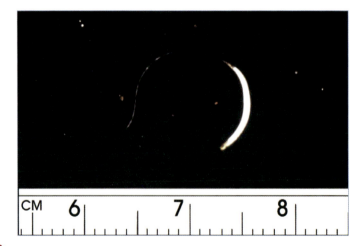

Image 152.3
This micrograph of an adult *Trichuris* female human whipworm reveals its size as approximately 4 cm. The female *Trichuris trichiura* worms begin to oviposit in the cecum and ascending colon 60–70 days after infection. Female worms in the cecum shed between 3,000 and 20,000 eggs per day. The life span of the adults is about 1 year. Courtesy of Centers for Disease Control and Prevention.

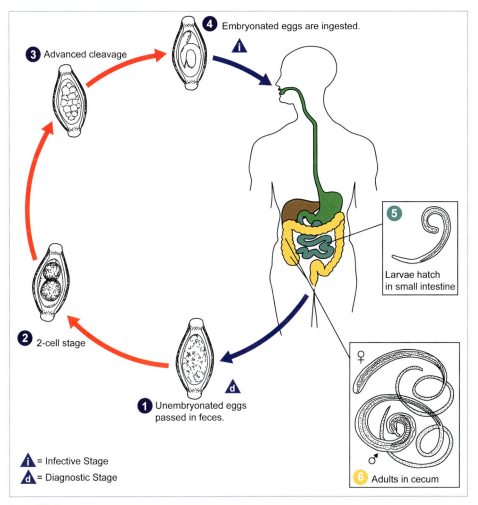

Image 152.4
Trichuris trichiura life cycle. The unembryonated eggs are passed with the stool (1). In the soil, the eggs develop into a 2-cell stage (2) and an advanced cleavage stage (3) and then embryonate (4); eggs become infective in 15–30 days. After ingestion (soil-contaminated hands or food), the eggs hatch in the small intestine and release larvae (5) that mature and establish themselves as adults in the colon (6). The adult worms (approximately 4 cm in length) live in the cecum and ascending colon. The adult worms are fixed in that location, with the anterior portions threaded into the mucosa. The females begin to oviposit 60–70 days after infection. Female worms in the cecum shed between 3,000 and 20,000 eggs per day. The life span of the adults is about 1 year. Courtesy of Centers for Disease Control and Prevention.

CHAPTER 153

African Trypanosomiasis
(African Sleeping Sickness)

CLINICAL MANIFESTATIONS

The clinical course of human African trypanosomiasis has 2 stages: the hemolymphatic stage, in which the parasite multiplies in subcutaneous tissues, lymph, and blood, and the neurological stage, after the parasite crosses the blood-brain barrier and infects the central nervous system (CNS). The rapidity of disease progression and clinical manifestations vary with the infecting subspecies. With *Trypanosoma bruceigambiense* infection (West African sleeping sickness), initial symptoms may be mild and include intermittent fever, headaches, muscle and joint aches, and malaise. Pruritus, rash, hepatosplenomegaly, weight loss, and lymphadenopathy (mainly posterior cervical [Winterbottom sign] but also possibly axillary, inguinal, and epitrochlear) can occur. CNS involvement typically develops after 1 to 2 years, with development of confusion, behavioral changes, cachexia, headache, sensory disturbances, poor coordination and movement disorders, seizures, tremors, speech disorders (eg, dysarthria, logorrhea), hallucinations, delusions, and daytime somnolence followed by nighttime insomnia. Trypanosome infiltration of endocrine organs (mainly thyroid and adrenal glands) and the heart may lead to disruptions of hormonal secretions and mild perimyocarditis.

Symptoms of *Trypanosoma brucei rhodesiense* infection (East African sleeping sickness) are similar to those of *T bruceigambiense* infection. An inoculation chancre may develop at the site of the tsetse fly bite. Initial manifestations include high fever, headaches, pruritis, lymphadenopathy (more often submandibular, axillary, and inguinal), rash, and muscle and joint aches. Thyroid dysfunction, adrenal insufficiency, and hypogonadism are found more frequently in *T brucei rhodesiense* infection, and myopericarditis may be more severe. Edema is reported more frequently in *T brucei rhodesiense* infection, and liver involvement with hepatomegaly is usually moderate, sometimes with ascites.

Clinical meningoencephalitis can develop after onset of the untreated systemic illness caused by both *Trypanosoma* subspecies. As the disease progresses, severe but less frequent complications can include renal failure requiring dialysis, multiorgan failure, disseminated intravascular coagulopathy, and coma. Both forms of African trypanosomiasis have high fatality rates; without treatment, infected patients usually die within 6 months after clinical onset of disease caused by *T brucei rhodesiense* and within 2 to 3 years from disease caused by *T brucei gambiense*.

ETIOLOGY

Human African trypanosomiasis (sleeping sickness) is caused by *Trypanosoma brucei* subspecies, which are protozoan parasites transmitted by blood-feeding tsetse flies. The West and Central African (Gambian) form is caused by *T brucei gambiense*, and the East and southern African (Rhodesian) form is caused by *T brucei rhodesiense*. Both are extracellular protozoan hemoflagellates that live in blood and tissue of the human host.

EPIDEMIOLOGY

The number of cases of human African trypanosomiasis is decreasing, with 977 cases reported to the World Health Organization in 2018, a greater than 90% reduction since 2000. Most of total reported cases worldwide (>95%) are caused by *T brucei gambiense*. There are occasional reported cases of African trypanosomiasis in the United States, typically in returning travelers who became infected with *T brucei rhodesiense* while on safari in East Africa. Transmission of *T brucei* subspecies is confined to an area in Africa between the latitudes of 14° north and 29° south, corresponding precisely with the distribution of the tsetse fly vector (*Glossina* species). In West and Central Africa, humans are the main reservoir of *T brucei gambiense*, although the parasite can sometimes be found in domestic animals, such as dogs and pigs. In East Africa, wild animals, such as antelope, bushbuck, and hartebeest, constitute the major reservoirs for sporadic infections with *T brucei rhodesiense*, although cattle serve as reservoir hosts in local outbreaks. *T brucei* subspecies can also be transmitted congenitally. Unintentional infections in laboratories caused by pricks with contaminated needles have occurred.

The **incubation period** for *T brucei rhodesiense* infection ranges from 3 to 21 days and for most cases is 5 to 14 days. For *T brucei gambiense* infection, the **incubation period** is usually longer; it is generally less than 1 month for travelers from countries without endemic disease.

DIAGNOSTIC TESTS

Diagnosis is made by identification of trypanosomes in specimens of blood, cerebrospinal fluid (CSF), or fluid aspirated from a chancre or lymph node or by inoculation of susceptible laboratory animals (mice) with heparinized blood in the case of *T brucei rhodesiense* infection. Examination of CSF is critical to management, and all patients diagnosed in the United States should undergo lumbar puncture; concentration methods (such as the double-centrifugation technique) should typically be used. Concentration and Giemsa staining of the buffy coat layer of peripheral blood is easier for *T brucei rhodesiense*, because the density of organisms in circulating blood is higher than for *T brucei gambiense*. Wet preparations of the buffy coat and of concentrated CSF sediment should be examined for motile trypanosomes. *T brucei gambiense* is more likely to be found in lymph node aspirates than in blood. The most widely used criteria for stage determination to assess CNS involvement include identification of trypanosomes in CSF or a CSF white blood cell count of 6 or higher; an elevated level of CSF neopterin and an increased level of intrathecal immunoglobulin M may also suggest second-stage disease. Serological testing for antibodies to *T brucei gambiense* is available outside the United States and is typically used only for screening purposes to help identify suspected cases; there is no comparable serological screening test for *T brucei rhodesiense*.

TREATMENT

The choice of drug(s) used for treatment depends on the type and stage of African trypanosomiasis (**www.cdc.gov/parasites/sleepingsickness/health_professionals/index.html#tx**). When no evidence of CNS involvement is present, the drug of choice for the acute hemolymphatic stage of infection is pentamidine for *T brucei gambiense* infection and suramin for *T brucei rhodesiense* infection. For treatment of infection with CNS involvement, the drug of choice is eflornithine alone or in combination with nifurtimox, if available, for *T brucei gambiense* infection; for *T brucei rhodesiense* infection, the drug of choice is melarsoprol (eflornithine is not effective for CNS treatment of *T brucei rhodesiense* infection). Melarsoprol encephalopathy may be reduced in severity by concomitant administration of corticosteroids. Suramin, eflornithine, and melarsoprol can be obtained from the Centers for Disease Control and Prevention (telephone: 404/718-4745). Consultation with a specialist familiar with the disease and its treatment is recommended. Patients who have had CNS involvement should undergo repeated CSF examinations every 6 months for 2 years because of the risk of relapse.

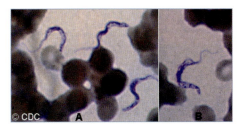

Image 153.1

A and B, Two areas from a thin blood smear (Giemsa stain) from a patient with African trypanosomiasis. Typical trypomastigote stages (the only stages found in patients) are a posterior kinetoplast, a centrally located nucleus, an undulating membrane, and an anterior flagellum. The 2 *Trypanosoma brucei* species that cause human trypanosomiasis, *T brucei gambiense* and *T brucei rhodesiense*, are indistinguishable morphologically. The trypanosomes length range is 14–33 μm. Courtesy of Centers for Disease Control and Prevention.

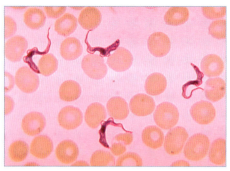

Image 153.2
Trypanosoma forms in blood smear from a patient with African trypanosomiasis (hematoxylin-eosin stain).

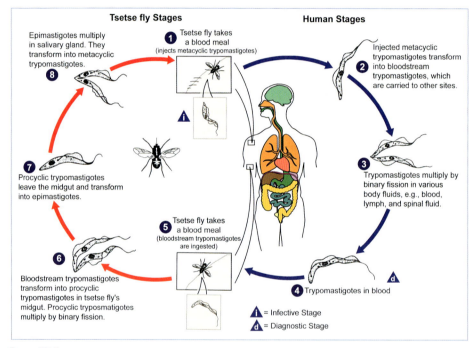

Image 153.3
Life cycle. During a blood meal on the mammalian host, an infected tsetse fly (genus *Glossina*) injects metacyclic trypomastigotes into skin tissue. The parasites enter the lymphatic system and pass into the bloodstream (1). Inside the host, they transform into bloodstream trypomastigotes (2), are carried to other sites throughout the body, reach other body fluids (eg, lymph, spinal fluid), and continue the replication by binary fission (3). The entire life cycle of African trypanosomes is represented by extracellular stages. The tsetse fly becomes infected with bloodstream trypomastigotes when taking a blood meal on an infected mammalian host (4, 5). In the fly's midgut, the parasites transform into procyclic trypomastigotes, multiply by binary fission (6), leave the midgut, and transform into epimastigotes (7). The epimastigotes reach the fly's salivary glands and continue multiplication by binary fission (8). The cycle in the fly takes approximately 3 weeks. Humans are the main reservoir for *Trypanosoma brucei gambiense*, but this species can also be found in animals. Wild game animals are the main reservoir of *Trypanosoma brucei rhodesiense*. Courtesy of Centers for Disease Control and Prevention.

CHAPTER 154

American Trypanosomiasis
(Chagas Disease)

CLINICAL MANIFESTATIONS

The acute phase of *Trypanosoma cruzi* infection (Chagas disease) lasts 2 to 3 months, followed by the chronic phase that, in the absence of successful antiparasitic treatment, is lifelong. The acute phase is commonly asymptomatic or characterized by mild, nonspecific symptoms. When disease is acquired by oral transmission, patients are more likely to exhibit symptoms of febrile illness. In the minority of patients with symptomatic acute-phase infection, fever, edema, cutaneous rash, myalgia, pallor, malaise, lymphadenopathy, and hepatosplenomegaly may develop. Meningoencephalitis and/or acute myocarditis are rare manifestations. Unilateral edema of the eyelids, known as the Romaña sign, may occur if the portal of entry is the conjunctiva. The edematous skin may be violaceous and associated with conjunctivitis and enlargement of the ipsilateral preauricular lymph node. In some patients, a red, indurated nodule known as a chagoma develops at the site of the original inoculation, usually on the face or arms.

Symptoms of acute Chagas disease can resolve without treatment within 3 months, and patients pass into the chronic phase of the infection. Most people with chronic *T cruzi* infection have no signs or symptoms and are said to have the indeterminate form of chronic Chagas disease. Serious progressive sequelae affecting the heart and/or gastrointestinal tract develop in 20% to 40% of cases years to decades after the initial infection (called *determinate* forms of chronic Chagas disease). Chagas cardiomyopathy is characterized by conduction system abnormalities, especially right bundle branch block and ventricular arrhythmias, and may progress to dilated cardiomyopathy and congestive heart failure. Patients with Chagas cardiomyopathy may die suddenly of ventricular arrhythmias, complete heart block, or embolic phenomena; death may also occur from intractable congestive heart failure. Less commonly, patients with chronic Chagas disease may develop digestive disease with dilatation of the colon and/or esophagus with swallowing difficulties accompanied by severe weight loss.

Congenital Chagas disease occurs in 1% to 10% of infants born to infected mothers and may be characterized by low birth weight, hepatosplenomegaly, and anemia; myocarditis and/or meningoencephalitis with seizures and tremors is rare. Most infants with congenital *T cruzi* infection have no signs or symptoms of disease.

Reactivation of chronic *T cruzi* infection with parasitemia may be life threatening and may occur in immunocompromised people, including people who are infected with HIV and those who are immunosuppressed after transplant.

ETIOLOGY

T cruzi, a protozoan hemoflagellate, causes American trypanosomiasis (Chagas disease).

EPIDEMIOLOGY

Parasites are transmitted in feces of infected triatomine insects (sometimes called "kissing bugs," a type of reduviid; local Spanish/Portuguese names include *vinchuca, chinche picuda*, or *barbeiro*). When found indoors, they tend to be found in pet areas, under bedding, and in rodent-infested areas. The bugs defecate during or after taking a blood meal. The bitten person is inoculated through inadvertent rubbing of insect feces containing the parasite into the site of the bite through the harmed skin or mucous membranes of the eye. The parasite can also be transmitted congenitally, during solid organ transplant, through blood transfusion, and by ingestion of food or drink contaminated by the vector's excreta. Unintentional laboratory infections can result from handling parasite cultures or blood from infected people or laboratory animals, usually through needlestick injuries. Vectorborne transmission of the disease is limited to the Western hemisphere, predominantly Mexico and Central and South America.

In the United States, 11 species of kissing bugs have been identified, and most have been found to be infected naturally with *T cruzi*. Triatomines have been found throughout the southern half of the United States, from California to Florida and as far north as Illinois and Pennsylvania. Significant numbers of wild animals are infected, including opossums, armadillos, wood rats, and raccoons. Animals usually acquire the parasite by eating infected triatomines. Rare vectorborne cases of

Chagas disease have been noted in the United States. Most *T cruzi*–infected individuals in the United States are immigrants from areas of Latin America with endemic infection.

An estimated 300,000 individuals with *T cruzi* infection live in the United States. Assuming a 1% to 5% risk of congenital transmission, based on estimates of maternal infection, approximately 63 to 315 infants are born with Chagas disease in the United States every year. Several transfusion- and transplant-associated cases have been documented in the United States.

The disease is an important cause of morbidity and death in Latin America, where an estimated 6 million people are infected, of whom approximately 20% to 40% either have or will develop cardiomyopathy and/or gastrointestinal tract disorders.

The **incubation period** for the acute phase of disease is 1 to 2 weeks or longer. Chronic manifestations do not appear for years to decades.

DIAGNOSTIC TESTS

During the acute phase of disease, the parasite is demonstrable in blood specimens by Giemsa staining after a concentration technique or in direct wet mounts or buffy-coat preparations. Molecular detection techniques (available at the Centers for Disease Control and Prevention) also have high sensitivity in the acute phase. The chronic phase of *T cruzi* infection is characterized by low-level intermittent parasitemia. Diagnosis in the chronic phase relies on serological tests to demonstrate immunoglobulin G (IgG) antibodies against *T cruzi*. Serological tests include indirect immunofluorescent and enzyme immunosorbent assays; no single serological test is sufficiently sensitive or specific to confirm a diagnosis of chronic *T cruzi* infection. The Pan American Health Organization and the World Health Organization recommend that samples be tested by using 2 diagnostic assays of different formats before treatment decisions are made.

The diagnosis of congenital Chagas disease can be made during the first 3 months after birth by identification of motile trypomastigotes by direct microscopy of fresh anticoagulated blood specimens or by polymerase chain reaction (PCR) testing, which is a useful tool in infants and has higher sensitivity than serological testing. If Chagas disease is not diagnosed earlier, serological testing should be performed after 9 months of age, once serum IgG measurements are expected to reflect infant response rather than maternal antibody. Some countries have congenital Chagas disease screening programs, which combine maternal screening with microscopic examination of cord blood from infants of seropositive mothers.

TREATMENT

The only drugs with proven efficacy are benznidazole and nifurtimox. Benznidazole was approved in 2017 by the US Food and Drug Administration (FDA) for treatment of Chagas disease in children 2 to 12 years of age. Nifurtimox was approved by the FDA on August 7, 2020, for the treatment of Chagas disease in children from birth to younger than 18 years.

Antitrypanosomal treatment is recommended for all cases of acute and congenital Chagas disease, reactivated infection attributable to immunosuppression, and chronic *T cruzi* infection in children and teens younger than 18 years. Treatment of chronic *T cruzi* infection in adults without advanced cardiomyopathy is generally recommended.

Trypanocidal therapy with benznidazole in patients with established Chagas cardiomyopathy significantly reduces serum parasite detection by PCR testing but does not significantly reduce cardiac clinical deterioration or death through 5 years of follow-up and is therefore not recommended. Both drugs have significant adverse event profiles. The recommended treatment courses are at least 60 days.

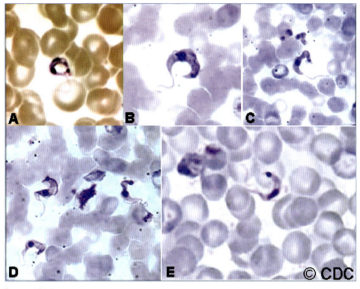

Image 154.1
A–E, *Trypanosoma cruzi* in blood smears (Giemsa stain). Courtesy of Centers for Disease Control and Prevention.

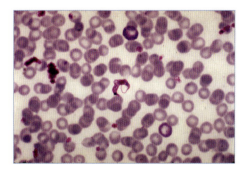

Image 154.2
This is a photomicrograph of *Trypanosoma cruzi* in a blood smear by use of Giemsa-staining technique. This protozoan parasite, *T cruzi*, is the causative agent for Chagas disease, also known as American trypanosomiasis. It is estimated that 16 million to 18 million people are infected with Chagas disease, and, of those infected, 50,000 die each year. Courtesy of Centers for Disease Control and Prevention.

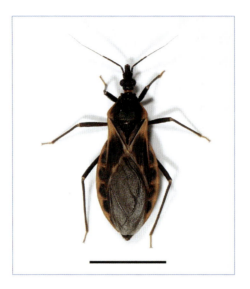

Image 154.3
Adult female "kissing bug" of the species *Triatoma rubida*, the most abundant triatomine species in southern Arizona (scale bar = 1 cm). Chagas disease is endemic throughout Mexico and Central and South America, with 7.7 million people infected, 108.6 million people considered to have risk, 33.3 million symptomatic cases, an annual incidence of 42,500 cases (through vectorial transmission), and 21,000 deaths every year. This disease is caused by the protozoan parasite *Trypanosoma cruzi*, which is transmitted to humans by bloodsucking insects of the family *Reduviidae* (*Triatominae*). Although mainly a vectorborne disease, Chagas disease can also be acquired by humans through blood transfusions and organ transplant, congenital acquisition (from a pregnant woman to her baby), and oral contamination (eg, foodborne).

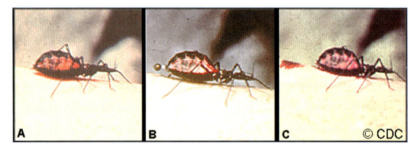

Image 154.4
A–C, Triatomine bug, *Trypanosoma cruzi* vector, defecating on the wound after taking a blood meal. Courtesy of Centers for Disease Control and Prevention.

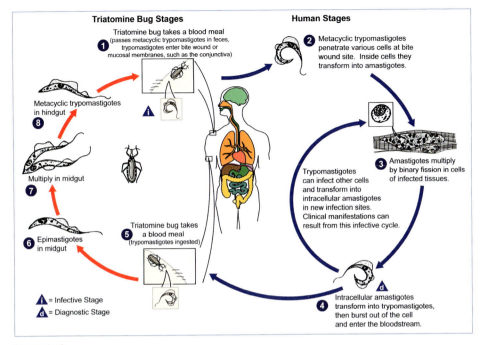

Image 154.5

Life cycle. An infected triatomine insect vector (or "kissing bug") takes a blood meal and releases trypomastigotes in its feces near the site of the bite wound. Trypomastigotes enter the host through the wound or through intact mucosal membranes, such as the conjunctiva (1). Common triatomine vector species for trypanosomiasis belong to the genera *Triatoma*, *Rhodnius*, and *Panstrongylus*. Inside the host, the trypomastigotes invade cells, where they differentiate into intracellular amastigotes (2). The amastigotes multiply by binary fission (3), differentiate into trypomastigotes, and are then released into the circulation as bloodstream trypomastigotes (4). Trypomastigotes infect cells from a variety of tissues and transform into intracellular amastigotes in new infection sites. Clinical manifestations can result from this infective cycle. The bloodstream trypomastigotes do not replicate (different from African trypanosomes). Replication resumes only when the parasites enter human or animal blood that contains circulating parasites (5). The ingested trypomastigotes transform into epimastigotes in the vector's midgut (6). The parasites multiply and differentiate in the midgut (7) and differentiate into infective metacyclic trypomastigotes in the hindgut (8). *Trypanosoma cruzi* can also be transmitted through blood transfusions, organ transplant, transplacental transmission, and laboratory accidents. Courtesy of Centers for Disease Control and Prevention.

CHAPTER 155

Tuberculosis

CLINICAL MANIFESTATIONS

Tuberculosis (TB) disease is caused by organisms of the *Mycobacterium tuberculosis* complex. Most infections caused by *M tuberculosis* complex in children and adolescents are asymptomatic. When pulmonary TB occurs, clinical manifestations most often appear 1 month to 2 years after infection and include fever, weight loss or poor weight gain, cough, night sweats, and chills. Chest radiographic findings are rarely specific for TB and include lymphadenopathy of the hilar, subcarinal, paratracheal, or mediastinal nodes; atelectasis or infiltrate of a segment or lobe; pleural effusion that can conceal small interstitial lesions; interstitial cavities; or miliary-pattern infiltrates. In selected instances, computed tomography or magnetic resonance imaging of the chest can clarify nonspecific or subtle radiographic findings. Although cavitation is a typical manifestation of reactivated TB in adults (and sometimes in adolescents) who were infected as children, cavitation is uncommon in childhood TB. Necrosis and cavitation, however, can result from a progressive primary focus in very young or immunocompromised patients and in patients with lymphobronchial disease. Extrapulmonary manifestations include meningitis and granulomatous inflammation of the lymph nodes, bones, joints, skin, and middle ear and mastoid. Gastrointestinal tract TB can mimic inflammatory bowel disease. Renal TB is unusual in younger children but can occur in adolescents. In addition, chronic abdominal pain with peritonitis and intermittent partial intestinal obstruction can be present in disease caused by *Mycobacterium bovis*. Congenital TB can mimic neonatal sepsis, or the infant may come to medical attention in the first 90 days after birth with bronchopneumonia and hepatosplenomegaly. Clinical findings in patients with drug-resistant TB disease are indistinguishable from manifestations in patients with drug-susceptible disease.

ETIOLOGY

The causative agent is *M tuberculosis* complex, a group of closely related acid-fast bacilli (AFB): *M tuberculosis, M bovis, Mycobacterium africanum,* and a few additional species infrequently associated with human infection. *M africanum* is rare in the United States, so clinical laboratories do not distinguish it routinely, and treatment recommendations are the same as for *M tuberculosis*. *M bovis* can be distinguished from *M tuberculosis* in reference laboratories, and although the spectrum of illness caused by *M bovis* is similar to that of *M tuberculosis*, the epidemiology, treatment, and prevention are different.

Definitions

- **BCG** is a live attenuated vaccine strain of *M bovis*. BCG vaccine is rarely administered to children in the United States but is one of the most widely used vaccines in the world. An isolate of BCG can be distinguished from wild-type *M bovis* only in a reference laboratory.

- **Positive tuberculin skin test (TST) result.** A positive TST result (Box 155.1) indicates possible infection with *M tuberculosis* complex. Tuberculin reactivity appears 2 to 10 weeks after initial infection; the median interval is 3 to 4 weeks. BCG immunization can produce a positive TST result.

- **Positive interferon-gamma release assay (IGRA) result.** A positive IGRA result indicates probable infection with *M tuberculosis* complex. IGRAs measure ex vivo interferon-gamma production from T lymphocytes in response to stimulation with antigens specific to *M tuberculosis* complex, including *M tuberculosis* and *M bovis*. The antigens used in IGRAs are not found in BCG or most pathogenic nontuberculous mycobacteria (eg, are not found in *Mycobacterium avium* complex but are found in *Mycobacterium kansasii*, *Mycobacterium szulgai,* and *Mycobacterium marinum*).

- **TB infection (TBI)** is *M tuberculosis* complex infection in a person who has no symptoms or signs of disease and chest radiograph findings that are normal or reveal evidence of healed infection (eg, calcification in the lung, the lymph nodes, or both) and a positive TST or IGRA result. Note that hilar adenopathy is evidence of TB disease, not TBI. TBI is also known as latent TB infection, or LTBI, but TBI is a more accurate term, because infection is not actually latent before manifesting as TB disease.

Box 155.1
Definitions of Positive Tuberculin Skin Test Results in Infants, Children, and Adolescents[a,b]

Induration ≥5 mm
Children in close contact with known or suspected contagious people with TB disease
Children suspected to have TB disease
- Findings on chest radiograph consistent with active or previous TB disease
- Clinical evidence of TB disease[c]

Children receiving immunosuppressive therapy[d] or with immunosuppressive conditions, including HIV infection

Induration ≥10 mm
Children with increased risk for disseminated TB disease
- Children younger than 4 years
- Children with other medical conditions, including Hodgkin disease, lymphoma, diabetes mellitus, chronic renal failure, or malnutrition (Box 155.2)
- Children born in high-prevalence regions of the world
- Children with significant travel to high-prevalence regions of the world[e]
- Children frequently exposed to adults who are living with HIV, experiencing homelessness, or incarcerated or to people who inject or use drugs or have alcohol use disorder

Induration ≥15 mm
Children without any risk factors

TB indicates tuberculosis; TST, tuberculin skin test.
[a] See www.cdc.gov/tb/publications/guidelines/pdf/ciw778.pdf.
[b] These definitions apply regardless of previous BCG immunization; erythema alone at the TST site does not indicate a positive test result. Tests should be read at 48–72 hours after placement.
[c] Evidence by physical examination or laboratory assessment that would include TB in the working differential diagnosis (eg, meningitis).
[d] Including immunosuppressive doses of corticosteroids or tumor necrosis factor-α antagonists or blockers or immunosuppressive drugs used in transplant recipients.
[e] Some experts define *significant travel* as travel or residence in a country with an elevated TB rate for at least 1 month.

- **TB disease** is illness in a person with infection in whom symptoms, signs, or radiographic manifestations caused by *M tuberculosis* complex are apparent; disease can be pulmonary, extrapulmonary, or both.
- **Multidrug-resistant TB (MDR TB)** is defined as infection or disease caused by a strain of *M tuberculosis* complex that is resistant to at least isoniazid and rifampin.
- **Extensively drug-resistant TB (XDR TB)** is defined as infection or disease caused by a strain of *M tuberculosis* complex that is resistant to isoniazid and rifampin, at least 1 fluoroquinolone, and at least 1 of the following parenteral drugs: amikacin, kanamycin, or capreomycin.
- **Drug-resistant TB (DR TB)** is infection or disease caused by a strain of *M tuberculosis* that is resistant to any drug used to treat drug-susceptible TB and includes isoniazid-resistant TB, rifampin-resistant TB, MDR TB, and XDR TB.
- **Directly observed therapy (DOT)** is an intervention by which medications are taken by the patient while a health care professional or trained third party (not a relative or friend) observes and documents that the patient ingests each dose of medication and assesses for possible adverse drug effects.
- **Exposed person** is anyone who has had recent (<3 months) contact with another person with suspected or confirmed contagious TB disease (pulmonary, laryngeal, tracheal, or endobronchial disease) and has a negative TST or IGRA result, normal physical examination findings, and chest radiographic findings that are normal or not compatible with TB. Some exposed people are or become infected (and subsequently develop a positive TST or IGRA result), and others do not become infected after exposure; the 2 groups cannot be distinguished initially.

- **Source person** is the person who has transmitted *M tuberculosis* complex to another person who subsequently develops TB infection or disease.

EPIDEMIOLOGY

Case rates of TB in all ages in North America are higher in urban, low-income areas and in non-white racial and ethnic groups; more than 87% of reported cases in the United States occur in Hispanic and nonwhite people. In recent years, more than 70% of all US cases have been in people born outside the United States. Almost 80% of childhood TB disease in the United States is associated with some form of foreign contact of the child, the parent, or a household member. Specific groups with greater rates of TB include immigrants, international adoptees, refugees from or travelers to high-prevalence regions (eg, Asia, Africa, Latin America, and countries of the former Soviet Union), people experiencing homelessness or those with unstable housing, people who inject or use drugs, people with alcohol use disorders, and residents of certain correctional facilities and other congregate settings. Secondhand smoke exposure increases the risk of TB disease developing in infected children.

Infants and postpubertal adolescents have increased risk for progression from TBI to TB disease. Other predictive factors for development of disease include recent infection (within the past 2 years); immunodeficiency, especially from HIV infection; use of immunosuppressive drugs, such as prolonged or high-dose corticosteroid therapy or chemotherapy and drugs for preventing transplant organ rejection; and certain diseases or medical conditions, including Hodgkin disease, lymphoma, diabetes mellitus, chronic renal failure, and malnutrition. Patients with TBI who are being treated with tumor necrosis factor-α (TNF-α) antagonists or blocking agents have higher risk for progressing to TB disease. A positive TST or IGRA result should be accepted as indicative of infection in individuals receiving or soon to receive these medications, and the patient should be evaluated and treated accordingly.

A diagnosis of TBI or TB disease in a young child is a public health sentinel event often representing recent transmission. Transmission of *M tuberculosis* complex is airborne, with inhalation of droplet nuclei usually produced by an adult or adolescent with contagious pulmonary, endobronchial, or laryngeal TB disease. The probability of transmission increases if the index person has a positive acid-fast sputum smear, productive cough, or pulmonary cavities or is a household contact. Although contagiousness usually lasts only a few days to weeks after initiation of effective drug therapy, it can last longer if the source person does not adhere to medical therapy or is infected with a drug-resistant strain. If the sputum smear becomes negative for AFB on 3 separate specimens at least 8 hours apart after treatment is initiated and the patient's condition has improved clinically, the treated patient can be considered to have low risk for transmitting *M tuberculosis*. Children younger than 10 years with only adenopathy in the chest or small pulmonary lesions (paucibacillary disease) and nonproductive cough are not contagious. Rare cases of pulmonary disease in young children, particularly with lung cavities or presence of AFB on sputum microscopy, and in infants with congenital TB can be contagious.

M bovis is transmitted most often by unpasteurized dairy products, but airborne human-to-human transmission can occur.

The **incubation period** from infection to development of a positive TST or IGRA result is 2 to 10 weeks. The risk of developing TB disease is highest during the 12 months after infection and remains high for 2 years; however, many years can elapse between initial *M tuberculosis* infection and subsequent disease.

DIAGNOSTIC TESTS

Testing for *M tuberculosis* Infection

Tuberculin Skin Test

The TST is 1 of 2 indirect methods for detecting *M tuberculosis* infection, with the other method being IGRA. Both methods rely on specific lymphocyte sensitization after infection. Conditions that decrease lymphocyte numbers or function, including severe TB disease, can reduce the sensitivity of these tests. Tuberculin is a purified protein derivative (PPD) from heat-inactivated *M tuberculosis*. The routine (ie, Mantoux) technique of administering the skin test consists of 5 tuberculin units of solution (PPD; 0.1 mL) injected intradermally by using a 27-gauge needle and a 1.0-mL syringe into the volar aspect of the forearm. Creation of a palpable wheal 6 to 10 mm in diameter is crucial to accurate testing.

Administration of TSTs and interpretation of results should be performed by trained and experienced health care personnel, because administration and interpretation by unskilled people or family members are unreliable. The standardized time for assessing the TST result is 48 to 72 hours after administration. The diameter of **induration** is measured transversely to the long axis of the forearm, and the result should be recorded in millimeters. Positive TST results, as defined in Box 155.1, can persist for several weeks.

Lack of reaction to a TST does not exclude TBI or TB disease. Approximately 10% to 40% of immunocompetent children with culture-documented TB disease do not react initially to a TST. Host factors, such as young age, poor nutrition, immunosuppression, viral infections (especially measles, varicella, and influenza), recent M tuberculosis infection, and disseminated TB disease, can decrease TST reactivity.

Classification of TST results is based on epidemiological and clinical factors. Interpretation of the size of induration (millimeters) as a positive result varies with the person's epidemiological risk of TBI and likelihood of progression to TB disease. Current guidelines from the Centers for Disease Control and Prevention (CDC), the American Thoracic Society, and the American Academy of Pediatrics recommend interpretation of TST findings on the basis of an individual's risk stratification and are summarized in Box 155.1. Prompt clinical and radiographic evaluation of all children and adolescents with a positive TST result is recommended.

BCG immunization, because of cross-reacting antigens present in the PPD, can result in induration of a TST. Distinguishing between a positive TST result caused by M tuberculosis complex infection and that caused by BCG requires a qualitative assessment of several factors. Reactivity of the TST (ie, millimeters of induration) attributable to prior BCG immunization may be absent or variable and depends on many factors, including age at BCG immunization, quality and strain of BCG vaccine used, number of doses of BCG vaccine received, nutritional and immunologic status of the vaccine recipient, frequency of TST administration, and time between immunization and TST. Evidence that increases the probability that a positive TST result is attributable to TBI includes known contact with a person with contagious TB, a family history of TB disease, more than 2 years since neonatal BCG immunization, and a TST reaction 15 mm or greater. Generally, interpretation of TST results in BCG recipients who are known contacts of a person with TB disease or who have high risk for developing TB disease is the same as for people who have not received BCG vaccine.

Blood-Based Testing With IGRAs

IGRAs measure ex vivo interferon-gamma production from T lymphocytes in response to stimulation with proprietary polypeptide mixtures that simulate antigens specific to M tuberculosis complex, which includes M tuberculosis and M bovis. The IGRA antigens used are not found in BCG or most pathogenic nontuberculous mycobacteria (eg, M avium complex) but are found in the nontuberculous mycobacteria M kansasii, M szulgai, and M marinum. Examples of IGRAs are the QuantiFERON-TB Gold Plus assay and the T-SPOT.TB assay. As with TSTs, IGRAs cannot distinguish between TBI and TB disease, and a negative result from these tests cannot exclude TBI or the possibility of TB disease in a patient with suggestive clinical findings. The sensitivity of IGRAs is similar to that of TSTs for detecting infection in adults and children who have untreated culture-confirmed TB. In many clinical settings, the specificity of IGRAs is higher than that for the TST, because the antigens used are not found in BCG or most pathogenic nontuberculous mycobacteria. IGRAs consistently perform well in children 2 years and older, and some data support their use for even younger children. The negative predictive value of IGRAs is unclear, but in general, if the IGRA result is negative and the TST result is positive in an asymptomatic, unexposed child, the diagnosis of TBI is unlikely, especially if the child has received a BCG vaccine. A negative result for either a TST or an IGRA should be considered especially unreliable in infants younger than 3 months.

TST Versus IGRA

For children younger than 2 years, TST is the preferred method for detection of M tuberculosis infection. For children 2 years and older, either TST or IGRA can be used, but in people previously vaccinated with BCG, IGRA is preferred to avoid a false-positive TST result caused by a previous vaccination with BCG. Low-grade, false-positive IGRA results occur in some individuals. A negative IGRA result cannot be interpreted universally as evidence of absence of infection. Indeterminate or invalid IGRA results have several possible causes that could be related to the patient, the assay itself, or its performance; these results do not exclude M tuberculosis infection and may necessitate repeated testing, possibly with a different test.

Specific recommendations for TST and IGRA use are provided in Box 155.2 and Figure 155.1.

Use of Tests for M tuberculosis Infection

The most reliable strategies for identifying TBI and preventing TB disease in children are based on identification of known risk factors for TBI and thorough and expedient contact tracing associated with cases of TB. Contact tracing is an intervention that should be coordinated through the local public health department. Universal testing with TST or IGRA, including programs based at schools, child care centers, and camps that include populations with low risk, is discouraged because it results in a low yield of positive results or a large proportion of false-positive results, leading to an inefficient use of health care resources. However, using a questionnaire to determine risk factors for TBI and identifying who should undergo a TST or an IGRA can be useful (Box 155.3). Risk assessment for TB should be performed at the first medical home encounter with a child and then annually if possible. Testing

---

Box 155.2
Tuberculin Skin Test and Interferon-Gamma Release Assay Recommendations for Infants, Children, and Adolescents[a]

Children for whom immediate TST or IGRA is indicated[b]
- Contacts of people with confirmed or suspected contagious TB (contact investigation)
- Children with radiographic or clinical findings suggesting TB disease
- Children immigrating from countries with endemic infection (eg, Asia, Middle East, Africa, Latin America, countries of the former Soviet Union), including international adoptees
- Children with history of significant[c] travel to countries with endemic infection who have substantial contact with the resident population[d]

Children who should undergo annual TST or IGRA
- Children living with HIV infection

Children with increased risk for progression of Mycobacterium tuberculosis *infection to TB disease:* Children with other medical conditions, including diabetes mellitus, chronic renal failure, malnutrition, or congenital or acquired immunodeficiencies, and children receiving TNF antagonists, deserve special consideration. Underlying immunodeficiencies associated with these conditions would theoretically enhance the possibility for progression to severe disease. Initial histories of potential exposure to TB should be included for all these patients. If these histories or local epidemiological factors suggest a possibility of exposure, immediate and periodic TST or IGRA should be considered. **A TST or an IGRA should be performed before initiation of immunosuppressive therapy, including prolonged systemic corticosteroid administration, organ transplant, use of TNF-α antagonists or blockers, or other immunosuppressive therapy in any child requiring these treatments.**

IGRA indicates interferon-gamma release assay; TB, tuberculosis; TNF, tumor necrosis factor; and TST, tuberculin skin test.
[a] BCG immunization is not a contraindication to a TST; IGRA is generally preferred for BCG-vaccinated children.
[b] Beginning as early as 3 months of age for TST and 2 years of age for IGRAs, for TBI and disease.
[c] Some experts define significant travel as birth, travel, or residence in a country with an elevated TB rate for at least 1 month.
[d] If the child is well and has no history of exposure, the TST or IGRA should be delayed for 8–10 weeks after return.

Figure 155.1
Guidance on Strategy for Use of Tuberculin Skin Test and Interferon-Gamma Release Assay for Diagnosis of *Mycobacterium tuberculosis* Infection in Children With at Least 1 Risk Factor, by Age and BCG Immunization Status

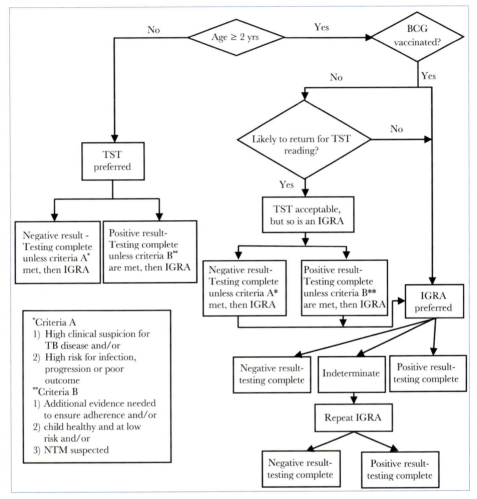

IGRA indicates interferon-gamma release assay; NTM, nontuberculous mycobacteria; TB, tuberculosis; and TST, tuberculin skin test.

Box 155.3
Validated Questions for Determining Risk of *Mycobacterium tuberculosis* Infection in Children in the United States

- Has a family member or contact had tuberculosis disease?
- Has a family member had a positive tuberculin skin test result?
- Was your child born in a high-risk country (countries other than the United States, Canada, Australia, New Zealand, or western and north European countries)?
- Has your child traveled to a high-risk country? How much contact did your child have with the resident population?

children for TBI and clinical evaluation for possible TB disease is indicated whenever a TST or IGRA result of a household member converts from a negative to positive result (indicating recent infection).

HIV Infection

Children living with HIV infection are considered to have high risk for TB and should be tested annually beginning at 3 through 12 months of age if perinatally infected or at the time of diagnosis of HIV infection in older children or adolescents. Conversely, children who have TB disease should be tested for HIV infection. The clinical manifestations and radiographic appearance of TB disease in children living with HIV infection tend to be like those in immunocompetent children, but manifestations in these children can be more severe, can be more unusual, and more often include extrapulmonary involvement of multiple organs. In HIV-infected patients, a TST induration of 5 mm or greater is considered a positive result (Box 155.1); however, a false-negative TST or IGRA result attributable to HIV-related immunosuppression can also occur. Diagnosing TB disease in an HIV-infected child with microbiological specimens is challenging, given the paucibacillary nature of TB in this population.

Organ Transplant Recipients

The risk of TB in organ transplant recipients is severalfold greater than in the general population. A careful history of previous exposure to TB should be taken from all transplant candidates, including details about previous TST or IGRA results and exposure to individuals with TB. All transplant candidates should undergo evaluation by TST or IGRA for TBI before the initiation of immunosuppressive therapy. A positive result of either test should be taken as evidence of *M tuberculosis* infection. In addition, donor-derived TB can be carried in an infected organ and should be considered as a possible cause of posttransplant fever and related symptoms.

Patients Receiving Immunosuppressive Therapies Including Biologic Response Modifiers

In addition to a detailed history of risk factors for *M tuberculosis* complex infection, all patients should undergo a TST or an IGRA before the initiation of therapy with high-dose systemic corticosteroids, antimetabolite agents, and TNF antagonists or blockers (eg, adalimumab, certolizumab pegol, etanercept, golimumab, and infliximab). Some experts recommend that if the child has at least 1 TB risk factor, both a TST and an IGRA should be performed to maximize sensitivity; a positive result of either test should be taken as evidence of *M tuberculosis* infection.

Other Considerations

Testing for TB at any age is not required before administration of live-virus vaccines. Live attenuated measles-mumps-rubella vaccines can temporarily suppress tuberculin reactivity for at least 4 to 6 weeks, and data suggest a similar suppression with varicella and yellow fever vaccines. The effect of live attenuated influenza vaccines on TST reactivity and IGRA results is unknown. If indicated, a TST can be performed or blood drawn for an IGRA at the same visit during which these vaccines are administered (ie, before substantial replication of the vaccine virus). The effects of live-virus vaccination on IGRA characteristics have not been determined; the same precautions as for TST should be followed.

Sensitivity to PPD tuberculin antigen persists for years in most instances, even after effective treatment. The durability of positive IGRA results has not been determined. Repeated testing with either TST or IGRA has no known clinical utility for assessing the effectiveness of treatment or for diagnosing newly acquired infection in patients who were previously infected with *M tuberculosis*.

Assessing for *M tuberculosis* Disease

Although both IGRA and TST provide evidence for infection with *M tuberculosis*, they cannot distinguish TBI from TB disease. Therefore, patients testing positive for *M tuberculosis* infection by IGRA or TST should be assessed for TB disease before any therapeutic intervention is initiated. This assessment should include (1) asking about symptoms of TB disease and exposure to TB patients; (2) physical examination for signs of TB disease; and (3) a chest radiograph. If radiographic signs of TB (eg, airspace opacities, pleural effusions, cavities, changes on serial radiographs) are visualized, then sputum or gastric aspirate sampling should be performed, as described below. Most experts recommend that children younger than 12 months who are suspected of having pulmonary or extrapulmonary TB disease (eg, have a positive TST result and symptoms, physical examination signs, or chest radiograph abnormalities consistent with TB disease), with or without neurological symptoms, should undergo a lumbar puncture (LP) to evaluate for tuberculous meningitis. Children 12 months and older with TB disease require an LP only if they have neurological signs or symptoms.

Laboratory Confirmation of *M tuberculosis*

Laboratory isolation of *M tuberculosis* complex by culture from a specimen of sputum, gastric aspirate, bronchial washing, pleural fluid, cerebrospinal fluid, urine, or other body fluid or a tissue biopsy specimen confirms the diagnosis of TB disease. Positive results from a rapid molecular method (eg, nucleic acid amplification tests [NAATs]) are also increasingly considered confirmatory, but culture isolation of the organism is still required after diagnosis with molecular methods for phenotypical susceptibility testing, genotyping, rapid molecular detection of drug-resistance genes, and species identification with the *M tuberculosis* complex. Children older than 2 years and adolescents frequently produce sputum spontaneously or by induction with aerosolized hypertonic saline. Studies have demonstrated successful collection of induced sputum from infants with pulmonary TB, but this requires special expertise. The best specimen for diagnosis of pulmonary TB in any child or adolescent in whom cough is absent or nonproductive and sputum cannot be induced is an early-morning gastric aspirate, which should be obtained with a nasogastric tube on awakening of the child and before ambulation or feeding. Aspirates collected on 3 separate mornings should be submitted for AFB staining and culture.

Fluorescent staining methods for specimen smears are more sensitive than the traditional Kinyoun acid-fast smears and are preferred. The overall diagnostic yield of microscopy of gastric aspirates and induced sputum is low in children with clinically suspected pulmonary TB, and false-positive stain results caused by the presence of nontuberculous mycobacteria occur rarely. Histological examination for and demonstration of AFB and granulomas in biopsy specimens from lymph node, pleura, mesentery, liver, bone marrow, or other tissues can be useful, but *M tuberculosis* complex organisms cannot be distinguished reliably from other mycobacteria in stained specimens. Regardless of results of the AFB smears, each specimen should be cultured.

Because *M tuberculosis* complex organisms are slow growing, detection of these organisms may take as long as 10 weeks by using solid media; use of liquid media and continuous monitoring systems allows detection within 1 to 6 weeks and usually within 3 weeks. Even with optimal culture techniques, *M tuberculosis* complex organisms are isolated from less than 75% of infants and 50% of children with pulmonary TB diagnosed by clinical criteria; the culture yields for most forms of extrapulmonary TB are even lower. Current methods for species identification of isolates from culture include molecular probes, NAATs, genetic sequencing, mass spectrometry, and biochemical tests. *M bovis* is usually suspected because of isolated pyrazinamide resistance, which is characteristic of almost all *M bovis* isolates, but further biochemical or molecular testing is required to distinguish *M bovis* from *M tuberculosis*.

For a child with clinically suspected TB disease, finding the culture-positive source person supports the child's presumptive diagnosis and provides the likely drug susceptibility of the child's organism. Culture material should be collected from children with evidence of TB disease, especially when (1) an isolate from a source person is unavailable; (2) the presumed source person has drug-resistant TB; (3) the child is immunocompromised or ill enough to require hospital admission; or (4) the child has extrapulmonary disease. Traditional methods of determining drug susceptibility require bacterial isolation. Several new molecular methods of rapidly determining drug resistance directly from clinical samples are now available.

NAATs are available for rapid detection of *M tuberculosis* complex organisms from smear-positive and smear-negative sputum specimens, and other laboratory-developed tests for rapid molecular detection are available locally. Some tests have been validated for specimens other than sputum: expert consultation is recommended for test availability and interpretation of results. Molecular methods that help find *M tuberculosis* genetic markers associated with drug resistance are supplementing the culture-based (ie, phenotypic) methods for drug susceptibility testing because they decrease the time to detection of drug resistance from weeks to hours, and in some instances, the results could be more reliable for patient care decisions. Some of the methods are verified for direct testing of patient specimens. However, culture-based results are still required for confirming susceptibility to each drug when drug resistance genes are not detected, because the absence of resistance genes is not entirely predictive of susceptibility. The molecular methods are constantly evolving, and expert consultation should be sought for a testing strategy when drug resistance is suspected.

TREATMENT (TABLE 155.1)

Specific Drugs

Regimen and dosage recommendations and the more commonly reported adverse reactions of first-line antituberculosis drugs are summarized in tables 155.1 to 155.3. The less commonly used (eg, second-line) antituberculosis drugs, their doses, and adverse effects are listed in Table 155.4. Some of these drugs have less effectiveness and greater toxicity; they should be used only in consultation with a specialist familiar with treatment of childhood TB. For treatment of TB disease, drugs must always be used in recommended combination and dosage to minimize emergence of drug-resistant strains. Use of nonstandard regimens for any reason (eg, drug allergy, drug resistance) should be undertaken only by an expert in treating TB.

Occasionally, a patient cannot tolerate oral medications. Isoniazid, rifampin, amikacin and related drugs, linezolid, and fluoroquinolones can be administered parenterally.

Treatment Regimens for TBI

Several regimens are recommended, depending on the circumstances for individual patients. Dosages and intervals are provided in Table 155.2.

Isoniazid-Rifapentine Therapy for TBI

A 12-week course, comprising a once-weekly dose of isoniazid and rifapentine, is a regimen that is safe, well tolerated, and at least as efficacious as 9 months of isoniazid taken daily. Most experts consider isoniazid-rifapentine to be the preferred regimen for treatment of TBI for children 2 years and older, although the pill burden in younger children is substantial and sometimes not well tolerated. Isoniazid-rifapentine should not be used in children younger than 2 years.

Rifampin Therapy for TBI

A 4-month course of rifampin given daily is also an acceptable regimen for the treatment of TBI. It is the preferred regimen when isoniazid resistance is likely, as judged from the exposure history. The regimen has been as effective as 9 months of daily isoniazid, the rates of adverse effects have been low, and the completion rates of therapy have been much higher than for 9 months of isoniazid.

Isoniazid-Rifampin Therapy for TBI

An additional possible regimen for treatment of TBI is 3 months of daily isoniazid and rifampin, with no age restriction on its use. This regimen is quite similar in principle to the isoniazid-rifapentine option; however, the medications are given daily because of the relatively short half-life of rifampin compared with that rifapentine. Efficacy and rates of completion of are comparable or better when compared with isoniazid monotherapy.

Isoniazid Therapy for TBI

Isoniazid monotherapy has been the most widely recommended and used treatment of pediatric TBI. The efficacy of isoniazid monotherapy reaches 98% against development of TB disease, but the long duration of isoniazid monotherapy results in poor adherence and low completion rates. The World Health Organization (WHO) recommends a treatment duration of 6 months to provide high coverage of the population in countries with a high disease burden. A 9-month regimen gives an additional 20% to 30% increase in efficacy. The CDC and National TB Controllers Association recommend 6- or 9-month durations of isoniazid monotherapy, if shorter-course rifamycin-based regimens cannot be used.

For infants, children, and adolescents, including those living with HIV infection or other immunocompromising conditions, the recommended duration of isoniazid therapy in the United States is 9 months. The WHO recommends a 6-month course of isoniazid, but modeling studies have shown that the efficacy of 6 months of treatment is approximately 30% less than that of a 9-month course. Many experts in North America accept

Table 155.1
Recommended Usual Treatment Regimens for Drug-Susceptible TB Infection and TB Disease in Infants, Children, and Adolescents

Infection or Disease Category	Regimen	Remarks
***Mycobacterium tuberculosis* infection** (positive TST or IGRA result, no disease)[a]		
• Isoniazid susceptible	12 weeks of isoniazid plus rifapentine, once a week	Most experts consider isoniazid-rifapentine to be the preferred regimen for treatment of TBI for children ≥2 years, and some experts prefer isoniazid-rifapentine therapy for TBI in children ≥2 years.
	OR	
	4 months of rifampin, once a day	Continuous daily therapy is required. Intermittent therapy even by DOT is not recommended.
	OR	
	3 months of isoniazid plus rifampin, once a day	To be considered if above 2 regimens are not feasible
	OR	
	6 or 9 months of isoniazid, once a day	If daily therapy is not possible, DOT twice a week can be used; medication doses differ with daily and twice-weekly regimens.
• Isoniazid resistant	4 months of rifampin, once a day	Continuous daily therapy is required. Intermittent therapy even by DOT is not recommended.
• Isoniazid-rifampin resistant	Consult a TB specialist.	Moxifloxacin or levofloxacin with or without ethambutol or pyrazinamide is most commonly given.
Pulmonary and extrapulmonary disease (except meningitis)[b]	2 months of RIPE daily or 3 times per week, followed by 4 months of isoniazid and rifampin[c] by DOT[d] for drug-susceptible *M tuberculosis*	Some experts recommend a 3-drug initial regimen (isoniazid, rifampin, and pyrazinamide) if the risk of drug resistance is low. DOT is highly desirable.
		If hilar adenopathy only and the risk of drug resistance is low, a 6-month course of isoniazid and rifampin is sufficient.
		DOT is required for intermittent regimens.
		Drugs can be given daily or 3 times per week; 2 times per week is acceptable if DOT resources are scarce.
	At least 9 months of isoniazid and rifampin for *Mycobacterium bovis* susceptible to these drugs	

(continues)

Table 155.1 (continued)

Infection or Disease Category	Regimen	Remarks
Meningitis	2 months of RIPE, if possible, or an aminoglycoside[e] or capreomycin, once a day[f,g]; followed by 4–10 months of isoniazid and rifampin, once a day or 3 times per week (9–12 months total) for drug-susceptible *M tuberculosis*	See text for information on corticosteroids.
	At least 12 months of therapy without pyrazinamide for *M bovis* susceptible to isoniazid and rifampin	

DOT indicates directly observed therapy; RIPE, rifampin, isoniazid, pyrazinamide, and ethambutol; TB, tuberculosis; and TBI, TB infection.
[a] See text for comments and additional acceptable/alternative regimens.
[b] Duration of therapy may be longer for people living with HIV infection, and additional drugs and dosing intervals may be indicated.
[c] Medications should be administered daily for the first 2 weeks–2 months of treatment and can then be administered daily or 3 times per week by DOT; twice weekly is acceptable if resources for DOT are limited. Intermittent therapy is not recommended for people living with HIV infection.
[d] If initial chest radiograph shows pulmonary cavities and/or if sputum culture after 2 months of therapy remains positive, the continuation phase is extended to 7 months, for a total treatment duration of 9 months.
[e] Parenteral streptomycin, kanamycin, or amikacin.
[f] Many experts add a fluoroquinolone to this initial regimen.
[g] When susceptibility to first-line drugs is established, the ethionamide, aminoglycoside (or capreomycin), and/or fluoroquinolone can be discontinued.

6 months of uninterrupted treatment as adequate. When adherence with daily therapy with isoniazid cannot be ensured, twice-a-week DOT can be considered, but each dose should be observed. Determination of serum aminotransferase concentrations before or during therapy is not indicated except in patients with underlying liver or biliary disease, during pregnancy or the first 12 weeks postpartum, with concurrent use of other potentially hepatotoxic drugs (eg, anticonvulsant or HIV agents), or if there is clinical concern of possible hepatotoxicity.

Therapy for TBI and Contacts of Patients With Isoniazid-Resistant *M tuberculosis* and When Isoniazid Cannot Be Administered

The incidence of isoniazid resistance among *M tuberculosis* complex isolates from US patients in 2017 was approximately 9%. Risk factors for drug resistance are listed in Box 155.4. If the source person is found to have isoniazid-resistant, rifampin-susceptible organisms, isoniazid should be discontinued and rifampin should be administered daily to contacts with TBI for a total course of 4 months. Optimal therapy for children with TBI caused by organisms with resistance to isoniazid and rifampin (ie, multidrug resistance) is unknown. In these circumstances, a fluoroquinolone alone and multidrug regimens have been used in observational studies. Drugs to consider include levofloxacin or moxifloxacin, with or without the addition of pyrazinamide or ethambutol, depending on susceptibility of the isolate. Consultation with a TB specialist is indicated.

Treatment of TB Disease

The goal of treatment is to achieve killing of replicating organisms in the tuberculous lesion in the shortest possible time. Achievement of this goal minimizes the possibility of development of resistant organisms. The major problem limiting successful treatment is poor adherence to prescribed treatment regimens. The use of DOT decreases the rates of relapse, treatment failures, and drug resistance; therefore, DOT is strongly recommended for treatment of all children and adolescents with TB disease in the United States.

Therapy for Presumed or Known Drug-Susceptible Pulmonary TB

A 6-month, 4-drug regimen consisting initially of rifampin, isoniazid, pyrazinamide, and ethambutol (RIPE) for the first 2 months and isoniazid and rifampin for the remaining 4 months is recommended for treatment of pulmonary disease, pulmonary disease with hilar adenopathy, and hilar adenopathy disease in infants, children, and adolescents when resistance to isoniazid, rifampin, or pyrazinamide is not suspected on the basis of exposure history or when favorable

Table 155.2
Regimens and Dosages Used in Pediatric Patients With TB Infection

Agent(s)	Dose and Age-group	Administration	Duration, mo	Age Restriction	Comments
Isoniazid + rifapentine (3HP)	**Age ≥12 y** Isoniazid: 15 mg/kg, rounded up to nearest 50 or 100 mg (max 900 mg) Rifapentine (by weight): 10–14 kg: 300 mg 14.1–25 kg: 450 mg 25.1–32 kg: 600 mg 32.1–49.9 kg: 750 mg ≥50.0 kg: 900 mg **Age 2–11 y** Isoniazid: 25 mg/kg, rounded up to nearest 50 or 100 mg (max 900 mg) Rifapentine: See above.	Weekly (SAT or DOT)	3	Not for children <2 y	Take with food, containing fat if possible; pyridoxine for selected patients.[a]
Rifampin (4R)	**Adult:** 10 mg/kg (max 600 mg) **Child:** 15–20 mg/kg (max 600 mg)	Daily (SAT)	4	None	Drug-drug interactions
Isoniazid + rifampin	Same doses as when drugs are used individually	Daily (SAT)	3	None	Not considered unless 3HP or 4R is not feasible
Isoniazid	**Adult:** 5 mg/kg (max dose 300 mg) **Child:** 10–15 mg/kg (max 300 mg)	Daily (SAT)	6 or 9	None	Seizures with overdose; pyridoxine for selected patients[a]
	Adult: 15 mg/kg (max dose 900 mg) **Child:** 20–30 mg/kg (max 900 mg)	Twice weekly (DOT)			

DOT indicates directly observed therapy; max, maximum; SAT, self-administrated therapy; TB, tuberculosis; and TBI, TB infection.

[a] For exclusively breastfed infants and for children and adolescents on meat- and milk-deficient diets; children with nutritional deficiencies, including all symptomatic children living with HIV infection; and pregnant adolescents and women.

Adapted from Nolt D, Starke JR; American Academy of Pediatrics Committee on Infectious Diseases. Tuberculosis infection in children: testing and treatment. *Pediatrics*. 2021;148(6):e2021054663.

Table 155.3
Drugs for Treatment of Drug-Susceptible TB Disease in Infants, Children, and Adolescents

Drugs	Dosage Forms	Daily Dosage (Range), mg/kg	Three Times per Week Dosage, mg/kg/dose	Maximum Dose	Most Common Adverse Reactions
Ethambutol	Tablets 100 mg 400 mg	20 (15–25)	50	Daily, 1 g Twice a week, 2.5 g	Optic neuritis (usually reversible), decreased red-green color discrimination, gastrointestinal tract disturbances, hypersensitivity
Isoniazid[a]	Scored tablets 100 mg	10 (10–15)[b]	20–30	Daily, 300 mg	Mild hepatic enzyme elevation, hepatitis,[b] peripheral neuritis, hypersensitivity
	300 mg			Twice a week, 900 mg	
Pyrazinamide[a]	Scored tablets, 500 mg	35 (30–40)	50	2 g	Hepatotoxic effects, hyperuricemia, arthralgia, gastrointestinal tract upset, pruritus, rash
Rifampin[a]	Capsules 150 mg 300 mg Syrup-formulated capsules	15–20[c]	15–20[c]	600 mg	Orange discoloration of secretions or urine, staining of contact lenses, vomiting, hepatitis, influenzalike reaction, thrombocytopenia, pruritus; oral contraceptives may be ineffective.

TB indicates tuberculosis.

[a] Rifamate is a capsule containing 150 mg of isoniazid and 300 mg of rifampin. Two capsules provide the usual adult (>50 kg) daily doses of each drug. Rifater, in the United States, is a capsule containing 50 mg of isoniazid, 120 mg of rifampin, and 300 mg of pyrazinamide. Isoniazid and rifampin are also available for parenteral administration.
[b] When isoniazid in a dosage exceeding 10 mg/kg/day is used in combination with rifampin, the incidence of hepatotoxic effects may be increased.
[c] Many experts recommend using a daily rifampin dose of 20–30 mg/kg/day for infants and toddlers and for serious forms of TB, such as meningitis and disseminated disease.

Table 155.4
Drugs for Treatment of Drug-Resistant TB Disease in Infants, Children, and Adolescents[a]

Drugs	Dosage, Forms	Daily Dosage	Maximum Dose	Adverse Reactions
Amikacin[b,c]	Vials 500 mg 1 g	15–30 mg/kg (IV or IM administration)	1 g	Auditory and vestibular toxic effects, nephrotoxic effects
Bedaquiline[d]	Tablets, 100 mg	Children ≥12 y: 400 mg daily for first 2 wk, then 200 mg 3 times/wk with 48 h between doses for wk 3–24	400 mg	Arthralgia, nausea, abdominal pain, headache; can prolong QTc interval, can elevate hepatic enzymes
Capreomycin[c]	Vials, 1 g	15–30 mg/kg (IM administration)	1 g	Auditory and vestibular toxicity and nephrotoxic effects
Cycloserine	Capsules, 250 mg	10–20 mg/kg, given in 2 divided doses	1 g	Psychosis, personality changes, seizures, rash
Ethionamide	Tablets, 250 mg	15–20 mg/kg, given in 2–3 divided doses	1 g	Gastrointestinal tract disturbances, hepatotoxic effects, hypersensitivity reactions, hypothyroidism
Kanamycin[b,c]	Vials 75 mg/2 mL 500 mg/2 mL 1 g/3 mL	15–30 mg/kg (IM or IV administration)	1 g	Auditory and vestibular toxic effects, nephrotoxic effects
Levofloxacin[b,e]	Tablets 250 mg 500 mg 750 mg Oral solution, 25 mg/mL	Adults: 750–1,000 mg (once daily) Children: 15–20 mg/kg	1 g	Hypersensitivity reactions; theoretical effect on growing cartilage, tendonitis, gastrointestinal tract disturbances, cardiac disturbances, peripheral neuropathy, rash, headache, restlessness, confusion; can prolong QTc interval
Linezolid[b,f]	Vials 5 mg/mL 25 mg/mL	Adults: 600 mg (once daily) Children <10 y: 10 mg/kg/dose, every 12 h Children ≥10 y: 10 mg/kg/dose daily	600 mg	Used for treatment of MDR TB; adverse events include bone marrow suppression.

(continues)

Table 155.4 (continued)

Drugs	Dosage, Forms	Daily Dosage	Maximum Dose	Adverse Reactions
Moxifloxacin[b,e]	Tablet, 400 mg IV, 400 mg/250 mL	Adults: 400 mg (once daily) Children: 10 mg/kg (once daily)	400 mg	Hypersensitivity reactions; theoretical effect on growing cartilage; tendonitis, gastrointestinal tract disturbances, cardiac disturbances, peripheral neuropathy, rash, headache, restlessness, confusion; can prolong QTc interval
Para-aminosalicylic acid	Packets, 3 g	200–300 mg/kg (2–4 times a day)	10 g	Gastrointestinal tract disturbances, hypersensitivity, hepatotoxic effects, hypothyroidism
Streptomycin[c]	Vials 1 g 4 g	20–40 mg/kg (IM administration)	1 g	Auditory and vestibular toxic effects, nephrotoxic effects and rash

FDA indicates US Food and Drug Administration; IM, intramuscular; IV, intravenous; MDR, multidrug-resistant; and TB, tuberculosis.

[a] These drugs should be used in consultation with a specialist in TB.
[b] These drugs do not have an indication from the FDA for treatment of TB.
[c] Dose adjustment in renal insufficiency; capreomycin and kanamycin are not approved for use in children <18 years. It has been used for children ≥12 years and ≥30 kg together with 4 other drugs for which the patient's MDR TB isolate is likely to be susceptible; safety and efficacy have not been established in children <12 years. Use with caution in end-stage renal impairment.
[d] Bedaquiline is not FDA approved for use in children <18 years. It has been used for children ≥12 years and ≥30 kg together with 4 other drugs for which the patient's MDR TB isolate is likely to be susceptible; safety and efficacy have not been established in children <12 years. Use with caution in end-stage renal impairment.
[e] Levofloxacin and moxifloxacin are not approved for use in children <18 years; their use in younger children necessitates assessment of the potential risks and benefits.
[f] Linezolid pharmacokinetics have not been well established in children. The doses listed yield a drug exposure approximately equal to that in adults taking 600 mg daily.

Box 155.4
People With Increased Risk for Drug-Resistant Tuberculosis (DR TB) Infection or Disease[a]

- People with a history of treatment of TB disease (or whose source case for the contact received such treatment)
- Contacts of a patient with contagious DR TB disease
- People from countries with high prevalence of DR TB, such as Russia and certain nations of the former Soviet Union, Asia, Africa, and Latin America
- Infected people whose source person has positive smears for acid-fast bacilli or cultures after 2 months of appropriate antituberculosis therapy and patients who do not respond to a standard treatment regimen
- Residence in geographic area with a high percentage of drug-resistant isolates

[a] See **wwwnc.cdc.gov/travel/page/yellowbook-home**.

drug-susceptibility results are available from the patient or the likely source person. If the chest radiograph shows one or more pulmonary cavities and/or the sputum culture result remains positive after 2 months of therapy, the duration of therapy should be extended to at least 9 months. Some experts administer 3 drugs (isoniazid, rifampin, and pyrazinamide) as the initial regimen if a presumed source person has been identified with known pan-susceptible *M tuberculosis* or has no risk factors for drug-resistant *M tuberculosis*. For children with only hilar adenopathy in whom drug resistance is not a consideration, a 6-month regimen of only isoniazid and rifampin is considered adequate by some experts.

In the 6-month regimen with 4-drug RIPE therapy, drugs are administered once a day for at least the first 2 weeks by DOT at least 5 days per week. An alternative to daily dosing between 2 weeks and 2 months of treatment is to administer these drugs 3 times a week by DOT (except in people living with HIV, in whom intermittent dosing is not recommended). After the initial 2-month period, a DOT regimen of isoniazid and rifampin is usually given daily or 3 times a week, although 2 times a week is acceptable. Several alternative regimens with differing durations of daily therapy and total therapy have been used successfully in adults and children. These alternative regimens should be prescribed and managed by a specialist in pediatric TB.

Therapy for Drug-Resistant Pulmonary TB Disease

Consultation with an expert in treating drug-resistant TB is strongly recommended when DR TB is suspected or occurs. Drug resistance is more common in certain groups (see Box 155.4). When resistance to drugs other than isoniazid is likely (see Box 155.4), initial therapy should be adjusted by adding at least 2 drugs to match the presumed drug susceptibility pattern until drug susceptibility results are available. If an isolate from the pediatric patient under treatment is unavailable, drug susceptibilities can be inferred by the drug susceptibility pattern of isolates from the presumed source person. Data for guiding drug selection may not be available for foreign-born children or in circumstances of international travel or adoption. If this information is unavailable, a 4- or 5-drug initial regimen should be strongly considered with close monitoring for clinical response.

Most cases of pulmonary TB in children that are caused by an isoniazid-resistant but rifampin- and pyrazinamide-susceptible strain of *M tuberculosis* complex can be treated with a 6-month regimen of rifampin, pyrazinamide, and ethambutol. If disease is extensive, many experts add a fluoroquinolone to this regimen. For cases of MDR TB disease, the treatment regimen needed for cure should include at least 4 or 5 antituberculosis drugs to which the organism is susceptible. Bedaquiline is approved by the US Food and Drug Administration as part of combination therapy in the treatment of adults with pulmonary MDR TB for whom an effective regimen could not be instituted; many experts recommend its use in children 12 years and older. The profile for delamanid is similar, but this drug is available only under a compassionate use protocol. Therapy for MDR TB is administered for 12 to 24 months from the time of culture conversion to negativity. An injectable drug initially administered 5 days per week, such as amikacin, kanamycin, or capreomycin, is often used for the first 4 to 6 months of treatment, as tolerated; some experts, however, are no longer recommending injectable drugs. Regimens in which drugs are administered intermittently are not recommended for drug-resistant disease (except for aminoglycosides and capreomycin, which are typically intermittent to limit toxicity); daily DOT is critical to prevent emergence of additional resistance. An expert in DR TB should be consulted for all drug-resistant cases.

Extrapulmonary TB Disease

In general, extrapulmonary TB, except for meningitis, can be treated with the same regimens as used for pulmonary TB. For suspected drug-susceptible tuberculous meningitis, daily treatment with isoniazid, rifampin, pyrazinamide, and ethionamide, if possible, or an aminoglycoside (parenteral streptomycin, kanamycin, or amikacin) or capreomycin should be initiated. Many experts add a fluoroquinolone to this initial regimen. When used to treat central nervous system (CNS) TB, rifampin should be given at a dose of 20 to 30 mg/kg/day to ensure adequate CNS penetration (see Table 155.3). When susceptibility to first-line drugs is established, the ethionamide, aminoglycoside (or capreomycin), and/or fluoroquinolone can be discontinued. Pyrazinamide is given for a total of 2 months, and isoniazid and rifampin are given for a total of 6 to 12 months. Isoniazid and rifampin can be given daily or 3 times per week after the first 2 months of treatment if the child has responded well.

Evaluation and Monitoring of Therapy in Children and Adolescents

Careful monthly monitoring of clinical and bacteriologic responses to therapy is important. With DOT, clinical evaluation is an integral component of each visit for drug administration. For patients with pulmonary TB, chest radiographs are often obtained after 2 months of therapy to evaluate response. After initiation of treatment, alveolar or interstitial infiltrates often start to decrease within 1 to 2 weeks but take much longer to resolve completely. Pleural effusions are slower to resolve and may require drainage for symptom relief; partial reaccumulation is common as an isolated finding but does not indicate treatment failure. Even with successful 6-month regimens, hilar adenopathy can persist for 2 to 3 years; normal radiographic findings are not necessary to discontinue therapy. Follow-up chest radiography beyond termination of successful therapy is not usually necessary unless clinical deterioration occurs.

If therapy has been interrupted, the date of completion should be extended. Although guidelines cannot be provided for every situation, factors to consider when establishing the date of completion include (1) length of interruption of therapy; (2) time during therapy (early or late) when interruption occurred; and (3) the patient's clinical, radiographic, and bacteriologic status before, during, and after interruption of therapy. The total doses administered by DOT should be calculated to guide the duration of therapy. Consultation with a specialist in TB is advised.

Untoward effects of TB therapy, including severe hepatitis in otherwise healthy infants, children, and adolescents, are rare. Routine determination of serum aminotransferase concentrations is not recommended during treatment of TBI or in most cases of TB disease unless the child develops symptoms suggestive of hepatotoxicity. Monthly clinical evaluations to observe for signs or symptoms of hepatitis and other adverse effects of drug therapy without routine monitoring of aminotransferase concentrations is appropriate follow-up. Regular physician-patient contact to assess drug adherence, efficacy, and adverse effects is an important aspect of management. DOT visits are also opportunities for checking on well-being and treatment tolerance. Patients should be provided with written instructions and advised to call a physician immediately if symptoms of adverse events, in particular hepatotoxicity (ie, nausea, vomiting, abdominal pain, jaundice), develop.

Other Treatment Considerations

Corticosteroids

The evidence supporting adjuvant treatment with corticosteroids for children with TB disease is incomplete. Corticosteroids are definitely indicated for children with tuberculous meningitis, because corticosteroids decrease rates of mortality and long-term neurological impairment. Corticosteroids can be considered for children with pleural and pericardial effusions (to hasten reabsorption of fluid), severe miliary disease (to mitigate alveolocapillary block), endobronchial disease (to relieve obstruction and atelectasis), and abdominal TB (to decrease the risk of strictures). Corticosteroids should be given only when accompanied by appropriate antituberculosis drug therapy. Most experts give 2 mg/kg/day of prednisone (maximum, 60 mg/day) or its equivalent for 4 to 6 weeks followed by tapering.

TB Disease and HIV Infection

Most adults living with HIV with drug-susceptible TB respond well to standard treatment regimens. However, optimal therapy for TB in children living with HIV infection has not been established. Treating TB in a child living with HIV infection is complicated by antiretroviral drug interactions with the rifamycins and overlapping toxicities. Therapy should always include at least 4 drugs initially, should be administered daily via DOT, and should be continued for at least 6 months. RIPE should be administered for at least the first 2 months. Ethambutol can be discontinued once DR TB disease is excluded. Rifampin may be contraindicated in people who are receiving antiretroviral therapy (ART). Rifabutin is substituted for rifampin in some circumstances. Consultation with a specialist who has experience in treating patients living with HIV infection with TB is strongly advised. If TB is diagnosed in an HIV-infected individual who is not yet receiving ART, even in the presence of severe immunosuppression, ART can be safely initiated within 2 weeks of antituberculosis therapy, despite the risk of inciting immune reconstitution syndrome.

Immunizations

Patients who are receiving treatment of TB can receive measles and other age-appropriate attenuated live-virus vaccines unless they are receiving high-dose systemic corticosteroids, are severely ill, or have other specific contraindications to immunization.

TB During Pregnancy and Breastfeeding

Pregnant women who have a positive TST or IGRA result, are asymptomatic, have normal chest radiograph findings, and had recent contact with a contagious person should be considered for therapy, which should usually begin after the first trimester. If there has been no recent contact with a contagious person, therapy can be delayed until after delivery. Pyridoxine supplementation is indicated for all pregnant and breastfeeding women receiving isoniazid.

If TB disease is diagnosed during pregnancy, a standard 6-month regimen for drug-susceptible TB is usually initiated; however, 9 months of therapy is indicated if pyrazinamide is not used initially. Prompt initiation of therapy is mandatory to protect mother and fetus.

Isoniazid, ethambutol, and rifampin are believed to be relatively safe for the fetus. The benefit of ethambutol and rifampin for therapy of TB disease in the mother outweighs the risk to the infant. Because aminoglycosides (streptomycin, kanamycin, or amikacin) or capreomycin may cause ototoxic effects in the fetus, they should not be used unless administration is essential for effective treatment. Ethionamide has been demonstrated to be teratogenic, so its use during pregnancy is contraindicated.

Women with TB who have been treated appropriately for 2 or more weeks and who are not considered contagious (smear-negative sputum) may breastfeed. Women with TB disease suspected of being contagious should refrain from breastfeeding and from other close contact with the infant because of potential spread of M tuberculosis through respiratory tract droplets or airborne transmission. However, expressed human milk can be fed to the infant, as long as there is no evidence of TB mastitis, which is rare. Although isoniazid is secreted in human milk, no adverse effects of isoniazid on breastfeeding infants have been demonstrated. Breastfed infants do not require pyridoxine supplementation unless they are receiving isoniazid, but breastfeeding mothers who are taking isoniazid should take pyridoxine. The isoniazid dosage of a breastfed infant whose mother is taking isoniazid does not require adjustment for the small amount of drug in the milk.

Congenital TB

Congenital TB is rare, but in utero infections can occur after maternal bacillemia and have been reported following in vitro fertilization of women from countries with endemic disease in whom infertility was likely related to subclinical maternal genitourinary tract TB.

None of the possible signs of congenital TB, such as fever, tachypnea, lethargy, organomegaly, or pulmonary infiltrates, distinguish it from other systemic infections of the newborn. The prognosis is poor without prompt treatment. If a newborn is suspected of having congenital TB, a TST and an IGRA, chest radiography, an LP, and appropriate cultures and radiography should be performed promptly. The TST result is usually negative in newborns with congenital or perinatally acquired infection; IGRA sensitivity in this context is unknown but is likely to be low. Regardless of the TST or IGRA results, treatment of the infant should be initiated promptly with rifampin, isoniazid, pyrazinamide, and either ethambutol (RIPE) or an aminoglycoside (streptomycin, kanamycin, or amikacin) or capreomycin. If meningitis is confirmed, corticosteroids should be added. The placenta should be examined histologically for granulomata and AFB, and a specimen should be cultured for *M tuberculosis* complex. The mother should be evaluated for presence of pulmonary or extrapulmonary disease, including genitourinary TB. HIV testing of the mother is essential.

Treatment of the Newborn Whose Mother Has TBI or TB Disease

Treatment of the newborn is based on categorization of the maternal infection. Although protection of the infant from exposure and infection is of paramount importance, contact between infant and mother should be allowed when possible. Differing circumstances and resulting recommendations are as follows:

- **Mother has a positive TST or IGRA result and normal chest radiographic findings.** If the mother is asymptomatic, no separation is required. The mother is usually a candidate for treatment of TBI after the initial postpartum period. The newborn needs no special evaluation or therapy. Because of the young infant's exquisite susceptibility and because the mother's positive TST or IGRA result could be a marker of an unrecognized case of contagious TB within the household, other household members should be questioned about having symptoms of TB and undergo a TST or an IGRA and further evaluation; this should not delay the infant's discharge from the hospital. These mothers can breastfeed their infants.

- **Mother has clinical signs and symptoms or abnormal findings on chest radiograph consistent with TB disease.** Cases of suspected or proven TB disease in mothers should be reported immediately to the local health department, and evaluation of all household members should be initiated as soon as possible. If the mother has TB disease, the infant should be evaluated for congenital TB, and the mother should be tested for HIV infection. The mother and the infant should be separated until the mother has been evaluated and, if TB disease is suspected, until the mother and infant are receiving appropriate antituberculosis therapy, the mother wears a mask, and the mother understands and is willing to adhere to infection-control measures. Women with TB who have been treated appropriately for 2 or more weeks and who are not considered contagious (smear-negative sputum) may breastfeed; women with TB disease suspected of being contagious should refrain from breastfeeding and from other close contact with the infant because of potential spread of *M tuberculosis* through respiratory tract droplets or airborne transmission. During separation, expressed human milk can be fed to the infant unless the mother has signs of tuberculous mastitis, which is rare. Once the infant is receiving isoniazid, separation is not necessary unless the mother has possible isoniazid-resistant TB disease or has poor adherence to treatment and DOT is not possible. If the mother is suspected of having isoniazid-resistant TB disease, an expert in TB disease management should be consulted.

- **Mother has a positive TST or IGRA result and abnormal findings on chest radiography but no evidence of TB disease.** If the chest radiograph of the mother appears abnormal but is not suggestive of TB disease and the history, physical examination, and sputum smear indicate no evidence of TB disease, the infant can be assumed to have low risk for *M tuberculosis* infection and need not be separated from the mother. The mother and her infant should receive follow-up care, and the mother should be treated for TBI. Other household members should undergo a TST or an IGRA and further evaluation.

TB Caused by *M Bovis*

Infections with *M bovis* account for approximately 1% to 2% of TB cases in the United States, with higher rates along the border with Mexico. Children who come from countries where *M bovis* is prevalent in cattle or whose parents come from those countries are more likely to be infected. Most infections in humans are transmitted from cattle by unpasteurized milk and its products, such as fresh cheese, although human-to-human transmission by the airborne route has been documented. In children, *M bovis* more commonly causes cervical lymphadenitis, intestinal TB disease and peritonitis, and meningitis. In adults, *M bovis* infection can progress to advanced pulmonary disease with a risk of transmission to others.

The TST result is typically positive in a person infected with *M bovis*; IGRAs have not been studied systematically for diagnosing *M bovis* infection in particular, but theoretically, they should have acceptable test characteristics. The definitive diagnosis of *M bovis* infection requires an isolate. The commonly used methods for identifying a microbial isolate as *M tuberculosis* complex do not distinguish *M bovis* from *M tuberculosis*, *M africanum*, and BCG, which is a live attenuated vaccine strain of *M bovis*; *M bovis* is suspected in clinical laboratories by its typical resistance to pyrazinamide. This approach can be unreliable, and species confirmation at a reference laboratory should be requested when *M bovis* is suspected. Molecular genotyping through the state health department may assist in identifying *M bovis*. BCG is rarely isolated from pediatric clinical specimens in the United States; however, it should be suspected from localized BCG suppuration or draining lymphadenitis in children who recently (within several months) received BCG vaccine or in infants with selected congenital immunodeficiency syndromes who received a BCG vaccine. Only a reference laboratory can distinguish an isolate of BCG from an isolate of *M bovis*.

Therapy for *M bovis* Disease

Controlled clinical trials for treatment of *M bovis* disease have not been conducted, and treatment recommendations for *M bovis* disease in adults and children are based on results from treatment trials for *M tuberculosis* disease. Although most strains of *M bovis* are pyrazinamide resistant and resistance to other first-line drugs has been reported, MDR strains are rare. Initial therapy for disease caused by *M bovis* should include 3 or 4 drugs, excluding pyrazinamide, that would be used to treat disease attributable to *M tuberculosis*.

For isoniazid- and rifampin-susceptible strains, a total treatment course of at least 9 months is recommended.

Parents should be counseled about the many infectious diseases transmitted by unpasteurized milk and its products, and parents who might import traditional, unpasteurized dairy products from countries where *M bovis* infection is prevalent in cattle should be advised against giving those products to their children. When people are exposed to an adult who has pulmonary disease caused by *M bovis* infection, they should be evaluated by the same methods as for *M tuberculosis*.

ISOLATION OF THE HOSPITALIZED PATIENT

Most children with TB disease, especially children younger than 10 years, are not contagious. Exceptions are (1) children with pulmonary cavities; (2) children with positive sputum AFB smears; (3) children with laryngeal involvement; (4) children with extensive pulmonary infection; or (5) neonates or infants with congenital TB undergoing procedures that involve the oropharyngeal airway (eg, endotracheal intubation). In these instances, airborne infection isolation precautions for TB are indicated until effective therapy has been initiated, sputum smears are negative, and coughing has abated. Additional criteria apply to suspected or known MDR TB.

Children with no cough and smear-negative sputum AFB can be hospitalized in an open ward. Infection prevention measures for hospital personnel and visitors exposed to contagious patients should include the use of personally "fit-tested" and "sealed" N95 particulate respirators for all patient contacts. If they have or are suspected to have DR TB, consultation regarding infection prevention and control should be made with public health authorities.

The major concern in infection control relates to adult household members and contacts who can be the source of infection. Visitation should be limited to people who have been evaluated by symptom screening and chest radiograph and do not have TB.

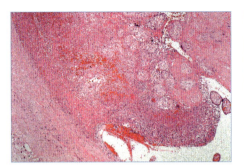

Image 155.1
A photomicrograph showing tuberculosis of the placenta. Although a rare circumstance, mother-to-child transmission of *Mycobacterium tuberculosis* can take place through the blood from different regions of the mother's body or originate from lesions within the placenta, as shown here. Courtesy of Centers for Disease Control and Prevention.

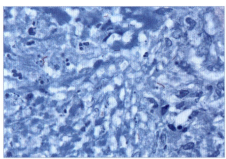

Image 155.2
Histopathologic features of placenta thrombus with inflammatory cells and acid-fast bacilli of *Mycobacterium tuberculosis* (Ziehl-Neelsen stain). Courtesy of Centers for Disease Control and Prevention.

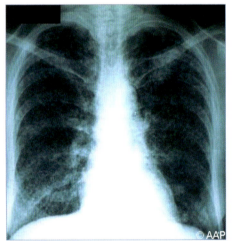

Image 155.3
Tuberculosis, miliary, in a 29-year-old woman 4 months after delivery. Tuberculosis may become exacerbated during pregnancy.

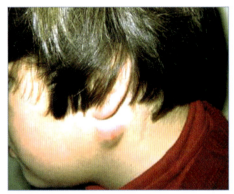

Image 155.4
Young man with *Mycobacterium tuberculosis* cervical lymphadenitis. Copyright Martin G. Myers, MD.

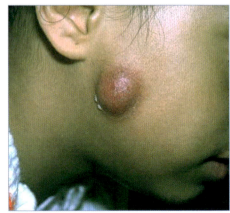

Image 155.5
Young woman with *Mycobacterium tuberculosis* cervical lymphadenitis. Copyright Martin G. Myers, MD.

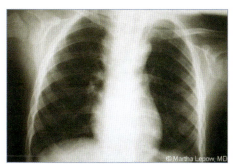

Image 155.6
Mycobacterium tuberculosis infection with paratracheal lymph nodes. Copyright Martha Lepow, MD.

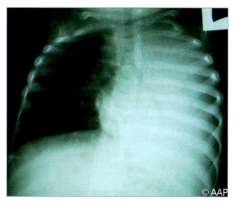

Image 155.7
A 1-year-old with endobronchial tuberculosis with pulmonary consolidation.

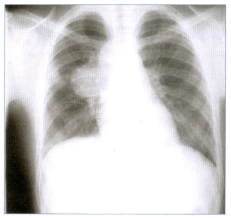

Image 155.8
A 13-year-old boy with tuberculosis. The patient had a 1-week history of shortness of breath and sharp pain on his right side while riding his bicycle. A purified protein derivative revealed 20 × 25 mm of induration at 72 hours. The chest computed tomographic scan revealed right hilar adenopathy and a primary complex in the right peripheral lung field. Copyright Barbara Jantausch, MD, FAAP.

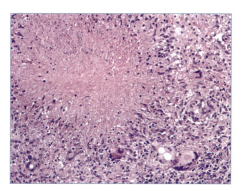

Image 155.9
Tuberculosis. Caseation and Langhans giant cells in a lymph node. Courtesy of Dimitris P. Agamanolis, MD.

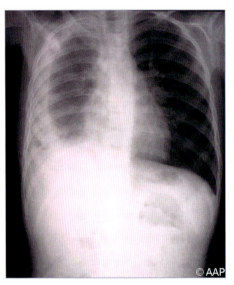

Image 155.10
Pulmonary tuberculosis with right pleural effusion.

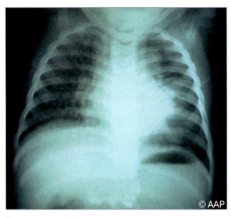

Image 155.11
A 10-month-old with radiographic changes of miliary tuberculosis.

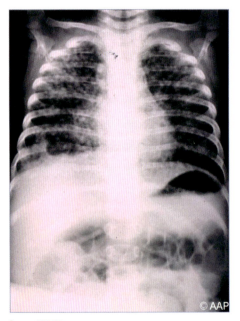

Image 155.12
Miliary tuberculosis with pulmonary cavitation (right lung).

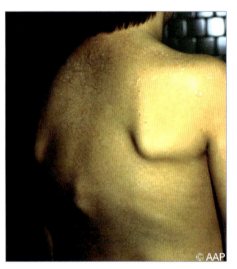

Image 155.13
Tuberculosis of the spine with paravertebral abscess (Pott disease).

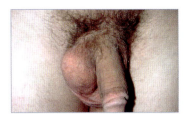

Image 155.14
A 15-year-old boy with tuberculous epididymitis. Copyright Martin G. Myers, MD.

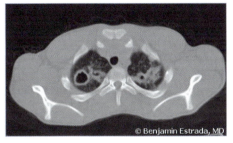

Image 155.16
Cavitary tuberculosis in a 15-year-old boy delineated by computed tomography. Courtesy of Benjamin Estrada, MD.

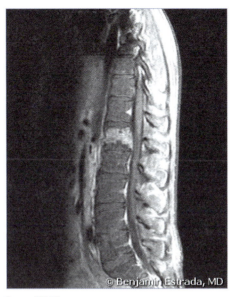

Image 155.15
Tuberculous spondylitis in a 14-year-old boy demonstrated by magnetic resonance imaging. Courtesy of Benjamin Estrada, MD.

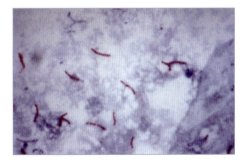

Image 155.17
This photomicrograph reveals *Mycobacterium tuberculosis* bacteria by use of acid-fast Ziehl-Neelsen stain (magnification ×1,000). The acid-fast stains depend on the ability of mycobacteria to retain dye when treated with mineral acid or an acid-alcohol solution, such as the Ziehl-Neelsen or Kinyoun stains that are carbolfuchsin methods specific for *M tuberculosis*. Courtesy of Centers for Disease Control and Prevention.

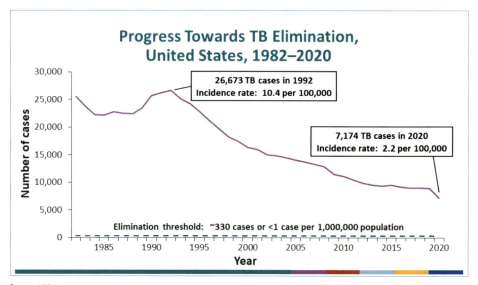

Image 155.18
Progress toward tuberculosis (TB) elimination, United States, 1982–2020. Courtesy of Centers for Disease Control and Prevention.

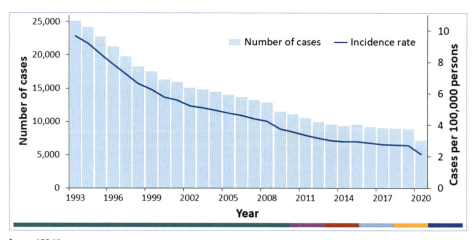

Image 155.19
Tuberculosis (TB) cases and incidence rates, United States, 1993–2020. Courtesy of Centers for Disease Control and Prevention.

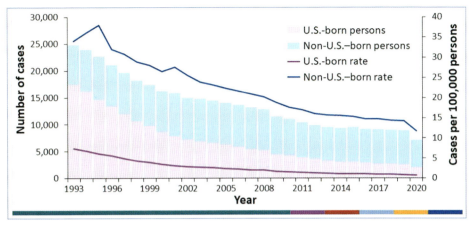

Image 155.20
Tuberculosis (TB) cases and incidence rates by origin of birth, United States, 1993–2020. Courtesy of Centers for Disease Control and Prevention.

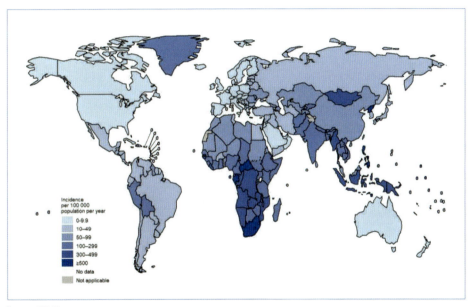

Image 155.21
Estimated tuberculosis incidence rates of 2020. Courtesy of World Health Organization.

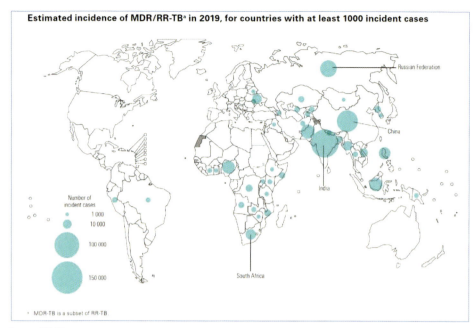

Image 155.22
Estimated incidence of multidrug-resistant (MDR)/rifampicin-resistant (RR) tuberculosis (TB) in 2019. Courtesy of World Health Organization.

CHAPTER 156

Nontuberculous Mycobacteria

(Environmental *Mycobacteria*, *Mycobacteria* other than *Mycobacterium tuberculosis*)

CLINICAL MANIFESTATIONS

Several syndromes are caused by nontuberculous mycobacteria (NTM).

- In children, the most common of these syndromes is cervical lymphadenitis.

- Cutaneous infection may follow soil- or water-contaminated traumatic wounds, surgeries, or cosmetic procedures (eg, tattoos, pedicures, body piercings).

- Less common syndromes include skin and soft tissue infection, osteomyelitis, otitis media, central catheter–associated bloodstream infections, and pulmonary infections, especially in adolescents with cystic fibrosis (CF).

- NTM, especially *Mycobacterium avium* complex (MAC [including *M avium* and *Mycobacterium avium-intracellulare*]) and *Mycobacterium abscessus*, can be recovered from sputum in 10% to 20% of adolescents and young adults with CF and can be associated with fever and declining clinical status.

- Disseminated infections are almost always associated with impaired cell-mediated immunity, as found in children with congenital immune defects (eg, interleukin-12 deficiency, JAK-STAT cytokine pathways abnormalities, NF-κB essential modulator mutation and related disorders, and interferon-gamma receptor defects), hematopoietic stem cell transplants, or advanced HIV infection. Disseminated NTM infection, most commonly MAC, is rare in children living with HIV during the first year after birth. The frequency of disseminated MAC increases with increasing age and declining $CD4^+$ T-lymphocyte counts, typically less than 50/µL, in children 6 years or older. Manifestations of disseminated NTM infections depend on the species and route of infection and include fever, night sweats, weight loss, abdominal pain, fatigue, diarrhea, and anemia. These signs and symptoms are also found in advanced immunosuppressed children living with HIV infection without disseminated MAC. For children living with HIV infection with disseminated MAC, respiratory symptoms and isolated pulmonary disease are uncommon. In patients living with HIV infection who develop immune restoration with initiation of combination antiretroviral therapy (ART), local NTM symptoms can worsen temporarily. This immune reconstitution syndrome usually occurs 2 to 4 weeks after initiation of ART. Symptoms can include worsening fever, swollen lymph nodes, local pain, and laboratory abnormalities.

ETIOLOGY

Of the close to 200 species of NTM that have been identified, only a few cause most human infections. The species most commonly infecting children in the United States are MAC, *Mycobacterium fortuitum, M abscessus,* and *Mycobacterium marinum* (Table 156.1). Several new species, which can be detected by nucleic acid amplification testing but cannot be grown by routine culture methods, have been identified in lymph nodes of children with cervical adenitis. NTM disease in patients living with HIV infection is usually caused by MAC. *M fortuitum, Mycobacterium chelonae, Mycobacterium smegmatis,* and *M abscessus* are commonly referred to as "rapidly growing" mycobacteria, because sufficient growth and identification can be achieved in the laboratory within 3 to 7 days on solid media, whereas MAC, *M marinum, Mycobacterium szulgai,* and most other NTM usually require several weeks before sufficient growth occurs for identification and are referred to as "slowly growing" mycobacteria. Rapidly growing mycobacteria have been implicated most often in wound, soft tissue, bone, pulmonary, central venous catheter, and middle-ear infections. Other mycobacterial species that are usually nonpathogenic have caused infections in immunocompromised hosts or have been associated with the presence of a foreign body.

EPIDEMIOLOGY

Many NTM species are ubiquitous in nature, being found in soil, food, water, and animals. Tap water is the major reservoir for *Mycobacterium kansasii, Mycobacterium lentiflavum, Mycobacterium*

Table 156.1
Diseases Caused by Nontuberculous *Mycobacterium* Species

Clinical Disease	Species
Cutaneous infection	Mycobacterium marinum Mycobacterium chelonae Mycobacterium fortuitum Mycobacterium abscessus Mycobacterium ulcerans[a]
Lymphadenitis	MAC Mycobacterium haemophilum Mycobacterium lentiflavum Mycobacterium kansasii M fortuitum M abscessus Mycobacterium malmoense[b]
Otologic infection	M abscessus M fortuitum
Pulmonary infection	MAC M kansasii M abscessus Mycobacterium xenopi M malmoense[b] Mycobacterium szulgai M fortuitum Mycobacterium simiae
Catheter-associated infection	M chelonae M fortuitum M abscessus
Prosthetic valve endocarditis	M chelonae M fortuitum Mycobacterium chimaera
Skeletal infection	MAC M kansasii M fortuitum M chelonae M marinum M abscessus M ulcerans[a]
Disseminated	MAC M kansasii Mycobacterium genavense M haemophilum M chelonae

MAC indicates *Mycobacterium avium* complex.
[a] Not endemic in the United States.
[b] Found primarily in northern Europe.

xenopi, Mycobacterium simiae, and health care–associated infections attributable to *M abscessus* and *M fortuitum*. Outbreaks have been associated with contaminated water used for acupuncture and pedicures and inks used for tattooing. Health care–associated outbreaks have occurred among children undergoing pulpotomy or other dental procedures associated with improperly maintained dental unit water lines. Outbreaks of otitis media caused by *M abscessus* have been associated with polyethylene ear tubes and use of contaminated equipment or water. Health care–associated outbreaks of *M chelonae* have been associated with use of commercial-grade misting humidifiers and nonsterile ice for invasive procedures. For *M marinum*, water in a fish tank or an aquarium or an injury in a saltwater environment are the major sources of infection. A waterborne route of transmission has been implicated for MAC infection in some immunocompromised hosts.

An international outbreak of *Mycobacterium chimaera* infection (including prosthetic valve endocarditis, vascular graft infection, and disseminated infection) was associated with heater-cooler devices used in heart surgery requiring cardiopulmonary bypass and was likely attributable to aerosolization of *M chimaera* from contaminated devices. Clinical manifestation was indolent and included fever, myalgia, arthralgia, fatigue, and weight loss, with diagnosis in patients occurring up to several years after exposure.

Although many people are exposed to NTM, it is unknown why some exposures result in acute or chronic infection. Usual portals of entry for NTM infection are believed to be abrasions in the skin, such as cutaneous lesions caused by *M marinum*; penetrating trauma, such as needles and organic material most often associated with *M abscessus* and *M fortuitum*; surgical sites, especially for cosmetic surgery and central vascular or peritoneal dialysis catheters; oropharyngeal mucosa, which is the presumed portal of entry for cervical lymphadenitis; tooth eruption, which is the presumed portal of entry for submandibular lymphadenitis; gastrointestinal or respiratory tract, for disseminated MAC; and respiratory tract, including tympanostomy tubes for otitis media. Pulmonary disease and rare cases of mediastinal adenitis and endobronchial disease occur. NTM are important pathogens in patients with CF and are emerging pathogens in individuals receiving biologic response modifiers, such as antitumor necrosis factor-α agents. Most infections remain localized at the portal of entry or in regional lymph nodes. Dissemination to distal sites occurs primarily in severely immunocompromised hosts.

No definitive evidence of person-to-person transmission of NTM exists outside of reports of possible occurrence in CF clinics.

Buruli ulcer disease is a skin and bone infection caused by *Mycobacterium ulcerans*, an emerging disease causing significant morbidity and disability in tropical areas such as Africa, Asia, South America, Australia, and the western Pacific.

The **incubation periods** are variable.

DIAGNOSTIC TESTS

Routine screening of respiratory or gastrointestinal tract specimens for MAC microorganisms is not recommended. Definitive diagnosis of NTM disease requires isolation of the organism. Consultation with the laboratory should occur to ensure that cultures and other specimens are handled correctly. For example, isolation of *Mycobacterium haemophilum* requires that the culture be maintained at 30 °C (86 °F) and that heme-containing medium is added for isolation. Because NTM are commonly found in the environment, contamination of cultures or transient colonization can occur. Caution must be exercised in interpretation of cultures obtained from nonsterile sites, such as gastric-washing specimens, endoscopy material, a single expectorated sputum sample, or urine specimens, and when the species cultured is usually nonpathogenic (eg, *Mycobacterium terrae* complex, *Mycobacterium gordonae*). An acid-fast bacilli smear-positive sample and repeated isolation on culture media of a single species from any site are more likely to indicate disease than culture contamination or transient colonization. Diagnostic criteria for NTM lung disease in adults include 2 or more separate sputum samples or 1 bronchial alveolar lavage specimen that grows NTM. These criteria have not been validated in children and apply best to MAC, *M kansasii*, and *M abscessus*. NTM isolates from draining sinus tracts or wounds are almost always significant clinically. Recovery of NTM from sites that are usually sterile, such as cerebrospinal fluid, pleural fluid, bone marrow, blood, lymph node aspirates, middle-ear or mastoid aspirates, or surgically excised tissue, is very likely to be significant. However, rare instances of sample or laboratory contamination leading to a false-positive culture result have been reported. With radiometric or nonradiometric broth techniques, blood cultures are highly sensitive in recovery of MAC and other bloodborne NTM species. If disseminated MAC disease is confirmed, the patient should be evaluated to identify an underlying immunodeficiency condition. Polymerase chain reaction–based assays for some NTM have been developed but are not yet widely available in commercial diagnostic laboratories.

Patients with NTM infection such as *M marinum*, *M kansasii*, or MAC cervical lymphadenitis can have a positive tuberculin skin test (TST) result, because the purified protein derivative preparation, derived from *Mycobacterium tuberculosis*, shares a number of antigens with these NTM species. These TST reactions usually measure less than 10 mm of induration but can measure more than 15 mm. The interferon-gamma release assays use 2 or 3 antigens specific to *M tuberculosis* complex and result in less cross-reactivity from *M avium-intracellulare* and most other NTM species than that of TST. However, cross-reactions can occur with infection caused by *M kansasii*, *M marinum*, and *M szulgai*.

TREATMENT

Many NTM are relatively resistant in vitro to antituberculosis drugs, but this does not necessarily correlate with clinical response, especially with MAC infections. Only limited controlled trials of drug treatment have been performed in adults with NTM infections. The approach to initial therapy should be directed by (1) the species causing the infection; (2) the results of drug-susceptibility testing, especially to macrolides; (3) the site(s) of infection; (4) the patient's immune status; and (5) the need to treat a patient presumptively for tuberculosis while awaiting culture reports that subsequently reveal NTM.

For NTM lymphadenitis in otherwise healthy children, especially when the disease is caused by MAC, complete surgical excision is curative and limits scar formation. Therapy with clarithromycin or azithromycin combined with ethambutol and/or rifampin or rifabutin may be beneficial for children in whom surgical excision is not possible or is incomplete and for children who have recurrent disease (Table 156.2), although published reports of antimicrobial therapy without surgical incision have shown variable success rates. The natural history of NTM lymphadenitis without curative surgical excision is slow resolution but with a high risk of spontaneous drainage through the skin and resulting scarring, even when antimicrobial management is used. Joint decision-making with the parent(s) and possibly the child, depending on age, and the surgeon is important in developing the best treatment plan for each patient.

The choice of drugs, dosages, and duration should be reviewed with a consultant experienced in the management of NTM infections but always includes 2 or more drugs (Table 156.2). Indwelling foreign bodies must be removed, and surgical debridement for serious localized disease is optimal. Clinical isolates of MAC are usually resistant to many of the approved antituberculosis drugs, including isoniazid, but are generally susceptible to clarithromycin and azithromycin and are often susceptible to combinations of ethambutol, rifabutin or rifampin, and amikacin or streptomycin. Secondary agents include moxifloxacin and linezolid. Susceptibility testing to these other agents has not been standardized and, thus, is not recommended routinely. Isolates of rapidly growing mycobacteria (*M fortuitum*, *M abscessus*, and *M chelonae*) should be tested in vitro against drugs to which they are commonly susceptible and drugs that have been used with some therapeutic success (eg, amikacin, imipenem, sulfamethoxazole or trimethoprim-sulfamethoxazole, cefoxitin, ciprofloxacin, clarithromycin, linezolid, clofazimine, doxycycline, and tigecycline).

The duration of therapy for NTM infections depends on host status, site(s) of involvement, and severity. Patients receiving therapy should be monitored. Patients receiving clarithromycin plus rifabutin or high-dose rifabutin (with another drug) should be observed for the rifabutin-related development of leukopenia, uveitis, polyarthralgia, and pseudojaundice.

Most patients who respond ultimately show substantial clinical improvement in the first 4 to 6 weeks of therapy. Elimination of the organisms

Table 156.2
Treatment of Nontuberculous Mycobacteria Infections in Children[a]

Organism	Disease	Initial Treatment
Slowly Growing Species		
Mycobacterium avium complex; Mycobacterium haemophilum; Mycobacterium lentiflavum	Lymphadenitis	Complete excision of lymph nodes; if excision is incomplete or disease recurs, clarithromycin or azithromycin plus ethambutol and/or rifampin (or rifabutin)
	Pulmonary infection	Clarithromycin or azithromycin plus ethambutol with rifampin or rifabutin (pulmonary resection in some patients whose drug therapy fails). For severe disease, an initial course of amikacin or streptomycin is often included. Clinical data in adults with mild to moderate disease support that 3-times-weekly therapy is as effective as daily therapy, with less toxicity. For patients with advanced or cavitary disease, drugs should be given daily.
Mycobacterium chimaera	Prosthetic valve endocarditis	Valve removal, prolonged antimicrobial therapy based on susceptibility testing
	Disseminated	See text.
Mycobacterium kansasii	Pulmonary infection	Rifampin plus ethambutol with isoniazid daily. If rifampin resistance is detected, a 3-drug regimen based on drug susceptibility testing should be used.
	Osteomyelitis	Surgical debridement and prolonged antimicrobial therapy by using rifampin plus ethambutol with isoniazid
Mycobacterium marinum	Cutaneous infection	None, if minor; rifampin, TMP-SMX, clarithromycin, or doxycycline[b] for moderate disease; extensive lesions may require surgical debridement. Susceptibility testing not routinely required.
Mycobacterium ulcerans	Cutaneous and bone infections	Daily intramuscular streptomycin and oral rifampin for 8 weeks; excision to remove necrotic tissue, if present; potential response to thermotherapy
Rapidly Growing Species		
Mycobacterium fortuitum group	Cutaneous infection	Initial therapy for serious disease is amikacin plus meropenem, IV, followed by clarithromycin, doxycycline[b] or TMP-SMX, or ciprofloxacin, orally, on the basis of in vitro susceptibility testing; may require surgical excision. Up to 50% of isolates are resistant to cefoxitin.
	Catheter infection	Catheter removal and amikacin plus meropenem, IV; clarithromycin, TMP-SMX, or ciprofloxacin, orally, on the basis of in vitro susceptibility testing
Mycobacterium abscessus	Otitis media; cutaneous infection	There is no reliable antimicrobial regimen because of variability in drug susceptibility. Clarithromycin plus initial course of amikacin plus cefoxitin or imipenem/meropenem; may require surgical debridement on the basis of in vitro susceptibility testing (50% are amikacin resistant).
	Pulmonary infection (in cystic fibrosis)	Serious disease, clarithromycin, amikacin, and cefoxitin or imipenem-meropenem on the basis of susceptibility testing; most isolates have very low minimum inhibitory concentrations to tigecycline; may require surgical resection.

(continues)

Table 156.2 (continued)

Organism	Disease	Initial Treatment
Rapidly Growing Species (continued)		
Mycobacterium chelonae	Catheter infection, prosthetic valve endocarditis	Catheter removal; debridement, removal of foreign material; valve replacement; and tobramycin (initially) plus clarithromycin, meropenem, and linezolid
	Disseminated cutaneous infection	Tobramycin and meropenem or linezolid (initially) plus clarithromycin

IV indicates intravenously; SMX, sulfamethoxazole; and TMP, trimethoprim.
[a] Treatment always includes ≥2 drugs.
[b] Doxycycline can be used for short durations (ie, ≤21 days) without regard to patient age but for longer treatment durations is not recommended for children <8 years. Only 50% of isolates of M marinum are susceptible to doxycycline.

from blood cultures can take longer, often up to 12 weeks. Most experts recommend a minimum treatment duration of 3 to 6 months or longer.

For patients with CF and isolation of MAC species, treatment is suggested only for those with clinical symptoms not attributable to other causes, worsening lung function, and chest radiographic progression. The decision to embark on therapy should include consideration of susceptibility testing results and should involve consultation with a specialist in CF care.

In patients living with HIV infection and in other immunocompromised people with disseminated MAC infection, multidrug therapy is recommended. Treatment of disseminated MAC infection should be undertaken in consultation with an expert because the infections are life threatening and drug-drug interactions may occur between medications used to treat disseminated MAC and HIV infections.

The optimal time to initiate ART in a child in whom HIV infection and disseminated MAC are newly diagnosed is not established. Many experts provide treatment of disseminated MAC for 2 weeks before initiating ART in an attempt to minimize occurrence of the immune reconstitution syndrome and minimize confusion relating to the cause of drug-associated toxicity.

Chemoprophylaxis

The most effective way to prevent disseminated MAC in children living with HIV infection is to preserve their immune function through use of combination ART. Children living with HIV infection who have advanced immunosuppression should be offered prophylaxis against disseminated MAC with azithromycin or clarithromycin on the basis of their $CD4^+$ T-lymphocyte counts, provided disseminated MAC has been excluded by 3 negative blood cultures in acid-fast bacilli–specific blood culture bottles. Combination therapy for prophylaxis should be avoided in children, if possible, because it has not been shown to be cost effective and increases rates of adverse events. Children with a history of disseminated MAC and continued immunosuppression should receive lifelong prophylaxis to prevent recurrence.

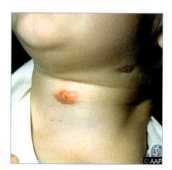

Image 156.1
Atypical mycobacterial tuberculous infection (lymphadenitis) with ulceration.

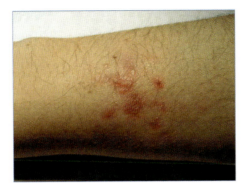

Image 156.2
Skin and soft tissue infections caused by nontuberculous mycobacteria (NTM) usually occur after traumatic injury, surgery, or cosmetic procedures, which may expose a wound to soil, water, or medical devices occasionally contaminated with environmental mycobacteria. Although the epidemiological factors and clinical manifestations of NTM responsible for skin and soft tissue infections differ, some species (*Mycobacterium avium* complex, *Mycobacterium kansasii, Mycobacterium xenopi,* and *Mycobacterium marinum*) have been reported worldwide, whereas others (*Mycobacterium ulcerans*) have limited geographic distribution. This figure shows *M marinum* infection of the arm of a fish-tank worker. *M marinum* causes diseases in many fish species and is distributed worldwide. It is an opportunistic pathogen of humans, in whom infection is infrequent and occurs by direct injury from fish fins or bites or after cutaneous trauma and subsequent exposure to contaminated water or other sources of infection (shrimp, shellfish, frogs, turtles, dolphin, eels, and oysters). Courtesy of Centers for Disease Control and Prevention/*Emerging Infectious Diseases*.

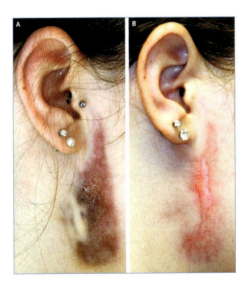

Image 156.3
An 18-year-old young woman presented with a large, fluctuant, violaceous plaque on her right cheek (A). Her right tragus had been professionally pierced 6 months earlier, and streaking had developed along the angle of her jaw 1 month after the piercing. A biopsy specimen showed granulomatous inflammation. The tissue culture grew *Mycobacterium fortuitum*. Copyright *New England Journal of Medicine*.

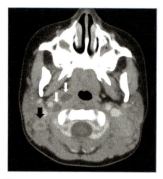

Image 156.4
Computed tomographic scan of the neck of a 3-year-old girl showing right lateral retropharyngeal abscess (white arrows) and enlarged bilateral posterior cervical lymph nodes with low attenuation of a right cervical lymph node (black arrow), consistent with atypical mycobacterium adenitis. Courtesy of *Emerging Infectious Diseases*.

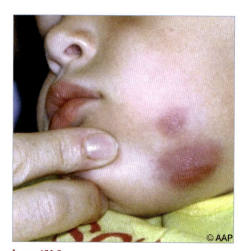

Image 156.5
Atypical mycobacterial tuberculosis (lymphadenitis) with ulceration.

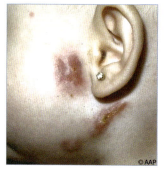

Image 156.6
Atypical mycobacterial lymphadenitis.

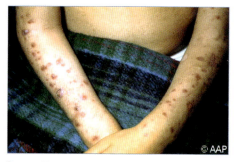

Image 156.7
Disseminated atypical mycobacterial tuberculosis with generalized cutaneous lesions in a boy with acute lymphoblastic leukemia in remission.

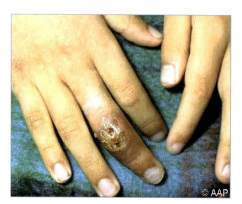

Image 156.8
The same patient as in Image 156.7 with atypical mycobacterial tuberculosis osteomyelitis of the right middle finger.

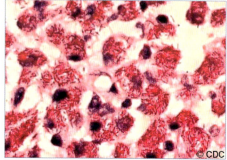

Image 156.9
Mycobacterium avium intracellulare infection of the lymph node in a patient with AIDS (Ziehl-Neelsen stain). Courtesy of Centers for Disease Control and Prevention.

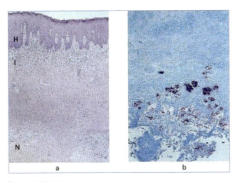

Image 156.10
a, Hematoxylin-eosin stain of a lesion specimen showing definitive Buruli ulcer disease in the pre-ulcerative stage (original magnification ×50). Notice the psoriasiform epidermal hyperplasia (H), superficial dermal lichenoid inflammatory infiltrate (I), and necrosis of subcutaneous tissues (N). b, Ziehl-Neelsen stain of the same nodule, showing abundant colonies of acid-fast bacilli in the necrotic subcutaneous tissues (original magnification ×100). Courtesy of *Emerging Infectious Diseases*.

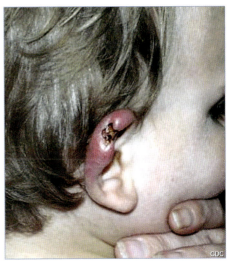

Image 156.11
An 18-month-old with culture- and polymerase chain reaction–confirmed Buruli ulcer of the right ear. She had briefly visited St Leonards, Australia. The initial lesion resembled a mosquito or another insect bite. Courtesy of Centers for Disease Control and Prevention/*Emerging Infectious Diseases* and Paul D. R. Johnson.

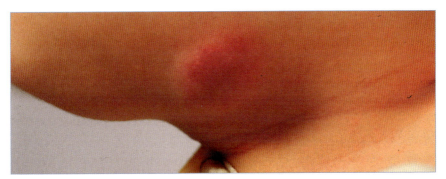

Image 156.12
A 2-year-old boy with a *Mycobacterium marinum* infection of submandibular lymphoid tissue. Courtesy of Larry Frenkel, MD.

CHAPTER 157
Tularemia

CLINICAL MANIFESTATIONS

There are several common manifestations of tularemia in children, with ulceroglandular disease being the most frequently identified. Characterized by a maculopapular lesion at the entry site with subsequent ulceration and slow healing, the ulceroglandular variant is associated with tender regional lymphadenopathy that can drain spontaneously. The glandular variant (regional lymphadenopathy with no ulcer) is also common. Less common disease variants include oculoglandular (severe conjunctivitis with preauricular lymphadenopathy), oropharyngeal (severe exudative stomatitis, pharyngitis, or tonsillitis with cervical lymphadenopathy), typhoidal (high fever, hepatomegaly, splenomegaly, or systemic infection including septicemia; pneumonia and/or meningitis may be found as complications), and secondary eruptions that can include vesicular skin lesions, which can be mistaken for herpes simplex virus or varicella-zoster virus cutaneous infections. Pneumonic tularemia, characterized by influenzalike symptoms often without chest radiograph abnormalities, manifests with fever, dry cough, chest pain, and hilar adenopathy and is normally associated with farming or lawn maintenance activities that create aerosols and dust. Pneumonic tularemia would also be the anticipated variant after intentional release of aerosolized organisms.

ETIOLOGY

Francisella tularensis is a small weakly staining gram-negative pleomorphic coccobacillus. Two subspecies (subsp) cause human infection in North America: *F tularensis* subsp *tularensis* (type A) and *F tularensis* subsp *holarctica* (type B). Type A is generally considered more virulent, although either can be lethal, especially if inhaled.

EPIDEMIOLOGY

F tularensis can infect more than 100 animal species; the vertebrate species considered most important in enzootic cycles are rabbits, hares, and rodents, especially muskrats, voles, beavers, and prairie dogs. Domestic cats and dogs are an additional but rare source of infection. In the United States, most human cases are attributed to tick bites but may also result from bites of other arthropod vectors, such as deer flies, or directly from contact with any of the aforementioned animal species. Infections attributable to tick and deer fly bites usually take the form of ulceroglandular or glandular tularemia. *F tularensis* bacteria can be transmitted to humans via the skin when handling infected animal tissue, as can occur when hunting or skinning infected rabbits, muskrats, prairie dogs, and other rodents. Infection has been reported in commercially traded hamsters and prairie dogs. Infection can also be acquired following ingestion of contaminated water or inadequately cooked meat or by inhalation of contaminated aerosols generated during lawn mowing, brush cutting, or certain farming activities (eg, baling contaminated hay). People have risk with occupational or recreational exposure to infected animals or their habitats; this group includes rabbit hunters and trappers, people exposed to certain ticks or biting insects, and laboratory technicians working with *F tularensis*, which is highly infectious and may be aerosolized when grown in culture. In the United States, most cases occur during May through September. Approximately two-thirds of cases occur in males, and one-quarter of cases occur in children younger than 15 years.

Tularemia has been reported in all US states except Hawaii. It is most common in central and western states and parts of Massachusetts (particularly Martha's Vineyard). In 2018, a total of 229 cases in the United States were reported.

Organisms can be present in blood during the first 2 weeks of disease and in cutaneous lesions for as long as 1 month if untreated. Person-to-person transmission has not been reported.

The **incubation period** is usually 3 to 5 days, with a range of 1 to 21 days.

DIAGNOSTIC TESTS

Diagnosis is established most often by serological testing. Patients do not develop antibodies until the second week of illness. A single serum antibody titer of 1:128 or greater determined by microagglutination (MA) or of 1:160 or greater determined by tube agglutination (TA) is consistent with recent or past infection and constitutes a presumptive diagnosis. For those with suspected disease and an initial nondiagnostic titer, a titer should be reobtained in 4 weeks. Confirmation by serological testing requires a 4-fold or greater titer change between serum samples obtained 4 weeks apart, with at least 1 of the specimens having a minimum titer of 1:128 or greater by MA or 1:160 or greater by TA. Nonspecific cross-reactions can occur with specimens containing heterophile antibodies or containing antibodies to *Brucella* species, *Legionella* species, or other gram-negative bacteria. However, cross-reactions rarely result in MA or TA titers that are diagnostic. Because of the propensity of *F tularensis* for causing laboratory-acquired infections, laboratory personnel should be alerted immediately when *F tularensis* infection is suspected.

F tularensis in ulcer exudate or aspirate material can be identified by laboratory-developed polymerase chain reaction assay or direct fluorescent antibody assay. Immunohistochemical staining is specific for detection of *F tularensis* in fixed tissues; however, this method is not available in most clinical laboratories. Isolation of *F tularensis* from specimens of blood, skin, ulcers, lymph node drainage, gastric washings, or respiratory tract secretions is best achieved by inoculation of cysteine-enriched media. Because *F tularensis* is a biosafety level–3 agent, if suspected on the basis of clinical and epidemiological history or Gram stain identification of tiny gram-negative coccobacillus, further work should be performed only in a certified Class II biosafety cabinet by using appropriate personal protective equipment (ie, back fastening gown, dual gloves, N95 respirator).

TREATMENT

Gentamicin (5 mg/kg/day, divided twice or 3 times/day, intravenously or intramuscularly, with the dose adjusted to maintain the desired peak serum concentrations of at least 5 μg/mL) is the drug of choice for the treatment of tularemia in children. Duration of therapy is usually 10 days. A 5- to 7-day course may be sufficient for mild disease, but a longer course is required for more severe illness (eg, meningitis). Ciprofloxacin is an alternative for mild disease (10- to 14-day course of oral ciprofloxacin; 20–40 mg/kg daily in 2 divided doses, maximum of 500 mg/dose). Doxycycline is associated with a higher rate of relapse than that of other therapies and is not recommended for definitive treatment. Suppuration of lymph nodes can occur despite antimicrobial therapy. *F tularensis* is nonsusceptible to β-lactam drugs, including carbapenems. Because of the difficulty in achieving adequate cerebrospinal fluid concentrations of gentamicin, combination therapy with doxycycline or ciprofloxacin plus gentamicin may be considered for patients with tularemic meningitis. Because treatment delay is associated with therapeutic failure, treatment should be initiated as soon as tularemia is suspected.

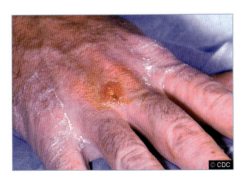

Image 157.1
A tularemic lesion on the dorsal skin of the right hand. Tularemia is caused by the bacterium *Francisella tularensis*. Symptoms vary depending on how the person was exposed to the disease; as shown, they can include skin ulcers. Courtesy of Centers for Disease Control and Prevention.

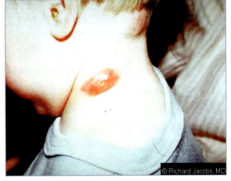

Image 157.2
An 8-year-old boy with 7 days of fever unresponsive to ceftriaxone was examined because of occipital and posterior cervical lymphadenitis. The cervical lymph node had spontaneously drained purulent material. A culture of the node aspirate was positive for *Francisella tularensis*. Courtesy of Richard Jacobs, MD.

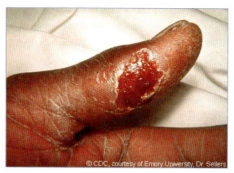

Image 157.3
Tularemic ulcer on the thumb. Irregular ulceration occurred at the site of entry of *Francisella tularensis*. Courtesy of Centers for Disease Control and Prevention/Emory University, Dr Sellers.

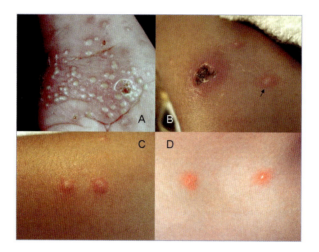

Image 157.4
A, A 6-week-old patient with vesicular tularemia initially diagnosed with herpes simplex. Findings from complete herpes evaluation were negative. B and C, A 10-year-old with vesicular lesions on arms and legs thought to be varicella. Arrow (B) shows a vesicle near the primary eschar. Evaluation was negative for varicella and herpes. Culture results of the eschar and vesicles confirmed tularemia. D, Varicella lesions shown for comparison. Courtesy of Centers for Disease Control and Prevention/Heinz F. Eichenwald, MD.

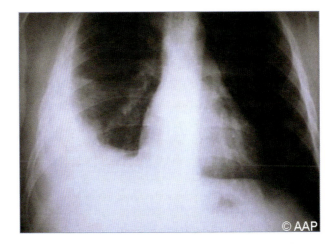

Image 157.5
Tularemia pneumonia. Posteroanterior chest radiograph showing pneumonia and pleural effusion in the lower lobe of the right lung; the pneumonia was unresponsive to ceftriaxone, azithromycin, and nafcillin. The patient had a history of tick bite and a high fever for 8 days, and his tularemia agglutinin titer was 1:2,048. An outbreak of pneumonic tularemia should prompt consideration of bioterrorism.

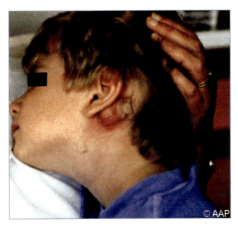

Image 157.6
Tularemia is a relatively rare infection that can manifest with painful cervical adenitis. This boy had a tick bite on his scalp that developed an ulcer followed by a large postauricular node. His tularemia titers were positive, and he responded to treatment with gentamycin.

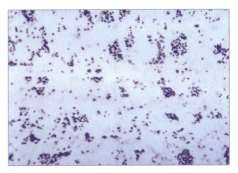

Image 157.7
This is a photomicrograph of *Francisella tularensis* bacteria with a methylene-blue stain. *F tularensis* is considered a potential biological weapon because of its extreme infectivity, ease of dissemination, and substantial capacity to cause illness and death. Courtesy of Centers for Disease Control and Prevention.

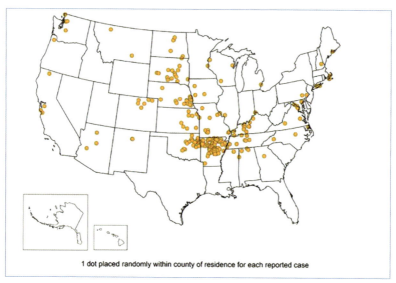

Image 157.8
Map of reported tularemia cases in the United States, 2019. Tularemia has been reported from all states except Hawaii but is most common in the south-central United States, the Pacific Northwest, and parts of Massachusetts, including Martha's Vineyard. Courtesy of Centers for Disease Control and Prevention.

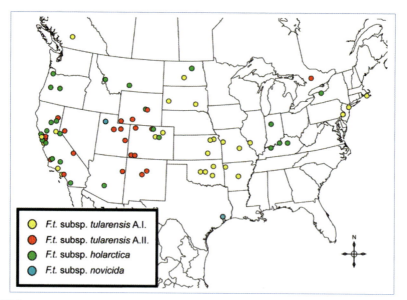

Image 157.9
Spatial distribution of 125 *Francisella tularensis* isolates for which information on originating county was available. Locations (colored circles) correspond to county centroids. >1 subspecies were isolated from some counties in California (Alameda, Contra Costa, Los Angeles, San Luis Obispo, and Santa Cruz) and Wyoming (Natrona). In some cases, a single circle may represent instances in which >1 sample of a given subspecies or genotypic group were isolated from a single county. Two isolates with county information, 1 from northern British Columbia and 1 from Alaska, are not shown. Courtesy of *Emerging Infectious Diseases*.

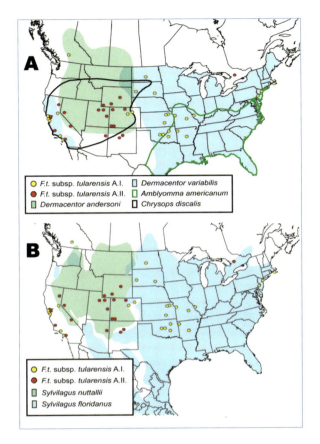

Image 157.10
Spatial distributions of isolates from the A1 and A2 subpopulations of *Francisella tularensis* subspecies (subsp) *tularensis* relative to (A) distribution of tularemia vectors *Dermacentor variabilis, Dermacentor andersoni, Amblyomma americanum,* and *Chrysops discalis* and (B) distribution of tularemia hosts *Sylvilagus nuttallii* and *Sylvilagus floridanus* species of rabbits. Courtesy of *Emerging Infectious Diseases*.

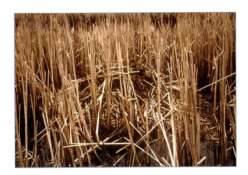

Image 157.11
This is a typical muskrat "house" camouflaged by reeds in Little Otter Creek, VT. The muskrat is a carrier of the bacterium *Francisella tularensis*, which is considered a dangerous potential biological weapon because of its extreme infectivity, ease of dissemination, and substantial capacity to cause illness and death. Courtesy of Centers for Disease Control and Prevention.

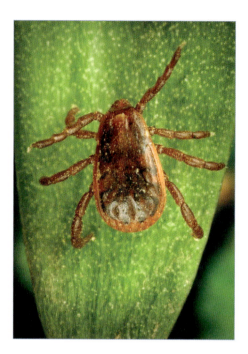

Image 157.12

This image depicts a male brown dog tick, *Rhipicephalus sanguineus*, from a superior, or dorsal, view looking down on this hard tick's scutum, or keratinized shield, which entirely covers its back, identifying it as a male. In the female, the dorsal abdomen is only partially covered, thereby offering room for abdominal expansion when she becomes engorged with blood while ingesting her blood meal obtained from her host. Courtesy of Centers for Disease Control and Prevention/James Gathany/William Nicholson.

CHAPTER 158

Louseborne Typhus
(Epidemic or Sylvatic Typhus)

CLINICAL MANIFESTATIONS

Louseborne or epidemic typhus is an uncommon disease that is spread through contact with infected human body lice. Patients develop abrupt onset of high fever, chills, and myalgia accompanied by severe headache and malaise. Rash often develops by day 4 to 7 after the start of illness but may not always be present and should not be relied on for diagnosis. When present, the rash usually begins on the trunk and axilla, spreads centrifugally to the limbs, and generally spares the face, palms, and soles. The rash is typically macular to maculopapular but, in advanced stages, can become petechial or hemorrhagic. The rash can be difficult to observe on patients with darkly pigmented skin and is absent in up to 40% of patients. There is no eschar, as might be present in many other rickettsial diseases. Abdominal concerns (ie, stomach pain, nausea) and changes in mental status are common, including delirium, drowsiness, seizures, and coma. Cough and tachypnea may be present. Myocardial and renal failure can occur when disease is severe. The fatality rate in untreated people can be as high as 30%. Mortality is less common in children and increases with advancing age. Untreated patients who recover typically have an illness lasting 2 weeks.

Brill-Zinsser disease is a relapse of epidemic typhus that can occur years after the initial episode and generally occurs when the body's immune system is weakened from illness, medications, or advanced age. The symptoms of Brill-Zinsser disease are generally milder and shorter than those of the initial infection. Factors that reactivate the rickettsiae are unknown.

Laboratory abnormalities in epidemic typhus may include thrombocytopenia, increased hepatic enzyme levels, hyperbilirubinemia, and elevated serum urea nitrogen level.

ETIOLOGY

Epidemic typhus is caused by *Rickettsia prowazekii*, which are gram-negative obligate intracellular bacteria.

EPIDEMIOLOGY

Epidemic typhus is transmitted by the human body louse (*Pediculus humanus corporis*), which is infected through feeding on patients with acute typhus fever. Humans are the primary reservoir of the organism. Infected lice excrete the bacteria in their feces and usually defecate at the time of feeding. Disease transmission can occur when infected louse feces are rubbed into broken skin or mucous membranes or are inhaled. People of all ages can be affected. Poverty, crowding, and poor sanitary conditions such as those found in war, famine, drought, and other natural disasters contribute to the spread of body lice and, hence, the disease. Cases have occurred throughout the world, including the colder, mountainous areas of Asia, Africa, some parts of Europe, and Central and South America, particularly in refugee camps and jails in resource-limited countries. Epidemic typhus is most common during winter, when conditions favor person-to-person transmission of the vector. Cases of epidemic typhus are rare in the United States, but there is no formal system for epidemic typhus surveillance. The last known epidemic in the United States occurred in 1921; sporadic human cases associated with close contact with infected flying squirrels (*Glaucomys volans*), their nests, or their ectoparasites are occasionally reported in the eastern United States. Cases have been reported in people who reside or work in flying squirrel–infested dwellings, even when direct contact is not reported. Flying squirrel–associated disease, called *sylvatic typhus*, typically manifests with a similar but generally milder illness than that observed with body louse–transmitted infection. Untreated illness can be severe, although no fatal cases of sylvatic typhus have been reported; the later development of Brill-Zinsser disease has been confirmed in at least 1 case of untreated sylvatic typhus.

People with Brill-Zinsser disease harbor active *R prowazekii* and, therefore, may pose a risk for reintroduction of the organism and new outbreaks. *Amblyomma* ticks in the Americas and in Ethiopia have been shown to carry *R prowazekii*, but their vector potential is unknown. Rickettsiae are present in the blood and tissues of patients during the early febrile phase but are not found in secretions. Direct person-to-person spread of the disease does not occur in the absence of the louse vector.

The **incubation period** is 1 to 2 weeks.

DIAGNOSTIC TESTS

Louseborne typhus may be diagnosed via indirect immunofluorescent antibody (IFA) assay; immunohistochemistry; polymerase chain reaction assay of blood, plasma, or tissue samples; or isolation by culture. Serological tests are the most common means of confirmation and can be used to detect either immunoglobulin G (IgG) or immunoglobulin M (IgM) antibodies. Preferably, the specimen should be obtained within the first week of symptoms and before (or within 24 hours of) doxycycline administration. The gold standard for serological diagnosis of louseborne typhus is a 4-fold increase in IgG antibody titer by the IFA test between acute sera obtained in the first week of illness and convalescent sera obtained 2 to 4 weeks later. A negative acute serological test result does not rule out a diagnosis of louseborne typhus, because detectable levels of IgG and IgM antibodies do not generally appear until around 7 to 10 days after onset of symptoms. An elevated acute titer may represent past infection rather than acute infection. Low-level elevated antibody titers can be an incidental finding in a significant proportion of the general population in some regions. IgM antibody titers may remain elevated for months and are not highly specific for acute louseborne typhus. Cross-reactivity may be observed to antibodies to *Rickettsia typhi* (the agent of endemic typhus), *Rickettsia rickettsii* (the agent of Rocky Mountain spotted fever), and other spotted fever group rickettsiae. *R prowazekii* may also be cultured and identified through submission to specific reference laboratories that are equipped to culture and identify epidemic typhus. Cell culture cultivation of the organism must be confirmed by molecular methods.

TREATMENT

Doxycycline is the drug of choice to treat louseborne typhus, regardless of patient age. The recommended dosage of doxycycline for adults is 100 mg twice per day, intravenously or orally, and the recommended dosage for children weighing less than 45 kg (<100 lb) is 2.2 mg/kg/dose, administered twice a day (maximum 100 mg/dose). Treatment should be continued for at least 3 days after defervescence and evidence of clinical improvement is documented, and the total treatment course is usually 7 to 10 days. Some patients may relapse if not treated for the full 7 to 10 days. Other broad-spectrum antimicrobial agents, including ciprofloxacin, are not recommended and may be more likely to result in fatal outcome. Chloramphenicol, where available, may be used in absolute contraindication of doxycycline (life-threatening allergy) but carries significant risks (ie, aplastic anemia). In epidemic settings where antimicrobial agents may be limited (eg, refugee camps), a single 200-mg dose of doxycycline in adults (or 4.4 mg/kg, maximum dose 200 mg as a single dose for children) may provide effective treatment and facilitate outbreak control when combined with delousing efforts.

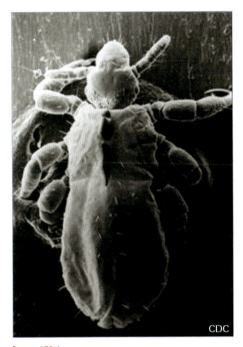

Image 158.1
Pediculus humanus humanus, the human body louse, viewed with an electron microscope (magnification ×120). Courtesy of Centers for Disease Control and Prevention/*Emerging Infectious Diseases* and Cédric Foucault.

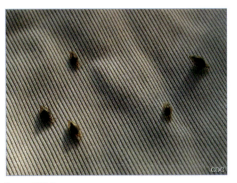

Image 158.2
Human body lice in clothes. Courtesy of Centers for Disease Control and Prevention/*Emerging Infectious Diseases* and Cédric Foucault.

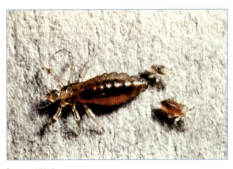

Image 158.3
This image depicts an adult female body louse, *Pediculus humanus*, and 2 larval young, which serve as the vector of epidemic typhus. Courtesy of Centers for Disease Control and Prevention.

CHAPTER 159

Murine Typhus
(Endemic or Fleaborne Typhus)

CLINICAL MANIFESTATIONS

Murine typhus, also known as endemic typhus or fleaborne typhus, resembles epidemic (louseborne) typhus but usually has a less abrupt onset with less severe systemic symptoms. The disease can be mild in young children. Fever, present in almost all patients, can be accompanied by myalgia and a persistent, usually severe, headache. Nausea, vomiting, anorexia, and abdominal pain and tenderness also develop in approximately half of patients. A macular or maculopapular rash appears by day 4 to 7 of illness in approximately 50% of patients, and it lasts 4 to 8 days. The rash is often distributed on the patient's trunk, although extremities can also be involved. Illness seldom lasts longer than 2 weeks. The clinical course is usually uncomplicated, but severe manifestations, such as central nervous system abnormalities, are possible. Laboratory findings include thrombocytopenia, elevated liver aminotransferase levels, hypoalbuminemia, hypocalcemia, and hyponatremia. Fatal outcome is rare but has been reported in up to 4% of hospitalized patients.

ETIOLOGY

Murine typhus is caused by *Rickettsia typhi*, which are gram-negative obligate intracellular bacteria.

EPIDEMIOLOGY

Rats, in which infection is inapparent, are the natural reservoirs for *R typhi*. The disease is worldwide in distribution and tends to occur most commonly in men; in children, boys and girls are affected equally. Outside the United States, the primary vector for transmission among rats and transmission to humans is the rat flea, *Xenopsylla cheopis*, although other fleas and mites have been implicated. A suburban cycle involving cat fleas (*Ctenocephalides felis*) and opossums (*Didelphis virginiana*) or feral cats has emerged as an important cause of murine typhus in the United States. Infection occurs when infected flea feces are rubbed into broken skin or mucous membranes or are inhaled. Murine typhus is rare in most of the United States, although it is likely underdiagnosed. Most diagnosed cases occur during the months of April to October and in southern California, southern Texas, the southeastern Gulf coast, and Hawaii.

The **incubation period** is 6 to 14 days.

DIAGNOSTIC TESTS

Antibody titers determined with *R typhi* antigen by an indirect fluorescent antibody assay are measured most commonly. Enzyme immunoassay or latex agglutination tests are also available. Antibody concentrations peak at around 4 weeks after infection, but results of antibody tests may be negative early in the course of illness. A 4-fold increase in immunoglobulin G (IgG) titer between acute and convalescent sera specimens obtained 2 to 4 weeks apart is confirmatory for laboratory diagnosis. Although more prone to false-positive results, immunoassays demonstrating increases in specific immunoglobulin M (IgM) antibody can aid in distinguishing clinical illness from previous exposure if interpreted with a concurrent IgG test result; use of IgM assays alone is not recommended. Because of cross-reactivity, standard serological tests might not differentiate murine typhus caused by *R typhi* from epidemic (louseborne) typhus (*Rickettsia prowazekii*) or from infection with spotted fever rickettsiae, such as *Rickettsia rickettsii*. More specific testing with antibody cross-absorption for immunofluorescent antibody assay or Western blot analyses is not available routinely. Isolation of the organism in cell culture is potentially hazardous and is performed best in specialized laboratories. Routine hospital blood cultures are not suitable for culture of *R typhi*. Molecular diagnostic assays on infected whole blood and skin biopsies can distinguish murine and epidemic typhus and other rickettsioses and are performed at the Centers for Disease Control and Prevention (CDC). Immunohistochemical procedures on formalin-fixed skin biopsy tissues can also be performed at the CDC.

TREATMENT

Doxycycline is the treatment of choice for murine typhus, regardless of patient age. The recommended dosage of doxycycline is 4.4 mg/kg per day, divided every 12 hours, intravenously or orally (maximum 100 mg/dose). Early diagnosis should be based on clinical suspicion and epidemiology. In a patient with disease that is clinically compatible with murine typhus, treatment should not be withheld because of a negative laboratory result or while awaiting laboratory confirmation, because severe or fatal infection can develop when treatment is delayed. Treatment should be continued for at least 3 days after defervescence and evidence of clinical improvement is documented. The total treatment course is usually 7 to 14 days. Fluoroquinolones or chloramphenicol is an alternative medication but may not be as effective.

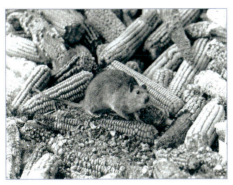

Image 159.1
A Norway rat, *Rattus norvegicus*, in a Kansas City, MO, corn storage bin. *R norvegicus* is known to be a reservoir of bubonic plague (transmitted to people by the bite of a flea or other insects), endemic typhus fever, rat-bite fever, and a few other dreaded diseases. Courtesy of Centers for Disease Control and Prevention.

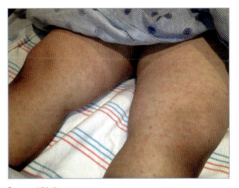

Image 159.2
A healthy 8-year-old boy had 5 days of fever, severe headache, and malaise before this rash began. He had been exposed to numerous cats with fleas before the onset of illness. Courtesy of Carol J. Baker, MD, FAAP.

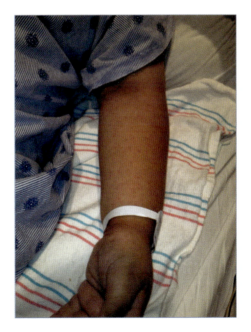

Image 159.3
The same boy as in Image 159.2 who had rash involving palms and soles as well as pancytopenia. He recovered completely with doxycycline therapy. Courtesy of Carol J. Baker, MD, FAAP.

CHAPTER 160

Ureaplasma urealyticum and *Ureaplasma parvum* Infections

CLINICAL MANIFESTATIONS

The role of *Ureaplasma* species in human disease is controversial. There has been an inconsistent association between presence of *Ureaplasma urealyticum* and nongonococcal urethritis. Without treatment, the urethritis usually resolves within 1 to 6 months. There has also been an inconsistent relationship of infection by *Ureaplasma* species with prostatitis and epididymitis in men and upper genital tract syndromes in women, including salpingitis, endometritis, and pelvic inflammatory disease. *Ureaplasma* organisms are commonly detected in placentas with histological chorioamnionitis (now known as intra-amniotic infection), and studies suggest that there is an association of upper genital tract infection by *Ureaplasma* species and adverse pregnancy outcomes. Some reports also describe an association between the presence of *Ureaplasma* in the vaginal flora and preterm birth.

U urealyticum and *Ureaplasma parvum* are frequently isolated from the lower respiratory tract and from lung biopsy specimens of preterm infants, and studies have demonstrated an association of *Ureaplasma* species with the development of bronchopulmonary dysplasia in preterm infants. These organisms have also been recovered from respiratory tract secretions of infants 3 months or younger with pneumonia, but their role in development of lower respiratory tract disease in otherwise healthy young infants is unclear. *Ureaplasma* species have been isolated from the bloodstream of newborns and from cerebrospinal fluid of infants with meningitis, intraventricular hemorrhage, and hydrocephalus. The contribution of *U urealyticum* to the outcome of infants with infections of the central nervous system (CNS) is unclear given the confounding effects of preterm birth and intraventricular hemorrhage.

Cases of *U urealyticum* or *U parvum* arthritis, osteomyelitis, pneumonia, pericarditis, meningitis, and progressive sinopulmonary disease have been reported, almost exclusively in immunocompromised patients. Patients with solid organ transplants appear to have major risk. A recently described syndrome of *Ureaplasma* sepsis with hyperammonemia (attributable to rapid hydrolysis of host urea by the organism) in lung transplant patients appears to be attributable to the introduction of the organism in the transplanted lung into naïve recipients who are immunosuppressed.

ETIOLOGY

Ureaplasma organisms are small pleomorphic bacteria that lack a cell wall. The genus contains 2 species capable of causing human infection, *U urealyticum* and *U parvum*. At least 14 serotypes have been described, 4 for *U parvum* and 10 for *U urealyticum*.

EPIDEMIOLOGY

The principal reservoir of human *Ureaplasma* species is the genital tract of sexually active adults. Colonization occurs in approximately half of sexually active women; the incidence among sexually active men is lower. Colonization is uncommon in prepubertal children and adolescents who are not sexually active, but a positive genital tract culture is not clearly definitive of sexual abuse. *Ureaplasma* species may colonize the throat, eyes, umbilicus, and perineum of newborns and may persist for several months after birth. *U parvum* is generally more common than *U urealyticum* as a colonizer in pregnant women and their offspring.

Because *Ureaplasma* species are commonly isolated from the female lower genital tract and neonatal respiratory tract in the absence of disease, a positive culture does not establish its causative role in acute infection. However, recovery of these organisms from an upper genital tract or lower respiratory tract specimen in the appropriate host who has evidence of clinical disease is much more indicative of true infection.

The **incubation period** after sexual transmission is 10 to 20 days.

DIAGNOSTIC TESTS

Specimens for culture require *Ureaplasma*-compatible transport media, with refrigeration at 4 °C (39 °F). If the specimen cannot be transported to the reference laboratory within 24 hours, the sample should be frozen at −70 °C

(−94 °F), not −20 °C (−4 °F). If a vaginal or urethral swab is used for collection, Dacron or calcium alginate swabs should be used to collect and inoculate transport media; cotton swabs should be avoided. Several rapid, sensitive real-time polymerase chain reaction (PCR) assays for detection of *U urealyticum* and *U parvum* have been developed. Many of these assays have greater sensitivity than culture, but they are not widely available outside of reference laboratories. Transport medium is not necessary for urine to be tested only by PCR assay. Such specimens can be concentrated 10-fold and frozen at −70 °C (−94 °F) immediately after collection and shipped on dry ice. *Ureaplasma* species can be cultured in urea-containing broth and agar in 2 to 4 days.

TREATMENT

A positive *Ureaplasma* culture or PCR assay result does not indicate need for therapy if the patient is asymptomatic. *Ureaplasma* species are generally susceptible to macrolides, tetracyclines, and quinolones, but because they lack a cell wall, they are nonsusceptible to penicillins or cephalosporins. They are also nonsusceptible to trimethoprim-sulfamethoxazole or clindamycin. For symptomatic children, adolescents, and adults, doxycycline can be used for treatment. Doxycycline can be used for short durations (ie, ≤21 days) without regard to patient age; azithromycin is the preferred antimicrobial agent for children younger than 8 years or people who are allergic to tetracyclines. Persistent urethritis after doxycycline treatment may be attributable to doxycycline-resistant *U urealyticum* or *Mycoplasma genitalium*. Recurrences are common, and tetracycline resistance may occur in up to 50% of *Ureaplasma* isolates in some patient populations. If tetracycline resistance is likely, azithromycin is indicated; a quinolone is an option if azithromycin resistance is also possible. Quinolone and macrolide coresistance remains uncommon, at less than 5% in the United States but up to 10% elsewhere including Australia and Southeast Asia. These infections are difficult to treat, and pristinamycin has proven effective.

In neonates, antimicrobial treatment with erythromycin has generally failed to prevent chronic pulmonary disease, possibly because erythromycin does not eliminate *Ureaplasma* organisms from the airways in a large proportion of infants. Bronchopulmonary dysplasia or death may be reduced by azithromycin (10 mg/kg/day for 7 days followed by 5 mg/kg/day for a maximum of 6 weeks). Definitive evidence of efficacy of antimicrobial agents in the treatment of CNS infections caused by *Ureaplasma* species in infants and children is lacking.

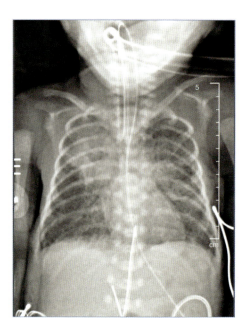

Image 160.1
This newborn, 23 weeks' gestation at birth, with maternal chorioamnionitis developed pneumonia 4 days after birth along with respiratory failure. Diagnosis was *Ureaplasma urealyticum* pneumonia on the basis of tracheal culture, which was positive for *U urealyticum*. The newborn was treated with azithromycin for 10 days with improvement in respiratory status. Copyright Mitali Sahni, MBBS, FAAP.

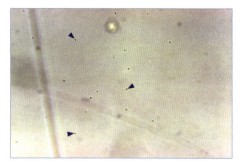

Image 160.2
Under a magnification of ×125, this photomicrograph revealed the presence of a number of small-sized *Ureaplasma urealyticum*, formerly known as T-strain mycoplasma bacterial colonies (arrowheads). This was described as heavy growth on 1 mL of agar. Courtesy of Centers for Disease Control and Prevention and Dr Francis Forrester.

CHAPTER 161

Varicella-Zoster Virus Infections

CLINICAL MANIFESTATIONS

Primary infection results in varicella (chickenpox), manifesting in unvaccinated people as a generalized, pruritic, erythematous vesicular rash typically consisting of 250 to 500 lesions in varying stages of development (ie, papules, vesicles) and resolution (crusting), low-grade fever, and other systemic symptoms. Complications include bacterial superinfection of skin lesions with or without bacterial sepsis, pneumonia, central nervous system (CNS) involvement (ie, acute cerebellar ataxia, encephalitis, stroke/vasculopathy), thrombocytopenia, and rarer complications such as glomerulonephritis, arthritis, and hepatitis. Primary viral pneumonia is an uncommon complication in immunocompetent children but is the most common complication in adults. Varicella tends to be more severe in adults, infants, and adolescents than in other children. Despite widespread use of varicella vaccine, breakthrough cases can occur in immunized children, but they are usually mild and rash manifestation is modified. Reye syndrome may follow varicella, although this outcome has become very rare with the recommendation not to use salicylate-containing compounds (eg, aspirin, bismuth subsalicylate) for children with chickenpox. In immunocompromised children, progressive, severe varicella may occur with continuing eruption of lesions (sometimes including hemorrhagic skin lesions) along with high fever persisting into the second week of illness and visceral dissemination (ie, encephalitis, hepatitis, and pneumonia). Severe and even fatal varicella has been reported in otherwise healthy children receiving high-dose corticosteroids (>2 mg/kg/day of prednisone or equivalent) for treatment of asthma and other illnesses.

Varicella-zoster virus (VZV) establishes latency in sensory (dorsal root, cranial nerve, and autonomic including enteric) ganglia during primary VZV infection. This latency occurs with both wild-type VZV and the vaccine strain. Reactivation results in herpes zoster (shingles), typically characterized by grouped vesicular skin lesions on an erythematous base in the unilateral distribution of 1 to 3 contiguous sensory dermatomes, most commonly in the thoracic and lumbar regions, frequently accompanied by localized pain and/or itching. Zoster may also result in cranial neuropathy, particularly in the fifth, seventh, and eighth cranial nerve distributions. Postherpetic neuralgia, pain that persists after resolution of the zoster rash, may last for weeks to months but is unusual in children. Zoster occasionally becomes disseminated in immunocompromised patients, with lesions appearing outside the primary dermatomes and/or visceral complications. VZV reactivation occurs less frequently in the absence of skin rash (zoster sine herpete); these patients may present with aseptic meningitis, encephalitis, stroke, acute retinal necrosis, or gastrointestinal tract involvement (visceral zoster). Recurrent zoster is rare and should prompt a consideration for an evaluation for immunodeficiency. A vesicular rash, especially in the distribution of the trigeminal ganglion or sacral sensory roots, may represent herpes simplex (so-called zosteriform herpes simplex) and should be assessed virologically (eg, by polymerase chain reaction [PCR] testing of swabbed material from the base of an unroofed vesicle) to distinguish this from zoster attributable to VZV.

Fetal infection after maternal varicella during the first or early second trimester of pregnancy occasionally results in fetal death or varicella embryopathy, characterized by limb hypoplasia, cutaneous scarring, eye abnormalities, and damage to the CNS (congenital varicella syndrome). The incidence of the congenital varicella syndrome among infants born to mothers who experience gestational varicella is approximately 2% when infection occurs between 8 and 20 weeks of gestation. Rarely, cases of congenital varicella syndrome have been reported in infants of women infected after 20 weeks of pregnancy, the latest occurring at 28 weeks' gestation. Children infected with VZV in utero may develop zoster early in life without having had extrauterine varicella.

Varicella infection has a higher case-fatality rate among infants when the mother develops varicella from 5 days before to 2 days after delivery, because there is little opportunity for development and transfer of maternal antibody across the placenta before delivery and the infant's cellular immune system is immature.

ETIOLOGY

VZV (also known as *human herpesvirus 3*) is a member of the *Herpesviridae* family, the subfamily *Alphaherpesvirinae*, and the genus *Varicellovirus*.

EPIDEMIOLOGY

Humans are the only source of infection for this highly contagious virus. Infection occurs when the virus comes into contact with the mucosa of the upper respiratory tract or the conjunctiva of a susceptible person. Person-to-person transmission occurs from direct contact with VZV lesions from varicella or herpes zoster or from airborne spread. Varicella is more contagious than herpes zoster. There is no evidence of VZV spread from fomites; the virus is extremely labile and is unable to survive for long in the environment. Varicella infection in a household member usually results in infection of almost all susceptible people in that household. Children who acquire their infection at home (secondary family members) often have more skin lesions than the index patient. Health care–associated transmission is well-documented.

In temperate climates in the prevaccine era, varicella was a disease with a marked seasonal distribution, with peak incidence during winter and spring mainly among children younger than 10 years. In tropical climates, acquisition of varicella often occurs later, resulting in a significant proportion of susceptible adults. High rates of vaccine coverage in the United States have eliminated discernible seasonality of varicella. Following implementation of universal immunization in the United States in 1995, varicella incidence declined by approximately 98% in all age-groups because of personal and herd immunity.

The age of peak incidence of varicella has shifted from children younger than 10 years to children 10 through 14 years of age. Immunity to wild-type varicella is generally lifelong. Symptomatic reinfection is uncommon in immunocompetent people. Asymptomatic primary infection is unusual.

Immunocompromised people with primary (varicella) or reactivated (herpes zoster) infection have increased risk for severe disease. Severe varicella and disseminated zoster are more likely to develop in children with congenital T-lymphocyte defects or AIDS than in people with B-lymphocyte abnormalities. Other groups of pediatric patients who may experience more severe or complicated varicella include infants, adolescents, patients with chronic cutaneous or pulmonary disorders, and patients receiving systemic corticosteroids or other immunosuppressive therapy or long-term salicylate therapy.

Patients are considered contagious from 1 to 2 days before onset of the rash until all lesions have dried/crusted.

The **incubation period** is usually 14 to 16 days, with a range of 10 to 21 days after exposure to rash. The **incubation period** may be prolonged for as long as 28 days after receipt of varicella-zoster immune globulin (VZIG) or immune globulin intravenous (IGIV) and may be shortened in immunocompromised patients. Varicella can develop after birth in infants born to mothers with active varicella around the time of delivery; the usual interval from onset of rash in a mother to onset in her neonate is 9 to 15 days.

DIAGNOSTIC TESTS

Diagnostic tests for VZV are summarized in Table 161.1. Vesicular fluid or a scab can be used to identify VZV with a PCR test, which is currently the diagnostic method of choice. During the acute phase of illness, VZV can also be identified by PCR assay of saliva or buccal swabs, although VZV is more likely to be detected in vesicular fluid or scabs. VZV can be demonstrated by direct fluorescent antibody (DFA) assay, by using scrapings of a vesicle base early in the eruption or by isolating the virus in cell culture from vesicular fluid. Viral culture and DFA assay are both much less sensitive than PCR assay. PCR testing that discriminates between vaccine and wild-type VZV is available free of charge through the specialized reference laboratory at the Centers for Disease Control and Prevention (404/639-0066), through a safety research program sponsored by Merck & Co (800/672-6372), and from 4 state public health laboratories serving as vaccine-preventable disease reference centers (Wisconsin, Minnesota, California, and New York).

A significant increase (4-fold increase in titer) in serum varicella immunoglobulin G antibody between acute and convalescent samples by any standard serological assay can confirm a diagnosis retrospectively, but this may not reliably occur in

Table 161.1
Diagnostic Tests for Varicella-Zoster Virus Infection

Test	Specimen	Comments
PCR	Vesicular swabs or scrapings, scabs from crusted lesions, biopsy tissue, CSF	Very sensitive method. Specific for VZV. Methods have been designed that distinguish vaccine strain from wild-type (see text).
Direct fluorescent antibody	Vesicle scraping, swab of lesion base (must include cells)	Specific for VZV. More rapid and more sensitive than culture, less sensitive than PCR.
Viral culture	Vesicular fluid, CSF, biopsy tissue	Distinguishes VZV from herpes simplex virus. High cost, limited availability; requires up to a week for result. Least sensitive.
Serology (IgG)	Acute and convalescent serum specimens for IgG	Specific for VZV. Commercial assays generally have low sensitivity to reliably detect vaccine-induced immunity.
Serology (IgM)	Acute serum specimens for IgM	IgM serology is less specific than IgG serology. IgM inconsistently detected. Not reliable method for routine confirmation.

CSF indicates cerebrospinal fluid; IgG, immunoglobulin G; IgM, immunoglobulin M; PCR, polymerase chain reaction; and VZV, varicella-zoster virus.

immunocompromised people. However, diagnosis of varicella by serological testing is seldom indicated. Commercially available enzyme immunoassay tests are not usually sufficiently sensitive to demonstrate reliably a vaccine-induced antibody response; therefore, routine postvaccination serological testing is not recommended. Commercial immunoglobulin M tests are not reliable for routine confirmation or ruling out of acute infection because of potential false-negative and false-positive results.

TREATMENT

Nonspecific therapies for varicella include keeping fingernails short to prevent trauma and secondary bacterial infection from scratching, frequent bathing, application of lotion to reduce pruritus, and acetaminophen for fever. Children with varicella should not receive salicylates or salicylate-containing products (eg, aspirin, bismuth subsalicylate) because these products increase the risk of Reye syndrome. Salicylate therapy should be stopped if possible in an unimmunized child who is exposed to varicella. Treatment with ibuprofen is controversial and should be avoided if possible.

The decision to use antiviral therapy and the route and duration of therapy should be determined by host factors and extent of infection. Antiviral drugs have a limited window of opportunity to affect the outcome of VZV infection. In immunocompetent hosts, most virus replication has stopped by 72 hours after onset of rash; the duration of replication may be extended in immunocompromised hosts. Oral acyclovir and valacyclovir are not recommended for routine use in otherwise healthy younger children with varicella, because their use results in only a modest decrease in symptoms. Antiviral therapy should be considered for otherwise healthy people with increased risk for moderate to severe varicella, such as unvaccinated people older than 12 years, those with chronic cutaneous or pulmonary disorders, those receiving long-term salicylate therapy, or those receiving short or intermittent courses of corticosteroids. Some experts also recommend use of oral acyclovir or valacyclovir for secondary household members in which the disease is usually more severe than in the primary patient or in children who have immunocompromised household contacts. Acyclovir therapy should also be considered for children with zoster and the continuing development of new lesions.

The American College of Obstetricians and Gynecology recommends that pregnant women with varicella be considered for treatment to minimize maternal morbidity. Intravenous acyclovir is recommended for pregnant patients with serious complications of varicella.

Intravenous acyclovir therapy is recommended for immunocompromised patients, including patients who have been treated with high-dose corticosteroid therapy for more than 14 days. Therapy initiated early in the course of the illness, especially within 24 hours of rash onset, maximizes benefit. Oral acyclovir should not be used to treat immunocompromised children with varicella, because of poor oral bioavailability. In the event of national shortages of intravenous acyclovir (as occurred in 2011–2012 and 2019), intravenous ganciclovir or foscarnet may be a reasonable alternative. Valacyclovir (20 mg/kg per dose, with a maximum dose of 1,000 mg, administered orally 3 times daily for 5 days) is licensed for treatment of varicella in children and teens 2 through 17 years of age. Some experts have used valacyclovir, with its improved bioavailability compared to that of oral acyclovir, in selected immunocompromised patients perceived to have low to moderate risk for developing severe varicella, such as HIV-infected patients with relatively normal concentrations of $CD4^+$ T lymphocytes and children with leukemia for whom careful follow-up is ensured. Famciclovir is available for treatment of VZV infections in adults, but its efficacy and safety have not been established for children. Although VZIG or IGIV, administered shortly after exposure, can prevent or modify the course of disease (Figure 161.1), immune globulin preparations are ineffective treatments once disease is established.

Antiviral susceptibility testing is not validated but can be considered in cases of poor response to standard therapy. Infections caused by acyclovir-resistant VZV strains, which are generally rare and limited to immunocompromised hosts with prior prolonged exposure to antiviral therapy or prophylaxis, have been successfully treated with parenteral foscarnet.

Figure 161.1
Management of Exposures to Varicella-Zoster Virus

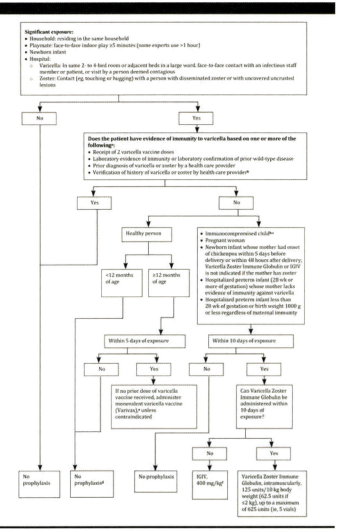

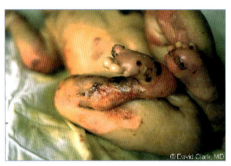

Image 161.1
Congenital varicella with short-limb syndrome and scarring of the skin. The mother had varicella during the first trimester of pregnancy. Courtesy of David Clark, MD.

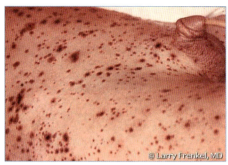

Image 161.2
A male toddler with hemorrhagic varicella complicating acute lymphocytic leukemia. Courtesy of Larry Frenkel, MD.

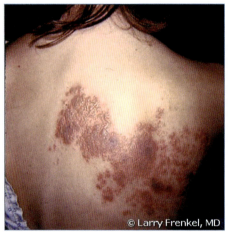

Image 161.3
Herpes zoster in an 18-year-old young woman, known to use illicit drugs, who also had an anaerobic lung abscess. Courtesy of Larry Frenkel, MD.

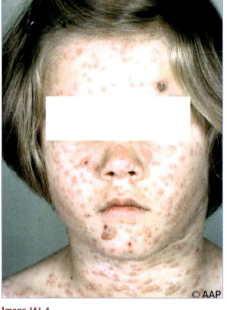

Image 161.4
School-aged girl with varicella who acquired it from a younger sibling, who had a milder clinical course with fewer lesions.

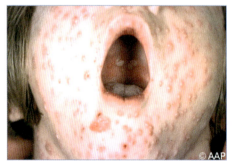

Image 161.5
This child acquired her varicella-zoster virus infection from a younger sibling. Varicella lesions are apparent on the palate. This is the same child as in Image 161.4.

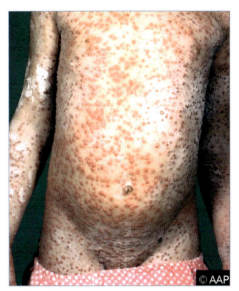

Image 161.6
School-aged child with varicella who acquired it from a younger sibling. This is the same child as in images 161.4 and 161.5 who had calamine lotion applied by the parents for itching. She recovered without incident.

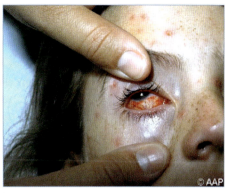

Image 161.7
Varicella with scleral lesions and bulbar conjunctivitis.

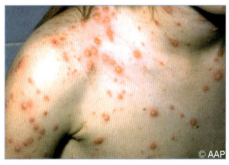

Image 161.8
An adolescent girl with varicella lesions in various stages. This is the same patient as in Image 161.7.

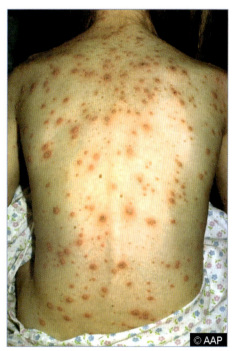

Image 161.9
An adolescent girl with varicella lesions in various stages. This is the same patient as in images 161.7 and 161.8.

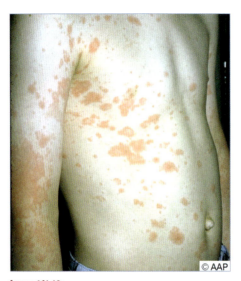

Image 161.10
Varicella with erythema multiforme.

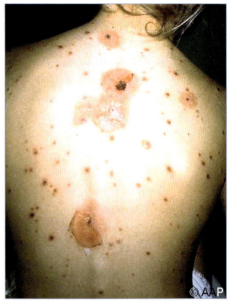

Image 161.11
Varicella with bullous lesions. Blood culture results were negative for bacteria. Cellulitis at sites of bullous lesions resolved while receiving oral dicloxacillin sodium. The child did not appear very ill.

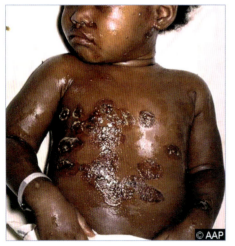

Image 161.12
Varicella with bullous lesions. Culture results of vesicle fluid were negative for bacteria.

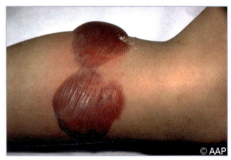

Image 161.13
Bullous varicella. *Staphylococcus aureus* organisms may be present in these large bullae.

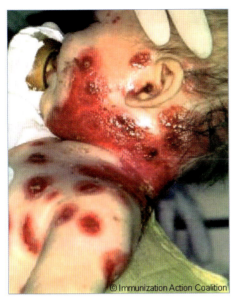

Image 161.14
A neonate with hemorrhagic varicella with cellulitis. This newborn contracted varicella at birth from his mother, who was infected. Copyright Immunization Action Coalition.

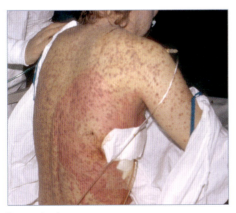

Image 161.16
Disseminated varicella in a 17-year-old girl with Hodgkin disease and failure to respond to intravenous acyclovir. Courtesy of George Nankervis, MD.

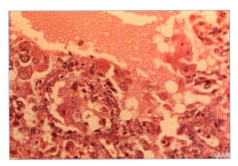

Image 161.15
Varicella (interstitial) pneumonia. Although rare in otherwise healthy children, this complication of varicella-zoster virus infection in adults accounts for much of the morbidity and mortality caused by the infection. Courtesy of Edgar O. Ledbetter, MD, FAAP.

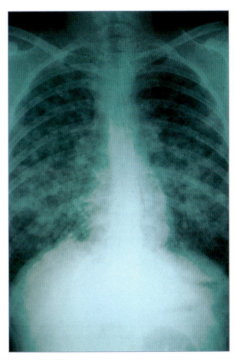

Image 161.17
Diffuse varicella pneumonia bilaterally shown in the chest radiograph of the patient in Image 161.16, with Hodgkin disease. Courtesy of George Nankervis, MD.

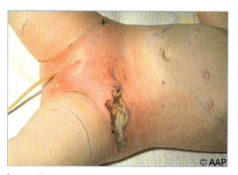

Image 161.18
Varicella complicated by necrotizing fasciitis. A blood culture result was positive for group A streptococci. The disease responded to antibiotics and surgical debridement followed by primary surgical closure.

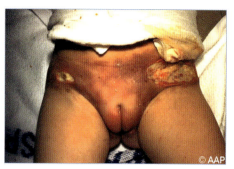

Image 161.19
Varicella and necrotizing fasciitis in the same patient as in Image 161.18 shortly after surgical debridement.

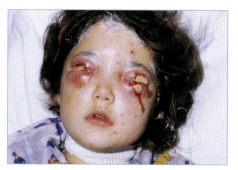

Image 161.20
A school-aged girl with bilateral periorbital cellulitis and necrotizing fasciitis caused by a group A β-hemolytic streptococcal infection complicating varicella. Courtesy of George Nankervis, MD.

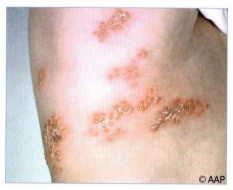

Image 161.21
Herpes zoster in an otherwise healthy child. Multiple dermatomes are involved.

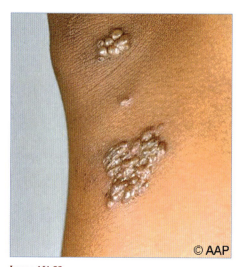

Image 161.22
Herpes zoster in an otherwise healthy child.

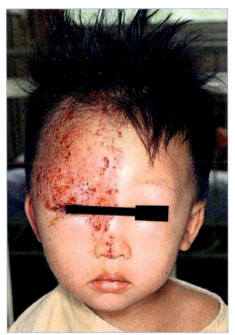

Image 161.23
Herpes zoster (shingles). Courtesy of C. W. Leung.

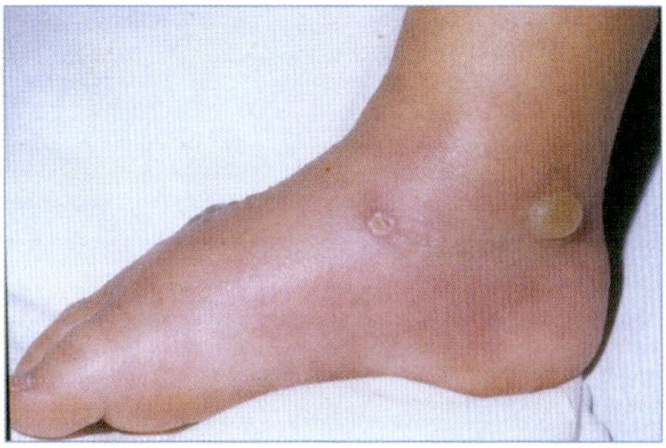

Image 161.24
Bullous varicella (uncomplicated) in a 1-year-old. Courtesy of George Nankervis, MD.

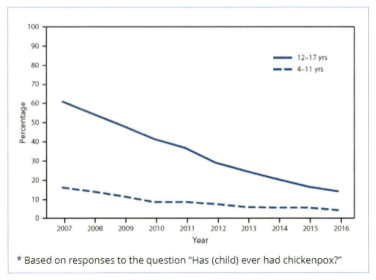

* Based on responses to the question "Has (child) ever had chickenpox?"

Image 161.25
Percentage of children and teens aged 4–17 years who had ever had varicella (chickenpox),* by age-group—National Health Interview Survey, 2007–2016. During 2007–2016, the percentage of children and teens aged 4–17 years who had ever had chickenpox decreased among both younger children (aged 4–11 years) and older children (aged 12–17 years). Among younger children, the percentage of children who had ever had chickenpox declined by 73.9%, from 16.1% in 2007 to 4.2% in 2016. Among older children, the percentage who had ever had chickenpox declined by 76.9%, from 61.4% in 2007 to 14.2% in 2016. During 2007–2016, older children were more likely than younger children to have ever had chickenpox. Courtesy of *Morbidity and Mortality Weekly Report.*

CHAPTER 162

Cholera
(*Vibrio cholerae*)

CLINICAL MANIFESTATIONS

Cholera is characterized by voluminous watery diarrhea and rapid onset of life-threatening dehydration. Hypovolemic shock may occur within hours of the onset of diarrhea. Stools have a characteristic rice-water appearance, are white tinged with small flecks of mucus, and contain high concentrations of sodium, potassium, chloride, and bicarbonate. Vomiting is a common feature of cholera. Fever and abdominal cramps are usually absent. In addition to dehydration and hypovolemia, common complications of cholera include hypokalemia, metabolic acidosis, and hypoglycemia, particularly in children. Although severe cholera is a distinctive illness characterized by profuse diarrhea and rapid dehydration, people infected with toxigenic *Vibrio cholerae* O1 may have either no symptoms or mild to moderate diarrhea lasting 3 to 7 days.

ETIOLOGY

V cholerae is a curved or comma-shaped motile gram-negative rod. There are more than 200 *V cholerae* serogroups, some of which carry the cholera toxin (CT) gene. Although those serogroups with the CT gene and others without the CT gene can cause acute watery diarrhea, only toxin-producing serogroups O1 and O139 have caused epidemic cholera, with O1 causing the vast majority of cases of cholera. *V cholerae* O1 is classified into 2 biotypes, classical and El Tor, and 2 major serotypes, Ogawa and Inaba. Since 1992, toxigenic *V cholerae* serogroup O139 has been recognized as a cause of epidemic cholera in Asia. Aside from the substitution of the O139 for the O1 antigen, the organism is almost identical to *V cholerae* O1 El Tor. All other serogroups of *V cholerae* are known collectively as *V cholerae* non-O1/non-O139. Toxin-producing strains of *V cholerae* non-O1/non-O139 can cause sporadic cases of severe dehydrating diarrheal illness but have not caused large outbreaks of cholera. Non–toxin-producing strains of *V cholerae* non-O1/non-O139 are associated with sporadic cases of gastroenteritis, sepsis, and rare cases of wound infection.

EPIDEMIOLOGY

Since the early 1800s, there have been 7 cholera pandemics. The current pandemic began in 1961 and is caused by *V cholerae* O1 El Tor. Molecular epidemiology shows that this pandemic has occurred in 3 successive waves, with each one spreading from South Asia to other regions in Asia, Africa, and the western Pacific Islands (Oceania). In 1991, epidemic cholera caused by toxigenic *V cholerae* O1 El Tor appeared in Peru and spread to most countries in South, Central, and North America, causing more than 1 million cases of cholera before subsiding. In 2010, *V cholerae* O1 El Tor was introduced into Haiti, on the island of Hispaniola, initiating a massive epidemic of cholera with more than 650,000 cases and 8,000 deaths. In the United States, sporadic cases resulting from travel to or ingestion of contaminated food transported from regions with endemic cholera are reported, including at least 40 cases imported from Hispaniola since 2010. Domestically acquired cases in the United States have been reported from eating Gulf coast seafood.

Humans are the only documented natural host, but free-living *V cholerae* organisms can persist in the aquatic environment. Infection is primarily acquired by ingestion of large numbers of organisms from contaminated water or food (particularly raw or undercooked shellfish, raw or partially dried fish, or moist grains or vegetables held at ambient temperature). People with low gastric acidity and with blood group O have increased risk for severe cholera infection.

The median **incubation period** is usually 1 to 2 days, with a range of a few hours to 5 days.

DIAGNOSTIC TESTS

V cholerae can be cultured from fecal specimens (preferred) or vomitus plated on thiosulfate citrate–bile salts–sucrose agar. Because most laboratories in the United States do not culture routinely for *V cholerae* or other *Vibrio* organisms, clinicians should request appropriate cultures for clinically suspected cases. Isolates of *V cholerae* should be sent to a state health department laboratory for confirmation and then forwarded to the Centers for Disease Control and Prevention (CDC) for confirmation, serogrouping, and detection of the CT gene (**www.cdc.gov/laboratory/specimen-submission/detail.html?CDCTestCode=CDC-10119**). Tests to detect serum antibodies to *V cholerae*, such as the vibriocidal assay and an anticholera toxin enzyme-linked immunoassay, are available at the CDC. Both assays require submission of acute and convalescent serum specimens and thus provide a retrospective diagnosis. A 4-fold increase in vibriocidal antibody titers between acute and convalescent sera suggests the diagnosis of cholera. Several commercial tests for rapid antigen detection of *V cholerae* O1 and O139 in stool specimens have been developed. These *V cholerae* O1 and O139 rapid diagnostic tests (RDTs) have sensitivities ranging from approximately 80% to 97% and specificities ranging from approximately 70% to 90% when compared with culture on thiosulfate citrate–bile salts–sucrose agar. RDTs are not a substitute for stool culture but potentially provide a rapid presumptive indication of a suspected cholera outbreak in regions where stool culture is not immediately available. Multiplex polymerase chain reaction panels can detect various bacteria, parasites, and viruses associated with gastrointestinal tract infections, and some can specifically detect *V cholerae* from unpreserved stool specimens and/or stool specimens preserved in Cary-Blair media.

TREATMENT

Timely and appropriate rehydration therapy is the cornerstone of management of cholera and reduces the mortality of severe cholera from greater than 10% to less than 0.5%. Rehydration therapy should be based on World Health Organization (WHO) standards, with the goal of replacing the estimated fluid deficit within 3 to 4 hours of initial manifestation. In patients with severe dehydration, isotonic intravenous fluids should be used, and lactated Ringer solution is the preferred commercially available option. For patients without severe dehydration, oral rehydration therapy by using the WHO reduced-osmolality oral rehydration solution (ORS) has been the standard, but data suggest that rice-based ORS or amylase-resistant starch ORS is more effective.

Antimicrobial therapy decreases the duration and volume of diarrhea and decreases the shedding of viable bacteria. Antimicrobial therapy should be considered for people who are moderately to severely ill. The choice of antimicrobial therapy should be made on the basis of the age of the patient (Table 162.1) as well as prevailing patterns of antimicrobial resistance. When prevailing patterns of resistance are unknown, antimicrobial susceptibility testing should be performed and monitored. Zinc supplementation should be considered as an adjunct to rehydration in children.

Table 162.1
Antibiotics for Suspected Cholera

Antibiotic	Pediatric Dose[a]	Adult Dose	Comment(s)
Doxycycline	4.4 mg/kg, single dose	300 mg, single dose	Use should be in epidemics caused by susceptible isolates. Not recommended for pregnant women.
Ciprofloxacin[b]	15 mg/kg, twice daily for 3 days (Single dose of 20 mg/kg has been used.)	500 mg, twice daily for 3 days	Decreased susceptibility to fluoroquinolones is associated with treatment failure. Ciprofloxacin is not recommended in children and pregnant women.
Azithromycin	20 mg/kg, single dose	1 g, single dose	
Erythromycin	12.5 mg/kg, 4 times/day for 3 days	250 mg, 4 times/day for 3 days	
Tetracycline[c]	12.5 mg/kg, 4 times/day for 3 days	500 mg, 4 times/day for 3 days	

[a] Not to exceed adult dose.
[b] Fluoroquinolones are not approved for children <18 years for this indication.
[c] For use in children ≥8 years.

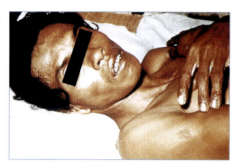

Image 162.1
An adult patient with cholera demonstrating "washerwoman's hand" sign. Because of severe dehydration, cholera manifests itself in decreased skin turgor, which produces the so-called washerwoman's hand sign. Courtesy of Centers for Disease Control and Prevention.

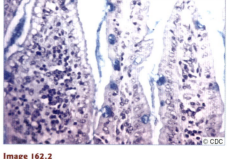

Image 162.2
Intestinal biopsy showing *Vibrio cholerae* causing increased mucus production. *V cholerae* is transmitted to humans through the ingestion of contaminated food or water and produces a cholera toxin that acts on the intestinal mucosa and causes severe diarrhea. Courtesy of Centers for Disease Control and Prevention.

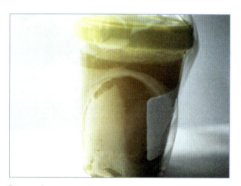

Image 162.3
Shown, a cup of typical rice-water stool from a patient with cholera shows flecks of mucus that have settled to the bottom. These stools are inoffensive, with a faint fishy odor. They are isotonic with plasma and contain high levels of sodium, potassium, and bicarbonate. They also contain extraordinary quantities of *Vibrio cholerae* bacterial organisms. Courtesy of Centers for Disease Control and Prevention.

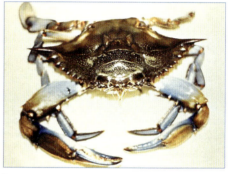

Image 162.4
Crabs have been a repeated source of cholera in the United States and elsewhere, even though they are rarely eaten raw. Crabs artificially inoculated with *Vibrio cholerae* O1 that have been boiled for <10 minutes or steamed for <30 minutes may still harbor viable vibrios, which can then multiply to high counts if the crabs are left at room temperature for several hours. Courtesy of Centers for Disease Control and Prevention.

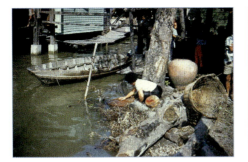

Image 162.5
Typical *Vibrio cholerae*–contaminated water supply. Ingestion of *V cholerae*–contaminated water is a typical mode of pathogen transmission. Courtesy of Centers for Disease Control and Prevention.

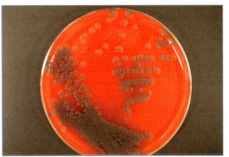

Image 162.7
Vibrio cholerae on blood agar. Colonies are nonhemolytic and opaque with a greenish cast. Courtesy of Julia Rosebush, DO; Robert Jerris, PhD; and Theresa Stanley, M(ASCP).

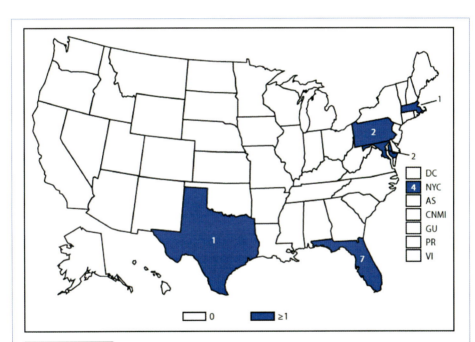

In 2012, as in 2010 and 2011, most cases of cholera reported the United States were in travelers who had recently arrived from Hispaniola. Of the 17 cholera infections in 2012, 16 were travel-associated (12 with travel to Hispaniola [nine to Haiti and three to the Dominican Republic] and four to other cholera-affected countries). One patient reported exposure to *Vibrio cholerae* in a laboratory.

Image 162.6
Number of reported cholera cases—United States and US territories, 2012. Courtesy of *Morbidity and Mortality Weekly Report*.

CHAPTER 163
Other *Vibrio* Infections

CLINICAL MANIFESTATIONS

Illness attributable to the following (mostly nontoxigenic) species of the *Vibrionaceae* family is known as vibriosis: (1) *Vibrio parahaemolyticus*, *Vibrio vulnificus*, and other *Vibrio* species; (2) nontoxigenic *Vibrio cholerae*; (3) toxigenic *V cholerae* O75 and O141; and (4) members of the *Vibrionaceae* family that are not in the genus *Vibrio* (eg, *Grimontia hollisae*). Associated clinical syndromes include gastroenteritis, wound infection, and septicemia. Gastroenteritis is the most common syndrome and is characterized by acute onset of watery nonbloody stools and crampy abdominal pain. Approximately half of affected people will have low-grade fever, headache, and chills; approximately 30% will have vomiting. Spontaneous recovery follows in 2 to 5 days. Wound infections typically start as cellulitis with vesicles and can progress to hemorrhagic bullae, necrosis, and/or necrotizing fasciitis. Septicemia can be primary or can follow gastroenteritis or wound infection and is often fulminant and accompanied by development of metastatic skin lesions within 36 hours. Risk factors for severe wound infections and for septicemia include liver disease, iron overload, hemolytic anemia, chronic renal failure, diabetes mellitus, low gastric acidity, and immunosuppression. Various otolaryngological manifestations attributable to *Vibrio alginolyticus* have been linked to swimming in salt water.

ETIOLOGY

Vibrio organisms are facultatively anaerobic, motile, gram-negative bacilli that are tolerant of salt. The most commonly reported nontoxigenic *Vibrio* species associated with diarrhea are *V parahaemolyticus* and *V cholerae* non-O1/non-O139. *V vulnificus* typically causes primary septicemia and severe wound infections, but the other species can also cause these syndromes. *V alginolyticus* typically causes wound and ear infections, with ear infections being more common in children.

EPIDEMIOLOGY

Vibrio species are natural inhabitants of marine and estuarine environments. In temperate climates, most noncholera *Vibrio* infections occur during summer and autumn months, when *Vibrio* populations in seawater are highest. Gastroenteritis usually follows ingestion of raw or undercooked seafood, especially oysters, clams, crabs, and shrimp. Wound infections are usually attributable to *V vulnificus* and can result from exposure of a preexisting wound to contaminated seawater or from punctures caused by handling of contaminated fish or shellfish. Exposure to contaminated water during natural disasters, such as hurricanes, has resulted in wound infections. Person-to-person transmission has not been reported. Infections associated with noncholera *Vibrio* organisms became nationally notifiable since January 2007. It is estimated that 80,000 cases, 500 hospitalizations, and 100 deaths from vibriosis occur each year in the United States.

The **incubation period** for gastroenteritis is typically 24 hours (with a range of 5–92 hours) and is 1 to 7 days for wound infections and septicemia.

DIAGNOSTIC TESTS

Depending on the clinical syndrome, *Vibrio* organisms can be isolated from stool, wound exudates, or blood. Because identification of the organism requires special techniques, laboratory personnel should be notified when infection with *Vibrio* species is suspected. Multiplex molecular panels are available, but the specificity in some diagnostic tests is poor. Infection should be confirmed by culture.

TREATMENT

Diarrhea is typically mild and self-limited and requires only oral rehydration. Wound infections require prompt surgical debridement of necrotic tissue, if present. Antimicrobial therapy is indicated for severe diarrhea, wound infection, and septicemia. Septicemia with or without hemorrhagic bullae and wound infections should be treated with a third-generation cephalosporin plus either doxycycline or ciprofloxacin. Severe diarrhea should be treated with doxycycline or ciprofloxacin. Doxycycline can be used for short durations (ie, ≤21 days) without regard to patient age. A combination of trimethoprim-sulfamethoxazole and an aminoglycoside is an alternative regimen.

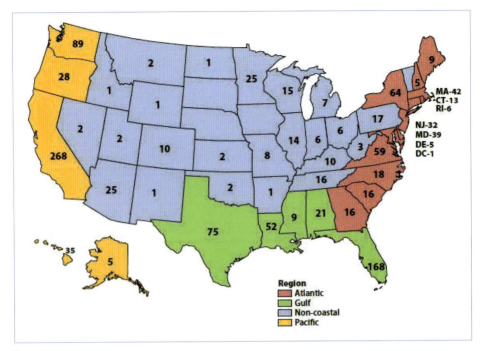

Image 163.1
Number of cases of *Vibrio* infections (excluding toxigenic *Vibrio cholerae* O1 and O139), by state, 2014 (N = 1,252 from 46 states and the District of Columbia). Of the 1,252 vibriosis cases, 325 (26%) were reported from Gulf coast states, 425 (34%) from Pacific coast states, 325 (26%) from Atlantic coast states, and 177 (14%) from non-coastal states. The *Vibrio* species reported most frequently from Gulf coast states were *Vibrio alginolyticus*, 91 (28%); *Vibrio vulnificus*, 64 (21%); and *Vibrio parahaemolyticus*, 62 (20%). The *Vibrio* species reported most frequently from non–Gulf coast states were *V parahaemolyticus*, 543 (59%); *V alginolyticus*, 148 (16%); and *V vulnificus*, 60 (7%). Courtesy of Centers for Disease Control and Prevention.

CHAPTER 164
West Nile Virus

CLINICAL MANIFESTATIONS

An estimated 70% to 80% of people infected with West Nile virus (WNV) are asymptomatic. Most symptomatic people experience an acute systemic febrile illness that often includes headache, myalgia, arthralgia, vomiting, diarrhea, or a transient maculopapular rash. Less than 1% of infected people develop neuroinvasive disease, which typically manifests as meningitis, encephalitis, or acute flaccid myelitis. WNV meningitis is indistinguishable clinically from aseptic meningitis caused by other viruses. Patients with WNV encephalitis usually present with fever, headache, seizures, mental status changes, focal neurological deficits, or movement disorders. WNV acute flaccid myelitis is often clinically and pathologically identical to poliovirus-associated poliomyelitis, with damage of anterior horn cells, and may progress to respiratory paralysis requiring mechanical ventilation. WNV-associated Guillain-Barré syndrome has also been reported and can be distinguished from WNV acute flaccid myelitis by clinical manifestations, findings on cerebrospinal fluid (CSF) analysis, and electrophysiological testing. Cardiac dysrhythmias, myocarditis, rhabdomyolysis, optic neuritis, uveitis, chorioretinitis, orchitis, pancreatitis, and hepatitis have rarely been described after WNV infection.

Routine clinical laboratory results are nonspecific in WNV infections. In patients with neuroinvasive disease, CSF examination generally shows lymphocytic pleocytosis, but neutrophils may predominate early in the illness. Brain magnetic resonance imaging findings are frequently normal, but signal abnormalities may be visualized in the basal ganglia, thalamus, and brainstem with WNV encephalitis and in the spinal cord with WNV acute flaccid myelitis.

Most patients with WNV nonneuroinvasive disease or meningitis recover completely, but fatigue, malaise, and weakness can linger for weeks or months. Recovery from WNV encephalitis or acute flaccid myelitis often takes weeks to months, and patients commonly have residual neurological deficits. Among patients with neuroinvasive disease, the overall case-fatality rate is approximately 10%, but it is significantly higher in WNV encephalitis and acute flaccid myelitis than in WNV meningitis.

Most women known to have been infected with WNV during pregnancy have delivered newborns without evidence of infection or clinical abnormalities. Rare cases of congenital infection and probable transmission via human milk have been reported. If WNV disease is diagnosed during pregnancy, a detailed examination of the fetus and of the newborn should be performed.

ETIOLOGY

WNV is an RNA virus of the *Flaviviridae* family (genus *Flavivirus*) that is related antigenically to St Louis encephalitis and Japanese encephalitis viruses.

EPIDEMIOLOGY

WNV is an arthropod borne virus (arbovirus) that is transmitted in an enzootic cycle between mosquitoes and amplifying vertebrate hosts, primarily birds. WNV is transmitted to humans primarily through bites of infected *Culex* mosquitoes. Humans do not usually develop a level or duration of viremia sufficient to infect mosquitoes and, therefore, are dead-end hosts. Person-to-person WNV transmission can occur through blood transfusion and solid organ transplant. Intrauterine and probable breastfeeding transmission have rarely been described. Transmission through percutaneous and mucosal exposure has occurred in laboratories and occupational settings.

WNV transmission has been documented on every continent except Antarctica. Since the 1990s, the largest outbreaks of WNV neuroinvasive disease have occurred in the Middle East, Europe, and North America. WNV was first detected in the Western hemisphere in New York City in 1999 and subsequently spread across the continental United States and Canada. From 1999 through 2018, there were 24,657 cases of WNV neuroinvasive disease reported in the United States, with peaks in national incidence in 2002, 2003, and 2012. WNV is the leading cause of neuroinvasive arboviral disease in the United States. In 2018, there were 1,658 cases of WNV neuroinvasive disease reported, more than 11 times the number of neuroinvasive disease cases reported for all other domestic arboviruses combined (eg, Eastern equine encephalitis; Jamestown Canyon, La Crosse, Powassan, and St Louis encephalitis viruses). Alaska and Hawaii are the only states without reported local transmission of WNV.

In temperate and subtropical regions, most human WNV infections occur in summer or early autumn. All age-groups and sexes are susceptible to WNV infection, but incidence of severe disease (eg, encephalitis and death) is highest among older adults. Chronic renal failure, history of cancer, history of alcohol use, diabetes, and hypertension have been associated with developing severe WNV disease.

The **incubation period** is usually 2 to 6 days but ranges from 2 to 14 days and can be up to 21 days in immunocompromised people and up to 37 days in solid organ transplant recipients.

DIAGNOSTIC TESTS

Detection of anti-WNV immunoglobulin M (IgM) antibodies in serum or CSF is the most common way to diagnose WNV infection. The presence of anti-WNV IgM is usually good evidence of recent WNV infection but may indicate infection with another closely related flavivirus. Because anti-WNV IgM can persist in the serum of some patients for longer than 1 year, a positive test result may occasionally reflect past infection. Detection of WNV IgM in CSF generally indicates recent neuroinvasive infection. WNV IgM antibodies are detectable in most WNV-infected patients within 3 to 8 days of symptom onset and typically remain detectable for 30 to 90 days. For patients from whom serum collected within 8 days of illness lacks detectable IgM, testing should be repeated on a convalescent-phase sample. Immunoglobulin G antibody is generally detectable shortly after IgM and can persist for years. Plaque-reduction neutralization tests can be performed to measure virus-specific neutralizing antibodies and to discriminate between cross-reacting antibodies from closely related flaviviruses. A 4-fold or greater increase in virus-specific neutralizing antibodies between acute- and convalescent-phase serum specimens collected 2 to 3 weeks apart may be used to confirm recent WNV infection.

Viral culture and WNV nucleic acid amplification tests (including reverse transcriptase–polymerase chain reaction [PCR]) can be performed on acute-phase serum, CSF, or tissue specimens. By the time most immunocompetent patients present with clinical symptoms, WNV RNA is usually no longer detectable; therefore, PCR assay is not recommended for diagnosis in immunocompetent hosts. Sensitivity of these tests is likely higher in immunocompromised patients. Immunohistochemical staining can detect WNV antigens in fixed tissue, but negative results are not definitive.

WNV disease should be considered in the differential diagnosis of febrile or acute neurological illnesses associated with recent exposure to mosquitoes, blood transfusion, or solid organ transplant and of illnesses in neonates whose mothers were infected with WNV during pregnancy or while breastfeeding. WNV and other arboviruses should be considered in the differential diagnosis of aseptic meningitis and encephalitis along with other causes such as herpes simplex virus and enteroviruses.

TREATMENT

No specific therapy is available; management of WNV disease is supportive. Although various therapies have been evaluated or used empirically for WNV disease, none has shown specific benefit.

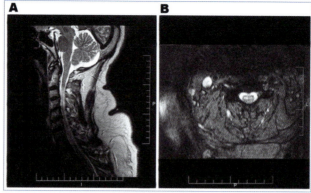

Image 164.1
West Nile virus–associated flaccid paralysis. Sagittal (A) and axial (B) T2-weighted magnetic resonance images of the cervical spinal cord in a patient with acute asymmetrical upper extremity weakness and subjective dyspnea. A, Diffuse cervical cord signal abnormality. B, Abnormal signal in the anterior horn region. Courtesy of *Emerging Infectious Diseases*.

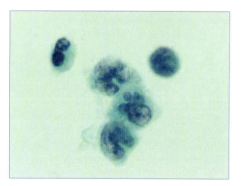

Image 164.2
Three Mollaret-like cells are present (center), with a neutrophil (upper left) and a lymphocyte (upper right) in cerebrospinal fluid from a patient with West Nile virus encephalitis, confirmed by reverse transcriptase–polymerase chain reaction and serological testing (Papanicolaou stain, magnification ×500). Courtesy of Centers for Disease Control and Prevention.

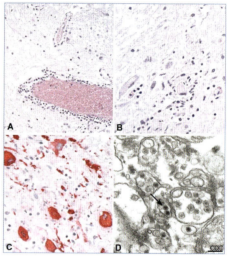

Image 164.3
Histopathologic features of West Nile virus (WNV) in human tissues. A and B, Inflammation, microglial nodules, and variable necrosis that occur during WNV encephalitis. C, WNV antigen (red) in neurons and neuronal processes with an immunohistochemical stain. D, Electron micrograph of WNV in the endoplasmic reticulum of a nerve cell (arrow) (bar = 100 nm). These 4 images are from a fatal case of WNV infection in a 39-year-old woman. Courtesy of *Emerging Infectious Diseases*.

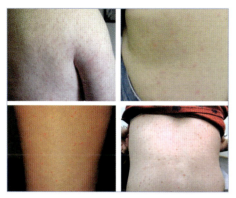

Image 164.4
Four patients with West Nile virus fever and erythematous, maculopapular rashes on the back (A), flank (B), posterior thigh (C), and back (D). Copyright *Clinical Infectious Diseases*.

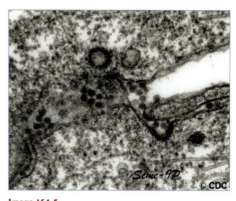

Image 164.5
Transmission electron micrograph of West Nile virus. This virus is transmitted between culicine mosquitoes and birds. Humans, horses, and other mammals are infected incidentally. Courtesy of Centers for Disease Control and Prevention.

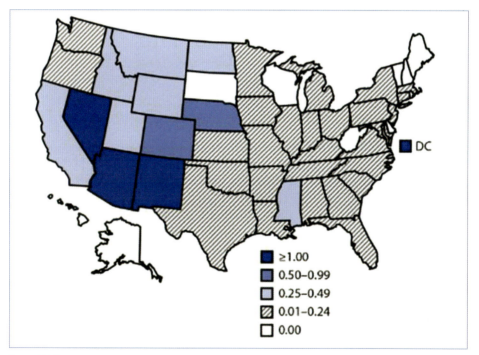

Image 164.6
Incidence of reported cases of West Nile virus neuroinvasive disease—United States, 2019. *Cases per 100,000 population. †No cases were reported from Alaska or Hawaii. Courtesy of Centers for Disease Control and Prevention.

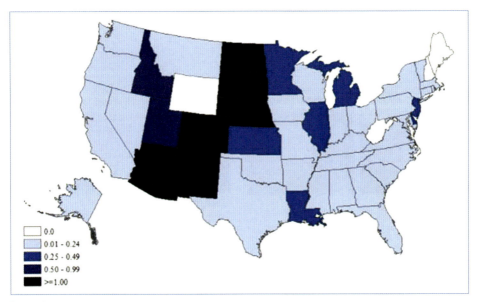

Image 164.7
West Nile Virus (WNV) neuroinvasive disease incidence by state—United States, 2021 (as of January 11, 2022). This map shows the incidence of human WNV neuroinvasive disease (eg, meningitis, encephalitis, or acute flaccid paralysis) by state for 2021 with shading ranging from 0.01–0.24, 0.25–0.49, 0.50–0.99, and >1.00 per 100,000 population. Courtesy of Centers for Disease Control and Prevention.

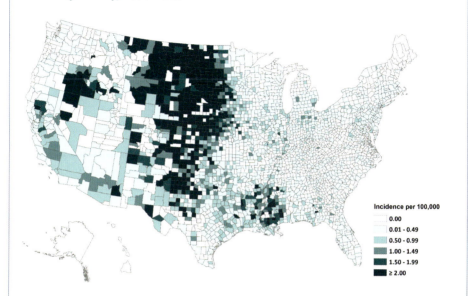

Image 164.8
Average annual incidence of West Nile virus neuroinvasive disease reported to the Centers for Disease Control and Prevention (CDC) by county, 1999–2020. Courtesy of Centers for Disease Control and Prevention.

CHAPTER 165

Yersinia enterocolitica and *Yersinia pseudotuberculosis* Infections
(Enteritis and Other Illnesses)

CLINICAL MANIFESTATIONS

Yersinia enterocolitica causes several age-specific syndromes and a variety of other less commonly reported clinical illnesses. Infection with *Y enterocolitica* typically manifests as fever, diarrhea, and abdominal pain in children younger than 5 years; stool often contains leukocytes, blood, and mucus. Diarrhea commonly persists for more than 2 weeks. Relapsing disease and, rarely, necrotizing enterocolitis have also been described. In older children and adults, a pseudoappendicitis syndrome attributable to mesenteric lymphadenitis (fever, abdominal pain, tenderness in the right lower quadrant of the abdomen, and leukocytosis) is common. Bacteremia is the major complication of *Y enterocolitica*–associated enteric infection occurring mostly in children younger than 1 year and in older children with predisposing conditions, such as excessive iron storage (eg, deferoxamine use, sickle cell disease, and β-thalassemia) and immunosuppressive states. Extraintestinal manifestations of *Y enterocolitica* are uncommon and include pharyngitis, meningitis, osteomyelitis, pyomyositis, conjunctivitis, pneumonia, empyema, endocarditis, acute peritonitis, abscesses of the liver and spleen, urinary tract infection, and primary cutaneous infection. Postinfectious sequelae with *Y enterocolitica* infection include erythema nodosum, reactive arthritis, uveitis, and glomerulonephritis. These sequelae occur most often in older children and adults, particularly people with HLA-B27 antigen.

Major manifestations of *Yersinia pseudotuberculosis* infection include fever, scarlatiniform rash, acute gastroenteritis, and abdominal symptoms. Acute pseudoappendiceal abdominal pain is common, resulting from ileocecal mesenteric adenitis or terminal ileitis. Other uncommon findings reported have been intestinal intussusception, erythema nodosum, septicemia mainly in individuals with underlying conditions, acute renal failure with nephritis, and sterile pleural and joint effusions. Clinical features can mimic those of Kawasaki disease; in Hiroshima, Japan, nearly 10% of children with a diagnosis of Kawasaki disease have serological or culture evidence of *Y pseudotuberculosis* infection.

ETIOLOGY

The genus *Yersinia* consists of 17 species of gram-negative bacilli belonging to the family Enterobacteriaceae. *Y. enterocolitica, Y pseudotuberculosis,* and *Yersinia pestis* are the 3 most recognized human pathogens; however, other *Yersinia* species have also been isolated from clinical specimens. Isolates of *Y enterocolitica* involved in human infections belong to several serotypes (O:3, O:8, O:9, and O:5.27) and are divided into 3 groups according to their pathogenic potential: nonpathogenic biotype 1A, weakly pathogenic biotypes 2 through 5, and highly pathogenic biotype 1B. Strains from biotype 1A can induce infections only in immunocompromised individuals. Serotype O:8, from biotype 1B, is the most virulent and has been responsible for several food poisoning outbreaks in the United States. At present, *Y enterocolitica* serotype O:3, found primarily in pigs, is the most frequent cause of yersiniosis in Europe and North America. The 3 *Yersinia* species have in common a tropism for lymphoid tissue and share factors that promote serum resistance, coordinate gene expression, and facilitate iron acquisition. Differences in virulence gene distribution exist among *Yersinia* species; for example, *Y enterocolitica* has a chromosomal gene encoding for an enterotoxin, and *Y pseudotuberculosis* produces a superantigen toxin among other factors. Virulence can be attributed to adhesion/invasion genes (ie, *ail, inv*), enterotoxins (ie, YstA, YstB), iron-scavenging genomic islands, and secretion systems. Highly pathogenic *Yersinia* are known to carry a 70 kilobase pYV virulence plasmid, which encodes a type III secretion system that is activated at human body temperatures and promotes entry into lymph tissues and subsequent evasion of host defense mechanisms.

EPIDEMIOLOGY

Yersinia infections are reported uncommonly in the United States. *Y enterocolitica* and *Y pseudotuberculosis* are isolated most often during the cool months of temperate climates. The Foodborne Diseases Active Surveillance Network

(FoodNet) conducts active surveillance for infections caused by 9 pathogens, including *Yersinia*. During 2018, FoodNet helped identify 465 *Yersinia* cases of infection, with an average incidence of 0.9 per 100,000 population, which represents a 58% increase in comparison to 2015–2017. This increased incidence likely resulted from increased use of culture-independent diagnostic tests that detect bacterial antigens and genes for *Y enterocolitica*. *Yersinia* incidence is highest among children younger than 5 years and among Black people; however, in recent years, a significant declining incidence among Black children has been observed. On the basis of FoodNet data from 1996–2007, compared with *Y enterocolitica* infection average annual incidence, *Y pseudotuberculosis* infection average annual incidence is much lower (0.04 cases per 1 million population), occurs in older people (median age was 47 years), and is more severe and invasive (72% were hospitalized, 11% died, and two-thirds of isolates were recovered from blood).

The principal reservoir of *Y enterocolitica* is swine, although it can be isolated from a variety of domestic and wildlife animals; *Y pseudotuberculosis* has been isolated from ungulates (ie, deer, elk, goats, sheep, cattle), rodents (ie, rats, squirrels, beaver), rabbits, and many bird species. Infection with *Y enterocolitica* is believed to be transmitted by ingestion of contaminated food (raw or incompletely cooked pork products, tofu, and unpasteurized or inadequately pasteurized milk), by contaminated surface or well water, by direct or indirect contact with animals, and, rarely, by transfusion with contaminated packed red blood cells and by person-to-person transmission. Cross-contamination has been documented to lead to infection in infants if their caregivers handle raw pork intestines (ie, chitterlings) and do not clean their hands or food preparation surfaces adequately before handling the infant or the infant's toys, bottles, or pacifiers. *Y pseudotuberculosis* can follow exposure to well and mountain waters contaminated with animal feces. Household pets can be a source of infection for children. Infections in Finland have been associated with eating fresh produce, presumably contaminated by wild animals carrying the organism.

The **incubation period** is typically 4 to 6 days, with a range of 1 to 14 days. Organisms are typically excreted for 2 to 3 weeks and up to 2 to 3 months in untreated cases. Prolonged asymptomatic carriage is possible.

DIAGNOSTIC TESTS

Y enterocolitica and *Y pseudotuberculosis* can be recovered from stool, throat swab specimens, mesenteric lymph nodes, peritoneal fluid, and blood. *Y enterocolitica* has also been isolated from synovial fluid, bile, urine, cerebrospinal fluid (CSF), sputum, pleural fluid, and wounds. Stool cultures generally yield bacteria during the first 2 weeks of illness, regardless of the nature of gastrointestinal tract manifestations. *Yersinia* organisms are not sought routinely in stool specimens by most laboratories in the United States. Laboratory personnel should be notified when *Yersinia* infection is suspected so stool can be cultured on suitable media (eg, CIN agar); however, strains of *Y enterocolitica* 3/O:3 and *Y pseudotuberculosis* may be inhibited on CIN agar, and MacConkey is preferred. DNA-based gastrointestinal syndrome panels that can reliably detect *Yersinia* are commercially available; these tests typically target only *Y enterocolitica* but may cross-react with other *Yersinia* species. Biotyping and serotyping for further identification of pathogenic strains are available through public health reference laboratories. Infection can also be confirmed by demonstrating increases in serum antibody titer after infection, but these tests are generally available only in reference or research laboratories. Cross-reactions of these antibodies with *Brucella, Vibrio, Salmonella, Rickettsia* organisms, and *Escherichia coli* can lead to false-positive *Y enterocolitica* and *Y pseudotuberculosis* titers. In patients with thyroid disease, persistently increased *Y enterocolitica* antibody titers can result from antigenic similarity of the organism with antigens of the thyroid epithelial cell membrane. Characteristic ultrasonographic features demonstrating edema of the wall of the terminal ileum and cecum with normal appendix help distinguish pseudoappendicitis from appendicitis and can help avoid exploratory surgery. Several DNA-based methods have been developed for both *Y enterocolitica* and *Y pseudotuberculosis* for use in clinical, food, and environmental samples.

TREATMENT

Neonates, immunocompromised hosts, and all patients with septicemia or extraintestinal disease require treatment of *Yersinia* infection. Parenteral therapy with a third-generation cephalosporin is appropriate, and evaluation of CSF should be performed for infected neonates. Otherwise healthy nonneonates with enterocolitis can be treated symptomatically. Although a clinical benefit of antimicrobial therapy for immunocompetent patients with enterocolitis, pseudoappendicitis syndrome, or mesenteric adenitis has not been established, some clinicians consider treatment because of its favorable effect on decreasing the duration of shedding of *Y enterocolitica* and *Y pseudotuberculosis*. In addition to third-generation cephalosporins, *Y enterocolitica* and *Y pseudotuberculosis* are usually susceptible to trimethoprim-sulfamethoxazole, aminoglycosides, fluoroquinolones, chloramphenicol, tetracycline, and doxycycline. *Y enterocolitica* isolates are usually resistant to first-generation cephalosporins and most penicillins.

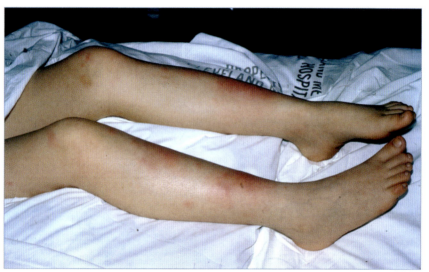

Image 165.1
Multiple erythema nodosum lesions over both lower extremities of a 10-year-old girl following a *Yersinia enterocolitica* infection. This immunoreactive complication may also occur in association with *Campylobacter jejuni* infections, tuberculosis, leprosy, coccidioidomycosis, histoplasmosis, and other infectious diseases. Courtesy of George Nankervis, MD.

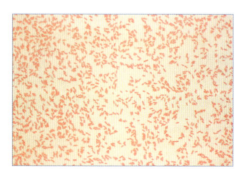

Image 165.2
A photomicrograph of *Yersinia enterocolitica* by use of Gram stain technique. Courtesy of Centers for Disease Control and Prevention.

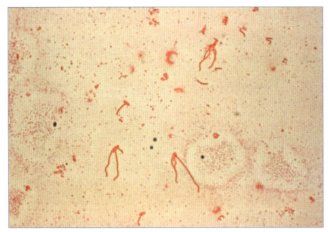

Image 165.3
A photomicrograph of *Yersinia enterocolitica* by use of flagella-staining technique. Symptoms of yersiniosis are fever, abdominal pain, and diarrhea (often bloody), and *Y enterocolitica* is the cause of most *Yersinia*-related illnesses in the United States (mostly in children). Courtesy of Centers for Disease Control and Prevention.

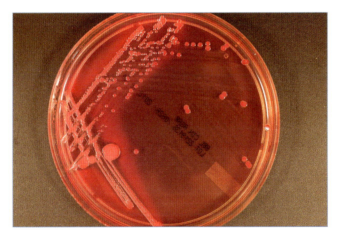

Image 165.4
Yersinia kristensenii on cefsulodin-irgasan-novobiocin agar. Colonies appear light rose in color with a darker, reddish center. Courtesy of Julia Rosebush, DO; Robert Jerris, PhD; and Theresa Stanley, M(ASCP).

CHAPTER 166
Zika

CLINICAL MANIFESTATIONS

Most Zika virus infections are asymptomatic. When infection is symptomatic, the clinical disease is usually mild, and symptoms last for a few days to a week. Commonly reported signs and symptoms include fever, pruritic maculopapular rash, arthralgia, and conjunctival hyperemia. Other findings include myalgia, headache, edema of the extremities, vomiting, retro-orbital pain, and lymphadenopathy. Clinical laboratory abnormalities are observed uncommonly in symptomatic patients but can include thrombocytopenia, leukopenia, and increased liver aminotransferase concentrations. Severe disease requiring hospitalization and deaths are rare. However, Guillain-Barré syndrome and rare reports of other neurological complications (eg, meningoencephalitis, myelitis, and uveitis) have been associated with Zika virus infection.

Congenital Zika virus infection can cause fetal loss as well as microcephaly and other serious neurological anomalies. Clinical findings reported in infants with confirmed congenital Zika virus infection include brain anomalies (eg, subcortical calcifications, ventriculomegaly, abnormal gyral patterns, corpus callosum agenesis, and cerebellar hypoplasia), ocular anomalies (eg, microphthalmia, cataracts, chorioretinal atrophy, and optic nerve hypoplasia), congenital contractures (eg, clubfoot and arthrogryposis), and neurological sequelae (eg, hypertonia, hypotonia, irritability, tremors, swallowing dysfunction, hearing loss, and visual impairment).

Rare cases of perinatal transmission from mothers who were viremic at delivery have been reported. These generally result in asymptomatic or mildly symptomatic illness in the neonate.

ETIOLOGY

Zika virus is a single-stranded RNA virus in the genus *Flavivirus* that is related antigenically to dengue, yellow fever, West Nile, St Louis encephalitis, and Japanese encephalitis viruses. Two major lineages, African and Asian, have been identified through phylogenetic analyses.

EPIDEMIOLOGY

Zika virus is transmitted to humans primarily by *Aedes aegypti* mosquitoes and less commonly by *Aedes albopictus* and possibly other *Aedes* (*Stegomyia*) species (eg, *Aedes polynesiensis* and *Aedes hensilli*). In the United States, *A aegypti* mosquitoes are found primarily in southern states. *A albopictus* mosquitoes have a wider distribution. Both *Aedes* species bite humans during the day and night. These are the same vectors that transmit dengue, chikungunya, and yellow fever viruses. Human and nonhuman primates are the main reservoirs of the virus, with humans acting as the primary host in which the virus multiplies, allowing spread to additional mosquitoes and then other humans. Additional modes of transmission have been identified, including perinatal, in utero, sexual, blood transfusion, and laboratory exposure. Although Zika virus has been detected in human milk, and a few probable cases of transmission of Zika virus by breastfeeding have been reported, to date there is no consistent evidence that infants acquire Zika virus through breastfeeding.

Zika virus was first identified in the Zika forest of Uganda in 1947. Before 2007, only sporadic human disease cases were reported from countries in Africa and Asia. In 2007, the first documented Zika virus disease outbreak was reported in the Federated States of Micronesia. In subsequent years, outbreaks of Zika virus disease were identified in countries in Southeast Asia and the western Pacific. In 2015, Zika virus was identified for the first time in the Western hemisphere, with large outbreaks reported in Brazil. Since then, the virus has spread throughout much of the Americas, with 48 countries and territories in the Americas reporting local transmission. During 2016 in the United States, large outbreaks occurred in Puerto Rico and the US Virgin Islands, and limited local transmission was identified in parts of Florida and Texas.

The **incubation period** is 3 to 14 days after the bite of an infected mosquito, with 50% of symptomatic cases developing symptoms 1 week after exposure.

DIAGNOSTIC TESTS

Zika virus infection should be considered in patients with acute onset of fever, maculopapular rash, arthralgia, or conjunctivitis who live in or have traveled to an area with ongoing transmission in the 2 weeks preceding illness onset. Because dengue and chikungunya virus infections share a similar geographic distribution and symptom complex with Zika virus infection, patients with suspected Zika virus infection should also be evaluated and treated for possible dengue or chikungunya virus infection. Other considerations in the differential diagnosis include malaria, rubella, measles, parvovirus infection, adenovirus infection, enterovirus infection, leptospirosis, rickettsiosis, and group A streptococcal infection.

Laboratory testing for Zika virus has a number of limitations. Zika virus RNA is only transiently present in body fluids; thus, a negative real-time reverse transcriptase–polymerase chain reaction (RT-PCR) result does not rule out infection. Likewise, a negative immunoglobulin M (IgM) serological test result does not rule out infection, because the serum specimen might have been collected before the development or after waning of IgM antibodies. Alternatively, IgM antibodies might be detectable for months after the initial infection, making it difficult to distinguish the timing of Zika acquisition. Cross-reactivity of the Zika virus IgM antibody tests with other flaviviruses can result in a false-positive test result. Recent epidemiological data indicate a declining prevalence of Zika virus infection in the Americas; this lower prevalence will result in a lower pretest probability of infection and a higher probability of false-positive test results.

Zika Laboratory Testing in Nonpregnant Symptomatic Individuals

For people with suspected Zika virus disease, Zika virus RT-PCR assay should be performed on serum and urine specimens collected less than 14 days after onset of symptoms. Serum IgM antibody testing should be performed if the RT-PCR result is negative or when 14 days or more has passed since illness onset.

Zika Laboratory Testing in Pregnant Women

Current recommendations from the Centers for Disease Control and Prevention take into account the decreasing prevalence of Zika virus disease cases in the Americas that occurred in 2017. Zika virus testing is not routinely recommended for asymptomatic pregnant women who have possible recent but not ongoing Zika virus exposure. Zika virus RT-PCR testing should be offered as part of routine obstetric care to asymptomatic pregnant women with ongoing possible Zika virus exposure (at the first prenatal visit and if negative at 2 other times during pregnancy). Because of the potential for persistence of IgM antibodies over several months, serological testing is no longer routinely recommended to screen asymptomatic women.

Zika Laboratory Testing for Congenital Infection

Zika virus testing is recommended for infants with clinical findings consistent with congenital Zika syndrome and possible maternal Zika virus exposure during pregnancy, regardless of maternal testing results, and for infants without clinical findings consistent with congenital Zika syndrome who are born to women with laboratory evidence of possible infection during pregnancy. Recommended laboratory testing for possible congenital Zika virus infection includes evaluation for Zika virus RNA in infant serum and urine and Zika virus IgM antibodies in serum. In addition, if cerebrospinal fluid (CSF) is obtained for other reasons, RT-PCR and IgM antibody testing should be performed on CSF, because CSF was the only sample that tested positive in a limited number of infants with congenital Zika virus infection.

Laboratory testing of infants should be performed as soon as possible after birth (within the first few days), although testing specimens within the first few weeks to months after birth might still be useful. If CSF was not collected for other reasons, testing CSF for Zika virus RNA and Zika virus IgM should be considered to improve the likelihood of diagnosis, especially if serum and urine testing are negative and another etiology has not been identified. Diagnosis of congenital Zika virus infection is confirmed by a positive Zika virus RT-PCR or by a positive Zika virus IgM and neutralizing antibody result. If neither Zika virus RNA nor Zika IgM antibodies are detected on the appropriate specimens obtained within the first few days after birth, congenital Zika virus infection is unlikely.

The plaque-reduction neutralization test (PRNT), which measures virus-specific neutralizing antibodies, can be used to help identify false-positive results. If the infant's initial sample is IgM nonnegative (nonnegative serology terminology varies by assay and might include *positive, equivocal, presumptive positive,* or *possible positive*) and RT-PCR negative, and PRNT was not performed on the mother's sample, PRNT for Zika and dengue viruses should be performed on the infant's initial sample. If the Zika virus PRNT result is negative, this suggests that the infant's Zika virus IgM test result is a false positive. For infants with clinical findings consistent with congenital Zika syndrome or maternal evidence of possible Zika virus infection during pregnancy who were not tested near birth, PRNT at the age of 18 months or older (after maternal antibodies have dissipated from the infant's system) might help confirm or rule out congenital Zika virus infection. If the PRNT result is negative at the age of 18 months or older, congenital Zika virus infection is unlikely.

TREATMENT

No specific antiviral treatment is currently available for Zika virus disease. Only supportive care is indicated, including rest, fluids, and symptomatic treatment (acetaminophen to relieve fever and antihistamines to treat pruritus). Aspirin and nonsteroidal anti-inflammatory drugs should be avoided until dengue can be ruled out, to reduce the risk of hemorrhagic complications.

Figure 166.1 outlines the current recommended evaluation of infants with possible maternal and congenital Zika virus exposure during pregnancy.

Clinical Treatment of Infants With Clinical Findings Consistent With Congenital Zika Infection

Zika virus testing is recommended, ultrasonography of the head should be performed, and a comprehensive ophthalmologic examination should be performed by the age of 1 month by an ophthalmologist experienced in assessment of infants. Referrals to a developmental specialist and for early intervention services are recommended. Additional consultation should be considered by infectious disease specialist (for evaluation of other congenital infections and assistance with Zika virus diagnosis and testing), clinical geneticist (for evaluation for other causes of microcephaly or congenital anomalies), and neurologist by the age of 1 month (for comprehensive neurological examination and consideration for other evaluations, such as advanced neuroimaging and electroencephalography). The initial clinical evaluation, including subspecialty consultations, can be performed before hospital discharge or in an outpatient setting. Ophthalmologic follow-up after the initial examination should be based on ophthalmology recommendations. Infants should be referred for automated auditory brainstem response (ABR) testing by the age of 1 month if the newborn hearing screening was passed via only otoacoustic emissions (OAE) methodology.

Clinical Treatment of Infants Without Clinical Findings Consistent With Congenital Zika Infection but Maternal Laboratory Evidence of Possible Zika Virus Infection During Pregnancy

Zika virus testing is recommended, and ultrasonography of the head should be performed by the age of 1 month to detect subclinical brain findings. All infants should undergo a comprehensive ophthalmologic examination by the age of 1 month to detect subclinical eye findings; further follow-up visits with an ophthalmologist after the initial examination should be based on ophthalmology recommendations. Infants should be referred for automated ABR testing by 1 month of age if the newborn screening was passed via only OAE methodology. Infants should be monitored for findings consistent with congenital Zika syndrome that could develop over time (eg, impaired visual acuity/function, hearing problems, developmental delay, delay in head growth).

Clinical Treatment of Infants Without Clinical Findings Consistent With Congenital Zika Infection Who Are Born to Mothers With Possible Zika Virus Infection During Pregnancy but Without Laboratory Evidence of Zika Virus During Pregnancy

Zika virus testing is not routinely recommended, and specialized clinical evaluation or follow-up is not routinely indicated. Health care professionals can consider additional evaluation in consultation with families. If findings suggestive of congenital Zika syndrome are identified at any time, referrals to the appropriate specialists should be made.

FIGURE 166.1

Recommendations for the Evaluation of Infants With Possible Congenital Zika Virus Infection Based on Infant Clinical Findings,[a,b] Maternal Testing Results,[c,d] and Infant Testing Results[e,f]—United States

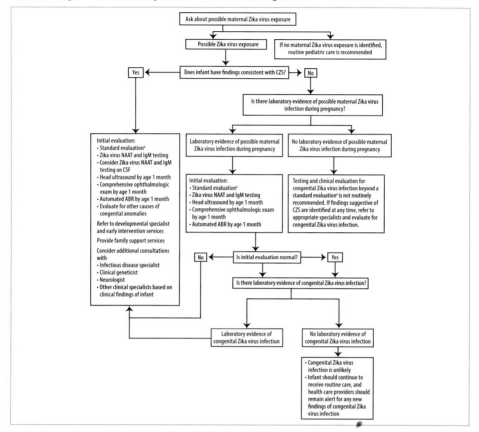

ABR indicates auditory brainstem response; CSF, cerebrospinal fluid; CZS, congenital Zika syndrome; exam, examination; IgM, immunoglobulin M; NAAT, nucleic acid amplification test; PRNT, plaque-reduction neutralization test; and RT-PCR, reverse transcriptase–polymerase chain reaction.

[a] All infants should undergo a standard evaluation at birth and at each subsequent health supervision visit by their health care professionals, including (1) comprehensive physical examination, including growth parameters, and (2) age-appropriate vision screening and developmental monitoring and screening with validated tools. Infants should undergo a standard newborn hearing screening at birth, preferably with ABR.

[b] Automated ABR by the age of 1 month if newborn hearing screening passed but performed with otoacoustic emission methodology.

[c] Laboratory evidence of possible Zika virus infection during pregnancy is defined as (1) Zika virus infection detected by a Zika virus RNA NAAT on any maternal, placental, or fetal specimen (referred to as *NAAT confirmed*) or (2) Zika virus infection diagnosed, timing of infection not determined or *Flavivirus* infection unspecified, timing of infection not determined by serological tests on a maternal specimen (ie, positive/equivocal Zika virus IgM and Zika virus PRNT titer ≥10, regardless of dengue virus PRNT value; or negative Zika virus IgM, and positive/equivocal dengue virus IgM, and Zika virus PRNT titer ≥10, regardless of dengue virus PRNT titer). The use of PRNT for confirmation of Zika virus infection, including in pregnant women, is not routinely recommended in Puerto Rico (**www.cdc.gov/zika/laboratories/lab-guidance.html**).

[d] This group includes women who were never tested during pregnancy as well as those whose test result was negative because of issues related to timing or sensitivity and specificity of the test. Because the latter issues are not easily discerned, all mothers with possible exposure to Zika virus during pregnancy who do not have laboratory evidence of possible Zika virus infection, including those whose test result was negative with currently available technology, should be considered in this group.

[e] Laboratory testing of infants for Zika virus should be performed as early as possible, preferably within the first few days after birth, and includes concurrent Zika virus NAAT in infant serum and urine and Zika virus IgM testing in serum. If CSF is obtained for other purposes, Zika virus NAAT and Zika virus IgM testing should be performed on CSF.

[f] Laboratory evidence of congenital Zika virus infection includes a positive Zika virus NAAT or a nonnegative Zika virus IgM with confirmatory neutralizing antibody testing result, if PRNT confirmation is performed.

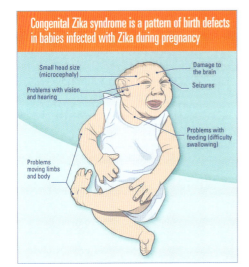

Image 166.1
Congenital Zika syndrome is a pattern of birth defects in babies infected with Zika virus during pregnancy.
Courtesy of Centers for Disease Control and Prevention.

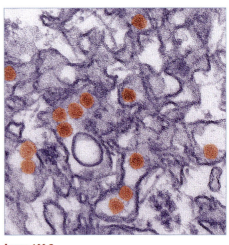

Image 166.2
Transmission electron micrograph of Zika virus, a member of the *Flaviviridae* family.

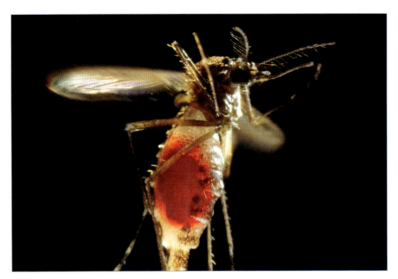

Image 166.3
A female *Aedes aegypti* mosquito takes flight as she leaves her host's skin surface. Courtesy of Centers for Disease Control and Prevention/James Gathany.

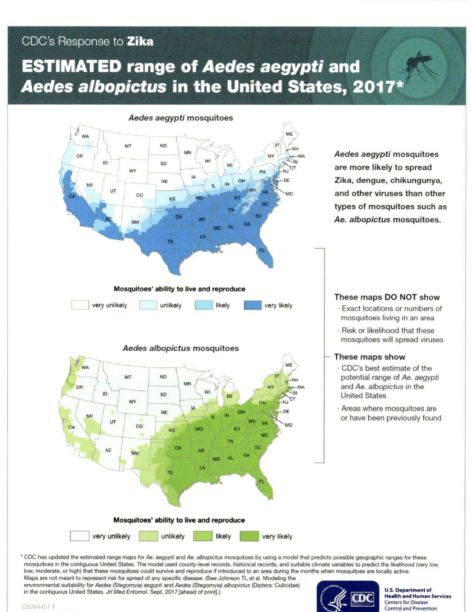

Image 166.4
Estimated range of *Aedes aegypti* and *Aedes albopictus* in the United States, 2017. Courtesy of Centers for Disease Control and Prevention.

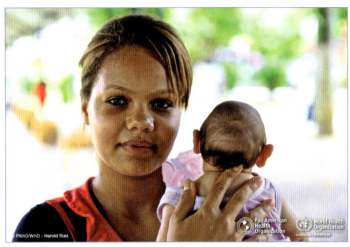

Image 166.5
Baby with microcephaly. Courtesy of Pan American Health Organization and World Health Organization.

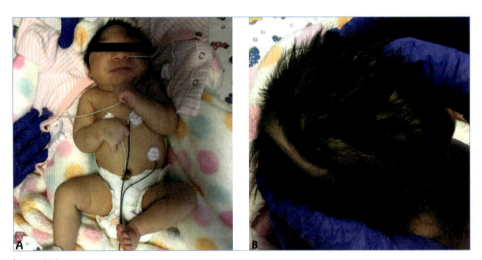

Image 166.6
A and B, This full-term newborn girl was delivered to a mother with a history of a positive result from serum Zika virus polymerase chain reaction assay at 23 weeks' gestation. At 29 weeks' gestation, the fetal head circumference was noted to be 203 mm (4–5 SD below the mean). Coarse calcifications at 37 weeks' gestation were noted on ultrasound. Postnatal testing results for other TORCH infections were negative. Head circumference at birth was 26.5 cm (6.23 SD below the mean). Physical examination was significant for craniofacial disproportion with narrow and laterally depressed frontal bone, upper wrist contractures, and redundant scalp skin with multiple rugae. Magnetic resonance imaging of the brain was significant for microcephaly with enlarged extra-axial spaces, smooth gyral pattern, dysgenesis of the corpus callosum, large bilateral posterior parietal and occipital lobe parenchymal cysts, and 5 small bilateral choroid plexus cysts. Copyright Ashley Howard, DO.

Index

Page numbers followed by *f* indicate a figure; *i*, an image; *t*, a table; and *b*, a box.

A

Abametapir, for pediculosis capitis, 491t, 492
Abdominal abscess
    actinomycosis, 1
    anaerobic gram-negative bacilli infections, 59
Abdominal actinomycosis, 1
Abdominal cramps and pain
    amebiasis, 7
    anthrax, 18
    arenaviruses, 253
    Bacillus cereus infections and intoxications, 54
    bacterial vaginosis, 54
    Balantidium coli infections, 61
    Blastocystis infections, 72
    brucellosis, 82
    bunyaviruses, 255
    Campylobacter infections, 88
    Chlamydia psittaci, 107
    Clostridioides difficile, 122
    coronaviruses, 137
    cryptosporidiosis, 146
    dengue, 166
    Diphyllobothrium, 695
    Dipylidium caninum, 695
    Enterobacteriaceae infections, 185
    enterovirus (nonpoliovirus), 192
    filoviruses, 259
    Giardia duodenalis infections, 219
    hepatitis E, 283
    hydatid disease, 695
    Hymenolepis nana, 695
    influenza, 335
    Kawasaki disease, 347
    louseborne typhus, 793
    malaria, 400
    microsporidia infections, 431
    murine typhus, 796
    norovirus and sapovirus infections, 453
    pelvic inflammatory disease (PID), 499
    Q fever, 543
    Rocky Mountain spotted fever (RMSF), 565
    Salmonella infections, 579
    schistosomiasis, 593
    Shigella infections, 599
    smallpox (variola), 603
    staphylococcal food poisoning, 614
    toxocariasis, 717
    trichinellosis, 730
    Trichomonas vaginalis infections, 734
    trichuriasis (whipworm infection), 739
    tuberculosis (TB), 750
    Vibrio infections, other, 816
    Yersinia enterocolitica and *Yersinia pseudotuberculosis* infections, 824
Abortion
    brucellosis, 82
    Listeria monocytogenes infections, 377
    lymphocytic choriomeningitis virus (LCMV), 398
    Zika virus, 828
Abscess
    Bartholin cyst, anaerobic gram-negative bacilli infections, 59
    brain
        amebic meningoencephalitis and keratitis, 14
        anaerobic gram-negative bacilli infections, 59
        Arcanobacterium haemolyticum infections, 35
        Fusobacterium infections, 216
        non–group A or B streptococcal and enterococcal infections, 652
        Pasteurella infections, 488
        Salmonella infections, 579
        Toxoplasma gondii infections, 720
    intra-abdominal
        actinomycosis, 1
        anaerobic gram-negative bacilli infections, 59
    liver, 82
        amebiasis, 7
        brucellosis, 82
        Pasteurella infections, 488
        Yersinia enterocolitica and *Yersinia pseudotuberculosis* infections, 824
    lungs
        anaerobic gram-negative bacilli infections, 59
        Burkholderia infections, 85
    lymph node, paracoccidioidomycosis, 460
    nocardiosis, 450
    orbital, *Staphylococcus aureus*, 616
    Pasteurella infections, 488
    peritonsillar
        anaerobic gram-negative bacilli infections, 59
        Fusobacterium infections, 216
        Staphylococcus aureus, 616
    pharyngeal, *Arcanobacterium haemolyticum* infections, 35

Abscess (*continued*)
  prostatic and scrotal, anaerobic gram-negative bacilli infections, 59
  rat-bite fever, 552
  skin, blastomycosis, 75
  spleen
    brucellosis, 82
    Yersinia enterocolitica and *Yersinia pseudotuberculosis* infections, 824
    Staphylococcus aureus, 616
Acanthamoeba, 14–16, 16–17*i*
Acidosis, rotavirus infections, 571
Acquired immunodeficiency syndrome (AIDS)
  amebic meningoencephalitis and keratitis and, 14
  cryptococcosis and, 143
  Cryptococcus neoformans and *Cryptococcus gattii* infections and, 145*i*
Acquired syphilis, 670, 678, 679*i*, 680
Acridine orange–stain, for relapsing fever, 80
Acrocyanosis, chikungunya, 103
Actinomyces, 1, 2–3*i*
Actinomyces israelii, 1, 2–3*i*
Actinomycetales, 449
Actinomycosis, 1–2, 2–3*i*
  abdominal, 1
  cervicofacial, 1
  clinical manifestations of, 1, 2*i*
  diagnostic tests for, 1
  epidemiology of, 1
  etiology of, 1
  incubation period of, 1
  other sites of, 1
  thoracic, 1
  treatment of, 2
Acute disseminated encephalomyelitis
  Mycoplasma pneumoniae and other *Mycoplasma* species infections, 444
  Toxoplasma gondii infections, 720
Acute flaccid myelitis (AFM), enterovirus (nonpoliovirus), 192
Acute kidney injury, coronaviruses, 137
Acute otitis media (AOM)
  Moraxella catarrhalis infections, 437
  Mycoplasma pneumoniae and other *Mycoplasma* species infections, 444
  Streptococcus pneumoniae (pneumococcal) infections, 657, 660
Acute respiratory distress syndrome (ARDS)
  blastomycosis, 75
  cryptococcosis, 143
  Ehrlichia, Anaplasma, and related infections, 177

Acute rheumatic fever (ARF), 639–642, 640*b*, 641*t*
Acute transient pneumonitis, *Ascaris lumbricoides* infections, 37
Acyclovir
  for herpes simplex virus (HSV), 288
  for varicella-zoster virus (VSV), 803
Adenitis, group B streptococcal (GBS) infections, 647
Adenoviridae, 4
Adenovirus infections, 4–5, 5–6*i*
  clinical manifestations of, 4, 5*i*
  diagnostic tests for, 4–5
  epidemiology of, 4
  etiology of, 4
  incubation period of, 4
  treatment of, 5
Adolescents
  candidiasis in, 94
  Chlamydia trachomatis in, 111
  gonococcal infections in, 228*i*
  herpes simplex virus (HSV) in, 285–286, 287
  HIV infection in, 318–319
  tuberculosis (TB) in, 765, 766
Aedes aegypti, 166–167
Aedes albopictus, 166–167
Aedes polynesiensis, 166
African trypanosomiasis, 742–743, 743–744*i*
  clinical manifestations of, 742
  diagnostic tests for, 743
  epidemiology of, 742–743
  etiology of, 742
  incubation period of, 743
  treatment of, 743
Ageusia, 137
Aggregatibacter (Actinobacillus) actinomycetemcomitans, 1
Agranulocytosis, Epstein-Barr virus, 197
AIDS. See Acquired immunodeficiency syndrome (AIDS)
Alanine aminotransferase
  coronaviruses and, 137
  dengue and, 166
  hepatitis C and, 277
Albendazole
  for *Ascaris lumbricoides* infections, 37
  for *Baylisascaris* infections, 68–69
  for cutaneous larva migrans, 151
  for hookworm infections, 302
  for lymphatic filariasis, 394
  for pinworm infection (*Enterobius vermicularis*), 510
  for strongyloidiasis, 668

for tapeworm diseases, 690
for toxocariasis, 717
for trichinellosis, 730
for trichuriasis (whipworm infection), 739
Alice in Wonderland syndrome, 197
Allergic bronchopulmonary aspergillosis, 41
Allergic sinusitis, 41
Alopecia
  syphilis, 670
  tinea capitis, 704
Alphaherpesviridae, 286, 802
Altered mental status
  African trypanosomiasis, 742
  amebic meningoencephalitis and keratitis, 14
  Baylisascaris infections, 68
  Chlamydia psittaci, 107
  Ehrlichia, Anaplasma, and related infections, 177
  louseborne typhus, 793
  relapsing fever, 79
  Rocky Mountain spotted fever (RMSF), 565
  Salmonella infections, 579
  West Nile virus (WNV), 818
Alternaria, 209t
Amblyomma americanum, 183i
Amebiasis, 7–9, 9–13i
  clinical manifestations of, 7, 9i, 11i
  control measures for, 9
  diagnostic tests for, 8, 10i
  epidemiology of, 7–8
  etiology of, 7
  incubation period of, 8
  isolation of hospitalized patient with, 9
  treatment of, 8–9
Amebic dysentery, 7
Amebic granuloma amebiasis, 7
Amebicides, 8
Amebic keratitis, 14–16, 16–17i
  clinical manifestations of, 14
  diagnostic tests for, 15
  epidemiology of, 14–15
  etiology of, 14
  incubation period of, 15
  treatment of, 15–16
Amebic meningoencephalitis, 14–16, 16–17i
  clinical manifestations of, 14
  diagnostic tests for, 15
  epidemiology of, 14–15
  etiology of, 14
  incubation period of, 15
  treatment of, 15–16
American trypanosomiasis, 745–746, 747–749i
  clinical manifestations of, 745
  diagnostic tests for, 746
  epidemiology of, 745–746
  etiology of, 745
  incubation period of, 746
  treatment of, 746
Aminoglycosides
  for *Enterobacteriaceae* infections, 186
  for *Giardia duodenalis* infections, 220
  for group B streptococcal (GBS) infections, 648
  for *Listeria monocytogenes* infections, 378
  for *Pseudomonas aeruginosa* infections, 540, 541
  for *Vibrio* infections, other, 816
Amoxicillin
  for actinomycosis, 2
  for group A streptococcal (GAS) infections, 636
  for *Helicobacter pylori* infections, 250–251, 250t, 251t
  for leptospirosis, 373
  for Lyme disease, 385–386, 385t
  for *Pasteurella* infections, 488
Amoxicillin-clavulanate
  for nocardiosis, 450
  for *Pasteurella* infections, 488–489
AmpC β-lactamases, 185
Amphotericin B deoxycholate
  for blastomycosis, 76
  for candidiasis, 92–94
  for coccidioidomycosis, 130–131
  for *Cryptococcus neoformans* and *Cryptococcus gattii* infections, 144
  for paracoccidioidomycosis, 460
  for sporotrichosis, 611
Amphotericin B lipid formulation
  for blastomycosis, 76
  for *Cryptococcus neoformans* and *Cryptococcus gattii* infections, 144
Ampicillin
  for actinomycosis, 2
  for *Enterobacteriaceae* infections, 186
  for group B streptococcal (GBS) infections, 648
  for *Haemophilus influenzae* type b (Hib) infections, 235
  for *Kingella kingae* infections, 354
  for leptospirosis, 373
  for *Listeria monocytogenes* infections, 378
  for meningococcal infections, 420
  for non–group A or B streptococcal and enterococcal infections, 653
  for *Pasteurella* infections, 488

Ampicillin (*continued*)
    for *Salmonella* infections, 581, 582
    for *Shigella* infections, 601
Ampicillin-sulbactam, for *Moraxella catarrhalis* infections, 437
Amsel criteria for bacterial vaginosis, 56–57
Anaerobic gram-negative bacilli infections, 59–60, 60*i*
    epidemiology of, 59
    etiology of, 59
    incubation period of, 59
    treatment of, 59–60
Anaplasma infections, 177–179, 177*t*, 180–184*i*, 561
    clinical manifestations of, 177
    diagnostic tests for, 179
    epidemiology of, 178, 178*t*
    etiology of, 177–178, 177*t*
    incubation period of, 178
    treatment of, 179
Anaplasma phagocytophilum, 49
Anaplasmataceae, 177–179
Ancylostoma braziliense, 151, 301
Ancylostoma caninum, 151, 301
Ancylostoma celanicum, 151
Ancylostoma ceylanicum, 301
Anemia
    brucellosis, 82
    Diphyllobothrium, 695
    malaria, 400
    trichuriasis (whipworm infection), 739
Angiostrongylus cantonensis, 471*t*, 479*i*
Angiostrongylus costaricensis, 471*t*, 473*i*
Anisakiasis, 471*t*, 478*i*
Anogenital warts, 331
Anorexia and weight loss
    African trypanosomiasis, 742
    amebiasis, 7
    arenaviruses, 253
    babesiosis, 49
    Balantidium coli infections, 61
    Blastocystis infections, 72
    brucellosis, 82
    coccidioidomycosis, 129
    cryptosporidiosis, 146
    Ehrlichia, *Anaplasma*, and related infections, 177
    Enterobacteriaceae infections, 185
    Giardia duodenalis infections, 219
    hepatitis A, 265
    hepatitis B, 269
    hepatitis E, 283
    leishmaniasis, 360

lymphocytic choriomeningitis virus (LCMV), 398
microsporidia infections, 431
murine typhus, 796
norovirus and sapovirus infections, 453
paracoccidioidomycosis, 460
pertussis (whooping cough), 503
Q fever, 543
rickettsialpox, 563
Salmonella infections, 579
tuberculosis (TB), 750
Anosmia, 137
Anthrax, 18–22, 22–25*i*
    case reporting, 22
    clinical manifestations of, 18, 22–23*i*
    control measures for, 21–22
    diagnostic tests for, 19–20
    epidemiology of, 18–19
    etiology of, 18
    incubation period of, 19
    isolation of hospitalized patient with, 21
    treatment of, 20–21
Antiretroviral therapy (ART)
    for *Cryptococcus neoformans* and *Cryptococcus gattii* infections, 144
    for cryptosporidiosis, 147
    for human herpesvirus 8, 312
    for HIV infection, 319
    for nontuberculous mycobacteria (NTM), 782
Anxiety, rabies, 546
Aplastic anemia, aspergillosis and, 41
Apnea
    Enterobacteriaceae infections, 185
    parechovirus infections, 480
    pertussis (whooping cough), 503
Appendicitis
    Pasteurella infections, 488
    pinworm infection (*Enterobius vermicularis*), 510
Appetite loss, coronaviruses, 137
Arboviruses, 26–28, 26*t*, 29*t*, 30–34*i*
    clinical manifestations of, 26–27, 26*t*, 30*i*
    diagnostic tests for, 27–28
    epidemiology of, 27
    etiology of, 27
    generalized febrile illness, 26
    genus, geographic location, and vectors for, 29*t*
    hemorrhagic fever, 27
    incubation period of, 27
    neuroinvasive disease, 26–27
    treatment of, 28

Arcanobacterium haemolyticum infections, 35, 36*i*
  clinical manifestations of, 35, 36*i*
  diagnostic tests for, 35
  epidemiology of, 35
  etiology of, 35
  incubation period of, 35
  treatment of, 35
Arenaviruses, 253–254, 254*i*
  clinical manifestations of, 253
  diagnostic tests for, 254
  epidemiology of, 253–254
  etiology of, 253
  incubation period of, 254
  treatment of, 254
Argentine hemorrhagic fever, 27, 253–254
Arrhythmias, tetanus, 700
Artesunate, 402
Arthralgia
  arboviruses, 26
  arenaviruses, 253
  babesiosis, 49
  brucellosis, 82
  Chlamydia psittaci, 107
  coccidioidomycosis, 129
  Ehrlichia, Anaplasma, and related infections, 177
  hepatitis B, 269
  hepatitis E, 283
  human herpesvirus 8, 311
  Kawasaki disease, 347
  Lyme disease, 381
  lymphocytic choriomeningitis virus (LCMV), 398
  malaria, 400
  parvovirus B19, 483
  syphilis, 670
  Toxoplasma gondii infections, 720
  West Nile virus (WNV), 818
  Zika virus, 828
Arthritis
  anaerobic gram-negative bacilli infections, 59
  brucellosis, 82
  chikungunya, 103
  Chlamydia psittaci, 107
  hepatitis B, 269
  Kawasaki disease, 347
  Kingella kingae infections, 353
  Lyme disease, 381
  lymphocytic choriomeningitis virus (LCMV), 398
  meningococcal infections, 419
  mumps, 439
  Mycoplasma pneumoniae and other
    Mycoplasma species infections, 444

  parvovirus B19, 483
  varicella-zoster virus (VSV) infections, 801
Ascaris lumbricoides infections, 37–38, 38–40*i*
  clinical manifestations of, 37
  control measures for, 38
  diagnostic tests for, 37
  epidemiology of, 37
  etiology of, 37
  incubation period of, 37
  isolation of hospitalized patient with, 38
  treatment of, 37–38
Ascites
  African trypanosomiasis, 742
  dengue, 166
  schistosomiasis, 593
Aspartate aminotransferase
  coronaviruses and, 137
  dengue and, 166
  lymphocytic choriomeningitis virus (LCMV)
    and, 398
Aspergillomas, 41
Aspergillosis, 41–44, 45–46*i*, 208
  allergic bronchopulmonary, 41
  allergic sinusitis, 41
  aspergillomas and otomycosis, 41
  chronic, 41
  clinical manifestations of, 41, 45*i*
  control measures for, 44
  cutaneous, 42
  diagnostic tests for, 42–43
  epidemiology of, 42
  etiology of, 41–42
  incubation period of, 42
  invasive, 41
  isolation of hospitalized patient with, 44
  treatment of, 43–44
Aspirin, for Kawasaki disease, 348–349
Asthma
  bocavirus and, 78
  human metapneumovirus (hMPV) and, 428
  parainfluenza viral infections and, 467
  rhinovirus infections and, 559
Astroviridae, 47
Astrovirus infections, 47, 48*i*
  clinical manifestations of, 47
  diagnostic tests for, 47
  epidemiology of, 47
  etiology of, 47
  incubation period of, 47
  treatment of, 47

Asymptomatic carriage of gonococcal infections, 224
Ataxia
    amebic meningoencephalitis and keratitis, 14
    prion diseases, 536
Atopobium vaginae, 56
Atovaquone, for babesiosis, 50
Azithromycin
    for *Arcanobacterium haemolyticum* infections, 35
    for babesiosis, 50
    for *Bartonella henselae* (cat-scratch disease), 64
    for *Campylobacter* infections, 89
    for chancroid and cutaneous ulcers, 100, 101
    for *Chlamydia psittaci*, 108
    for cholera, 813*t*
    for *Escherichia coli* diarrhea, 205
    for granuloma inguinale, 232
    for group A streptococcal (GAS) infections, 637
    for *Legionella pneumophila* infections, 356
    for leptospirosis, 373
    for Lyme disease, 385*t*
    for *Mycoplasma pneumoniae* and other *Mycoplasma* species infections, 445
    for nontuberculous mycobacteria (NTM), 780
    for pertussis (whooping cough), 504, 505*t*
    for *Salmonella* infections, 581, 582
    for *Shigella* infections, 600
Aztreonam, for *Pseudomonas aeruginosa* infections, 541

B

Babesia divergens, 49, 50
Babesia duncani, 49, 50
Babesia microti, 49
Babesiosis, 49–50, 50–53*i*
    clinical manifestations of, 49
    diagnostic tests for, 49–50
    epidemiology of, 49
    etiology of, 49
    incubation period of, 49
    treatment of, 50
Bacillus anthracis, 18–19
Bacillus cereus infections and intoxications, 54–55, 55*i*
    clinical manifestations of, 54
    diagnostic tests for, 54–55
    diarrheal syndrome, 54
    emetic syndrome, 54
    epidemiology of, 54
    etiology of, 54
    incubation period of, 54
    invasive extraintestinal infection, 54
    treatment of, 55
Back pain
    brucellosis, 82
    bunyaviruses, 255
    Listeria monocytogenes infections, 377
    malaria, 400
    smallpox (variola), 603
Bacteremia
    anthrax, 18
    Arcanobacterium haemolyticum infections, 35
    Bacillus cereus infections and intoxications, 54
    Campylobacter infections, 88
    Clostridioides difficile, 122
    group B streptococcal (GBS) infections, 647
    Haemophilus influenzae type b (Hib) infections, 234
    Kingella kingae infections, 353
    meningococcal infections, 419
    Moraxella catarrhalis infections, 437
    non–group A or B streptococcal and enterococcal infections, 652
    Pseudomonas aeruginosa infections, 540
    Salmonella infections, 579
    Staphylococcus aureus, 616
Bacterial vaginosis, 56–57, 58*i*
    clinical manifestations of, 56
    diagnostic tests for, 56–57
    epidemiology of, 56
    etiology of, 56
    incubation period of, 56
    treatment of, 57
Bacteroides fragilis, 60*i*
Bacteroides infections, 59–60, 60*i*
    clinical manifestations of, 59
    epidemiology of, 59
    etiology of, 59
    incubation period of, 59
    treatment of, 59–60
Balamuthia mandrillaris, 14–16, 16–17*i*
Balantidium coli infections, 61, 61–62*i*
    clinical manifestations of, 61
    diagnostic tests for, 61
    epidemiology of, 61
    etiology of, 61
    incubation period of, 61
    treatment of, 61
Baloxavir marboxil, for influenza, 338, 338*t*
Bartonella clarridgeiae, 63
Bartonella henselae (cat-scratch disease), 63–64, 65–67*i*

clinical manifestations of, 63, 65*i*
diagnostic tests for, 64
epidemiology of, 63–64
etiology of, 63
incubation period of, 64
treatment of, 64–65
Bartonella quintana, 63
Bartholin cyst abscess, anaerobic gram-negative bacilli infections, 59
Baylisascaris infections, 68–69, 69–71*i*
clinical manifestations of, 68
diagnostic tests for, 68
epidemiology of, 68
etiology of, 68
incubation period of, 68
treatment of, 68–69
Baylisascaris procyonis, 68
BCG vaccine, 750
Bell palsy, relapsing fever, 79
Benznidazole, for American trypanosomiasis, 746
β-lactam/β-lactamase inhibitor combinations
for *Burkholderia* infections, 86
for *Kingella kingae* infections, 354
for Lyme disease, 385*t*
for non–group A or B streptococcal and enterococcal infections, 653
for *Pseudomonas aeruginosa* infections, 540
Biopsy
Baylisascaris infections, 68
cyclosporiasis, 153
Helicobacter pylori infections, 249, 252*i*
leishmaniasis, 361
leprosy, 368
microsporidia infections, 431
rickettsialpox, 563
Bioterrorism
anthrax, 19, 21, 25*i*
smallpox (variola), 603
BioThrax, 21
Bipolaris, 209*t*, 212*i*
Bismuth, for *Helicobacter pylori* infections, 250*t*, 251
BK virus, 533–534, 535*i*
clinical manifestations of, 533
diagnostic tests for, 534
epidemiology of, 533–534
etiology of, 533
treatment of, 534
Bladder cancer, schistosomiasis and, 593
Blastocystis infections, 72, 73–74*i*
clinical manifestations of, 72
diagnostic tests for, 72

epidemiology of, 72
etiology of, 72
incubation period of, 72
Blastomyces dermatitidis, 75
Blastomyces gilchristii, 75
Blastomyces helicus, 75
Blastomycosis, 75–76, 76–77*i*, 208
clinical manifestations of, 75, 76*i*
diagnostic tests for, 75
epidemiology of, 75
etiology of, 75
incubation period of, 75
treatment of, 76
Bloating
Blastocystis infections, 72
Giardia duodenalis infections, 219
Blood-brain barrier, African trypanosomiasis and, 742
Blood pressure, labile, tetanus, 700
Bloody nasal discharge, diphtheria, 171
Bloody stools
amebiasis, 7
Balantidium coli infections, 61
Campylobacter infections, 88
Escherichia coli diarrhea, 202, 202*t*
schistosomiasis, 593
Shigella infections, 599
staphylococcal food poisoning, 615*i*
trichuriasis (whipworm infection), 739
Yersinia enterocolitica and *Yersinia pseudotuberculosis* infections, 824
Bocavirus, 78
clinical manifestations of, 78
diagnostic tests for, 78
epidemiology of, 78
etiology of, 78
treatment of, 78
Body lice (pediculosis corporis), 495, 496*i*
clinical manifestations of, 495
diagnostic tests for, 495
epidemiology of, 495
etiology, 495
incubation period of, 495
treatment of, 495
Bolivian hemorrhagic fever, 27, 253–254
Bordetella bronchiseptica, 503
Bordetella holmesii, 503
Bordetella parapertussis, 503
Bordetella pertussis, 503
Borrelia afzelii, 381
Borrelia burgdorferi, 49, 50, 80, 184*i*, 381–386
Borrelia garinii, 381–382

Borrelia hermsii, 79
Borrelia infections other than Lyme disease, 79–80, 81*i*
 clinical manifestations of, 79
 diagnostic tests for, 80
 epidemiology of, 79–80
 etiology of, 79
 incubation period of, 80
 treatment of, 80
Borrelia mayonii, 381, 382
Borrelia miyamotoi, 381
Borrelia parkeri, 79
Borrelia recurrentis, 79
Borrelia turicatae, 79
Botulism and infant botulism, 115–117, 117–119*i*
 clinical manifestations of, 115, 117–118*i*
 diagnostic tests for, 116
 epidemiology of, 115–116
 etiology of, 115
 incubation period of, 115–116
 treatment of, 116–117
Bowel dilation, *Balantidium coli* infections, 61
Bowel perforation, *Balantidium coli* infections, 61
Bowel ulceration, *Balantidium coli* infections, 61
Bradycardia
 pertussis (whooping cough), 503
 Salmonella infections, 579
Brain
 abscess
  amebic meningoencephalitis and keratitis, 14
  anaerobic gram-negative bacilli infections, 59
  Arcanobacterium haemolyticum infections, 35
  Fusobacterium infections, 216
  non–group A or B streptococcal and enterococcal infections, 652
  Pasteurella infections, 488
  Salmonella infections, 579
  Toxoplasma gondii infections, 720
 actinomycosis infection and, 1
 lesions, amebic meningoencephalitis and keratitis, 14
 nocardiosis and, 449
 paragonimiasis and, 463
 parechovirus infections and, 480
 prion diseases, 536–538, 538–539*i*
 West Nile virus (WNV) and, 818
Breathing difficulty
 Ascaris lumbricoides infections, 37
 coronaviruses, 137
 Enterobacteriaceae infections, 185

 pertussis (whooping cough), 503
 Q fever, 543
Brill-Zinsser disease, 793
Brincidofovir, for smallpox (variola), 604
Bronchiolitis
 adenovirus infections, 4
 bocavirus, 78
 enterovirus (nonpoliovirus), 192
 human metapneumovirus (hMPV), 428
 influenza, 335
 parainfluenza viral infections, 467
 respiratory syncytial virus (RSV), 555
Bronchitis, *Mycoplasma pneumoniae* and other *Mycoplasma* species infections, 444
Bronchopneumonia, measles, 411
Bronchospasm, enterovirus (nonpoliovirus), 192
Brucella abortus, 82
Brucella canis, 82
Brucella ceti, 82
Brucella inopinata, 82
Brucella melitensis, 82
Brucella neotomae, 82
Brucella pinnipedialis, 82
Brucella suis, 82
Brucellosis, 82–83, 84*i*
 clinical manifestations of, 82
 diagnostic tests for, 82–83
 epidemiology of, 82
 etiology of, 82
 incubation period of, 82
 treatment of, 83
Brugia malayi, 393
Brugia timori, 393
Bruising, filoviruses, 259
Bubonic plague, 516, 517
Buffered charcoal–yeast extract (BCYE) media, 355, 449
Bullous myringitis, *Mycoplasma pneumoniae* and other *Mycoplasma* species infections, 444
Bullous skin lesions
 chikungunya, 103
 clostridial myonecrosis, 120
 cutaneous larva migrans, 151
 scabies, 588
Bunyaviruses, 255–256, 256*t*, 257–258*i*
 clinical manifestations of, 255, 257*i*
 diagnostic tests for, 256, 256*t*
 epidemiology of, 255
 etiology of, 255
 incubation period of, 256
 treatment of, 256

Burkholderia cepacia, 87*i*
Burkholderia infections, 85–86, 87*i*
    clinical manifestations of, 85
    diagnostic tests for, 86
    epidemiology of, 85–86
    etiology of, 85
    incubation period of, 86
    treatment of, 86
Burkholderia pseudomallei, 85, 87*i*
Burns, anaerobic gram-negative bacilli infections, 59

C

California encephalitis, 34*i*
Campylobacter coli, 89
Campylobacter fetus, 88–89
Campylobacter hyointestinalis, 88
Campylobacter infections, 88–89, 89–90*i*
    clinical manifestations of, 88
    diagnostic tests for, 89
    epidemiology of, 88–89
    etiology of, 88
    incubation period of, 89
    treatment of, 89
Campylobacter jejuni, 88–89
Campylobacter lari, 88
Campylobacter upsaliensis, 88
Cancer
    human papillomavirus (HPV) infections, 331, 333
    non–group A or B streptococcal and
        enterococcal infections, 652
Candida albicans, 92–95
Candida auris, 93
Candida dubliniensis, 92
Candida glabrata, 92, 93
Candida guilliermondii, 92
Candida krusei, 92, 93
Candida lusitaniae, 92, 93
Candida parapsilosis, 92, 93
Candida tropicalis, 92
Candidatus Neoehrlichia mikurensis, 561
Candidiasis, 91–95, 95–99*i*, 208
    chemoprophylaxis for, 94–95
    clinical manifestations of, 91, 95–98*i*
    diagnostic tests for, 91–92
    epidemiology of, 91
    etiology of, 91
    incubation period of, 91
    invasive disease, 93–94
    treatment of, 92–95
Capillariasis of intestine, 471*t*

Capillary leak syndrome, bunyaviruses, 255
Carbapenem
    for *Burkholderia* infections, 86
    for *Enterobacteriaceae* infections, 187
    for *Fusobacterium* infections, 217
    for *Salmonella* infections, 582
Carbapenemase-producing *Enterobacteriaceae*, 186
Carbapenem-cilastatin, for nocardiosis, 450
Carbuncles, *Staphylococcus aureus*, 616
Cardiac injury
    American trypanosomiasis, 745
    coronaviruses, 137
    dengue, 166
    Kawasaki disease, 349–350
    louseborne typhus, 793
Carditis, Lyme disease, 381
Case reporting, anthrax, 22
Cat-scratch disease. *See Bartonella henselae* (cat-scratch disease)
Cat-scratch disease (*Bartonella henselae*), 63–64, 65–67*i*
    clinical manifestations of, 63, 65*i*
    diagnostic tests for, 64
    epidemiology of, 63–64
    etiology of, 63
    incubation period of, 64
    treatment of, 64–65
Cefepime
    for *Pseudomonas aeruginosa* infections, 541
    for *Streptococcus pneumoniae* (pneumococcal)
        infections, 659
Cefixime, for *Pasteurella* infections, 488
Cefotaxime
    for *Enterobacteriaceae* infections, 186
    for group B streptococcal (GBS) infections, 648
    for *Haemophilus influenzae* type b (Hib)
        infections, 235
    for leptospirosis, 373
    for meningococcal infections, 420
    for nocardiosis, 450
    for *Pasteurella* infections, 488
    for *Streptococcus pneumoniae* (pneumococcal)
        infections, 659
Cefoxitin, for *Fusobacterium* infections, 217
Cefpodoxime, for *Pasteurella* infections, 488
Ceftaroline, for coagulase-negative staphylococcal
    (CoNS) infections, 632
Ceftazidime
    for *Burkholderia* infections, 86
    for *Pseudomonas aeruginosa* infections, 541
    for *Streptococcus pneumoniae* (pneumococcal)
        infections, 659

Ceftriaxone
- for chancroid and cutaneous ulcers, 100
- for *Fusobacterium* infections, 217
- for gonococcal infections, 226
- for *Haemophilus influenzae* type b (Hib) infections, 235
- for leptospirosis, 373
- for Lyme disease, 385t
- for meningococcal infections, 420
- for nocardiosis, 450
- for *Pasteurella* infections, 488
- for *Salmonella* infections, 581
- for *Shigella* infections, 600

Cefuroxime
- for Lyme disease, 385t
- for *Pasteurella* infections, 488

Cellulitis
- anaerobic gram-negative bacilli infections, 59
- *Enterobacteriaceae* infections, 185
- group B streptococcal (GBS) infections, 647
- *Haemophilus influenzae* type b (Hib) infections, 234, 236–238i
- *Moraxella catarrhalis* infections, 437
- *Pasteurella* infections, 488
- *Pseudomonas aeruginosa* infections, 540
- *Staphylococcus aureus*, 616
- *Vibrio* infections, other, 816

Central catheter–associated bloodstream infection
- *Bacillus cereus* infections and intoxications, 54
- nontuberculous mycobacteria (NTM), 777

Central nervous system (CNS)
- African trypanosomiasis and, 742
- amebic meningoencephalitis and keratitis and, 14
- anthrax and, 20
- arboviruses and, 26–27
- *Baylisascaris* infections and, 68
- candidiasis and, 93–94
- coccidioidomycosis and, 129
- cryptococcosis and, 143
- *Enterobacteriaceae* infections and, 185
- Epstein-Barr virus and, 197
- filoviruses and, 259
- herpes simplex virus (HSV) and, 285, 289
- *Legionella pneumophila* infections and, 355
- paragonimiasis and, 463
- parechovirus infections and, 480
- *Pasteurella* infections and, 488
- rabies and, 546
- schistosomiasis and, 593
- syphilis and, 670
- varicella-zoster virus (VSV) infections and, 801

Cephalic tetanus, 700
Cephalosporins
- for chancroid and cutaneous ulcers, 100
- for *Enterobacteriaceae* infections, 186
- for group A streptococcal (GAS) infections, 637
- for *Kingella kingae* infections, 353, 354
- for *Moraxella catarrhalis* infections, 437
- for non–group A or B streptococcal and enterococcal infections, 653
- for *Pasteurella* infections, 488–489
- for *Salmonella* infections, 582
- for *Staphylococcus aureus*, 619
- for *Streptococcus pneumoniae* (pneumococcal) infections, 659
- for *Ureaplasma urealyticum* and *Ureaplasma parvum* infections, 799
- for *Vibrio* infections, other, 816
- for *Yersinia enterocolitica* and *Yersinia pseudotuberculosis* infections, 826

Cerebellar ataxia
- mumps, 439
- *Mycoplasma pneumoniae* and other *Mycoplasma* species infections, 444

Cerebellitis, Q fever, 543
Cerebral malaria, 400
Cerebral vasculitis, toxocariasis, 717
Cerebrospinal fluid (CSF)
- African trypanosomiasis and, 743
- amebic meningoencephalitis and keratitis and, 15
- arboviruses and, 27
- *Baylisascaris* infections and, 68
- coccidioidomycosis and, 130
- *Cryptococcus neoformans* and *Cryptococcus gattii* infections and, 143–144
- *Enterobacteriaceae* infections and, 186
- enterovirus (nonpoliovirus) and, 193
- *Haemophilus influenzae* type b (Hib) infections and, 235
- leptospirosis and, 373
- *Listeria monocytogenes* infections and, 378
- lymphocytic choriomeningitis virus (LCMV) and, 398–399
- meningococcal infections and, 420
- mumps and, 439
- pleocytosis, Kawasaki disease, 347
- poliovirus infections and, 528
- prion diseases and, 538
- syphilis and, 672
- West Nile virus (WNV) and, 818, 819

Cervical adenitis, anaerobic gram-negative bacilli infections, 59

Cervical lymphadenopathy
   Arcanobacterium haemolyticum infections, 35
   diphtheria, 171
   Kawasaki disease, 346
   Legionella pneumophila infections, 355
   nontuberculous mycobacteria (NTM), 777
   tularemia, 786
Cervicitis, *Chlamydia trachomatis*, 110
Cervicofacial actinomycosis, 1
Chagas disease, 470, 745–746, 747–749*i*
   clinical manifestations of, 745
   diagnostic tests for, 746
   epidemiology of, 745–746
   etiology of, 745
   incubation period of, 746
   treatment of, 746
Chancroid and cutaneous ulcers, 100–101, 101–102*i*
   clinical manifestations of, 100, 101–102*i*
   diagnostic tests for, 100
   epidemiology of, 100
   etiology of, 100
   incubation period of, 100
   syphilis, 670
   treatment of, 100–101
Chemiluminescent immunoassays, hepatitis C, 278
Chemoprophylaxis, for *Pneumocystis jirovecii* infections and, 524–525, 525*b*
Chemotherapy
   for human herpesvirus 8, 312
   for lymphatic filariasis, 394
Chest pain
   anthrax, 18
   Ascaris lumbricoides infections, 37
   blastomycosis, 75
   coccidioidomycosis, 129
   cryptococcosis, 143
   Legionella pneumophila infections, 355
   nocardiosis, 449
   tularemia, 786
Chickenpox. *See* Varicella-zoster virus (VSV) infections
Chikungunya, 29*t*, 30*i*, 32*i*, 103–104, 104*i*
   clinical manifestations of, 103, 104*i*
   diagnostic tests for, 103–104
   epidemiology of, 103
   etiology of, 103
   incubation period of, 103
   treatment of, 104
Chills and sweats
   anthrax, 18

babesiosis, 49
brucellosis, 82
Chlamydia psittaci, 107
Ehrlichia, *Anaplasma*, and related infections, 177
hantavirus pulmonary syndrome (HPS), 245
influenza, 335
louseborne typhus, 793
malaria, 400
meningococcal infections, 419
Pasteurella infections, 488
Pneumocystis jirovecii infections, 522
Q fever, 543
rat-bite fever, 552
relapsing fever, 79
Toxoplasma gondii infections, 720
tuberculosis (TB), 750
Vibrio infections, other, 816
Chlamydia pneumoniae, 105–106, 106*i*
   clinical manifestations of, 105
   diagnostic tests for, 105–106
   epidemiology of, 105
   etiology of, 105
   incubation period of, 105
   treatment of, 106
Chlamydia psittaci, 107–108, 108–109*i*
   clinical manifestations of, 107
   diagnostic tests for, 107–108
   epidemiology of, 107
   etiology of, 107
   incubation period of, 107
   treatment of, 108
Chlamydia trachomatis, 110–113, 113–114*i*, 444
   bacterial vaginosis, 56
   clinical manifestations of, 110, 113*i*, 114*i*
   diagnostic tests for, 111–112
   epidemiology of, 110–111
   etiology of, 110
   incubation period of, 111
   pelvic inflammatory disease (PID), 499–501
   treatment of, 112–113
Chloramphenicol
   for *Fusobacterium* infections, 217
   for louseborne typhus, 794
   for plague, 517
   for Rocky Mountain spotted fever (RMSF), 566
Cholecystitis, Q fever, 543
Cholelithiasis, *Salmonella* infections, 579
Cholera, 812–813, 813*t*, 814–815*i*
   clinical manifestations of, 812, 814*f*
   diagnostic tests for, 812–813
   epidemiology of, 812

Cholera (*continued*)
    etiology of, 812
    incubation period of, 812
    treatment of, 813, 813*t*
Chorioamnionitis
    bacterial vaginosis, 54
    Haemophilus influenzae type b (Hib)
        infections, 234
Chorioretinitis, *Toxoplasma gondii* infections, 720
Chronic aspergillosis, 41
Chronic asymptomatic parasitemia, 400
Chronic granulomatous disease (CGD)
    Burkholderia infections and, 85
    nocardiosis and, 449
Chronic obstructive pulmonary disease (COPD)
    blastomycosis and, 75
    human metapneumovirus (hMPV) and, 428
    nocardiosis and, 449
    rhinovirus infections and, 559
Ciclopirox
    for tinea corporis, 709
    for tinea pedis and tinea unguium, 715
Cidofovir
    for molluscum contagiosum, 434
    for polyomaviruses, 534
    for smallpox (variola), 604
Ciprofloxacin
    for anthrax, 20, 22
    for cholera, 813*t*
    for louseborne typhus, 794
    for plague, 517
    for *Pseudomonas aeruginosa* infections, 541
    for *Salmonella* infections, 582
    for tularemia, 787
Cladophialophora, 210*t*
Clarithromycin
    for *Helicobacter pylori* infections, 250*t*, 251*t*
    for *Mycoplasma pneumoniae* and other
        Mycoplasma species infections, 445
    for nocardiosis, 450
    for nontuberculous mycobacteria (NTM), 780
    for pertussis (whooping cough), 505*t*
Clindamycin
    for anthrax, 20, 22
    for babesiosis, 50
    for bacterial vaginosis, 57
    for *Fusobacterium* infections, 217
    for group A streptococcal (GAS) infections,
        637, 638
    for *Ureaplasma urealyticum* and *Ureaplasma
        parvum* infections, 799

Clofazimine, for leprosy, 369
Clonorchis sinensis, 471*t*
Clostridial myonecrosis, 120–121, 121*i*
    clinical manifestations of, 120, 121*i*
    epidemiology of, 120
    etiology of, 120
    incubation period of, 120
    treatment of, 120–121
Clostridioides difficile, 122–125, 124*t*, 125–126*i*
    clinical manifestations of, 122
    diagnostic tests for, 122–123
    epidemiology of, 122
    etiology of, 122
    incubation period of, 122
    treatment of, 123–125, 124*t*
Clostridium baratii, 115
Clostridium botulinum, 115
Clostridium butyricum, 115
Clostridium novyi, 120
Clostridium perfringens, 120, 127, 128*i*
    clinical manifestations of, 127
    epidemiology of, 127
    etiology of, 127
    incubation period of, 127
    treatment of, 127
Clostridium septicum, 120
Clostridium sordellii, 120
Clostridium tetani, 700–701
Clotrimazole
    for candidiasis, 92
    for pityriasis versicolor, 513
    for tinea corporis, 709
Coagulase-negative staphylococcal (CoNS)
        infections, 631–632, 632*i*
    clinical manifestations of, 631
    diagnostic tests for, 631–632
    epidemiology of, 631
    etiology of, 631
    incubation period of, 631
    treatment of, 632
Coagulopathy
    coronaviruses, 137
    enterovirus (nonpoliovirus), 192
    meningococcal infections, 419
    parechovirus infections, 480
Coccidioides immitis, 129
Coccidioides posadasii, 129
Coccidioidomycosis, 129–131, 131–136*i*, 208
    clinical manifestations of, 129, 132–134*i*, 136*i*
    diagnostic tests for, 130
    epidemiology of, 129

etiology of, 129
incubation period of, 129
treatment of, 130–131
Colitis
  amebiasis, 7
  Balantidium coli infections, 61
  cytomegalovirus (CMV) infection, 158
  Shigella infections, 599
  trichuriasis (whipworm infection), 739
Colon ulceration amebiasis, 7
Colorado tick fever, 26, 26t, 29t
Coma
  meningococcal infections, 419
  Rocky Mountain spotted fever (RMSF), 565
Common cold
  adenovirus infections and, 4
  bocavirus and, 78
  rhinovirus infections and, 559
Community-acquired pneumonia, *Streptococcus pneumoniae* (pneumococcal) infections, 657
Community-associated MRSA, 618
Computed tomography (CT)
  amebiasis, 10*i*
  amebic meningoencephalitis and keratitis, 15, 16*i*
  aspergillosis, 46*i*
  Enterobacteriaceae infections, 189*i*
  herpes simplex, 292*i*
  histoplasmosis, 298*i*, 299*i*
  HIV infection, 325*i*
  Legionella pneumophila infections, 359*i*
  non–group A or B streptococcal and enterococcal infections, 656*i*
  nontuberculous mycobacteria (NTM), 784*i*
  Salmonella infections, 584*i*
  tapeworm diseases, 691*i*
  Toxoplasma gondii infections, 727*i*
  tuberculosis (TB), 773*i*
Condylomata acuminata, 331
Congenital cytomegalovirus (CMV) infection, 158, 161
Congenital rubella syndrome, 573, 574
Congenital syphilis, 670, 675
Congenital *Toxoplasma gondii* infections, 720, 722–723
Congenital tuberculosis, 767–768
Congestive heart failure, Kawasaki disease, 347
Conjunctival problems
  American trypanosomiasis, 745
  arenaviruses, 253
  bunyaviruses, 255
  leptospirosis, 372
  tularemia, 786

Conjunctivitis
  Bartonella henselae (cat-scratch disease), 63
  bunyaviruses, 255
  chikungunya, 103
  coronaviruses, 137
  enterovirus (nonpoliovirus), 192
  Lyme disease, 381
  measles, 411
  meningococcal infections, 419
  neonatal
    anaerobic gram-negative bacilli infections, 59
    Chlamydia trachomatis, 110
  rickettsialpox, 563
  rubella, 573
  Streptococcus pneumoniae (pneumococcal) infections, 657
  Yersinia enterocolitica and *Yersinia pseudotuberculosis* infections, 824
Constipation
  Blastocystis infections, 72
  Chlamydia psittaci, 107
  poliovirus infections, 528
  Salmonella infections, 579
Control measures
  for amebiasis, 9
  for anthrax, 21–22
  for *Ascaris lumbricoides* infections, 38
  for aspergillosis, 44
Corneal perforation, *Pseudomonas aeruginosa* infections, 540
Coronary artery disease, Kawasaki disease, 346–347
Coronaviruses, including SARS-CoV-2 and MERS-CoV, 137–139, 140–142*i*
  clinical manifestations of, 137–138
  diagnostic tests for, 139
  epidemiology of, 138–139
  etiology of, 138
  incubation period of, 139
  treatment of, 139
Corticosteroids
  for African trypanosomiasis, 743
  for *Baylisascaris* infections, 68
  cryptococcosis and, 143
  for Kawasaki disease, 349
  for parainfluenza viral infections, 468
  for respiratory syncytial virus (RSV), 557
  for *Salmonella* infections, 582
  for scabies, 589
  for toxocariasis, 717
  for trichinellosis, 730

Corticosteroids (*continued*)
    for tuberculosis (TB), 766–767
    for varicella-zoster virus (VSV) infections, 803, 804
Corynebacterium diphtheriae, 171
Corynebacterium ulcerans, 171
Coryza
    enterovirus (nonpoliovirus), 192
    measles, 411
    rubella, 573
Cough
    Ascaris lumbricoides infections, 37
    blastomycosis, 75
    bocavirus, 78
    Chlamydia psittaci, 107
    coccidioidomycosis, 129
    coronaviruses, 137
    cryptococcosis, 143
    Ehrlichia, *Anaplasma*, and related infections, 177
    hantavirus pulmonary syndrome (HPS), 245
    influenza, 335
    Legionella pneumophila infections, 355
    louseborne typhus, 793
    lymphocytic choriomeningitis virus (LCMV), 398
    malaria, 400
    measles, 411
    Mycoplasma pneumoniae and other *Mycoplasma* species infections, 444
    nocardiosis, 449
    paragonimiasis, 463
    pertussis (whooping cough), 503
    Pneumocystis jirovecii infections, 522
    Q fever, 543
    relapsing fever, 79
    respiratory syncytial virus (RSV), 555
    rhinovirus infections, 559
    rubella, 573
    toxocariasis, 717
    tuberculosis (TB), 750
    tularemia, 786
Covert toxocariasis, 717
COVID-19. *See* Coronaviruses, including SARS-CoV-2 and MERS-CoV
Coxiella burnetti infection, 543–544, 544–545*i*
    clinical manifestations of, 543
    diagnostic tests for, 543–544
    epidemiology of, 543
    etiology of, 543
    incubation period of, 543
    treatment of, 544
Crackles, respiratory syncytial virus (RSV), 555

Cranial nerve palsies
    amebic meningoencephalitis and keratitis, 14
    chikungunya, 103
    Chlamydia psittaci, 107
    Epstein-Barr virus, 197
    Kawasaki disease, 347
    Lyme disease, 381
    tetanus, 700
    varicella-zoster virus (VSV) infections and, 801
C-reactive protein level, elevated, coronaviruses, 137
Creatinine levels, elevated, chikungunya, 103
Creeping eruption, cutaneous larva migrans, 151
Crepitus, clostridial myonecrosis, 120
Creutzfeldt-Jakob disease (CJD), 536
Crimean-Congo hemorrhagic fever (CCHF), 255, 256*t*, 257*i*
Croup
    adenovirus infections, 4
    enterovirus (nonpoliovirus), 192
    human metapneumovirus (hMPV), 428
    influenza, 335
    measles, 411
    Mycoplasma pneumoniae and other *Mycoplasma* species infections, 444
    parainfluenza viral infections, 467
Cryptococcal antigen (CRAG) detection methods, 143–144
Cryptococcosis, 143–144, 208
Cryptococcus gattii infections, 143–144, 145*i*
    clinical manifestations of, 143
    diagnostic tests for, 143–144
    epidemiology of, 143
    etiology of, 143
    treatment of, 144
Cryptococcus neoformans infections, 143–144, 145*i*
    clinical manifestations of, 143
    diagnostic tests for, 143–144
    epidemiology of, 143
    etiology of, 143
    treatment of, 144
Cryptosporidiosis, 146–147, 147–150*i*
    clinical manifestations of, 146
    diagnostic tests for, 146–147
    epidemiology of, 146
    etiology of, 146
    incubation period of, 146
    treatment of, 147
Cryptosporidium hominis, 146
Cryptosporidium parvum, 72, 146
Culex tarsalis mosquito, 34*i*
Cunninghamella, 211*t*

Curvularia, 210t
Cutaneous anthrax, 18
Cutaneous diphtheria, 171, 172
Cutaneous larva migrans, 151, 151–152i
    clinical manifestations of, 151, 151–152i
    diagnostic tests for, 151
    epidemiology of, 151
    etiology of, 151
    incubation period of, 151
    treatment of, 151
Cutaneous leishmaniasis, 360
Cutaneous plague, 516
Cyanosis
    anthrax, 18
    Enterobacteriaceae infections, 185
Cyclosporiasis, 153, 154i
    clinical manifestations of, 153
    diagnostic tests for, 153
    epidemiology of, 153
    etiology of, 153
    incubation period of, 153
    treatment of, 153
Cysticercosis, 689–691, 691–694i
    clinical manifestations of, 689
    diagnosis of, 689–690
    epidemiology of, 689
    etiology of, 689
    incubation period of, 689
    treatment of, 690–691
Cystic fibrosis (CF)
    Burkholderia infections and, 85
    nocardiosis and, 449
    nontuberculous mycobacteria (NTM) and, 777
    Pseudomonas aeruginosa infections and, 540, 541
Cystitis, polyomaviruses, 534
Cystoisosporiasis, 155, 156–157i
Cytomegalovirus (CMV) infection, 158–161, 162–164i
    clinical manifestations of, 158, 162–163i, 165i
    diagnostic tests for, 160
    epidemiology of, 158–159
    etiology of, 158
    incubation period of, 159
    treatment of, 160–161

D

Dactylitis, *Salmonella* infections, 579
Dapsone, for leprosy, 369
Daptomycin, for coagulase-negative staphylococcal (CoNS) infections, 632

Death
    amebic meningoencephalitis and keratitis, 14
    Baylisascaris, 68
    Burkholderia, 85
    cholera, 812
    Clostridioides difficile, 122
    coccidioidomycosis, 129
    cryptosporidiosis, 146
    dengue, 167
    human metapneumovirus (hMPV), 428
    Kawasaki disease, 347
    Legionella pneumophila infections, 355
    leishmaniasis, 360
    louseborne typhus, 793
    malaria, 400
    measles, 411
    meningococcal infections, 419
    murine typhus, 796
    parechovirus infections, 480
    pertussis (whooping cough), 503
    plague, 516
    prion diseases, 536
    relapsing fever, 79
    Rocky Mountain spotted fever (RMSF), 565
    varicella-zoster virus (VSV) infections, 801
Decubitus ulcers, anaerobic gram-negative bacilli infections, 59
Deep neck space infection, *Fusobacterium* infections, 216
Dehydration
    astrovirus infections, 47
    cholera, 812
    Giardia duodenalis infections, 219
    rotavirus infections, 571
    Shigella infections, 600
    staphylococcal food poisoning, 615i
Deltavirus, 281
Dementia
    prion diseases, 536
    syphilis, 670
Dengue, 26t, 27, 29t, 166–167, 168–170i
    clinical manifestations of, 166
    diagnostic tests for, 167
    epidemiology of, 166–167
    etiology of, 166
    incubation period of, 167
    treatment of, 167
Dental infection, anaerobic gram-negative bacilli infections, 59
Dermacentor andersoni, 565
Dermacentor variabilis, 565

Dermatitis
　lymphocytic choriomeningitis virus (LCMV), 398
　molluscum contagiosum, 434
　onchocerciasis, 456
　schistosomiasis, 593
Dermatophytic reaction
　tinea capitis, 704
　tinea corporis, 708
　tinea cruris, 712
　tinea pedis and tinea unguium, 714
Dexamethasone
　for coronaviruses, 144
　for *Haemophilus influenzae* type b (Hib) infections, 235
　for *Streptococcus pneumoniae* (pneumococcal) infections, 659
Diabetic ketoacidosis, coronaviruses, 137
Diaphoresis
　clostridial myonecrosis, 120
　tetanus, 700
Diarrhea
　amebiasis, 7
　arenaviruses, 253
　astrovirus infections, 47
　Bacillus cereus infections and intoxications, 54
　Balantidium coli infections, 61
　Blastocystis infections, 72
　Campylobacter infections, 88
　Chlamydia psittaci, 107
　cholera, 812
　Clostridioides difficile, 122
　Clostridium perfringens, 127
　coronaviruses, 137
　cryptosporidiosis, 146
　Diphyllobothrium, 695
　Dipylidium caninum, 695
　Ehrlichia, Anaplasma, and related infections, 177
　Enterobacteriaceae infections, 185
　enterovirus (nonpoliovirus), 192
　filoviruses, 259
　Giardia duodenalis infections, 219
　hantavirus pulmonary syndrome (HPS), 245
　human herpesvirus 8, 311
　hydatid disease, 695
　Hymenolepis nana, 695
　influenza, 335
　Kawasaki disease, 347
　malaria, 400
　measles, 411
　microsporidia infections, 431
　norovirus and sapovirus infections, 453

Q fever, 543
Rocky Mountain spotted fever (RMSF), 565
rotavirus infections, 571
Salmonella infections, 579
schistosomiasis, 593
Shigella infections, 599
staphylococcal food poisoning, 614, 615*i*
tapeworm diseases, 689
trichinellosis, 730
trichuriasis (whipworm infection), 739
Vibrio infections, other, 816
West Nile virus (WNV), 818
Yersinia enterocolitica and *Yersinia pseudotuberculosis* infections, 824
Dientamoeba fragilis, 7
Diethylcarbamazine
　for lymphatic filariasis, 394
　for onchocerciasis, 457
Dilated cardiomyopathy, *Chlamydia psittaci*, 107
Diphtheria, 171–172, 173–176*i*
　clinical manifestations of, 171, 173–175*i*
　diagnostic tests for, 172
　epidemiology of, 171
　etiology of, 171
　incubation period of, 171
　treatment of, 172
Diphtheria (equine) antitoxin (DAT), 172
Diphyllobothrium, 695
Dipylidium caninum, 695
Direct fluorescent antibody (DFA) antibody test
　rabies, 546
　varicella-zoster virus (VSV) infections, 802
Directly observed therapy (DOT), 751
Diskitis, *Kingella kingae* infections, 353
Disseminated infection
　adenovirus infections, 4
　Bartonella henselae (cat-scratch disease), 63
　coccidioidomycosis, 129
　gonococcal infections (DGIs), 224
　herpes simplex virus (HSV), 285
　human herpesvirus 8, 311
　Lyme disease, 381
　nontuberculous mycobacteria (NTM), 777
　sporotrichosis, 610
Disseminated intravascular coagulation
　babesiosis, 49
　bunyaviruses, 255
　Ehrlichia, Anaplasma, and related infections, 177
Dizziness, hantavirus pulmonary syndrome (HPS), 245
Donovanosis, 232, 233*i*

Doxycycline
- for actinomycosis, 2
- for anthrax, 20, 22
- for *Bartonella henselae* (cat-scratch disease), 64
- for brucellosis, 83
- for *Chlamydia pneumoniae*, 106
- for *Chlamydia psittaci*, 108
- for cholera, 813*t*
- for *Ehrlichia*, *Anaplasma*, and related infections, 179
- for *Legionella pneumophila* infections, 356
- for leptospirosis, 373
- for louseborne typhus, 794
- for Lyme disease, 385–386, 385*t*
- for lymphatic filariasis, 394
- for murine typhus, 796
- for *Mycoplasma pneumoniae* and other *Mycoplasma* species infections, 445
- for onchocerciasis, 457
- for *Pasteurella* infections, 488
- for plague, 517
- for Q fever, 544
- for relapsing fever, 80
- for rickettsial diseases, 562
- for rickettsialpox, 563
- for Rocky Mountain spotted fever (RMSF), 566
- for *Ureaplasma urealyticum* and *Ureaplasma parvum* infections, 799
- for *Vibrio* infections, other, 816

Dracunculiasis, 472*t*, 473*i*, 476*i*
Drug-resistant tuberculosis (DR TB), 751, 765–766
Dural sinus venous thrombosis, *Fusobacterium* infections, 216
Dysarthria, prion diseases, 536
Dysautonomia, rabies, 546
Dysesthesia, rabies, 546
Dyspnea
- anthrax, 18
- *Chlamydia psittaci*, 107
- hantavirus pulmonary syndrome (HPS), 245
- paragonimiasis, 463
- *Pneumocystis jirovecii* infections, 522

Dysuria
- bacterial vaginosis, 54
- *Trichomonas vaginalis* infections, 734

E

Eastern equine encephalitis, 26, 26*t*, 29*t*, 30*i*, 31*i*
Ebola Rapid Antigen Test, 261
Ebola virus disease (EVD), 27, 259–261, 261–264*i*
- clinical manifestations of, 259
- diagnostic tests for, 260–261
- epidemiology of, 260
- etiology of, 259
- incubation period of, 260
- treatment of, 261

Echinocandins, for candidiasis, 92–93
Echinococcus granulosis, 695–696
Echinococcus multilocularis, 695–696
Echoviruses. *See* Enterovirus (nonpoliovirus)
Ecthyma gangrenosum
- *Pseudomonas aeruginosa* infections, 540
- *Staphylococcus aureus*, 616

Eczema herpeticum, 286
Edema
- American trypanosomiasis, 745
- chikungunya, 103
- clostridial myonecrosis, 120
- syphilis, 670
- Zika virus, 828

Eflornithine, for African trypanosomiasis, 743
Ehrlichia chaffeensis, 177–178
Ehrlichia infections, 177–179, 177*t*, 180–184*i*, 561
- clinical manifestations of, 177, 180*i*
- diagnostic tests for, 179
- epidemiology of, 178, 178*t*
- etiology of, 177–178, 177*t*
- incubation period of, 178
- treatment of, 179

Electrolyte abnormalities
- rotavirus infections, 571
- *Shigella* infections, 599

Emetic syndrome, *Bacillus cereus* infections and intoxications, 54
Empyema
- coccidioidomycosis, 129
- *Pasteurella* infections, 488
- *Yersinia enterocolitica* and *Yersinia pseudotuberculosis* infections, 824

Encephalitis
- adenovirus infections, 4
- astrovirus infections, 47
- bunyaviruses, 255
- *Chlamydia psittaci*, 107
- enterovirus (nonpoliovirus), 192
- Epstein-Barr virus, 197
- lymphocytic choriomeningitis virus (LCMV), 398
- measles, 411
- mumps, 439
- *Mycoplasma pneumoniae* and other *Mycoplasma* species infections, 444

Encephalitis (*continued*)
   parainfluenza viral infections, 467
   parechovirus infections, 480
   Q fever, 543
   rubella, 573
   Toxoplasma gondii infections, 720
   West Nile virus (WNV), 818
Encephalitozoon intestinalis, 431
Encephalopathy
   Bartonella henselae (cat-scratch disease), 63
   Ehrlichia, Anaplasma, and related infections, 177
Endemic typhus, 796–797, 797*i*
   clinical manifestations of, 796, 797*i*
   diagnostic tests for, 796
   epidemiology of, 796
   etiology of, 796
   incubation period of, 796
   treatment of, 796–797
Endocardia fibroelastosis, mumps, 439
Endocarditis
   anaerobic gram-negative bacilli infections, 59
   Arcanobacterium haemolyticum infections, 35
   aspergillosis, 37
   Bacillus cereus infections and intoxications, 54
   Bartonella henselae (cat-scratch disease), 63
   brucellosis, 82
   Chlamydia psittaci, 107
   Haemophilus influenzae type b (Hib) infections, 234
   Kingella kingae infections, 353
   Legionella pneumophila infections, 355
   Moraxella catarrhalis infections, 437
   non–group A or B streptococcal and enterococcal infections, 652
   Pasteurella infections, 488
   Pseudomonas aeruginosa infections, 540
   rat-bite fever, 552
   Salmonella infections, 579
   Staphylococcus aureus, 616
   Streptococcus pneumoniae (pneumococcal) infections, 657
   Yersinia enterocolitica and *Yersinia pseudotuberculosis* infections, 824
Endometritis
   anaerobic gram-negative bacilli infections, 59
   Chlamydia trachomatis, 110
   Ureaplasma urealyticum and *Ureaplasma parvum* infections, 798
Endophthalmitis
   Haemophilus influenzae type b (Hib) infections, 234
   meningococcal infections, 419
   Pseudomonas aeruginosa infections, 540
Entamoeba bangladeshi, 7, 9
Entamoeba dispar, 7, 9, 13*i*
Entamoeba histolytica, 7, 8, 12*i*, 13*i*
Entamoeba moshkouskii, 7, 9
Enteric fever, 579–582
Enteroaggregative *E coli* (EAEC), 203
Enterobacteriaceae infections in newborns, 185–187, 187–191*i*, 599
   clinical manifestations of, 185, 187–190*i*
   diagnostic tests for, 186
   epidemiology of, 185–186
   etiology of, 185
   incubation period of, 186
   treatment of, 186–187
Enterobius vermicularis (pinworm infection), 510–511, 511–512*i*
   clinical manifestations of, 510, 511*i*
   diagnostic tests for, 510
   epidemiology of, 510
   etiology of, 510
   incubation period of, 510
   treatment of, 510–511
Enterocytozoon bieneusi, 431
Enteroinvasive *E coli* (EIEC), 203
Enteropathogenic *E coli* (EPEC), 202
Enterotoxigenic *E coli* (ETEC), 202
Enterovirus (nonpoliovirus), 192–193, 194–196*i*
   clinical manifestations of, 192, 194–196*i*
   diagnostic tests for, 193
   epidemiology of, 192–193
   etiology of, 192
   incubation period of, 193
   treatment of, 193
Enzyme immunoassay (EIA)
   adenovirus infections, 4–5
   amebiasis, 8
   anthrax, 19
   aspergillosis, 42
   Bartonella henselae (cat-scratch disease), 64
   blastomycosis, 75
   brucellosis, 82–83
   coccidioidomycosis, 130
   cryptosporidiosis, 146
   Escherichia coli diarrhea, 204
   hepatitis C, 278
   herpes simplex virus (HSV), 287
   histoplasmosis, 297
   Lyme disease, 383
   murine typhus, 796

rotavirus infections, 572
Salmonella infections, 580–581
Enzyme-linked immunosorbent assay (ELISA), Lyme disease, 383
Eosinophilia
   Ascaris lumbricoides infections, 37
   schistosomiasis, 594
   toxocariasis, 717
Eosinophilic enteritis, cutaneous larva migrans, 151
Eosinophilic enterocolitis, pinworm infection (*Enterobius vermicularis*), 510
Eosin stain, leishmaniasis, 361
Epidemic typhus, 793–794, 795*i*
   clinical manifestations of, 793
   diagnostic tests for, 794
   epidemiology of, 793–794
   etiology of, 793
   incubation period of, 794
   treatment of, 794
Epidermodysplasia verruciformis, 331
Epidermophyton floccosum, 708, 712
Epididymitis
   Chlamydia trachomatis, 110
   Trichomonas vaginalis infections, 734
   Ureaplasma urealyticum and *Ureaplasma parvum* infections, 798
Epididymo-orchitis, brucellosis, 82
Epiglottitis, *Haemophilus influenzae* type b (Hib) infections, 234, 235
Epstein-Barr virus, 197–200, 198*t*, 199*f*, 200–201*i*
   clinical manifestations of, 197, 200–201*i*
   diagnostic tests for, 198–199, 198*t*, 199*f*
   epidemiology of, 198
   etiology of, 198
   false-positive nontreponemal results and, 672
   Fusobacterium infections and, 216
   incubation period of, 198
   as opportunistic infection, 313
   treatment of, 199–200
Erythema
   Kawasaki disease, 345
   parechovirus infections, 480
   Pasteurella infections, 488
   tinea capitis, 704
   tinea corporis, 708
   tinea cruris, 712
Erythema infectiosum, 483–484, 483*t*, 485–487*i*
   clinical manifestations of, 483, 483*t*, 485–487*i*
   diagnostic tests for, 484
   epidemiology of, 484
   etiology of, 483–484
   incubation period of, 484
   treatment of, 484
Erythema migrans, Lyme disease, 381, 384, 385*t*
Erythema multiforme
   coccidioidomycosis, 129
Erythema nodosum
   Bartonella henselae (cat-scratch disease), 63
   blastomycosis, 75
   Campylobacter infections, 88
   coccidioidomycosis, 129
   Mycoplasma pneumoniae and other *Mycoplasma* species infections, 444
   Yersinia enterocolitica and *Yersinia pseudotuberculosis* infections, 824
Erythromycin
   for *Arcanobacterium haemolyticum* infections, 35
   for *Campylobacter* infections, 89
   for chancroid and cutaneous ulcers, 100
   for *Chlamydia psittaci*, 108
   for *Chlamydia trachomatis*, 112
   for cholera, 813*t*
   for diphtheria, 172
   for *Mycoplasma pneumoniae* and other *Mycoplasma* species infections, 445
   for pertussis (whooping cough), 504, 505*t*
Escherichia coli diarrhea, 199, 202–205, 202*t*, 205–207*i*
   amebiasis, 9
   bacterial vaginosis, 56
   clinical manifestations of, 202–203, 202*t*
   diagnostic tests for, 204
   epidemiology of, 203–204
   etiology of, 203
   incubation period of, 204
   neonatal infections, 185–187, 187–191*i*
   treatment of, 204–205
Esophageal varices, schistosomiasis, 593
Esophagitis, aspergillosis, 37
Espundia, 360
Ethambutol
   for nontuberculous mycobacteria (NTM), 780
   for tuberculosis (TB) disease, 760
Ethylsuccinate, for *Chlamydia trachomatis*, 112
Exophiala, 210*t*
Exposed person, tuberculosis (TB), 751
Exserohilum, 210*t*, 212*i*, 214*i*
Extended-spectrum β-lactamases (ESBLs), 185
Extensively drug-resistant tuberculosis (XDR TB), 751

F

Facial flushing
  arenaviruses, 253
  bunyaviruses, 255
Failure to thrive
  Giardia duodenalis infections, 219
  microsporidia infections, 431
Fasciola hepatica, 474–475i
Fascioliasis, 472t
Fasciolopsiasis, 472t
Fatal familial insomnia, 536
Fatal sporadic insomnia, 536
Fatigue and malaise
  African trypanosomiasis, 742
  American trypanosomiasis, 745
  arboviruses, 26
  arenaviruses, 253
  astrovirus infections, 47
  babesiosis, 49
  blastomycosis, 75
  brucellosis, 82
  Campylobacter infections, 88
  Chlamydia psittaci, 107
  coccidioidomycosis, 129
  coronaviruses, 137
  cryptosporidiosis, 146
  dengue, 166
  Ehrlichia, Anaplasma, and related infections, 177
  Enterobacteriaceae infections, 185
  filoviruses, 259
  Giardia duodenalis infections, 219
  hepatitis A, 265
  hepatitis B, 269
  hepatitis E, 283
  influenza, 335
  louseborne typhus, 793
  Lyme disease, 381
  lymphocytic choriomeningitis virus (LCMV), 398
  meningococcal infections, 419
  Mycoplasma pneumoniae and other
    Mycoplasma species infections, 444
  norovirus and sapovirus infections, 453
  paracoccidioidomycosis, 460
  parvovirus B19, 483
  Pneumocystis jirovecii infections, 522
  poliovirus infections, 528
  rhinovirus infections, 559
  rickettsialpox, 563
  Rocky Mountain spotted fever (RMSF), 565
  Salmonella infections, 579
  smallpox (variola), 603
  syphilis, 670
  toxocariasis, 717
  Toxoplasma gondii infections, 720
  West Nile virus (WNV), 818
Fecal transplant for *Clostridioides difficile*, 125
  diphtheria, 171
Fetal death. *See* Abortion
Fever
  adenovirus infections, 4
  African trypanosomiasis, 742
  amebiasis, 7
  amebic meningoencephalitis and keratitis, 14
  American trypanosomiasis, 745
  anthrax, 18
  arboviruses, 26
  Arcanobacterium haemolyticum infections, 35
  Ascaris lumbricoides infections, 37
  astrovirus infections, 47
  babesiosis, 49
  Bacillus cereus infections and intoxications, 54
  Bartonella henselae (cat-scratch disease), 63
  blastomycosis, 75
  bocavirus, 78
  brucellosis, 82
  bunyaviruses, 255
  Burkholderia infections, 85
  Campylobacter infections, 88
  chikungunya, 103
  Chlamydia psittaci, 107
  clostridial myonecrosis, 120
  Clostridioides difficile, 122
  coccidioidomycosis, 129
  coronaviruses, 137
  cryptosporidiosis, 146
  cytomegalovirus (CMV) infection, 158
  dengue, 166
  Ehrlichia, Anaplasma, and related infections, 177
  Enterobacteriaceae infections, 185
  Epstein-Barr virus, 197
  filoviruses, 259
  hantavirus pulmonary syndrome (HPS), 245
  hepatitis A, 265
  hepatitis E, 283
  human herpesvirus 8, 311
  human metapneumovirus (hMPV), 428
  influenza, 335
  Kawasaki disease, 347
  leishmaniasis, 360
  leptospirosis, 372
  Listeria monocytogenes infections, 377
  louseborne typhus, 793

Lyme disease, 381
lymphatic filariasis, 393
lymphocytic choriomeningitis virus (LCMV), 398
malaria, 400
measles, 411
meningococcal infections, 419
murine typhus, 796
Mycoplasma pneumoniae and other *Mycoplasma* species infections, 444
nocardiosis, 449
norovirus and sapovirus infections, 453
paracoccidioidomycosis, 460
parvovirus B19, 483
Pasteurella infections, 488
pelvic inflammatory disease (PID), 499
Pneumocystis jirovecii infections, 522
poliovirus infections, 528
Q fever, 543
rat-bite fever, 552
relapsing fever, 79
respiratory syncytial virus (RSV), 555
rhinovirus infections, 559
rickettsial diseases, 561
rickettsialpox, 563
Rocky Mountain spotted fever (RMSF), 565
rubella, 573
Salmonella infections, 579
Shigella infections, 599
smallpox (variola), 603
staphylococcal food poisoning, 614, 615i
syphilis, 670
toxocariasis, 717
Toxoplasma gondii infections, 720
trichinellosis, 730
tuberculosis (TB), 750
tularemia, 786
varicella-zoster virus (VSV) infections, 801
Vibrio infections, other, 816
West Nile virus (WNV), 818
Yersinia enterocolitica and *Yersinia pseudotuberculosis* infections, 824
Zika virus, 828
Fidaxomicin, for *Clostridioides difficile*, 123
Fifth disease, 483–484, 483t, 485–487i
 clinical manifestations of, 483, 483t, 485–487i
 diagnostic tests for, 484
 epidemiology of, 484
 etiology of, 483–484
 incubation period of, 484
 treatment of, 484
Filariasis, 456–457, 457–459i

Filiform warts, 331
Filoviruses, 259–261, 261–264i
 clinical manifestations of, 259
 diagnostic tests for, 260–261
 epidemiology of, 260
 etiology of, 259
 incubation period of, 260
 treatment of, 261
Flatulence
 Blastocystis infections, 72
 Giardia duodenalis infections, 219
Flat warts, 331
Flaviviridae, 27
Flavivirus, 166
Fleaborne typhus, 796–797, 797i
 clinical manifestations of, 796, 797i
 diagnostic tests for, 796
 epidemiology of, 796
 etiology of, 796
 incubation period of, 796
 treatment of, 796–797
FLOTAC method, 739
Fluconazole
 for candidiasis, 92–93, 94, 95
 for coccidioidomycosis, 130
 for *Cryptococcus neoformans* and *Cryptococcus gattii* infections, 144
 for tinea capitis, 705t, 706
 for tinea cruris, 712
Fluoroquinolones
 for anthrax, 20
 for *Burkholderia* infections, 86
 for *Chlamydia pneumoniae*, 106
 for *Enterobacteriaceae* infections, 187
 for *Escherichia coli* diarrhea, 205
 for *Listeria monocytogenes* infections, 378
 for *Moraxella catarrhalis* infections, 437
 for *Mycoplasma pneumoniae* and other *Mycoplasma* species infections, 445
 for *Pasteurella* infections, 488
 for polyomaviruses, 534
 for *Salmonella* infections, 581
 for *Shigella* infections, 600
Folliculitis
 Pseudomonas aeruginosa infections, 540
 tinea capitis, 704
Foodborne illness
 Bacillus cereus infections and intoxications, 54
 botulism, 115–116
 Campylobacter infections, 88–89
 Clostridium perfringens, 127

Foodborne illness (*continued*)
   cyclosporiasis, 153
   Escherichia coli diarrhea, 203–204
   Listeria monocytogenes infections, 377
   staphylococcal food poisoning, 614, 615*i*
   tapeworm diseases, 695
   trichinellosis, 730, 731–732*i*
Francisella tularensis, 786–787
Fungal diseases, other, 208, 209–211*t*, 212–215*i*
Fungemia, cryptococcal, 143
Furuncles, *Staphylococcus aureus*, 616
Fusariosis, 208
Fusarium, 209*t*
Fusobacterium infections, 59, 216–217, 218*i*
   clinical manifestations of, 216, 218*i*
   diagnostic tests for, 217
   epidemiology of, 216–217
   etiology of, 216
   treatment of, 217
Fusobacterium necrophorum, 216
Fusobacterium nucleatum, 216

G

Galactomannan test, 42–43
Gammaherpesvirinae, 311
Ganciclovir
   for cytomegalovirus (CMV) infection, 160–161
   for human herpesviruses 6 and 7, 308
Gangrene
   anaerobic gram-negative bacilli infections, 59
   Haemophilus influenzae type b (Hib) infections, 234
Gardnerella vaginalis, 56, 57, 58*i*, 499
Gas gangrene, 120–121, 121*i*
Gastroenteritis
   adenovirus infections, 4
   astrovirus infections, 47
   Campylobacter infections, 88
   norovirus and sapovirus infections, 453
   Salmonella infections, 579
   Vibrio infections, other, 816
Gastrointestinal plague, 516
Gastrointestinal tract symptoms
   Legionella pneumophila infections, 355
   Listeria monocytogenes infections, 377
   norovirus and sapovirus infections, 453
   Q fever, 543
Generalized febrile illness arboviruses, 26

Gentamicin
   for brucellosis, 83
   for group B streptococcal (GBS) infections, 648
   for *Listeria monocytogenes* infections, 378
   for non–group A or B streptococcal and enterococcal infections, 653
   for plague, 517
   for tularemia, 787
Gerstmann-Sträussler-Scheinker disease, 536
Gianotti-Crosti syndrome, 269
Giardia duodenalis infections, 72, 146, 219–220, 221–223*i*
   clinical manifestations of, 219
   diagnostic tests for, 219–220
   epidemiology of, 219
   etiology of, 219
   incubation period of, 219
   treatment of, 220
Giemsa stain
   American trypanosomiasis, 746
   babesiosis, 49
   Ehrlichia, Anaplasma, and related infections, 179
   leishmaniasis, 361
   lymphatic filariasis, 393
   molluscum contagiosum, 434
   plague, 516
   relapsing fever, 80
Gingivitis, *Fusobacterium* infections, 216
Gingivostomatitis, herpes simplex virus (HSV), 285
Glomerulonephritis
   Bartonella henselae (cat-scratch disease), 63
   hepatitis B, 269
   mumps, 439
   varicella-zoster virus (VSV) infections, 801
   Yersinia enterocolitica and *Yersinia pseudotuberculosis* infections, 824
Glucocorticoid therapy. *See* Corticosteroids
Gnathostoma spinigerum, 473*i*
Gonococcal infections, 224–226, 227–231*i*
   clinical manifestations of, 224, 227–230*i*
   diagnostic tests for, 225–226
   etiology of, 224
   incubation period of, 225
   neonatal, 226
   treatment of, 226
Graft infections, *Legionella pneumophila* infections, 355
Gram-negative bacilli infections, 59–60, 60*i*
   Enterobacteriaceae infections, 185–187, 187–191*i*
   Moraxella catarrhalis infections, 437

Gram stain
- actinomycosis, 1
- amebic meningoencephalitis and keratitis, 15
- anthrax, 19
- bacterial vaginosis, 57
- brucellosis, 84*i*
- *Campylobacter* infections, 89*i*
- clostridial myonecrosis, 120, 121*i*
- *Fusobacterium* infections, 217
- *Haemophilus influenzae* type b (Hib) infections, 235
- *Listeria monocytogenes* infections, 378
- *Staphylococcus aureus*, 618–619

Granuloma inguinale, 232, 233*i*
- clinical manifestations of, 232, 233*i*
- diagnostic tests for, 232
- epidemiology of, 232
- etiology of, 232
- incubation period of, 232
- treatment of, 232

Granulomatosis infantisepticum, 377
Granulomatous amebic encephalitis (GAE), 14
Griseofulvin
- for tinea capitis, 705, 705*t*
- for tinea cruris, 712

Grocott-Gomori methenamine–silver nitrate stain, 42
Group A coxsackieviruses. *See* Enterovirus (nonpoliovirus)
Group A streptococcal (GAS) infections, 632, 633–642, 637*b*, 639–640*b*, 641*t*, 642–646*i*
- acute rheumatic fever (ARF), 639–642, 640*b*, 641*t*
- bacterial vaginosis, 56
- clinical manifestations of, 633
- diagnostic tests for, 635–636
- epidemiology of, 634–635
- etiology of, 634
- incubation period of, 635
- pharyngitis, 636–638
- toxic shock syndrome, 638–639, 639*b*
- treatment of, 636–642, 639–640*b*, 641*t*

Group B coxsackievirus. *See* Enterovirus (nonpoliovirus)
Group B streptococcal (GBS) infections, 647–649, 649–651*i*, 649*f*
- clinical manifestations of, 647, 649–651*i*
- diagnostic tests for, 647–648
- epidemiology of, 647
- etiology of, 647
- incubation period of, 647
- treatment of, 648–649

Growth delay
- *Ascaris lumbricoides* infections, 37
- *Blastocystis* infections, 72
- trichuriasis (whipworm infection), 739

Grunting, respiratory syncytial virus (RSV), 555
Guillain-Barré syndrome
- *Campylobacter* infections, 88
- chikungunya, 103
- Epstein-Barr virus, 197
- lymphocytic choriomeningitis virus (LCMV), 398
- parainfluenza viral infections, 467
- rabies, 546
- West Nile virus (WNV), 818
- Zika virus, 828

H

Haemophilus ducreyi, 100
Haemophilus influenzae type b (Hib) infections, 234–235, 236–244*i*, 499
- clinical manifestations of, 234, 236–238*i*, 240*i*, 242*i*
- diagnostic tests for, 235
- epidemiology of, 234
- etiology of, 234
- incubation period of, 234
- treatment of, 235

Hand-foot-and-mouth disease, 192, 194–196*i*
Hansen disease. *See* Leprosy
Hantaviridae, 245, 255
Hantavirus pulmonary syndrome (HPS), 245–246, 247–248*i*
- clinical manifestations of, 245
- diagnostic tests for, 246
- epidemiology of, 245–246
- etiology of, 245
- treatment of, 246

Haverhill fever, 552
Headache
- African trypanosomiasis, 742
- amebic meningoencephalitis and keratitis, 14
- anthrax, 18
- arboviruses, 26
- arenaviruses, 253
- babesiosis, 49
- brucellosis, 82
- bunyaviruses, 255
- chikungunya, 103
- *Chlamydia psittaci*, 107
- coccidioidomycosis, 129
- coronaviruses, 137

Headache (*continued*)
  Ehrlichia, Anaplasma, and related infections, 177
  filoviruses, 259
  hantavirus pulmonary syndrome (HPS), 245
  influenza, 335
  Legionella pneumophila infections, 355
  leptospirosis, 372
  louseborne typhus, 793
  Lyme disease, 381
  lymphatic filariasis, 393
  lymphocytic choriomeningitis virus (LCMV), 398
  malaria, 400
  murine typhus, 796
  Mycoplasma pneumoniae and other *Mycoplasma* species infections, 444
  nocardiosis, 449
  norovirus and sapovirus infections, 453
  parvovirus B19, 483
  poliovirus infections, 528
  Q fever, 543
  rat-bite fever, 552
  relapsing fever, 79
  rhinovirus infections, 559
  rickettsial diseases, 561
  rickettsialpox, 563
  Rocky Mountain spotted fever (RMSF), 565
  rubella, 573
  Salmonella infections, 579
  smallpox (variola), 603
  syphilis, 670
  Toxoplasma gondii infections, 720
  Vibrio infections, other, 816
  West Nile virus (WNV), 818
  Zika virus, 828
Head lice (pediculosis capitis), 490–492, 491*t*, 493–494*i*
  clinical manifestations of, 490, 493*i*
  diagnostic tests for, 490
  epidemiology of, 490
  etiology of, 490
  incubation period of, 490
  treatment of, 490–492, 491*t*
Health care–associated MRSA, 618
Hearing loss
  cytomegalovirus (CMV) infection, 158
  mumps, 439
  syphilis, 670
Heart, actinomycosis infection, 1
Heartland virus, 26, 26*t*, 29*t*
Heart rate instabilities, *Enterobacteriaceae* infections, 185

Helicobacter pylori infections, 249–251, 250*t*, 251*t*, 252*i*
  clinical manifestations of, 249
  diagnostic tests for, 249–250
  epidemiology of, 249
  etiology of, 249
  incubation period of, 249
  treatment of, 250–251, 250*t*, 251*t*
Hematemesis, schistosomiasis, 593
Hematospermia, schistosomiasis, 593
Hematuria
  polyomaviruses, 534
  schistosomiasis, 593
Hemiparesis, amebic meningoencephalitis and keratitis, 14
Hemolysis, *Shigella* infections, 599
Hemolytic anemia
  babesiosis, 49
  Epstein-Barr virus, 197
  Mycoplasma pneumoniae and other *Mycoplasma* species infections, 444
  syphilis, 670
Hemolytic-uremic syndrome
  Q fever, 543
  Shigella infections, 599
  Streptococcus pneumoniae (pneumococcal) infections, 657
Hemophagocytic lymphohistiocytosis (HLH)
  dengue, 166
  Epstein-Barr virus, 197, 199
  leishmaniasis, 360
Hemophagocytosis
  brucellosis, 82
  Q fever, 543
Hemorrhage
  chikungunya, 103
  leptospirosis, 372
  malaria, 400
  polyomaviruses, 534
  Salmonella infections, 579
  smallpox (variola), 603
  trichinellosis, 730
Hemorrhagic cystitis adenovirus infections, 4
Hemorrhagic fevers
  arboviruses, 27
  arenaviruses, 253–254, 254*i*
  bunyaviruses, 255–256, 256*t*, 257–258*i*
  filoviruses, 259–261, 261–264*i*
Hemorrhagic fever with renal syndrome (HFRS), 255, 256*t*
Hepadnaviridae, 270

Hepatic abscess
  amebiasis, 9
  brucellosis, 82
  Pasteurella infections, 488
Hepatic aminotransferase levels
  chikungunya and, 103
  Kawasaki disease and, 347
  murine typhus and, 796
  Zika virus and, 828
Hepatitis
  adenovirus infections, 4
  bunyaviruses, 255
  chikungunya, 103
  Chlamydia psittaci, 107
  cytomegalovirus (CMV) infection, 158
  dengue, 166
  enterovirus (nonpoliovirus), 192
  parechovirus infections, 480
  Q fever, 543
  rickettsialpox, 563
  syphilis, 670
  varicella-zoster virus (VSV) infections, 801
Hepatitis A, 265–266, 266–268*i*
  clinical manifestations of, 265, 266*i*
  diagnostic tests for, 265–266
  epidemiology of, 265
  etiology of, 265
  incubation period of, 265
  treatment of, 266
Hepatitis B, 269–274, 271*f*, 272–273*f*, 272*t*, 274–276*i*
  clinical manifestations of, 269–270, 274*i*
  diagnostic tests for, 271, 271*f*, 272–273*f*, 272*t*
  epidemiology of, 270–271
  etiology of, 270
  incubation period of, 271
  resolved, 270
  treatment of, 273–274
Hepatitis C, 277–279, 279–280*i*
  clinical manifestations of, 277
  diagnostic tests for, 278–279
  epidemiology of, 277–278
  etiology of, 277
  incubation period of, 278
  treatment of, 279
Hepatitis D, 281, 282*i*
  clinical manifestations of, 281
  diagnostic tests for, 281
  epidemiology of, 281
  etiology of, 281
  incubation period of, 281
  treatment of, 281

Hepatitis E, 283, 284*i*
  clinical manifestations of, 283
  diagnostic tests for, 283
  epidemiology of, 283
  etiology of, 283
  incubation period of, 283
  treatment of, 283
Hepatomegaly
  amebiasis, 7
  Baylisascaris infections, 68
  Salmonella infections, 579
  tularemia, 786
Hepatosplenomegaly
  African trypanosomiasis, 742
  American trypanosomiasis, 745
  brucellosis, 82
  Epstein-Barr virus, 197
  leishmaniasis, 360
  malaria, 400
  relapsing fever, 79
  schistosomiasis, 593
  syphilis, 670
Herpangina, enterovirus (nonpoliovirus), 192
Herpes simplex virus (HSV), 285–289, 289–295*i*
  bacterial vaginosis, 56
  clinical manifestations of, 285–286, 289–295*i*
  diagnostic tests for, 287–288
  epidemiology of, 286–287
  etiology of, 286
  incubation period of, 287
  neonatal, 285–286, 288
  treatment of, 288–289
Herpes simplex virus encephalitis (HSE), 286
Herpesviridae, 286, 311, 802
Heterophyes heterophyes, 477*i*
Hilar adenopathy, tularemia, 786
Histoplasmosis, 208, 296–298, 298–300*i*
  clinical manifestations of, 296
  diagnostic tests for, 296–297
  epidemiology of, 296
  etiology of, 296
  incubation period of, 296
  treatment of, 297–298
HIV. *See* Human immunodeficiency virus (HIV) infection
Hookworm infections, 301–302, 302–305*i*
  clinical manifestations of, 301, 302–303*i*
  diagnostic tests for, 301–302
  epidemiology of, 301
  etiology of, 301
  incubation period of, 301
  treatment of, 302

Hordeola, *Staphylococcus aureus*, 616
Human bite wounds, anaerobic gram-negative bacilli infections, 59
Human bocavirus (HBoV), 78
  clinical manifestations of, 78
  diagnostic tests for, 78
  epidemiology of, 78
  etiology of, 78
  treatment of, 78
Human coronaviruses (HCoVs). *See* Coronaviruses, including SARS-CoV-2 and MERS-CoV
Human herpesvirus 4. *See* Epstein-Barr virus
Human herpesvirus 8, 311–312, 312*i*
  clinical manifestations of, 311, 312*i*
  diagnostic tests for, 311–312
  epidemiology of, 311
  etiology of, 311
  incubation period of, 311
  treatment of, 312
Human herpesviruses 6 and 7, 306–308, 308–310*i*
  clinical manifestations of, 306, 308–310*i*
  diagnostic tests for, 307–308
  epidemiology of, 306–307
  etiology of, 306
  incubation period of, 307
  treatment of, 308
Human immunodeficiency virus (HIV) infection, 313–320, 315*t*, 316–318*f*, 321–330*i*
  Bartonella henselae (cat-scratch disease) and, 63
  candidiasis and, 91
  chancroid and cutaneous ulcers and, 100
  clinical manifestations of, 313, 321–327*i*
  cryptococcosis and, 143, 147
  Cryptococcus neoformans and *Cryptococcus gattii* infections and, 144
  cryptosporidiosis and, 146
  cytomegalovirus (CMV) infection and, 158
  diagnostic tests for, 314–319, 315*t*, 316–318*f*
  etiology of, 313–314
  human herpesvirus 8 and, 311–312
  incubation period of, 314
  leishmaniasis and, 360
  microsporidia infections and, 431
  molluscum contagiosum and, 434
  nocardiosis and, 449
  nontuberculous mycobacteria (NTM) and, 782
  Pneumocystis jirovecii infections and, 522, 523*t*
  syphilis and, 670
  tuberculosis (TB) and, 756, 767
Human metapneumovirus (hMPV), 428, 429*i*
  clinical manifestations of, 428
  diagnostic tests for, 428
  epidemiology of, 428
  etiology of, 428
  incubation period of, 428
  treatment of, 428
Human papillomavirus (HPV) infections, 331–333, 333–334*i*
  clinical manifestations of, 331, 333–334*i*
  diagnostic tests for, 332–333
  epidemiology of, 332
  etiology of, 332
  incubation period of, 332
  treatment of, 333
Human tetanus immune globulin (TIG), 701
Hyalohyphomycosis, 209*t*
Hydatid disease, 695–696, 696–699*i*
  etiologies, diagnosis, and treatment of, 695–696
Hydrocephalus, lymphocytic choriomeningitis virus (LCMV), 398
Hydronephrosis, schistosomiasis, 593
Hydrophobia, rabies, 546
Hydrops of the gallbladder, Kawasaki disease, 347
Hydroxychloroquine, for Q fever, 544
Hymenolepis nana, 695
Hyperbaric oxygen, for clostridial myonecrosis, 121
Hypergammaglobulinemia, 360
  toxocariasis, 717
Hypersplenism, malaria, 400
Hypertension, schistosomiasis, 593
Hypoalbuminemia
  leishmaniasis, 360
  murine typhus, 796
Hypocalcemia, murine typhus, 796
Hypoglycemia, 400
Hyponatremia
  murine typhus, 796
  Rocky Mountain spotted fever (RMSF), 565
Hypotension
  anthrax, 18
  bunyaviruses, 255
  Clostridioides difficile, 122
  hantavirus pulmonary syndrome (HPS), 245
  Moraxella catarrhalis infections, 437
Hypothermia, staphylococcal food poisoning, 614
Hypovolemia, cholera, 812
Hypoxemia
  hantavirus pulmonary syndrome (HPS), 245
  Pneumocystis jirovecii infections, 522
Hypoxia, anthrax, 18

I

Id reaction
  tinea capitis, 704
  tinea corporis, 708
  tinea cruris, 712
  tinea pedis and tinea unguium, 714
Imipenem-cilastatin, for *Pseudomonas aeruginosa* infections, 541
Immune globulin intravenous (IGIV)
  for enterovirus (nonpoliovirus), 193
  for group A streptococcal (GAS) infections, 639
  for Kawasaki disease, 348, 349
  for parechovirus infections, 481
  for parvovirus B19, 484
  for polyomaviruses, 534
  for *Staphylococcus aureus*, 623
Immunization
  23-valent pneumococcal polysaccharide vaccine (PPSV23), 657, 658t
  BCG, 750
  diphtheria, 172
  Haemophilus influenzae type b (Hib), 234
  for HIV-exposed children, 319–320
  measles, 320, 350, 411–412
  mumps, 439
  pertussis (whooping cough), 503
  poliovirus, 528–529
  tetanus, 320, 700, 701
  tuberculosis (TB) and, 767
  varicella, 320, 350, 801
Immunofluorescent antibody (IFA)
  Bartonella henselae (cat-scratch disease), 64
  influenza, 336, 337t
  Legionella pneumophila infections, 356
  leptospirosis, 373
  louseborne typhus, 794
  Lyme disease, 383
  Rocky Mountain spotted fever (RMSF), 566
Immunoglobulin G (IgG) antibody
  arboviruses and, 28
  arenaviruses and, 254
  Bartonella henselae (cat-scratch disease) and, 64
  bocavirus and, 78
  brucellosis and, 83
  bunyaviruses and, 256
  cytomegalovirus (CMV) infection and, 160
  hepatitis A and, 265–266
  Legionella pneumophila infections and, 356
  louseborne typhus and, 794
  measles and, 412
  mumps and, 440
  murine typhus and, 796
  Mycoplasma pneumoniae and other *Mycoplasma* species infections and, 445
  parvovirus B19 and, 484
  Q fever and, 544
  Rocky Mountain spotted fever (RMSF) and, 566
  Toxoplasma gondii infections and, 721–722
  varicella-zoster virus (VSV) infections, 802
  West Nile virus (WNV) and, 819
Immunoglobulin M (IgM) antibody
  arboviruses and, 27–28
  Bartonella henselae (cat-scratch disease) and, 64
  bocavirus and, 78
  brucellosis and, 83
  bunyaviruses and, 256
  chikungunya and, 103–104
  coccidioidomycosis and, 130
  cytomegalovirus (CMV) infection and, 160
  hepatitis A and, 265–266
  human herpesviruses 6 and 7 and, 308
  louseborne typhus and, 794
  measles and, 412
  mumps and, 440
  murine typhus and, 796
  Mycoplasma pneumoniae and other *Mycoplasma* species infections and, 445
  parvovirus B19 and, 484
  Rocky Mountain spotted fever (RMSF) and, 566
  rubella and, 574
  Toxoplasma gondii infections and, 721–722
  West Nile virus (WNV) and, 819
Immunohistochemical assays
  leptospirosis, 373
  prion diseases, 538
  smallpox (variola), 604
Immunosuppressive therapies and tuberculosis (TB), 756
Impetigo
  group A streptococcal (GAS) infections, 638
  Staphylococcus aureus, 616
Inactive chronic hepatitis B, 269–270
Incontinence, pertussis (whooping cough), 503
Increased intracranial pressure, meningococcal infections, 419
Indirect fluorescent antibody assay, murine typhus, 796
Indirect hemagglutination test, amebiasis, 8
Indwelling catheter, candidiasis and, 94
Infectious mononucleosis. *See* Epstein-Barr virus

Influenza, 335–338, 337–338t, 339–344i
  clinical manifestations of, 335
  diagnostic tests for, 336–337, 337t
  epidemiology of, 336
  etiology of, 335
  incubation period of, 336
  treatment of, 337–338, 338t
Influenzalike illness
  adenovirus infections, 4
  Legionella pneumophila infections, 355
  Toxoplasma gondii infections, 720
  tularemia, 786
Inhalation anthrax, 18
Injection anthrax, 18
Intercostal and subcostal retractions, respiratory syncytial virus (RSV), 555
Interferon-gamma release assay (IGRA) result, 750, 753–754, 754b, 755f
Intestinal obstruction
  Ascaris lumbricoides infections, 37
  tuberculosis (TB), 750
Intestinal perforation
  Clostridioides difficile, 122
  Shigella infections, 599
Intrauterine infection, brucellosis, 82
Intussusception, coronaviruses, 137
Invasive aspergillosis, 41
Invasive colitis, amebiasis, 8
Invasive extraintestinal infection, *Bacillus cereus*, 54
Iodoquinol, for *Balantidium coli* infections, 61
Iridocyclitis, relapsing fever, 79
Iron lungs, 531–532i
Irritability
  Enterobacteriaceae infections, 185
  Hymenolepis nana, 695
  Kawasaki disease, 347
Irritable bowel syndrome (IBS)
  after *Blastocystis* infections, 72
  after *Giardia duodenalis* infections, 220
  after *Shigella* infections, 599
Isavuconazole, for paracoccidioidomycosis, 460
Isolation of hospitalized patient
  with amebiasis, 9
  with anthrax, 21
  with *Ascaris lumbricoides* infections, 38
  with aspergillosis, 44
  with tuberculosis (TB), 769
Isoniazid
  for tuberculosis (TB) disease, 760
  for tuberculosis infection (TBI), 758, 760
Isoniazid-rifampin, for tuberculosis infection (TBI), 758
Isoniazid-rifapentine, for tuberculosis infection (TBI), 758
Itraconazole
  for blastomycosis, 76
  for candidiasis, 92–93
  for coccidioidomycosis, 130
  for histoplasmosis, 297–298
  for paracoccidioidomycosis, 460
  for sporotrichosis, 611
  for tinea capitis, 705t
  for tinea cruris, 712
Ivermectin
  for *Ascaris lumbricoides* infections, 37
  for cutaneous larva migrans, 151
  for lymphatic filariasis, 394
  for onchocerciasis, 456
  for pediculosis capitis, 491t, 492
  for pediculosis pubis, 497
  for scabies, 589
  for strongyloidiasis, 668
Ixodes pacificus, 184i, 382
Ixodes scapularis, 49, 382

J

Jamestown Canyon virus, 26, 26t, 29t
Japanese encephalitis, 26, 26t, 29t
Jarisch-Herxheimer reaction, 80, 373
Jaundice
  arboviruses, 26
  Enterobacteriaceae infections, 185
  hepatitis A, 265
  hepatitis B, 269
  hepatitis C, 277
  hepatitis E, 283
  leptospirosis, 372
  malaria, 400
  relapsing fever, 79
JC virus, 533–534, 535i
  clinical manifestations of, 533
  diagnostic tests for, 534
  epidemiology of, 533–534
  etiology of, 533
  treatment of, 534
Jock itch, 712–713, 713i
  clinical manifestations of, 712, 713i
  diagnostic tests for, 712
  epidemiology of, 712
  etiology of, 712

incubation period of, 712
treatment of, 712–713
Joint infections, *Legionella pneumophila* infections, 355
Jugular venous thrombosis (JVT), 216

K

Kala-azar, 360
Kaposi sarcoma (KS), 311
Kaposi sarcoma–associated herpesvirus, 311–312, 312*i*
Kaposi sarcoma herpesvirus-associated inflammatory cytokine syndrome (KICS), 311
Kato-Katz method, 739
Kawasaki disease, 345–350, 346*f*, 350–352*i*
   clinical manifestations of, 345–347, 346*f*, 350–352*i*
   diagnostic tests for, 348
   epidemiology of, 348
   etiology of, 347
   incubation period of, 348
   treatment of, 348–350
Keratitis, Lyme disease, 381
Kidney
   failure
      Ehrlichia, *Anaplasma*, and related infections, 177
      leptospirosis, 372
      louseborne typhus, 793
      malaria, 400
   Legionella pneumophila infections and, 355
Kingella kingae infections, 353–354, 354*i*
   clinical manifestations of, 353
   diagnostic tests for, 353
   epidemiology of, 353
   etiology of, 353
   incubation period of, 353
   treatment of, 353–354
KI polyomavirus, 534
Klebsiella granulomatis, 232
Kuru, 536

L

Lacelike rash, parvovirus B19, 483
La Crosse virus, 26, 26*t*, 29*t*
Lactate dehydrogenase, lymphocytic choriomeningitis virus (LCMV) and, 398
Lactobacillus, bacterial vaginosis, 56
Lactobacillus crispatus, 56

Laryngotracheobronchitis. *See* Croup
Larval migrans
   Baylisascaris infections, 68
   paragonimiasis, 463
Laryngospasm, tetanus, 700
Laryngotracheitis, diphtheria, 171
Laryngotracheobronchitis. *See* Croup
Lassa virus (LASV), 27, 253
Latex agglutination tests, murine typhus, 796
Legionellaceae, 355
Legionella pneumophila infections, 355–356, 356–359*i*
   clinical manifestations of, 355
   diagnostic tests for, 355–356
   epidemiology of, 355
   etiology of, 355
   incubation period of, 355
   treatment of, 356
Legionnaires' disease, 355
Leishmania (Viannia) braziliensis, 360
Leishmania (Viannia) guyanensis, 360–361
Leishmania (Viannia) panamensis, 360
Leishmania (Viannia) peruviana, 360
Leishmania aethiopica, 360
Leishmania amazonensis, 360
Leishmania donovani, 361
Leishmania enrietti, 361
Leishmania infantum, 361
Leishmania major, 360
Leishmania mexicana, 360
Leishmaniasis, 360–362, 362–366*i*
   clinical manifestations of, 360, 362–364*i*
   cutaneous, 360
   diagnostic tests for, 361–362
   epidemiology of, 361
   etiology of, 360–361
   incubation period of, 361
   mucosal, 360
   post–kala-azar dermal, 360
   treatment of, 362
   visceral, 360
Leishmania tropica, 360
Lemierre syndrome, 216–217, 218*i*
   Arcanobacterium haemolyticum infections, 35
Leprosy, 367–369, 369–371*i*
   clinical manifestations of, 367, 369–371*i*
   diagnostic tests for, 368
   epidemiology of, 368
   etiology of, 367
   incubation period of, 368
   treatment of, 368–369

Leptospira, 80, 372–373
Leptospirosis, 372–373, 374–376*i*
  clinical manifestations of, 372, 375*i*
  diagnostic tests for, 373
  epidemiology of, 372
  etiology of, 372
  incubation period of, 373
  treatment of, 373
Lesions. *See also* Rash
  actinomycosis, 1, 2–3*i*
  amebic meningoencephalitis and keratitis, 14
  anthrax, 18, 22–23*i*
  Bartonella henselae (cat-scratch disease), 63, 65*i*
  blastomycosis, 75, 76*i*
  candidiasis, 91, 95–98
  chancroid and cutaneous ulcers, 100, 101–102*i*
  chikungunya, 103, 104*i*
  coccidioidomycosis, 129, 132–134*i*, 136*i*
  cytomegalovirus (CMV) infection, 158, 162–163*i*, 165*i*
  diphtheria, 171, 173–175*i*
  enterovirus (nonpoliovirus), 192, 194–196*i*
  gram-negative bacilli infections, 59–60, 60*i*
  granuloma inguinale, 232, 233*i*
  Lyme disease, 381, 382–383
  molluscum contagiosum, 434
  nocardiosis, 449
  paracoccidioidomycosis, 460
  pityriasis versicolor, 513
  rickettsialpox, 563, 564*i*
  scabies, 588
  schistosomiasis, 593
  smallpox (variola), 603
  sporotrichosis, 610
  syphilis, 670
  tinea corporis, 708
  tinea cruris, 712
  tinea pedis and tinea unguium, 714
  tularemia, 786
  varicella-zoster virus (VSV) infections, 801
  Vibrio infections, other, 816
Leukemia
  aspergillosis and, 41
  non–group A or B streptococcal and enterococcal infections and, 652
Leukocytosis, toxocariasis, 717
Leukopenia
  arboviruses, 26
  arenaviruses, 253
  brucellosis, 82
  coronaviruses, 137
  cytomegalovirus (CMV) infection, 158
  dengue, 166
  filoviruses, 259
  lymphocytic choriomeningitis virus (LCMV), 398
  Zika virus, 828
Levofloxacin
  for anthrax, 22
  for *Legionella pneumophila* infections, 356
  for plague, 517
  for *Pseudomonas aeruginosa* infections, 541
Limb ischemia, meningococcal infections, 419
Limb pain, meningococcal infections, 419
Linezolid
  for coagulase-negative staphylococcal (CoNS) infections, 632
  for *Listeria monocytogenes* infections, 378
  for nocardiosis, 450
  for non–group A or B streptococcal and enterococcal infections, 653
Liposomal amphotericin B
  for *Cryptococcus neoformans* and *Cryptococcus gattii* infections, 144
  for leishmaniasis, 362
Listeria monocytogenes infections, 377–378, 379–380*i*
  clinical manifestations of, 377, 379*i*
  diagnostic tests for, 378
  epidemiology of, 377–378
  etiology of, 377
  incubation period of, 378
  treatment of, 378
Liver
  abscess
    amebiasis, 7
    brucellosis, 82
    Pasteurella infections, 488
    Yersinia enterocolitica and *Yersinia pseudotuberculosis* infections, 824
  actinomycosis infection and, 1
  cryptococcosis and, 145*i*
  enlarged, dengue, 166
  failure
    Bacillus cereus infections and intoxications, 54
    Ehrlichia, *Anaplasma*, and related infections, 177
    hepatitis C, 277
  granulomata, *Bartonella henselae* (cat-scratch disease), 63
  paragonimiasis and, 463

Rocky Mountain spotted fever (RMSF) and, 565
Toxoplasma gondii infections and, 720
Localized gonococcal infections, 224
Local tetanus, 700
Lockjaw. *See* Tetanus
Lomentospora prolificans, 209t
Louseborne relapsing fever, 79–80, 81*i*
    clinical manifestations of, 79
    diagnostic tests for, 80
    epidemiology of, 79–80
    etiology of, 79
    incubation period of, 80
    treatment of, 80
Louseborne typhus, 793–794, 795*i*
    clinical manifestations of, 793
    diagnostic tests for, 794
    epidemiology of, 793–794
    etiology of, 793
    incubation period of, 794
    treatment of, 794
Lungs
    abscess
        anaerobic gram-negative bacilli infections, 59
        Burkholderia infections, 85
    coronaviruses and, 137
    cryptococcosis and, 145*i*
    paracoccidioidomycosis and, 460
    paragonimiasis and, 463
    parainfluenza viral infections and, 467
    schistosomiasis and, 593
    tuberculosis (TB) and, 750
Lyme disease, 381–386, 385t, 387–392*i*
    clinical manifestations of, 381, 387–389*i*
    diagnostic tests for, 382–384
    epidemiology of, 382
    etiology of, 381–382
    incubation period of, 382
    treatment of, 384–386, 385t
Lymphadenitis
    Burkholderia infections, 85
    coccidioidomycosis, 129
    Kawasaki disease, 346
    plague, 516
    Q fever, 543
    Staphylococcus aureus, 616
Lymphadenopathy
    African trypanosomiasis, 742
    American trypanosomiasis, 745
    arenaviruses, 253
    Bartonella henselae (cat-scratch disease), 63, 65–66*i*
    brucellosis, 82
    Epstein-Barr virus, 197
    human herpesvirus 8, 311
    leishmaniasis, 360
    lymphatic filariasis, 393
    Pasteurella infections, 488
    pediculosis capitis, 490
    rat-bite fever, 552
    rubella, 573
    syphilis, 670
    tinea capitis, 704
    Toxoplasma gondii infections, 720
    tularemia, 786
    Zika virus, 828
Lymphatic filariasis, 393–394, 394–397*i*
    clinical manifestations of, 393, 395–396*i*
    diagnostic tests for, 393–394
    epidemiology of, 393
    etiology of, 393
    incubation period of, 393
    treatment of, 394
Lymphedema
    lymphatic filariasis, 393
    rickettsialpox, 563
Lymphocytic choriomeningitis virus (LCMV), 253, 398–399, 399*i*
    clinical manifestations of, 398
    diagnostic tests for, 398–399
    epidemiology of, 398
    etiology of, 398
    incubation period of, 398
    treatment of, 399
Lymphocytic meningitis, Lyme disease, 381
Lymphocytosis
    Epstein-Barr virus, 197
    Toxoplasma gondii infections, 720
Lymphogranuloma venereum (LGV), *Chlamydia trachomatis*, 110–113
Lymphopenia
    chikungunya, 103
    coronaviruses, 137
    filoviruses, 259
    lymphocytic choriomeningitis virus (LCMV), 398
Lyssavirus, 546

M

Macrolides
    for chancroid and cutaneous ulcers, 100
    for *Chlamydia pneumoniae*, 106
    for group A streptococcal (GAS) infections, 637

Macrolides (*continued*)
    for *Moraxella catarrhalis* infections, 437
    for *Mycoplasma pneumoniae* and other
        Mycoplasma species infections, 445
    for *Ureaplasma urealyticum* and *Ureaplasma*
        parvum infections, 799
Magnetic resonance imaging (MRI)
    Baylisascaris infections, 69–70*i*
    influenza, 340*i*
    measles, 416
    Streptococcus pneumoniae (pneumococcal)
        infections, 665*i*
    tapeworm diseases, 692*i*
    tuberculosis (TB), 773*i*
    West Nile virus (WNV), 820*i*
Majocchi granuloma, 708, 709, 713
Malabsorption, *Giardia duodenalis* infections, 219
Malaria, 400–402, 403–409*i*, 470
    clinical manifestations of, 400–401, 403*i*
    diagnostic tests for, 402
    epidemiology of, 401–402
    etiology of, 401
    incubation period of, 402
    treatment of, 402
Malathion
    for pediculosis capitis, 491, 491*t*
    for pediculosis pubis, 497
Malazzesia, 208, 211*t*, 215*i*
MALDI-TOF (matrix-assisted laser desorption/
        ionization–time-of-flight) test
    clostridial myonecrosis, 120
    Cryptococcus neoformans and *Cryptococcus*
        gattii infections, 144
    nocardiosis, 450
    rat-bite fever, 552
    Staphylococcus aureus, 619
Malnutrition
    Ascaris lumbricoides infections, 37
    cryptosporidiosis, 146
    Giardia duodenalis infections, 219
    microsporidia infections, 431
Mamastrovirus (MAstV), 47
Marburg fever, 27
Marburg virus disease, 259–261, 261–264*i*
    clinical manifestations of, 259, 264*i*
    diagnostic tests for, 260–261
    epidemiology of, 260
    etiology of, 259
    incubation period of, 260
    treatment of, 261
Mastadenovirus, 4

Mastitis
    mumps, 439
    Staphylococcus aureus, 616
Mastoiditis
    Fusobacterium infections, 216
    Moraxella catarrhalis infections, 437
    Pseudomonas aeruginosa infections, 540
    Streptococcus pneumoniae (pneumococcal)
        infections, 657
McMaster method, 739
Measles, 320, 350, 411–412, 413–418*i*
    clinical manifestations of, 411, 413–418*i*
    diagnostic tests for, 412–413
    epidemiology of, 411–412
    etiology of, 411
    incubation period of, 412
    treatment of, 413
Mebendazole
    for *Ascaris lumbricoides* infections, 37
    for hookworm infections, 302
    for pinworm infection (*Enterobius*
        vermicularis), 510–511
    for toxocariasis, 717
    for trichinellosis, 730
    for trichuriasis (whipworm infection), 739
Megasphaera, 56
Melioidosis, 86, 87*i*
Meningismus, Rocky Mountain spotted fever
        (RMSF), 565
Meningitic plague, 516, 517
Meningitis
    adenovirus infections, 4
    anaerobic gram-negative bacilli infections, 59
    aspergillosis, 37
    astrovirus infections, 47
    brucellosis, 82
    Chlamydia psittaci, 107
    coccidioidomycosis, 129
    cryptococcosis, 143
    Cryptococcus neoformans and *Cryptococcus*
        gattii infections, 145*i*
    Ehrlichia, Anaplasma, and related infections, 177
    Enterobacteriaceae infections, 185
    enterovirus (nonpoliovirus), 192
    Epstein-Barr virus, 197
    Fusobacterium infections, 216
    group B streptococcal (GBS) infections, 647
    Haemophilus influenzae type b (Hib)
        infections, 234
    Kingella kingae infections, 353
    leptospirosis, 372

for *Listeria monocytogenes* infections, 378
Lyme disease, 381
lymphocytic choriomeningitis virus (LCMV), 398
meningococcal infections, 419
Moraxella catarrhalis infections, 437
Mycoplasma pneumoniae and other
    Mycoplasma species infections, 444
  clinical manifestations of, 185, 187–190*i*
  diagnostic tests for, 186
  epidemiology of, 185–186
  etiology of, 185
  incubation period of, 186
  neonatal, 185–187, 187–191*i*
  treatment of, 186–187
non–group A or B streptococcal and
    enterococcal infections, 652
parainfluenza viral infections, 467
parechovirus infections, 480
Pasteurella infections, 488
poliovirus infections, 528
Pseudomonas aeruginosa infections, 540
Q fever, 543
rat-bite fever, 552
relapsing fever, 79
Salmonella infections, 579
Staphylococcus aureus, 616
Streptococcus pneumoniae (pneumococcal)
    infections, 657
syphilis, 670
tularemia, 786
West Nile virus (WNV), 818
Yersinia enterocolitica and *Yersinia*
    pseudotuberculosis infections, 824
Meningococcal infections, 419–420, 421–427*i*, 421*b*
  clinical manifestations of, 419, 421–425*i*, 427*i*
  diagnostic tests for, 420, 421*t*
  epidemiology of, 419–420
  etiology of, 419
  incubation period of, 420
  treatment of, 420
Meningoencephalitis
  African trypanosomiasis, 742
  American trypanosomiasis, 745
  chikungunya, 103
  Cryptococcus neoformans and *Cryptococcus*
    gattii infections, 143
  cytomegalovirus (CMV) infection, 158
  dengue, 166
  enterovirus (nonpoliovirus), 192
  paragonimiasis, 463
  parechovirus infections, 480

  toxocariasis, 717
  Toxoplasma gondii infections, 720
Merkel cell polyomavirus (MCPyV), 534
Meropenem
  for *Burkholderia* infections, 86
  for *Pseudomonas aeruginosa* infections, 541
MERS-CoV. *See* Coronaviruses, including SARS-
    CoV-2 and MERS-CoV
Metabolic acidosis, malaria, 400
Metapneumovirus, 428
Methicillin-resistant *Staphylococcus aureus*
    (MRSA), 618–620
Methicillin-susceptible *Staphylococcus aureus*
    (MSSA), 619–620
Methotrexate, for Lyme disease, 386
Methylprednisolone, for Kawasaki disease, 349
Metronidazole
  for amebiasis, 8
  for bacterial vaginosis, 57
  for *Balantidium coli* infections, 61
  for *Blastocystis* infections, 72
  for *Clostridioides difficile*, 124
  for *Fusobacterium* infections, 217
  for *Giardia duodenalis* infections, 220
  for *Helicobacter pylori* infections, 250*t*, 251*t*
  for *Trichomonas vaginalis* infections, 735
Miconazole
  for candidiasis, 92
  for tinea corporis, 709
  for tinea cruris, 712
Microagglutination (MA), tularemia, 786–787
Microimmunofluorescence (MIF), for *Chlamydia*
    psittaci, 107
Microsporidia infections, 430–431, 430*t*, 432–433*i*
  clinical manifestations of, 430, 430*t*
  diagnostic tests for, 431
  epidemiology of, 430–431
  etiology of, 430
  incubation period of, 431
  treatment of, 431
Microsporum audouinii, 704
Microsporum canis, 704, 708
Middle East respiratory syndrome (MERS), 137
Miltefosine, for leishmaniasis, 362
Minocycline, for *Burkholderia* infections, 86
Multisystem inflammatory syndrome in children
    (MIS-C), 137
Mobiluncus, 56, 58*i*
Molluscum contagiosum, 434, 435–436*i*
  clinical manifestations of, 434, 435–436*i*
  diagnostic tests for, 434

Molluscum contagiosum (*continued*)
    epidemiology of, 434
    etiology of, 434
    incubation period of, 434
    treatment of, 434
Moraxella catarrhalis infections, 437, 438*i*
    clinical manifestations of, 437
    diagnostic tests for, 437
    epidemiology of, 437
    etiology of, 437
    treatment of, 437
Morbillivirus, 411
Moxidectin, for onchocerciasis, 456
Moxifloxacin
    for anaerobic infections, 60
    for plague, 517
Mucormycosis, 208, 211*t*, 213*i*, 215*i*
Mucosal bleeding, dengue, 166
Mucosal leishmaniasis, 360
Multicentric Castleman disease (MCD), 311
Multidrug-resistant tuberculosis (MDR TB), 751
Multiorgan failure, coronaviruses, 137
Multiplex nucleic acid–based assays
    for astrovirus infections, 47
    for coronaviruses, 139
    for *Enterobacteriaceae* infections, 186
Multisystem inflammatory syndrome in children (MIS-C), 137–139
Mumps, 439–440, 440–443*i*
    clinical manifestations of, 439, 440–442*i*
    diagnostic tests for, 439–440
    epidemiology of, 439
    etiology of, 439
    incubation period of, 439
    treatment of, 440
Mupirocin, for *Staphylococcus aureus*, 619
Murine typhus, 796–797, 797*i*
    clinical manifestations of, 796, 797*i*
    diagnostic tests for, 796
    epidemiology of, 796
    etiology of, 796
    incubation period of, 796
    treatment of, 796–797
Muscle and joint pain
    African trypanosomiasis, 742
    chikungunya, 103
    rat-bite fever, 552
    relapsing fever, 79
    syphilis, 670
Muscle spasms, tetanus, 700

Myalgia
    American trypanosomiasis, 745
    arboviruses, 26
    arenaviruses, 253
    babesiosis, 49
    blastomycosis, 75
    brucellosis, 82
    bunyaviruses, 255
    chikungunya, 103
    Chlamydia psittaci, 107
    coccidioidomycosis, 129
    coronaviruses, 137
    Ehrlichia, Anaplasma, and related infections, 177
    filoviruses, 259
    hantavirus pulmonary syndrome (HPS), 245
    influenza, 335
    Legionella pneumophila infections, 355
    leptospirosis, 372
    Listeria monocytogenes infections, 377
    louseborne typhus, 793
    Lyme disease, 381
    lymphocytic choriomeningitis virus (LCMV), 398
    malaria, 400
    meningococcal infections, 419
    murine typhus, 796
    norovirus and sapovirus infections, 453
    parvovirus B19, 483
    rhinovirus infections, 559
    rickettsial diseases, 561
    rickettsialpox, 563
    Rocky Mountain spotted fever (RMSF), 565
    Toxoplasma gondii infections, 720
    trichinellosis, 730
    West Nile virus (WNV), 818
    Zika virus, 828
Mycobacterium africanum, 750
Mycobacterium bovis, 750, 752, 768–769
Mycobacterium leprae, 367–368
Mycobacterium tuberculosis, 750, 752, 756–758
Mycoplasma genitalium, 56, 444, 499
Mycoplasma hominis, 56, 444, 499
Mycoplasma pneumoniae and other *Mycoplasma* species infections, 444–445, 446–448*i*
    clinical manifestations of, 444, 447–448*i*
    diagnostic tests for, 445
    epidemiology of, 444
    etiology of, 444
    incubation period of, 444
    neonatal, 185–187, 187–191*i*
    treatment of, 445
Mycoplasmataceae, 444

Myelitis/transverse myelitis
  chikungunya, 103
  Chlamydia psittaci, 107
  cytomegalovirus (CMV) infection, 158
  Epstein-Barr virus, 197
  lymphocytic choriomeningitis virus (LCMV), 398
  mumps, 439
  Mycoplasma pneumoniae and other
      Mycoplasma species infections, 444
  toxocariasis, 717
  Toxoplasma gondii infections, 720
  West Nile virus (WNV), 818
Myocarditis
  American trypanosomiasis, 745
  Campylobacter infections, 88
  chikungunya, 103
  Chlamydia psittaci, 107
  dengue, 166
  diphtheria, 171
  enterovirus (nonpoliovirus), 192
  Epstein-Barr virus, 197
  Kawasaki disease, 347
  leptospirosis, 372
  lymphocytic choriomeningitis virus (LCMV), 398
  meningococcal infections, 419
  mumps, 439
  Mycoplasma pneumoniae and other
      Mycoplasma species infections, 444
  parechovirus infections, 480
  Q fever, 543
  rat-bite fever, 552
  relapsing fever, 79
  Salmonella infections, 579
  toxocariasis, 717
  Toxoplasma gondii infections, 720
Myoclonus, prion diseases, 536
Myopericarditis
  enterovirus (nonpoliovirus), 192
  parainfluenza viral infections, 467
Myositis
  influenza, 335
  Toxoplasma gondii infections, 720

N

Naegleria fowleri, 14–16, 16–17*i*
Nairoviridae, 255
Nasal congestion
  influenza, 335
  rhinovirus infections, 559

Nasal flaring, respiratory syncytial virus (RSV), 555
Nasopharyngitis
  Chlamydia trachomatis, 110
  diphtheria, 171
Nausea
  anthrax, 18
  astrovirus infections, 47
  babesiosis, 49
  Bacillus cereus infections and intoxications, 54
  Blastocystis infections, 72
  chikungunya, 103
  Chlamydia psittaci, 107
  coronaviruses, 137
  dengue, 166
  Ehrlichia, Anaplasma, and related infections, 177
  hantavirus pulmonary syndrome (HPS), 245
  hepatitis A, 265
  hepatitis B, 269
  hydatid disease, 695
  influenza, 335
  leptospirosis, 372
  lymphocytic choriomeningitis virus (LCMV), 398
  malaria, 400
  microsporidia infections, 431
  murine typhus, 796
  norovirus and sapovirus infections, 453
  poliovirus infections, 528
  relapsing fever, 79
  Rocky Mountain spotted fever (RMSF), 565
  staphylococcal food poisoning, 614
  tapeworm diseases, 689
  trichinellosis, 730
Neck stiffness, Lyme disease, 381
Necrotizing fasciitis
  anaerobic gram-negative bacilli infections, 59
  group B streptococcal (GBS) infections, 647
Neisseria gonorrhoeae, 224–225
  bacterial vaginosis, 56
  pelvic inflammatory disease (PID), 499–501
Neisseria meningitidis, 419–420
Neoehrlichia, 561
Neonatal candidiasis, 93–94
Neonatal chlamydial conjunctivitis, 110
Neonatal gonococcal infections, 226, 227*i*
Neonatal herpes simplex virus (HSV), 285, 286, 288
Neonatal HIV infection, 315, 318, 318*f*
Neonatal meningitis, 185–187, 187–191*i*
  clinical manifestations of, 185, 187–190*i*
  diagnostic tests for, 186
  epidemiology of, 185–186

Neonatal meningitis (*continued*)
   etiology of, 185
   incubation period of, 186
   treatment of, 186–187
Neonatal septicemia, 185–187, 187–191*i*
   clinical manifestations of, 185, 187–190*i*
   diagnostic tests for, 186
   epidemiology of, 185–186
   etiology of, 185
   incubation period of, 186
   treatment of, 186–187
Neorickettsia, 561
Nephritis
   chikungunya, 103
   Chlamydia psittaci, 107
Nephropathy, polyomaviruses, 534
Nephrotic syndrome, malaria, 400
Neural larval migrans, *Baylisascaris* infections, 68
Neurocysticercosis, 470
Neuroinvasive disease
   arboviruses, 26–27
   dengue, 166
Neuroretinitis, *Bartonella henselae* (cat-scratch disease), 63
Neurotoxocariasis, 717
Newborns and infants
   American trypanosomiasis in, 745
   bacterial infections in, caused by *Enterobacteriaceae*, 185
   botulism and infant botulism in, 115–117, 117–118*i*
   Chlamydia trachomatis in, 110–112
   congenital cytomegalovirus (CMV) infection in, 158
   gonococcal infections in, 224, 226
   group B streptococcal (GBS) infections in, 647–649, 649–651*i*, 649*f*
   respiratory syncytial virus (RSV) in, 555
   syphilis in, 670, 673, 675, 676–677*t*
   Toxoplasma gondii infections in, 720–721, 722–723
   Trichomonas vaginalis infections in, 735
   tuberculosis in, 767–768
   Zika virus in, 828–830, 831*f*, 832–834*i*
Niclosamide
   for *Dipylidium caninum*, 695
   for *Hymenolepis nana*, 695
   for tapeworm diseases, 690
Nifurtimox
   for African trypanosomiasis, 743
   for American trypanosomiasis, 746

Nitazoxanide
   for *Ascaris lumbricoides* infections, 37
   for *Balantidium coli* infections, 61
   for *Blastocystis* infections, 72
   for *Clostridioides difficile*, 125
   for cryptosporidiosis, 147
   for *Giardia duodenalis* infections, 220
Nitroimidazole, for *Giardia duodenalis* infections, 220
Nocardia abscessus, 449
Nocardia brasiliensis, 449
Nocardia brevicatena-paucivorans complex, 449
Nocardia cyriacigeorgica, 449
Nocardia farcinica, 449
Nocardia nova, 449
Nocardia pseudobrasiliensis, 449
Nocardia transvalensis complex, 449
Nocardia veterana, 449
Nocardiosis, 449–450, 450–452*i*
   clinical manifestations of, 449, 450–451*i*
   diagnostic tests for, 449–450
   epidemiology of, 449
   etiology of, 449
   incubation period of, 449
   treatment of, 450
Non–group A or B streptococcal and enterococcal infections, 652–654, 653*t*, 654–656*i*
   clinical manifestations of, 652, 654–655*i*
   diagnostic tests for, 653
   epidemiology of, 652–653
   etiology of, 652, 653*t*
   incubation period of, 653
   treatment of, 653–654
Nonpoliovirus. *See* Enterovirus (nonpoliovirus)
Nontuberculous mycobacteria (NTM), 777–782, 778*t*, 781–782*t*, 782–785*i*
   clinical manifestations of, 777, 782–785*i*
   diagnostic test for, 779–780
   epidemiology of, 777, 779
   etiology of, 777, 778*t*
   incubation period of, 779
   treatment of, 780–782, 781–782*t*
Nontyphoidal *Salmonella* (NTS) infection, 579–582
Norfloxacin, for *Salmonella* infections, 582
Norovirus infections, 453–454, 454–455*i*
   clinical manifestations of, 453
   diagnostic tests for, 453–454
   epidemiology of, 453
   etiology of, 453
   incubation period of, 453
   treatment of, 454

Nuchal rigidity, rickettsialpox, 563
Nucleic acid amplification tests (NAATs)
   arboviruses, 28
   Chlamydia pneumoniae, 105
   Chlamydia psittaci, 108
   Chlamydia trachomatis, 111
   Clostridioides difficile, 123
   hepatitis C, 278–279
   human herpesvirus 8, 311
   HIV infection, 315
   influenza, 336, 337*t*
   Mycoplasma pneumoniae and other *Mycoplasma* species infections, 445
   pertussis (whooping cough), 503–504
   rat-bite fever, 552
   Staphylococcus aureus, 619
   Streptococcus pneumoniae (pneumococcal) infections, 658
   Trichomonas vaginalis infections, 734–735
Nugent score for bacterial vaginosis, 57
Numbered enteroviruses. *See* Enterovirus (nonpoliovirus)
Nystatin, for candidiasis, 92

O

Ocular infections
   adenovirus, 4
   amebic keratitis, 14–15
   aspergillosis, 37
   Bacillus cereus, 54
   Bartonella henselae (cat-scratch disease), 63
   brucellosis, 82
   Kingella kingae infections, 353
   Pasteurella infections, 488
   Pseudomonas aeruginosa infections, 540
   toxocariasis, 717
   trachoma, 112
Ocular larval migrans, 717
   Baylisascaris infections, 68
Ocular lesions, herpes simplex virus (HSV), 289
Ocular plague, 516
Ocular trauma, *Bacillus cereus* infections and, 54
Old World arenaviruses, 253–254
Old World hantaviruses, 255
Oliguria, bunyaviruses, 255
Omphalitis
   anaerobic gram-negative bacilli infections, 59
   Staphylococcus aureus, 616
Onchocerciasis ("river blindness"), 456–457, 457–459*i*
   clinical manifestations of, 456
   diagnostic tests for, 456
   epidemiology of, 456
   etiology of, 456
   incubation period of, 456
   treatment of, 456–457
Onychomadesis, 192
Oophoritis, mumps, 439
Opisthorchis felineus, 471*t*
Opisthorchis sinensis, 474*i*
Opisthorchis viverrini, 471*t*
Optic atrophy, syphilis, 670
Optic neuritis
   Epstein-Barr virus, 197
   Lyme disease, 381
Orbital cellulitis
   Arcanobacterium haemolyticum infections, 35
   Staphylococcus aureus, 616
Orchitis
   enterovirus (nonpoliovirus), 192
   Epstein-Barr virus, 197
   lymphocytic choriomeningitis virus (LCMV), 398
   mumps, 439
Organ transplant recipients and tuberculosis (TB), 756
Orientia, 561
Ornithodoros tholozani, 81*i*
Ornithosis, 107–108, 108–109*i*
   clinical manifestations of, 107
   diagnostic tests for, 107–108
   epidemiology of, 107
   etiology of, 107
   incubation period of, 107
   treatment of, 108
Orthopneumovirus, 555
Oseltamivir, for influenza, 337–338, 338*t*
Osteochondritis, syphilis, 670
Osteolytic lesions, *Bartonella henselae* (cat-scratch disease), 63
Osteomyelitis
   anaerobic gram-negative bacilli infections, 59
   aspergillosis, 37
   Bacillus cereus infections and intoxications, 54
   brucellosis, 82
   group B streptococcal (GBS) infections, 647
   Haemophilus influenzae type b (Hib) infections, 234
   Kingella kingae infections, 353
   Moraxella catarrhalis infections, 437
   non–group A or B streptococcal and enterococcal infections, 652
   nontuberculous mycobacteria (NTM), 777

Osteomyelitis (*continued*)
    Pasteurella infections, 488
    Pseudomonas aeruginosa infections, 540
    Q fever, 543
    Salmonella infections, 579
    Staphylococcus aureus, 616
    Streptococcus pneumoniae (pneumococcal) infections, 657
    Yersinia enterocolitica and *Yersinia pseudotuberculosis* infections, 824
Otitis externa, *Pseudomonas aeruginosa* infections, 540
Otitis media
    adenovirus infections, 4
    anaerobic gram-negative bacilli infections, 59
    bocavirus, 78
    Fusobacterium infections, 216
    Haemophilus influenzae type b (Hib) infections, 234, 235
    human metapneumovirus (hMPV), 428
    influenza, 335
    measles, 411
    Moraxella catarrhalis infections, 437
    Mycoplasma pneumoniae and other *Mycoplasma* species infections, 444
    nontuberculous mycobacteria (NTM), 777
    rhinovirus infections, 559
Otomycosis, 41
Oxacillin, for *Kingella kingae* infections, 353
Oxamniquine, for schistosomiasis, 594

P

Palatal palsy, diphtheria, 171
Pallor
    American trypanosomiasis, 745
    clostridial myonecrosis, 120
    parvovirus B19, 483
Pancreatitis
    dengue, 166
    enterovirus (nonpoliovirus), 192
    mumps, 439
Pancytopenia
    brucellosis, 82
    human herpesvirus 8, 311
    leishmaniasis, 360
Papillomaviridae, 332
Paracoccidioidomycosis, 208, 460–461, 461–462*i*
    clinical manifestations of, 460
    diagnostic tests for, 460
    epidemiology of, 460
    etiology of, 460
    incubation period of, 460
    treatment of, 460–461
Paragonimiasis, 463–464, 464–466*i*
    clinical manifestations of, 463
    diagnostic tests for, 464
    epidemiology of, 463
    etiology of, 463
    incubation period of, 463
    treatment of, 464
Paragonimus africanus, 463
Paragonimus heterotremus, 463
Paragonimus kellicotti, 463
Paragonimus uterobilateralis, 463
Paragonimus westermani, 463
Parainfluenza viral infections, 467–468, 468–469*i*
    clinical manifestations of, 467, 469*i*
    diagnostic tests for, 468
    epidemiology of, 467
    etiology of, 467
    incubation period of, 467
    treatment of, 468
Paralysis
    poliovirus infections, 528
    rabies, 546
Paramyxoviridae, 411
Parasitic diseases, 470, 471–472*t*, 473–479*i*
Parechovirus infections, 480–481, 481–482*i*
    clinical manifestations of, 480, 481–482*i*
    diagnostic tests for, 480–481
    epidemiology of, 480
    etiology of, 480
    incubation period of, 480
    treatment of, 481
Paresthesias, poliovirus infections, 528
Parinaud oculoglandular syndrome, 63, 65*i*
Paronychia, *Staphylococcus aureus*, 616
Parotitis
    anaerobic gram-negative bacilli infections, 59
    enterovirus (nonpoliovirus), 192
    Epstein-Barr virus, 439
    mumps, 439
    parainfluenza viral infections, 467
    Staphylococcus aureus, 616
Parrot fever, 107–108, 108–109*i*
    clinical manifestations of, 107
    diagnostic tests for, 107–108
    epidemiology of, 107
    etiology of, 107
    incubation period of, 107
    treatment of, 108

Parvoviridae, 78
Parvovirus B19, 483–484, 483t, 485–487i
　clinical manifestations of, 483, 483t, 485–487i
　diagnostic tests for, 484
　epidemiology of, 484
　etiology of, 483–484
　incubation period of, 484
　treatment of, 484
Pasteurella infections, 488–489, 489i
　clinical manifestations of, 488, 489i
　diagnostic tests for, 488
　epidemiology of, 488
　etiology of, 488
　incubation period of, 488
　treatment of, 488–489
Paul-Bunnell test, 198
Pediculicides
　for pediculosis capitis, 490
　for pediculosis corporis, 495
　for pediculosis pubis, 497
Pediculosis capitis (head lice), 490–492, 491t, 493–494i
　clinical manifestations of, 490, 493i
　diagnostic tests for, 490
　epidemiology of, 490
　etiology of, 490
　incubation period of, 490
　treatment of, 490–492, 491t
Pediculosis corporis (body lice), 495, 496i
　clinical manifestations of, 495
　diagnostic tests for, 495
　epidemiology of, 495
　etiology, 495
　incubation period of, 495
　treatment of, 495
Pediculosis pubis (pubic lice, crab lice), 497, 498i
　clinical manifestations of, 497, 498i
　diagnostic tests for, 497
　epidemiology of, 497
　etiology of, 497
　incubation period of, 497
　treatment of, 497
Pediculus humanus, 80, 81i
Pediculus humanus capitis, 490
Pediculus humanus corporis, 495
Pegylated interferon alfa
　for hepatitis B, 274
　for hepatitis D, 281
Pelvic inflammatory disease (PID), 499–501, 500t, 502i
　anaerobic gram-negative bacilli infections, 59
　Chlamydia trachomatis, 110
　clinical manifestations of, 499
　diagnostic tests for, 500–501, 500t
　epidemiology of, 499–500
　etiology of, 499
　incubation period of, 500
　treatment of, 501
　Ureaplasma urealyticum and *Ureaplasma parvum* infections, 798
Pelvic pain, schistosomiasis, 593
Pelvic peritonitis, pinworm infection (*Enterobius vermicularis*), 510
Penicillin
　for *Kingella kingae* infections, 353
　for leptospirosis, 373
　for *Pasteurella* infections, 488–489
　for pertussis (whooping cough), 504
Penicillin G
　for actinomycosis, 2
　for *Bacteroides* infections, 59–60
　for clostridial myonecrosis, 121
　for diphtheria, 172
　for group A streptococcal (GAS) infections, 637
　for leptospirosis, 373
　for meningococcal infections, 420
　for non–group A or B streptococcal and enterococcal infections, 653
　for rat-bite fever, 552
　for relapsing fever, 80
　for syphilis, 673, 675
Penicillin V, for group A streptococcal (GAS) infections, 636–637
Penicillin with β-lactamase inhibitor combinations, for *Fusobacterium* infections, 217
Penicilliosis, 212i
Penicillium marneffei, 212i, 213i
Pentamidine, for *Pneumocystis jirovecii* infections and, 524
Peramivir, for influenza, 337, 338t
Perianal infections, anaerobic gram-negative bacilli infections, 59
Perianal ulceration amebiasis, 7
Peribunyaviridae, 27
Pericardial effusion, Kawasaki disease, 347
Pericarditis
　Campylobacter infections, 88
　Chlamydia psittaci, 107
　Haemophilus influenzae type b (Hib) infections, 234
　meningococcal infections, 419

Pericarditis (*continued*)
   Mycoplasma pneumoniae and other
      Mycoplasma species infections, 444
   non–group A or B streptococcal and
      enterococcal infections, 652
   Q fever, 543
   rat-bite fever, 552
   Staphylococcus aureus, 616
   Streptococcus pneumoniae (pneumococcal)
      infections, 657
Perihepatitis, pelvic inflammatory disease (PID), 499
Periorbital cellulitis
   Haemophilus influenzae type b (Hib)
      infections, 236–237*i*
   Streptococcus pneumoniae (pneumococcal)
      infections, 657
Periorbital edema, trichinellosis, 730
Periostitis, syphilis, 670
Peripheral neuropathy, *Mycoplasma pneumoniae*
      and other *Mycoplasma* species
      infections, 444
Peritonitis
   anaerobic gram-negative bacilli infections, 59
   Ascaris lumbricoides infections, 37
   aspergillosis, 37
   candidiasis, 91
   Haemophilus influenzae type b (Hib)
      infections, 234
   Moraxella catarrhalis infections, 437
   Pasteurella infections, 488
   Streptococcus pneumoniae (pneumococcal)
      infections, 657
   tuberculosis (TB), 750
   Yersinia enterocolitica and *Yersinia*
      pseudotuberculosis infections, 824
Peritonsillar abscess
   anaerobic gram-negative bacilli infections, 59
   Fusobacterium infections, 216
   Staphylococcus aureus, 616
Permethrin
   for pediculosis capitis, 490, 491, 491*t*
   for pediculosis pubis, 497
   for scabies, 589
Personality changes, amebic meningoencephalitis
      and keratitis, 14
Pertussis (whooping cough), 503–505, 505*t*, 506–509*i*
   clinical manifestations of, 503, 506*i*, 508*i*
   diagnostic tests for, 503–504
   epidemiology of, 503
   etiology of, 503
   incubation period of, 503
   treatment of, 504–505, 505*t*
Pertussis-like syndrome
   adenovirus infections, 4
   influenza, 335
Petechiae
   arenaviruses, 253
   bunyaviruses, 255
Phaeohyphomycoses, 208, 209–210*t*, 212*i*
Pharyngeal erythema, *Arcanobacterium*
      haemolyticum infections, 35
Pharyngeal plague, 516, 517
Pharyngitis
   adenovirus infections, 4
   Arcanobacterium haemolyticum infections, 35
   Chlamydia psittaci, 107
   enterovirus (nonpoliovirus), 192
   Epstein-Barr virus, 197
   group A streptococcal (GAS) infections,
      636–638
   Mycoplasma pneumoniae and other
      Mycoplasma species infections, 444
   non–group A or B streptococcal and
      enterococcal infections, 652
   tularemia, 786
   Yersinia enterocolitica and *Yersinia*
      pseudotuberculosis infections, 824
Phenuiviridae, 27, 255
Photophobia
   lymphocytic choriomeningitis virus (LCMV), 398
   rickettsialpox, 563
Phthirus pubis, 498*i*
Picornaviridae, 192
Pinworm infection (*Enterobius vermicularis*), 510–
      511, 511–512*i*
   clinical manifestations of, 510, 511*i*
   diagnostic tests for, 510
   epidemiology of, 510
   etiology of, 510
   incubation period of, 510
   treatment of, 510–511
Piperacillin-tazobactam
   for *Pasteurella* infections, 489
   for *Pseudomonas aeruginosa* infections, 541
Piperonyl butoxide
   for pediculosis capitis, 490, 491*t*
   for pediculosis pubis, 497
Pityriasis versicolor, 513–514, 514–515*i*
   clinical manifestations of, 513, 514–515*i*
   diagnostic tests for, 513
   epidemiology of, 513

etiology of, 513
incubation period of, 513
treatment of, 513–514
Plague, 516–517, 517–521*i*
  clinical manifestations of, 516, 517–518*i*
  diagnostic tests for, 516
  epidemiology of, 516
  etiology of, 516
  incubation period of, 516
  treatment of, 516–517
Palatal enanthema, rubella, 573
Plantar warts, 331
Plasmodium falciparum, 400, 401
Plasmodium knowlesi, 400–401
Plasmodium malariae, 400
Plasmodium ovale, 400, 401
Plasmodium vivax, 400, 401
Pleconaril, for enterovirus (nonpoliovirus), 193
Pleural effusion
  Burkholderia infections, 85
  coccidioidomycosis, 129
  dengue, 166
  Mycoplasma pneumoniae and other
    Mycoplasma species infections, 444
Pleural empyema
  anaerobic gram-negative bacilli infections, 59
  Staphylococcus aureus, 616
  Streptococcus pneumoniae (pneumococcal) infections, 657
Pleurodynia, enterovirus (nonpoliovirus), 192
Pnemoviridae, 428
Pneumocystis jirovecii infections, 522–525, 523*t*, 525*b*, 526–527*i*
  clinical manifestations of, 522
  diagnostic tests for, 523
  epidemiology of, 522, 523*t*
  etiology of, 522
  incubation period of, 522
  treatment, 524–525, 525*b*
Pneumonia
  actinomycosis, 1
  anaerobic gram-negative bacilli infections, 59
  Bacillus cereus infections and intoxications, 54
  Bartonella henselae (cat-scratch disease), 63
  bocavirus, 78
  Burkholderia infections, 85
  Chlamydia psittaci, 107
  Chlamydia trachomatis, 110
  cytomegalovirus (CMV) infection, 158
  enterovirus (nonpoliovirus), 192
  Epstein-Barr virus, 197
  group B streptococcal (GBS) infections, 647

Haemophilus influenzae type b (Hib) infections, 234
human metapneumovirus (hMPV), 428
influenza, 335
Kingella kingae infections, 353
Legionella pneumophila infections, 355
meningococcal infections, 419
Moraxella catarrhalis infections, 437
Mycoplasma pneumoniae and other
  Mycoplasma species infections, 444
non–group A or B streptococcal and
  enterococcal infections, 652
parainfluenza viral infections, 467
parechovirus infections, 480
pertussis (whooping cough), 503
Pseudomonas aeruginosa infections, 540
Q fever, 543
rat-bite fever, 552
Staphylococcus aureus, 616
Streptococcus pneumoniae (pneumococcal)
  infections, 657, 660–661
syphilis, 670
tetanus, 700
Toxoplasma gondii infections, 720
tularemia, 786
varicella-zoster virus (VSV) infections, 801
Yersinia enterocolitica and *Yersinia
  pseudotuberculosis* infections, 824
Pneumonic plague, 516, 517
Pneumonitis
  Baylisascaris infections, 68
  blastomycosis, 75
  brucellosis, 82
  cutaneous larva migrans, 151
  enterovirus (nonpoliovirus), 192
  relapsing fever, 79
  Toxoplasma gondii infections, 720
Pneumoviridae, 555
Pocapavir, for enterovirus (nonpoliovirus), 193
Poliovirus infections, 528–529, 530–532*i*
  clinical manifestations of, 528, 530–531*i*
  diagnostic tests for, 529
  epidemiology of, 528–529
  etiology of, 528
  incubation period of, 529
  treatment of, 529
Polyarteritis nodosa, hepatitis B, 269
Polyarthralgia
  arboviruses, 26
  chikungunya, 103
  rubella, 573

Polyarthritis
    rat-bite fever, 552
    rubella, 573
Polymerase chain reaction (PCR)
    actinomycosis, 1
    adenovirus infections, 4
    amebiasis, 8
    amebic meningoencephalitis and keratitis, 15
    anthrax, 19
    babesiosis, 50
    Bartonella henselae (cat-scratch disease), 64
    bocavirus, 78
    Chlamydia pneumoniae, 105
    Chlamydia psittaci, 108
    coronaviruses, 139, 140*i*
    cytomegalovirus (CMV) infection, 160
    Ehrlichia, Anaplasma, and related infections, 179
    Epstein-Barr virus, 199
    Escherichia coli diarrhea, 204
    herpes simplex virus (HSV), 287
    human herpesvirus 8, 311
    human herpesviruses 6 and 7, 307
    Legionella pneumophila infections, 356
    leishmaniasis, 361
    leprosy, 368
    Listeria monocytogenes infections, 378
    Lyme disease, 384
    malaria, 402
    Mycoplasma pneumoniae and other *Mycoplasma* species infections, 445
    pertussis (whooping cough), 504
    Pneumocystis jirovecii infections and, 523
    polyomaviruses, 534
    Q fever, 544
    relapsing fever, 80
    rickettsial diseases, 562
    Rocky Mountain spotted fever (RMSF), 566
    rotavirus infections, 572
    smallpox (variola), 604
    Streptococcus pneumoniae (pneumococcal) infections, 658
    syphilis, 671
    Ureaplasma urealyticum and *Ureaplasma parvum* infections, 799
    varicella-zoster virus (VSV) infections, 802
Polymyositis, *Toxoplasma gondii* infections, 720
Polyomaviruses, 533–534, 535*i*
    clinical manifestations of, 533
    diagnostic tests for, 534
    epidemiology of, 533–534
    etiology of, 533
    treatment of, 534

Polyuria, bunyaviruses, 255
Pontiac fever, 355
Porphyromonas, 59
Posaconazole
    for aspergillosis, 44
    for candidiasis, 92
Postanginal sepsis, *Fusobacterium* infections, 216
Post-dengue acute disseminated encephalomyelitis, 166
Postexposure prophylaxis (PEP), for anthrax, 20, 21
Post–kala-azar dermal leishmaniasis, 360
Postnatal rubella, 573
Postpartum endometritis bacterial vaginosis, 54
Poststreptococcal reactive arthritis (PSRA), 642
Powassan virus, 26, 26*t*, 29*t*
Poxviridae, 604
Praziquantel
    for *Dipylidium caninum*, 695
    for *Hymenolepis nana*, 695
    for paragonimiasis, 464
    for schistosomiasis, 594
    for tapeworm diseases, 690
Pregnancy and breastfeeding
    bacterial vaginosis during, 57
    brucellosis during, 82
    candidiasis during, 93
    Chlamydia psittaci during, 107
    Chlamydia trachomatis during, 113
    coccidioidomycosis during, 130
    Giardia duodenalis infections during, 220
    hepatitis C during, 278
    Listeria monocytogenes infections during, 377
    Lyme disease during, 386
    plague during, 517
    relapsing fever during, 80
    syphilis during, 673, 674*f*, 675
    Trichomonas vaginalis infections during, 734, 735
    tuberculosis (TB) during, 767, 768
    Ureaplasma urealyticum and *Ureaplasma parvum* infections during, 798
    varicella-zoster virus (VSV) infections during, 801
    West Nile virus (WNV) during, 818
    Zika virus during, 828–830, 831*f*, 832–834*i*
Premature rupture of membranes, bacterial vaginosis, 54
Preterm delivery
    bacterial vaginosis and, 54
    brucellosis and, 82
    cytomegalovirus (CMV) infection and, 161
    human metapneumovirus (hMPV) and, 428
    Listeria monocytogenes infections and, 377

Staphylococcus aureus and, 616
syphilis and, 670
Ureaplasma urealyticum and *Ureaplasma parvum* infections and, 798
Prevotella bivia, 56
Prevotella infections, 59–60, 60i
    epidemiology of, 59
    etiology of, 59
    incubation period of, 59
    treatment of, 59–60
Prevotella melaninogenica, 59
Prevotella oralis, 59
Primary amebic meningoencephalitis (PAM), 14
Primary effusion lymphoma, 311
Prion diseases, 536–538, 538–539i
    clinical manifestations of, 536–537
    diagnostic tests for, 538
    epidemiology of, 537
    etiology of, 537
    incubation period of, 538
    treatment of, 538
Procalcitonin level, elevated, coronaviruses, 137
Progressive multifocal leukoencephalopathy (PML), 534
Progressive respiratory distress, *Legionella pneumophila* infections, 355
Prostatic abscess, anaerobic gram-negative bacilli infections, 59
Prostatitis
    anaerobic gram-negative bacilli infections, 59
    schistosomiasis, 593
    Trichomonas vaginalis infections, 734
    Ureaplasma urealyticum and *Ureaplasma parvum* infections, 798
Prostration
    meningococcal infections, 419
    smallpox (variola), 603
    staphylococcal food poisoning, 614
Proteinuria, bunyaviruses, 255
Proton pump inhibitor, for *Helicobacter pylori* infections, 250t, 251t
Pruritis
    African trypanosomiasis, 742
    bacterial vaginosis, 54
    cutaneous larva migrans, 151
    Dipylidium caninum, 695
    Hymenolepis nana, 695
    onchocerciasis, 456
    pediculosis corporis (body lice), 495
    pinworm infection (*Enterobius vermicularis*), 510
    rabies, 546
    scabies, 588

schistosomiasis, 593
tinea cruris, 712
tinea pedis and tinea unguium, 714
Trichomonas vaginalis infections, 734
Pseudallescheria boydii/Scedosporium apiospermum complex, 209t, 213–214i
Pseudomonas aeruginosa infections, 540–541, 541–542i
    clinical manifestations of, 540, 541–542i
    diagnostic tests for, 540
    epidemiology of, 540
    etiology of, 540
    incubation period of, 540
    treatment of, 540–541
Pseudoparalysis, syphilis, 670
Psittacosis, 107–108, 108–109i
    clinical manifestations of, 107
    diagnostic tests for, 107–108
    epidemiology of, 107
    etiology of, 107
    incubation period of, 107
    treatment of, 108
Pulmonary edema, meningococcal infections, 419
Pulmonary embolism, tetanus, 700
Purpura
    bunyaviruses, 255
    hepatitis B, 269
    meningococcal infections, 419
    Mycoplasma pneumoniae and other *Mycoplasma* species infections, 444
Purulent meningitis, *Bacillus cereus* infections and intoxications, 54
Purulent pericarditis, *Haemophilus influenzae* type b (Hib) infections, 234
Pustulosis, *Staphylococcus aureus*, 616
Pyoderma, pediculosis corporis (body lice), 495
Pyogenic arthritis
    Arcanobacterium haemolyticum infections, 35
    Streptococcus pneumoniae (pneumococcal) infections, 657
Pyomyositis, *Yersinia enterocolitica* and *Yersinia pseudotuberculosis* infections, 824
Pyrantel pamoate
    for *Ascaris lumbricoides* infections, 37
    for pinworm infection (*Enterobius vermicularis*), 510
Pyrazinamide
    for drug-resistant tuberculosis (DR TB), 765
    for tuberculosis (TB) disease, 760
Pyrethrins
    for pediculosis capitis, 491, 491t
    for pediculosis pubis, 497

Pyrimethamine, sulfadiazine, and folinic acid (P/S/FA), for *Toxoplasma gondii* infections, 723, 724t, 725b, 726t

Q

Q fever, 543–544, 544–545i
   clinical manifestations of, 543
   diagnostic tests for, 543–544
   epidemiology of, 543
   etiology of, 543
   incubation period of, 543
   treatment of, 544
Quinine, for babesiosis, 50
Quinolones, for chancroid and cutaneous ulcers, 100

R

Rabies, 546–547, 547–551i
   clinical manifestations of, 546
   diagnostic tests for, 546–547
   epidemiology of, 546
   etiology of, 546
   incubation period of, 546
   treatment of, 547
Racemic epinephrine aerosol, for parainfluenza viral infections, 468
Radicular pain, rabies, 546
Radiculitis, Lyme disease, 381
Radiography
   Anthrax, 24i
   Chlamydia psittaci, 107, 108i
   Chlamydia trachomatis, 110, 113i
   coagulase-negative staphylococcal (CoNS) infections, 632i
   coccidioidomycosis, 129–133i, 135i–136i
   coronaviruses, 140i
   cytomegalovirus (CMV) infection, 163i
   diphtheria, 174i
   Enterobacteriaceae infections, 189i
   group B streptococcal (GBS) infections, 649–650i
   Haemophilus influenzae type b (Hib) infections, 238–240i
   hantavirus pulmonary syndrome (HPS), 247i
   histoplasmosis, 296, 298–299i
   HIV infection, 325i
   human metapneumovirus (hMPV), 429i
   hydatid disease, 697i
   influenza, 340–341i
   Legionella pneumophila infections, 356–357i, 359i
   measles, 415i
   Mycoplasma pneumoniae and other *Mycoplasma* species infections, 444, 446i
   nocardiosis, 451i
   other tapeworm infections, 697i
   paragonimiasis, 464
   parainfluenza viral infections, 468–469i
   pertussis (whooping cough), 506i, 507i, 509i
   plague, 518i
   Pneumocystis jirovecii infections, 522, 526i, 527i
   Q fever, 543, 544i
   respiratory syncytial virus (RSV), 557i
   rubella, 577i
   Salmonella infections, 583i, 584i
   Staphylococcus aureus, 626–628i
   Streptococcus pneumoniae (pneumococcal) infections, 662–666i
   syphilis, 673, 676t, 680–681i, 688i
   tuberculosis (TB), 768, 770–772i
   tularemia, 789i
   Ureaplasma urealyticum infection, 800i
   varicella-zoster virus (VSV) infections, 809i
Rales, respiratory syncytial virus (RSV), 555
Rapid cell culture
   influenza, 336, 337t
   malaria, 402
Rapid influenza diagnostic tests, 336, 337t
Rapid molecular assays, influenza, 336, 337t
Rapid plasma reagin (RPR) test, syphilis, 671–672
Rash. *See also* Lesions
   African trypanosomiasis, 742
   American trypanosomiasis, 745
   arboviruses, 26
   Arcanobacterium haemolyticum infections, 35, 36i
   Baylisascaris infections, 68
   chikungunya, 103
   Chlamydia psittaci, 107
   coccidioidomycosis, 129
   coronaviruses, 137
   dengue, 166
   Ehrlichia chaffeensis, 177
   Epstein-Barr virus, 197
   filoviruses, 259
   hepatitis B, 269
   herpes simplex virus (HSV), 285
   human herpesvirus 8, 311
   leptospirosis, 372
   louseborne typhus, 793

measles, 411
meningococcal infections, 419
Moraxella catarrhalis infections, 437
murine typhus, 796
Mycoplasma pneumoniae and other
    Mycoplasma species infections, 444
parvovirus B19, 483
Q fever, 543
rat-bite fever, 552
relapsing fever, 79
rickettsial diseases, 561
rickettsialpox, 563, 564*i*
Rocky Mountain spotted fever (RMSF), 565
rubella, 573
SARS-CoV-2, 140*i*
smallpox (variola), 603
syphilis, 670
toxocariasis, 717
trichinellosis, 730
varicella-zoster virus (VSV) infections, 801
West Nile virus (WNV), 818
Zika virus, 828
Rat-bite fever, 552–553, 553–554*i*
    clinical manifestations of, 552, 553–554*i*
    diagnostic tests for, 552
    epidemiology of, 552
    etiology of, 552
    incubation period of, 552
    treatment of, 552–553
Reactive arthritis
    Campylobacter infections, 88
    Chlamydia trachomatis, 110
    Clostridioides difficile, 122
    poststreptococcal, 642
    Shigella infections, 599
    Yersinia enterocolitica and *Yersinia*
        pseudotuberculosis infections, 824
Reactive gliosis, 536
Real-time quaking-induced conversion (RT-QuIC), 538
Recurrent respiratory papillomatosis (RRP), 331
Refractory shock, leptospirosis, 372
Rehydration
    for *Bacillus cereus* infections and intoxications, 55
    for *Campylobacter* infections, 89
    for cholera, 813
    for *Clostridium perfringens*, 127
    for dengue, 167
    for rotavirus infections, 572
    for *Shigella* infections, 600
    for *Vibrio* infections, other, 816
Relapsing fever, 79–80, 81*i*
    clinical manifestations of, 79
    diagnostic tests for, 80
    epidemiology of, 79–80
    etiology of, 79
    incubation period of, 80
    treatment of, 80
Remdesivir, for coronaviruses, 144
Renal failure. *See* Kidney
Reoviridae, 27, 571
Respiratory failure
    coronaviruses, 137
    dengue, 166
    malaria, 400
Respiratory syncytial virus (RSV), 555–557, 557–558*i*
    clinical manifestations of, 555
    diagnostic tests for, 556
    epidemiology of, 556
    etiology of, 555–556
    incubation period of, 556
    treatment of, 556–557
Retinitis
    bunyaviruses, 255
    chikungunya, 103
    cytomegalovirus (CMV) infection, 158
Retro-orbital pain
    arenaviruses, 253
    Zika virus, 828
Retropharyngeal space infection, anaerobic gram-negative bacilli infections, 59
Reverse transcriptase–polymerase chain reaction (RT-PCR)
    bunyaviruses, 256
    coronaviruses, 139, 140*i*
    dengue, 167
    enterovirus (nonpoliovirus), 193
    filoviruses, 261
    human metapneumovirus (hMPV), 428
    influenza, 336, 337*t*
    measles, 412
    mumps, 439–440
    norovirus and sapovirus infections, 453
    parainfluenza viral infections, 468
    parechovirus infections, 480–481
    poliovirus infections, 529
    rabies, 546–547
    respiratory syncytial virus (RSV), 556
    rhinovirus infections, 559
    Zika virus, 829
Reye syndrome, 335, 801
Rhabdomyolysis, Q fever, 543

Rhabdoviridae, 546
Rhadinovirus, 311
Rhinitis
　influenza, 335
　respiratory syncytial virus (RSV), 555
　rhinovirus infections, 559
　syphilis, 670
Rhinorrhea
　bocavirus, 78
　coronaviruses, 137
Rhinovirus infections, 559, 560*i*
　clinical manifestations of, 559, 560*i*
　diagnostic tests for, 559
　epidemiology of, 559
　etiology of, 559
　incubation period of, 559
　treatment of, 559
Rhipicephalus sanguineus, 565
Rhizomucor pusillus, 212*i*
Rhizopus, 211*t*
Rhodotorula, 208
Ribavirin
　for arenaviruses, 254
　for bunyaviruses, 256
　for hantavirus pulmonary syndrome (HPS), 246
　for respiratory syncytial virus (RSV), 556
Rib fractures, pertussis (whooping cough), 503
Rickettsia, 561
Rickettsia akari, 563
Rickettsia australis, 563
Rickettsia felis, 563
Rickettsial diseases, 561–562
　clinical manifestations of, 561
　diagnostic tests for, 562
　epidemiology of, 561–562
　etiology of, 561
　incubation period of, 561
　treatment of, 562
Rickettsialpox, 563, 564*i*
　clinical manifestations of, 563, 564*i*
　diagnostic tests for, 563
　epidemiology of, 563
　etiology of, 563
　incubation period of, 563
　treatment of, 563
Rickettsia prowazekii, 793–794, 796
Rickettsia rickettsii, 794
Rickettsia typhi, 794, 796
Rifabutin, for nontuberculous mycobacteria (NTM), 780

Rifampin
　for brucellosis, 83
　for drug-resistant tuberculosis (DR TB), 765
　for *Ehrlichia*, *Anaplasma*, and related infections, 179
　isoniazid, pyrazinamide, and ethambutol (RIPE) therapy, 760, 761–764*t*, 765
　for leprosy, 369
　for *Listeria monocytogenes* infections, 378
　for nontuberculous mycobacteria (NTM), 780
　for tuberculosis (TB) disease, 760
　for tuberculosis infection (TBI), 758
Rift Valley fever (RVF), 255, 256*t*, 258*i*
Rigors
　Ehrlichia, *Anaplasma*, and related infections, 177
　influenza, 335
　Legionella pneumophila infections, 355
　malaria, 400
Ringworm
　of the body (tinea corporis), 708–709, 709–711*i*
　　clinical manifestations of, 708, 709–711*i*
　　diagnostic tests for, 708
　　epidemiology of, 708
　　etiology of, 708
　　incubation period of, 708
　　treatment of, 709
　of the feet (tinea pedis and tinea unguium), 714–715, 715–716*i*
　　clinical manifestations of, 714, 716*i*
　　diagnostic tests for, 714
　　epidemiology of, 714
　　etiology of, 714
　　incubation period of, 714
　　treatment of, 714–715
　of the scalp (tinea capitis), 704–706, 705*t*, 706–707*i*
　　clinical manifestations of, 704, 706–707*i*
　　diagnostic tests for, 704–705
　　epidemiology of, 704
　　etiology of, 704
　　incubation period of, 704
　　treatment of, 705–706, 705*t*
"River blindness" (onchocerciasis), 456–457, 457–459*i*
　clinical manifestations of, 456
　diagnostic tests for, 456
　epidemiology of, 456
　etiology of, 456
　incubation period of, 456
　treatment of, 456–457

Rocky Mountain spotted fever (RMSF), 561–562, 565–566, 567–570i
   clinical manifestations of, 565, 567–568i
   diagnostic tests for, 566
   epidemiology of, 565–566
   etiology of, 565
   incubation period of, 566
   treatment of, 566
Roseola. *See* Human herpesviruses 6 and 7
Rose spots, 579
Rotavirus infections, 571–572, 572i
   clinical manifestations of, 571, 572i
   diagnostic tests for, 572
   epidemiology of, 571
   etiology of, 571
   incubation period of, 572
   treatment of, 572
Roundworms. *See Ascaris lumbricoides* infections
Rubella, 573–574, 575–578i
   clinical manifestations of, 573, 575–577i
   congenital rubella syndrome, 573, 574
   diagnostic tests for, 574
   epidemiology of, 573–574
   etiology of, 573
   incubation period of, 574
   postnatal, 573
   treatment of, 574
Rubivirus, 573

S

Salmonella infections, 579–582, 582–587i
   clinical manifestations of, 579, 582–583i
   diagnostic tests for, 580–581
   epidemiology of, 579–580
   etiology of, 579
   incubation period of, 580
   treatment of, 581–582
Salpingitis
   Chlamydia trachomatis, 110
   pinworm infection (*Enterobius vermicularis*), 510
   Ureaplasma urealyticum and *Ureaplasma parvum* infections, 798
Sapovirus infections, 453–454, 454–455i
   clinical manifestations of, 453
   diagnostic tests for, 453–454
   epidemiology of, 453
   etiology of, 453
   incubation period of, 453
   treatment of, 454
Sarcoptes scabiei, 588

SARS-CoV-2. *See* Coronaviruses, including SARS-CoV-2 and MERS-CoV
Scabies, 588–589, 589–592i
   clinical manifestations of, 588, 589–591i
   diagnostic tests for, 589
   epidemiology of, 588
   etiology of, 588
   incubation period of, 588
   treatment of, 589
Scaling
   tinea capitis, 704
   tinea corporis, 708
Scedosporiosis, 208
Schistosoma guineensis, 594
Schistosoma intercalatum, 594
Schistosoma japonicum, 593–594
Schistosoma mansoni, 593–594
Schistosomiasis, 593–594, 595–598i
   clinical manifestations of, 593, 595–596i
   diagnostic tests for, 594
   epidemiology of, 593–594
   etiology of, 593
   incubation period of, 594
   treatment of, 594
Scrotal abscess, anaerobic gram-negative bacilli infections, 59
Scrotal gangrene, anaerobic gram-negative bacilli infections, 59
Secnidazole, for bacterial vaginosis, 57
Seizures
   African trypanosomiasis, 742
   amebic meningoencephalitis and keratitis, 14
   arboviruses, 26, 30i
   Baylisascaris infections, 68
   Campylobacter infections, 88
   chikungunya, 104i
   cysticercosis, 689, 692i
   Haemophilus influenzae, 242
   hemorrhagic fevers, 253
   herpes simplex, 286
   human herpesvirus 7, 306
   influenza, 335
   louseborne typhus, 793
   paragonimiasis, 463
   parainfluenza viral infections, 467
   parechovirus infections, 480
   pertussis, 503
   roseola, 310i
   Shigella infections, 599
   smallpox (variola), 603
   syphilis, 670

Seizures (*continued*)
   toxocariasis, 717
   Toxoplasma gondii infections, 720, 727*i*
   West Nile virus (WNV), 818
Selenium sulfide, for pityriasis versicolor, 513
Sensorineural hearing loss (SNHL), cytomegalovirus (CMV) infection, 158
Sepsis
   anthrax, 18
   Arcanobacterium haemolyticum infections, 35
   Bacillus cereus infections and intoxications, 54
   Ehrlichia, Anaplasma, and related infections, 177
   enterovirus (nonpoliovirus), 192
   herpes simplex virus (HSV), 285
   parechovirus infections, 480
   plague, 516
   postanginal, *Fusobacterium* infections, 216
   Pseudomonas aeruginosa infections, 540–542*i*
   rat-bite fever, 552
   Toxoplasma gondii infections, 720
   varicella-zoster virus (VSV) infections, 801
Septic arthritis
   group B streptococcal (GBS) infections, 647
   Haemophilus influenzae type b (Hib) infections, 234
   Moraxella catarrhalis infections, 437
   non–group A or B streptococcal and enterococcal infections, 652
   Pasteurella infections, 488
   rat-bite fever, 552
   Staphylococcus aureus, 616
Septicemia
   leptospirosis, 372
   meningococcal infections, 419
   neonatal, 185–187, 187–191*i*
      clinical manifestations of, 185, 187–190*i*
      diagnostic tests for, 186
      epidemiology of, 185–186
      etiology of, 185
      Haemophilus influenzae type b (Hib) infections, 234
      incubation period of, 186
      treatment of, 186–187
      non–group A or B streptococcal and enterococcal infections, 652
   Pasteurella infections, 488
   Shigella infections, 599
   Streptococcus pneumoniae (pneumococcal) infections, 657
   tularemia, 786
   Vibrio infections, other, 816

Septicemic plague, 516, 517
Septic pulmonary emboli, *Staphylococcus aureus*, 616
Septic thrombophlebitis, *Staphylococcus aureus*, 616
Serological tests
   amebiasis, 8
   arbovirus infections, 28
   babesiosis, 50
   Baylisascaris infections, 68
   brucellosis, 82, 83
   bunyaviruses, 256
   chikungunya, 104
   Chlamydia psittaci, 107
   Chlamydia trachomatis, 112
   coccidioidomycosis, 130
   cytomegalovirus (CMV) infection, 160
   Ehrlichia, Anaplasma, and related infections, 179
   hantavirus pulmonary syndrome (HPS), 246
   hepatitis A, 265–266
   hepatitis B, 271
   HIV infection, 314–315
   human herpesvirus 8, 312
   human herpesviruses 6 and 7, 307–308
   Listeria monocytogenes infections, 378
   louseborne typhus, 794
   Lyme disease, 383
   parainfluenza viral infections, 468
   Q fever, 543
   relapsing fever, 80
   rickettsial diseases, 562
   schistosomiasis, 594
   strongyloidiasis, 667–668
   Toxoplasma gondii infections, 721
   tularemia, 786–787
Severe acute respiratory syndrome (SARS). *See* Coronaviruses, including SARS-CoV-2 and MERS-CoV
Severe anemia, 400
Sexually transmitted infections (STIs)
   bacterial vaginosis and, 54
   chancroid and cutaneous ulcers, 100–101
   Chlamydia trachomatis, 110–111
   gonococcal infections, 224–225
   granuloma inguinale, 232
   herpes simplex, 285
   HIV, 313
   human papillomavirus (HPV) infections, 332
   pelvic inflammatory disease (PID) and, 499–500
   syphilis, 670–671
   Trichomonas vaginalis infections, 734–735

Shiga toxin–producing *E coli* (STEC), 202
Shigella infections, 599–601, 601–602i
    bacterial vaginosis, 56
    clinical manifestations of, 599
    diagnostic tests for, 600
    epidemiology of, 599–600
    etiology of, 599
    incubation period of, 600
    treatment of, 600–601
Shock
    anthrax, 18
    arboviruses, 27
    arenaviruses, 253
    bunyaviruses, 255
    cholera, 812
    Clostridioides difficile, 122
    coronaviruses, 137
    dengue, 166
    Kawasaki disease, 346
    malaria, 400
    meningococcal infections, 419
    Rocky Mountain spotted fever (RMSF), 565
    Salmonella infections, 579
    Toxoplasma gondii infections, 720
Shortness of breath. *See* Breathing difficulty
Sickle cell disease
    Mycoplasma pneumoniae and other
        Mycoplasma species infections and, 444
    Salmonella infections and, 579
    Yersinia enterocolitica and *Yersinia*
        pseudotuberculosis infections and, 824
Silver stain
    Bartonella henselae (cat-scratch disease), 64, 66i
    blastomycosis, 75
    Pneumocystis jirovecii infections and, 523
Sinusitis
    anaerobic gram-negative bacilli infections, 59
    Fusobacterium infections, 216
    Moraxella catarrhalis infections, 437
    Mycoplasma pneumoniae and other
        Mycoplasma species infections, 444
    non–group A or B streptococcal and
        enterococcal infections, 652
    Staphylococcus aureus, 616
    Streptococcus pneumoniae (pneumococcal)
        infections, 660
Skin discoloration
    leishmaniasis, 360
    leprosy, 367
    louseborne typhus, 793
    onchocerciasis, 456

    pediculosis corporis (body lice), 495
    tinea cruris, 712
Sleep disturbances
    Hymenolepis nana, 695
    pertussis (whooping cough), 503
    pinworm infection (*Enterobius vermicularis*), 510
Sleeping sickness, 742–743, 743–744i
    clinical manifestations of, 742
    diagnostic tests for, 743
    epidemiology of, 742–743
    etiology of, 742
    incubation period of, 743
    treatment of, 743
Smallpox (variola), 603–604, 605–609i
    clinical manifestations of, 603–604, 605–609i
    diagnostic tests for, 604
    epidemiology of, 604
    etiology of, 604
    incubation period of, 604
    treatment of, 604
Sneezing, rhinovirus infections, 559
Sodium stibogluconate, leishmaniasis, 362
Sore throat
    coronaviruses, 137
    influenza, 335
    lymphocytic choriomeningitis virus (LCMV), 398
    poliovirus infections, 528
    rhinovirus infections, 559
    syphilis, 670
Source person, tuberculosis (TB), 752
Spinal cord degeneration, syphilis, 670
Spinosad, for pediculosis capitis, 491t, 492
Spirillum minus, 552
Spirochaetaceae, 382, 670
Spleen
    abscess
        brucellosis, 82
        Yersinia enterocolitica and *Yersinia*
            pseudotuberculosis infections, 824
    granulomata, *Bartonella henselae* (cat-scratch
        disease), 63
    paragonimiasis and, 463
    rupture, Epstein-Barr virus, 197
    Streptococcus pneumoniae (pneumococcal)
        infections and, 657
Splenomegaly
    human herpesvirus 8, 311
    Salmonella infections, 579
    syphilis, 670
    tularemia, 786
Spondylitis, brucellosis, 82

Spontaneous abortion. *See* Abortion
Sporothrix brasiliensis, 610
Sporothrix globosa, 610
Sporothrix schenckii, 610
Sporothrix schenckii sensu stricto, 610
Sporotrichosis, 208, 610–611, 611–613*i*
    clinical manifestations of, 610, 611–612*i*
    diagnostic tests for, 610–611
    epidemiology of, 610
    etiology of, 610
    incubation period of, 610
    treatment of, 611
Spotted fever rickettsiosis (SFR), 565–566
Staphylococcal food poisoning, 614, 615*i*
    clinical manifestations of, 614
    diagnostic tests for, 614
    epidemiology of, 614
    etiology of, 614
    incubation period of, 614
    treatment of, 614
Staphylococcal scalded skin syndrome (SSSS), 616
Staphylococcal toxic shock syndrome (TSS), 616–617, 617*b*, 619, 623
Staphylococcus aureus, 614, 615*i*, 616–623, 617*b*, 621–622*t*, 624–630*i*
    clinical manifestations of, 616, 617*b*, 624–628*i*
    diagnostic tests for, 618–619
    epidemiology of, 616–618
    etiology of, 616
    incubation period of, 618
    treatment of, 619–623, 621–622*t*
Staphylococcus epidermidis, 614
Staphylococcus intermedius, 614
Streptobacillus moniliformis, 552
St Louis encephalitis, 26, 26*t*, 29*t*, 34*i*
Stomatitis, enterovirus (nonpoliovirus), 192
Stool tests
    amebiasis, 8–9
    anthrax, 19
    Ascaris lumbricoides infections, 37
    astrovirus infections, 47
    Bacillus cereus infections, 54–55
    Balantidium coli infections, 61
    Blastocystis infections, 72
    Clostridioides difficile, 123
    Clostridium perfringens, 127
    cryptosporidiosis, 146–147
    cyclosporiasis, 153
    Escherichia coli diarrhea, 204
    Giardia duodenalis infections, 219
    hookworm infections, 301

    microsporidia infections, 431
    poliovirus infections, 529
    Salmonella infections, 580
    Shigella infections, 600
    tapeworm diseases, 689, 695–696
Strawberry cervix, 734
Streptococcus agalactiae, 499
Streptococcus pneumoniae (pneumococcal) infections, 657–661, 658*t*, 659*t*, 661–666*i*
    clinical manifestations of, 651–652*i*, 657
    diagnostic tests for, 658
    epidemiology of, 657
    etiology of, 657
    incubation period of, 657
    treatment of, 659–661, 659*t*
Streptomycin, for plague, 517
Strongyloides stercoralis, 667–668
Strongyloidiasis, 470, 667–668, 668–669*i*
    clinical manifestations of, 667, 668*i*
    diagnostic tests for, 667–668
    epidemiology of, 667
    etiology of, 667
    incubation period of, 667
    treatment of, 668
Subacute sclerosing panencephalitis (SSPE), 411
Supportive treatment
    Bacillus cereus infections and intoxications, 55
    Bartonella henselae (cat-scratch disease), 64
    botulism and infant botulism, 116
    chikungunya, 104
    Escherichia coli diarrhea, 204
    human metapneumovirus (hMPV), 428
    lymphocytic choriomeningitis virus (LCMV), 399
    mumps, 440
    norovirus and sapovirus infections, 454
    parvovirus B19, 484
    rubella, 574
    staphylococcal food poisoning, 614
    West Nile virus (WNV), 819
    Zika virus, 830
Surgical interventions
    actinomycosis, 2
    clostridial myonecrosis, 120
    coccidioidomycosis, 131
    Q fever, 544
    tapeworm diseases, 690–691
    toxocariasis, 717
    Ureaplasma urealyticum and *Ureaplasma parvum* infections, 799

Swelling
  Pasteurella infections, 488
  plague, 516
Swimmer's itch, 594
Sylvatic typhus, 793–794, 795*i*
  clinical manifestations of, 793
  diagnostic tests for, 794
  epidemiology of, 793–794
  etiology of, 793
  incubation period of, 794
  treatment of, 794
Syncope, pertussis (whooping cough), 503
Syphilis, 100, 670–680, 674*f*, 676–677*t*, 679*t*, 680–688*i*
  acquired, 670, 678, 679*i*, 680
  clinical manifestations of, 670, 680–684*i*, 687–688*i*
  congenital, 670, 675
  diagnostic tests for, 671–673
  epidemiology of, 670–671
  etiology of, 670
  incubation period of, 671
  treatment of, 673–680, 674*f*, 676–677*t*, 679*t*

T

Tachycardia
  clostridial myonecrosis, 120
  tetanus, 700
Tachypnea
  louseborne typhus, 793
  malaria, 400
  Pneumocystis jirovecii infections, 522
  respiratory syncytial virus (RSV), 555
Taenia asiatica, 689
Taenia saginata, 689
Taeniasis, 689–691, 691–694*i*
  clinical manifestations of, 689
  diagnosis of, 689–690
  epidemiology of, 689
  etiology of, 689
  incubation period of, 689
  treatment of, 690–691
Taenia solium, 689–690
Talaromyces (Penicillium) marneffei, 209*t*
Talaromycosis, 209*t*
Tapeworm diseases, 689–691, 691–694*i*
  clinical manifestations of, 689
  diagnosis of, 689–690
  Diphyllobothrium, 695
  Dipylidium caninum, 695

Echinococcus granulosus and *Echinococcus multilocularis*, 695–696
  epidemiology of, 689
  etiology of, 689
  Hymenolepis nana, 695
  incubation period of, 689
  treatment of, 690–691
TB disease, 751
Tecovirimat, for smallpox (variola), 604
Tenderness, *Pasteurella* infections, 488
Tenesmus
  Shigella infections, 599
  trichuriasis (whipworm infection), 739
Tenosynovitis, *Pasteurella* infections, 488
Terbinafine
  for tinea capitis, 705*t*, 706
  for tinea cruris, 712
Testicles, actinomycosis infection, 1
Tetanus, 320, 700–701, 701–703*i*
  clinical manifestations of, 700, 701–703*i*
  diagnostic tests for, 701
  epidemiology of, 700
  etiology of, 700
  incubation period of, 700–701
  treatment of, 701
Tetracycline
  for *Balantidium coli* infections, 61
  for *Chlamydia pneumoniae*, 106
  for cholera, 813*t*
  for *Helicobacter pylori* infections, 250*t*
  for *Ureaplasma urealyticum* and *Ureaplasma parvum* infections, 799
Thoracic actinomycosis, 1
Thrombocytopenia
  arboviruses, 26
  arenaviruses, 253
  babesiosis, 49
  brucellosis, 82
  chikungunya, 103
  cytomegalovirus (CMV) infection, 158
  Epstein-Barr virus, 197
  hepatitis B, 269
  lymphocytic choriomeningitis virus (LCMV), 398
  malaria, 400
  mumps, 439
  murine typhus, 796
  Mycoplasma pneumoniae and other *Mycoplasma* species infections, 444
  relapsing fever, 79
  Rocky Mountain spotted fever (RMSF), 565
  rubella, 573

Thrombocytopenia (*continued*)
  syphilis, 670
  varicella-zoster virus (VSV) infections, 801
  Zika virus, 828
Thrombocytopenic purpura, *Bartonella henselae* (cat-scratch disease), 63
Thrombophlebitis, *Chlamydia psittaci*, 107
Thrush. *See* Candidiasis
Thyroiditis, mumps, 439
Thyroid dysfunction, African trypanosomiasis, 742
Tickborne encephalitis, 26, 26t, 29t
Tickborne relapsing fever, 79–80, 81*i*
  clinical manifestations of, 79
  diagnostic tests for, 80
  epidemiology of, 79–80
  etiology of, 79
  incubation period of, 80
  treatment of, 80
Tigecycline, for *Prevotella* infections, 60
Tinea capitis, 704–706, 705t, 706–707*i*
  clinical manifestations of, 704, 706–707*i*
  diagnostic tests for, 704–705
  epidemiology of, 704
  etiology of, 704
  incubation period of, 704
  treatment of, 705–706, 705t
Tinea corporis, 708–709, 709–711*i*
  clinical manifestations of, 708, 709–711*i*
  diagnostic tests for, 708
  epidemiology of, 708
  etiology of, 708
  incubation period of, 708
  treatment of, 709
Tinea cruris, 712–713, 713*i*
  clinical manifestations of, 712, 713*i*
  diagnostic tests for, 712
  epidemiology of, 712
  etiology of, 712
  incubation period of, 712
  treatment of, 712–713
Tinea pedis, 714–715, 715–716*i*
  clinical manifestations of, 714, 715–716*i*
  diagnostic tests for, 714
  epidemiology of, 714
  etiology of, 714
  incubation period of, 714
  treatment of, 714–715
Tinea unguium, 714–715, 715–716*i*
  clinical manifestations of, 714, 716*i*
  diagnostic tests for, 714
  epidemiology of, 714
  etiology of, 714
  incubation period of, 714
  treatment of, 714–715
Tinidazole
  for amebiasis, 8
  for bacterial vaginosis, 57
  for *Blastocystis* infections, 72
  for *Giardia duodenalis* infections, 220
  for *Trichomonas vaginalis* infections, 735
Tissue cell culture, for influenza, 336, 337t
Togaviridae, 27, 573
Tolnaftate
  for tinea corporis, 709
  for tinea cruris, 712
Tonsillitis
  actinomycosis, 1
  adenovirus infections, 4
  Fusobacterium infections, 216
  tularemia, 786
Toxic megacolon
  amebiasis, 7
  Clostridioides difficile, 122
  Shigella infections, 599
Toxic shock syndrome
  Ehrlichia, *Anaplasma*, and related infections, 177
  non–group A or B streptococcal and enterococcal infections, 652
  staphylococcal toxic shock syndrome (TSS), 616–617, 617b, 619, 623
Toxocara canis, 717
Toxocara cati, 717
Toxocariasis, 470, 717, 718–719*i*
  clinical manifestations of, 717
  diagnostic tests for, 717
  epidemiology of, 717
  etiology of, 717
  incubation period of, 717
  treatment of, 717
Toxoplasma gondii infections, 720–723, 724t, 725b, 726–729*i*, 726t
  clinical manifestations of, 720–721, 726*i*
  diagnostic tests for, 721–723
  epidemiology of, 721
  etiology of, 721
  incubation period of, 721
  treatment of, 723, 724t, 725b, 726t
Toxoplasmic encephalitis (TE), 721
Tracheitis, *Moraxella catarrhalis* infections, 437
Trachoma, 110–113
Transmissible spongiform encephalopathies (TSEs), 536–538, 538–539*i*
  clinical manifestations of, 536–537
  diagnostic tests for, 538

epidemiology of, 537
etiology of, 537
incubation period of, 538
treatment of, 538
Treponema carateum, 670
Treponema pallidum, 80, 100, 670
Trichinella spiralis, 730
Trichinellosis, 730, 731–733*i*
  clinical manifestations of, 730, 731*i*
  diagnostic tests for, 730
  epidemiology of, 730
  etiology of, 730
  incubation period of, 730
  treatment of, 730
Trichodysplasia spinulosa–associated
    polyomavirus (TSPyV), 534
Trichomonas vaginalis infections, 56, 734–735,
    736–738*i*
  clinical manifestations of, 734
  diagnostic tests for, 734–735
  epidemiology of, 734
  etiology of, 734
  incubation period of, 734
  treatment of, 735
Trichophyton interdigitale, 712
Trichophyton mentagrophytes, 708, 712
Trichophyton rubrum, 708, 712
Trichophyton tonsurans, 704, 708, 712
Trichophyton verrucosum, 712
Trichophyton violaceum, 704
Trichosporon, 208, 210*t*
Trichuriasis (whipworm infection), 739, 740–741*i*
  clinical manifestations of, 739
  diagnostic tests for, 739
  epidemiology of, 739
  etiology of, 739
  incubation period of, 739
  treatment of, 739
Trichuris trichiura, 739
Triclabendazole, for paragonimiasis, 464
Trimethoprim-sulfamethoxazole
  for brucellosis, 83
  for *Burkholderia* infections, 86
  for cyclosporiasis, 153
  for *Enterobacteriaceae* infections, 187
  for *Listeria monocytogenes* infections, 378
  for *Moraxella catarrhalis* infections, 437
  for nocardiosis, 450
  for paracoccidioidomycosis, 460
  for pertussis (whooping cough), 504, 505*t*
  for *Pneumocystis jirovecii* infections, 524

for *Salmonella* infections, 581, 582
for *Shigella* infections, 601
for *Ureaplasma urealyticum* and *Ureaplasma
    parvum* infections, 799
for *Vibrio* infections, other, 816
Trismus, tetanus, 700
Trypanosoma, 360
Trypanosoma brucei gambiense, 742–743
Trypanosoma brucei rhodesiense, 158, 742–743
Trypanosoma cruzi, 745–746
Tube agglutination (TA), tularemia, 786–787
Tuberculin skin test (TST), 750, 751*b*, 752–754,
    754*b*, 755*f*
Tuberculosis (TB), 750–769, 751*b*, 754–755*b*, 755*f*,
    759–764*t*, 765*b*, 770–776*i*
  clinical manifestations of, 750, 770*i*, 772–773*i*
  diagnostic tests for, 752–758, 754*b*, 755*b*, 755*f*
  epidemiology of, 752
  etiology of, 750–752, 751*b*
  incubation period of, 752
  isolation of hospitalized patient with, 769
  treatment of, 758–769, 759–760*t*, 761–764*t*, 765*b*
Tuberculosis (TB) disease, 751, 760, 761–764*t*,
    765–766, 765*b*
Tuberculosis infection (TBI), 750, 758, 759–760*t*, 760
Tubo-ovarian disease, anaerobic gram-negative
    bacilli infections, 59
Tularemia, 786–787, 787–792*i*
  clinical manifestations of, 786, 787–789*i*
  diagnostic tests for, 786–787
  epidemiology of, 786
  etiology of, 786
  incubation period of, 786
  treatment of, 787
23-valent pneumococcal polysaccharide vaccine
    (PPSV23), 657, 658*t*

u

Ulcerative lesions
  leishmaniasis, 360
  leprosy, 367
  syphilis, 670
Ultrasonography
  amebiasis, 8
  Escherichia coli diarrhea, 205*i*
Uncinaria stenocephala, 151, 301
Ureaplasma, 444
Ureaplasma parvum infection, 798–799, 800*i*
  clinical manifestations of, 798
  diagnostic tests for, 798–799

Ureaplasma parvum infection (*continued*)
  epidemiology of, 798
  etiology of, 798
  incubation period of, 798
  treatment of, 799
Ureaplasma urealyticum infection, 499, 798–799, 800*i*
  clinical manifestations of, 798
  diagnostic tests for, 798–799
  epidemiology of, 798
  etiology of, 798
  incubation period of, 798
  treatment of, 799
Urethritis
  Chlamydia trachomatis, 110
  Kawasaki disease, 347
  meningococcal infections, 419
  Moraxella catarrhalis infections, 437
  pinworm infection (*Enterobius vermicularis*), 510
  Trichomonas vaginalis infections, 734
  Ureaplasma urealyticum and *Ureaplasma parvum* infections, 798
Urinary tract infection (UTI)
  Burkholderia, 85
  Pseudomonas aeruginosa infections, 540
  Salmonella infections, 579
  schistosomiasis, 593
  Yersinia enterocolitica and *Yersinia pseudotuberculosis* infections, 824
Urticaria
  Blastocystis infections, 72
  hepatitis B, 269
Uveitis
  chikungunya, 103
  enterovirus (nonpoliovirus), 192
  Kawasaki disease, 347
  leptospirosis, 372
  Lyme disease, 381
  syphilis, 670
  Yersinia enterocolitica and *Yersinia pseudotuberculosis* infections, 824

V

Vaginal bleeding, irregular, pelvic inflammatory disease (PID), 499
Vaginal discharge
  pelvic inflammatory disease (PID), 499
  Trichomonas vaginalis infections, 734
Vaginitis, 56
  Chlamydia trachomatis, 110
  pinworm infection (*Enterobius vermicularis*), 510

Valacyclovir, for varicella-zoster virus (VSV) infections, 803, 804
Valganciclovir, for cytomegalovirus (CMV) infection, 160–161
Vancomycin
  for *Clostridioides difficile*, 124
  for coagulase-negative staphylococcal (CoNS) infections, 632
  for non–group A or B streptococcal and enterococcal infections, 653
  for *Staphylococcus aureus*, 623
  for *Streptococcus pneumoniae* (pneumococcal) infections, 659, 660
Vancomycin–intermediately susceptible *Staphylococcus aureus*, 618
Vancomycin-resistant *Staphylococcus aureus*, 618
Variant CJD, 536
Varicella-zoster virus (VSV) infections, 320, 350, 603–604, 801–804, 805*f*, 806–811*i*
  clinical manifestations of, 801, 806–811*i*
  diagnostic tests for, 802–803, 803*t*
  epidemiology of, 802
  etiology of, 802
  incubation period of, 802
  treatment of, 803–804, 805*f*
Varicellovirus, 802
Variola (smallpox), 603–604, 605–609*i*
  clinical manifestations of, 603–604, 605–609*i*
  diagnostic tests for, 604
  epidemiology of, 604
  etiology of, 604
  incubation period of, 604
  treatment of, 604
Vascular collapse, malaria, 400
Venereal Disease Research Laboratory (VDRL) slide test, syphilis, 671–672
Venezuelan equine encephalomyelitis, 34*i*
Venezuelan hemorrhagic fever, 253–254
Ventricular shunt infection
  Bacillus cereus infections and intoxications, 54
  Moraxella catarrhalis infections, 437
Viannia, 360
Vibrio cholerae, 812–813, 813*t*, 814–815*i*, 816
  clinical manifestations of, 812, 814*f*
  diagnostic tests for, 812–813
  epidemiology of, 812
  etiology of, 812
  incubation period of, 812
  treatment of, 813, 813*t*
Vibrio infections, other, 816, 817*i*
  clinical manifestations of, 816
  diagnostic tests for, 816

epidemiology of, 816
etiology of, 816
incubation period of, 816
treatment of, 816
Vibrionaceae, 816
Vibrio vulnificus, 816
Visceral larval migrans, 717
  Baylisascaris infections, 68
Visceral leishmaniasis, 360
Visual disturbances
  bunyaviruses, 255
  onchocerciasis, 456
  toxocariasis, 717
Vitamin A
  for measles, 413
  for *Shigella* infections, 601
Vomiting
  anthrax, 18
  arenaviruses, 253
  astrovirus infections, 47
  Bacillus cereus infections and intoxications, 54
  chikungunya, 103
  Chlamydia psittaci, 107
  cholera, 812
  coronaviruses, 137
  cryptosporidiosis, 146
  dengue, 166
  Ehrlichia, Anaplasma, and related infections, 177
  Enterobacteriaceae infections, 185
  enterovirus (nonpoliovirus), 192
  filoviruses, 259
  hantavirus pulmonary syndrome (HPS), 245
  influenza, 335
  Kawasaki disease, 347
  leptospirosis, 372
  lymphocytic choriomeningitis virus (LCMV), 398
  malaria, 400
  murine typhus, 796
  pelvic inflammatory disease (PID), 499
  pertussis (whooping cough), 503
  Q fever, 543
  rat-bite fever, 552
  rickettsialpox, 563
  Rocky Mountain spotted fever (RMSF), 565
  rotavirus infections, 571
  smallpox (variola), 603
  staphylococcal food poisoning, 614, 615*i*
  trichinellosis, 730
  Vibrio infections, other, 816
  West Nile virus (WNV), 818
  Zika virus, 828

Voriconazole
  for aspergillosis, 43
  for candidiasis, 92–93
  for paracoccidioidomycosis, 460
Vulvitis, 56
Vulvovaginal infections, anaerobic gram-negative bacilli infections, 59

W

Warts, human papillomavirus (HPV) infections, 331
Wayson stain, plague, 516
Weakness
  arenaviruses, 253
  brucellosis, 82
  filoviruses, 259
  Q fever, 543
  West Nile virus (WNV), 818
Weight loss. *See* Anorexia and weight loss
Western equine encephalomyelitis, 34*i*
West Nile virus (WNV), 26–28, 26*t*, 29*t*, 34*i*, 818–819, 820–823*i*
  clinical manifestations of, 818, 821*i*
  diagnostic tests for, 819
  epidemiology of, 818–819
  etiology of, 818
  incubation period of, 819
  treatment of, 819
Wheezing
  bocavirus, 78
  respiratory syncytial virus (RSV), 555
  toxocariasis, 717
Whipworm infection (trichuriasis), 739, 740–741*i*
  clinical manifestations of, 739
  diagnostic tests for, 739
  epidemiology of, 739
  etiology of, 739
  incubation period of, 739
  treatment of, 739
Whooping cough (pertussis), 503–505, 505*t*, 506–509*i*
  clinical manifestations of, 503, 506*i*, 508*i*
  diagnostic tests for, 503–504
  epidemiology of, 503
  etiology of, 503
  incubation period of, 503
  treatment of, 504–505, 505*t*
Wound infections
  Burkholderia, 85
  clostridial myonecrosis, 120–121, 121*i*
  Clostridioides difficile, 122

Wound infections (*continued*)
    Legionella pneumophila infections, 355
    postoperative, anaerobic gram-negative bacilli infections, 59
    Pseudomonas aeruginosa infections, 540
    Staphylococcus aureus, 616
    tetanus, 700
    Vibrio infections, other, 816
Wright stain
    for babesiosis, 49
    for *Ehrlichia*, *Anaplasma*, and related infections, 179
    for molluscum contagiosum, 434
    plague, 516
    for relapsing fever, 80
Wuchereria bancrofti, 393
WU polyomavirus, 534

Y

Yeasts, invasive, 210–211t
Yellow fever, 26, 26t, 27, 29t, 31i, 33i
Yellow fever virus, 33i
Yersinia enterocolitica infections, 824–826, 826–827i
    clinical manifestations of, 824, 826i
    diagnostic tests for, 825
    epidemiology of, 824–825
    etiology of, 824
    incubation period of, 825
    treatment of, 826
Yersinia pestis, 516
Yersinia pseudotuberculosis infections, 824–826, 826–827i
    clinical manifestations of, 824, 826i
    diagnostic tests for, 825
    epidemiology of, 824–825
    etiology of, 824
    incubation period of, 825
    treatment of, 826

Z

Zanamivir, for influenza, 337, 338, 338t
Zika virus, 26t, 28, 29t, 828–830, 831f, 832–834i
    clinical manifestations of, 828, 832i, 834i
    diagnostic tests for, 829–830
    epidemiology of, 828
    etiology of, 828
    incubation period of, 828
    treatment of, 830, 831f
Zygomycosis, 212i, 213i